KEY FACTS TO REMEMBER

ESSENTIAL PRECAUTIONS FOR PRACTICE

PROCEDURES

CONTENTS IN BRIEF

Maternal-Newborn Nursing Care

The Nurse, the Family, and the Community

FOURTH EDITION

Patricia Wieland Ladewig, RNC, PhD
Professor and Dean, School
for Health Care Professsions
Regis University
Denver, Colorado

Marcia L. London, RNC, MSN, NNP
Associate Professor and
Director, Neonatal Nurse
Practitioner Program
Beth-El College of Nursing
Colorado Springs, Colorado

Sally B. Olds, RNC, MS
Associate Professor
Beth-El College
of Nursing
Colorado Springs,
Colorado

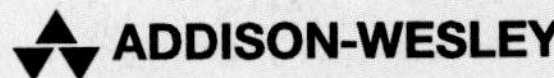

An imprint of Addison Wesley Longman, Inc.

Menlo Park, California • Reading, Massachusetts • New York • Harlow, England
Don Mills, Ontario • Sydney • Mexico City • Madrid • Amsterdam

Executive Editor: Patricia Cleary
Project Editor: Virginia Simione Jutson
Managing Editor: Wendy Earl
Production Editor: David Rich
Editor: Laura M. Bonazzoli
Art and Photo Supervisor: Bradley Burch
Editorial Assistant: Marla Nowick
Text Designer: Andrew Ogus ■ Andrew Ogus Book Design
Cover Designer: Yvo Riezebos
Manufacturing Supervisor: Merry Free Osborn

Art and photography credits appear on pages 822–823.

Library of Congress Cataloging-in-Publication Data

Ladewig, Patricia W.
Maternal-newborn nursing care : the nurse, the family, and the community / Patricia Wieland Ladewig, Marcia L. London, Sally B. Olds.—4th ed.
p. cm.
Rev. ed. of: Essentials of maternal-newborn nursing / Patricia Wieland Ladewig, Marcia L. London, Sally B. Olds. 3rd ed. © 1994.
Includes bibliographical references and index.
ISBN 0-8053-5622-3
1. Maternity nursing. 2. Neonatology. 3. Pediatric nursing. I. London, Marcia L., II. Olds, Sally B., 1940– . III. Ladewig, Patricia W. Essentials of maternal-newborn nursing. IV. Title.
[DNLM: 1. Maternal-Child Nursing. WY 157.3 L154m 1998]
R0951.L33 1998
610.73'67—dc21
DNLM/DLC
for Library of Congress 97-37686
CIP

ISBN 0-8053-5622-3

1 2 3 4 5 6 7 8 9 10—RNV—01 00 99 98 97

Addison Wesley Longman, Inc.
2725 Sand Hill Road
Menlo Park, California 94025

The authors and publishers have exerted every effort to ensure that drug selections and dosages set forth in this text are in accord with current recommendations and practice at the time of publication. However, in view of ongoing research, changes in government regulations, and the constant flow of information relating to drug therapy and drug reactions, the reader is urged to check the package insert for each drug for any change in indications of dosage and for added warnings and precautions. This is particularly important where the recommended agent is a new and/or infrequently employed drug. Mention of a particular generic or brand name drug is not an endorsement, nor an implication that it is preferable to other named or unnamed agents.

The quilt on the cover, "Pool," was designed and pieced by Angela Holland.

We dedicate this book to courage.

To the courage of parents who nurture their children and protect them, who stand fast through the struggles of guiding their children, and who hold fast to hope.

To the courage of the family to nurture, to love, to hold on through adversity, to stay together, and to set each other free when it is time.

To the courage of those who seek to know themselves and who journey to find truth, strength, and finally peace.

To the courage of those who seek knowledge so they can touch lives.

To the courage of students, mothers, fathers, teachers, friends, who hold onto dreams and make them real.

PWL
MLL
SBO

CONTRIBUTORS AND REVIEWERS

Kathy Marvel, RNC, MSN, Contributor
Columbia Rose Medical Center
Denver, Colorado

Reviewers

Louise Aurilio, RNC, BSAS, MSN, CNA
Youngstown State University
Girard, Ohio

Constance Bobik, RN, MSN
Brevard Community College
Cocoa, Florida

Deborah A. Blackwell, RNC, PhD
Clemson University
Clemson, South Carolina

Julie Boozer, RN, PhD, ACCE
Wesley College
Dover, Delaware

Deborah Cameron, RN, BAAN, MEd
Centennial College
Scarborough, Ontario, Canada

Sandra K. Cesario, RNC, MS
University of Oklahoma
Tulsa, Oklahoma

Nancy Darland, RNC, MSN, CNS
Louisiana Tech University
Ruston, Louisiana

Debra J. Drake, RN, BSN, MSN, CCE
Ivy Tech State College
Indianapolis, Indiana

Nancy Duphily, RNC, MS, CCE
Mount Wachusett Community College
Gardner, Massachusetts

Cynthia C. Eubank, RN, MEd, MSN
Des Moines Area Community College
Ankeny, Iowa

Patricia A. Jamerson, RNC, MSN, PhD(c)
Avila College
Kansas City, Missouri

Catherine L. Juve, RN, MN, MPH, PhD
University of San Francisco
San Francisco, California

Marilyn Lowe, RNC, MSN, CNM
Methodist Hospital
Omaha, Nebraska

Jane McAteer, RN, BSN, MN
College of San Mateo
San Mateo, California

Julia Stuart Monaghan, RN, RM, BNS(c), MHM, MRCNA
Townsville, Australia

Marie Rogers, RNC, MSN, MA
Kalamazoo Valley Community College
Kalamazoo, Michigan

Ida L. Slusher, RN, DSN
Berea College
Berea, Kentucky

Betsy Stetson, RN, EdD, FACCE
University of San Francisco
San Francisco, California

Reid Smith Suchanec, RN, MSN
Delaware Technical and Community College
Newark, Delaware

Linda Salsman Ungerleider, RN, MSN, FACCE
North Park University
Chicago, Illinois

Elizabeth K. Wajdowicz, RN, BSN, MA, PhD
St. Petersburg Junior College
St. Petersburg, Florida

Barbara J. West, RN, BSN, MSN, ARNP, SNM
Broward Community College
Ft. Lauderdale, Florida

Susan Karm Wieczorek, MSN, CNS, CETN
St. Francis Hospital
Columbus, Georgia

Julie M. Wismont, RN, BSN, MS, PhD
University of Michigan
Ann Arbor, Michigan

Marybeth Young, RN, PhD
Loyola University
Chicago, Illinois

Student Reviewers

Lori Aiken, RN
Clemson University
Clemson, South Carolina

Matt Santangelo, RN
Broward Community College
Davie, Florida

Torry E. Simmons, RN
Des Moines Area Community College
Indianola, Iowa

PREFACE

Now, more than ever before, nurses play a central role in planning for and during the experience of birth, and in how families feel about the experience afterward. In addition, nurses working with childbearing families today are challenged by a variety of forces affecting the provision of nursing care. Shortened lengths of stay, the trend toward greater use of community-based and home care, the impact of HIV/AIDS, the increased use of unlicensed assistive personnel, downsizing and mergers of health care systems, the increased number of for-profit systems, and the general aging of the population all alter the way we practice nursing today and in the future.

The underlying philosophy of *Maternal-Newborn Nursing Care: The Nurse, the Family, and the Community* (formerly *Essentials of Maternal-Newborn Nursing*) remains unchanged. We believe that pregnancy and childbirth are normal life processes and that family members are co-participants in care. We remain committed to providing a text that is accurate and readable, a text that helps students develop the skills and abilities they need now and in the future in an ever-changing health care environment.

Community-Based Nursing Care

Although pregnancy, birth, and the postpartal period cover a period of months, in reality most women spend only two to three days in an acute care facility if at all. Thus, by its very nature, maternal-newborn nursing is primarily community-based nursing. Moreover, because of the changes resulting from managed care, even women with high-risk pregnancies are receiving more care in their homes and in the community and spending less time in hospital settings.

This greater emphasis on nursing care provided in community-based settings is a driving force in health care today and, consequently, forms a dominant theme throughout this edition. The new title is a reflection of the important role the nurse plays within the community. In addition, we have addressed this topic in focused, user-friendly ways. **Community-Based Nursing Care** is a heading used throughout the text to assist students in identifying specific aspects of this content. Because we consider home care to be one form of community-based care, it often has a separate heading under community-based nursing care. Even more importantly, a new chapter, **Home Care of the Postpartal Family,** provides a thorough explanation of home care both from a theoretical perspective and as a significant tool in caring for childbearing families.

Community in Focus boxes are an exciting new feature in this addition. These boxes describe innovative community nursing programs in operation in different parts of the United States. For example, "Community in Focus: The SANE Program" on page 119 describes the Sexual Assault Nurse Examiner program, a nurse-implemented program designed to provide better care to survivors of sexual assault.

Emphasis on Client/Family Teaching

Client and family teaching remains a critical element of effective nursing care, one that we continue to emphasize and highlight in the new edition. Again our focus is on the teaching that nurses do at all stages of pregnancy and the childbearing process—including the important postpartal teaching that is done before and after families are discharged. Throughout the text, discussion of client/family teaching is highlighted by an apple logo in the margin. In several places a more detailed discussion of client/family teaching is summarized in **Teaching Guides** such as the one on Sexual Activity During Pregnancy, which starts on page 216. These Teaching Guides help students plan and organize their client teaching. The tear-out **Client-Family Teaching Cards** are also handy tools for the student to use while studying or as a quick reference in the clinical setting. In addition, a fold-out, full-color **Fetal Development Chart** depicts maternal/fetal development by month and provides specific teaching guidelines for each stage of pregnancy. Students can use this as another study tool or as a quick clinical reference.

Critical Thinking and the Nursing Process

We firmly believe that now, more than ever, nurses must be creative, flexible, and open to change. They must also be able to think critically and problem solve effectively. For these reasons, we have organized the text around the five steps of the nursing process: assessment, diagnosis, planning, implementation, and evaluation. Within this framework the nurse's role is clearly delineated.

In addition to organizing each chapter using the nursing process, numerous special features reinforce the nursing process as the framework for providing nursing care and for thinking critically about nursing action.

The **Assessment Guides** incorporate expected findings, possible alterations and causes, and guidelines for nursing interventions. Procedures such as the one on page 113 describe actions specific to maternal-newborn nursing care in step-by-step fashion.

In keeping with the changing approaches to nursing care management, **Critical Pathways** are featured throughout the text. Four critical pathways—intrapartal, newborn, postpartal, and cesarean birth—are designed to help students plan and manage care within normally anticipated timeframes. In addition, critical pathways are provided that address nursing care for women with complications such as pregnancy-induced hypertension and diabetes mellitus as well as for high-risk newborns. This information will help students become familiar with this approach to managing care so that they are better prepared in the clinical setting.

To further support the development of critical thinking skills, **Critical Thinking in Action** boxes provide brief scenarios that ask students to determine the appropriate response. Suggested answers to the scenarios are provided in Appendix H so students will have immediate feedback on their decision-making skills.

State of the Art Teaching/ Learning Tools

Instructors and students alike value the in-text learning aids included in our textbooks. With this edition, we have once again created a text that is easy to learn from and easy to use as a reference. Each chapter begins with Objectives and a list of Key Terms, and ends with a summary of Chapter Highlights as well as a list of References. When appropriate, we have included **Drug Guides** for those medications commonly used in maternal-newborn nursing to guide students in correctly administering the medications. **Key Facts to Remember** provide a quick review of important content in a convenient boxed format, while **Essential Precautions in Practice** remind students of important precautions to take in order to practice safely. Finally, a Glossary of terms commonly used in the field of maternal-newborn nursing can be found at the back of the text.

Enhanced Visual Appeal

Because today's students are more visually oriented than ever, we have developed an exciting new four-color design and art program to command their interest and emphasize the key information they need to learn. Students are brought closer to the childbearing experience through the dramatic photographs of women and families from many cultures and backgrounds.

Commitment to Diversity

With this edition, we attempt to make our text even more inclusive through a commitment to diversity and multiculturalism. We realize such an approach is difficult at best, but feel its success cannot be measured simply in terms of specific photos, charts, or tables. Instead, we believe that with its subtle integration of a variety of issues and scenarios affecting maternal-newborn nursing care—beyond the emphasis on ethnicity alone—our approach is more accessible overall.

Complete Teaching/ Learning Package

Student Tutorial Disk. A new addition to the teaching/learning package is a Student Tutorial Disk. This disk contains approximately 250 NCLEX-style multiple-choice questions which emphasize the application of nursing care. Students are able to test their knowledge and gain immediate feedback through rationales for right and wrong answers. This disk is packaged with every copy of the textbook and is free to students.

Student Workbook. This useful workbook has been revised, streamlined, and updated in keeping with the changes made in this edition. It provides a concise review of essential content and includes exercises and strategies to help students focus their study.

Clinical Handbook. This portable handbook provides students with a succinct quick-reference guide for use in the clinical setting. Content is organized by each stage of the childbirth process and includes normal and at risk information. Procedures, tables, photos, and illustrations are integrated throughout.

800-Item Test Bank. Available printed or as computer software for the IBM, this updated test bank helps faculty quickly and easily create numerous unique examinations. Test items follow the NCLEX two-column format and are classified by cognitive level, nursing process step, and client need.

Instructor's Manual. This effective and time-saving aid has been revised and streamlined. It provides suggestions for covering important content and is organized by topics according to subject matter. The Instructor's Manual is available via e-mail or on disk.

Transparency Acetates. A set of 40 full-color transparency acetates, including illustrations not otherwise included in the text, provide visual support for your lectures.

The full complement of supplemental teaching materials in available to qualified instructors.

Acknowledgments

Our field, maternal-newborn nursing, is consistently changing and evolving. Thus our goal for each new edition is to ensure that our text reflects the most current research and the latest information about nursing. We are grateful for our colleagues in nursing education and clinical practice who help us achieve this goal through their suggestions, contributions, and words of encouragement. Whenever a nurse takes the time to write or speak to one of us at a professional gathering, we recognize again the intense commitment of nurses to excellence in practice. And so we thank our colleagues.

In publishing as in health care, quality assurance is an essential part of the process; this is the dimension reviewers add. Some reviewers assist us by validating the content, some by their attention to detail, and some by challenging us to examine our ways of thinking to develop a new awareness. Thus we extend our sincere thanks to all of those who reviewed the manuscript for this text; their names and affiliations are listed before this preface.

We are also grateful to the contributors to the fifth edition of our other text, *Maternal-Newborn Nursing: A Family-Centered Approach*. They include:

Tsulan Balka, RNC, MA, ACCE
Saint Joseph Hospital
Denver, Colorado

S. Robin Barca, RNC, MS, CCE
Houston Valley Hospital and Medical Center
Kingsport, Tennessee

Emily Coogan Bennett, RNC, MS
Medical College of Virginia
Richmond, Virginia

Barbara E. Carey, RNC, MN, NNP, CPNP
University of California, Los Angeles
Los Angeles, California

Nancy Kiernan Case, RN, PhD
Regis University
Denver, Colorado

Jane E. Congleton, RN, BSN, MS, CGC
Memorial Hospital
Colorado Springs, Colorado

Mary English, RNC, MSN
Pennsylvania Reproductive Associates
Philadelphia, Pennsylvania

Vicky Flanagan, RN, MSN
Dartmouth-Hitchcock Medical Center
Lebanon, New Hampshire

Mary Hagedorn, RN, PhD, CPNP
Beth-El College of Nursing and Health Sciences
Colorado Springs, Colorado

Mary Ellen Honeyfield, RNC, MS, NNP
Innovative Health Care Incorporated
Denver, Colorado

Jeanne M. Howell, RN, MS, CNM
Alexandria OB/GYN Associates
Alexandria, Minnesota

Sara L. Jarrett, RN, MA, MS
Regis University
Denver, Colorado

Virginia Gramzow Kinnick, BSN, MSN, EdD, CNM
University of Northern Colorado
Greeley, Colorado

Cheryl Pope Kish, RN, MSN, EdD
Georgia College
Milledgeville, Georgia

Ruth Likler, RNC, BSN
Presbyterian/Saint Lukes Medical Center
Denver, Colorado

Marilyn Lowe, RNC, MSN
Nebraska Methodist Hospital
Omaha, Nebraska

Vicki A. Lucas, RNC, PhD
Memorial Hospital Southwest
Houston, Texas

Deborah Cooper McGee, RNC, MSN, PNNP
Presbyterian/Saint Lukes Medical Center
Denver, Colorado

Patricia Budd Moores, RN, PhD
Beth-El College of Nursing and Health Sciences
Colorado Springs, Colorado

Carol Myers, RNC, BSN
Toledo Hospital
Toledo, Ohio

Candace Layn Polzella, MSS, RD
Schwenksville, Pennsylvania

Diane Roth, RNC, BSN, RD, MS
Health One/Swedish Medical Center
Englewood, Colorado

Victoria Stetson, CNM, MS
Lovelace Medical Center
Albuquerque, New Mexico

Catherine E. Theorell, RNC, MSN, NNP
Rush-Presbyterian Saint Lukes Medical Center
Chicago, Illinois

Candice J. Tolve, RNC, MS
Regis University
Denver, Colorado

Susan Thompson Voss, RN, MSN
Blessing-Rieman College of Nursing
Quincy, Illinois

Helen B. Walker, RNC, MSN, CNS
Mobile Infirmary Medical Center
Mobile, Alabama

A project of this scope requires the skill and expertise of many people. We would personally like to thank the following people:

Patti Cleary, Executive Editor, is someone we feel privileged to know. She is an exceptional individual—witty, wise, and caring. She is a woman of great personal integrity whose friendship and guidance we treasure. She has never let us down.

Ginnie Simione Jutson, Associate Editor and our newest friend at Addison Wesley Longman, brought warmth, skill, and incredible patience to this effort. This is the first time we have worked with Ginnie but we look forward to a long partnership. She shares our vision for the text and is always available to lend her support and assistance.

Many thanks to Laura Bonazzoli, Developmental Editor, who brought her skill and eye for detail to bear in assisting us to revise several chapters. It was wonderful working with her again.

Dave Rich, Production Editor, is a rock! He has an incredible eye for detail and the patience of a saint. Unflappable, he guided us through the myriad of details and crises that inevitably accompany the production phase of a textbook. We would be lost without him!

Bradley Burch of Wendy Earl Productions coordinated all the art for the manuscript. We have worked with Bradley several times and are always awed by his expertise, commitment to the project, and patience. It is a pleasure to work with him.

Marla Nowick, Administrative Assistant, has committed hours to this text converting manuscript from our disks to Production's format. She also provided support for many aspects of the project. She is truly amazing.

Finally, we extend a special word of thanks to Kathy Marvel, RN, MSN, Nurse Manager, Women's and Children's Services, Columbia Rose Medical Center, Denver, Colorado. Kathy brought her exceptional clinical expertise to bear in developing the critical pathways found in this edition. Her knowledge and commitment to nursing are exemplary. Thanks, Kathy!

During these times of uncertainty and change in health care we are sustained by our passion for nursing and our vision of what family-centered childbirth truly means. Time and again we have seen the difference a skilled nurse can make in the lives of people in need. We, like you, are committed to helping all nurses recognize and take pride in that fact. Thank you for your letters, your comments, and your suggestions. We are renewed by your support.

Patricia Wieland Ladewig
Marcia L. London
Sally B. Olds

DEAR STUDENTS:

We believe that working with childbearing families gives you the opportunity to experience the essence of nursing at its best. You can play a vital role in helping families learn what they need to know in order to be as independent as possible; you can improve and refine your assessment skills as you work with essentially healthy women and infants, and those with complications; and you can also use the other nursing skills you have learned in a variety of acute care settings.

We love this field and we know that many of you will as well. Some of you, on the other hand, may find that this area of nursing is not your first interest, and that's OK, too. We would have a real problem if every nurse loved the same area!

We do hope that you will use this opportunity to grow in professional ability and to appreciate the importance of all you do as nurses—not just the technical and organizational tasks, although they are undoubtedly crucial, but also the caring you bring to the role of nurse. When you hold the hand of a laboring woman or help an adolescent plan a way to tell her parents of her pregnancy; when you provide accepting care to a woman with AIDS or gently stroke the skin of a preterm infant; when you rejoice with a delighted father or console a grieving one; you are practicing the heart of nursing.

Caring in an optimal environment is not difficult, but caring in today's practice setting is more of a challenge. Finding a way to maintain a caring environment when you are overworked and stretched by fiscal constraints and a lack of adequate staffing requires great dedication, creativity, and personal resolve. We have attempted to help you translate caring into practice throughout this text through the tone of the book, the photos and art work, the personal quotes, and the content itself with its emphasis on holistic care.

As you work to translate what you learn into practice, please take care of yourselves as well. Providing excellent nursing care is infinitely rewarding and can be energizing, but it is also draining both physically and emotionally. Make time to play, rest, exercise, be with loved ones, and participate in things that rejuvenate you.

We think that nurses are very special people and we are proud to be counted among them. Good luck with your studies! We wish you well.

PAT W. LADEWIG
MARCIA L. LONDON
SALLY B. OLDS

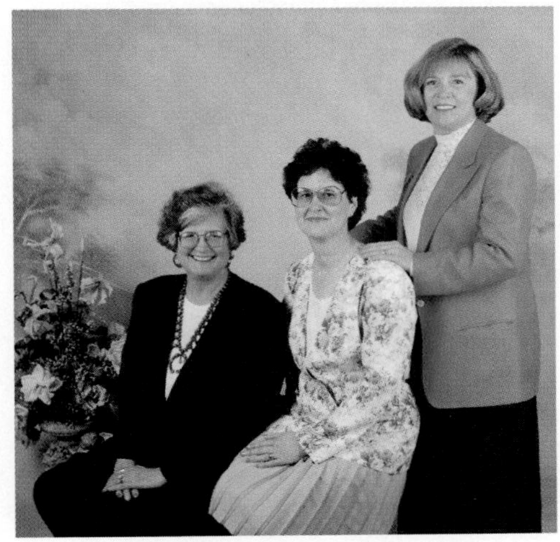

Left to right: Sally Olds; Marcia London; Pat Ladewig

CONTENTS

PART TWO: PREGNANCY 151

continued

A VISUAL GUIDE TO *MATERNAL-NEWBORN NURSING CARE*

INCREASED EMPHASIS ON COMMUNITY

A new chapter, "Home Care of the Postpartal Family," discusses assessment, teaching, and physical care of the postpartal family in the home.

Community in Focus boxes describe innovative community-based nursing programs in operation today throughout the United States.

Chapter 5: Women's Health Care 119

COMMUNITY IN FOCUS The SANE Program

In many communities, the treatment of a woman immediately following a rape has been almost as traumatic as the rape itself. Often the woman is taken to the local emergency room accompanied by a police officer, and sits in the waiting room while others speculate as to why she requires a police escort. She may have to wait 4–8 hours or more to be seen by the physician, who first has to treat life-threatening emergencies. During this period, she is not allowed to urinate, shower, eat or drink anything, or change her clothes, because these activities might destroy or alter physical evidence. The police officer who accompanies the rape victim is also detained, unable to leave the victim until the examination is completed and specimens obtained, thus preserving the chain of evidence.

In Tulsa, Oklahoma, the Sexual Assault Nurse Examiner (SANE) Program is designed to address this problem. SANE is coordinated by the police department and provides a seamless program of post-rape health care, personal counseling, and prosecution by combining the resources of seven community organizations: the police department, the District Attorney's office, Call Rape (rape crisis center), the Victim/Witness Center, the Tulsa City/County Health Department, the University of Oklahoma College of Medicine, and Hillcrest Medical Center (Kauffold 1996).

Following the report of a rape, provided the woman's physical injuries are not severe, a police officer brings the rape victim to a special examination suite, away from the busy emergency room. They are met there by a specially trained female sexual assault nurse examiner and a rape crisis counselor. The victim is examined immediately by the SANE nurse, who completes the lengthy examination and gathers all necessary forensic evidence. The hospital ob/gyn resident is available to the nurse if there is a need for further examination and treatment.

Because the evidence collected by the SANE nurses has been of such high quality, the Tulsa District Attorney has designated SANE nurses as expert witnesses in rape trials. Each SANE nurse participates in an extensive training program, agrees to serve as an expert witness if necessary, and takes calls so that nurses are always available to respond when a rape occurs.

Similar programs exist elsewhere. The Sexual Assault Response Team (SART), which started in San Diego, is a multidisciplinary approach that also makes use of SANE nurses. The SART Program is designed to ensure that victims receive necessary health care, emotional support, evidentiary examinations, and referral information. The International Association of Forensic Nurses (the terms *sexual assault nurse examiner* and *forensic nurse* are comparable) estimates that 30–40 new SART programs have started in the United States in the past year (Voelker 1996).

These programs are highly effective in addressing a real community need. In Tulsa, for example, successful convictions of accused rapists are up significantly (Kauffold 1996). Equally important, however, the victim of a rape is treated with care and compassion and not victimized a second time.

values to which they ascribe. Many families or mates blame the survivor for the assault and feel angry with her for not having been more careful. They may also incorrectly view the rape as a sexual act rather than an act

Prosecution of the Rapist

Legally, rape is considered a crime against the state and prosecution of the assailant is a community responsibility. The survivor, however, ...

230 Part II: Pregnancy

of the effects of these substances on her development as well as on the development of the fetus.

Ongoing care should include the same assessments that the older pregnant woman receives. The nurse should pay special attention to evaluating fetal growth by determining when quickening occurs and by measuring fundal height, fetal heart tones, and fetal movement. Corresponding dates of auscultating fetal heart tones with the date of last menstrual period and quickening can be helpful in determining correct estimations of time of birth. If there is a question of size–date discrepancy by 2 cm either way, an ultrasound is warranted to establish fetal age so that instances of intrauterine growth retardation (IUGR) can be diagnosed and treated early.

For adolescents, the incidence of a subsequent pregnancy is very high. Thus, despite the pregnant teen's strong assertion that she will not be sexually active again, contraception is an important consideration during the postpartal period. Because of the risks of thrombophlebitis associated with immediate postpartum use of oral contraceptives, many caregivers recommend that the adolescent use barrier methods of contraception (foam and condoms). Postpartal visits are then scheduled at 2 weeks to assess for problems and at 4 weeks to discuss and initiate contraception if it is acceptable to her, often using oral contraceptives (Reedy 1991).

Promotion of Family Adaptation

The nurse assesses the family situation during the first prenatal visit and determines what level of involvement the adolescent desires from each of her family members and from the father of the child, as well as her perception of their present support. A sensitive approach to the daughter-mother relationship helps motivate their communication. If the mother and daughter agree, the mother should be included in the client's care. Encouraging the mother to become part of the maternity team, join grandmother crisis support groups, and obtain counseling helps the mother adapt to her role and support her daughter.

The nurse should also help the mother assess and meet her daughter's needs. Some adolescents become more dependent during pregnancy, and some become more independent. The mother can ease and encourage her daughter's self-growth by understanding how to respond to and support her.

The adolescent's relationship with her father will also be affected by her pregnancy. The nurse can provide information to the father and encourage his involvement to whatever degree is acceptable to both daughter and father.

The father of the adolescent's infant should not be forgotten in promoting the family's adaptation to the pregnancy. He should be included to the extent that he wishes and the teenage mother finds acceptable.

Community-Based Nursing Care

Educational programs for adolescents address two areas: pregnancy prevention and, if pregnancy occurs, prenatal education. Ideally these programs are community based and include the clinic or the caregiver's office, community agencies, and the school system. Many adolescents cite school as the preferred agency for education.

Effective pregnancy prevention programs generally include a focus on abstinence or on delaying sexual initiation, information about human sexuality and contraceptive options, and training in negotiation and decision-making skills. Research suggests that the programs are most effective when they target early adolescents (Frost and Forrest 1995).

The most effective method for education during pregnancy and early parenting appears to be mainstreaming the pregnant adolescent in academic classes with her peers and adding classes appropriate to her needs. Classes about growth and development beginning with the newborn and early infancy can help teenage parents have more realistic expectations of their infants and may help decrease child abuse. Mainstreaming pregnant adolescents in school is also an ideal way to help them complete their education while learning the skills they need to cope with childbearing and parenting. Vocational guidance in this setting is also most beneficial to their future.

Regardless of the sponsorship or setting of prenatal classes for pregnant teenagers and adolescent fathers, the adolescent's developmental tasks must be considered. For example, methods for teaching this age group should be somewhat different from regular prenatal classes (Figure 10–2). The younger adolescent tends to be a more concrete thinker than the older, more mature pregnant adult. Increased use of audiovisuals appropriate to their social situation and age is helpful. More demonstrations may be required, and they need to be simple and direct.

Areas that might be included in prenatal classes are anatomy and physiology, sex education, exercises for pregnancy and after birth, maternal and infant nutrition, growth and development of the fetus, labor and birth, family planning, and infant development. Adolescents may want to participate in the teaching of these classes and should be encouraged to do so. Peer support and friendships can blossom among these young women, helping them all to mature.

The clinic can offer rap sessions, pamphlets, or films in the waiting room. Giving the clients something to do while they wait for their appointments may encourage them to return and also help them learn. Decorating the clinic with attractive educational posters and creating an

Community-Based Nursing Care is described in key sections of the text to help you understand how therapeutic care of maternal-newborn conditions is given in the community. Because we consider home care to be one form of community-based care, it often appears as a separate heading under Community-Based Nursing Care.

LEARNING TOOLS

Procedures describe actions specific to maternal-newborn nursing care in step-by-step fashion.

Drug Guides describe the action, use, administration, and nursing considerations for the most important medications used in maternal-newborn nursing.

PROCEDURE 17–1 Performing Nasal Pharyngeal Suctioning

Nursing Action	Rationale
Objective: Clear secretions from the newborn's nose and/or oropharynx if respirations are depressed and/or if amniotic fluid was meconium-stained.	
• Tighten the lid on the DeLee mucus trap or other suction device collection bottle.	This avoids spillage of secretions and prevents air from leaking out of the lid.
• Connect one end of the DeLee tubing to low suction.	
• Insert the other end of the tubing 3 to 5 inches in the newborn's nose or mouth (Figure 17–10).	

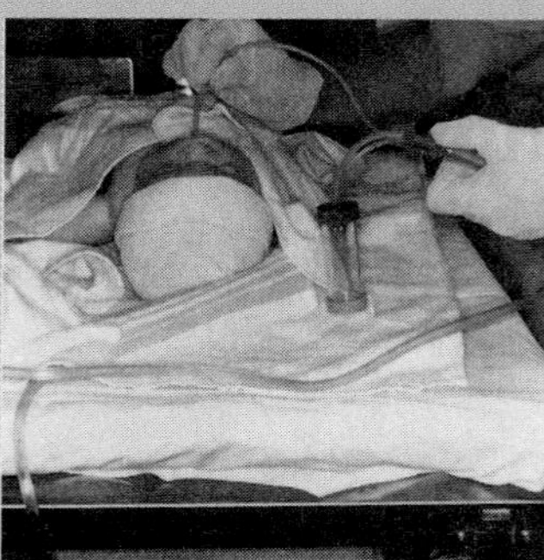

FIGURE 17–10 DeLee mucus trap.

Nursing Action	Rationale
• Continue suction as you remove the tube.	This avoids redepositing secretions in the newborn's nasopharynx.
• Continue to reinsert the tube and provide suction for as long as fluid is aspirated. *Note: Excessive suctioning can cause vagal stimulation, which causes decreased heart rate.*	
• If it is necessary to pass the tube into the newborn's stomach to remove meconium secretions that the newborn swallowed before birth, insert the tube into the newborn's mouth and then into the stomach. Provide suction and continue suction as you remove the tube.	
Objective: Record relevant information on the newborn's chart.	
• Document completion of the procedure and the amount and type of secretions.	This provides documentation

DRUG GUIDE Dinoprostone (Cervidil) Vaginal Insert

Pregnancy Risk Category: C

Overview of Maternal-Fetal Action

Dinoprostone is a naturally occurring form of prostaglandin E_2. Dinoprostone can be used at term to ripen the cervix and can stimulate the smooth muscle of the uterus to enhance uterine contractions. A single vaginal insert may be used to ripen the cervix and then oxytocin can be administered 30 minutes later (Zatuchni and Slupik 1996; Forest Pharmaceuticals, Inc. Drug Insert 1995).

Route, Dosage, Frequency

The vaginal insert contains 10 mg of Dinoprostone. The insert is placed transversely in the posterior fornix of the vagina and the patient is kept supine for two hours but then may ambulate. The Dinoprostone is released at approximately 0.3 mg/hour over a 12 hour period. The vaginal insert should be removed by pulling on the retrieval string upon onset of uterine contractions or after 12 hours (Forest Pharmaceuticals, Inc. Drug Insert 1995).

Contraindications

Patient with known sensitivity to prostaglandins.

Presence of fetal distress.

Patient who has had unexplained bleeding during pregnancy.

Patient with strong suspicion of cephalopelvic disproportion.

Patient already receiving oxytocin.

Patient with 6 or more previous term pregnancies.

Patient who is not anticipated to be able to give birth vaginally.

Dinoprostone Vaginal Insert should be used with CAUTION in patients with ruptured membranes, a fetus in breech presentation, presence of glaucoma or history of asthma (Forest Pharmaceuticals, Inc. 1995).

Maternal Side Effects

Uterine hyperstimulation with or without fetal distress has occurred in a very small number (2.8–4.7%) of patients. Less than 1% of patients have experienced fever, nausea, vomiting, diarrhea, or abdominal pain (Forest Pharmaceuticals, Inc. 1995).

Effects on Fetus/Neonate

Fetal distress (Zatuchni and Slupik 1996).

Nursing Considerations

Assess for presence of contraindications.

Monitor maternal vital signs, cervical dilatation and effacement carefully.

Monitor fetal status for presence of reassuring fetal heart rate pattern (baseline 120–160 bpm, presence of short-term variability, average variability, presence of accelerations with fetal movement, absence of late or variable decelerations).

Remove vaginal insert if uterine hyperstimulation, sustained uterine contractions, fetal distress, or any other maternal adverse actions occur.

Relative maternal contraindications include but are not limited to the following (ACOG 1991):

- Client refusal
- Placenta previa or vasa previa
- Abnormal fetal presentation
- Cord presentation
- Presenting part above the pelvic inlet
- Prior classic uterine incision
- Active genital herpes infection
- Pelvic structural deformities or cephalopelvic disproportion (CPD)
- Invasive cervical carcinoma

Before an induction is attempted, assessment must indicate that both the woman and the unborn child are ready for labor. This assessment includes evaluation of fetal maturity and cervical readiness.

Labor Readiness

Fetal Maturity

Gestational age of the fetus can be determined throughout the gestational period by ultrasound examination. Amniotic fluid studies also provide important information on fetal maturity. (See Chapter 14 for a discussion of methods to assess fetal maturity.)

Cervical Readiness

The findings of vaginal examinations help determine whether cervical changes favorable to induction have occurred. Bishop (1964) developed a prelabor scoring system that has proved helpful in predicting the inducibility of women (Table 20–1). Components evaluated are cervical dilatation, effacement, consistency, and position, as well as the station of the fetal presenting part. A score of 0, 1, 2, or 3 is given to each assessed characteristic. The higher the total score for all the criteria, the more likely it is that labor will ensue. The lower the total score, the higher the failure rate. A favorable cervix is the most important criterion for a successful induction.

The presence of a cervix that is anterior, soft, more than 50 percent effaced, and dilated at least 3 cm, with the fetal head at +1 station or lower is favorable for a successful induction (Dunn 1990).

Procedure for Oxytocin Infusion

The most frequently used methods of induction are amniotomy, described earlier, and intravenous oxytocin infusion, or both.

Intravenous administration of oxytocin is an effective method of initiating uterine contractions (inducing

CRITICAL THINKING EXERCISES

Critical Thinking in Action boxes teach problem-solving and decision-making skills by asking you to determine appropriate responses to real-life clinical situations.

quish the child. The nurse can encourage the young woman to share her feelings about each alternative and the projected consequences as they relate to her situation in life. The nurse can also provide information about community resources available with help for each alternative. The nurse should provide information in an open, nonjudgmental way without imposing personal values on the teen. Once the adolescent has decided on a course, health care providers should respect her decision and support her efforts to achieve her goals.

If the adolescent chooses to maintain her pregnancy, the nurse should give her an overview of what she will experience over the course of her pregnancy and should provide a thorough explanation and rationale for each procedure as it occurs. If she elects to terminate the pregnancy, the nurse should give her information about abortions, including what to expect, costs, applicable state laws about parental notification, and so forth. This approach fosters the adolescent's understanding and gives her some measure of control.

Early adolescents tend to be egocentric and oriented to the present. They may not regard as important the fact that their health and habits affect the fetus. Consequently, it is often useful to emphasize the effects of these practices on the client herself. The young woman will also need help in problem solving and in visualizing the future so she can plan effectively.

The middle adolescent is developing the ability to think abstractly and can recognize that actions may ... may not yet have ac... ...kills, however, and ...rses should antic... ...s and initiate dis... ...she has any con...

CRITICAL THINKING IN ACTION

Cindy Lenz, a 15-year-old Gr1P0, is 16 weeks pregnant when she arrives for her second prenatal visit. She is drinking diet soda and eating potato chips as she waits for her appointment. Her 18-year-old boyfriend is with her. In reviewing her history the nurse remembers that Cindy had tried to get pregnant for several months. Her boyfriend, a high school dropout, has a part-time job. As a result Cindy is still living at home, although she does not get along with her mother or sister. Cindy plans to stay in school until her baby is born because she has two other friends at school who are also pregnant. As the nurse weighs Cindy she asks a few questions about her nutritional habits and finds that Cindy eats lots of junk food and very few vegetables or fruits. How should the nurse discuss Cindy's nutritional needs with her?

Answers can be found in Appendix H.

portance of iron in her diet. A nutritional consultation is indicated for all adolescents. Group classes are helpful because peer pressure is strong among this age group.

Adolescents may fear laboratory tests, which can evoke early childhood memories of being "stuck" with needles or hurt. Explanations help relieve anxiety and coordination of services will avoid multiple venous punctures.

Pregnancy-induced hypertension represents the most prevalent medical complication of pregnant adolescents. The criteria of blood pressure readings of 140/90 mm Hg are not acceptable as the determinant of PIH in adolescents. Women aged 14 to 20 years without evidence of high blood pressure usually have diastolic readings between 50 and 66 mm H...

KEY FACTS TO REMEMBER

What Women Need to Know About Pain Relief Medications

Before receiving medications, the woman should understand the following:

- Type of medication administered
- Route of administration
- Expected effects of medication
- Implications for fetus/neonate
- Safety measures needed (for example, remain in bed with side rails up)

- The fetal presenting part is engaged.
- There is progressive descent of the fetal presenting part. No complications are present.

If normal parameters are not present, the nurse may need to complete further assessments with the physician/certified nurse-midwife.

Before administering the medication, the nurse once again validates whether the woman has a history of any drug reactions or allergies and provides information about the medication. See Key Facts to Remember: What Women Need to Know About Pain Relief Medications. After giving the medication, the nurse records the drug name, dose, route, and site, and the woman's B/P and pulse, on the FHR monitor strip and on the woman's records. If the woman is ... side rails should be raised ...

ESSENTIAL PRECAUTIONS FOR PRACTICE

During Administration of Analgesia and Anesthesia

Examples of times when disposable gloves should be worn include:

- Administering intravenous medications for analgesia to prevent exposure to blood.
- Starting intravenous fluids prior to regional blocks.
- Assisting the woman into position for an epidural or spinal. While the nurse assists the woman into position, the nurse may inadvertently be exposed to vaginal fluids or amniotic fluid.

REMEMBER to wash your hands prior to putting on the disposable gloves and AGAIN immediately after you remove the gloves.

For further information consult OSHA and CDC guidelines.

Narcotic Analgesics

Meperidine Hydrochloride (Demerol)

Meperidine hydrochloride (Demerol) is a narcotic analgesic that is effective for alleviating pain during the first stage of labor. It may be given by the intravenous or intramuscular route. The IV route provides effective analgesia within 5 to 10 m... 3 hours; the usual IV... given intramuscularly... and 75 mg; the durati...

Neonatal depress...

GUIDE FOR UNIVERSAL PRECAUTIONS

Essential Precautions for Practice boxes, integrated throughout the text, illustrate the application of appropriate infection control practices in a variety of situations.

KEY FACTS TO REMEMBER

Preeclampsia-Eclampsia

- Preeclampsia, which occurs after the 20th week of pregnancy, involves elevated BP, edema, and proteinuria. It may be mild or severe.
- A woman with preeclampsia who has a seizure is said to have eclampsia.
- The exact cause of preeclampsia is unknown.
- Vasospasm is responsible for most of the clinical manifestations, including the CNS signs of headache, hyperreflexia, and convulsion. Vasospasm also causes poor placental perfusion, which leads to IUGR.
- The only known cure for preeclampsia is birth of the infant, but symptoms may develop up to 48 hours postpartum.
- Management is supportive and includes anticonvulsant therapy, generally with $MgSO_4$; prevention of renal, hepatic, and hematologic complications; and careful assessment of fetal well-being.
- Nursing care focuses on implementing appropriate interventions based on the data gathered from regular assessment of vital signs, reflexes, degree of edema and proteinuria, response to therapy, fetal status, detection of developing complications, knowledge level and psychologic state of the woman and her family.

the second trimester, chronic hypertension should be suspected. The cause of chronic hypertension has not been determined. In most chronic hypertensive women the disease is mild...

Chronic Hypertension with Superimposed Preeclampsia

Preeclampsia may develop in a woman previously found to have chronic hypertension. Close monitoring and careful management are indicated if the following signs develop:

- Elevations of systolic blood pressure 30 mm Hg above the baseline or diastolic blood pressure 15–20 mm Hg above the baseline, on two occasions at least 6 hours apart
- Proteinuria
- Edema occurring in the upper half of the body

A woman with chronic hypertension who develops superimposed preeclampsia often progresses quickly to eclampsia, sometimes before 30 weeks of pregnancy.

Late or Transient Hypertension

Late hypertension exists when transient elevation of blood pressure occurs during labor or in the early postpartal period, returning to normal within 10 days after birth.

Care of the Woman at Risk for Rh Sensitization

The Rh blood group is present on the surface of erythrocytes of a majority of the population. When it is present, a person is designated as Rh-positive. Those without the factor are de... ...egative. If an ...

EMPHASIS ON KEY CONCEPTS

Key Facts to Remember provides quick review of chapter content crucial to effective nursing practice.

DYNAMIC VISUAL PROGRAM

Full-Color Format enhances visual learning of anatomy and physiologic processes and highlights key information. Dramatic photographs and personal reflections of childbearing women bring you closer to the childbearing experience.

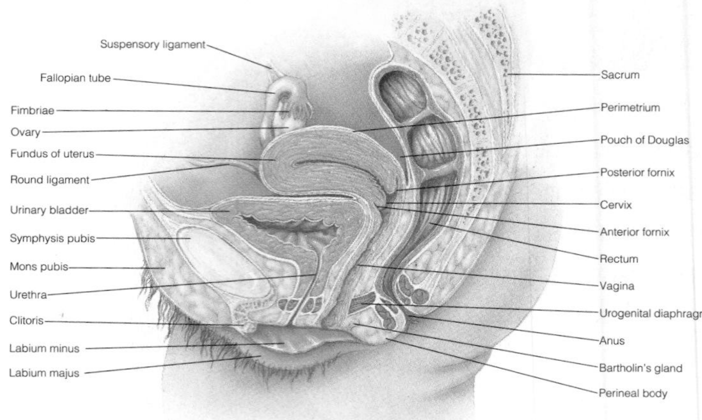

FIGURE 2–2 Female internal reproductive organs.

lies on her back after intercourse, the space in the fornix permits the pooling of semen near the cervix and increases the chances of impregnation.

The walls of the vagina are covered with ridges, or *rugae,* crisscrossing each other. These rugae allow the vagina to stretch during the descent of the fetal head.

During a woman's reproductive life, an acidic vaginal environment is normal (pH 4–5). The acidic environment is maintained by a symbiotic relationship between lactic acid–producing bacilli (Döderlein bacillus or lactobacillus) and the vaginal epithelial cells. These cells contain glycogen, which is broken down by the bacilli into lactic acid. The amount of glycogen is regu-

y interruption of this
lf-cleaning action of
caused by antibi-
eal sprays or de-
ssues for women,

normal only dur-
n the first days of
ting in the infant.
l from infancy

until puberty and after menopause. The vagina's blood and lymphatic supplies are extensive (Figure 2–3).

The pudendal nerve supplies what relatively little somatic innervation there is to the lower third of the vagina. Thus sensation during sexual excitement and coitus is minimal, as is vaginal pain during the second stage of labor.

The vagina has three functions:

- To serve as the passage for sperm and for the fetus during birth
- To provide passage for the menstrual products from the uterine endometrium to the outside of the body
- To protect against trauma from sexual intercourse and infection from pathogenic organisms

Uterus

Throughout the ages, the uterus, or womb, has been endowed with a mystical aura. Numerous customs, taboos, mores, and values have evolved about women and their reproductive function. Although scientific knowledge has replaced much of this folklore, remnants of old ideas and superstitions persist. The nurse must be

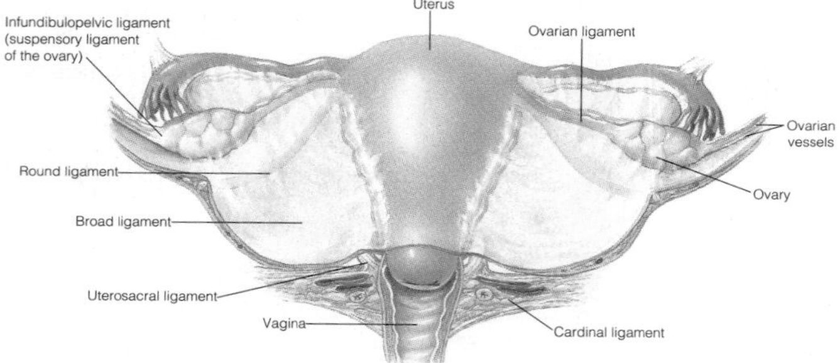

FIGURE 2–6 Uterine ligaments.

contractions of labor are responsible for the dilatation of the cervix and provide the major force for the passage of the fetus through the pelvic axis and vaginal canal at birth. The mucosal layer, or **endometrium,** of the uterine corpus is the innermost layer. This single layer is composed of columnar epithelium, glands, and stroma. From menarche to menopause, the endometrium undergoes monthly degeneration and renewal in the absence of pregnancy. As it responds to the governing hormonal cycle and prostaglandin influence, the endometrium varies in thickness from 0.5 to 5 mm.

The glands of the endometrium produce a thin, watery, alkaline secretion that keeps the uterine cavity moist. This *endometrial milk* not only helps sperm travel to the fallopian tubes but also nourishes the developing embryo before it lodges in the endometrium (Chapter 3).

The blood supply to the endometrium is unique. Some of the blood vessels are not sensitive to cyclic hormonal control, whereas others are extremely sensitive to it. These differing responses allow part of the endometrium to remain intact while other endometrial tissue is shed during menstruation.

The Cervix The narrow neck of the uterus is the cervix. It meets the body of the uterus at the internal os and descends about 2.5 cm to connect with the vagina at the external os (Figure 2–4). Thus it provides a protective portal for the body of the uterus. The cervix is divided by its line of attachment into the vaginal and supravaginal areas. The *vaginal cervix* projects into the vagina at an angle of from 45 to 90 degrees. The *supravaginal cervix* is surrounded by the attachments that give the uterus its main support: the uterosacral ligaments, the transverse ligaments of the cervix (Mackenrodt's ligaments), and the pubocervical ligaments.

The vaginal cervix appears pink and ends at the external os. The cervical canal appears rosy red and is lined with columnar ciliated epithelium, which contains mucus-secreting glands. Most cervical cancer begins at this squamocolumnar junction. The specific location of the junction varies with age and number of pregnancies. Elasticity is the chief characteristic of the cervix. Its ability to stretch is due to the high fibrous and collagenous content of the supportive tissues and also to the vast number of folds in the cervical lining.

The cervical mucus has three functions:

- To lubricate the vaginal canal
- To act as a bacteriostatic agent
- To provide an alkaline environment to shelter deposited sperm from the acidic vagina

At ovulation, cervical mucus is clearer, thinner, more profuse, and more alkaline than at other times.

Uterine Ligaments The uterine ligaments support and stabilize the various reproductive organs. The ligaments shown in Figure 2–6 are described as follows:

1. The **broad ligament** keeps the uterus centrally placed and provides stability within the pelvic cavity. It is a double layer that is continuous with the abdominal peritoneum. The broad ligament covers the uterus anteriorly and posteriorly and extends outward from the uterus to enfold the fallopian tubes. The round and ovarian ligaments are at the

GUIDES TO CARE PLANNING AND MANAGEMENT

Critical Pathways are provided for the intrapartal client, the newborn, and the postpartal client, as well as for women with complications and high-risk newborns. These pathways are designed to help you plan and manage care within normally anticipated time lines.

CRITICAL PATHWAY FOR FETAL STRESS continued

Category	
Family involvement	• Keep woman and family well informed through factual information
Teaching/ psychosocial	• Inform woman of fetal status • Explain treatment plan. Provide accurate information. • Assess the emotional status of patient and family • Reassure woman and family
Date	

the mother, her partner, and the health team members contributes to a more realistic understanding of the medical condition and its associated treatments. The nurse may discuss prior experiences the family has had with stress and what they feel were their coping abilities at that time. Identifying the family's social supports and resources is also important.

Nursing Diagnosis

Nursing diagnoses that may apply include the following:

- Grief related to an actual loss
- Alteration in family process related to loss of a family member
- Ineffective individual and family coping related to depression in response to loss of a child
- Ineffective family coping related to death of a child
- Anxiety related to death of a child

Nursing Plan and Implementation

The parents of a stillborn infant suffer a devastating experience, precipitating an intense emotional trauma. During the pregnancy, the couple has already begun the attachment process, which now must be terminated through the grieving process. The behaviors that couples exhibit while mourning may be associated with the five stages of grieving described by Elizabeth Kübler-Ross (1969). Often the first stage is *denial* of the death of the ... care provider suspects ... a second opinion ... t be convinced of ... stillborn infant. ... m the feelings of ... e anger may be ... h team members, ... f the fetus is sud- ... ird stage, may or ... couple's prepara- ... ath is unantici

pated, the couple may have no time for bargaining. In the fourth stage, *depression* is evidenced by preoccupation, weeping, and withdrawal. Physiologic postpartal depression appearing 24–48 hours after birth may compound the depression of grief. The final stage is *acceptance,* which involves the process of resolution. This is a highly individualized process that may take months to complete.

Some facilities use a checklist to ensure that caregivers address important aspects of working with the parents. The checklist becomes a communication tool between staff members to share information particular to this couple (Brown 1992). Such a checklist might include the following items:

- When the fetal death is known before admission, inform the admission department and nursing staff so they can avoid making inappropriate remarks.
- Allow the woman and her partner to remain together as much as they wish. Provide privacy by assigning them a private room.
- Stay with the couple; do not leave them alone and isolated.
- As much as possible, have the same nurse provide care to increase the support for the couple. Develop a care plan to provide for continuity of care. Encourage family members to visit support persons.
- Have the most experienced labor and birth nurse auscultate for fetal heart tones. This avoids the searching that a more inexperienced nurse might feel compelled to do. Avoid the temptation to listen again "to make sure."
- Listen to the couple; do not offer explanations. They require solace without minimizing the situation.
- Facilitate the woman and her partner's participation in the labor and birth process. When possible, allow them to make decisions about who will be present and what ritual will occur during the birth process. Allow the woman to make the decision whether to have sedation during labor and birth. Provide a

CRITICAL PATHWAY FOR FETAL STRESS

Category		
Referral	• Physician • Neonatologist	
Assessment	• Preexisting maternal diseases • Maternal hypotension, bleeding • Placental abnormalities • Diagnostic studies 1. Maternal hemoglobin and hematocrit 2. Urinalysis	• Nursing assessment: • Determine FHR baseline • Assess variability • Monitor decelerations • Monitor accelerations • Evaluate contraction pattern • Monitor uterine resting tone • Take maternal vital signs • Evaluate amniotic fluid
Comfort	• Assess comfort level	
Nursing interventions and report	• Decreased variability of fetal heart rate • Late decelerations in FHR • Fetal hyperactivity • Presence of meconium in the amniotic fluid If any of the above are found, initiate the following interventions: 1. Administer oxygen to the woman with tight face mask at 7–10 L/minute, per physician order 2. Notify physician of maternal and fetal assessment findings. Document assessment and specific information relayed to physician 3. Assess maternal vital signs 4. Institute emergency measures for prolapse of cord: • Manually exert pressure on the presenting part. This must be done continuously. Woman may be maintained in supine position, Trendelenburg position, knee-chest position, or on her side with a pillow to elevate her hips • If occult prolapse is suspected, change maternal position to side-lying • Notify physician/certified nurse-midwife immediately • Potential fetal stress if: • Tachycardia > 160 bpm; bradycardia < 110 bpm • Decreased long-term variability; short-term variability absent • Persistent late decelerations; prolonged variable decelerations • Absence of accelerations with fetal movement or scalp stimulation • Temperature 100.4F or >; hypotension • Meconium stained amniotic fluid • Contractions closer than every 2 minutes lasting > 90 seconds • Inadequate resting tone between contractions • Ripe cervix feels soft to the examining finger, is located in a medial to anterior position, is more than 50% effaced, and is 2–3 cm dilated • Unripe cervix feels firm to the examining finger, is long and thick, is perhaps in a posterior position, and is dilated little or not at all	
Activity	• Change maternal position (lateral, left side preference)	
Nutrition	• IV infusion • Ice chips	
Elimination	• Encourage voiding q2h • Monitor and record I/O	
Medications	• Increase IV fluid (as per institutional protocol) • Discontinue oxytocin if infusing	
Discharge planning/ home care	• Plan for home care visits after discharge from birthing facility • Introduce the home care nurse to the family before discharge	

GUIDES FOR ASSESSMENT AND EVALUATION

Assessment Guides summarize assessment findings, alterations and possible causes, and nursing responses to assessment data to help you make distinctions between normal and abnormal clinical findings.

178 Part II: Pregnancy

INITIAL PRENATAL ASSESSMENT GUIDE

Physical Assessment/ Normal Findings	Alterations and Possible Causes*	Nursing Responses to Data†
Vital Signs		
Blood pressure (BP): 90–140/60–90	High BP (essential hypertension; renal disease; pregestational hypertension; apprehension or anxiety associated with pregnancy diagnosis, exam, or other crises; PIH if initial assessment not done until after 20 weeks' gestation)	BP > 140/90 requires immediate consideration; establish woman's BP; refer to physician if necessary. Assess woman's knowledge about high BP; counsel on self-care and medical management.
Pulse: 60–90 beats/min. Rate may increase 10 beats/min during pregnancy	Increased pulse rate (excitement or anxiety, cardiac disorders)	Count for 1 full minute; note irregularities.
Respiration: 16–24 breaths/min (or pulse rate divided by four). Pregnancy may induce a degree of hyperventilation; thoracic breathing predominant	Marked tachypnea or abnormal patterns	Assess for respiratory disease.
Temperature: 36.2–37.6C (98–99.6F)	Elevated temperature (infection)	Assess for infection process or disease state if temperature is elevated; refer to physician/CNM.
Weight		
Depends on body build	Weight < 45 kg (100 lb) or > 91 kg (200 lb); rapid, sudden weight gain (PIH)	Evaluate need for nutritional counseling; obtain information on eating habits, cooking practices, foods regularly eaten, income limitations, need for food supplements, pica and other abnormal food habits. Note initial weight to establish baseline for weight gain throughout pregnancy.
Skin		
Color: Consistent with racial background; pink nail beds	Pallor (anemia); bronze, yellow (hepatic disease, other causes of jaundice)	The following tests should be performed: complete blood count (CBC), bilirubin level, urinalysis, and blood urea nitrogen (BUN).
	Bluish, reddish, mottled; dusky appearance or pallor of palms and nail beds in dark-skinned women (anemia)	If abnormal, refer to physician.
Condition: Absence of edema (slight edema of lower extremities is normal during pregnancy)	Edema (PIH); rashes, dermatitis (allergic response)	Counsel on relief measures for slight edema. Initiate PIH assessment; refer to physician.
Lesions: Absence of lesions	Ulceration (varicose veins, decreased circulation)	Further assess circulatory status; refer to physician if lesion severe.
Spider nevi common in pregnancy	Petechiae, multiple bruises, ecchymosis (hemorrhagic disorders; abuse)	Evaluate for bleeding or clotting disorder. Provide oportunities to discuss abuse if suspected.
	Change in size or color (carcinoma)	Refer to physician.

*Possible causes of alterations are placed in parentheses.

†This column provides guidelines for further assessment and initial nursing intervention.

Teaching Guides help you understand how to assess common teaching needs in maternity care situations, create a particular teaching session, and evaluate the session's success.

394 Part III: Birth

TEACHING GUIDE | What to Expect During Labor

Assessment
As each woman is admitted into the birthing area the nurse assesses the woman's knowledge regarding the childbirth experience. The woman's knowledge base will be affected by previous births, attendance at childbirth education classes, and the amount of information she has been able to gather during her pregnancy by asking questions or reading. The nurse also assesses the factors that affect communication and anxiety level. Labor progress is assessed so that decisions regarding what to teach and the time available for teaching can be ascertained. If the woman is in early labor and she needs additional information, the nurse proceeds with teaching.

Nursing Diagnosis
The key nursing diagnosis probably will be: Knowledge deficit related to lack of information about nursing care during labor.

Nursing Plan and Implementation
The teaching focuses on information regarding the assessments and support the woman will receive during labor.

Client Goals
At the completion of the teaching the woman will be able to do the following:

- Verbalize the assessments the nurse will complete during labor
- Discuss the support/comfort measures that are available

Teaching Plan

Content	Teaching Method
Aspects of the admission process include the following: • Abbreviated history • Physical assessment (maternal vital signs [VS], fetal heart rate [FHR], contraction status, status of membranes) • Assessment of uterine contractions (frequency, duration, intensity) • Orientation to surroundings • Introductions to other staff who will be assisting her • Determination of woman's and family support person's expectations of the nurse Present aspects of ongoing physical care, such as when to expect assessment of maternal VS, FHR, and contractions.	Provide information on the basic assessment and care activities. Allow time for questions and discussion as labor progress permits.
If electronic fetal monitor is used, orient the woman to how it works and the information it provides. Orient woman to sights and sounds of monitor. Explain what "normal" data will look like and what characteristics are being watched for.	Demonstrate fetal monitor.
Be sure to note that assessments will increase as the labor progresses; about the time the woman would like to be left alone (transition phase), the assessments increase in order to help keep the mother and baby safe by noting any changes from the normal course.	
Explain the vaginal examination and what information can be obtained.	Use cervical dilatation chart to illustrate the amount of dilatation.
Review comfort techniques that may be used in labor, and ascertain what the woman thinks will be effective in promoting comfort.	Discussion.
Review breathing techniques the woman has learned so the nurse will be able to support her technique.	Ask woman to demonstrate technique.
Review comfort/support measures such as: positioning, back rub, effleurage, touch, distraction techniques, ambulation.	Discussion.
If woman is in early labor, offer to give her a tour of the birthing area.	Provide a tour of birthing area, explaining equipment and routines. Include partner.

Evaluation
At the end of this teaching session, the woman will be able to verbalize assessments that will occur during her labor and to discuss comfort/support measures that may be used.

DISCUSSIONS ON CLIENT/FAMILY TEACHING

Throughout the text, discussion of client/family teaching is highlighted by an apple logo in the margin.

USEFUL REFERENCE CARDS

Teaching Cards, which you can tear out, provide a handy study tool or useful reference for the clinical setting.

Part One | Basic Concepts

It seems that I knew the moment you began. We had been planning and wanting the pregnancy for months. We carefully kept track of my menstrual periods and calculated the time of ovulation, and yet pregnancy kept eluding us. Then suddenly one night, I knew that you were there. This had been the moment, and even as I lay quietly I somehow could sense your presence. That feeling never changed, it just grew stronger as you grew inside me.

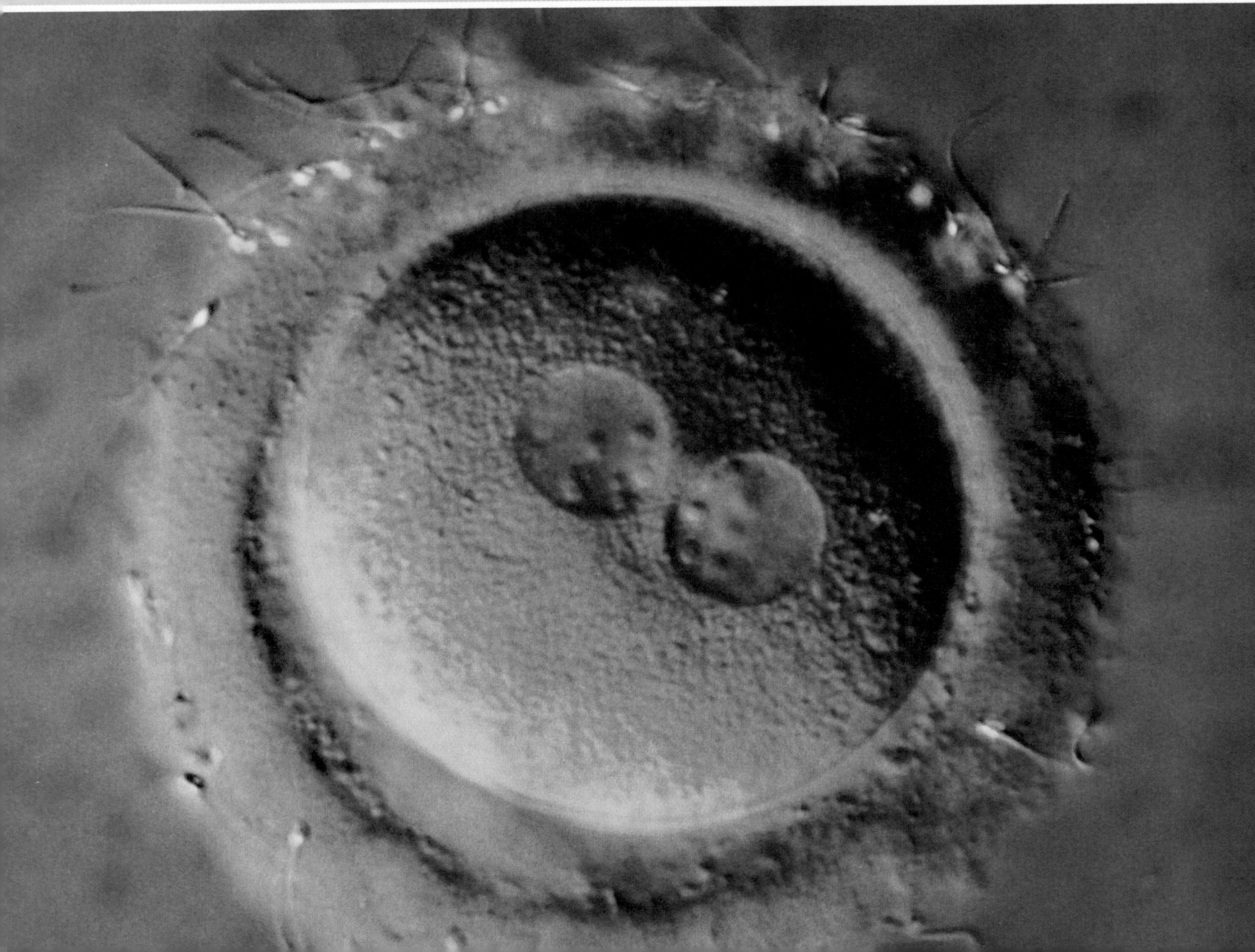

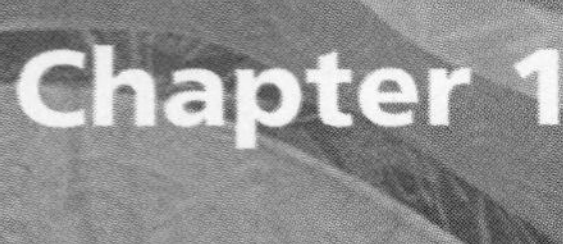

Chapter 1 Contemporary Maternal-Newborn Care

OBJECTIVES

- Relate the concept of the expert nurse to nurses caring for childbearing families.
- Identify the nursing roles available to the maternal-newborn nurse.
- Delineate significant legal and ethical issues that influence the practice of maternal-newborn nursing.
- Describe the Human Genome Project.
- Summarize selected tools used for critical thinking in maternal-newborn nursing practice.
- Discuss the application of the nursing process in the maternal-newborn setting.
- Contrast descriptive and inferential statistics.
- Relate the availability of statistical data to the formulation of further research questions.

KEY TERMS

Assisted reproductive technology (ART)
Birth rate
Certified nurse-midwife (CNM)
Certified registered nurse (RNC)
Clinical nurse specialist (CNS)
Infant mortality rate
Informed consent
Intrauterine fetal surgery
Maternal mortality rate
Nurse practitioner (NP)
Nursing process
Professional nurse

The practice of most nurses is filled with special moments, shared experiences, times in which they know they have practiced the essence of nursing and, in so doing, touched a life. What is the essence of nursing? Simply stated, nurses care *for* people, care *about* people, and use their expertise to help people help themselves, as the following situation demonstrates.

I like working with students. I enjoy their enthusiasm, the questions they ask, and the ways in which they cause me to examine my practice. I love being a nurse, I am passionate about the importance of what I do, and I want to seize every chance to influence those who will be practicing beside me someday. An incident that took place last week is a perfect example. I had a Junior nursing student working with me in one of our birthing rooms. It was her first day caring for laboring women, and she was scared and excited at the same time. We were taking care of a healthy woman who had two boys at home and really wanted a girl. As labor progressed, the student and I worked closely together, monitoring contractions, teaching the woman and her husband, doing what we could to ease her discomfort. Sometimes the student asked how I knew when to do something—a vaginal check, for example—and each time I'd try to think beyond "I just do" to give her some clues. During the birth the student stayed close to the mother, coaching and helping with breathing. The student felt she had an important role to play and she handled it beautifully. At the moment of birth the student and dad leaned forward, watching as the baby just slipped into the world. There wasn't a sound until the student said in a voice filled with awe, "Ooh, it's a girl!" Then we all laughed and hugged each other. What a day—using my expertise to help others and helping a future nurse recognize the importance of what we do!

All nurses who provide care and support to childbearing women and their families can make a difference. But how does this happen? How do nurses develop expertise and become skilled, caring practitioners?

In her classic work, Benner (1984) suggests that, as nurses develop their skills in making clinical judgments and intervening appropriately, they progress through five levels of competence. Beginning as a novice, the new nurse progresses to advanced beginner and then to competent, proficient, and, finally, expert nurse.

The student discussed above was clearly a novice. Lacking in experience, the novice relies on rules to guide actions. Gaining experience, the nurse begins to draw on that experience to view situations more holistically, becoming increasingly aware of subtle cues that indicate physiologic and psychologic changes. Expert nurses, like the nurse in the preceding situation, have a clear vision of what is possible in a given situation. This holistic perspective is based on a wealth of knowledge bred of experience and enables the nurse to act intuitively to provide effective care. In reality, "intuition" reflects the nurse's internalization of information. When faced with a clinical situation, nurses draw almost subconsciously on their stored knowledge and judgment.

The use of intuitive perception is especially important to the "art of nursing" in areas such as maternal-newborn nursing, where change occurs quickly and families look to the nurse for help and guidance. Labor nurses become attuned to a woman's progress or lack of progress; nursery nurses detect subtle changes in their small charges; antepartal and postpartal nurses become adept at assessing and teaching. Thus skilled nursing practice depends on a solid base of knowledge and clinical expertise delivered in a caring, holistic manner.

Empowerment is an important concept for nurses today. Empowerment may be viewed as both a process and an outcome. As an internal process, empowerment results as individuals develop ever-increasing awareness of competence, mastery, and control over their own lives. An empowered self develops as a result of five processes—control, competence, credibility, confidence, and comfort. For nurses, these attributes evolve as they mature in the profession (Moores 1997).

Control develops as nurses learn to handle their own emotions and as they participate in the control of clinical situations by learning to make and act on client care decisions. Control issues are often difficult for advanced beginners (Benner 1984), and they may look to expert nurses for guidance (Moores 1997). As nurses provide good nursing care and develop a sound knowledge base, they gain competence. From this competence flows credibility as others begin to trust and believe in them. Nurses in turn become self-reliant, learning to have confidence in their judgments, which is critical to feelings of empowerment. Finally a sense of comfort develops and nurses feel able to predict probable outcomes (Moores 1997).

Empowered nurses are better able to approach client care situations effectively with full knowledge that they are legally, ethically, and morally accountable for their actions. Empowered nurses are able to interact as equals with other health care providers and collaborate with them to resolve problems and accomplish goals (Moores 1997). When empowered nurses practice proactively they anticipate problems before they develop and avoid undesirable client outcomes (Hagedorn et al 1997). Empowered nurses share responsibility and accountability with each childbearing family, thereby helping the family become self-determining.

We believe that many nurses who work with childbearing families are experts: They are sensitive, intuitive, and technically skilled. They are empowered professionals who can collaborate effectively with others and advocate for those individuals and families who need their support. They can support the efforts of childbearing families to make decisions about their needs and desires. They can foster independence and self-reliance. Such nurses do make a difference in the quality of care childbearing families receive.

Contemporary Childbirth

The scope of practice of the maternal-newborn nurse has changed dramatically in the past 25 years. Today's maternal-newborn nurses have far broader responsibilities and focus more on the specific goals of the individual childbearing woman and her family.

Contemporary childbirth is characterized by an emphasis on the family and the family's choices about the birth experience. Today the concept of family-centered childbirth is accepted and encouraged. Fathers are active participants, not simply bystanders; siblings are encouraged to visit and meet the newest family member, and they may even attend the birth.

In addition, new definitions of family are evolving that include the family of the single mother—which may be her mother, sister, another relative, a close friend, or the father of the child. Recognition is given as well to the importance of extended families in many cultures, and support is not necessarily limited to one person.

The family can make choices about the place of birth (hospital, birthing center, or home), the primary caregiver (physician, certified nurse-midwife, or even lay midwife), and birth-related experiences (position for birth, use of analgesia and anesthesia, and methods of childbirth preparation, for example).

As recently as the early 1990s women who gave birth vaginally remained in the hospital approximately three days. This provided ample time for nurses to assess the family's knowledge and skill and to complete essential teaching. In an effort to control costs, discharge within 12 to 24 hours after birth became the norm. This practice may not cause problems for women with supportive families, thorough prenatal preparation, and adequate resources for necessary follow-up care. However, because early discharge severely limits the time available for client teaching, women with little knowledge, experience, or support may be inadequately prepared to care for themselves and their newborn infants. The negative impact of this practice has gained recognition nationwide and drawn a variety of responses, from legislation to education.

Community-Based Nursing Care

Cost, access, and quality of health care are major issues facing society today. The health care reform movement reflects efforts to deal with these pressing issues realistically and effectively. The current health care system still emphasizes high-technology care, however. Approximately 75 percent of third-party payments are for hospital-based acute care. Furthermore, 5 percent of the population spends 58 percent of US health care resources (ANA 1993).

Changing the current system requires new ways of thinking and providing services. Many advocates of a new direction for health care support the increasing emphasis on primary care. They believe that primary health care services should be the base upon which all other services are built. Primary care includes a focus on health promotion, illness prevention, and individual responsibility for one's own health. These services are best provided in community-based settings. Third-party payers and managed care organizations are beginning to recognize the importance of primary care in containing costs and maintaining health. Estimates suggest that by the turn of the century only 40 percent of nurses will work in a traditional hospital setting. Community-based health care systems providing primary care and some secondary care will be available in schools, workplaces, homes, churches, clinics, transitional care programs, and other ambulatory settings.

Weisman (1996) suggests that the growth and diversity of managed care plans offers both opportunities and challenges for women's health care. The potential exists for managed care organizations to work with consumers to provide a model for coordinated and comprehensive well woman care that includes improved delivery of screening and preventive services. One challenge managed care organizations will face is how to relate to essential community providers of care, such as family-planning clinics or women's health centers, that offer a unique service or serve groups of women with special needs (adolescents, disabled women, and ethnic or racial minorities). "The extent to which satisfactory contractual relationships are negotiated between managed care plans and community providers may in turn have profound effects on the survival of some of these providers and their future availability to women" (Weisman 1996, p 3).

Community-based care remains an essential element of health care for uninsured or underinsured individuals, as well as for individuals who benefit from programs such as Medicare or state-sponsored health-related programs. While some of these programs, such as those offered through public health departments, are broad based, others, such as parenting classes for adolescents, are geared to the needs of a specific population.

Community-based care is also part of a trend initiated by consumers, who are asking for a "seamless" system of family-centered, comprehensive, coordinated health care, health education, and social services (Plotnick and Presler 1996). This seamless system requires coordination as clients move from primary care services to acute care facilities and then back into the community. The shortened length of hospital stays further mandates the coordination of services. Nurses can assume this care management role and perform an important service for individuals and families.

Maternal-child nurses are especially sensitive to these changes in health care delivery because the vast majority of health care provided to childbearing women and their families takes place outside of hospitals in clinics, offices, and community-based organizations. In addition, maternal-child nurses offer specialized services such as childbirth preparation classes or postpartal exercise classes. In essence, we are already expert at providing community-based nursing care. However, it is important that we remain knowledgeable about current practices and trends and open to new ways of meeting the needs of women and children. "Opportunities exist to redirect our efforts in homes, in child care and early intervention centers, in schools, and in managed care settings" (Plotnik and Presler 1996).

HOME CARE

Providing health care in the home is an especially important dimension of community-based nursing care. Shorter hospital stays end in the discharge of individuals who still require support, assistance, and teaching. Home care helps fill this gap. Conversely, home care also enables individuals to remain at home with conditions that formerly would have required hospitalization.

Nurses are the major providers of home care services. Home care nurses perform direct nursing care and also supervise unlicensed assistive personnel who provide less skilled levels of service. In a home setting nurses use their skills in assessment, therapeutics, communication, teaching, problem solving, and organization to meet the needs of childbearing women and their families. They also play a major role in coordinating services from other providers, such as physical therapists or lactation consultants.

Postpartal and newborn home visits are becoming a recognized way of ensuring a satisfactory transition from the birthing center to the home. This is a positive trend, and this method of meeting the needs of childbearing families should become standard practice.

We believe that home care offers nurses the opportunity to function in an autonomous role and make a significant difference for individuals and families. Chapter 29 discusses home care in more detail and provides guidance about making a home visit. Throughout the text there is further information on the use of home care to meet the needs of pregnant women with health problems, such as diabetes or preterm labor.

Nursing Roles

The depth of care provided by nurses caring for women and for childbearing families depends on their education, qualifications, and scope of practice. A **professional nurse** has graduated from an accredited basic program in nursing, has successfully completed the nursing licensure examination (NCLEX), and is currently licensed as a registered nurse (RN). A **certified registered nurse (RNC)** has shown expertise in a field by taking a national certification exam. A **nurse practitioner** (NP) has received specialized education in a master's degree program or a certificate program and thus can function in an advanced practice role. Nurse practitioners often provide ambulatory care services to the expectant family, and some NPs also function in acute care settings. They focus on physical and psychosocial assessments, including health history, physical examination, and certain diagnostic tests and procedures. The nurse practitioner makes clinical judgments and begins appropriate treatments, seeking physician consultation when necessary. The emerging emphasis on community-based care has greatly increased opportunities for NPs.

The **clinical nurse specialist (CNS)** has a master's degree and specialized knowledge and competence in a specific clinical area. The **certified nurse-midwife (CNM)** is educated in the two disciplines of nursing and midwifery and is certified by the American College of Nurse-Midwives. The CNM is prepared to manage independently the care of women at low risk for complications during pregnancy and birth and the care of normal newborns (Figure 1–1).

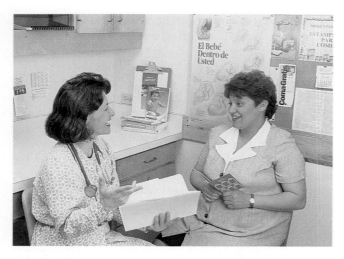

FIGURE 1–1 A certified nurse-midwife confers with her client.

Legal Considerations

Scope of Practice

The *scope of practice* is defined as the limits of nursing practice set forth in state statutes. Although some state practice acts continue to limit nursing practice to the traditional responsibilities of providing client care related to health maintenance and disease prevention, most state practice acts cover expanded practice roles that include collaboration with other health professionals in planning and providing care, physician-delegated diagnosis and prescriptive privilege, and the delegation of client care tasks to other specified licensed and unlicensed personnel. Specified care activities for certified nurse-midwives and women's health, perinatal, and neonatal nurse practitioners may include diagnosis and prenatal management of uncomplicated pregnancies (CNMs may also manage births) and prescribing and dispensing medications under protocols in specified circumstances. A nurse must function within the scope of practice or risk being accused of practicing medicine without a license.

Standards of Nursing Care

Standards of care establish minimum criteria for competent, proficient delivery of nursing care. Such standards are designed to protect the public and are used to judge the quality of care provided. Legal interpretation of actions within standards of care is based on what a reasonably prudent nurse with similar education and experience would do in similar circumstances.

A number of different sources publish written standards of care. The American Nurses' Association (ANA) has published standards of professional practice written by the ANA Congress for Nursing Practice. The ANA Divisions of Practice have also published standards, including the standards of practice for maternal-child health. Specialty organizations, such as the Association of Women's Health, Obstetrics, and Neonatal Nurses (AWHONN); the National Association of Neonatal Nurses (NANN); and the Association of Operating Room Nurses (AORN) have developed standards for specialty practice. Agency policies, procedures, and protocols also provide appropriate guidelines for care standards. The Joint Commission on the Accreditation of Healthcare Organizations (JCAHO), a nongovernmental agency that audits the operation of hospitals and health care facilities, has also contributed to the development of nursing standards.

Some standards carry the force of law; others, although not legally binding, carry important legal significance. Any nurse who fails to meet appropriate standards of care invites allegations of negligence or malpractice. However, any nurse who practices within the guidelines established by an agency, or follows local or national standards, is assured of providing clients with competent nursing care and therefore decreases the potential for litigation.

Informed Consent

Informed consent is a legal concept that protects a client's right to autonomy and self-determination by specifying that no action may be taken without that person's prior understanding and freely given consent. While this policy is usually enforced for such major procedures as surgery or regional anesthesia, it pertains to any nursing, medical, or surgical intervention. To touch a person without consent (except in an emergency) constitutes battery. In a normal, uncomplicated labor, when the woman has time to give consent, consent must be obtained. Consent is not informed unless the woman understands the usual procedures, their rationales, and any associated risks. To be a truly active participant in decision making about her care, she should also understand possible alternatives.

The person who is ultimately responsible for the treatment or procedure should provide the information necessary to obtain informed consent. In most instances this is the physician. In such cases the nurse's role is to witness the client's signature giving consent. If the nurse determines that the client does not understand the procedure or risks, he or she must notify the physician, who must then provide additional information to ensure that the consent is "informed." Anxiety, fear, pain, and medications that alter consciousness may influence an individual's ability to give informed consent. An oral consent is legal, but written consent is easier to defend in a court of law.

When a medication or procedure is indicated, a client who makes an informed choice to refuse the medication or treatment is usually required to sign a form releasing the doctor and clinical facility from liability resulting from the effects of such a refusal. (For example, Jehovah's Witnesses, who commonly refuse blood transfusions, are required to sign such release forms.)

Nurses are responsible for educating clients about any nursing care provided. Before each nursing intervention, the maternal-newborn nurse lets the woman know what to expect, thus ensuring her cooperation and obtaining her consent. Afterward, the nurse documents the teaching and the learning outcomes in the woman's record.

The importance of clear, concise, and complete nursing records cannot be overemphasized. These records are evidence that the nurse obtained consent, performed prescribed treatments, reported important observations to the appropriate staff, and adhered to acceptable standards of care.

Right to Privacy

The right to privacy is the right of a person to keep her or his person and property free from public scrutiny. Maternity nurses must remember that this includes avoiding unnecessary exposure of the childbearing woman's body. To protect the woman, only those responsible for her care should examine her or discuss her case.

The right to privacy is protected by state constitutions, statutes, and common law. The ANA, the National League for Nursing (NLN), and JCAHO have adopted professional standards protecting the privacy of clients. Health care agencies should also have written policies dealing with client privacy.

Laws, standards, and policies about privacy specify that information about clients' treatment, condition, and prognosis can be shared only by health professionals responsible for their care. Information considered "vital statistics" (name, age, occupation, and so on) may be revealed legally, but is often withheld because of ethical considerations. The client should be consulted regarding what information may be released and to whom. When the client is a celebrity or is considered newsworthy, inquiries by the media are best handled by the public relations department of the agency.

Ethical Issues

Although ethical dilemmas confront nurses in all areas of practice, those related to pregnancy, birth, and the newborn seem especially difficult to resolve. These dilemmas result from conflicting social, cultural, and religious values and beliefs held by individuals.

Maternal-Fetal Conflict

Until fairly recently, the fetus was viewed legally as a nonperson. However, advances in technology have permitted the physician to treat the fetus and monitor fetal development. The fetus is increasingly viewed as a client separate from the mother, although treatment of the fetus necessarily involves the mother.

Most women are strongly motivated to protect the health and well-being of their fetus. In some instances, however, women have refused interventions on behalf of the fetus, and forced interventions have occurred. These include forced cesarean birth; coercion of mothers who practice high-risk behaviors such as substance abuse to enter treatment; and, perhaps most controversial, mandating experimental in utero therapy or surgery in an attempt to correct a specific birth defect. Each of these interventions infringes on the autonomy of the mother. Attempts have also been made to criminalize the behavior of women who fail to follow a physician's advice or who engage in behaviors (such as substance abuse) that are considered harmful to the fetus.

The American College of Obstetricians and Gynecologists (ACOG) Committee on Ethics (1987), the American Academy of Pediatrics (1988), and the American Medical Association Board of Trustees (1990) all reaffirm the fundamental right of pregnant women to make informed, uncoerced decisions about medical interventions. All three groups also recognize that cases of maternal-fetal conflict involve two clients, both of whom deserve respect and treatment. All agree that such cases "are best resolved through the use of internal hospital mechanisms including counseling, the intervention of specialists, and the utilization of ethics committees . . . and that a resort to judicial intervention is rarely, if ever, appropriate" (Mitchell 1994, p 94).

Abortion

Since the 1973 Supreme Court decision in *Roe v Wade,* abortion has been legal in the United States. Abortion can be performed until the period of viability. After that time abortion is permissible only when the life or health of the mother is threatened. Before viability, the rights of the mother are paramount; after viability, the rights of the fetus take precedence. There are continuing efforts by individuals and states to limit or abolish abortion by prohibiting Medicaid funding of abortions and putting other restrictions on the procedure. These include restricting abortions to hospitals (which significantly increases the cost of the procedure) and requiring agencies to provide graphic details of the procedure, ostensibly to obtain informed consent.

In 1993, shortly after taking the oath of office, President Clinton signed executive orders that (a) lifted the "gag rule" prohibiting most health care providers at federally funded clinics from discussing abortion with pregnant women; (b) permitted the use of fetal tissue in federally funded research, even if the tissue was obtained from an abortion; and (c) permitted overseas US military personnel and their dependents to receive abortions at military hospitals at their own expense. Thus the controversy continues.

At present the decision for abortion is to be made by the woman and her physician. Caregivers have the right to refuse to perform an abortion or to assist with the procedure if abortion is contrary to their moral and ethical beliefs. However, a nurse who refuses to participate in an abortion because of moral or ethical beliefs must be certain that a qualified person is available to provide appropriate care for the client. Clients must never be abandoned, regardless of the nurse's beliefs.

Intrauterine Fetal Surgery

Intrauterine fetal surgery, an example of therapeutic research, is a therapy for anatomic lesions that can be corrected surgically and are incompatible with life if not treated. The procedure involves opening the uterus during the second trimester (before viability), performing the planned surgery, and replacing the fetus in the uterus. The risks to the fetus are substantial, and the mother is committed to cesarean births for this and subsequent pregnancies (because the upper, active segment of the uterus is entered). The parents must be informed of the experimental nature of the treatment, the risks of the surgery, the commitment to cesarean birth, and alternatives to the treatment. The parents must have the opportunity to ask questions and time to make a considered choice.

As in other aspects of maternity care, caregivers must respect the pregnant woman's autonomy. The procedure involves health risks to the woman, and she retains the right to refuse any surgical procedure. In such cases health care providers must ensure that their zeal for new technology does not lead them to focus on the fetus at the expense of the mother (Contemporary OB/GYN 1994).

Reproductive Assistance

Assisted reproductive technology (ART) is the term used to describe highly technologic approaches used to produce pregnancy. In vitro fertilization and embryo transfer (IVF-ET), a therapy offered to selected infertile couples, is perhaps the best known ART technique. In this process, ovulation is induced and one or more oocytes are retrieved by transvaginal ultrasound scanning in conjunction with transvaginal aspiration. The oocytes are then fertilized with sperm from the partner or a donor. Three to four embryos are transferred to the woman's uterus when they reach the four- to six-cell stage (Stillman and Gindoff 1994). Zygote intrafallopian transfer (ZIFT) is similar to IVF-ET, except that the developing embryo is implanted in the fallopian tube. The success rates of these procedures are low; births resulted in approximately 16 percent of IVF-ET procedures and in 22 percent of ZIFT procedures (Hurst and Schlaff 1994). Researchers have also begun to use natural cycle IVF. This approach does not use fertility drugs (with their associated risks) to stimulate ovulation and results in the implantation of a single oocyte instead of multiple oocytes (Levy and Gindoff 1994).

Gamete intrafallopian transfer (GIFT) is used in women with at least one functioning tube whose infertility is due to unknown causes or male factors such as low sperm count. In GIFT, multiple oocytes are retrieved by laparoscopy from the woman or a donor and transferred with sperm directly into the fallopian tubes. A resulting pregnancy is considered in vivo fertilization.

Some legislative efforts have been made to address consumer concerns about ART. In the United States the Federal Fertility Clinic Success Rate and Certification Act (FCSRCA) of 1992 requires standardized reporting of pregnancy success rates associated with ART programs and addresses issues related to laboratory quality. However, it does not deal with unethical practices that may occur or false reporting of success rates (Wilcox and Marks 1996).

In Canada the Royal Commission on New Reproductive Technologies was charged with examining the range of technologies related to reproduction. Among its most important recommendations, the commission advocated legislation to prohibit several aspects of technology, such as selling human eggs, zygotes, sperm, fetuses, or fetal tissue. It also recommended that the government establish a national regulatory body to license and regulate the provision of reproductive technology services in Canada (Baird 1996).

Surrogate childbearing is another approach to infertility. Surrogate childbearing occurs when a woman agrees to become pregnant for a childless couple. She may be artificially inseminated with the male partner's sperm or a donor's sperm or may receive a gamete transfer, depending on the infertile couple's needs. If fertilization occurs, the woman carries the fetus to term and releases the infant to the couple after birth.

These methods of resolving infertility raise many ethical issues, including religious objections to artificial conception, financial and moral responsibility for a child born with a congenital defect, candidate selection, and the threat of genetic engineering. Other ethical questions include: What should be done with surplus fertilized oocytes? To whom do frozen embryos belong? Parents together or separately? The hospital or infertility clinic? Who is liable if a woman or her offspring contracts HIV disease from donated sperm? Should children be told the method of their conception?

Cord Blood Banking

Cord blood, taken from a newborn's umbilical cord by the physician or nurse-midwife assisting with the birth, may play a role in combating leukemia, certain other cancers, and immune and blood system disorders. This is possible because cord blood, like bone marrow, contains regenerative stem cells, which can replace diseased cells in the affected individual. The value of bone marrow transplants is recognized, and there is a national registry of potential bone marrow donors. The process of collecting bone marrow is expensive and uncomfortable, however, and the National Marrow Donor Registry is able to find a matching bone marrow donor only 20 to 30 percent of the time (Randal 1995).

According to Stephenson (1995), cord blood has numerous advantages over bone marrow: (1) Collecting it involves no risk to mother or infant. (2) Large-scale cord blood banking would promote better availability of stem cells for racial and minority groups, who are seriously underrepresented in bone marrow registries. (3) It is less likely than bone marrow to trigger a potentially fatal rejection response. (4) It seems to be more tolerant of slight mismatches between donor and recipient. (5) There is less probability that it will contain infectious agents.

Blood banks that process and store cord blood have now been established in the United States. Two options are available for families:

1. They can elect to register their infant's cord blood privately. The blood is collected at birth, and the family assumes all costs for analyzing, preparing, and storing the blood. The blood is quickly available for use by the donor, a sibling, or the mother. (During pregnancy mother and infant seem to become immunologically tolerant of each other). This option is especially useful in families with a history of malignancy or genetic blood disease.
2. They can elect to donate the cord blood to an established registry for use by others.

Sugarman and colleagues (1995) have identified several ethical issues associated with cord blood banking:

- Who owns the blood? The donor? The parents? Private blood banks? Society?
- How can caregivers ensure that informed consent is correctly obtained? The family must understand that, if they choose to donate, the mother will be asked to provide a blood sample and a detailed history about her health and infectious disease status.
- How will obligations to notify the family and donor be addressed if testing of the blood reveals infectious diseases or genetic disorders? Should there be any ongoing assessment of donors so that recipients can be notified if health problems develop?
- How can the system be set up to maintain privacy and confidentiality?
- How will issues of distribution of the harvested blood be addressed to ensure fairness and availability to individuals from all races, ethnic groups, and income levels?

The timing for collecting cord blood is discussed in Chapter 17.

The Human Genome Project

The Human Genome Project (HGP) is an international, multidisciplinary effort to explore and map human genetic material. In the United States the Human Genome Project is a coordinated, 15-year national research program to identify all human genetic material—the genome—by developing a human genetic map of all chromosomes, by improving existing genetic maps, and by determining the complete sequence of human DNA. Jointly sponsored by the US Department of Energy and the National Institutes of Health (NIH), the project is also designed to develop new technologies and techniques to support the effort (US Department of Energy 1996). In addition, the HGP is charged with analyzing the legal, ethical, and social implications arising from the availability of genetic information about individuals; developing public policy options to deal with those issues; and identifying advanced ways of sharing the information that emerges with researchers, scientists, physicians, and others so that the data can be used for the public good (National Center for Human Genome Research 1996). As part of the effort the HGP has also established research training programs for pre- and postdoctoral fellows.

The implications of the effort are staggering. For example, in 1989 the gene involved in cystic fibrosis was identified. Subsequently a diagnostic test was developed to identify gene carriers of cystic fibrosis in high-risk individuals and families. Currently the first human gene therapy approaches are being evaluated in federally funded clinical trials. More recently researchers located two genes implicated in a hereditary form of colon cancer. With the genes identified, it is now possible to develop a blood test to detect high-risk individuals (National Center for Human Genome Research 1996).

As more genetic information becomes available, questions arise regarding the use and protection of such information. Gene manipulation and gene therapy, once limited to science fiction novels, now present a reality that adds to the complex ethical questions of use and control of technology. Other emerging issues include the question of payment for genetic testing; appropriate counseling following testing; confidentiality; qualifications of individuals engaged in testing, counseling, and interventions; mandated testing; and the right to refuse genetic information.

Implications for Nursing Practice

The complex ethical issues facing maternal-newborn nurses have many social, cultural, legal, and professional ramifications. Ethical decisions in maternal-child nursing are often complicated by moral obligations to more than one client. Straightforward solutions to the ethical dilemmas encountered in caring for childbearing families are often, quite simply, not available.

Nurses must learn to anticipate ethical dilemmas, clarify their own positions and values related to the issues, understand the legal implications of the issues, and develop appropriate strategies for ethical decision making. To accomplish these tasks, they may read about bioethical issues, participate in discussion groups, or attend courses and workshops on ethical topics pertinent to their areas of practice. Nurses also need to develop skills in logical thinking and critical analysis.

Tools for Critical Thinking in Maternal-Newborn Nursing Practice

Critical thinking is a complex mental process that involves separating fact from opinion, identifying stereotypes and prejudices that may influence information, exploring differing ideas and views, and developing new insights or conclusions. Maternal-newborn nurses use critical thinking in all aspects of their nursing practice. Indeed, the hallmark of effective professional nursing is the application of theory to practice in a logical, individualized way to analyze data and make decisions.

Nurses draw on several tools for practice in providing thoughtful, effective nursing care. The nursing process is one of these tools. It provides a systematic approach to clinical decision making. Other tools, such as communication skills, help the nurse gather information; still others, such as a comprehensive knowledge base, standards of care, statistical data, and nursing research, provide information for decision making.

This section is not designed to give a complete explanation of nursing tools but to highlight them and explore ways in which the maternal-newborn nurse uses them in practice.

Critical Thinking

In nursing, as in all aspects of health care, decision making has become more complex. Nurses have a myriad of data at their disposal and must be able to sort out the relevant information. They analyze information by mentally asking questions: What is important? Which data cluster together? What pieces of information are missing? Does the picture I see make sense intellectually? What other experiences have I had that I can draw on?

But what exactly is critical thinking? The National Council for Excellence in Critical Thinking Instruction (1992, p 2) has defined it as "the intellectually disciplined process of actively and skillfully conceptualizing, applying, analyzing, synthesizing, and evaluating information gathered from or generated by observation, experience, reflection, reasoning, or communication, as a guide to belief and action." Critical thinking skills enable the nurse to recognize and evaluate taken-for-granted assumptions that shape practice in order to identify valid information and seek out alternative courses of action when necessary (Brookfield 1993). It is a learned ability.

Experts stress that critical thinking has cognitive, psychomotor, and affective elements that must all be addressed. Nurses learn the cognitive and psychomotor elements as they have opportunities to apply knowledge from classroom experiences, seminars, and readings to client situations in a variety of settings (Bowers and McCarthy 1993). Less easily taught, but critically important, the affective element focuses on moral reasoning, awareness of self and personal beliefs, and the development of values and standards that guide activities and decisions (Woods 1993).

The Critical Thinking in Action scenarios in this text provide clinical vignettes designed to challenge the reader to address a specific clinical situation by drawing on material presented in the chapter. Because this problem-solving approach is very specific, we have provided possible solutions at the end of this text, in Appendix H.

Knowledge Base

Current knowledge and theories from a variety of disciplines form the basis for nursing actions. Maternal-newborn nurses build their practice on a comprehensive knowledge base that includes information about pregnancy, labor, and birth; the postpartal period; and the newborn period. Nursing theories such as those related to adaptation, stress, human caring, locus of control, and care of individuals may also be part of the nurse's knowledge base. In addition, nurses synthesize knowledge from other disciplines, including psychology, sociology, biology, chemistry, and business.

Acquisition of knowledge is a lifelong process for today's professional nurse. New technology is being developed and implemented at a rapid rate; change and progress are inevitable. Specialization has become prevalent as nurses work to keep their knowledge base current. Specialization provides a narrower focus and helps direct the learning process.

Nursing Process

The **nursing process,** built on a comprehensive knowledge base, represents a logical approach to problem identification and resolution, and is the foundation for nursing practice. The nursing process consists of five steps—assessment, nursing diagnosis, planning, implementation, and evaluation—and is an analog of the problem-solving process used by nurses since Florence Nightingale.

In the assessment phase of the nursing process the maternal-newborn nurse gathers both subjective and objective data about the health status of the childbearing woman. The nurse obtains subjective information from the woman and family members, including their perceptions of the woman's health status and of any health impairment or problem and its management. Objective data are measurable and include physical assessment findings and laboratory test results.

The second step in the process is the analysis, assimilation, and clustering of assessment data into relevant categories from which nursing diagnoses are derived. Each nursing diagnosis describes a specific actual or potential health problem, its etiology, and the associated signs and symptoms. The formulation of a nursing diagnosis is the crucial step in the process, for the resulting plan of care is based on the problems as the nurse perceives them. In contrast to the medical diagnosis, which generally remains the same throughout the woman's health problem, the nursing diagnosis will reflect the changing response of the woman as her condition improves or worsens, and as she and her family adjust to those changes.

Once the analysis is completed and nursing diagnoses are formulated, the nurse moves to the third step of the nursing process: planning. In this phase, the nurse establishes outcome goals, identifies interventions that will help the client meet the established goals, develops outcome criteria that will signify that the goals have been met, and prioritizes the care needed. The beginning nurse usually works through this process step by step, while the more experienced nurse is frequently able to develop an intricate plan of care covering all the steps simultaneously.

In the fourth step of the nursing process, the maternal-newborn nurse implements the identified plan of care and specific nursing interventions. The nurse uses many skills that are common to other areas of nursing and many skills specific to the maternal-newborn setting. Common interventions include, for example, auscultating fetal heart rate, providing comfort measures for a laboring woman, changing maternal position to improve a fetal-monitor tracing, using nursing techniques to help a postpartum woman void, and teaching a new family about infant care.

The woman's progress or lack of progress toward the identified expected outcomes (goals) is evaluated by the woman and the nurse. These questions are asked: Have expected outcomes been met? Is reassessment needed? Are new problems present? Are changes in any part of the process necessary? Do new priorities need to be identified? Is revision of the plan of care required?

Evaluation is a logical end step, but it also is used throughout the entire nursing process. The nurse continually evaluates the assessments that have been made, the priorities of care, and the effectiveness of the nursing interventions as nursing care is delivered.

Critical Pathways

One result of the nursing process is the creation of critical pathways. Critical pathways specify essential nursing activities and provide basic guidelines about expected outcomes at specified time intervals. This enables the nurse to determine whether a client's responses meet general norms at any given time. In the text we have provided critical pathways for a woman experiencing a normal vaginal birth and a cesarean birth. We have also provided critical pathways for the normal newborn, for a woman in the postpartal period, and for selected conditions or problems.

Communication Skills

Communication is a major tool in critical thinking. Effective communication directly influences the quality of information available for nurses to use in decision making. It most often involves verbal and nonverbal interactions between the nurse and other health care providers or the nurse and the client and her family. The maternal-newborn nurse uses communication skills in all interactions with the childbearing woman and her family. The nurse begins by establishing rapport and a sense of trust with the client. Rapport and trust are enhanced when the nurse respects the woman's individuality and beliefs, provides privacy, and is nonjudgmental.

The nurse uses therapeutic communication techniques (Table 1–1) during assessment, interventions, and all teaching activities. To ensure successful communication, the nurse may need to use a variety of techniques.

Standards of Care

As discussed on page 6, nursing standards of care identify the basic expectations and functions of a particular nursing role and provide a framework of accountability and guidelines for ethical nursing practice. They also provide a basis for identifying quality in specific health care settings and direction and guidance for the practicing nurse. Because health care settings vary from one region to another, the standards are used as a foundation

TABLE 1–1 Examples of Therapeutic Communication Techniques in Maternal-Newborn Nursing

Technique	Example
Listening attentively	The nurse faces the client, maintains eye contact, and leans slightly toward her. The nurse concentrates attention on the interaction with the client.
Using open-ended questions	The nurse asks questions such as: "How do you feel about exercise during pregnancy?"
Clarifying	The nurse confirms the meaning of a comment.
	Client: "One person said to do exercises this way, and another person said I was not doing them right."
	Nurse: "So you feel you are getting conflicting instructions from us?"
	Client: "Yes, it's hard not knowing what to do."
Paraphrasing	The nurse restates the client's message in the nurse's own words.
	Client: "I can't exercise in the morning, and the evening seems so full, and..."
	Nurse: "You are having difficulty exercising."
Focusing	The nurse helps the woman focus on a particular aspect of the conversation.
	Client: "I am having strange feelings in my body, mostly in my abdomen."
	Nurse: "Describe the feeling."

for developing individualized policies and protocols. The Association of Women's Health, Obstetrics, and Neonatal Nurses (AWHONN) has assumed a leadership role in developing standards for nurses who care for childbearing families.

Statistics

Nurses often overlook or underestimate the usefulness of statistics. Health-related statistics provide an objective basis for projecting client needs, planning the use of resources, and determining the effectiveness of specific treatments.

There are two major types of statistics: descriptive and inferential. Descriptive statistics describe or summarize a set of data. They report the facts—what is—in a concise and easily retrievable way. An example of a descriptive statistic is the birth rate in the United States. Although these statistics support no conclusions about why some phenomenon has occurred, they do identify certain trends and high-risk "target groups" and generate possible research questions. Inferential statistics allow the investigator to draw conclusions or inferences about what is happening between two or more variables in a population and to suggest or refute causal relationships between them.

TABLE 1–2 Live Birth Rates and Infant Mortality Rates in Selected Countries, 1993

Country	Birth Rate	Infant Mortality Rate
Japan	11	4
Canada	14	7
United States	15	8
Brazil	21	57
Egypt	29	74
Pakistan	42	99
Sierra Leone	45	139

*Live births per 1000 population.

Source: *World Almanac and Book of Facts* (1996). New York: Pharos Books.

Descriptive statistics are the starting point for the formation of research questions. Inferential statistics answer specific questions and generate theories to explain relationships between variables. Theory applied in nursing practice can help change the specific variables that may be causing or at least contributing to certain health problems.

The following sections discuss descriptive statistics that are particularly important to maternal-newborn health care. Inferential considerations are addressed as possible research questions that may assist in identifying relevant variables.

Birth Rate

Birth rate refers to the number of live births per 1000 people. In 1990, 4,158,212 babies were born in the US, a birth rate of 17.5. Since 1990 the overall birth rate in the United States has declined each year. In 1994, 3,952,767 babies were born in the United States, and the birth rate dropped to 15.2 (Ventura et al 1996). This is the fourth straight year in which the overall birth rate has decreased.

In 1990, there were 450,486 live births in Canada, a birth rate of 15.3. In 1992, the birth rate dropped to 14. Internationally, birth rates vary significantly. Table 1–2 compares the 1993 birth rates of selected countries.

Research questions that can be posed about birth rates include the following:

- Is there an association between birth rates and changing social values?
- Do the differences in birth rates among various countries reflect cultural differences? Availability of contraceptive information? Other factors?

Infant Mortality

The **infant mortality rate** is the number of deaths of infants under 1 year of age per 1000 live births in a given population. In 1993, 33,466 infant deaths were reported, resulting in an infant mortality rate of 8.4, the lowest rate ever recorded for the United States (Gardner and Hudson 1996). (Neonatal mortality is the number of deaths of infants less than 28 days of age per 1000 live births; perinatal mortality includes both neonatal deaths and fetal deaths per 1000 live births; and fetal death is death in utero at 20 weeks or more gestation.)

The US infant mortality rate continues to be an area of concern because the United States has fallen to 22nd place in infant mortality rankings among industrialized nations. Health care professionals, policy makers, and the public continue to stress the need for better prenatal care, coordination of health services, and provision of comprehensive maternal-child services in the United States. However, as many as one-fourth of pregnant women in some US communities do not receive prenatal care (Moore and Paul 1992).

Table 1–2 identifies infant mortality rates for selected countries for 1992. As the data indicate, the range is dramatic among the countries listed. Information about birth rates and mortality rates is limited for some countries because of a lack of organized reporting mechanisms.

The information raises questions about access to health care during pregnancy and after birth and about standards of living, nutrition, and sociocultural factors. Additional factors affecting the infant mortality rate may be identified by considering the following research questions:

- Does infant mortality correlate with a specific maternal age?
- What are the leading causes of infant mortality in each country?
- Do mortality rates differ among racial groups? If so, are the differences associated with the availability of prenatal care? With the educational level of the mother or father?

Maternal Mortality

Maternal mortality is the number of deaths from any cause during the pregnancy cycle (including the 42-day postpartal period) per 100,000 live births. The **maternal mortality rate** in the United States has decreased steadily in the last 30 years to 7.5 in 1993 (Gardner and Hudson 1996). Factors influencing the decrease in maternal mortality include the increased use of hospitals and specialized health care personnel by maternity clients; the establishment of care centers for high-risk mothers and infants; the prevention and control of infection with antibiotics and improved techniques; the availability of blood and blood products for transfusions; and the lowered rates of anesthesia-related deaths.

Additional factors may be identified by asking the following research questions:

- Is there a correlation between maternal mortality and age?
- Is there a correlation with availability of health care? Economic status?

Implications for Nursing Practice

Nurses can use statistics in a number of ways. For example, they can use statistical data to

- Determine populations at risk
- Assess the relationship between specific factors
- Help establish databases for specific client populations
- Determine the levels of care needed by particular client populations
- Evaluate the success of specific nursing interventions
- Determine priorities in case loads
- Estimate staffing and equipment needs of hospital units and clinics

Statistical information is available through many sources, including professional literature; state and city health departments; vital statistics sections of private, county, state, and federal agencies; special programs or agencies (such as family planning); and demographic profiles of specific geographic areas. Nurses who use this information will be better prepared to promote the health needs of maternal-newborn clients and their families.

Nursing Research

Research is a vital step in expanding the science of nursing. It is also a means of improving client care and continuing to advance the profession of nursing.

Research by nurses can help clarify the relationships between the health professional and the client. Nursing research can also help determine the psychosocial and physical risks and benefits of both nursing and medical interventions.

The gap between research and practice is being narrowed by the publication of research findings in popular nursing journals, the establishment of departments of nursing research in hospitals, and collaborative research efforts by nurse researchers and clinical practitioners. In addition, numerous nursing journal articles give "how-to" information for translating research into practice.

Critical Thinking: A Case Study

Each of the tools of critical thinking—knowledge base, nursing process, communication skills, standards of care, statistics, and nursing research—can exist separately, but in practice they overlap and build upon each other as illustrated in the following case study.

Two birthing unit nurses express concerns to each other about the seemingly high numbers of adolescents who have been giving birth in their unit. At the next staff meeting they voice their concerns and raise questions about whether the number of teenage mothers seen in their unit is higher than normal. After discussion the nurses decide they need to formulate a plan to gather more information. Each nurse volunteers to pursue a particular aspect of the plan of action. Their plan includes contacting the local public health department for local and national statistics on this age group; looking at the availability of health care for adolescents in their community; investigating the particular health problems of pregnant teenagers and risks to their infants; checking the availability of prenatal education groups for adolescents; finding out whether their community has school health programs and what the program content is; looking at national statistics identifying when adolescents seek prenatal care; talking with local CNMs, physicians, and prenatal clinic personnel to see if the national statistics apply to their community; collecting information about current legislative issues affecting adolescent health care; seeking further information about the needs of adolescents during pregnancy and birth by doing a library search; and looking for continuing education programs dealing with the pregnant adolescent client.

At subsequent staff meetings, nurses share information and identify other areas to investigate. How they evaluate the data and apply them will depend on the requirements of their maternal-newborn unit and the unique needs of their community.

Possible outcomes may include developing a research study, volunteering in local adolescent clinics, developing and teaching prenatal classes for adolescents, volunteering to teach in community school health programs, organizing a continuing education program on the adolescent mother for community hospitals, and forming a network within their professional nursing organization to stay informed about legislative issues pertaining to adolescents.

As this example illustrates, the application of critical thinking tools helps the nurse analyze data and plan a course of action.

CHAPTER HIGHLIGHTS

- Many nurses working with childbearing families are expert practitioners who are able to serve as role models for nurses who have not yet attained the same level of competence.
- Contemporary childbirth is family centered, offers choices about birth, and recognizes the needs of siblings and other family members.
- A nurse must practice within the scope of practice or be open to the accusation of practicing medicine without a license. The standard of care against which individual nursing practice is compared is that of a reasonably prudent nurse.
- Informed consent—based on knowledge of a procedure and its benefits, risks, and alternatives—must be secured before providing treatment.
- Assisted reproductive technology (ART) is the term used to describe highly technologic approaches used to produce pregnancy, including in vitro fertilization and embryo transfer (IVF-ET), zygote intrafallopian transfer (ZIFT), and gamete intrafallopian transfer (GIFT).
- Abortion can legally be performed until the age of viability. The decision to have an abortion is made by the woman in consultation with her physician. Caregivers have the right to refuse to perform an abortion or assist with the procedure.
- Cord blood banking provides the opportunity to have stem cells available to treat a variety of cancers and blood system disorders. Its growing popularity has revealed several ethical issues.
- Today's nurse uses a variety of nursing skills in applying the critical thinking process in the setting of maternal-newborn nursing.
- The nursing process, composed of assessment, nursing diagnosis, planning, implementation, and evaluation, provides a systematic method of approaching nursing practice.
- Nursing standards provide information and guidelines for nurses in their own practice, in developing policies and protocols in health care settings, and in directing the development of quality nursing care.
- Descriptive statistics describe or summarize a set of data. Inferential statistics allow the investigator to draw conclusions about what is happening between two or more variables in a population.
- Nursing research is vital to add to the nursing knowledge base, expand clinical practice, and expand nursing theory.

REFERENCES

American Academy of Pediatrics, Committee on Bioethics: Fetal therapy: Ethical considerations. *Pediatrics* 1988; 88:898.

American College of Obstetricians and Gynecologists, Committee on Ethics: *Opinion No. 55: Patient Choices: Maternal-Fetal Conflict.* Washington, DC: ACOG, 1987.

American Medical Association, Board of Trustees: Legal interventions during pregnancy. *JAMA* 1990; 264:2663.

American Nurses Association: Primary Health Care: The nurse solution. In: *Nursing Facts.* Washington, DC: Author, 1993.

Arnold LS et al: Lessons from the past. *MCN* March/April 1989; 14(2):75.

Baird PA: New reproductive technologies: The Canadian perspective. *Women Health Issues* May/June 1996; 6(3):156.

Benner P: *From Novice to Expert.* Redwood City, CA: Addison-Wesley, 1984.

Bowers B, McCarthy D: Developing analytical thinking skills in early undergraduate education. *J Nurs Educ* March 1993; 32(3):107.

Brookfield S: On impostership, cultural suicide, and other dangers: How nurses learn critical thinking. *J Continuing Educ Nurs* September/October 1993; 24(5):197.

Fetal surgery: Past, present, and future work in this frontier. *Contemp OB/GYN* April 15, 1994; 39(s):59.

Gardner P, Hudson BL: Advance report of final mortality statistics, 1993. *Monthly Vital Statistics Report* February 29, 1996; 44(7):1.

Hagedorn MIE et al: A model for professional nursing practice. In: *Legal Aspects of Maternal-Child Nursing Practice.* Gardner SL, Hagedorn MIE (editors). Menlo Park, CA: Addison Wesley Longman, 1997.

Hurst BS, Schlaff WD: Assisted reproduction: What role for ZIFT? *Contemp OB/GYN* October 15, 1994; 39(s):9.

Levy MJ, Gindoff PR: Who benefits most from natural-cycle IVF? *Contemp OB/GYN* February 1994; 39(2):11.

Mitchell JJ: Maternal-fetal conflict: A role for the healthcare ethics committee. *Healthcare Ethics Comm Forum* 1994; 6(2):93.

Moore ML, Paul NW: *Improving Access to Prenatal Care: Innovative Responses to a National Dilemma.* White Plains, NY: March of Dimes Birth Defects Foundation. Birth Defects: Original article series, Vol 28, No 4, 1992.

Moores P: Empowering women in the practice setting. In: *Legal Aspects of Maternal-Child Nursing Practice.* Gardner SL, Hagedorn MIE (editors). Menlo Park, CA: Addison Wesley Longman, 1997.

National Center for Human Genome Research: *About the Human Genome Project.* 1996; http://www.nchgr.nih.gov/.

National Council for Excellence in Critical Thinking: *Critical Thinking: Shaping the Mind of the 21st Century.* Rohnert Park, CA: Sonoma State University, Center for Critical Thinking and Moral Critique, 1992.

Plotnick J, Presler B: Rugged individualism and compassion: The foundation of public policy. *MCN* January/February 1996; 21(1):20.

Randal J: Cord blood offers patients new blood cell source. *J National Cancer Inst* February 1, 1995; 87(3):164.

Stephenson J: Terms of engraftment: Umbilical cord blood transplants arouse enthusiasm. *JAMA* June 21, 1995; 273(23):1813.

Sugarman J et al: Ethical aspects of banking placental blood for transplantation. *JAMA* December 13, 1995; 274(22):1783.

US Department of Energy: *An Introduction to the Human Genome Program.* 1996; http://www.er.doe.gov/...on/oher/hug_intro.html.

Ventura SJ et al: Advance report of final natality statistics, 1994. *Monthly Vital Statistics Report* June 24, 1996; 44(11):1.

Weisman CS: Proceedings of women's health and managed care: Balancing cost, access, and quality. Introduction to the proceedings. *Women Health Issues* January/February 1996; 6(1):1.

Wilcox LS, Marks JS: Regulating assisted reproductive technologies: Public health, consumer protection, and public resources. *Women Health Issues* May/June 1996; 6(3):175.

Woods JH: Affective learning: One door to critical thinking. *Holistic Nurs Pract* 1993; 7(3):64.

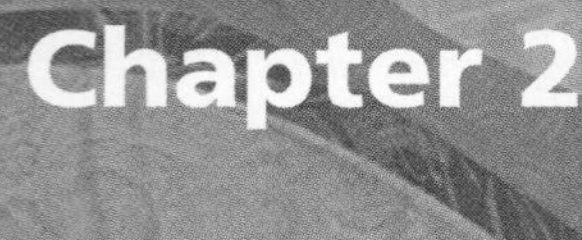

Chapter 2 Reproductive Anatomy and Physiology

OBJECTIVES

- Identify the structures and functions of the female and male reproductive systems.
- Summarize the actions of the hormones that affect reproductive functioning.
- Identify the two phases of the ovarian cycle and the changes that occur in each phase.
- Describe the phases of the menstrual cycle, their dominant hormones, and the changes that occur in each phase.
- Discuss the significance of specific female reproductive structures during childbirth.

KEY TERMS

Ampulla
Areola
Breasts
Broad ligament
Cardinal ligaments
Cervix
Conjugate vera
Cornua
Corpus
Corpus luteum
Diagonal conjugate
Endometrium
Estrogens
Fallopian tubes
False pelvis
Female reproductive cycle (FRC)
Fimbria
Follicle-stimulating hormone (FSH)
Fundus
Gonadotropin-releasing hormone (GnRH)
Graafian follicle
Human chorionic gonadotropin (hCG)
Infundibulopelvic ligament
Innominate bones
Ischial spines
Isthmus
Luteinizing hormone (LH)
Myometrium
Nidation
Obstetric conjugate
Ovarian ligaments
Ovulation
Pelvic cavity
Pelvic diaphragm
Pelvic inlet
Pelvic outlet
Perimetrium
Perineal body
Progesterone
Prostaglandins
Round ligaments
Sacral promontory
Spermatogenesis
Symphysis pubis
Testosterone
Transverse diameter
True pelvis
Uterosacral ligaments
Uterus
Vagina
Vulva
Zona pellucida

Understanding childbearing requires more than understanding sexual intercourse or the process by which the female and male sex cells unite. The nurse must also become familiar with the structures and functions that make childbearing possible and the phenomena that initiate it. This chapter concerns the anatomic, physiologic, and sexual aspects of the female and male reproductive systems. Chapter 5 discusses the psychosocial aspects of human sexuality.

The male and female reproductive organs are *homologous;* that is, they are fundamentally similar in structure and function. The primary functions of both male and female reproductive systems are to produce sex cells and transport them to locations where their union can occur. The sex cells, called *gametes,* are produced by specialized organs called *gonads.* A series of ducts and glands within both male and female reproductive systems contributes to the production and transport of the gametes.

Female Reproductive System

The female reproductive system consists of the external and internal genitals and the accessory organs of the breasts. Because of its importance to childbearing, the bony pelvis is also discussed in this chapter.

External Genitals

All the external reproductive organs except the glandular structures can be directly inspected. The size, color, and shape of these structures vary extensively among races and individuals. The female external genitals, referred to as the **vulva** or *pudendum,* include the following structures (Figure 2–1):

- Mons pubis
- Labia majora
- Labia minora
- Clitoris
- Urethral meatus and opening of the paraurethral (Skene's) glands
- Vaginal vestibule (vaginal orifice, vulvovaginal glands, hymen, and fossa navicularis)
- Perineal body

Although they are not true parts of the female reproductive system, the urethral meatus and perineal body are considered here because of their proximity and relationship to the vulva. The vulva has a generous supply of blood and nerves. As a woman ages, estrogen secretions decrease, causing the vulvar organs to atrophy and become subject to a variety of lesions.

Mons Pubis

The *mons pubis* is a softly rounded mound of subcutaneous fatty tissue beginning at the lowest portion of the anterior abdominal wall (Figure 2–1). Also known as the mons veneris, this structure covers the front portion of the symphysis pubis. The mons pubis is covered with pubic hair, typically with the hairline forming a transverse line across the lower abdomen. The hair is short and varies from sparse and fine in Asian women to heavy, coarse, and curly in African women. The mons pubis protects the pelvic bones, especially during coitus.

Labia Majora

The *labia majora* are longitudinal, raised folds of pigmented skin, one on either side of the vulvar cleft. As the pair descend, they narrow and merge to form the posterior junction of the perineal skin. Their chief function is to protect the structures lying between them.

The labia majora are covered by stratified squamous epithelium containing hair follicles and sebaceous glands with underlying adipose and muscle tissue. Under the skin, the dartos muscle sheet is responsible for the wrinkled appearance of the labia majora as well as for their sensitivity to heat and cold. The inner surface of the labia majora in women who have not had children is moist and looks like mucous membrane, whereas after many births it is more skinlike (Cunningham et al 1997). With each pregnancy, the labia majora become less prominent. Because of the extensive venous network in the labia majora, varicosities may occur during pregnancy, and obstetric or sexual trauma may cause hematomas. The labia majora share an extensive lymphatic supply with the other structures of the vulva, which can facilitate the spread of cancer in the female reproductive organs. Because of the nerves supplying the labia majora (from the first lumbar and third sacral segment of the spinal cord), certain regional anesthesia blocks will affect them.

Labia Minora

The *labia minora* are soft folds of skin within the labia majora that converge near the anus, forming the *fourchette.* Each labium minus has the appearance of shiny mucous membrane, moist and devoid of hair follicles. The labia minora are rich in sebaceous glands, which lubricate and waterproof the vulvar skin and provide bactericidal secretions. Because the sebaceous glands do not open into hair follicles but open directly onto the surface of the skin, sebaceous cysts commonly occur in this area. Vulvovaginitis in this area is very irritating because the labia minora have many tactile nerve endings. The labia minora increase in size at puberty and decrease after menopause because of changes in estrogen levels.

Clitoris

The *clitoris,* located between the labia minora, is about 5 to 6 mm long and 6 to 8 mm across. Its tissue is essentially erectile, and it is extremely sensitive to touch. The glans of the clitoris is partly covered by a fold of skin called the *prepuce.* This area resembles an opening to an orifice, and may be confused with the urethral meatus. Accidental attempts to insert a catheter in this area produce extreme discomfort. The clitoris has very rich blood and nerve supplies and exists primarily for female sexual enjoyment. In addition, it secretes *smegma,* the odor of which may be sexually stimulating to the male.

Urethral Meatus and Paraurethral Glands

The *urethral meatus* is located 1 to 2.5 cm beneath the clitoris in the midline of the vestibule; it often appears as a puckered, slitlike opening. The paraurethral glands, or *Skene's ducts,* open into the posterior wall of the urethra close to its orifice. Their secretions lubricate the vaginal vestibule, facilitating sexual intercourse.

Vaginal Vestibule

The vaginal vestibule is a boat-shaped depression enclosed by the labia majora and visible when they are separated. The vestibule contains the vaginal opening, or *introitus,* which is the border between the external and internal genitals.

The *hymen* is a thin, elastic membrane that partly closes the vaginal opening. Its strength, shape, and size vary greatly among women. The hymen is essentially avascular. The belief that the intact hymen is a sign of virginity and that it is ruptured only with the first sexual intercourse is not valid. The hymen may be broken through strenuous physical activity, masturbation, menstruation, or the use of tampons. Occasionally a woman about to give birth still has an intact hymen.

External to the hymenal ring at the base of the vestibule are two small papular elevations containing the openings of the ducts of the *vulvovaginal (Bartholin's) glands.* They lie under the constrictor muscle of the vagina. These glands secrete a mucus that is clear and thick, with an alkaline pH, all of which enhance the viability and motility of the sperm deposited in the vaginal vestibule. These gland ducts can harbor *Neisseria gonorrhea* and other bacteria, which can cause pus formation and Bartholin's gland abscesses (Davies 1990).

Perineal Body

The perineal body is a wedge-shaped mass of fibromuscular tissue found between the lower part of the vagina and the anus. This area is also called the *perineum.*

The muscles that meet at the perineal body are the external sphincter ani, both levator ani, the superficial and deep transverse perineal, and the bulbocavernosus.

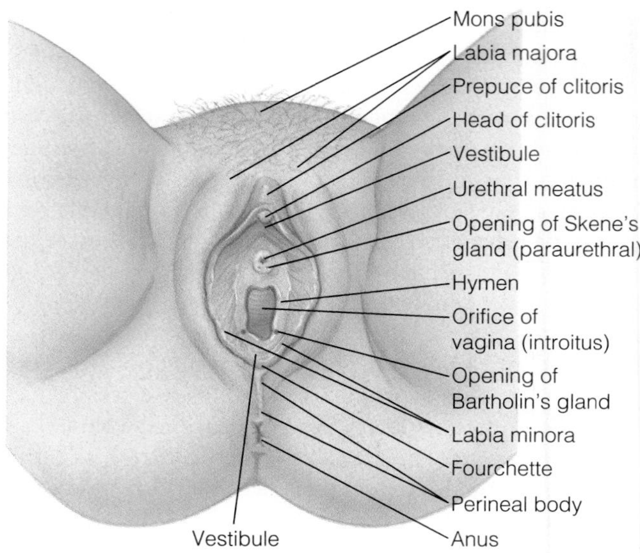

FIGURE 2–1 Female external genitals, longitudinal view.

These muscles mingle with elastic fibers and connective tissue in an arrangement that allows a remarkable amount of stretching. The perineal body is subject to laceration during childbirth. It is the site of episiotomy during birth (see Chapter 19).

Female Internal Reproductive Organs

The female internal reproductive organs are the vagina, uterus, fallopian tubes, and ovaries (Figure 2–2). These are target organs for estrogenic hormones, and they play a unique part in the reproductive cycle. The internal reproductive organs can be palpated during vaginal examination and assessed with various instruments.

Vagina

The **vagina** is a muscular and membranous tube that connects the external genitals with the uterus. It extends from the vulva to the uterus in a position nearly parallel to the plane of the pelvic brim. The vagina is often called the *birth canal* because it forms the lower part of the axis through which the fetus must pass during birth.

Because the cervix of the uterus projects into the upper part of the anterior wall of the vagina, the anterior wall is approximately 2.5 cm shorter than the posterior wall. Measurements range from 6 to 8 cm for the anterior wall and from 7 to 10 cm for the posterior wall.

In the upper part of the vagina, which is called the vaginal *vault,* there is a recess or hollow around the cervix. This area is called the vaginal *fornix.* Since the walls of the vaginal vault are very thin, various structures can be palpated through the walls, including the uterus, a distended bladder, the ovaries, the appendix, the cecum, the colon, and the ureters. When a woman

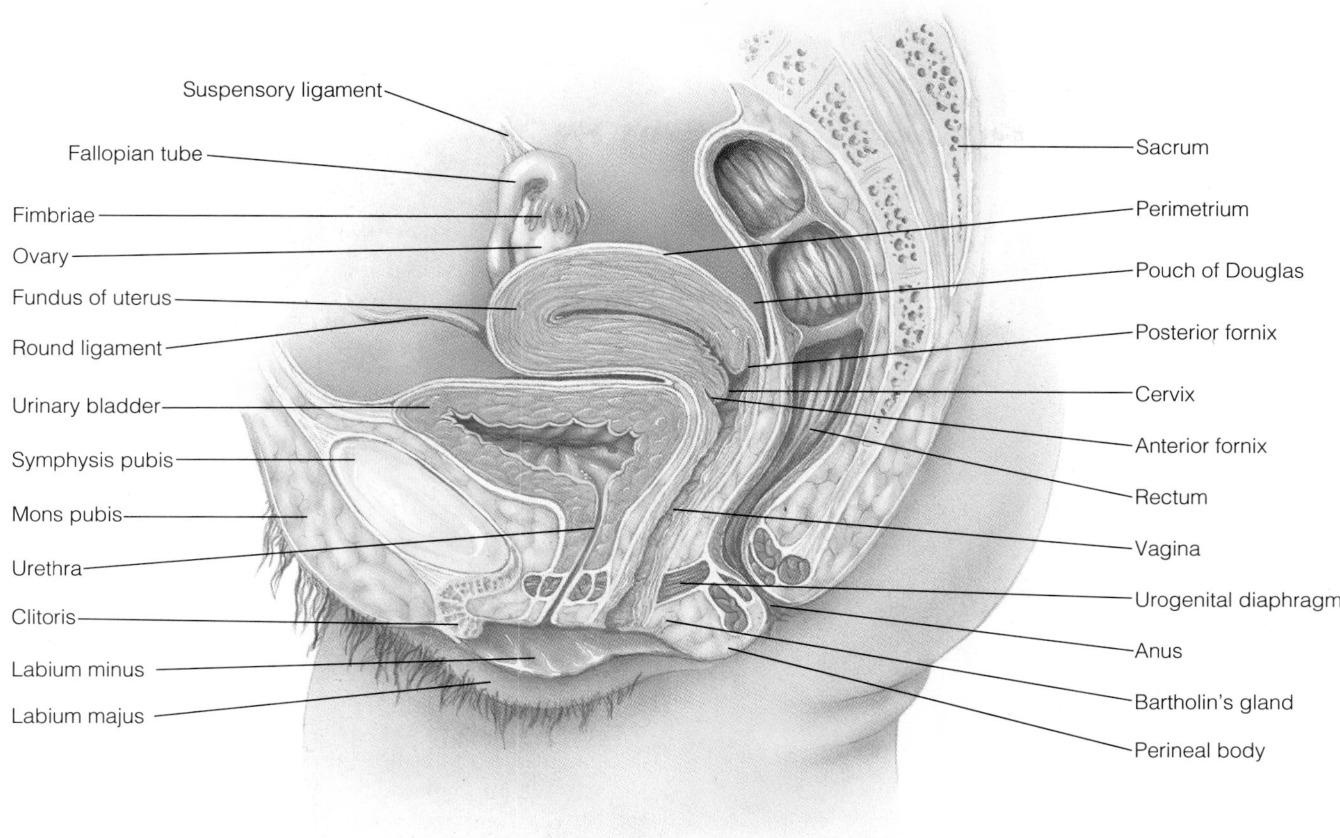

FIGURE 2–2 Female internal reproductive organs.

lies on her back after intercourse, the space in the fornix permits the pooling of semen near the cervix and increases the chances of impregnation.

The walls of the vagina are covered with ridges, or *rugae,* crisscrossing each other. These rugae allow the vagina to stretch during the descent of the fetal head.

During a woman's reproductive life, an acidic vaginal environment is normal (pH 4–5). The acidic environment is maintained by a symbiotic relationship between lactic acid–producing bacilli (Döderlein bacillus or lactobacillus) and the vaginal epithelial cells. These cells contain glycogen, which is broken down by the bacilli into lactic acid. The amount of glycogen is regulated by the ovarian hormones. Any interruption of this process can destroy the normal self-cleaning action of the vagina. Such interruption may be caused by antibiotic therapy, douching, or use of perineal sprays or deodorants. For discussion of comfort issues for women, see Chapter 5.

The acidic vaginal environment is normal only during the mature reproductive years and in the first days of life when maternal hormones are operating in the infant. A relatively neutral pH of 7.5 is normal from infancy until puberty and after menopause. The vagina's blood and lymphatic supplies are extensive (Figure 2–3).

The pudendal nerve supplies what relatively little somatic innervation there is to the lower third of the vagina. Thus sensation during sexual excitement and coitus is minimal, as is vaginal pain during the second stage of labor.

The vagina has three functions:

- To serve as the passage for sperm and for the fetus during birth
- To provide passage for the menstrual products from the uterine endometrium to the outside of the body
- To protect against trauma from sexual intercourse and infection from pathogenic organisms

Uterus

Throughout the ages, the uterus, or womb, has been endowed with a mystical aura. Numerous customs, taboos, mores, and values have evolved about women and their reproductive function. Although scientific knowledge has replaced much of this folklore, remnants of old ideas and superstitions persist. The nurse must be

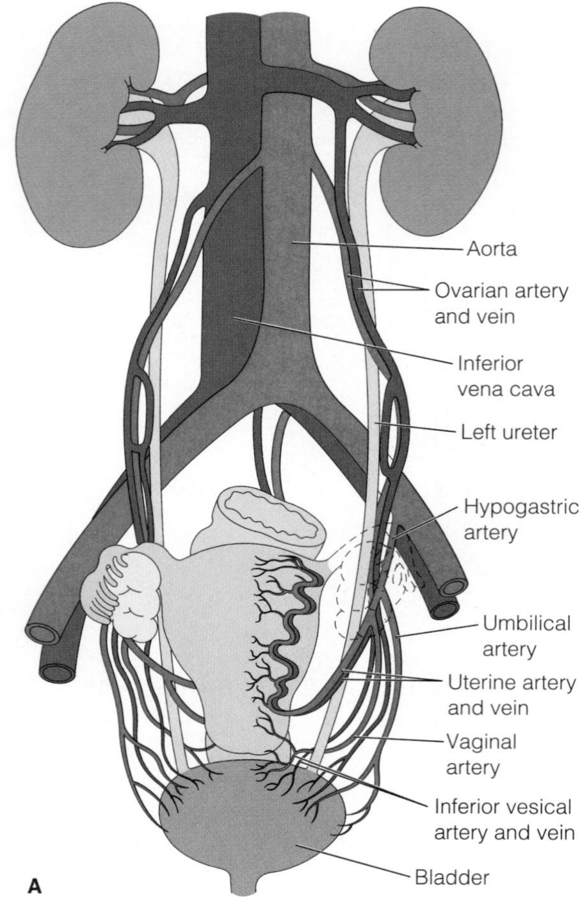

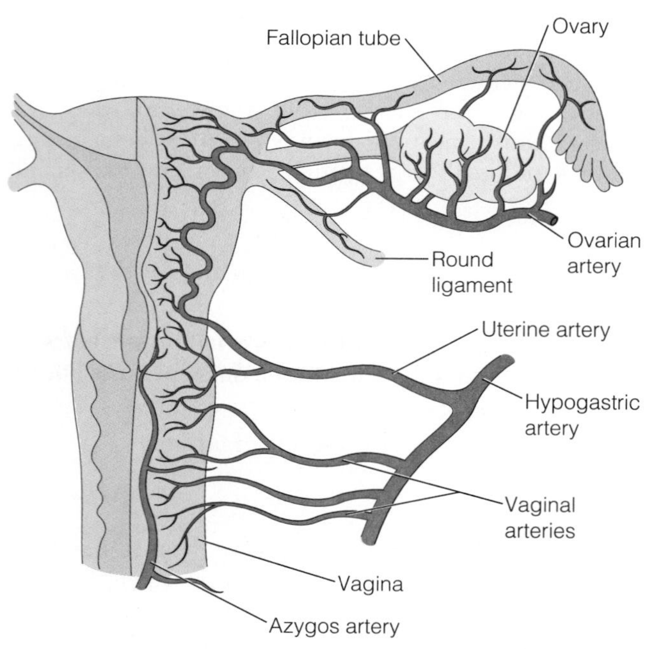

FIGURE 2–3 Blood supply to internal reproductive organs. ***A*** Pelvic blood supply. ***B*** Blood supply to vagina, ovaries, uterus, and fallopian tube.

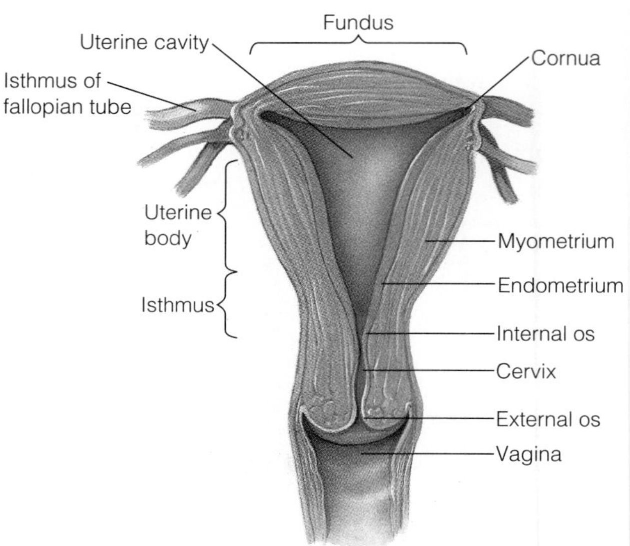

FIGURE 2–4 Structures of the uterus.

able to recognize and deal with such attitudes and beliefs so that nursing care can be effective.

The **uterus** is a hollow, muscular, thick-walled organ shaped like an upside-down pear. It lies in the center of the pelvic cavity between the base of the bladder and the rectum and above the vagina (Figure 2–4). It is level with or slightly below the brim of the pelvis, with the external opening of the cervix (external os) about the level of the ischial spines. The mature organ weighs about 50 to 70 g and is approximately 7.5 cm long, 5 cm wide, and 1 to 2.5 cm thick (Resnik 1994).

The position of the uterus can vary, depending on a woman's posture, number of children borne, bladder and rectal fullness, and even normal respiratory patterns. Only the cervix is anchored laterally. The body of the uterus can move freely forward or backward. The axis also varies. Generally, the uterus bends forward, forming a sharp angle with the vagina. There is a bend in the area of the isthmus of the uterus; from there the cervix points downward. The uterus is said to be *anteverted* when it is in this position. The anteverted position is considered normal.

The uterus is kept in place by three sets of supports. The upper supports are the broad and round ligaments. The middle supports are the cardinal, pubocervical, and uterosacral ligaments. The lower supports are those structures considered to make up the pelvic muscular floor.

The isthmus is a slight constriction in the uterus that divides it into two unequal parts. The upper two-thirds of the uterus is the **corpus,** or *body,* composed mainly of a smooth muscle layer (myometrium). The lower third is the cervix or neck. The rounded uppermost portion of

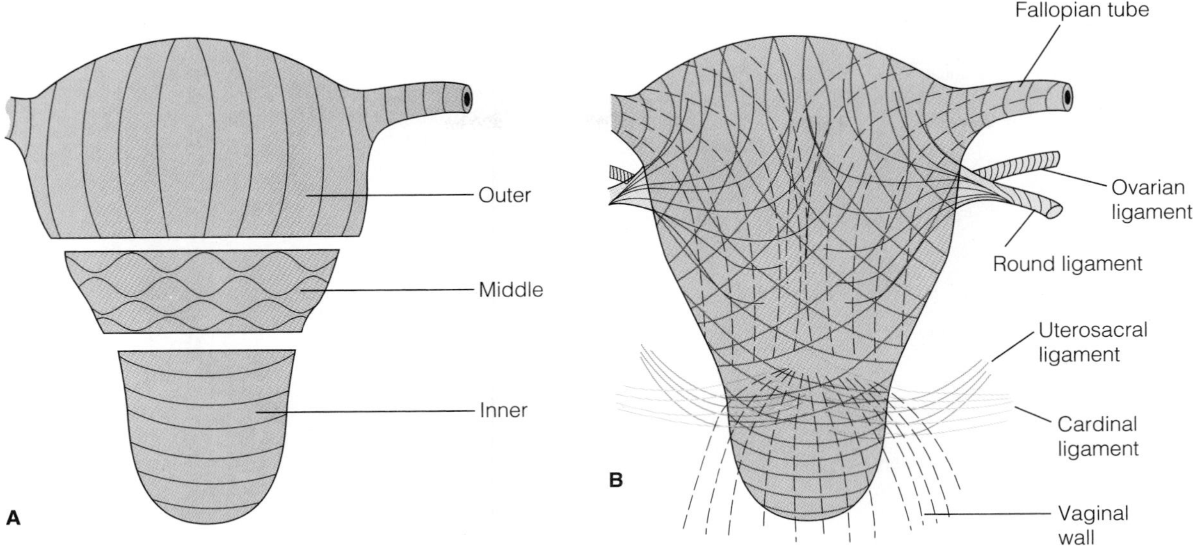

FIGURE 2–5 Uterine muscle layers. ***A*** Muscle fiber placement. ***B*** Interlacing of uterine muscle layers.

the corpus that extends above the points of attachment of the fallopian tubes is called the **fundus.** The elongated portion of the uterus where the fallopian tubes enter is called the **cornua.**

The isthmus is about 6 mm above the uterine opening of the cervix (the internal os), and it is in this area that the uterine lining changes into the mucous membrane of the cervix; it joins the corpus to the cervix. The isthmus takes on importance in pregnancy because it becomes the lower uterine segment. With the cervix, it is a passive segment and not part of the contractile uterus. At birth, this thin lower segment, situated behind the bladder, is the site for lower-segment cesarean births (see Chapter 20).

The blood and lymphatic supplies to the uterus are extensive (see Figure 2–3). Innervation of the uterus is entirely by the autonomic nervous system. Even without an intact nerve supply, the uterus can contract adequately for birth; for example, hemiplegic women have adequate uterine contractions.

The function of the uterus is to provide a safe environment for fetal development. The uterine lining is cyclically prepared by steroid hormones for implantation of the embryo (**nidation**). Once the embryo is implanted, the developing fetus is protected until it is expelled.

Both the body of the uterus and the cervix are changed permanently by pregnancy. The body never returns to its prepregnant size, and the external os changes from a circular opening of about 3 mm to a transverse slit with irregular edges.

The Corpus The uterine corpus is made up of three layers. The outermost layer is the *serosal layer* or **perimetrium,** which is composed of peritoneum. The middle layer is the *muscular uterine layer* or **myometrium.** This muscular uterine layer is continuous with the muscle layers of the fallopian tubes and the vagina. This helps these organs present a unified reaction to various stimuli—ovulation, orgasm, or the deposit of sperm in the vagina. These muscle fibers also extend into the ovarian, round, and cardinal ligaments and minimally into the uterosacral ligaments, which helps explain the vague but disturbing pelvic "aches and pains" reported by many pregnant women.

The myometrium has three distinct layers of uterine (smooth) involuntary muscles (Figure 2–5). The outer layer, found mainly over the fundus, is made up of longitudinal muscles, which cause cervical effacement and expel the fetus during birth. The thick middle layer is made up of interlacing muscle fibers in figure eight patterns. These muscle fibers surround large blood vessels, and their contraction produces a hemostatic action (a tourniquetlike action on blood vessels to stop bleeding after birth). The inner muscle layer is composed of circular fibers that form sphincters at the fallopian tube attachment sites and at the internal os. The internal os sphincter inhibits the expulsion of the uterine contents during pregnancy but stretches in labor as cervical dilatation occurs. An incompetent cervical os can be caused by a torn, weak, or absent sphincter at the internal os. The sphincters at the fallopian tubes prevent menstrual blood from flowing backward into the fallopian tubes from the uterus.

Although each layer of muscle has been discussed as having a unique function, it must be remembered that the uterine musculature works as a whole. The uterine

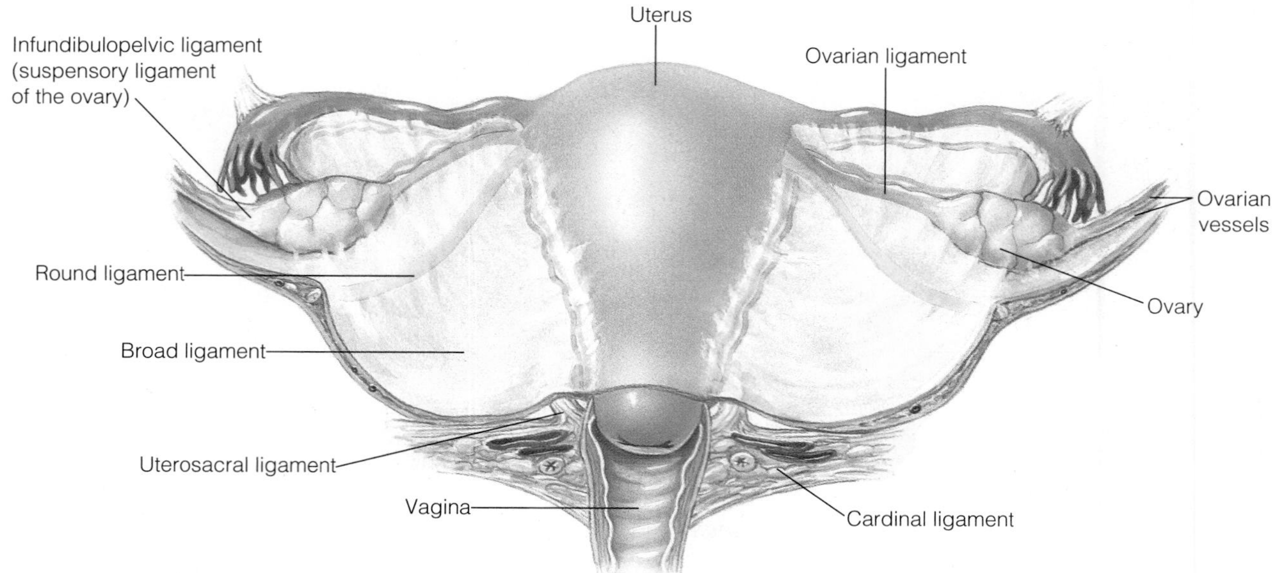

FIGURE 2–6 Uterine ligaments.

contractions of labor are responsible for the dilatation of the cervix and provide the major force for the passage of the fetus through the pelvic axis and vaginal canal at birth. The mucosal layer, or **endometrium,** of the uterine corpus is the innermost layer. This single layer is composed of columnar epithelium, glands, and stroma. From menarche to menopause, the endometrium undergoes monthly degeneration and renewal in the absence of pregnancy. As it responds to the governing hormonal cycle and prostaglandin influence, the endometrium varies in thickness from 0.5 to 5 mm.

The glands of the endometrium produce a thin, watery, alkaline secretion that keeps the uterine cavity moist. This *endometrial milk* not only helps sperm travel to the fallopian tubes but also nourishes the developing embryo before it lodges in the endometrium (Chapter 3).

The blood supply to the endometrium is unique. Some of the blood vessels are not sensitive to cyclic hormonal control, whereas others are extremely sensitive to it. These differing responses allow part of the endometrium to remain intact while other endometrial tissue is shed during menstruation.

The Cervix The narrow neck of the uterus is the cervix. It meets the body of the uterus at the internal os and descends about 2.5 cm to connect with the vagina at the external os (Figure 2–4). Thus it provides a protective portal for the body of the uterus. The cervix is divided by its line of attachment into the vaginal and supravaginal areas. The *vaginal cervix* projects into the vagina at an angle of from 45 to 90 degrees. The *supravaginal cervix* is surrounded by the attachments that give the uterus its main support: the uterosacral ligaments, the transverse ligaments of the cervix (Mackenrodt's ligaments), and the pubocervical ligaments.

The vaginal cervix appears pink and ends at the external os. The cervical canal appears rosy red and is lined with columnar ciliated epithelium, which contains mucus-secreting glands. Most cervical cancer begins at this squamocolumnar junction. The specific location of the junction varies with age and number of pregnancies. Elasticity is the chief characteristic of the cervix. Its ability to stretch is due to the high fibrous and collagenous content of the supportive tissues and also to the vast number of folds in the cervical lining.

The cervical mucus has three functions:

- To lubricate the vaginal canal
- To act as a bacteriostatic agent
- To provide an alkaline environment to shelter deposited sperm from the acidic vagina

At ovulation, cervical mucus is clearer, thinner, more profuse, and more alkaline than at other times.

Uterine Ligaments The uterine ligaments support and stabilize the various reproductive organs. The ligaments shown in Figure 2–6 are described as follows:

1. The **broad ligament** keeps the uterus centrally placed and provides stability within the pelvic cavity. It is a double layer that is continuous with the abdominal peritoneum. The broad ligament covers the uterus anteriorly and posteriorly and extends outward from the uterus to enfold the fallopian tubes. The round and ovarian ligaments are at the

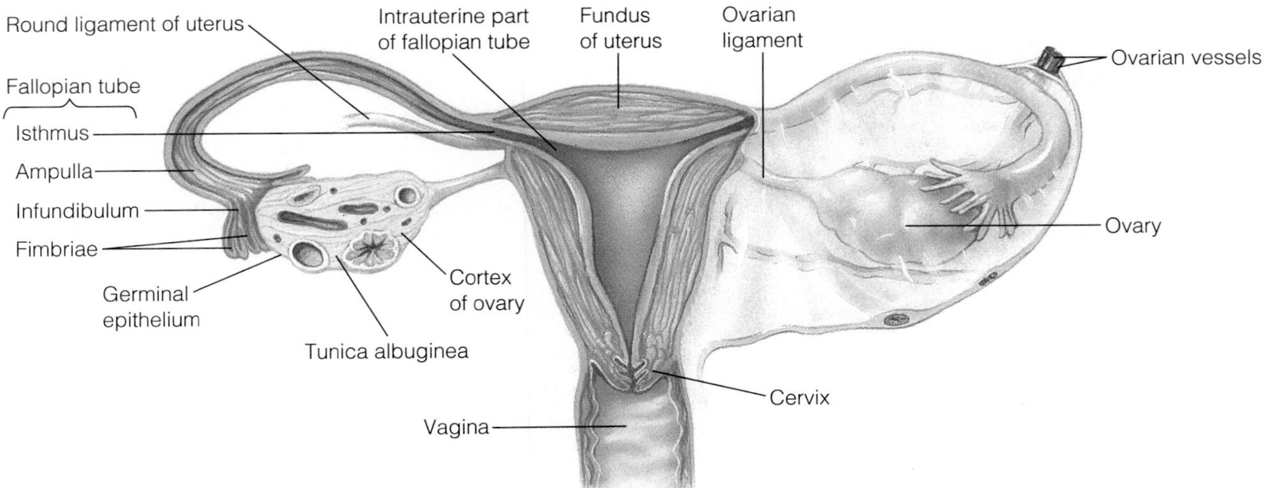

FIGURE 2–7 Fallopian tube and ovary.

upper border of the broad ligament. At its lower border, it forms the cardinal ligaments. Between the folds of the broad ligament are connective tissue, involuntary muscle, blood and lymph vessels, and nerves.

2. The **round ligaments** help the broad ligament keep the uterus in place. The round ligaments arise from the sides of the uterus near the fallopian tube insertions. They extend outward between the folds of the broad ligament, passing through the inguinal ring and canals and eventually fusing with the connective tissue of the labia majora. Made up of longitudinal muscle, the round ligaments enlarge during pregnancy. During labor the round ligaments steady the uterus, pulling downward and forward so that the presenting part of the fetus is forced into the cervix.
3. The **ovarian ligaments** anchor the lower pole of the ovary to the cornua of the uterus. They are composed of muscle fibers, which allow the ligaments to contract. This contractile ability influences the position of the ovary to some extent, thus helping the fimbriae of the fallopian tubes to "catch" the ovum as it is released each month.
4. The **cardinal ligaments** are the chief uterine supports, suspending the uterus from the side walls of the true pelvis. These ligaments, also known as Mackenrodt's or transverse cervical ligaments, arise from the sides of the pelvic walls and attach to the cervix in the upper vagina. These ligaments prevent uterine prolapse and also support the upper vagina (Figure 2–6).
5. The **infundibulopelvic ligament** suspends and supports the ovaries (Figure 2–6). Arising from the outer third of the broad ligament, the infundibulopelvic ligament contains the ovarian vessels and nerves.
6. The **uterosacral ligaments** provide support for the uterus and cervix at the level of the ischial spines (Figure 2–6). Arising on each side of the pelvis from the posterior wall of the uterus, the uterosacral ligaments sweep back around the rectum and insert on the sides of the first and second sacral vertebras. The uterosacral ligaments contain smooth muscle fibers, connective tissue, blood and lymph vessels, and nerves. They also contain sensory nerve fibers that contribute to dysmenorrhea (painful menstruation) (see Chapter 5).

Fallopian Tubes

The **fallopian tubes,** also known as the *oviducts* or *uterine tubes,* arise from each side of the uterus and reach almost to the sides of the pelvis, where they turn toward the ovaries (Figure 2–7). Each tube is approximately 8–13.5 cm long. The fallopian tubes link the peritoneal cavity with the uterus and vagina. This linkage increases a woman's biologic vulnerability to disease processes. A short section of each fallopian tube is inside the uterus; its opening into the uterus is only 1 mm in diameter.

Each fallopian tube may be divided into three parts: the **isthmus,** the ampulla, and the infundibulum or fimbria. The isthmus is straight and narrow, with a thick muscular wall and an opening (lumen) 2 to 3 mm in diameter. It is the site of tubal ligation, a surgical procedure to prevent pregnancy.

Next to the isthmus is the curved **ampulla,** which comprises the outer two-thirds of the tube. Fertilization of the secondary oocyte by a spermatozoon usually occurs here. The ampulla ends at the **fimbria,** which is a funnel-shaped enlargement with many projections, called *fimbriae,* reaching out to the ovary. The longest of these, the *fimbria ovarica,* is attached to the ovary to increase the chances of intercepting the ovum as it is released.

The wall of the fallopian tube is made up of four layers: peritoneal (serous), subserous (adventitial), muscular, and mucous tissues. The peritoneum covers the tubes. The subserous layer contains the blood and nerve supply, and the muscular layer is responsible for the peristaltic movement of the tube. The mucosal layer, immediately next to the muscular layer, is composed of ciliated and nonciliated cells, with the number of ciliated cells more abundant at the fimbria. Nonciliated cells secrete a protein-rich, serous fluid that nourishes the ovum. The constantly moving tubal cilia propel the ovum toward the uterus. Because the ovum is a large cell, this ciliary action is needed to assist the tube's muscular-layer peristalsis. Any malformation or malfunction of the tubes can result in infertility, ectopic pregnancy, or even sterility.

A rich blood and lymphatic supply serves each fallopian tube (see Figure 2–3). Thus the tubes have an unusual ability to recover from an inflammatory process.

The fallopian tubes have three functions:

- To provide transport for the ovum from the ovary to the uterus (transport time through the fallopian tubes varies from 3 to 4 days)
- To provide a site for fertilization
- To serve as a warm, moist, nourishing environment for the ovum or zygote (fertilized egg) (see Chapter 3 for further discussion)

Ovaries

The ovaries are two almond-shaped structures just below the pelvic brim. One ovary is located on either side of the pelvic cavity. Their size varies among women and with the stage of the menstrual cycle. Each ovary weighs approximately 6 to 10 g and is 1.5 to 3 cm wide, 2 to 5 cm long, and 1 to 1.5 cm thick. The ovaries of girls are small, but they become larger after puberty. They also change in appearance from a dull white, smooth-surfaced organ to a pitted gray organ. The pitting is caused by scarring due to ovulation.

The ovaries are held in place by the broad, ovarian, and infundibulopelvic ligaments.

There is no peritoneal covering for the ovaries. Although this lack of covering assists the mature ovum to erupt, it also allows easier spread of malignant cells from cancer of the ovaries. A single layer of cuboidal epithelial cells, called the germinal epithelium, covers the ovaries. The ovaries are composed of three layers: the tunica albuginea, the cortex, and the medulla. The *tunica albuginea* is a dense, dull white, protective layer. The *cortex* is the main functional part because it contains ova, graafian follicles, corpora lutea, degenerated corpora lutea (corpora albicantia), and degenerated follicles. The *medulla* is completely surrounded by the cortex and contains the nerves and the blood and lymphatic vessels.

The ovaries are the primary source of two important hormones: the estrogens and progesterone. *Estrogens* are associated with those characteristics contributing to femaleness, including breast alveolar lobule growth and duct development. The ovaries secrete large amounts of estrogen, while the adrenal cortex (extraglandular sites) produces minute amounts of estrogen in nonpregnant women.

Progesterone is often called the *hormone of pregnancy* because its effects on the uterus allow pregnancy to be maintained. The placenta is the primary source of progesterone during pregnancy. This hormone also inhibits the action of prolactin, thereby preventing lactation during pregnancy (Cunningham et al 1997). The interplay between the ovarian hormones and other hormones such as FSH and LH is responsible for the cyclic changes that allow pregnancy. The hormonal and physical changes that occur during the female reproductive cycle are discussed in depth later in this chapter.

Between the ages of 45 and 55, a woman's ovaries secrete decreasing amounts of estrogen. Eventually, ovulatory activity ceases and menopause occurs.

Bony Pelvis

The female bony *pelvis* has two unique functions:

- To support and protect the pelvic contents.
- To form the relatively fixed axis of the birth passage.

Because the pelvis is so important to childbearing, its structure must be understood clearly.

Bony Structure

The pelvis is made up of four bones: two innominate bones, the sacrum, and the coccyx. The pelvis resembles a bowl or basin; its sides are the innominate bones, and its back is the sacrum and coccyx. Lined with fibrocartilage and held tightly together by ligaments, the four bones join at the symphysis pubis, the two sacroiliac joints, and the sacrococcygeal joints (Figure 2–8).

The **innominate bones,** popularly known as the *hip bones,* are made up of three separate bones: the ilium, ischium, and pubis. These bones fuse to form a circular cavity, the *acetabulum,* which articulates with the femur.

The *ilium* is the broad, upper prominence of the hip. The *iliac crest* is the margin of the ilium. The *iliac spine,* the foremost projection nearest the groin, is the site of attachment for ligaments and muscles.

The *ischium,* the strongest bone, is under the ilium and below the acetabulum. The L-shaped ischium ends

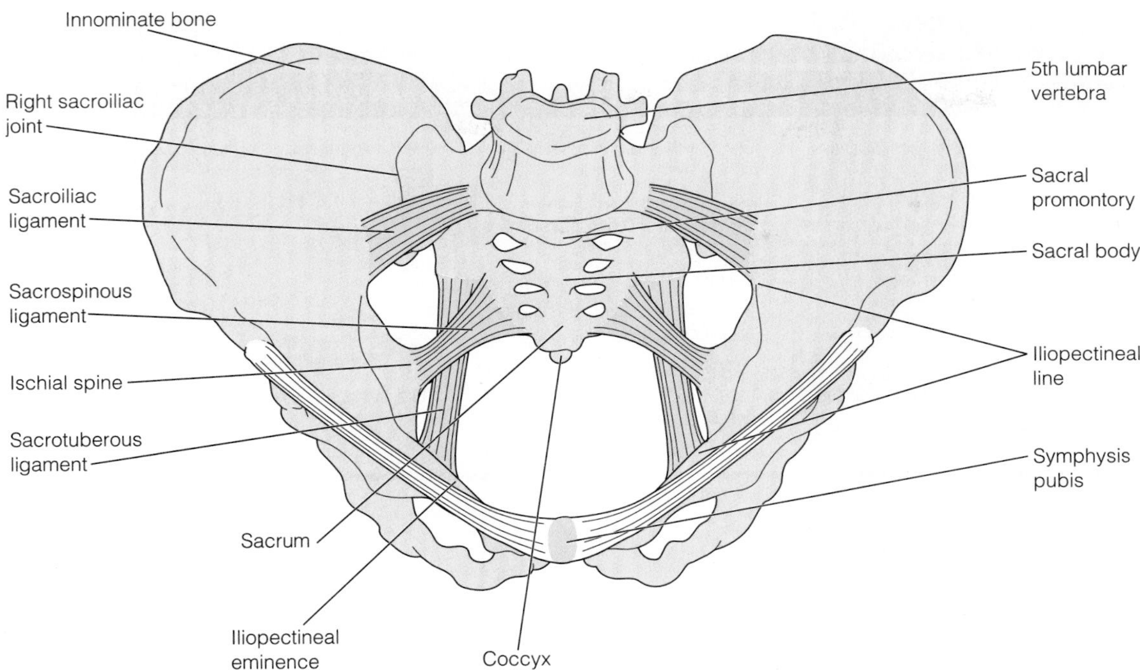

FIGURE 2–8 Pelvic bones with supporting ligaments.

in a marked protuberance, the *ischial tuberosity,* on which the weight of a seated body rests. The **ischial spines** arise near the junction of the ilium and ischium and jut into the pelvic cavity. The shortest diameter of the pelvic cavity is between the ischial spines. The ischial spines serve as reference points during labor to evaluate the descent of the fetal head into the birth canal (see Chapter 15 and Figure 15–7).

The **pubis** forms the slightly bowed front portion of the innominate bone. Extending medially from the acetabulum to the midpoint of the bony pelvis, the pubis meets the other pubis to form a joint called the **symphysis pubis.** The triangular space below this junction is known as the *pubic arch.* The fetal head passes under this arch during birth. The symphysis pubis is formed by heavy fibrocartilage and the superior and inferior pubic ligaments. The mobility of the inferior ligament increases during a first pregnancy and to a greater extent in subsequent pregnancies.

The sacroiliac joints also have a degree of mobility that increases near the end of pregnancy as the result of an upward, gliding movement. The pelvic outlet may be increased by 1.5 to 2 cm in the squatting, sitting, and dorsal lithotomy positions. These relaxations of the joints are induced by the hormones of pregnancy.

The *sacrum* is a wedge-shaped bone formed by the fusion of five vertebras. On the anterior upper portion of the sacrum is a projection into the pelvic cavity known as the **sacral promontory.** This projection is another obstetric guide in determining pelvic measurements. (For a discussion of pelvic measurements, see Chapter 8.)

The small triangular bone last on the vertebral column is the *coccyx.* It articulates with the sacrum at the sacrococcygeal joint. The coccyx usually moves backward during labor to provide more room for the fetus.

Pelvic Floor

The muscular *pelvic floor* of the bony pelvis is designed to overcome the force of gravity exerted on the pelvic organs. It acts as a buttress to the irregularly shaped pelvic outlet, thereby providing stability and support for surrounding structures.

Deep fascia, the levator ani, and coccygeal muscles form the part of the pelvic floor known as the **pelvic diaphragm.** Above it is the pelvic cavity; below and behind it is the perineum.

The levator ani muscle makes up the major portion of the pelvic diaphragm and consists of four muscles: ileococcygeus, pubococcygeus, puborectalis, and pubovaginalis. The ileococcygeal muscle, a thin muscular sheet underlying the sacrospinous ligament, helps the levator ani support the pelvic organs. Muscles of the pelvic floor are shown in Figure 2–9 and discussed in Table 2–1, both on page 26.

TABLE 2–1 Muscles of the Pelvic Floor

Muscle	Origin	Insertion	Innervation	Action
Levator ani	Pubis, lateral pelvic wall, and ischial spine	Blends with organs in pelvic cavity	Inferior rectal, second and third sacral nerves, plus anterior rami of third and fourth sacral nerves	Supports pelvic viscera; helps form pelvic diaphragm
Iliococcygeus	Pelvic surface of ischial spine and pelvic fascia	Central point of perineum, coccygeal raphe, and coccyx		Assists in supporting abdominal and pelvic viscera
Pubococcygeus	Pubis and pelvic fascia	Coccyx		
Puborectalis	Pubis	Blends with rectum; meets similar fibers from opposite side		Forms sling for rectum, just posterior to it; raises anus
Pubovaginalis	Pubis	Blends into vagina		Supports vagina
Coccygeus	Ischial spine and sacrospinous ligament	Lateral border of lower sacrum and upper coccyx	Third and fourth sacral nerves	Supports pelvic viscera; helps form pelvic diaphragm; flexes and abducts coccyx

Pelvic Division

The pelvic cavity is divided into the false pelvis and the true pelvis (Figure 2–10*A*). The **false pelvis** is the portion above the pelvic brim or linea terminalis. Its primary function is to support the weight of the enlarged pregnant uterus and direct the presenting fetal part into the true pelvis below.

The **true pelvis** is the portion that lies below the linea terminalis. The bony circumference of the true pelvis is made up of the sacrum, coccyx, and innominate bones and represents the bony limits of the birth canal.

This area is of paramount importance in obstetrics because its size and shape must be adequate for normal fetal passage during labor and at birth. The relationship of the fetal head to this cavity is of critical importance.

The true pelvis consists of three parts: the inlet, the pelvic cavity, and the outlet (Figure 2–10*B*). Associated with each part are distinct measurements that aid in evaluating the adequacy of the pelvis for childbirth. (For further discussion, see Chapter 8.)

The **pelvic inlet** is the upper border of the true pelvis. The female pelvic inlet is typically rounded. Its size and shape are determined by assessing three anteroposterior diameters. The diagonal conjugate extends from the subpubic angle to the middle of the sacral promontory

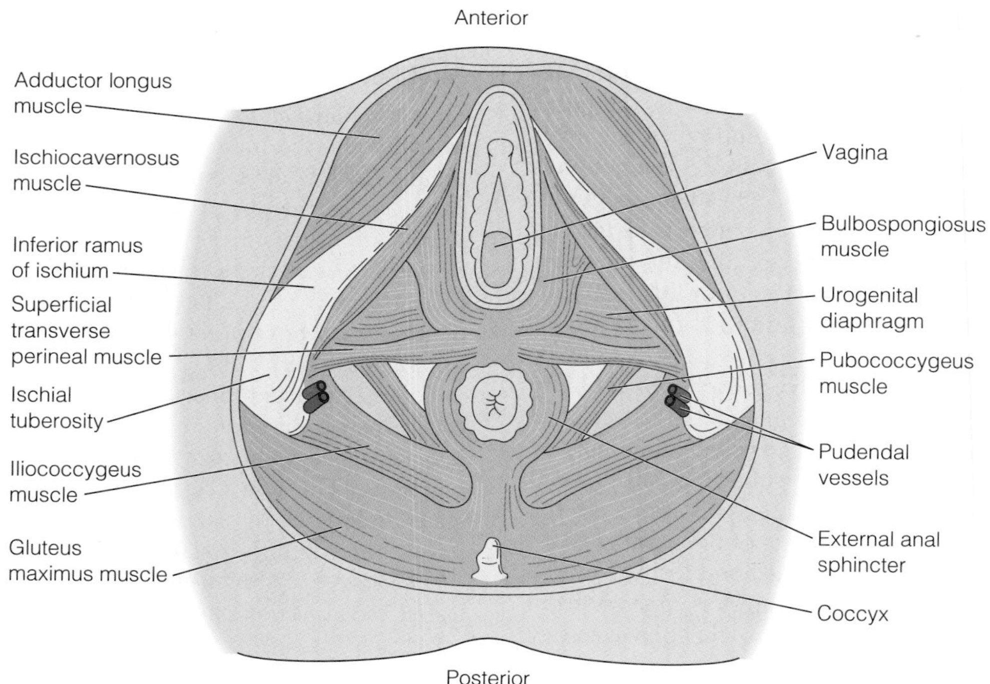

FIGURE 2–9 Muscles of the pelvic floor. (The puborectalis, pubovaginalis, and coccygeal muscles cannot be seen from this view.)

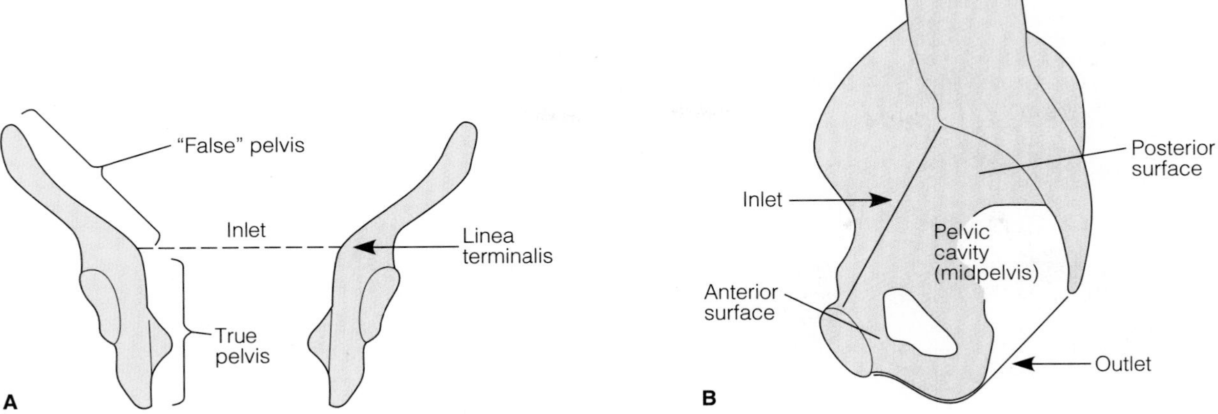

FIGURE 2–10 Female pelvis: *A* False pelvis is shallow cavity above inlet; true pelvis is deeper portion of the cavity below inlet. *B* True pelvis consists of inlet, cavity (midpelvis), and outlet.

and is typically 12.5 cm. The diagonal conjugate can be measured manually during a pelvic examination. The **obstetric conjugate** extends from the middle of the sacral promontory to an area approximately 1 cm below the pubic crest. Its length is estimated by subtracting 1.5 cm from the diagonal conjugate (Figure 2–11). The fetus passes through the obstetric conjugate, and the size of this diameter determines whether the fetus can move down into the birth canal in order for engagement to occur. The true (anatomic) conjugate, or **conjugate vera,** extends from the middle of the sacral promontory to the middle of the pubic crest (superior surface of the symphysis). One additional measurement, the transverse diameter, helps determine the shape of the inlet. The **transverse diameter** is the largest diameter of the inlet and is measured by using the linea terminalis as the point of reference.

The **pelvic cavity** (canal) is a curved canal with a longer posterior than anterior wall. The curvature of the lumbar spine influences the shape and tilt (inclination) of the pelvic cavity (Figure 2–10*B*).

The **pelvic outlet** is at the lower border of the true pelvis. The size of the pelvic outlet can be determined by assessing the *transverse diameter,* which is also called

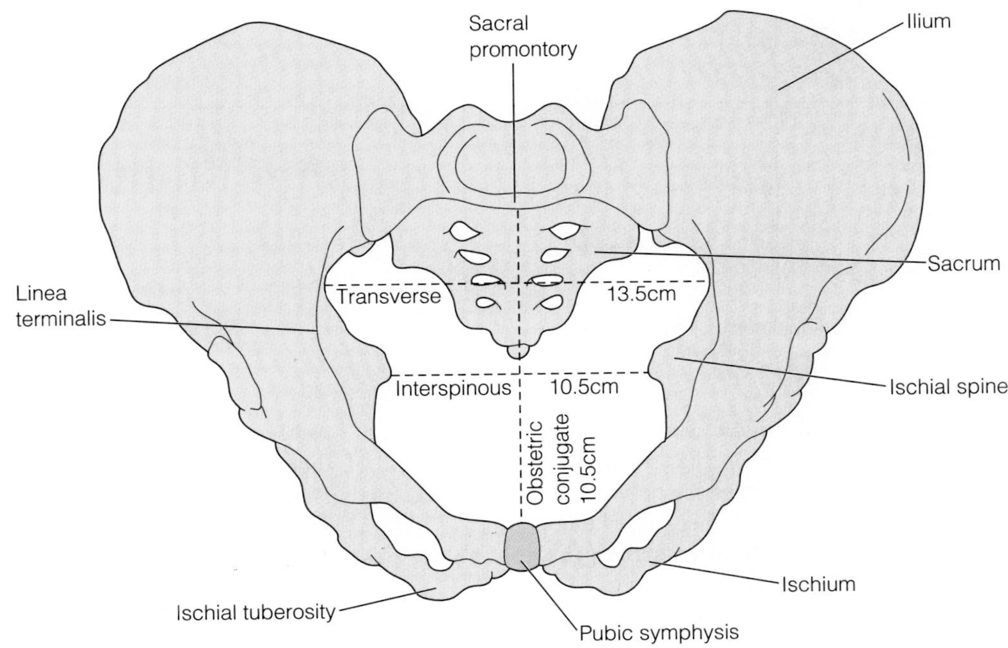

FIGURE 2–11 Pelvic planes: coronal section and diameters of the bony pelvis.

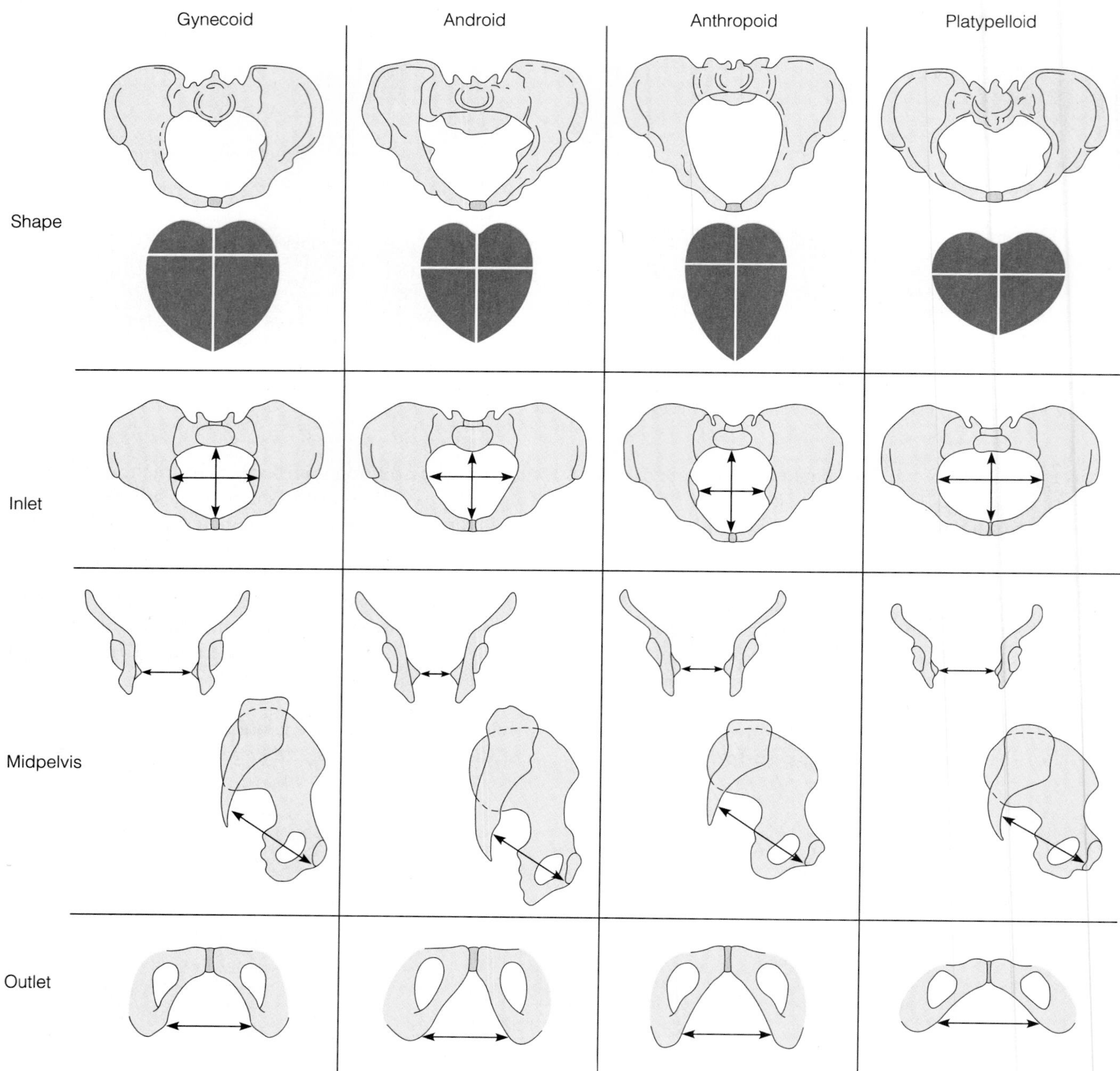

FIGURE 2–12 Comparison of Caldwell-Moloy pelvic types.

the *bi-ischial,* or *intertuberous, diameter.* This diameter extends from the inner surface of one ischial tuberosity to the other. The pubic arch is also part of the pelvic cavity. The pubic arch has great importance because the fetus must pass under it during birth. If it is narrow, the baby's head may be pushed backward toward the coccyx, making extension of the head difficult. The shoulders of a large baby may also get stuck under the pubic arch, making birth more difficult. This situation is known as "outlet dystocia," and forceps (outlet) assisted birth is required (see Chapter 20). The clinical assessment of each of these obstetrical diameters is discussed further in Chapter 8.

Pelvic Types

The Caldwell-Moloy classification of pelves is widely used to differentiate bony pelvic types (Caldwell and Moloy 1933). The four basic types are *gynecoid, android, anthropoid,* and *platypelloid* (Figure 2–12). The type of pelvis is determined by assessing the posterior segment of the pelvic inlet. Each type has a characteristic shape, and each shape has implications for labor and birth. See Chapter 15 for further discussion.

Breasts

The **breasts,** or *mammary glands,* considered accessories of the reproductive system, are specialized sebaceous glands. They are conical and symmetrically placed on the sides of the chest. The greater pectoral and anterior serratus muscles underlie each breast. Suspending the breasts are fibrous tissues, called *Cooper's ligaments,* that extend from the deep fascia in the chest outward to just under the skin covering the breast. Frequently, the left breast is larger than the right.

The biologic function of the breasts is to provide nourishment and protective maternal antibodies to infants. They also are a source of pleasurable sexual sensation.

In the center of each mature breast is the *nipple,* a protrusion about 0.5 to 1.3 cm in diameter. The nipple is composed mainly of erectile tissue, which becomes more rigid and prominent during the menstrual cycle, sexual excitement, pregnancy, and lactation. The nipple is surrounded by the heavily pigmented **areola,** 2.5 to 10 cm in diameter. Both the nipple and the areola are roughened by small papillae called *tubercles of Montgomery.* As an infant suckles, these tubercles secrete a fatty substance that helps lubricate and protect the breasts.

The breasts are composed of glandular, fibrous, and adipose tissue. The glandular tissue is arranged in a series of 15 to 24 lobes separated by fibrous and adipose tissue. Each lobe is made up of several lobules composed of many alveoli clustered around tiny ducts. The lining of these ducts secretes the various components of milk. The ducts from several lobules merge to form the larger *lactiferous ducts,* which open on the surface of the nipple (Figure 2–13).

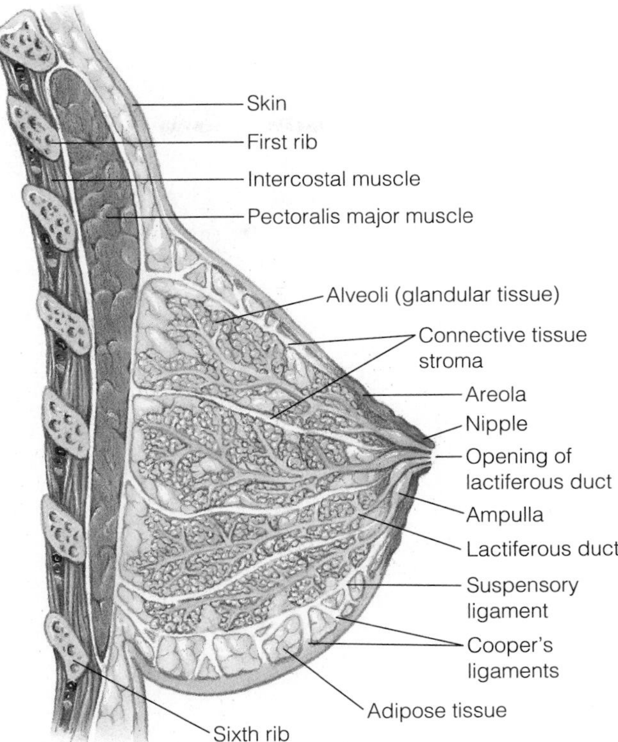

FIGURE 2–13 Anatomy of the breast: sagittal view of partially dissected left breast.

The Female Reproductive Cycle

The **female reproductive cycle (FRC)** is composed of the ovarian cycle, during which ovulation occurs, and the menstrual cycle, during which menstruation occurs. These two cycles take place simultaneously (Figure 2–14).

Effects of Female Hormones

After menarche, a female undergoes a cyclic pattern of ovulation and menstruation (if pregnancy does not occur) for a period of 30 to 40 years. This cycle is an orderly process under neurohormonal control. Each month one oocyte matures, ruptures from the ovary, and enters the fallopian tube. The ovary, vagina, uterus, and fallopian tubes are major target organs for female hormones.

The ovaries not only produce mature gametes but also secrete hormones. Ovarian hormones include the estrogens, progesterone, and testosterone. The ovary is sensitive to FSH and LH. The uterus is sensitive to estrogen and progesterone. The relative proportion of these hormones to each other controls the events of both ovarian and menstrual cycles (Wallach 1996).

Estrogens

Estrogens are secreted in large amounts by the ovaries in nonpregnant women. The major estrogenic effects are due primarily to three classical estrogens: estrone, β-estradiol, and estriol. The major estrogen is β-estradiol.

Estrogens are associated with the characteristics contributing to "femaleness." They control the development of the female secondary sex characteristics: breast development, widening of the hips, and adipose deposits in the buttocks and mons pubis. Estrogens also assist in the maturation of the ovarian follicles and cause the endometrial mucosa to proliferate following menstruation. The amount of estrogens is greatest during the proliferative (follicular or estrogenic) phase of the

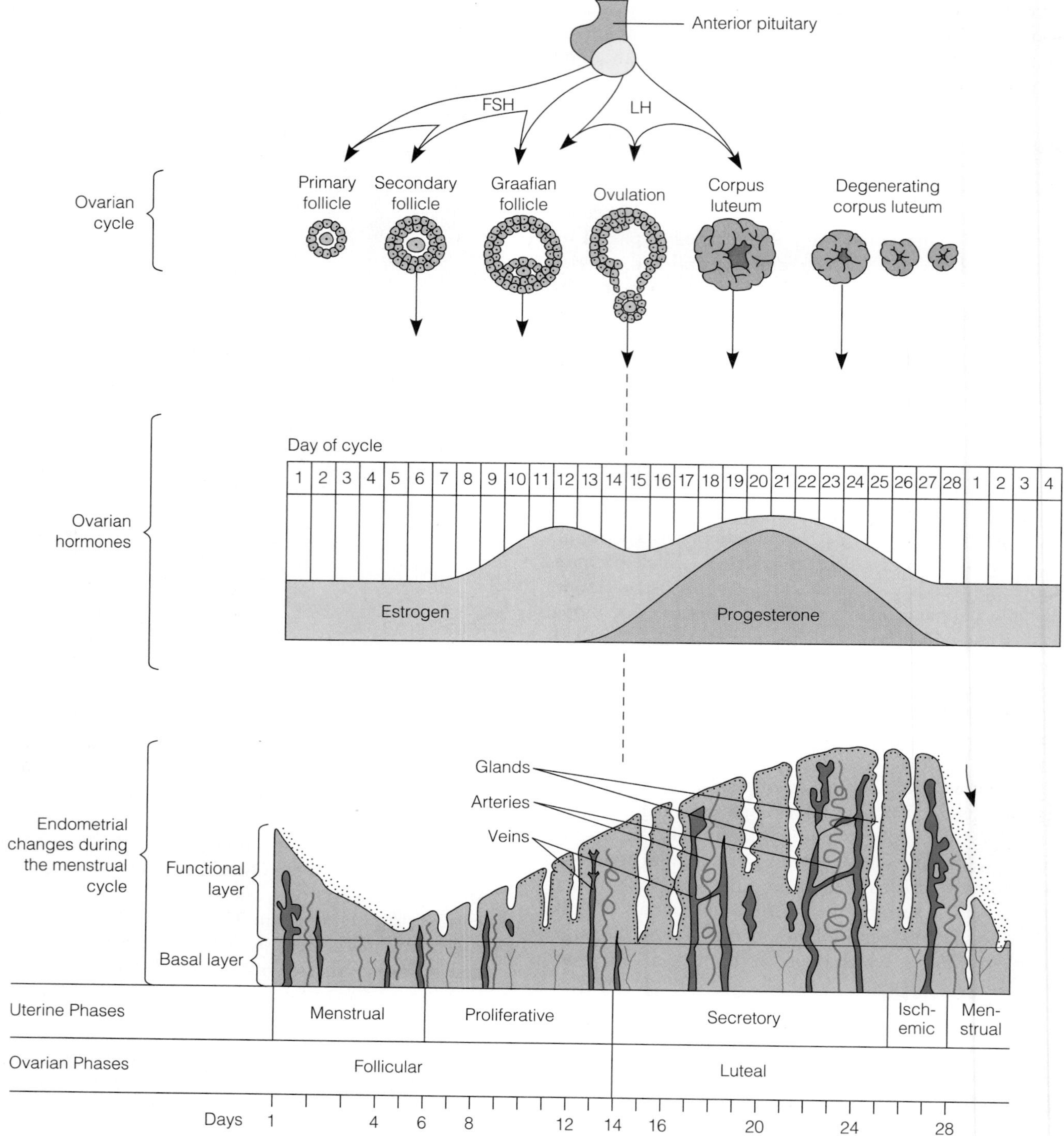

FIGURE 2–14 Female reproductive cycle: interrelationships of hormones with the four phases of the uterine cycle and the two phases of the ovarian cycle.

menstrual cycle. Estrogens also cause the uterus to increase in size and weight because of increased glycogen, amino acids, electrolytes, and water. Blood supply is augmented as well. Under the influence of estrogens, myometrial contractility increases in both the uterus and the fallopian tubes, and there is increased uterine sensitivity to oxytocin. Estrogens inhibit FSH production and stimulate LH production.

Estrogens have effects on many hormones and other carrier proteins. This explains, for example, the increased amount of protein-bound iodine in pregnant women and women who use oral contraceptives containing estrogen. Estrogens may increase libidinal feelings in humans. They decrease the excitability of the hypothalamus, which may cause an increase in sexual desire.

Progesterone

Progesterone is secreted by the corpus luteum and is found in greatest amounts during the secretory (luteal or progestational) phase of the menstrual cycle. It decreases the motility and contractility of the uterus caused by estrogens, thereby preparing the uterus for implantation after fertilization of the ovum. The endometrial mucosa is in a ready state as a result of estrogenic influence. Progesterone causes the uterine endometrium to further increase its supply of glycogen, arterial blood, secretory glands, amino acids, and water.

Under the influence of progesterone, the vaginal epithelium proliferates and the cervix secretes thick, viscous mucus. Breast glandular tissue increases in size and complexity. Progesterone also prepares the breasts for lactation.

The temperature rise of about 0.35C (0.5F) that accompanies ovulation and persists throughout the secretory phase of the menstrual cycle is probably due to progesterone.

Prostaglandins (PGs)

Prostaglandins (oxygenated fatty acids), which are produced by the cells of the endometrium and are also classified as hormones, have a varied action in the body. The different types of prostaglandins (PGs) are indicated by Roman letters and either numbers (PGE_2) or Greek letters ($PGF_{2\alpha}$). Generally PGEs relax smooth muscles and are potent vasodilators; PGFs are potent vasoconstrictors and increase the contractility of muscles and arteries. While their primary actions seem antagonistic, they achieve their basic regulatory functions in cells through an intricate pattern of reciprocal events. The discussion here will summarize their role in ovulation and menstruation.

Prostaglandin production increases during follicular maturation, is dependent on gonadotropins, and is essential to ovulation. Extrusion of the ovum, resulting from the increased contractility of the smooth muscle in the theca layer of the mature follicle, is thought to be caused by $PGF_{2\alpha}$ (Speroff et al 1994). Significant amounts of PGs are found in and around the follicle at the time of ovulation.

While the exact mechanism by which the corpus luteum degenerates in the absence of pregnancy remains obscure, $PGF_{2\alpha}$ is thought to induce progesterone withdrawal, the lowest point of which coincides with the onset of early menses.

During the late secretory phase, the level of $PGF_{2\alpha}$ is higher than that of PGE. This event increases vasoconstriction and contractility of the myometrium, which contributes to the ischemia preceding menstruation. High concentration of PGs may also account for the vasoconstriction of the endometrium venous lacunae allowing for platelet aggregation at vascular rupture points, thereby preventing a rapid blood loss during menstruation. The menstrual flow's high concentration of PGs may also facilitate the process of tissue digestion, which allows for an orderly shedding of the endometrium during menstruation.

Neurohumoral Basis of the Female Reproductive Cycle

The FRC is controlled by complex interactions between the nervous and endocrine systems and their target tissues. These interactions involve the hypothalamus, anterior pituitary, and ovaries.

The hypothalamus secretes gonadotropin-releasing hormone (GnRH) to the pituitary gland in response to signals received from the central nervous system. This releasing hormone is often called both luteinizing hormone–releasing hormone (LHRH) and follicle-stimulating hormone–releasing hormone (FSHRH) (Derman et al 1996).

In response to GnRH, the anterior pituitary secretes the gonadotropic hormones **follicle-stimulating hormone (FSH)** and **luteinizing hormone (LH)**. FSH is primarily responsible for the maturation of the ovarian follicle. As the follicle matures, it secretes increasing amounts of estrogen, which enhance the development of the follicle (Shoham and Schachter 1996). (This estrogen is also responsible for the rebuilding/proliferation phase of the endometrium after it is shed during menstruation.)

Final maturation of the follicle will not come about without the action of LH. The anterior pituitary's production of LH increases six- to tenfold as the follicle matures. About 10 to 12 hours after the peak production of LH, ovulation occurs (Speroff et al 1994).

The LH is also responsible for the "luteinizing" of the theca and granulosa cells of the ruptured follicle. As a result, estrogen production is reduced and progesterone secretion continues. Thus estrogen levels fall a day before ovulation; tiny amounts of progesterone are

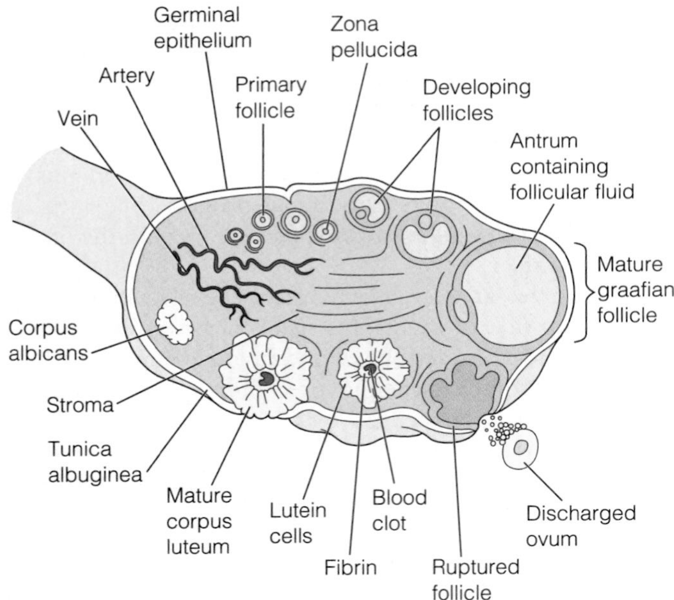

FIGURE 2–15 Various stages of development of the ovarian follicles.

in evidence. Ovulation takes place following the very rapid growth of the follicle—as the sustained high level of estrogen diminishes and progesterone secretion begins.

The ruptured follicle undergoes rapid change and complete luteinization is accomplished and the mass of cells becomes the corpus luteum. The lutein cells secrete large amounts of progesterone with smaller amounts of estrogen. (At the same time, the excessive amounts of progesterone are responsible for the secretory phase of the uterine cycle.) Seven or eight days following ovulation, the corpus luteum begins to involute, losing its secretory function. The production of both progesterone and estrogen is severely diminished. The anterior pituitary responds with increasingly large amounts of FSH; a few days later LH production begins. As a result, new follicles become responsive to another ovarian cycle and begin maturing.

The Ovarian Cycle

The ovarian cycle has two phases: the *follicular phase* (days 1–14) and the *luteal phase* (days 15–28) in a 28-day cycle. Figure 2–15 depicts the changes that the follicle undergoes during the ovarian cycle. Usually only the length of the follicular phase varies in menstrual cycles of varying duration; the luteal phase is of fixed length. During the follicular phase, the immature follicle matures as a result of FSH. The oocyte grows within the follicle. A mature **graafian follicle** appears about the 14th day under dual control of FSH and LH. It is a large structure, measuring about 5 to 10 mm. In the fully mature graafian follicle, the oocyte is surrounded by fluid and enclosed in a thick elastic capsule called the **zona pellucida.**

Just before ovulation, the mature oocyte completes its first meiotic division (see Chapter 3 for a description of meiosis). As a result of this division, two cells are formed: a small cell called a *polar body* and a larger cell called the *secondary oocyte.* The secondary oocyte matures into the ovum (see Figure 3–2).

As the graafian follicle matures and enlarges, it comes close to the surface of the ovary. The ovary surface forms a blisterlike protrusion, and the follicle walls become thin. The secondary oocyte, polar body, and follicular fluid are pushed out. The ovum is discharged near the fimbria of the fallopian tube and is pulled into the tube to begin its journey toward the uterus.

Occasionally, ovulation is accompanied by midcycle pain known as *mittelschmerz.* This pain may be caused by a thick tunica albuginea or by a local peritoneal reaction to the expelling of the follicular contents. Vaginal discharge may increase during ovulation, and a small amount of blood (midcycle spotting) may be discharged as well.

The body temperature increases about 0.3 to 0.6C (0.5–1.0F) 24 to 48 hours after the time of ovulation. It remains elevated until the day before menstruation begins. There may be an accompanying sharp basal body temperature drop before the increase. These temperature changes are useful clinically in determining the approximate time ovulation occurs.

Generally the ovum takes several minutes to travel through the ruptured follicle to the fallopian tube opening. The contractions of the tube's smooth muscle and its ciliary action propel the ovum through the tube. The ovum remains in the ampulla where, if it is fertilized, cleavage can begin. The ovum is thought to be fertile for only 6 to 24 hours. It reaches the uterus 72 to 96 hours after its release from the ovary.

The luteal phase begins when the ovum leaves its follicle. Under the influence of LH, the **corpus luteum** develops from the ruptured follicle. Within 2 or 3 days, the corpus luteum becomes yellowish and spherical and increases in vascularity. If the ovum is fertilized and implants in the endometrium, the fertilized egg begins to secrete **human chorionic gonadotropin (hCG),** which is needed to maintain the corpus luteum. If fertilization does not occur, within about a week after ovulation the corpus luteum begins to degenerate, eventually becoming a connective tissue scar called the *corpus albicans.* With degeneration comes a decrease in estrogen and progesterone. This allows for an increase in LH and FSH, which trigger the hypothalamus. Approximately 14 days after ovulation (in a 28-day cycle), in the absence of pregnancy, menstruation begins.

TABLE 2–2 Characteristics of Menstrual Cycle and Ovulation

Menstrual phase (days 1–5)	Estrogen levels are low. Cervical mucus is scanty, viscous, and opaque. Endometrium is shed.
Proliferative phase (days 6–14)	Endometrium and myometrium thickness increases. Estrogen peaks just before ovulation. Cervical mucosa at ovulation: Is clear, thin, watery, and alkaline Is more favorable to sperm Has elasticity *(spinnbarkheit)* greater than 5 cm Shows ferning pattern on microscopic exam Just before ovulation, body temperature drops; at ovulation, basal body temperature increases 0.3 to 0.6C, and *mittelschmerz* and/or midcycle spotting may occur.
Secretory phase (days 15–26)	Estrogen drops sharply, and progesterone dominates. Vascularity of entire uterus increases. Tissue glycogen increases, and the uterus is made ready for implantation.
Ischemic phase (days 27–28)	Both estrogen and progesterone levels fall. Spiral arteries undergo vasoconstriction. Endometrium becomes pale. Blood vessels rupture. Blood escapes into uterine stromal cells.

The Menstrual Cycle

Menstruation is cyclic uterine bleeding in response to cyclic hormonal changes. Menstruation occurs when the ovum is not fertilized and begins about 14 days after ovulation in a 28-day cycle. The menstrual discharge, also referred to as the *menses,* or *menstrual flow,* is composed of blood mixed with fluid, cervical and vaginal secretions, bacteria, mucus, leukocytes, and other cellular debris. The menstrual discharge is dark red and has a distinctive odor.

Menstrual parameters vary greatly among individuals. Generally, menstruation occurs every 28 days, plus or minus 5 to 10 days. Emotional and physical factors such as illness, excessive fatigue, stress or anxiety, and vigorous exercise programs can alter the cycle interval. Certain environmental factors such as temperature and altitude may also affect the cycle. The duration of menses is from 2 to 8 days, with the blood loss averaging 30 to 80 mL and the loss of iron averaging 0.5 to 1 mg daily.

The menstrual cycle has four phases: menstrual, proliferative, secretory, and ischemic (see Table 2–2) (Ferenczy 1996). Menstruation occurs during the *menstrual phase.* Some endometrial areas are shed, while others remain. Some of the remaining tips of the endometrial glands begin to regenerate. The endometrium is in a resting state following menstruation. Estrogen levels are low, and the endometrium is 1 to 2 mm deep. During this part of the cycle, the cervical mucosa is scanty, viscous, and opaque.

KEY FACTS TO REMEMBER

Summary of Female Reproductive Cycle

Ovarian Cycle

Follicular phase (days 1–14): Primordial follicle matures under influence of FSH and LH up to the time of ovulation.

Luteal phase (days 15–28): Ovum leaves follicle; corpus luteum develops under LH influence and produces high levels of progesterone and low levels of estrogen.

Menstrual Cycle

Menstrual phase (days 1–5)

Proliferative phase (days 6–14): Estrogen peaks just prior to ovulation. Cervical mucus at ovulation is clear, thin, watery, alkaline, and more favorable to sperm; shows ferning pattern; and has *spinnbarkheit* greater than 5 cm. At ovulation, body temperature drops, then rises sharply and remains elevated.

Secretory phase (days 15–26): Estrogen drops sharply and progesterone dominates.

Ischemic phase (days 27–28): Both estrogen and progesterone levels drop.

The *proliferative phase* begins when the endometrial glands enlarge, becoming twisted and longer in response to increasing amounts of estrogen. The blood vessels become prominent and dilated, and the endometrium increases in thickness six- to eightfold. This gradual process reaches its peak just before ovulation. The cervical mucosa becomes thin, clear, watery, and more alkaline, making the mucosa more favorable to spermatozoa. As ovulation nears, the cervical mucosa shows increased elasticity, called *spinnbarkeit.* At ovulation, the mucus will stretch more than 5 cm. The cervical mucosa pH increases from below 7.0 to 7.5 at the time of ovulation. On microscopic examination, the mucosa shows a characteristic ferning pattern (see Figure 4–3). This fern pattern is a useful aid in assessing ovulation time. For further discussion, see Key Facts to Remember: Summary of Female Reproductive Cycle.

The *secretory phase* follows ovulation. The endometrium, under estrogenic influence, undergoes slight cellular growth. Progesterone, however, causes such marked swelling and growth that the epithelium is warped into folds. The amount of tissue glycogen increases. The glandular epithelial cells begin to fill with cellular debris, become twisted, and dilate. The glands

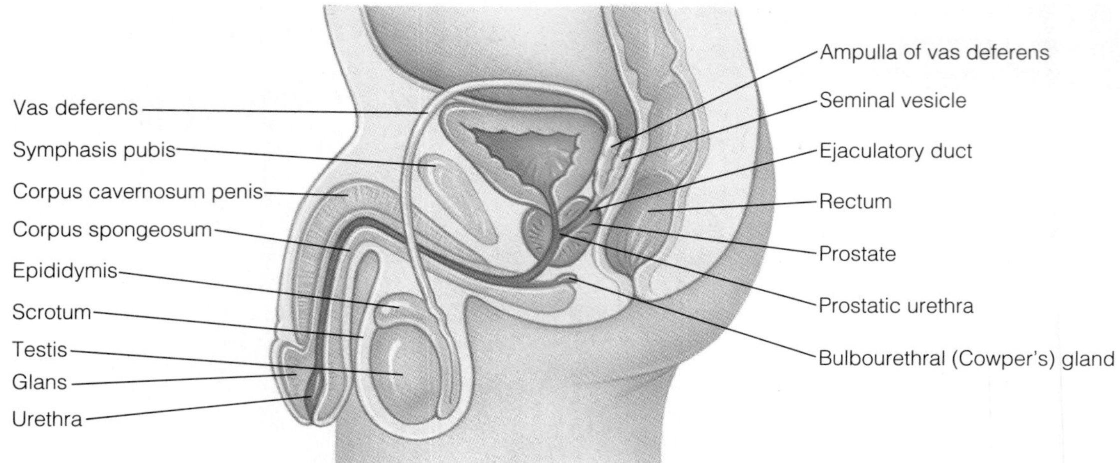

FIGURE 2–16 Male reproductive system, sagittal view.

secrete small quantities of endometrial fluid in preparation for a fertilized ovum. The vascularity of the entire uterus increases greatly, providing a nourishing bed for implantation. If implantation occurs, the endometrium, under the influence of progesterone, continues to develop and become even thicker (see Chapter 3 for a discussion of implantation).

If fertilization does not occur, the *ischemic phase* begins. The corpus luteum begins to degenerate, and as a result both estrogen and progesterone levels fall. Areas of necrosis appear under the epithelial lining. Extensive vascular changes also occur. Small blood vessels rupture, and the spiral arteries constrict and retract, causing a deficiency of blood in the endometrium, which becomes pale. This ischemic phase is characterized by the escape of blood into the stromal cells of the uterus. The menstrual flow begins, and the menstrual cycle is launched again. After menstruation the basal layer remains, so that the tips of the glands can regenerate the new functional endometrial layer.

Male Reproductive System

The primary reproductive functions of the male genitals are to produce and transport sex cells (sperm) through and eventually out of the genital tract into the female genital tract. The external and internal genitals of the male reproductive system are shown in Figure 2–16.

External Genitals

The two external reproductive organs are the penis and scrotum. The *penis* is an elongated, cylindrical structure consisting of a body, called the *shaft,* and a cone-shaped end, called the *glans.* The penis lies in front of the scrotum.

The shaft of the penis is made up of three longitudinal columns of erectile tissue: the paired *corpora cavernosa* and a third, the *corpus spongiosum.* These columns are covered by dense fibrous connective tissue and then enclosed by elastic tissue. The penis is covered by a thin outer layer of skin.

The corpus spongiosum contains the urethra. The urethra terminates in a slitlike opening, located in the tip of the glans, called the *urethral meatus.* A circular fold of skin arises just behind the glans and covers it. Known as the *prepuce,* or *foreskin,* it is frequently removed by the surgical procedure of circumcision (see Chapter 23).

If the corpus spongiosum does not surround the urethra completely, the urethral meatus may occur on the ventral aspect of the penile shaft (hypospadias) or on the dorsal aspect (epispadias).

Sexual stimulation causes the penis to elongate, thicken, and stiffen, a process called *erection.* The penis becomes erect when its blood vessels become engorged, a consequence of parasympathetic nerve stimulation. If stimulation is intense enough, the forceful and sudden expulsion of semen occurs through the rhythmic contractions of the penile muscles. This phenomenon is called *ejaculation.*

The penis serves both the urinary and the reproductive systems. Urine is expelled through the urethral meatus. The reproductive function of the penis is to deposit sperm in the vagina so that fertilization of the ovum can occur.

The *scrotum* is a pouchlike structure that hangs in front of the anus and behind the penis. Composed of skin and the *dartos muscle,* the scrotum shows increased pigmentation and scattered hairs. The sebaceous glands open directly onto the scrotal surface; their secretion has a distinctive odor. Contraction of the dartos and cremasteric muscles shortens the scrotum and draws it closer to the body, thus wrinkling its outer surface. The degree of wrinkling is greatest in young men and at cold temperatures and is least in older men and at warm temperatures.

Inside the scrotum are two lateral compartments, each containing a testis with its related structures. The left testis and its scrotal sac usually hang lower than the right.

The function of the scrotum is to protect the testes and the sperm by maintaining a temperature lower than that of the body. Spermatogenesis will not occur if the testes fail to descend and thus remain at body temperature. Because it is sensitive to touch, pressure, temperature, and pain, the scrotum defends against potential harm to the testes.

Internal Reproductive Organs

The male internal reproductive organs include the gonads (testes or testicles), a system of ducts (epididymides, vas deferens, ejaculatory duct, and urethra), and accessory glands (seminal vesicles, prostate gland, bulbourethral glands, and urethral glands). See Key Facts to Remember: Summary of Male Reproductive Organ Functions.

Testes

The *testes* are a pair of oval glandular organs contained in the scrotum. In the sexually mature male, they are the site of spermatozoa production and the secretion of several male sex hormones.

Each testis is 4–6 cm long, 2–3 cm wide, and 3–4 cm thick. Each weighs about 10–15 g. The testis is covered by an outer serous membrane and an inner capsule that is tough, white, and fibrous. The connective tissue sends projections inward to form septa, dividing the testis into 250 to 400 lobules. Each lobule contains 1 to 3 tightly packed, convoluted *seminiferous tubules* containing sperm cells in all stages of development.

The seminiferous tubules are surrounded by loose connective tissue, which houses abundant blood and lymph vessels and *interstitial (Leydig's) cells*. The interstitial cells produce testosterone, the primary male sex hormone.

The seminiferous tubules come together to form 20 to 30 straight tubules, which in turn form an anastomotic network of thin-walled spaces, the *rete testis*. The rete testis forms 10 to 15 efferent ducts that empty into the duct of the epididymis.

Most of the cells lining the seminiferous tubules undergo **spermatogenesis,** a process of maturation in which spermatocytes become spermatozoa. (Chapter 3 further discusses the process of spermatogenesis.) Sperm production varies among and within the tubules, with cells in different areas of the same tubule undergoing different stages of spermatogenesis. The tubules also contain *Sertoli's cells,* which nourish and protect the spermatocytes. The sperm are eventually released from the tubules into the epididymis, where they continue to mature.

Like the female reproductive cycle, the process of spermatogenesis and other functions of the testes are the result of complex neural and hormonal controls. The hypothalamus secretes releasing factors, which stimulate the anterior pituitary to release the gonadotropins—FSH and LH. These hormones cause the testes to produce testosterone, which maintains spermatogenesis, increases sperm production by the seminiferous tubules, and stimulates production of seminal fluid.

KEY FACTS TO REMEMBER

Summary of Male Reproductive Organ Functions

The testes house seminiferous tubules and gonads.

- Seminiferous tubules contain sperm cells in various stages of development and undergoing meiosis.
- Sertoli's cells nourish and protect spermatocytes (phase between spermatids and spermatozoa).
- Leydig's cells are the main source of testosterone.
- Epididymides provide an area for maturation of sperm and a reservoir for mature spermatozoa.
- The vas deferens connects the epididymis with the prostate gland, then connects with ducts from the seminal vesicle to become an ejaculatory duct.
- Ejaculatory ducts provide a passageway for semen and seminal fluid into the urethra.
- Seminal vesicles secrete yellowish fluid rich in fructose, prostaglandins, and fibrinogen. This provides nutrition that increases motility and fertilizing ability of sperm. Prostaglandins also aid fertilization by making the cervical mucus more receptive to sperm.
- The prostate gland secretes thin, alkaline fluid containing calcium, citric acid, and other substances. Alkalinity counteracts acidity of ductus and seminal vesicle secretions.
- Bulbourethral (Cowper's) glands secrete alkaline, viscous fluid into semen, aiding in neutralization of acidic vaginal secretions.

Testosterone is the most prevalent and potent of the testicular hormones. Its target organs are the testes, prostate, and seminal vesicles. In addition, testosterone is responsible for the development of secondary male characteristics and certain behavioral patterns. The effects of testosterone include structural and functional development of the male genital tract, emission and ejaculation of seminal fluid, distribution of body hair, promotion of growth and strength of long bones, increased muscle mass, and enlargement of the vocal cords. The action of testosterone on the central nervous system is thought to produce aggressiveness and sexual drive. The action of testosterone is constant, not cyclic like that of the female hormones. Its production is not limited to a certain number of years, but it is thought to decrease in quantity with age.

The testes have two primary functions:

- To serve as the site of spermatogenesis
- To produce testosterone

Epididymis

The *epididymis* is a duct about 5.6 m long, although it is convoluted into a compact structure about 3.75 cm long. An epididymis lies behind each testis. It arises from the top of the testis, courses downward, and then passes upward, where it becomes the vas deferens.

The epididymis provides a reservoir where maturing spermatozoa can survive for a long period. When discharged from the seminiferous tubules into the epididymis, the sperm are immotile and incapable of fertilizing an ovum. The spermatozoa remain in the epididymis for 2–10 days. As the sperm move along the tortuous course of the epididymis they become both motile and fertile (Marieb and Mallatt 1992).

Vas Deferens and Ejaculatory Ducts

The *vas deferens,* also known as the *ductus deferens,* is about 40 cm long and connects the epididymis with the prostate. One vas deferens arises from the posterior border of each testis. It joins the spermatic cord and weaves over and between several pelvic structures until it meets the vas deferens from the opposite side. Each vas deferens then unites with a seminal vesicle duct to form the ejaculatory duct's *terminal ampulla.* It then unites with the seminal vesicle duct (a gland) to form the *ejaculatory duct,* which enters the prostate gland and ends in the prostatic urethra. The ejaculatory ducts serve as passageways for semen and fluid secreted by the seminal vesicles. The main function of the vas deferens is to rapidly squeeze the sperm from their storage sites (the epididymis and distal part of the vas deferens) into the urethra.

Urethra

The male *urethra* is the passageway for both urine and semen. The urethra begins in the bladder and passes through the prostate gland, where it is called the *prostatic urethra.* The urethra emerges from the prostate gland to become the *membranous urethra.* It terminates in the penis, where it is called the *penile urethra.*

Accessory Glands

The male accessory glands secrete a unique and essential component of the total seminal fluid in an ordered sequence.

The *seminal vesicles* are two glands composed of many lobes. Each vesicle is about 7.5 cm long. They are situated between the bladder and the rectum immediately above the base of the prostate. The epithelium lining the seminal vesicles secretes an alkaline, viscid, clear fluid rich in high-energy fructose, prostaglandins, fibrinogen, and proteins. During ejaculation, this fluid mixes with the sperm in the ejaculatory ducts. This fluid helps provide an environment favorable to sperm motility and metabolism (Aumüller and Riva 1992).

The *prostate gland* encircles the upper part of the urethra and lies below the neck of the urinary bladder. Made up of several lobes, it measures about 4 cm in diameter and weighs 20–30 g. The prostate is made up of both glandular and muscular tissue. It secretes a thin, milky, alkaline fluid containing high levels of zinc, calcium, citric acid, and acid phosphatase (Marieb and Mallatt 1992). This fluid protects the sperm from the acidic environment of the vagina and the male urethra, which could be spermicidal.

The *bulbourethral (Cowper's) glands* are a pair of small round structures on either side of the membranous urethra. The glands secrete a clear, viscous, thick alkaline fluid rich in mucoproteins that becomes part of the semen. This secretion also lubricates the penile urethra during sexual excitement and neutralizes the acid in the male urethra and vagina, thereby enhancing sperm motility.

The *urethral (Littre's) glands* are tiny mucus-secreting glands found throughout the membranous lining of the penile urethra. Their secretions add to those of the bulbourethral glands.

Semen

The male ejaculate, *semen* or *seminal fluid,* is made up of spermatozoa and the secretions of all the accessory glands. The seminal fluid transports viable and motile sperm to the female reproductive tract. Effective transportation of sperm requires adequate nutrients, an adequate pH (about 7.5), a specific concentration of sperm to fluid, and an optimal osmolarity.

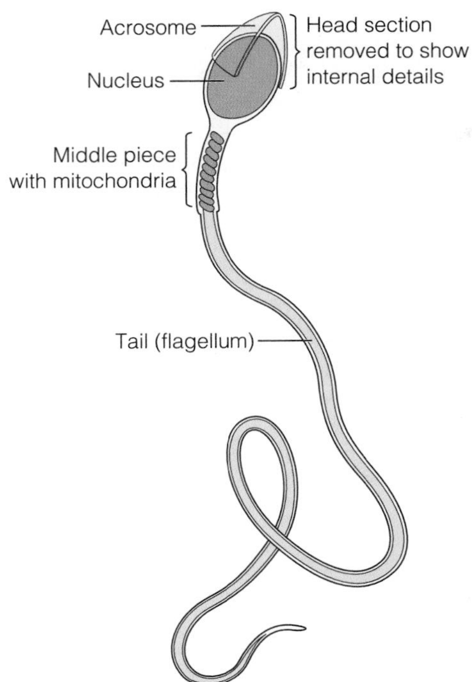

FIGURE 2–17 Schematic representation of a mature spermatozoon.

A spermatozoon is made up of a *head* and a *tail.* The tail is divided into the middle piece and end piece (Figure 2–17). The head's main components are the *acrosome* and *nucleus.* The head carries the male's haploid number of chromosomes (23), and it is the part that enters the ovum at fertilization (Chapter 3). The tail, or *flagellum,* is specialized for motility.

Sperm may be stored in the male genital system for up to 42 days, depending primarily on the frequency of ejaculations. The average volume of ejaculate following abstinence for several days is 2 to 5 mL, but may vary from 1 to 10 mL. Repeated ejaculation results in decreased volume. Once ejaculated, sperm can live only two or three days in the female genital tract.

KEY CONCEPTS

- Reproductive activities require a complex interaction between the reproductive structures, the central nervous system, and such endocrine glands as the pituitary, hypothalamus, testes, and ovaries.
- The female reproductive system consists of the ovaries, where female germ cells and female sex hormones are formed; the fallopian tubes, which capture the ovum and allow transport to the uterus; the uterus, which is the implantation site for the fertilized ovum (blastocyst); the cervix, which is a protective portal for the body of the uterus and the connection between the vagina and the uterus; and the vagina, which is the passageway from the external genitals to the uterus and provides for discharge of menstrual products to the outside of the body.
- The female reproductive cycle is composed of the ovarian cycle, during which ovulation occurs, and the menstrual cycle, during which menstruation occurs. These two cycles take place simultaneously and are under neurohumoral control.
- The ovarian cycle has two phases: the follicular phase and the luteal phase. During the follicular phase, the primordial follicle matures under the influence of FSH and LH until ovulation occurs. The luteal phase begins when the ovum leaves the follicle and the corpus luteum develops under the influence of LH. The corpus luteum produces high levels of progesterone and low levels of estrogen.
- The menstrual cycle has four phases: menstrual, proliferative, secretory, and ischemic. Menstruation is the actual shedding of the endometrial lining, when estrogen levels are low. The proliferative phase begins when the endometrial glands begin to enlarge under the influence of estrogen and cervical mucosal changes occur; the changes peak at ovulation. The secretory phase follows ovulation and, influenced primarily by progesterone, the uterus increases its vascularity to make ready for possible implantation. The ischemic phase is characterized by degeneration of the corpus luteum, decreases in both estrogen and progesterone levels, constriction of the spiral arteries, and escape of blood into the stromal cells of the endometrium.
- The male reproductive system consists of the testes, where male germ cells and male sex hormones are formed; a series of continuous ducts through which spermatozoa are transported outside the body; accessory glands that produce secretions important to sperm nutrition, survival, and transport; and the penis, which serves as the reproductive organ of intercourse.

REFERENCES

Aumüller G, Riva A: Morphology and functions of the human seminal vesicle. *Andrologia* 1992; 24:183.

Caldwell WE, Moloy HC: Anatomical variations in the female pelvis and their effect on labor with a suggested classification. *Am J Obstet Gynecol* 1933; 26:479.

Cunningham FG et al (editors). *Williams Obstetrics,* 20th ed. Stamford, CT: Appleton & Lange, 1997.

Davies J: Anatomy of the female genital tract. In: *Danforth's Obstetrics and Gynecology,* 6th ed. Scott JR et al (editors). Philadelphia: Lippincott, 1990.

Derman SG, McClamrock HD, Adashi EY: Regulation of the pituitary response to gonadotropin-releasing hormone. In: *Gynecology and Obstetrics, Vol. 5.* Sciarri JJ et al (editors). Hagerstown, MD: Harper & Row, 1996.

Ferenczy A: The endometrial cycle. In: *Gynecology and Obstetrics, Vol. 5.* Sciarri JJ et al (editors). Hagerstown, MD: Harper & Row, 1996.

Marieb EN, Mallatt J: *Human Anatomy.* Redwood City, CA: Benjamin/Cummings, 1992.

Resnik R: Anatomic alterations in the reproductive tract. In: *Maternal-Fetal Medicine: Principles and Practice,* 3rd ed. Creasy RK, Resnik R (editors). Philadelphia: Saunders, 1994.

Shoham Z, Schachter M: Estrogen biosynthesis: Regulation, action, remote effects, and value of monitoring in ovarian stimulation cycles. *Fertil Steril* 1996; 65(4):687.

Speroff L et al: *Clinical Gynecologic Endocrinology and Infertility,* 5th ed. Baltimore: Williams & Wilkins, 1994.

Wallach EE: The mechanism of ovulation. In: *Gynecology and Obstetrics, Vol. 5.* Sciarri JJ et al (editors). Hagerstown, MD: Harper & Row, 1996.

Chapter 3 Conception and Fetal Development

OBJECTIVES

- Identify the difference between meiotic cellular division and mitotic cellular division.
- Compare the processes by which ova and sperm are produced.
- Describe the components of the process of fertilization.
- Identify the differing processes by which fraternal (dizygotic) and identical (monozygotic) twins are formed.
- Describe in order of increasing complexity the structures that form during the cellular multiplication and differentiation stages of intrauterine development.
- Describe the development, structure, and functions of the placenta and umbilical cord during intrauterine life.
- Summarize the significant changes in growth and development of the fetus in utero at 4, 6, 12, 16, 20, 24, 28, 36, and 40 weeks' gestation.
- Identify the vulnerable periods during which malformations of the various organ systems may occur, and describe the resulting congenital malformations.

KEY TERMS

Amnion
Amniotic fluid
Bag of waters (BOW)
Blastocyst
Body stalk
Capacitation
Chorion
Cleavage
Cotyledons
Decidua basalis
Decidua capsularis
Decidua vera (parietalis)
Diploid number of chromosomes
Ductus arteriosus
Ductus venosus
Ectoderm
Embryo
Embryonic membranes
Endoderm
Fertilization
Fetus
Foramen ovale
Gametes
Gametogenesis
Haploid number of chromosomes
Lanugo
Meiosis
Mesoderm
Mitosis
Morula
Placenta
Postconception age periods
Teratogen
Trophoblast
Umbilical cord
Vernix caseosa
Wharton's jelly
Zygote

Each person is unique. Yet our bodies are very similar, both in structure and function. Even our chromosomes are made of the same biochemical substances. What, then, makes each of us unique? The answer lies in the physiologic mechanisms of heredity, the processes of cellular division, and the environmental factors that influence our development from the moment we are conceived. This chapter explores the processes involved in conception and fetal development—the basis of uniqueness.

Cellular Division

All humans begin life as a single cell (fertilized ovum or **zygote**). This single cell reproduces itself, and each resulting cell also reproduces itself in a continuing process. The new cells are similar to the cells from which they came. Cells are reproduced either by mitosis or meiosis, two different but related processes. **Mitosis** produces exact copies of the original cell, making growth and development possible, and in mature individuals it is the process by which our body cells continue to divide and replace themselves. **Meiosis** is the cell division leading to the development of eggs and sperm needed to produce a new organism.

Mitosis

During mitosis, the cell undergoes several changes ending in cell division. As the last phase of cell division nears completion, a furrow develops in the cell cytoplasm, which divides it into two *daughter cells,* each with its own nucleus. Daughter cells have the same **diploid number of chromosomes** (46) and same genetic makeup as the cell from which they came. When a cell with 46 chromosomes undergoes mitosis, the result is two identical cells, each with 46 chromosomes.

Meiosis

Meiosis consists of two successive cell divisions. In the first division, the chromosomes replicate, doubling the structure of each of the 46 chromosomes. Next, a pairing takes place between homologous chromosomes (Sadler 1990). Instead of separating immediately, as in mitosis, the chromosomes become closely intertwined. At each point of contact, there is a physical exchange of genetic material between the chromatids (the arms of the chromosomes). New combinations are provided by the newly formed chromosomes; these combinations account for the wide variation of traits in people (eg, hair or eye color). The chromosome pairs then separate, and the members of the pair move to opposite sides of the cell. The cell divides, forming two daughter cells, each with 23 double-structured chromosomes—the same amount of DNA as a normal somatic cell. In the second division, the chromatids of each chromosome separate and move to opposite poles of each of the daughter cells. Cell division occurs, resulting in the formation of four cells, each containing 23 single chromosomes (the **haploid number of chromosomes**). These daughter cells contain only half the DNA of a normal somatic cell (Moore and Persaud, 1993). See Key Facts to Remember: Comparison of Meiosis and Mitosis.

During the second meiotic division, two of the chromatids may not move apart rapidly enough when the cell divides. The still-paired chromatids are carried into one of the daughter cells and eventually form an extra chromosome. This condition, *autosomal nondisjunction* (chromosomal mutation), is harmful to the offspring should fertilization occur.

Another type of chromosomal mutation can occur if chromosomes break during meiosis. If the broken segment is lost, the result is a shorter chromosome; this situation is known as *deletion.* If the broken segment becomes attached to another chromosome, it is called *translocation,* which often results in harmful structural mutations (Thompson et al 1991). The effects of translocation and autosomal nondisjunction are described in Chapter 4.

Gametogenesis

Meiosis occurs during **gametogenesis,** the process by which germ cells, or **gametes,** are produced. The gametes must have a haploid number (23) of chromosomes so that when the female gamete (the egg or ovum) and the male gamete (sperm or spermatozoon) unite to form the zygote (the fertilized ovum), the normal human diploid number of chromosomes (46) is reestablished.

Oogenesis

Oogenesis is the process by which the female gametes, or ova, are produced. The ovaries begin to develop early in the fetal life of the female. All the ova that the female will produce are formed by the sixth month of fetal life. The ovary gives rise to oogonial cells, which develop into oocytes. Meiosis begins in all oocytes before the female fetus is born, but stops before the first division is complete and remains in this arrested phase until puberty. During puberty, the mature primary oocyte proceeds (by oogenesis) through the first meiotic division in the graafian follicle of the ovary.

KEY FACTS TO REMEMBER

Comparison of Meiosis and Mitosis

Meiosis

Purpose

Produce reproductive cells (gametes). Reduction of chromosome number by half (from diploid [46] to haploid [23]), so that when fertilization occurs the normal diploid number is restored. Introduces genetic variability.

Cell division

Two-stage reduction.

Number of daughter cells

Four daughter cells, each containing one-half the number of chromosomes as the mother cell, or 23 chromosomes. Nonidentical to original cell.

Mitosis

Purpose

Produce cells for growth and tissue repair. Cell division characteristic of all somatic cells.

Cell division

One-stage cell division.

Number of daughter cells

Two daughter cells identical to the mother cell, each with the diploid number (46 chromosomes).

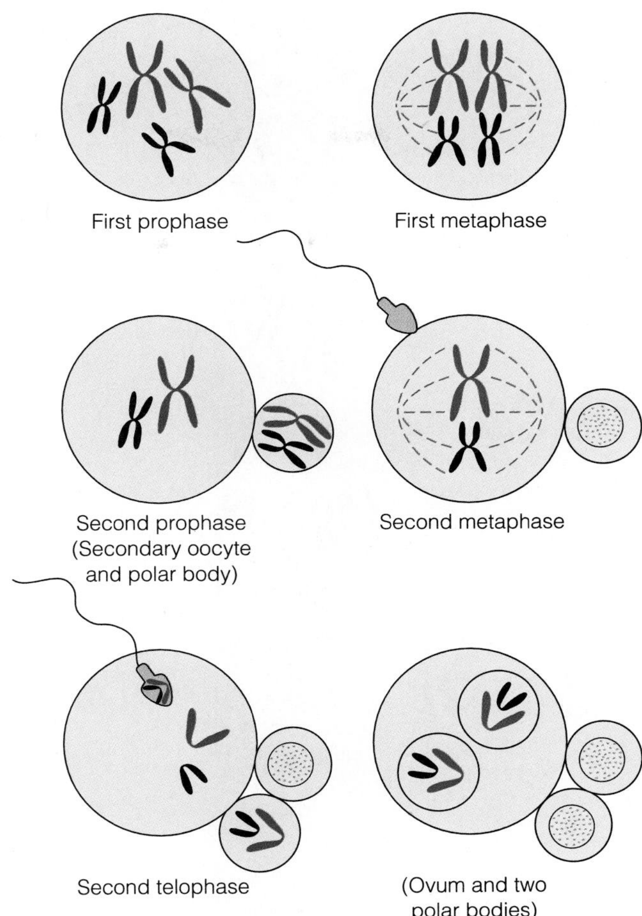

FIGURE 3–1 Human oogenesis and fertilization.

The first meiotic division produces two cells of unequal size with different amounts of cytoplasm, but with the same number of chromosomes. These two cells are the *secondary oocyte* and a minute *polar body.* Both the secondary oocyte and the polar body contain 22 double-structured autosomal chromosomes and one double-structured sex chromosome (X). At the time of ovulation, a second meiotic division begins immediately and proceeds as the oocyte moves down the fallopian tube. Division is again not equal, and the secondary oocyte proceeds to metaphase where its meiotic division is arrested.

Only when fertilized by the sperm does the secondary oocyte complete the second meiotic division, forming a mature ovum with the haploid number of chromosomes and a second polar body (also haploid) (Figure 3–1). The first polar body has also divided in two, producing two additional polar bodies. Thus, at the completion of meiosis, four haploid cells have been produced: the three polar bodies, which eventually disintegrate, and one ovum (Sadler 1990) (Figure 3–2).

Spermatogenesis

During puberty, the germinal epithelium in the seminiferous tubules of the testes begins the process of spermatogenesis, which produces the male gamete (sperm). The (diploid number) spermatogonium replicates before it enters the first meiotic division, during which it is called the *primary spermatocyte.* During this first meiotic division, the spermatogonium forms two cells called *secondary spermatocytes,* each of which contains 22 double-structured autosomal chromosomes and either a double-structured X sex chromosome or a double-structured Y sex chromosome. During the second meiotic division, they divide to form four spermatids, each with the haploid number of chromosomes. The spermatids undergo a series of changes during which they lose most of their cytoplasm and become sperm (spermatozoa).

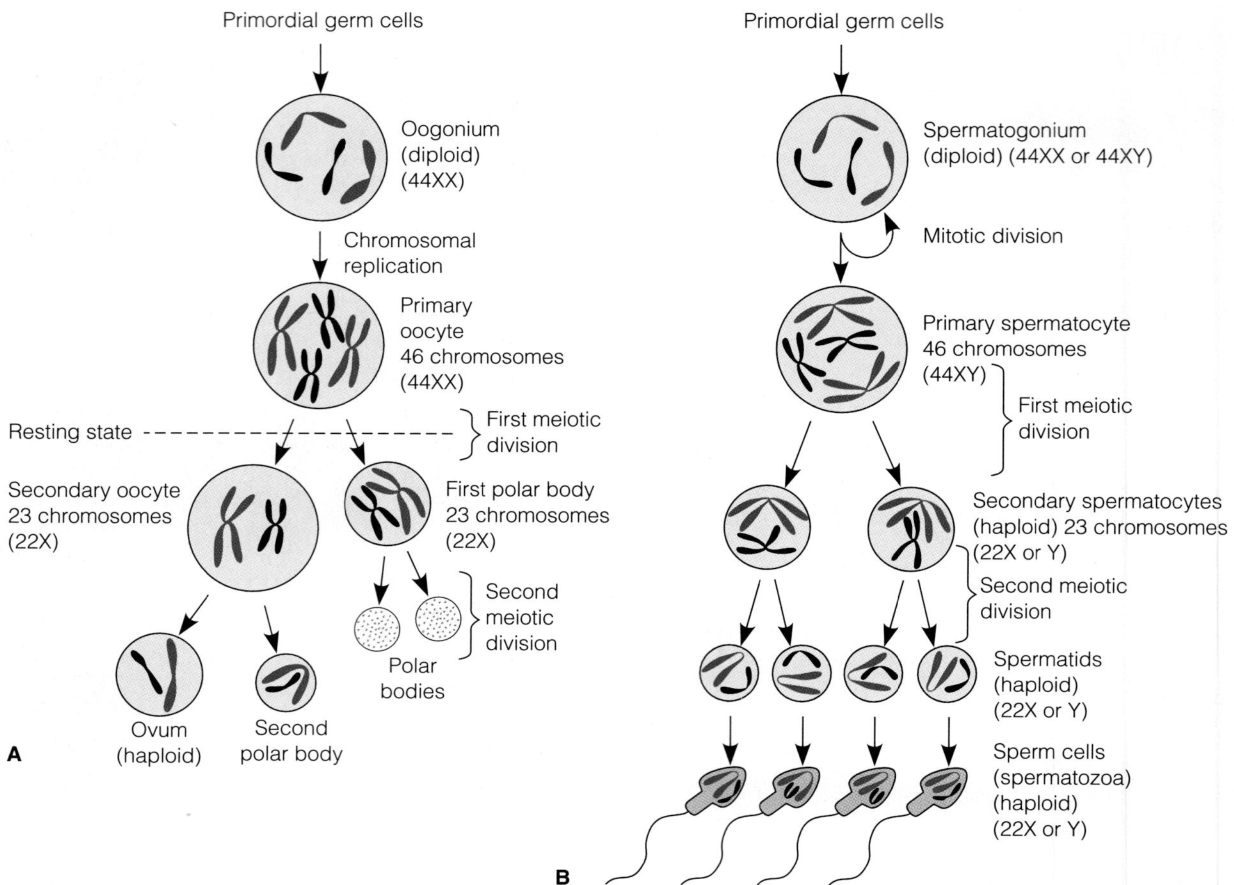

FIGURE 3–2 Gametogenesis involves meiosis within the ovary and testis. ***A*** During meiosis each oogonium produces a single haploid ovum once some cytoplasm moves into the polar bodies. ***B*** Each spermatogonium produces four haploid spermatozoa.

The Process of Fertilization

Fertilization is the process by which a sperm fuses with an ovum to form a new diploid cell, or zygote. Following are the events that lead to fertilization.

Preparation for Fertilization

The process of fertilization takes place in the ampulla (outer third) of the fallopian tube. During ovulation, high estrogen levels increase peristalsis within the fallopian tubes, which helps move the ovum (which has no inherent power of movement) down the tube. The high estrogen levels also cause a thinning of the cervical mucus, facilitating movement of the sperm through the cervix, into the uterus, and up the fallopian tube.

The ovum's cell membrane is surrounded by two layers of tissue. The layer closest to the cell membrane is called the *zona pellucida.* It is a clear, noncellular layer whose function is not known. Surrounding the zona pellucida is a ring of elongated cells, called the *corona radiata* because they radiate from the ovum like the gaseous corona around the sun. These cells are held together by hyaluronic acid.

The mature ovum and spermatozoa have only a brief time to unite. Ova are considered fertile for about 24 hours after ovulation. Sperm can survive in the female reproductive tract for up to 72 hours, but are believed to be healthy and highly fertile for only about 24 hours (Moore and Persaud 1993).

In a single ejaculation, the male deposits approximately 200 to 400 million spermatozoa in the vagina, of which fewer than 200 actually reach the ampulla (Moore and Persaud 1993). The spermatozoa propel themselves up the female tract by the flagellar movement of their tails. Transit time from the cervix into the fallopian tube can be as short as 5 minutes but usually takes an average of 4 to 6 hours after ejaculation (Cunningham et al 1997). Prostaglandins in the semen may increase uterine smooth muscle contractions, which help transport the sperm. The fallopian tubes have a dual ciliary action that facilitates movement of the ovum toward the uterus and movement of the sperm from the uterus toward the ovary.

The sperm's nucleus, which contains its genetic material, is compacted into the head of the sperm and cov-

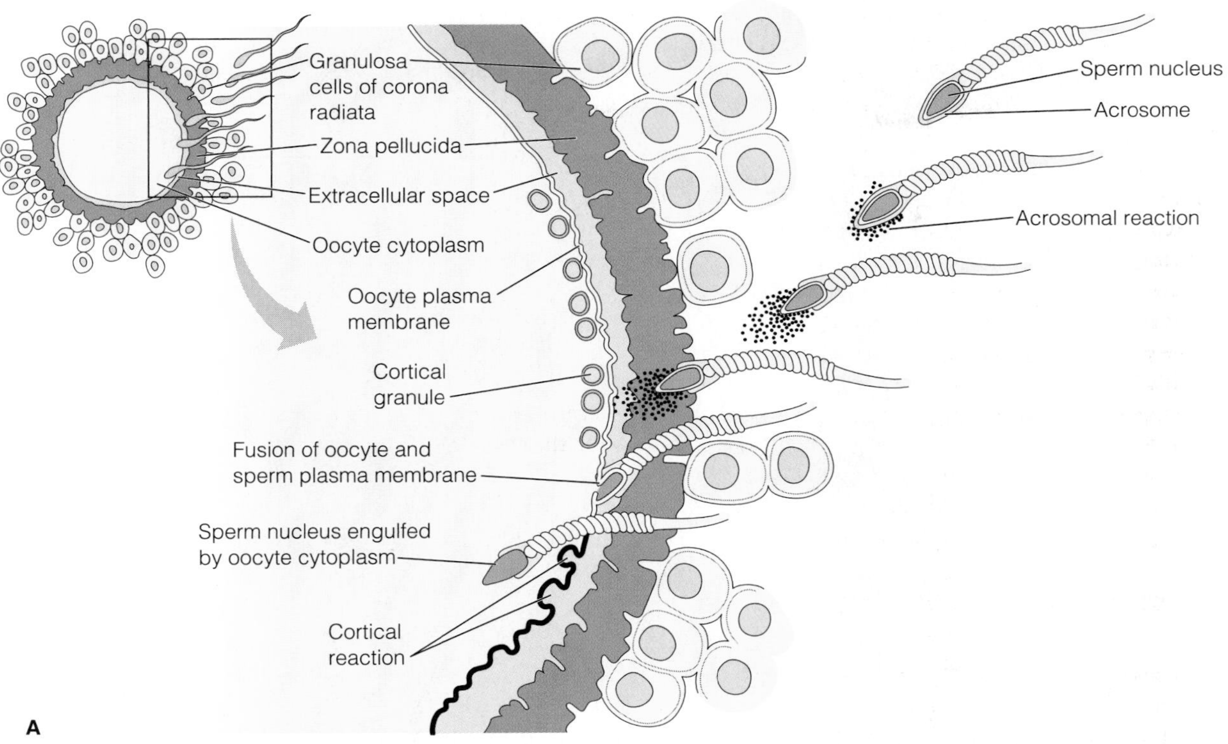

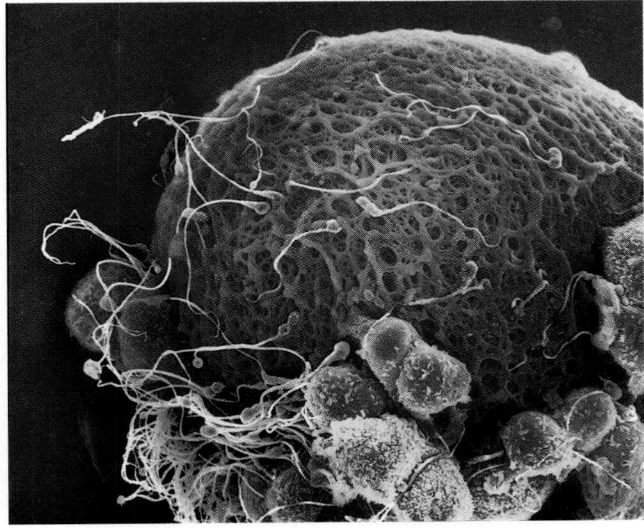

FIGURE 3–3 Sperm penetration of an ovum. ***A*** The sequential steps of oocyte penetration by a sperm are depicted moving from top to bottom. ***B*** Scanning electron micrograph of a human sperm surrounding a human ovum (750×). The smaller spherical cells are granulosa cells of the corona radiata.

Source: Scanning electron micrograph from Nisson L: *A Child Is Born.* New York: Dell Publishing, 1990.

ered by a protective cap called an *acrosome,* which is in turn covered by a plasma membrane. Before fertilization can be achieved, the sperm must undergo **capacitation,** a process that removes the plasma membrane, exposes the acrosome to the acidic environment of the ovum's corona radiata, and induces an attraction to the ovum (Ben-Shlomo and Shalev 1996). Capacitation occurs in the female reproductive tract (aided by uterine enzymes) and is thought to take about 7 hours.

Following capacitation, the *acrosomal reaction* occurs: The acrosomes of the millions of sperm surrounding the ovum release their enzymes (hyaluronidase, a protease called acrosin, and corona-dispersing enzymes) and thus break down the hyaluronic acid in the ovum's corona radiata (Speroff et al 1994). Hundreds of acrosomes must rupture before enough hyaluronic acid is cleared for a single sperm to penetrate the ovum's zona pellucida successfully.

At the moment of penetration, a cellular change occurs in the ovum that renders it impenetrable by other sperm. This event is called the *block to polyspermy.* The cellular change is mediated by release of cortical granules, organelles found just below the ovum's surface, and is called the *cortical reaction* (Speroff et al 1994) (Figure 3–3).

The Moment of Fertilization

After the sperm enters the ovum, a chemical signal prompts the secondary oocyte to complete the second meiotic division, forming the nucleus of the ovum and ejecting the second polar body. Then the nuclei of the ovum and sperm swell and approach each other. The true moment of fertilization occurs as the nuclei unite. Their individual nuclear membranes disappear, and

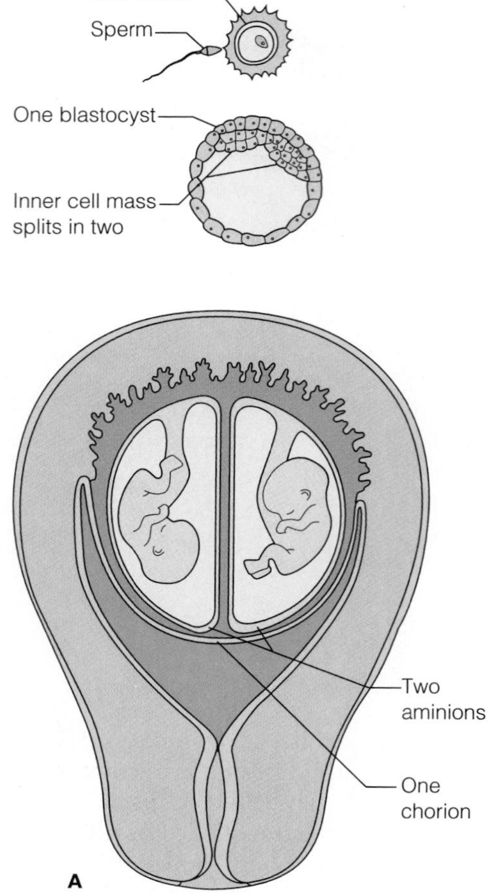

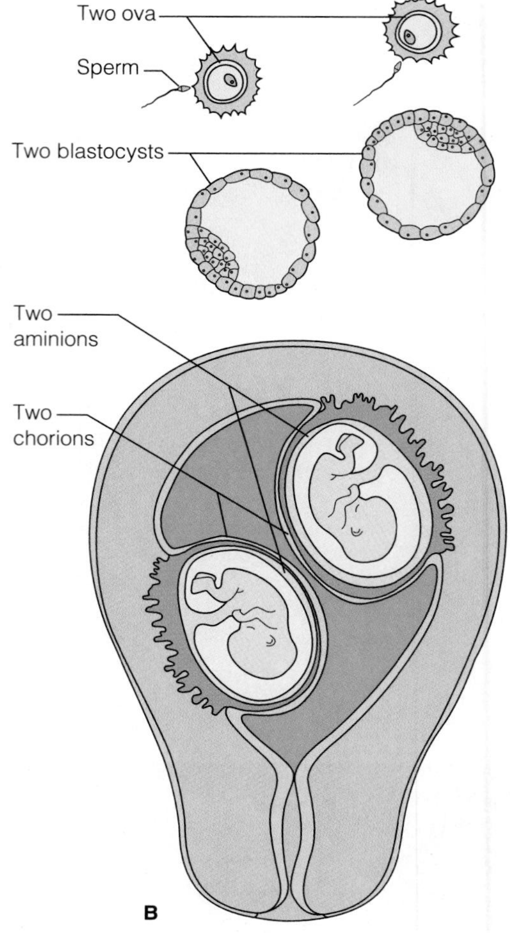

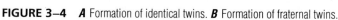

FIGURE 3–4 ***A*** Formation of identical twins. ***B*** Formation of fraternal twins.

their chromosomes pair up to produce the diploid zygote. Since each nucleus contains a haploid number of chromosomes (23), this union restores the diploid number (46). The zygote contains a new combination of genetic material that results in an individual different from either parent or anyone else.

It is also at the moment of fertilization that the sex of the zygote is determined. As discussed in Chapter 4, the two chromosomes (the *sex chromosomes*) of the 23rd pair—either XX or XY—determine the sex of an individual. X chromosomes are larger and bear more genes than Y chromosomes. Females have two X chromosomes, and males have an X and a Y chromosome. While the mature ovum produced by oogenesis can have only one type of sex chromosome—an X—spermatogenesis produces two sperm with an X chromosome and two sperm with a Y chromosome. When each gamete contributes an X chromosome, the resulting zygote is female. When the ovum contributes an X and the sperm contributes a Y chromosome, the resulting zygote is male. Certain traits are termed *sex linked* because they are controlled by the genes on the X sex chromosome.

Twins

Twins have been reported to occur more often among black women than among white women, and more often among white women than among women of Asian origin (Benirschke 1995). Among all groups, as parity (having given birth to a viable infant) increases, so does the chance for multiple births.

Twins may be either *fraternal* or *identical*. If they are fraternal, they are *dizygotic,* which means they arise from two separate ova fertilized by two separate spermatozoa (Figure 3–4). There are two placentas, two chorions, and two amnions; however, the placentas sometimes fuse and appear to be one. Despite their birth relationship, fraternal twins are no more similar to each other than they would be to siblings born singly. They may be of the same or different sex.

Dizygotic twinning increases with maternal age up to about age 35 and then decreases abruptly. The chance of dizygotic twins increases with parity in conceptions that occur in the first 3 months of marriage and also with coital frequency; the chance of dizygotic twinning decreases during periods of malnutrition and during winter and spring for women living in the northern hemisphere. Studies indicate dizygotic twins occur in certain families, perhaps because of genetic factors that result in elevated serum gonadotropin levels leading to double ovulation (Benirschke 1994).

Identical, or *monozygotic,* twins develop from a single fertilized ovum. They are of the same sex and have the same genotype (appearance). Identical twins usually have a common placenta (Figure 3–4).

Monozygotic twins originate from division of the fertilized ovum at different stages of early development, after the zygote consists of thousands of cells. Complete separation of the cellular mass into two parts is necessary for twin formation. The number of amnions and chorions present depends on the timing of the division:

1. If division occurs within 3 days of fertilization (before the inner cell mass and chorion are formed), two embryos, two amnions, and two chorions will develop. This dichorionic-diamniotic situation occurs about 20 percent to 30 percent of the time, and there may be two distinct placentas or a single fused placenta.
2. If division occurs about 5 days after fertilization, two embryos develop with separate amnionic sacs. These sacs will eventually be covered by a common chorion—thus there will be a monochorionic-diamniotic placenta.
3. If the amnion has already developed approximately 7–13 days after fertilization, division results in two embryos with a common amnionic sac and a common chorion (a monochorionic-monoamniotic placenta). This type occurs about 1 percent of the time (Revenis and Johnson 1994).

Monozygotic twinning is considered a random event and occurs in approximately 3.5 per 1000 live births. The survival rate of monozygotic twins is 10 percent lower than that of dizygotic twins, and congenital anomalies are more prevalent. Both twins may have the same malformation.

Intrauterine Development

Development after fertilization can be divided into two phases: cellular multiplication and cellular (embryonic membrane) differentiation. These phases and the process of implantation (nidation), which occurs between them, are discussed next.

Cellular Multiplication

Cellular multiplication begins as the zygote moves through the fallopian tube toward the cavity of the uterus. This transport takes 3 days or more (Cunningham et al 1993).

The zygote now enters a period of rapid mitotic divisions called **cleavage,** during which it divides into two cells, four cells, eight cells, and so on. These cells, called *blastomeres,* are so small that the developing cell mass is only slightly larger than the original zygote. The blastomeres are held together by the zona pellucida, which is under the corona radiata. The blastomeres will eventually form a solid ball of cells called the **morula.** As the morula enters the uterus, its intracellular fluid increases, and a cavity begins to form within it. The inner solid mass of cells is called the **blastocyst.** The outer layer of cells that surrounds the cavity and replaces the zona pellucida is the **trophoblast.** Eventually, the trophoblast develops into one of the embryonic membranes, the chorion. The blastocyst develops into a double layer of cells called the embryonic disc and the other embryonic membrane (the amnion). The journey of the fertilized ovum to its destination in the uterus is illustrated in Figure 3–5.

Implantation (Nidation)

While floating in the uterine cavity, the blastocyst is nourished by the uterine glands, which secrete a mixture of lipids, mucopolysaccharides, and glycogen. The trophoblast attaches itself to the surface of the endometrium for further nourishment. The most frequent site of attachment is the upper part of the posterior uterine wall. Between days 7 and 9 after fertilization, the zona pellucida disappears and the blastocyst implants itself by burrowing into the uterine lining. It penetrates down toward the maternal capillaries until it is completely covered (Moore and Persaud 1993, Navot and Bergh 1996). The lining of the uterus thickens below the implanted blastocyst, and the cells of the trophoblast grow down into the thickened lining, forming processes called *villi.*

Under the influence of progesterone, the endometrium increases in thickness and vascularity in preparation for implantation and nutrition of the ovum. After implantation, the endometrium is called the *decidua.* The portion of the decidua that covers the blastocyst is called the **decidua capsularis;** the portion directly under the implanted blastocyst is the **decidua basalis;** and the portion that lines the rest of the uterine cavity is the **decidua vera (parietalis).** The maternal part of the placenta develops from the decidua basalis, which contains large numbers of blood vessels (see magnified insert in Figure 3–5).

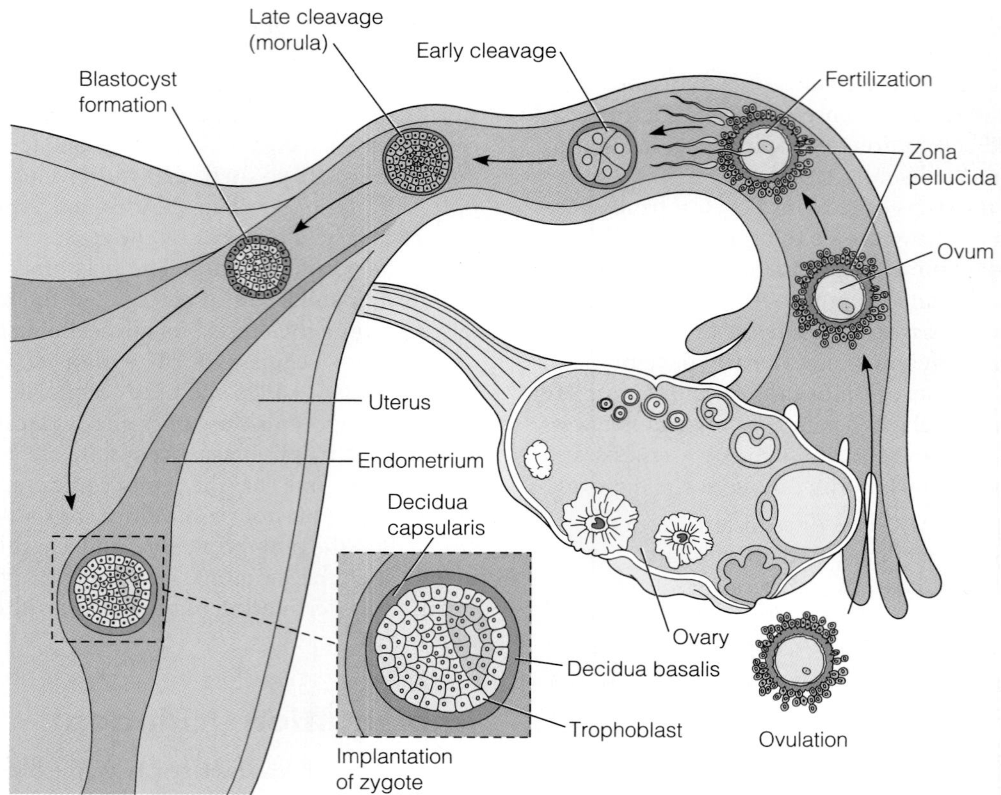

FIGURE 3–5 During ovulation, the ovum leaves the ovary and enters the fallopian tube. Fertilization generally occurs in the outer third of the fallopian tube. Subsequent changes in the fertilized ovum from conception to implantation are depicted.

Cellular Differentiation

Primary Germ Layers

About the 10th to 14th day after conception, the homogenous mass of blastocyst cells differentiates into the primary germ layers (Figure 3–6). These three layers, the **ectoderm, mesoderm,** and **endoderm,** are formed at the same time as the embryonic membranes, and all tissues, organs, and organ systems will develop from these layers (Figure 3–7 on page 47 and Table 3–1 on page 48).

Embryonic Membranes

The **embryonic membranes** begin to form at the time of implantation (Figure 3–8). These membranes protect and support the embryo as it grows and develops inside the uterus. The first membrane to form is the **chorion,** the outermost embryonic membrane that encloses the amnion, embryo, and yolk sac. The chorion is a thick membrane that develops from the trophoblast and has many fingerlike projections *(chorionic villi)* on its surface. These chorionic villi that can be used for early genetic testing of the embryo at 8 to 10 weeks' gestation by choronic villi sampling (see Chapters 4 and 19). The villi begin to degenerate, except for those just under the embryo, which grow and branch into depressions in the uterine wall, forming the fetal portion of the placenta. By the fourth month of pregnancy, the surface of the chorion is smooth except at the place of attachment to the uterine wall.

The second membrane, the **amnion,** originates from the ectoderm, a primary germ layer, during the early stages of embryonic development. The amnion is a thin protective membrane that contains amniotic fluid. The space between the membrane and the embryo is the *amniotic cavity.* This cavity surrounds the embryo and yolk sac, except where the developing embryo (germ-layer disc) attaches to the trophoblast via the umbilical cord. As the embryo grows, the amnion expands until it comes in contact with the chorion. These two slightly adherent fetal membranes form the fluid-filled amniotic sac or **bag of waters (BOW)** that protects the floating embryo.

Amniotic Fluid

Amniotic fluid functions as a cushion to protect against mechanical injury. It also helps control the embryo's temperature, permits symmetrical external growth of

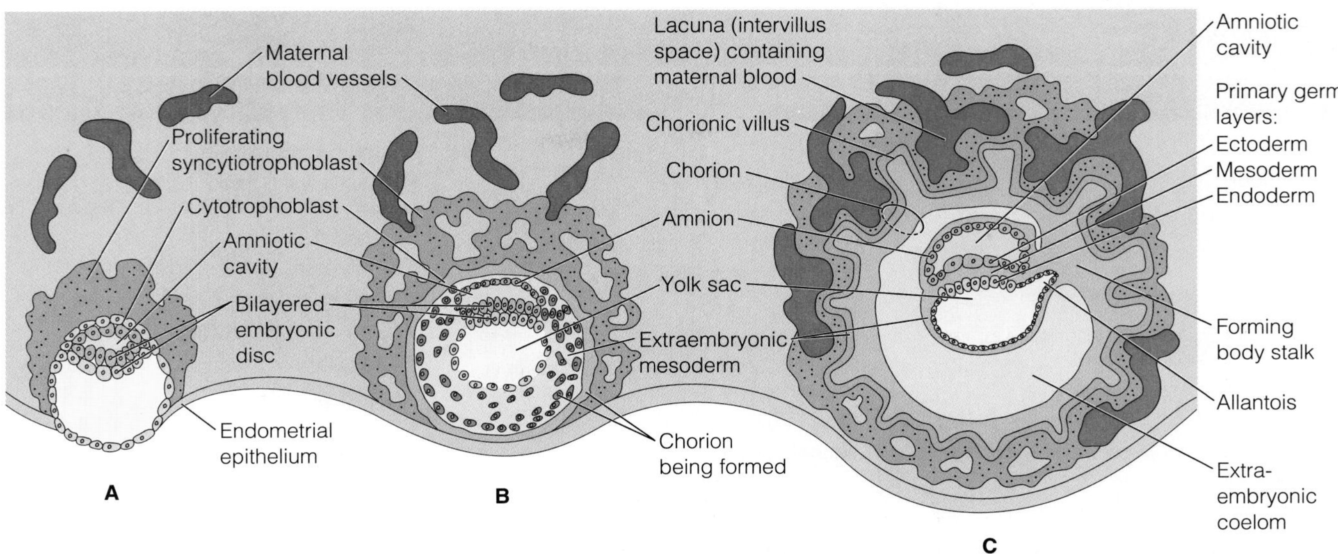

FIGURE 3–6 Formation of primary germ layers. ***A*** Implantation of a 7½-day blastocyst in which the cells of the embryonic disc are separated from the amnion by a fluid-filled space. The erosion of the endometrium by the syncytiotrophoblast is ongoing. ***B*** Implantation is completed by day 9 and extraembryonic mesoderm is beginning to form a discrete layer beneath the cyctotrophoblast. ***C*** By day 16 the embryo shows all three germ layers, a yolk sac, and an allantois (an outpouching of the yolk sac that forms the structural basis of the body stalk, or umbilical cord). The cytotrophoblast and associated mesoderm have become the chorion, and choronic villi are developing.

Source: Adapted from Marieb EN: *Human Anatomy and Physiology,* 3rd ed. Redwood City, CA: Benjamin/Cummings, 1995, p 1008.

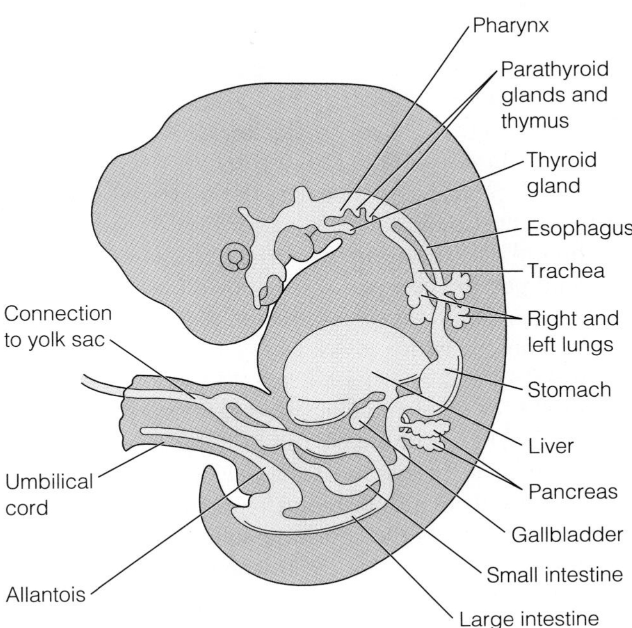

FIGURE 3–7 Endoderm differentiates to form the epithelial lining of the digestive and respiratory tracts and associated glands.

Source: Adapted from Marieb EN: *Human Anatomy and Physiology,* 3rd ed. Redwood City, CA: Benjamin/Cummings, 1995, p 1013.

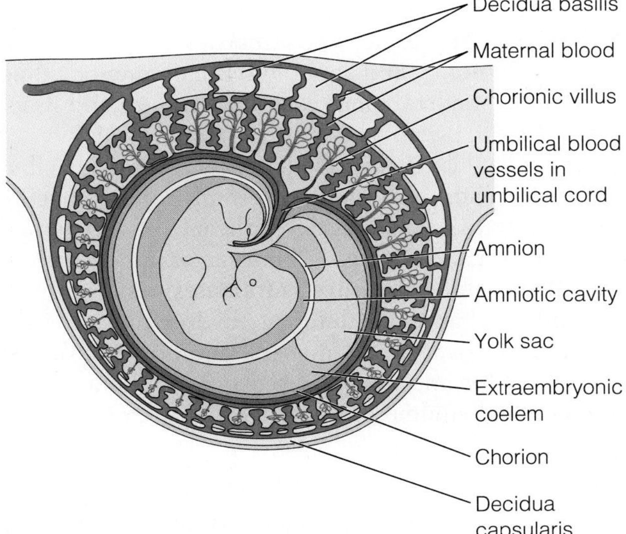

FIGURE 3–8 Early development of primary embryonic membranes. At 4½ weeks, the decidua capsularis (placental portion enclosing the embryo on the uterine surface) and decidua basalis (placental portion encompassing the elaborate chorionic villi and maternal endometrium) are well formed. The chorionic villi lie in blood-filled intervillus spaces within the endometrium. The amnion and yolk sac are well developed.

Source: Adapted from Marieb EN: *Human Anatomy and Physiology,* 3rd ed. Redwood City, CA: Benjamin/Cummings, 1995, p 1008.

TABLE 3–1 Derivation of Body Structures from Primary Cell Layers

Ectoderm	Mesoderm	Endoderm
Epidermis	Dermis	Respiratory tract epithelium
Sweat glands	Wall of digestive tract	Epithelium (except nasal), including pharynx, tongue, tonsils, thyroid, parathyroid, thymus, tympanic cavity
Sebaceous glands	Kidneys and ureter (suprarenal cortex)	Lining of digestive tract
Nails	Reproductive organs (gonads, genital ducts)	Primary tissue of liver and pancreas
Hair follicles	Connective tissue (cartilage, bone, joint cavities)	Urethra and associated glands
Lens of eye	Skeleton	Urinary bladder (except trigone)
Sensory epithelium of internal and external ear, nasal cavity, sinuses, mouth, anal canal	Muscles (all types)	Vagina (parts)
Central and peripheral nervous systems	Cardiovascular system (heart, arteries, veins, blood, bone marrow)	
Nasal cavity	Pleura	
Oral glands and tooth enamel	Lymphatic tissue and cells	
Pituitary glands	Spleen	
Mammary glands		

the embryo, prevents adherence of the amnion, and allows freedom of movement so that the embryo-fetus can change position, thus aiding in musculoskeletal development. The amount of amniotic fluid at 10 weeks is about 30 mL, and it increases to 350 mL at 20 weeks. After 20 weeks, the volume ranges from 700 to 1000 mL (Moore and Persaud 1993). The amniotic fluid volume is constantly changing as the fluid moves back and forth across the placental membrane. As the pregnancy continues, the fetus contributes to the volume of amniotic fluid by excreting urine. The fetus swallows up to 600 mL every 24 hours, and about 400 mL of amniotic fluid flows out of the fetal lungs each day (Gilbert and Brace 1993).

Amniotic fluid is slightly alkaline and contains albumin, uric acid, creatinine, lecithin, sphingomyelin, bilirubin, vernix, leukocytes, epithelial cells, enzymes, and fine hair called **lanugo.** Abnormal variations in amniotic fluid volume are oligohydramnios (less than normal amount of amniotic fluid) and hydramnios, or polyhydramnios (over 2000 mL of amniotic fluid). See Chapter 19 for an in-depth discussion of alterations in amniotic fluid volume.

Yolk Sac

In humans, the yolk sac is small and functions early in embryonic life. It develops as a second cavity in the blastocyst on about day 8 or 9 after conception. It forms primitive red blood cells during the first 6 weeks of development until the embryo's liver takes over the process. As the embryo develops, the yolk sac is incorporated into the umbilical cord, where it can be seen as a degenerated structure after birth.

Placenta

The **placenta** is the means of metabolic and nutrient exchange between the embryonic and maternal circulations. Placental development and circulation do not begin until the third week of embryonic development. The placenta develops at the site where the embryo attaches to the uterine wall. Expansion of the placenta continues until about the 20th week, when it covers approximately one-half of the internal surface of the uterus. After 20 weeks' gestation, the placenta becomes thicker but not wider. At 40 weeks' gestation, the placenta is about 15–20 cm (5.9–7.9 in) in diameter and 2.5–3.0 cm (1.0–1.2 in) in thickness. At that time, it weighs about 400–600 g (14–21 oz).

The placenta has two parts: the maternal and fetal portions. The maternal portion consists of the decidua basalis and its circulation. Its surface is red and fleshlike. The fetal portion consists of the chorionic villi and their circulation. The fetal surface of the placenta is covered by the amnion, which gives it a shiny, gray appearance (Figures 3–9 and 3–10).

Development of the placenta begins with the chorionic villi. The trophoblast cells of the chorionic villi form spaces in the tissue of the decidua basalis. These spaces fill with maternal blood, and the chorionic villi grow into them. As the chorionic villi differentiate, two trophoblastic layers appear: an outer layer, called the *syncytium* (consisting of syncytiotrophoblasts), and an inner layer, known as the cytotrophoblast (Figure 3–6). The cytotrophoblast thins out and disappears about the fifth month, leaving only a single layer of syncytium covering the chorionic villi. The syncytium is in direct contact with the maternal blood in the intervillous spaces. It

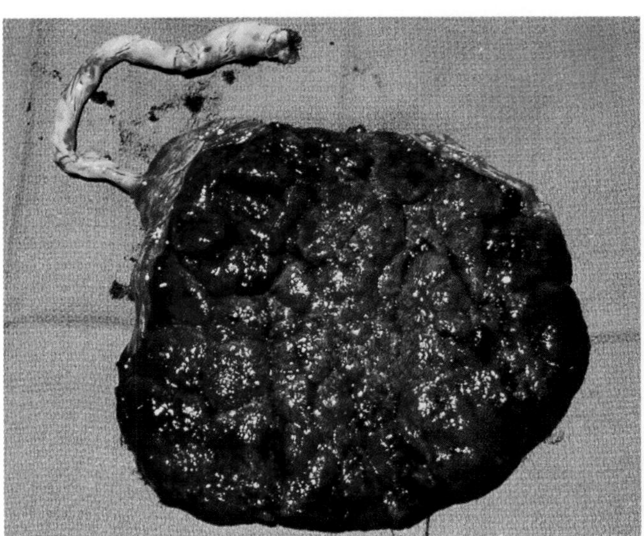

FIGURE 3–9 Maternal side of placenta.

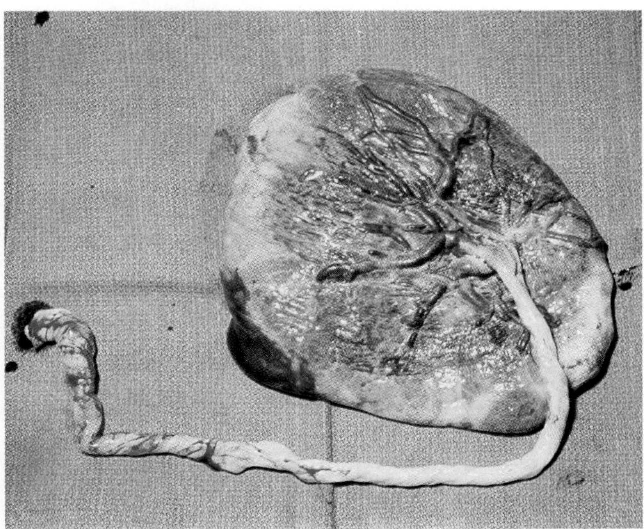

FIGURE 3–10 Fetal side of placenta.

is the functional layer of the placenta and secretes the placental hormones of pregnancy.

A third, inner layer of connective mesoderm develops in the chorionic villi, forming *anchoring villi.* These anchoring villi eventually form the *septa* (partitions) of the placenta. The septa divide the mature placenta into 15 to 20 segments called **cotyledons** (subdivisions of the placenta made up of anchoring villi and decidual tissue). In each cotyledon, the *branching villi* form a highly complex vascular system that allows compartmentalization of the uteroplacental circulation. The exchange of gases and nutrients takes place across these vascular systems.

Exchange of substances across the placenta is minimal during the first 3 to 5 months of development because of limited permeability. The villous membrane is initially too thick. As the villous membrane thins, placental permeability increases until about the last month of pregnancy, when permeability begins to decrease as the placenta ages.

In the fully developed placenta, fetal blood in the villi and maternal blood in the intervillous spaces are separated by three to four thin layers of tissue.

Placental Circulation After implantation of the blastocyst, the cells distinguish themselves into fetal cells and trophoblastic cells. The proliferating trophoblast successfully invades the decidua basalis of the endometrium, first opening the uterine capillaries and later opening the larger uterine vessels. The chorionic villi are an outgrowth of the blastocystic tissue. As these villi continue to grow and divide, the fetal vessels begin to form. The intervillous spaces in the decidua basalis develop as the endometrial spiral arteries are opened.

By the fourth week, the placenta has begun to function as a means of metabolic exchange between embryo and mother. The completion of the maternal–placental–fetal circulation occurs about 17 days after conception, when the embryonic heart begins functioning (Cunningham et al 1997). By 14 weeks, the placenta is a discrete organ. It has grown in thickness as a result of growth in the length and size of the chorionic villi and accompanying expansion of the intervillous space.

In the fully developed placenta's umbilical cord, fetal blood flows through the two umbilical arteries to the capillaries of the villi, becomes oxygen enriched, and then flows back through the umbilical vein into the fetus (Figure 3–11 on page 50). Late in pregnancy, a soft blowing sound *(funic souffle)* can be heard over the area of the umbilical cord. The sound is synchronous with the fetal heartbeat and fetal blood flow through the umbilical arteries.

Maternal blood, rich in oxygen and nutrients, spurts from the spiral uterine arteries into the intervillous spaces. These spurts are produced by the maternal blood pressure. The blood is directed toward the chorionic plate, and as the spurt loses pressure, it becomes lateral (spreads out). Fresh blood enters continuously and exerts pressure on the contents of the intervillous spaces, pushing blood toward the exits in the basal plate. The blood then drains through the uterine and other pelvic veins. A *uterine souffle,* timed precisely with the mother's pulse, is also heard just above the mother's symphysis pubis during the last months of pregnancy. This souffle is caused by the augmented blood flow entering the dilated uterine arteries.

Braxton Hicks contractions (Chapter 15) are believed to facilitate placental circulation by enhancing the

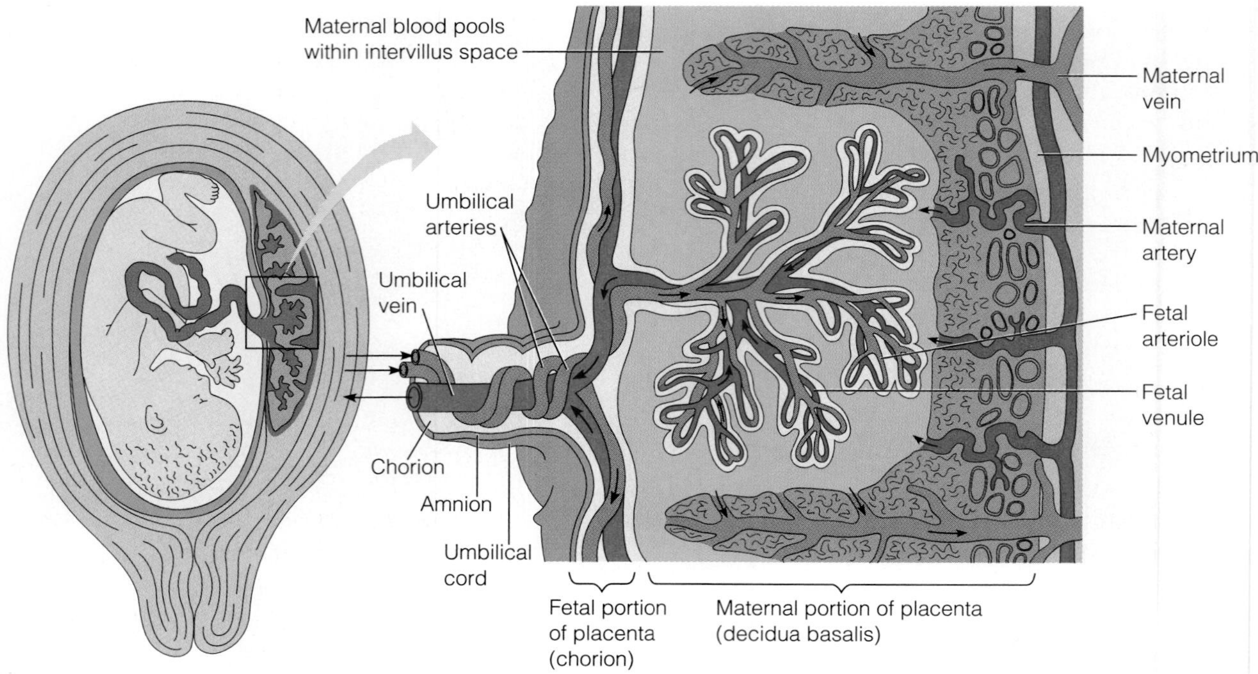

FIGURE 3–11 Vascular arrangement of the placenta. Arrows indicate the direction of blood flow. Maternal blood flows through the uterine arteries to the intervillous spaces of the placenta and returns through the uterine veins to maternal circulation. Fetal blood flows through the umbilical arteries into the villous capillaries of the placenta and returns through the umbilical vein to the fetal circulation.

movement of blood from the center of the cotyledon through the intervillous space. Placental blood flow is enhanced when the woman is lying on her left side because the vena cava is not compromised.

Placental Functions Placental exchange functions occur only in those fetal vessels that are in intimate contact with the covering syncytial membrane. The syncytium villi have brush borders containing many microvilli, which greatly increases the exchange rate between maternal and fetal circulation (Sadler 1990).

The placental functions, many of which begin soon after implantation, include fetal respiration, nutrition, and excretion. To carry out these functions, the placenta is involved in metabolic and transfer activities. In addition, it has endocrine functions and special immunologic properties.

Metabolic Activities The placenta continuously produces glycogen, cholesterol, and fatty acids for fetal use and hormone production. The placenta also produces numerous enzymes required for fetoplacental transfer; breaks down certain substances, such as epinephrine and histamine; and stores glycogen and iron.

Transport Function The placental membranes actively control the transfer of a wide range of substances by five major mechanisms:

1. *Simple diffusion* moves substances from an area of higher concentration to an area of lower concentration. Substances that move across the placenta by simple diffusion include water, oxygen, carbon dioxide, electrolytes (sodium and chloride), anesthetic gases, and drugs. Insulin and steroid hormones originating from the adrenals and thyroid hormones also cross the placenta, but at a very slow rate. The rate of oxygen transfer across the placental membrane is greater than that allowed by simple diffusion, indicating that oxygen is also transferred by facilitated diffusion of some type.
2. *Facilitated transport* involves a carrier system to move molecules from an area of greater concentration to an area of lower concentration at a more rapid rate than by simple diffusion. Molecules such as glucose, galactose, and some oxygen are transported by this method. The glucose level in the fetal blood ordinarily is approximately 20–30

percent lower than the glucose level in the maternal blood, because the fetus is metabolizing glucose rapidly. This in turn causes rapid transport of additional glucose from the maternal blood into the fetal blood.

3. *Active transport* can work against a concentration gradient and allows molecules to move from areas of lower concentration to areas of higher concentration. Amino acids, calcium, iron, iodine, water-soluble vitamins, and glucose are transferred across the placenta this way (Eden and Boehm 1990).
4. *Pinocytosis* is important for transferring large molecules such as albumin and gamma-globulin. Materials are engulfed by amebalike cells, forming plasma droplets.
5. *Hydrostatic* and *osmotic pressures* allow the bulk flow of water and some solutes.

Other modes of transfer also exist. For example, fetal red blood cells pass into the maternal circulation through breaks in the placental membrane, particularly during labor and birth. Certain cells, such as maternal leukocytes, and microorganisms, such as viruses (eg, the human immunodeficiency virus [HIV], which causes acquired immunodeficiency syndrome [AIDS]) and the bacterium *Treponema pallidum,* which causes syphilis, can also cross the placental membrane under their own power (Moore and Persaud 1993). Some bacteria and protozoa infect the placenta by causing lesions and then entering the fetal blood system.

Reduction of the placental surface area, as with abruptio placentae (partial or complete premature separation of abnormally implanted placenta), lessens the area that is functional for exchange. Placental diffusion distance also affects exchange. In conditions such as diabetes and placental infection, edema of the villi increases the diffusion distance, thus increasing the distance the substance has to be transferred. Blood flow alteration changes the transfer rate of substances. Decreased blood flow in the intervillous space is seen in labor and with certain maternal diseases such as hypertension. Mild fetal hypoxia increases the umbilical blood flow, but severe hypoxia results in decreased blood flow.

As the maternal blood picks up fetal waste products and carbon dioxide, it drains back into the maternal circulation through the veins in the basal plate. Fetal blood is hypoxic by comparison; it therefore attracts oxygen from the mother's blood. Affinity for oxygen increases as the fetal blood gives up its carbon dioxide, which also decreases its acidity.

Endocrine Functions The placenta produces hormones that are vital to the survival of the fetus. These include human chorionic gonadotropin (hCG); human placental lactogen (hPL); and two steroid hormones, estrogen and progesterone.

The hormone hCG is similar to luteinizing hormone (LH) and prevents the normal involution of the corpus luteum at the end of the menstrual cycle. If the corpus luteum stops functioning before the 11th week of pregnancy, spontaneous abortion occurs. The hCG also causes the corpus luteum to secrete increased amounts of estrogen and progesterone.

After the 11th week, the placenta produces enough progesterone and estrogen to maintain pregnancy. In the male fetus, hCG also exerts an interstitial cell-stimulating effect on the testes, resulting in the production of testosterone. This small secretion of testosterone during embryonic development is the factor that causes male sex organs to grow. Human chorionic gonadotropin may play a role in the trophoblasts' immunologic capabilities (ability to exempt the placenta and embryo from rejection by the mother's system). Human chorionic gonadotropin is used as a basis for pregnancy tests (see Chapter 7).

Human chorionic gonadotropin is present in maternal blood serum 8 to 10 days after fertilization, just as soon as implantation has occurred, and is detectable in maternal urine at the time of missed menses. It reaches its maximum level at 50 to 70 days' gestation and then begins to decrease as placental hormone production increases.

Progesterone is a hormone essential for pregnancy. It increases the secretions of the fallopian tubes and uterus to provide appropriate nutritive matter for the developing morula and blastocyst. It also appears to aid in ovum transport through the fallopian tube (Moore and Persaud 1993). Progesterone causes decidual cells to develop in the uterine endometrium, and it must be present in high levels for implantation to occur. Progesterone also decreases the contractility of the uterus, thus preventing uterine contractions from causing spontaneous abortion.

Prior to stimulation by hCG, the production of progesterone by the corpus luteum reaches a peak about 7 to 10 days after ovulation. Implantation occurs at about the same time as this peak. At 16 days after ovulation, progesterone reaches a level between 25 and 50 mg per day and continues to rise slowly in subsequent weeks (Cunningham et al 1997). After 10 weeks, the placenta (specifically, the syncytiotrophoblast) takes over the production of progesterone and secretes it in tremendous quantities, reaching levels late in pregnancy of more than 250 mg per day.

By 7 weeks, the placenta produces more than 50 percent of the estrogens in the maternal circulation. Estrogens serve mainly a proliferative function, causing enlargement of the uterus, breasts, and breast glandular tissue. Estrogens also have a significant role in increasing vascularity and vasodilation, particularly in the villous capillaries toward the end of pregnancy. Placental estrogens increase markedly toward the end of pregnancy, to as much as 30 times the daily production in the middle of a normal monthly menstrual cycle. The primary estrogen secreted by the placenta is different from that secreted by the ovaries. The placenta secretes mainly *estriol,* whereas the ovaries secrete primarily *estradiol.* The placenta cannot synthesize estriol by itself. Essential precursors are provided by the fetal adrenal glands and are transported to the placenta for the final conversion to estriol.

The hormone *human placental lactogen (hPL),* sometimes referred to as human chorionic somatomammotropin (hCS), is similar to human pituitary growth hormone; hPL stimulates certain changes in the mother's metabolic processes, which ensure that more protein, glucose, and minerals are available for the fetus. Secretion of hPL can be detected by about 4 weeks. New placental proteins have been identified that may have clinical uses. These include SP 1 (Schwangerschafts protein 1), PP 5 (placental protein 5), and others (Eden and Boehm 1990).

Immunologic Properties The placenta and embryo are transplants of living tissue within the same species, and are therefore considered *homografts.* Unlike other homografts, the placenta and embryo appear exempt from immunologic reaction by the host. Most recent data suggest that there is a suppression of cellular immunity by the placental hormones (progesterone and hCG) during pregnancy. One theory suggests that trophoblastic tissue is immunologically inert. It may contain a cell coating that masks transplantation antigens, repels sensitized lymphocytes, and protects against antibody formation.

Umbilical Cord

As the placenta is developing, the **umbilical cord** is also being formed from the amnion. The **body stalk,** which attaches the embryo to the yolk sac, contains blood vessels that extend into the chorionic villi. The body stalk fuses with the embryonic portion of the placenta to provide a circulatory pathway from the chorionic villi to the embryo (see Figure 3.11). As the body stalk elongates to become the umbilical cord, the vessels in the cord decrease to one large vein and two smaller arteries. About 1 percent of umbilical cords have only two vessels, an artery and a vein; this condition may be associated with congenital malformations primarily of the renal and cardiovascular systems. A specialized connective tissue known as **Wharton's jelly** surrounds the blood vessels. This tissue, plus the high blood volume pulsating through the vessels, prevents compression of the umbilical cord in utero. At term (38–42 weeks' gestation), the average cord is 2 cm (0.8 in) across and about 55 cm (22 in) long. The cord can attach itself to the placenta in various sites. Central insertion into the placenta is considered normal. (See Chapter 19 for a discussion of the various attachment sites.)

Umbilical cords appear twisted or spiraled. This is most likely caused by fetal movement. A true knot in the umbilical cord rarely occurs; if it does, the cord is usually long. More common are so-called false knots, caused by the folding of cord vessels. A *nuchal cord* is said to exist when the umbilical cord encircles the fetal neck.

Fetal Circulatory System

Because the fetus must maintain the blood flow to the placenta to obtain oxygen and nutrients and to remove carbon dioxide and other waste products, the circulatory system of the fetus has several unique features.

Most of the blood supply bypasses the fetal lungs, since they do not carry out respiratory gas exchange. The placenta assumes the function of the fetal lungs by supplying oxygen and allowing the fetus to excrete carbon dioxide into the maternal bloodstream. Figure 3–12 shows the fetal circulatory system. The blood from the placenta flows through the umbilical vein, which enters the fetus at the site that, after birth, is the umbilicus (belly button). It divides into two branches, one of which circulates a small amount of blood through the fetal liver and empties into the inferior vena cava through the hepatic vein. The second and larger branch, called the **ductus venosus,** empties directly into the fetal vena cava. This blood then enters the right atrium, passes through the **foramen ovale** into the left atrium, and pours into the left ventricle, which pumps it into the aorta. Some blood returning from the head and upper extremities by way of the superior vena cava is emptied into the right atrium and passes through the tricuspid valve into the right ventricle. This blood is pumped into the pulmonary artery, and a small amount passes to the lungs for nourishment only. The larger portion of blood passes from the pulmonary artery through the **ductus arteriosus** into the descending aorta, bypassing the lungs. Finally, blood returns to the placenta through the two umbilical arteries, and the process is repeated.

The fetus obtains oxygen via diffusion from the maternal circulation because of the gradient difference of Po_2 of 50 mm Hg in maternal blood in the placenta to 30 mm Hg Po_2 in the fetus. At term the fetus receives oxygen from the mother's circulation at a rate of 20 to 30 mL per min (Sadler 1990). Fetal hemoglobin facilitates obtaining oxygen from the maternal circulation,

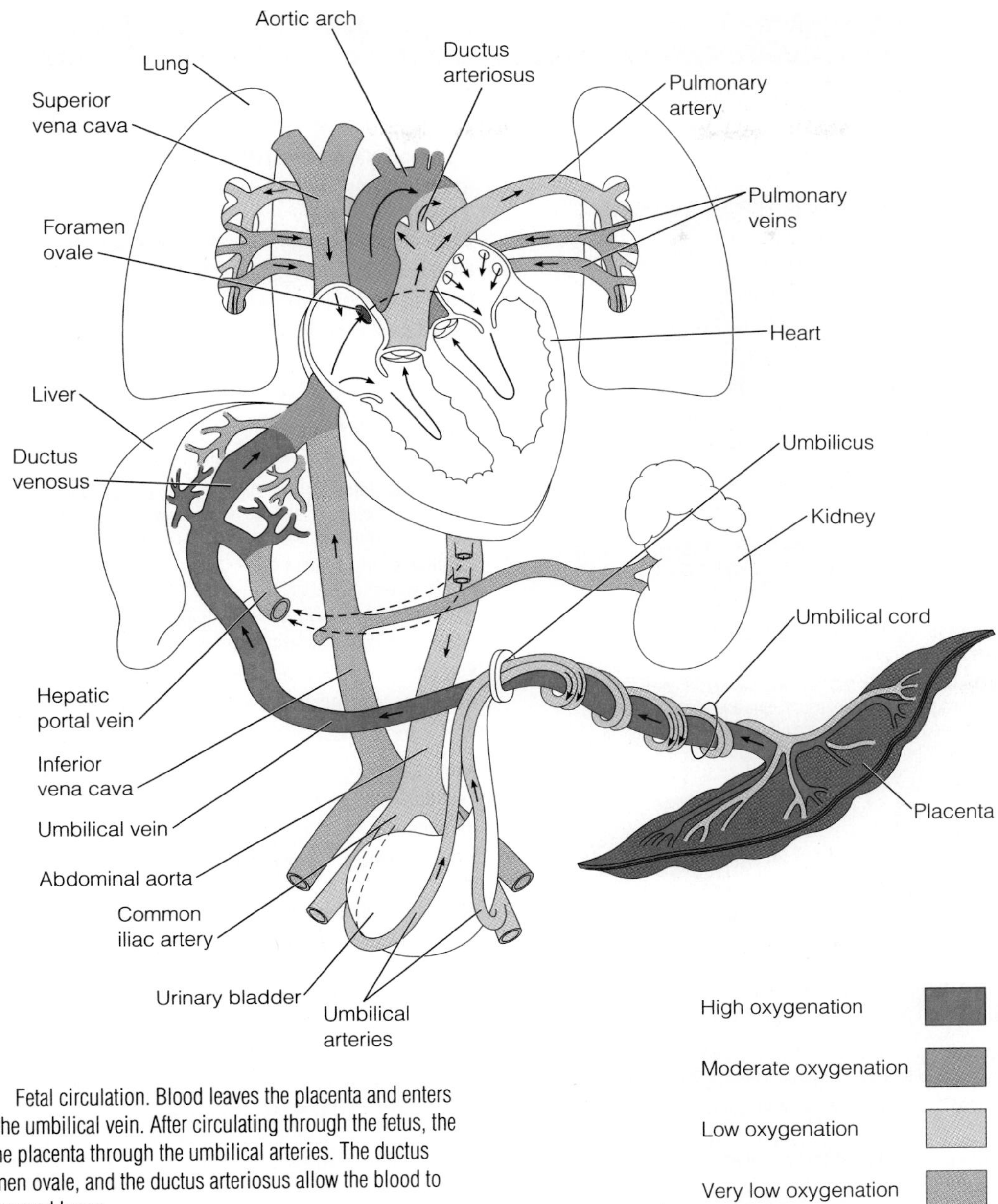

FIGURE 3–12 Fetal circulation. Blood leaves the placenta and enters the fetus through the umbilical vein. After circulating through the fetus, the blood returns to the placenta through the umbilical arteries. The ductus venosus, the foramen ovale, and the ductus arteriosus allow the blood to bypass the fetal liver and lungs.

since it carries as much as 20 to 30 percent more oxygen than adult hemoglobin. For further discussion, see Chapter 21.

Fetal circulation delivers the highest available oxygen concentration to the head, neck, brain, and heart (coronary circulation) and a lesser amount of oxygenated blood to the abdominal organs and the lower body. This circulatory pattern leads to *cephalocaudal* (head-to-tail) development in the fetus.

Embryo and Fetal Development and Organ Formation

Pregnancy is calculated to last an average of 10 lunar months: 40 weeks, or 280 days. This period of 280 days is calculated from the beginning of the last menstrual period to the time of birth. Estimated date of birth (EDB)

TABLE 3–2 Summary of Organ System Development

Age: 2–3 weeks

Length: 2 mm C–R (Crown-to-Rump)

Nervous system: Groove forms along middle back as cells thicken; neural tube forms from closure of neural groove.

Cardiovascular system: Beginning of blood circulation; tubular heart begins to form during third week.

Gastrointestinal system: Liver begins to function.

Genitourinary system: Formation of kidneys beginning.

Respiratory system: Nasal pits forming.

Endocrine system: Thyroid tissue appears.

Eyes: Optic cup and lens pit have formed; pigment in eyes.

Ear: Auditory pit is now enclosed structure.

Age: 4 weeks

Length: 4–6 mm C–R

Weight: 0.4 g

Nervous system: Anterior portion of neural tube closes to form brain; closure of posterior end forms spinal cord.

Musculoskeletal system: Noticeable limb buds.

Cardiovascular system: Tubular heart beats at 28 days and primitive red blood cells circulate through fetus and chorionic villi.

Gastrointestinal system: Mouth: formation of oral cavity; primitive jaws present; esophagotracheal septum begins division of esophagus and trachea. Digestive tract: stomach forms; esophagus and intestine become tubular; ducts of pancreas and liver forming.

Age: 5 weeks

Length: 8 mm C–R

Weight: Only 0.5% of total body weight is fat (to 20 weeks).

Nervous system: Brain has differentiated and cranial nerves are present.

Musculoskeletal system: Developing muscles have innervation.

Cardiovascular system: Atrial division has occurred.

Age: 6 weeks

Length: 12 mm C–R

Musculoskeletal system: Bone rudiments present; primitive skeletal shape forming; muscle mass begins to develop; ossification of skull and jaws begins.

Cardiovascular system: Chambers present in heart; groups of blood cells can be identified.

Gastrointestinal system: Oral and nasal cavities and upper lip formed; liver begins to form red blood cells.

Respiratory system: Trachea, bronchi, and lung buds present.

Ear: Formation of external, middle, and inner ear continues.

Sexual development: Embryonic sex glands appear.

Age: 7 weeks

Length: 18 mm C–R

Cardiovascular system: Fetal heartbeats can be detected.

Gastrointestinal system: Mouth: tongue separates; palate folds. Digestive tract: stomach attains final form.

Genitourinary system: Separation of bladder and urethra from rectum.

Respiratory system: Diaphragm separates abdominal and thoracic cavities.

Eyes: Optic nerve formed; eyelids appear, thickening of lens.

Sexual development: Differentiation of sex glands into ovaries and testes begins.

Age: 8 weeks

Length: 2.5–3 cm C–R

Weight: 2 g

Musculoskeletal system: Digits formed; further differentiation of cells in primitive skeleton; cartilaginous bones show first signs of ossification; development of muscles in trunk, limbs, and head; some movement of fetus now possible.

Cardiovascular system: Development of heart essentially complete; fetal circulation follows two circuits—four extraembryonic and two intraembryonic.

Gastrointestinal system: Mouth: completion of lip fusion. Digestive tract: rotation in midgut; anal membrane has perforated.

Ear: External, middle, and inner ear assuming final forms.

Sexual development: Male and female external genitals appear similar until end of ninth week.

Age: 10 weeks

Length: 5–6 cm C–H (Crown-to-Heel)

Weight: 14 g

Nervous system: Neurons appear at caudal end of spinal cord; basic divisions of brain present.

Musculoskeletal system: Fingers and toes begin nail growth.

Gastrointestinal system: Mouth: separation of lips from jaw; fusion of palate folds. Digestive tract: developing intestines enclosed in abdomen.

Genitourinary system: Bladder sac formed.

Endocrine system: Islets of Langerhans differentiated.

Eyes: Eyelids fused closed; development of lacrimal duct.

Sexual development: Males: production of testosterone and physical characteristics between 8 and 12 weeks.

Age: 12 weeks

Length: 8 cm C–R; 11.5 cm C–H

Weight: 45 g

Musculoskeletal system: Clear outlining of miniature bones (12–20 weeks); process of ossification is established throughout fetal body; appearance of involuntary muscles in viscera.

Note: Age refers to gestational age of fetus/conceptus; fertilization age.

Sources: Sadler TW: *Langman's Medical Embryology,* 6th ed. Baltimore: Williams & Wilkins, 1990; and Moore KL, Persaud TVN: *The Developing Human: Clinically Oriented Embryology,* 5th ed. Philadelphia: Saunders, 1993.

is usually calculated by this method. The fertilization age, or postconception age, of the fetus is calculated to be about two weeks less, or 266 days (38 weeks). The latter measurement is more accurate because it measures time from the fertilization of the ovum, or conception. The basic events of organ development in the embryo and fetus are outlined in Table 3–2. The time periods in the table are **postconception age periods.** For detailed discussion of the development of each body system, see Chapter 21.

TABLE 3–2 continued

Age: 12 weeks *continued*

Gastrointestinal system: Mouth: completion of palate. Digestive tract: appearance of muscles in gut; bile secretion begins; liver is major producer of red blood cells.

Respiratory system: Lungs acquire definitive shape.

Skin: Pink and delicate.

Endocrine system: Hormonal secretion from thyroid; insulin present in pancreas.

Immunologic system: Appearance of lymphoid tissue in fetal thymus gland.

Age: 16 weeks

Length: 13.5 cm C–R; 15 cm C–H

Weight: 200 g

Musculoskeletal system: Teeth beginning to form hard tissue that will become central incisors.

Gastrointestinal system: Mouth: differentiation of hard and soft palate. Digestive tract: development of gastric and intestinal glands; intestines begin to collect meconium.

Genitourinary system: Kidneys assume typical shape and organization.

Skin: Appearance of scalp hair; lanugo present on body; transparent skin with visible blood vessels; sweat glands developing.

Eye, ear, and nose: Formed.

Sexual development: Sex determination possible.

Age: 18 weeks

Musculoskeletal system: Teeth beginning to form hard tissue (enamel and dentine) that will become lateral incisors.

Cardiovascular system: Fetal heart tones audible with fetoscope at 16–20 weeks.

Age: 20 weeks

Length: 19 cm C–R; 25 cm C–H

Weight: 435 g (6% of total body weight is fat)

Nervous system: Myelination of spinal cord begins.

Musculoskeletal system: Teeth beginning to form hard tissue that will become canine and first molar. Lower limbs are of final relative proportions.

Gastrointestinal system: Fetus actively sucks and swallows amniotic fluid; peristaltic movements begin.

Skin: Lanugo covers entire body; brown fat begins to form; vernix caseosa begins to form.

Immunologic system: Detectable levels of fetal antibodies (IgG type).

Blood formation: Iron is stored and bone marrow is increasingly important.

Age: 24 weeks

Length: 23 cm C–R; 28 cm C–H

Weight: 780 g

Nervous system: Brain looks like mature brain.

Musculoskeletal system: Teeth are beginning to form hard tissue that will become the second molar.

Age: 24 weeks *continued*

Respiratory system: Respiratory movements may occur (24–40 weeks). Nostrils reopen. Alveoli appear in lungs and begin production of surfactant; gas exchange possible.

Skin: Reddish and wrinkled, vernix caseosa present.

Immunologic system: IgG levels reach maternal levels.

Eyes: Structurally complete.

Age: 28 weeks

Length: 27 cm C–R; 35 cm C–H

Weight: 1200–1250 g

Nervous system: Begins regulation of some body functions.

Skin: Adipose tissue accumulates rapidly; nails appear; eyebrows and eyelashes present.

Eyes: Eyelids open (28–32 weeks).

Sexual development: Males: testes descend into inguinal canal and upper scrotum.

Age: 32 weeks

Length: 31 cm C–R; 38–43 cm C–H

Weight: 2000 g

Nervous system: More reflexes present.

Age: 36 weeks

Length: 35 cm C–R; 42–48 cm C–H

Weight: 2500–2750 g

Musculoskeletal system: Distal femoral ossification centers present.

Skin: Pale; body rounded, lanugo disappearing, hair fuzzy or woolly; few sole creases; sebaceous glands active and helping to produce vernix caseosa (36–40 weeks).

Ears: Ear lobes soft with little cartilage.

Sexual development: Males: scrotum small and few rugae present; descent of testes into upper scrotum to stay (36–40 weeks). Females: labia majora and minora equally prominent.

Age: 40 weeks

Length: 40 cm C–R; 48–52 cm C–H

Weight: 3200+ g (16% of total body weight is fat)

Respiratory system: At 38 weeks, lecithin-spingomyelin (L/S) ratio approaches 2:1 (indicates decreased risk of respiratory distress from inadequate surfactant production if born now).

Skin: Smooth and pink; vernix present in skinfolds; moderate to profuse silky hair; lanugo hair on shoulders and upper back; nails extend over tips of digits; creases cover sole.

Ears: Ear lobes firmer due to increased cartilage.

Sexual development: Males: rugous scrotum. Females: labia majora well developed and minora small or completely covered.

Human development follows three stages. The preembryonic stage consists of the first 14 days of development after the ovum is fertilized; the embryonic stage covers the period from day 15 until approximately the 8th week, and the fetal stage extends from the end of the 8th week until birth.

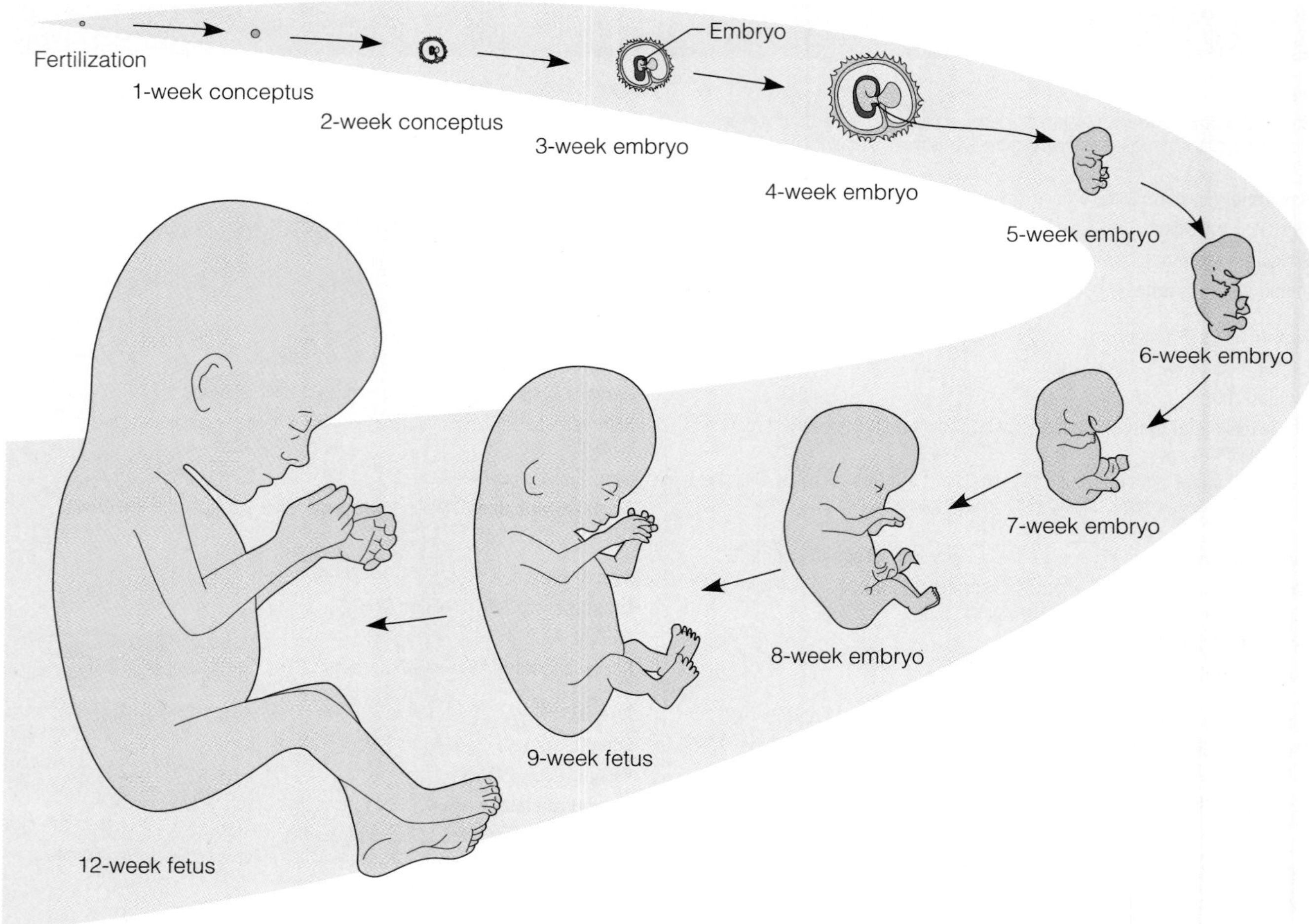

FIGURE 3–13 The actual size of a human conceptus from fertilization to the early fetal stage. The embryonic stage begins in the 3rd week after fertilization; the fetal stage begins in the 9th week.
Source: Adapted from Marieb EN: *Human Anatomy and Physiology*, 3rd ed. Redwood City, CA: Benjamin/Cummings, 1995, p 1000.

Preembryonic Stage

The first 14 days of development, starting the day the ovum is fertilized (conception), are called the *preembryonic stage* or the *stage of the ovum*. This period is characterized by rapid cellular multiplication and differentiation and the establishment of the embryonic membranes and primary germ layers, discussed earlier.

Embryonic Stage

The stage of the **embryo** starts on day 15 (the beginning of the third week after conception) and continues until approximately the eighth week, or until the embryo reaches a *crown-to-rump (C–R)* length of 3 cm or 1.2 in. This length is usually reached about 56 days after fertilization (the end of the 8th gestational week). During the embryonic stage, tissues differentiate into essential organs and the main external features develop (Figure 3–13). The embryo is the most vulnerable to teratogens during this period.

Third Week

In the third week, the embryonic disk becomes elongated and pear-shaped, with a broad cephalic end and a narrow caudal end. The ectoderm has formed a long cylindrical tube for brain and spinal cord development. The gastrointestinal tract, created from the endoderm, appears as another tubelike structure communicating with the yolk sac. The most advanced organ is the heart. At 3 weeks, a single tubular heart forms just outside the body cavity of the embryo.

Fourth to Fifth Week

During days 21 to 32, *somites* (a series of mesodermal blocks) form on either side of the embryo's midline. The vertebrae that form the spinal column will develop from these somites. Prior to 28 days, arm and leg buds are not visible, but the tail bud is present. The pharyngeal arches—which will form the lower jaw, hyoid bone, and larynx—develop at this time. The pharyngeal pouches appear now; these pouches will form the eustachian

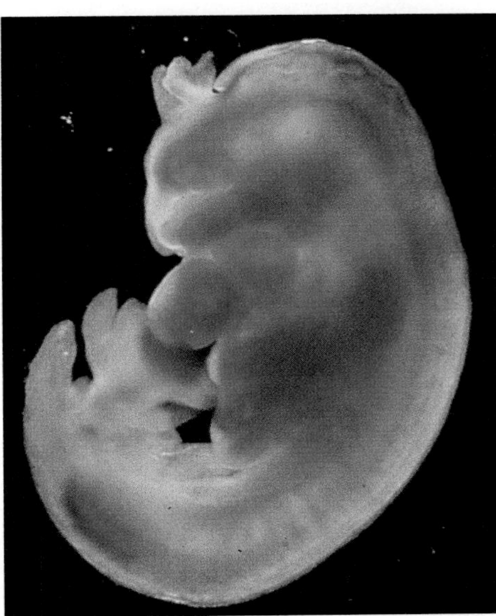

FIGURE 3–14 The embryo at 5 weeks. The embryo has a marked C-shaped body and a rudimentary tail.

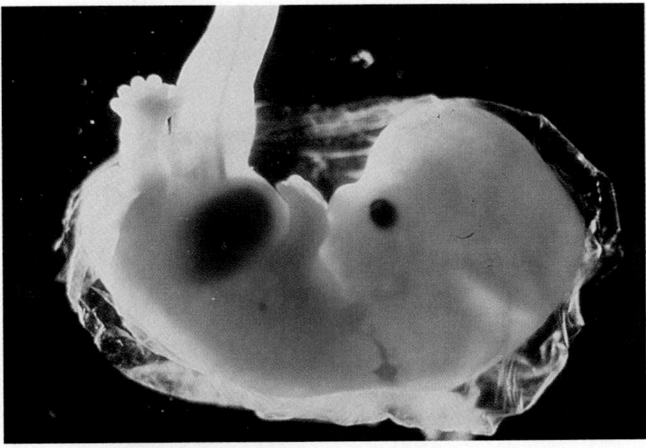

FIGURE 3–15 The embryo at 7 weeks. The head is rounded and nearly erect. The eyes have shifted forward and closer together, and the eyelids begin to form.

tube and cavity of the middle ear, the tonsils, and the parathyroid and thymus glands. The primordia of the ear and eye are also present. By the end of 28 days, the tubular heart is beating at a regular rhythm and pushing its own primitive blood cells through the main blood vessels.

During the fifth week, the optic cups and lens vessels of the eye form and the nasal pits develop. Partitioning in the heart occurs with the dividing of the atrium. The embryo has a marked C-shaped body, accentuated by the rudimentary tail and the large head folded over a protuberant trunk (Figure 3–14). By day 35, the arm and leg buds are well developed, with paddle-shaped hand and foot plates. The heart, circulatory system, and brain show the most advanced development. The brain has differentiated into five areas, and ten pairs of cranial nerves are recognizable.

Sixth to Seventh Week

At 6 weeks the head structures are more highly developed and the trunk is straighter than in earlier stages. The upper and lower jaws are recognizable, and the external nares are well formed. The trachea has developed, and its caudal end is bifurcated for beginning lung formation. The upper lip has formed, and the palate is developing. The ears are developing rapidly. The arms have begun to extend ventrally across the chest, and both arms and legs have digits, although they may still be webbed. There is a slight elbow bend in the arms, which are more advanced in development than the legs. Beginning at this stage, the prominent tail will recede. The heart now has most of its definitive characteristics, and fetal circulation begins to be established. The liver starts to produce blood cells. At 7 weeks the head of the embryo is rounded and nearly erect (Figure 3–15). The eyes have shifted and are closer together and the eyelids are beginning to form. Prior to this time the rectal and urogenital passages formed one tube that ended in a blind pouch; they now separate into two tubular structures. The intestines enter the extraembryonic coelom in the area of the umbilical cord (called umbilical herniation) (Moore and Persaud 1993). At this point the beginnings of all essential external and internal structures are present.

Eighth Week

At 8 weeks the embryo is approximately 3 cm (1.2 in) long C–R and clearly resembles a human being. Facial features continue to develop. The eyelids begin to fuse. Auricles of the external ears begin to assume their final shape, but they are still set low (Moore and Persaud 1993). External genitals appear, but sex is not discernible, and the rectal passage opens with the perforation of the anal membrane. The circulatory system through the umbilical cord is well established. Long bones are beginning to form, and the large muscles are now capable of contracting.

Fetal Stage

By the end of the eighth week, the embryo is sufficiently developed to be called a **fetus.** Every organ system and external structure that will be found in the full-term newborn is present. The remainder of gestation is devoted to refining structures and perfecting function.

Ninth to Twelfth Week

By the end of the ninth week the fetus reaches a C–R length of 5 cm (2 in) and weighs about 14 g. The head is large and comprises almost half of the fetus's entire size

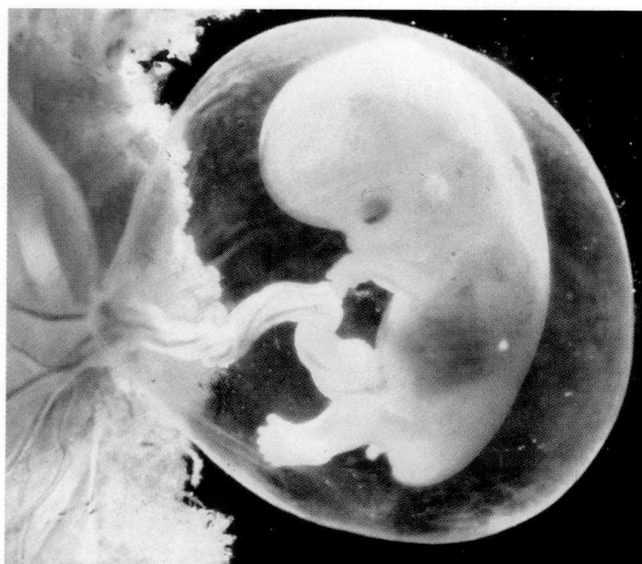

FIGURE 3–16 The fetus at 9 weeks. Every organ system and external structure is present.

Source: Nilsson L: A Child Is Born. New York: Dell Publishing, 1990.

(Figure 3–16). At 12 weeks, the fetus reaches 8 cm (3.2 in) C–R and weighs about 45 g (1.6 oz). The face is well formed, with the nose protruding, the chin small and receding, and the ear acquiring a more adult shape. The eyelids close at about the 10th week and will not reopen until about 28 weeks. Some reflex movement of the lips suggestive of the sucking reflex has been observed at 3 months. Tooth buds now appear for all 20 of the child's first teeth (baby teeth). The limbs are long and slender, with well-formed digits. The fetus can curl the fingers toward the palm and begins to make a tiny fist. The legs are still shorter and less developed than the arms. The urogenital tract completes its development, well-differentiated genitals appear, and the kidneys begin to produce urine. Red blood cells are produced primarily by the liver. Fetal heart tones can be ascertained by electronic devices between 8 and 12 weeks. The rate is 120–160 beats per minute.

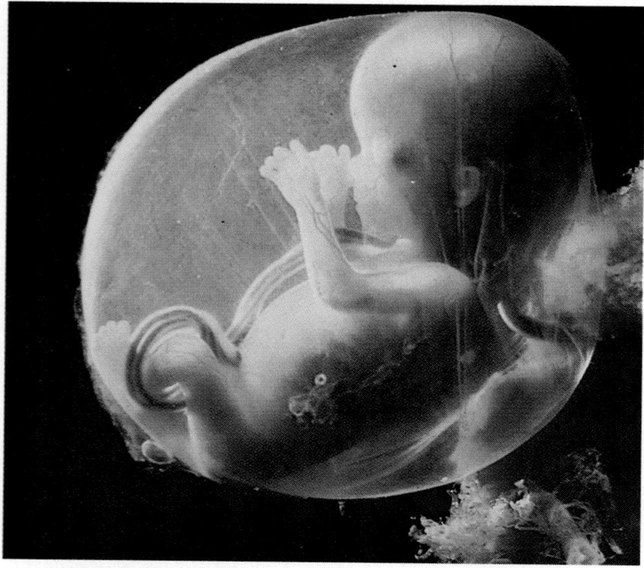

FIGURE 3–17 The fetus at 14 weeks. During this period of rapid growth the skin is so transparent that blood vessels are visible beneath it. More muscle tissue and body skeleton have developed, which holds the fetus more erect.

Source: Nilsson L: *A Child Is Born.* New York: Dell Publishing, 1990.

Between 13 and 16 weeks is a period of rapid growth. **Lanugo,** or fine hair, begins to develop, especially on the head. The skin is so transparent that blood vessels are clearly visible beneath it. More muscle tissue and body skeleton have developed and hold the fetus more erect (Figure 3–17). Active movements are present; the fetus stretches and exercises its arms and legs. It makes sucking motions, swallows amniotic fluid, and produces meconium in the intestinal tract.

Twentieth Week

The fetus doubles its C–R length and now measures 19 cm (8 in). Fetal weight is between 435 and 465 g (15.2–16.3 oz). Lanugo covers the entire body and is especially prominent on the shoulders. Subcutaneous deposits of brown fat, which has a rich blood supply, make the skin less transparent. Nipples now appear over the mammary glands. The head is covered with fine, woolly hair, and the eyebrows and eyelashes are beginning to form. Nails are present on both fingers and toes. Muscles are well developed, and the fetus is active (Figure 3–18). The mother feels fetal movement known as *quickening.* The fetal heartbeat is audible through a fetoscope. Quickening and fetal heartbeat can help in validating the estimated date of birth.

Twenty-Fourth Week

The fetus at 24 weeks reaches a *crown-to-heel (C–H)* length of 28 cm (11.2 in). It weighs about 780 g (1 lb, 10 oz). The hair on the head is growing long, and eyebrows and eyelashes have formed. The eye is structurally complete and will soon open. The fetus has a reflex hand grip (grasp reflex) and, by the end of 6 months, a startle reflex. Skin covering the body is reddish and wrinkled, with little subcutaneous fat. Skin on the hands and feet has thickened, with skin ridges on palms and soles forming distinct foot- and fingerprints. The skin over the entire body is covered with **vernix caseosa,** a protective cheeselike, fatty substance secreted by the sebaceous glands. The alveoli in the lungs are just beginning to form.

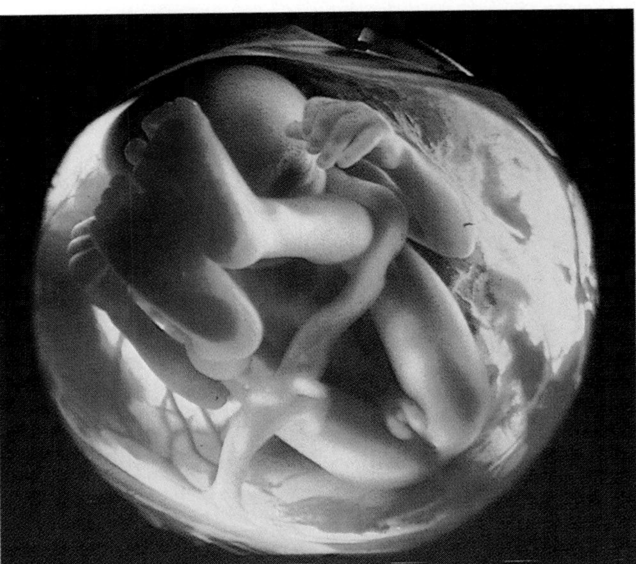

FIGURE 3–18 The fetus at 20 weeks. The fetus now weighs 435–465 g and measures about 19 cm. Subcutaneous deposits of brown fat make the skin a little less transparent. "Wooly" hair covers the head, and nails have developed on the fingers and toes.

Source: Nilsson L: *A Child Is Born*. New York: Dell Publishing, 1990.

Twenty-Fifth to Twenty-Eighth Week

At 6 months the fetal skin is still red, wrinkled, and covered with vernix caseosa. During this time the brain is developing rapidly, and the nervous system is complete enough to provide some degree of regulation of body functions. The eyelids open and close under neural control. In the male fetus, the testes begin to descend into the scrotal sac. Respiratory and circulatory systems have developed; even though the lungs are still physiologically immature, they are sufficiently developed to provide gas exchange. A fetus born at this time will require immediate and prolonged intensive care to survive, and then to decrease the risk of major handicap. The fetus at 28 weeks is about 35–38 cm (14–15 in) long C–H and weighs about 1200–1250 g (2 lb, 10.5 oz–2 lb, 12 oz).

Twenty-Ninth to Thirty-Second Week

At 30 weeks the pupillary light reflex is present (Moore and Persaud 1993). The fetus is gaining weight from an increase in body muscle and fat and weighs about 2000 g (4 lb, 6.5 oz) with a length of about 38–43 cm (15–17 in) by 32 weeks of age. The central nervous system (CNS) has matured enough to direct rhythmic breathing movements and partially control body temperature. However, the lungs are not yet fully mature. Bones are fully developed, but soft and flexible. The fetus begins storing iron, calcium, and phosphorous. In males the testicles may be located in the scrotal sac, but are often still high in the inguinal canal.

Thirty-Sixth Week

The fetus begins to get plump, with less wrinkled skin covering the deposits of subcutaneous fat. Lanugo begins to disappear, and the nails reach the edge of the fingertips. By 35 weeks of age the fetus has a firm grasp and exhibits spontaneous orientation to light. By 36 weeks of age the weight is usually 2500–2750 g (5 lb, 12 oz–6 lb, 11.5 oz), and the C–H length of the fetus is about 42–48 cm (16–19 in). An infant born at this time has a good chance of surviving but may require some special care, especially if there is intrauterine growth retardation.

Thirty-Eighth to Fortieth Week

The fetus is considered full term 38 weeks after conception. The C–H length varies from 48–52 cm (19–21 in), with males usually longer than females. Generally males also weigh more than females. The weight at term is about 3000–3600 g (6 lb, 10 oz–7 lb, 15 oz). The skin is pink and has a smooth, polished look. The only lanugo left is on the upper arms and shoulders. The hair on the head is no longer woolly but is coarse and about an inch long. Vernix caseosa is present, with heavier deposits remaining in creases and folds of the skin. The body and extremities are plump, with good skin turgor, and the fingernails extend beyond the fingertips. The chest is prominent but still a little smaller than the head, and mammary glands protrude in both sexes. The testes are in the scrotum or palpable in the inguinal canals.

As the fetus enlarges, amniotic fluid diminishes to about 500 mL or less, and the fetal body mass fills the uterine cavity. The fetus assumes what is called its *position of comfort,* or *lie*. The head is generally pointed downward following the shape of the uterus (and possibly because the head is heavier than the feet). The extremities, and often the head, are well flexed. After five months, feeding patterns, sleeping patterns, and activity patterns become established, so at term the fetus has its own body rhythms and individual style of response.

Key Facts to Remember (Fetal Development: What Parents Want to Know) on page 60 lists some important developmental milestones.

Factors Influencing Embryonic and Fetal Development

Among factors that may affect embryonic development are the quality of the sperm or ovum from which the zygote was formed, the genetic code established at fertilization, and the adequacy of the intrauterine environment. If the environment is unsuitable before cellular

KEY FACTS TO REMEMBER

Fetal Development: What Parents Want to Know

4 weeks:	The fetal heart begins to beat.
8 weeks:	All body organs are formed.
8–12 weeks:	Fetal heart tones can be heard by Doppler device.
16 weeks:	Baby's sex can be seen. Although thin, the fetus looks like a baby.
20 weeks:	Heartbeat can be heard with fetoscope. Mother feels movement (quickening). Baby develops a regular schedule of sleeping, sucking, and kicking. Hands can grasp. Baby assumes a favorite position in utero. Vernix (lanolinlike covering) protects the body and lanugo (fine hair) keeps oil on skin. Head hair, eyebrows, and eyelashes present.
24 weeks:	Weighs 1 lb, 10 oz. Activity is increasing. Fetal respiratory movements begin.
28 weeks:	Eyes begin to open and close. Baby can breathe at this time. Surfactant needed for breathing at birth is formed. Baby is two-thirds its final size.
32 weeks:	Baby has fingernails and toenails. Subcutaneous fat is being laid down. Baby appears less red and wrinkled.
38–40 weeks:	Baby fills total uterus. Baby gets antibodies from mother.

differentiation occurs, all the cells of the zygote are affected. The cells may die, which causes spontaneous abortion, or growth may be slowed, depending on the severity of the situation. When differentiation is complete and the fetal membranes have formed, an injurious agent has the greatest effect on those cells undergoing the most rapid growth. Thus the time of injury is critical in the development of anomalies.

Because organs are formed primarily during embryonic development, the growing organism is considered most vulnerable to noxious agents during the first months of pregnancy; therefore it is important to know the gestational age of the embryo or fetus to determine the potential effects of teratogens. Any agent, such as a drug, virus, or radiation, that can cause development of abnormal structures in an embryo is called a **teratogen.** Chapter 9 discusses the effects of specific teratogenic agents on the developing fetus.

Adequacy of the maternal environment is also important during the periods of rapid embryonic and fetal development. Maternal nutrition can affect brain development. The period of maximum brain growth and myelination begins with the fifth lunar month before birth and continues during the first 6 months after birth, when there is a twofold increase in myelination. In the second 6 months after birth to 2 years of age there is about a 50 percent further increase (Volpe 1995). Amino acids, glucose, and fatty acids are considered to be the primary dietary factors in brain growth. A subtle type of damage that affects the associative capacity of the brain, possibly leading to learning disabilities, may be caused by nutritional deficiency at this stage. Maternal nutrition may also predispose to the development of adult coronary heart disease, hypertension, and diabetes in babies who were small or disproportionate at birth (Godfrey and Barker 1995). (Maternal nutrition is discussed in depth in Chapter 11.)

Another prenatal influence on the intrauterine environment is maternal hyperthermia associated with sauna or hot tub use. Studies of the effects of maternal hyperthermia during the first trimester have raised concern about possible CNS defects and failure of neural tube closure. Maternal substance abuse also affects the intrauterine environment and is discussed in Chapters 12 and 25.

CHAPTER HIGHLIGHTS

- Humans have 46 chromosomes, which are divided into 23 pairs—22 pairs of autosomes and one pair of sex chromosomes.
- Mitosis is the process by which additional somatic (body) cells are formed. It provides growth and development of the organisms and replacement of body cells.
- Meiosis is the process by which new organisms are formed. It occurs during gametogenesis (oogenesis and spermatogenesis) and consists of two successive cell divisions (reduction division), which produce a gamete with 23 chromosomes (22 chromosomes and 1 sex chromosome), the haploid number of chromosomes.
- Gametes must have a haploid number (23) of chromosomes so that when the female gamete (ovum) and the male gamete (spermatozoon) unite (fertilization) to form the zygote, the normal human diploid number of chromosomes (46) is reestablished.

- An ovum is considered fertile for about 24 hours after ovulation, and the sperm is capable of fertilizing the ovum for only about 24 hours after it is deposited in the female reproductive tract.
- Fertilization usually takes place in the ampulla (outer third) of the fallopian tube.
- Both capacitation and acrosomal reaction must occur for the sperm to fertilize the ovum. Capacitation is the removal of the plasma membrane, which exposes the acrosomal covering of the sperm head. Acrosomal reaction is the deposit of hyaluronidase in the corona radiata, which allows the sperm head to penetrate the ovum.
- Sex chromosomes are referred to as X and Y. Females have two X chromosomes and males have an X and a Y chromosome. Y chromosomes are carried only by the sperm. To produce a male child, the mother contributes an X chromosome and the father contributes a Y chromosome.
- Twins are either monozygotic (identical) or dizygotic (fraternal). Dizygotic twins arise from two separate ova fertilized by two separate spermatozoa. Monozygotic twins develop from a single ovum fertilized by a single spermatozoon.
- Intrauterine development first proceeds via cellular multiplication in which the zygote undergoes rapid mitotic division called cleavage. As a result of cleavage, the zygote divides and multiplies into cell groupings called blastomeres, which are held together by the zona pellucida. The blastomeres eventually become a solid ball of cells called the morula. When a cavity forms in the morula cell mass, the inner solid cell mass is called the blastocyst.
- Implantation usually occurs in the upper part of the posterior uterine wall when the blastocyst burrows into the uterine lining.
- After implantation the endometrium is called the decidua. Decidua capsularis is the portion that covers the blastocyst. Decidua basalis is the portion that is directly under the blastocyst. Decidua vera is the portion that lines the rest of the uterine cavity.
- Embryonic membranes are called the amnion and the chorion. The amnion is formed from the ectoderm and is a thin protective membrane that contains the amniotic fluid and the embryo. The chorion is a thick membrane that develops from the trophoblast and encloses the amnion, embryo, and yolk sac.
- Amniotic fluid cushions the fetus against mechanical injury, controls the embryo's temperature, allows symmetrical external growth, prevents adherence to the amnion, and permits freedom of movement.
- Primary germ layers will give rise to all tissues, organs, and organ systems. The three primary germ cell layers are ectoderm, endoderm, and mesoderm.
- The placenta develops from the chorionic villi and decidua basalis has two parts: The maternal portion, consisting of the decidua basalis, is red and fresh-looking; the fetal portion, consisting of chorionic villi, is covered by the amnion and appears shiny and gray. The placenta is made up of 15–20 segments called cotyledons.
- The placenta serves endocrine (production of hPL, hCG, estrogen, and progesterone), metabolic, and immunologic functions. It acts as the fetus's respiratory organ, is an organ of excretion, and aids in the exchange of nutrients.
- The umbilical cord contains two umbilical arteries, which carry deoxygenated blood from the fetus to the placenta, and one umbilical vein, which carries oxygenated blood from the placenta to the fetus. The umbilical cord normally has a central insertion into the placenta. Wharton's jelly, a specialized connective tissue, helps prevent compression of the umbilical cord in utero.
- Fetal circulation is a specially designed circulatory system that provides for oxygenation of the fetus while bypassing the fetal lungs.
- Stages of fetal development include the preembryonic stage (the first 14 days of human development starting at the time of fertilization), the embryonic stage (from day 15 after fertilization, or the beginning of the 3rd week, until approximately 8 weeks after conception), and the fetal stage (from 8 weeks until birth at approximately 40 weeks postconception).
- Significant events that occur during the embryonic stage are that the fetal heart begins to beat at 4 weeks and fetal circulation is established at 6 weeks.
- The fetal stage is devoted to refining structures and perfecting function. Some significant developments during the fetal stage are:
  - At 8–12 weeks, all organ systems are formed and simply require maturation.
  - At 16 weeks, sex can be determined visually.
  - At 20 weeks, fetal heartbeat can be auscultated by a fetoscope, and the mother can feel movement (quickening).
  - At 24 weeks, vernix caseosa covers the entire body.
  - At 26–28 weeks, the eyes reopen.
  - At 32 weeks, skin appears less wrinkled and red, since subcutaneous fat has been laid down.

    - At 36 weeks, fingernails reach the ends of fingers.
    - At 40 weeks, vernix caseosa is apparent only in creases and folds of skin, and lanugo remains only on upper arms and shoulders.
- The embryo is particularly vulnerable to teratogenesis during the first 8 weeks of cell differentiation and organ system development.

REFERENCES

Ben-Shlomo I, Shalev E: The chemotactic attraction of human sperms to the oocyte: A maturing concept. *Fertil Steril* 1996; 66(1):13.

Benirschke K: The biology of the twinning process: How placentation influences outcome. *Semin Perinatol* 1995; 19(5):342.

Benirschke K: Normal development. In: *Maternal-Fetal Medicine: Principles and Practice,* 3rd ed. Creasy RK, Resnik R (editors). Philadelphia: Saunders, 1994.

Cunningham FG, MacDonald PC, Gant NG: *Williams' Obstetrics,* 20th ed. Stamford, CT: Appleton & Lange, 1997.

Eden RD, Boehm FH (editors): *Assessment and Care of the Fetus: Physiological, Clinical, and Medicolegal Principles.* Norwalk, CT: Appleton & Lange, 1990.

Gilbert WM, Brace RA: Amniotic fluid volume and normal flows to and from the amniotic cavity. *Semin Perinatol* 1993; 17(3):150.

Godfrey KM, Barker DJP: Maternal nutrition in relation to fetal and placental growth. *Euro J Obstet Gynecol and Repro Biol* 1995; 61:15.

Moore KL, Persaud TVN: *The Developing Human: Clinically Oriented Embryology,* 5th ed. Philadelphia: Saunders, 1993.

Navot D, Bergh PA: Implantation. In: *Gynecology and Obstetrics, Vol. 5.* Sciarra JJ et al (editors). Hagerstown, MD: Harper & Row, 1996.

Revenis ME, Johnson LA: Multiple gestations. In: *Neonatology: Pathophysiology and Management of the Newborn,* 4th ed. Avery GB, Fletcher M, MacDonald MG. Philadelphia: Lippincott, 1994.

Sadler TW: *Langman's Medical Embryology,* 6th ed. Baltimore: Williams & Wilkins, 1990.

Speroff L, Glass RH, Kase NG: *Clinical Gynecologic Endocrinology and Infertility,* 5th ed. Baltimore: Williams & Wilkins, 1994.

Thompson MW, McInnes RR, Willard HF: *Thompson & Thompson's Genetics in Medicine,* 5th ed. Philadelphia: Saunders, 1991.

Volpe JJ: *Neurology of the Newborn,* 3rd ed. Philadelphia: Saunders, 1995.

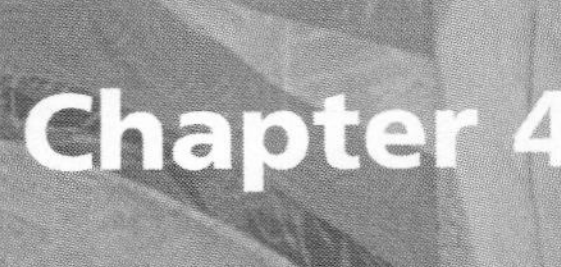

Chapter 4 Families with Special Reproductive Concerns

OBJECTIVES

- Identify the essential components of fertility.
- Describe the elements of the preliminary investigation of infertility.
- Summarize the indications for the tests and associated treatments, including assisted reproductive technologies, that are done in an infertility workup.
- Identify the physiologic and psychologic effects of infertility on a couple.
- Describe the nurse's role as counselor, educator, and advocate for couples during infertility evaluation and treatment.
- Discuss the indications for preconceptual chromosomal analysis and prenatal testing.
- Identify the general characteristics of an autosomal dominant disorder.
- Compare autosomal recessive disorders with X-linked (sex-linked) recessive disorders.
- Compare prenatal and postnatal diagnostic procedures used to determine the presence of genetic disease.
- Explore the emotional impact on a couple undergoing genetic testing or coping with the birth of a baby with a genetic disorder, and explain the nurse's role in genetic counseling.

KEY TERMS

Artificial insemination
Autosomes
Basal body temperature recording (BBT)
Chromosomes
Endometrial biopsy
Ferning capacity
Gamete intrafallopian transfer (GIFT)
Genotype
Huhner test
Hysterosalpingography (HSG)
Hysteroscopy
In vitro fertilization (IVF)
Infertility
Karyotype
Laparoscopy
Mendelian (single-gene) inheritance
Monosomies
Mosaicism
Non-Mendelian (multifactorial) inheritance
Pedigree
Phenotype
Sex chromosomes
Spinnbarkeit
Sterility
Subfertility
TORCH syndrome
Trisomies
Ultrasound
Zygote intrafallopian transfer (ZIFT)

Most couples who want children are able to have them with little trouble. Pregnancy and childbirth usually take their normal course, and a healthy baby is born without problems. But some less fortunate couples are unable to fulfill their dream of having the desired baby because of infertility or genetic problems.

This chapter explores two particularly troubling reproductive problems: the inability to conceive and the risk of bearing babies with genetic abnormalities.

Infertility

Infertility is defined as lack of conception despite unprotected sexual intercourse for at least 12 months (Hatcher et al 1994). Infertility has a profound emotional, psychologic, and economic impact on both the affected couples and society. Approximately 8 percent of couples in their reproductive years are infertile (Speroff et al 1994). **Sterility** is the term applied when there is an absolute factor preventing reproduction. **Subfertility** is used to describe a couple having difficulty conceiving because both partners have reduced fecundity (Hatcher et al 1994).

Primary infertility identifies women who have never conceived, whereas *secondary infertility* indicates those who have formerly been pregnant but have not conceived during one or more years of unprotected intercourse (Speroff et al 1994) or cannot sustain a pregnancy.

It is the public perception that the incidence of infertility is increasing, but in fact it may be decreasing (Mosher and Pratt 1993). What has changed is the composition of the infertile population; the infertility diagnosis has increased in age group 25–44 because of delayed childbearing and the entry of the baby boom cohort into this age range. The perception that infertility is on the rise may be related to the following factors:

- The increase in open discussion about reproductive issues
- The increase in assisted reproduction techniques
- The increase in availability and use of infertility services
- The increase in insurance coverage of diagnosis of and treatment for infertility
- The increased number of childless women over 35 seeking medical attention for infertility (Speroff et al 1994)
- The increased incidence of sexually transmitted disease (Wilcox and Mosher 1993)
- The decreasing population of adoptable babies

Essential Components of Fertility

Understanding the elements essential for normal fertility can help the nurse identify the many factors that may cause infertility. The following components must be present for normal fertility:

- Female partner:
  - The cervical mucus must be favorable to ensure survival of spermatozoa and facilitate passage to the upper genital tract.
  - The fallopian tubes must be patent and have normal fimbria with peristaltic movements toward the uterus to facilitate transport and interaction of ovum and sperm.
  - The ovaries must produce and release normal ova in a regular cyclic fashion.
  - There must be no obstruction between the ovaries and the uterus.
  - The endometrium must be in a physiologic state that allows implantation of the blastocyst and sustains normal growth.
  - Adequate reproductive hormones must be present.
- Male partner:
  - The testes must produce spermatozoa of normal quality, quantity, and motility.
  - The male genital tract must not be obstructed.
  - The male genital tract secretions must be normal.
  - Ejaculated spermatozoa must be deposited in the female genital tract in such a manner that they reach the cervix.

These normal findings are correlated with possible causes of deviation in Table 4–1.

With intricacies of timing and environment playing such a crucial role, it is an impressive natural phenomenon that approximately 92 percent of couples in the United States are able to conceive. The remaining 8 percent of couples suffer infertility due to a male factor (40%), a female factor (40%), or either an unknown cause or a problem with both partners (10–20%) (Speroff et al 1994). In 35 percent of infertile couples there are multiple etiologies. Professional intervention can help approximately half of infertile couples achieve pregnancy (Hill 1992).

Couples should be referred for infertility evaluation if they have been unable to conceive after at least one year of attempting to achieve pregnancy. If the woman is over 35, it may be appropriate to refer the couple after only six to nine months of unprotected intercourse without conception. At 25 years of age, the age at which couples are the most fertile, the average length of time needed to achieve conception is 5.3 months. The average 20- to 30-year-old American couple has intercourse

TABLE 4–1 Possible Causes of Infertility

Normal Findings	Deviations from Normal
Female	
Favorable cervical mucus	Cervicitis, cervical stenosis, use of coital lubricants, antisperm antibodies (immunologic response)
Clear passage between cervix and tubes	Myomas, adenomyosis, polyps, endometritis, cervical stenosis, congenital anomalies (eg, septate uterus, DES exposure)
Patent tubes with normal motility	Pelvic inflammatory disease, peritubal adhesions, endometriosis, IUD, salpingitis (eg, chlamydia, recurrent STIs), neoplasm, ectopic pregnancy, tubal ligation
Ovulation and release of ova	Primary ovarian failure, polycystic ovarian disease, hypothyroidism, pituitary tumor, lactation, periovarian adhesions, endometriosis, premature ovarian failure, hyperprolactinemia, Turner syndrome
No obstruction between ovary and tubes	Adhesions, endometriosis, pelvic inflammatory disease
Endometrial preparation	Anovulation, luteal phase defect, malformation, uterine infection, Asherman's syndrome
Male	
Normal semen analysis	Abnormalities of sperm or semen, polyspermia, congenital defect in testicular development, mumps after adolescence, cryptorchidism, infections, gonadal exposure to x-rays, chemotherapy, smoking, alcohol abuse, malnutrition, chronic or acute metabolic disease, medications (eg, morphine, ASA, ibuprofen), cocaine, marijuana use, constrictive underclothing, heat
Unobstructed genital tract	Infections, tumors, congenital anomalies, vasectomy, strictures, trauma, varicocele
Normal genital tract secretions	Infections, autoimmunity to semen, tumors
Ejaculate deposited at the cervix	Premature ejaculation, impotence, hypospadias, retrograde ejaculation (eg, diabetic), neurologic cord lesions, obesity (inhibiting adequate penetration)

one to three times a week, a frequency that should be sufficient to achieve pregnancy if all other factors are satisfactory. In about 20 percent of cases, conception occurs within the first month of unprotected intercourse (Speroff et al 1994). Delaying parenthood appears to increase the possibility that one or more of the physiologic processes necessary for conception will be adversely affected (Speroff et al 1994).

Preliminary Investigation

The easiest and least intrusive infertility testing approach is used first. Extensive testing is avoided until data confirm that the timing of intercourse and length of coital exposure have been adequate. The nurse informs the couple of the most fertile times to have intercourse during the menstrual cycle. Teaching the couple the signs and timing of ovulation and most effective times for intercourse within the cycle may solve the problem before extensive testing needs to be initiated (see Table 4–2). Primary assessment, including a comprehensive history and physical examination for any obvious causes of infertility, is done before a costly, time-consuming, and emotionally trying investigation is initiated. During the first visit for the preliminary investigation, the nurse explains the basic infertility workup. The basic investigation for the couple depends on the individuals' history and usually includes assessment of ovarian function, cervical mucosal adequacy and receptivity to sperm, sperm adequacy, tubal patency, and the general condition of the pelvic organs. Since about 40 percent of infertility is related to a male factor, a semen analysis should be one of the first diagnostic tests before moving on to the more invasive diagnostic procedures involving the woman.

TABLE 4–2 Fertility Awareness

Avoid douching and artificial lubricants. Prevent alteration of pH of vagina and introduction of spermicidal agents.

Promote retention of sperm. The male superior position with female remaining recumbent for at least 1 hour after intercourse maximizes the number of sperm reaching the cervix.

Avoid leakage of sperm. Elevate the woman's hips with a pillow after intercourse. Avoid getting up to urinate for 1 hour after intercourse.

Maximize the potential for fertilization. Have intercourse 1 to 3 times per week at intervals of no less than 48 hours.

Avoid emphasizing conception during sexual encounters to decrease anxiety and potential sexual dysfunction.

Maintain adequate nutrition and reduce stress. Using stress-reduction techniques and good nutritional habits increases sperm production.

Explore other methods to increase fertility awareness, such as home assessment of cervical mucus and basal body temperature (BBT) recordings.

It is never easy to discuss one's own sexual activity, especially when potentially irreversible problems with fertility may exist. The mutual desire to have children is a cornerstone of many marriages. A fertility problem is a deeply personal, emotion-laden area in a couple's life (Blenner 1991). The self-esteem of one or both partners may be threatened if the inability to conceive is perceived as a lack of virility or femininity. The nurse can provide comfort to the client by offering a sympathetic ear, a nonjudgmental atmosphere, and appropriate

TABLE 4–3 Initial Infertility Physical Workup and Laboratory Evaluations

Female	Male
Physical examination Assessment of height, weight, blood pressure, temperature, and general health status Endocrine evaluation of thyroid for exophthalmos, lid lag, tremor, or palpable gland Optic fundi evaluation for presence of increased intracranial pressure, especially in oligomenorrheal or amenorrheal women (possible pituitary tumor) Reproductive features (including breast and external genital area) Physical ability to tolerate pregnancy Pelvic examination Papanicolaou smear Culture for gonorrhea if indicated and possibly chlamydia or mycoplasma culture (opinions vary) Signs of vaginal infections (Chapter 10) Shape of escutcheon (eg, Does pubic hair distribution resemble that of a male?) Size of clitoris (enlargement caused by endocrine disorders) Evaluation of cervix: old lacerations, tears, erosion, polyps, condition and shape of os, signs of infections, cervical mucus (evaluate for estrogen effect of spinnbarkeit and cervical ferning) Bimanual examination Size, shape, position, and motility of uterus Presence of congenital anomalies Presence of endometriosis Evaluation of adnexa: ovarian size, cysts, fixations, or tumors Rectovaginal examination Presence of retroflexed or retroverted uterus Presence of rectouterine pouch masses Presence of possible endometriosis Laboratory examination Complete blood count Sedimentation rate if indicated Serology Urinalysis Rh factor and blood grouping If indicated, thyroid function tests, prolactin levels, glucose tolerance test, 17-ketosteroid assay, 17-hydrocorticoid assay, testosterone or dehydroepiandrosterone levels	Physical examination General health (assessment of height, weight, blood pressure) Endocrine evaluation (eg, presence of gynecomastia) Visual fields evaluation for bitemporal hemianopia Abnormal hair patterns Urologic examination (includes presence or absence of phimosis; location of urethral meatus; size and consistency of each testis, vas deferens, and epididymis; presence of varicocele) Rectal examination Size and consistency of the prostate with microscopic evaluation of prostate fluid for signs of infection Size and consistency of seminal vesicles Laboratory examination Complete blood count Sedimentation rate if indicated Serology Urinalysis Rh factor and blood grouping Semen analysis If indicated, testicular biopsy, buccal smear

information and instructions throughout the diagnostic and therapeutic process. Since counseling includes discussion of very personal matters, nurses who are comfortable with their own sexuality are more capable of establishing rapport and eliciting relevant information.

The first interview should be with both partners and should include a comprehensive history of both partners and a physical and pelvic examination of the woman. Table 4–3 outlines what is entailed in a complete infertility physical workup and laboratory evaluation for both partners. Figure 4–1 outlines the historical database, diagnostic tests usually performed, and health care interventions in cases of infertility.

Tests for Infertility

After a thorough history and physical examination of both partners, tests may be initiated to identify causes of infertility (Stansberry 1996).

Due to the high incidence of multifactorial infertility, it is important to assess both partners. A thorough female evaluation includes assessment of ovulatory function, as well as structure and function of the cervix, uterus, fallopian tubes, and ovaries. See Chapter 3 for an in-depth discussion of the fertility cycle. Evaluation of the male may include at least two semen analyses to confirm or rule out a seminal deficiency. Functional tests such as the hamster sperm penetration assay (SPA) or serum and semen immunobead testing for the presence of antisperm antibody (immunologic infertility) may be performed.

Female Assessment

Evaluation of Ovulatory Factors Ovulation problems account for approximately 15 percent of female infertility (Speroff et al 1994). For a review of female reproductive cycle characteristics see Chapter 2.

One basic test of ovulatory function is the **basal body temperature (BBT)** recording, which aids in identification of follicular and luteal phase abnormalities. At the initial visit, the nurse instructs the woman in the technique of recording basal body temperature, which may be taken with a BBT thermometer. This special kind of thermometer measures temperatures between 96F and 100F and is calibrated by tenths of a degree, making

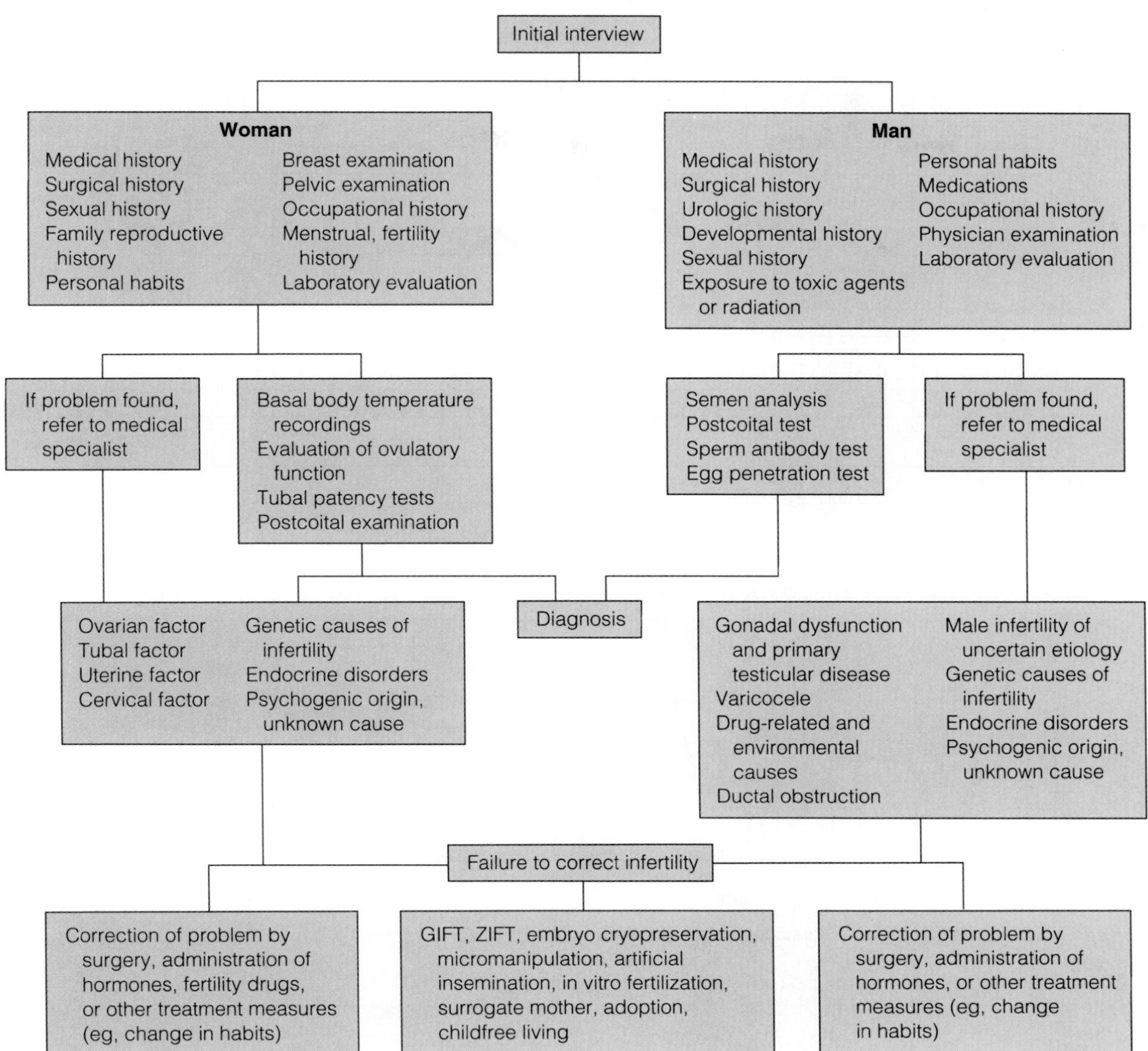

FIGURE 4–1 Flow chart for management of the infertile couple.

slight temperature changes readily apparent. The BBT should be taken every morning before getting out of bed and after at least 3 hours of sleep (Hatcher et al 1994). Studies have shown that in addition to the traditional glass/mercury BBT thermometer, tympanic thermometry is a valid method to obtain basal body temperatures and has the advantage of being simple and taking less than 2 minutes to get a reading (Wolf and Baker 1993).

The woman records daily variations on the temperature graph. The graph shows a typical biphasic pattern during ovulatory cycles, whereas in anovulatory cycles it remains monophasic. The woman uses the readings on the temperature graph to detect ovulation and timing of intercourse (Figure 4–2).

Basal temperature for females in the preovulatory phase is usually below 98F (36.7C). As ovulation approaches, production of estrogen increases, which at its peak causes a slight drop, then a rise, in the basal temperature. When ovulation occurs, there is a surge of luteinizing hormone (LH), and progesterone is produced by the corpus luteum, causing a 0.5F to 1.0F (0.3C to 0.6C) rise in basal temperature and an atypical biphasic pattern. Figure 4–2*B* shows a biphasic ovulatory BBT chart. Progesterone is thermogenic (produces heat); therefore it maintains the temperature increase during the second half of the menstrual cycle (luteal phase). Temperature elevation does not predict the day of ovulation, but it does provide supportive evidence of ovulation about a day after it has occurred. Actual release of the ovum probably occurs 24–36 hours before the first temperature elevation (Speroff et al 1994).

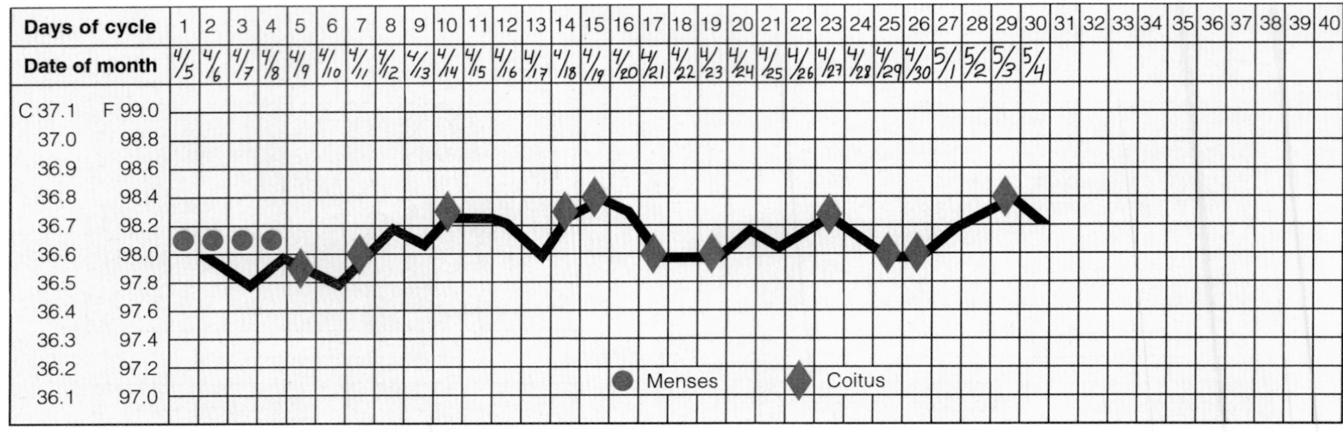

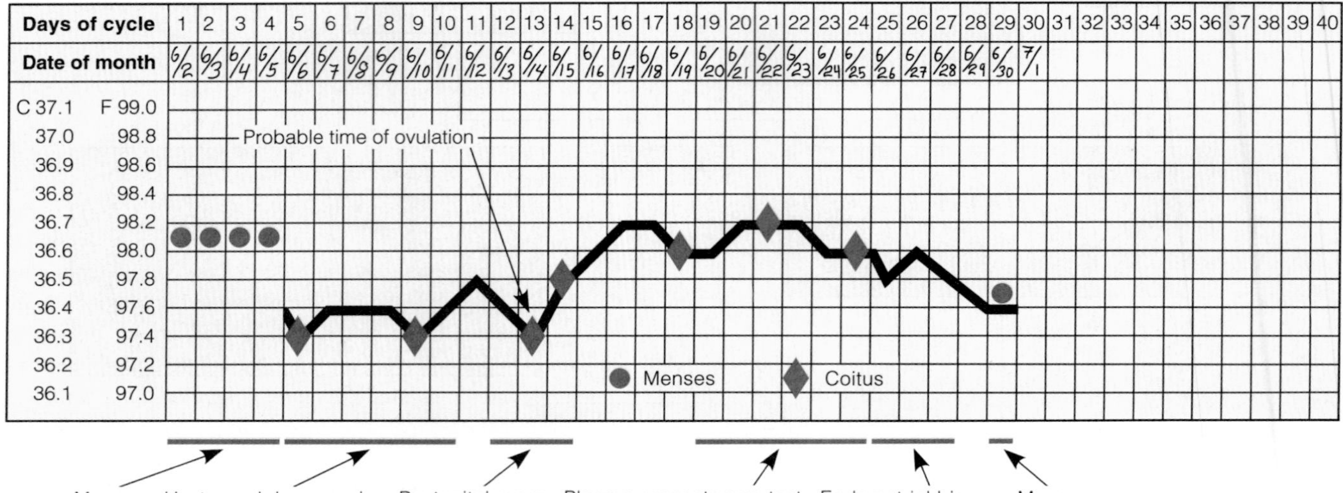

FIGURE 4–2 ***A*** A monophasic, anovulatory basal body temperature (BBT) chart. ***B*** A biphasic BBT chart illustrating probable time of ovulation, the different types of testing, and the time in the cycle that each would be performed.

With the additional documentation of coitus, serial BBT charts can be used to indicate approximately when the woman is ovulating and if intercourse is occurring at the proper time to achieve conception. A proposed schedule for intercourse based on serial BBT charts might be to recommend sexual intercourse *every other day* beginning 3–4 days before, and continuing for 2–3 days after, the expected time of ovulation. See Teaching Guide: Self-Care Methods of Determining Ovulation on pages 70 and 71.

Hormonal assessments of ovulatory function fall into the following categories:

1. *Gonadotropin levels (FSH, LH).* Baseline hormonal assessment of FSH and LH provides valuable information about normal ovulatory function. Measured on cycle day 3, FSH is the single most valuable test of ovarian reserve and function. FSH should always be measured, particularly in women over 35, to predict the potential for successful treatment with ovulation induction treatment cycles. High levels predict a very poor outcome for conception and pregnancy. LH levels may be measured early in the cycle to rule out androgen excess disorders, causing a disruption in normal follicular development and oocyte maturation. Daily sampling of LH at midcycle can detect the LH surge. The day of the LH surge is believed to be the day of maximum fertility. Urine LH ovulation prediction kits are also available for home use to better time postcoital testing, insemination, and coitus.
2. *Progesterone assays.* Progesterone levels furnish the best evidence of ovulation and corpus luteum functioning. Serum levels begin to rise with the LH surge and peak about 8 days later. A level of 3 ng/mL 3 days after the LH surge confirms ovulation. On day 21 (7 days postovulation) a level of

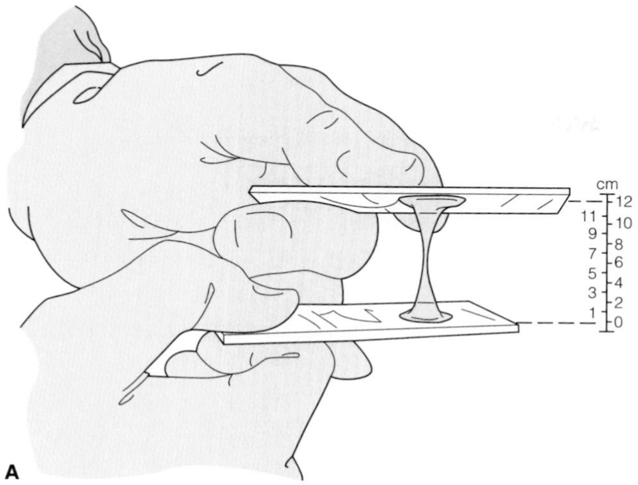

A

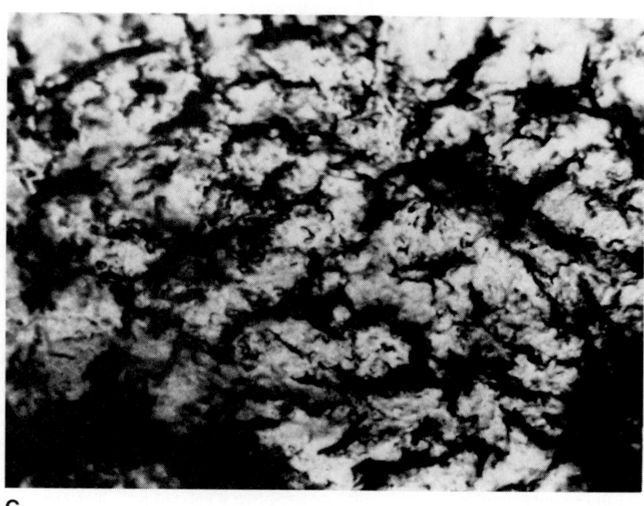

C

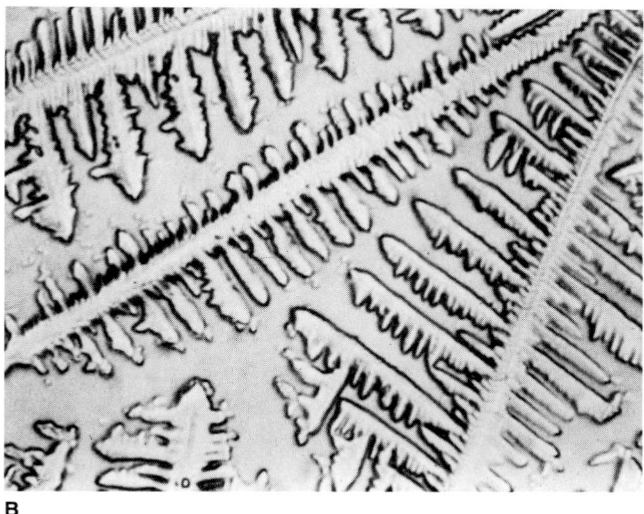

B

FIGURE 4–3 ***A*** Spinnbarkeit (elasticity). ***B*** Ferning pattern. ***C*** Lack of ferning.

Source: Speroff L et al: *Clinical Gynecologic Endocrinology and Infertility,* 5th ed. Baltimore: Williams & Wilkins, 1994, p. 818.

10 ng/mL or higher indicates an adequate luteal phase.

Endometrial biopsy provides information about the effects of progesterone produced by the corpus luteum after ovulation and endometrial receptivity. The biopsy is performed not earlier than 10–12 days after ovulation using a paracervical block. The simple procedure requires only a little cervical dilatation (3 mm diameter) and consists of removing a sample of endometrium with a small pipette attached to suction (Speroff et al 1994). The patient should be informed that some pelvic discomfort, cramping, and vaginal spotting is normal during and following the procedure. The onset of menses following biopsy should be reported for accurate interpretation of the report.

A dysfunction may exist if the endometrial lining does not show the expected amount of secretory tissue for that day of the woman's menstrual cycle. Endometrial biopsies and serum progesterone assay may both be necessary to confirm luteal phase dysfunction.

Ultrasound is now an invaluable adjunct in infertility diagnosis and treatment. Transvaginal ultrasound is the method of choice for follicular monitoring of patients undergoing induction cycles, for timing ovulation for insemination and intercourse, for IVF oocycte retrieval, and for monitoring early pregnancy.

Evaluation of Cervical Factors The cervical mucous cells of the endocervix consist predominantly of water. As ovulation approaches, the ovary increases its secretion of estrogen and produces changes in the cervical mucus. The amount of mucus increases tenfold, and the water content rises significantly.

Mucus elasticity (**spinnbarkeit**) increases and viscosity decreases at ovulation. Excellent spinnbarkeit exists when the mucus can be stretched 8 to 10 cm or longer (Jaffe and Jewelewicz 1991). This is accomplished by using two glass slides (Figure 4–3*A*) or by grasping some mucus at the external os and stretching it through the vagina toward the introitus. (See Teaching Guide: Self-Care Methods of Determining Ovulation.)

The **ferning capacity** (crystallization) (Figure 4–3*B*) of the cervical mucus also increases as ovulation approaches. Ferning is caused by *decreased* levels of salt and water interacting with the glycoproteins in the mucus during the ovulatory period and is thus an indirect indication of estrogen production. To test for ferning, mucus is obtained from the cervical os, spread on a glass

TEACHING GUIDE Self-Care Methods of Determining Ovulation

Assessment
The nurse focuses on the woman's knowledge of her own body functions, mucus secretions, and menstrual cycle.

Nursing Diagnosis
The essential nursing diagnoses will probably be: Self-care deficit related to lack of knowledge of normal body changes occurring with menstruation and ovulation; Ineffective individual coping related to inexperience with self-care measures for determining fertile days.

Nursing Plan and Implementation
The teaching plan will include information on expected changes in cervical mucus and body temperature related to menstrual cycle, how to recognize that ovulation has occurred, and self-care methods for determining fertility days.

Client Goals
At the completion of the teaching session the woman will be able to:

1. Accurately identify cervical mucus changes
2. Accurately take and record BBT
3. Discuss the changes in BBT and cervical mucus that indicate ovulation has occurred
4. Summarize physical symptoms that may indicate ovulation has occurred.

Teaching Plan

Content

BASAL BODY TEMPERATURE (BBT) Expected findings: The BBT can sometimes drop 12 to 24 hours before ovulation, but a sustained rise *almost always* follows for several days. Or a biphasic pattern with temperature elevation for 12 to 14 days prior to menstruation can be seen. At ovulation, temperature will rise 0.4–0.8F above baseline preovulatory level. Some women notice a drop in temperature 24 hours prior to ovulation. Once a 0.4–0.8F rise has occurred for 3 consecutive days, a woman who does not desire pregnancy can safely have intercourse because her fertile days have passed. All 3 days should have higher temperature readings than any of the previous days in the cycle. A woman needs to take her BBT for 3 to 4 months to develop a consistent pattern.

Procedure: For accurate results the woman should take her temperature for 5 minutes every morning before she gets out of bed (needs at least 3 hours of sleep) and before starting any activity (including smoking). She should choose one site (oral, vaginal, rectal) and use same site each time. A BBT thermometer is preferable. After 5 minutes she should record her temperature on special BBT chart (with 0.1 markings). She connects the temperature dots for each day to see baseline temperature readings.

After taking her temperature, the woman must shake down the thermometer to prepare for the next day. This is important because even the activity of shaking the thermometer before use can cause a small increase in basal temperature.

Special considerations include situations that can disturb body temperature: large alcohol intake, sleeplessness, gastrointestinal or other febrile illness, immunization, warm or hot climate, jet lag, shift work, or use of electric blanket.

Teaching Method

Discuss BBT changes.

Demonstrate BBT thermometer and chart.

Provide pictures of anovulation cycle and biphasic cycle.

slide, allowed to air dry, and examined under the microscope. Within 24 to 48 hours postovulation, rising levels of progesterone markedly decrease the quantity of cervical mucus and increase its viscosity and cellularity. The resulting absence of spinnbarkeit and ferning capacity promotes sperm survival.

To be receptive to sperm, cervical mucus must be thin, clear, watery, profuse, alkaline, and acellular

TEACHING GUIDE continued

Teaching Plan *continued*

CERVICAL MUCUS METHOD Expected findings: Pre- and postovulatory mucus is yellow, thick, and dry; absent; or white and cloudy. Close to or during ovulation mucus is clear, slippery (like egg whites), and elastic (can be stretched between two fingers—*spinnbarkeit*). Ovulation most likely occurs about 24 hours after the last day of abundant, slippery discharge (Hatcher et al 1994). Four days after peak mucus or when it is again dry, thick, and cloudy, the woman has passed her fertile days and may resume intercourse.

Show woman posters of mucus changes, spinnbarkeit of different elasticity.

Discuss feelings about actual procedure.

Mucus changes: During menstruation blood covers up sensation of wetness or mucus. For a few days after menstruation the vagina feels moist but is not distinctly wet (called "dry" days). The next mucus stage is thick, cloudy, whitish or yellowish, and sticky mucus. Vagina still doesn't feel wet, and this lasts for several days. As ovulation nears, mucus usually becomes more abundant, accompanied by an increasingly wet sensation. Next the clear slippery mucus decreases until it is no longer detectable, and either the thick, cloudy, sticky mucus returns or there is no mucus at all until the next menstrual period.

Procedure: The woman should check her vagina each day when she uses the bathroom, either by dabbing the vaginal opening with toilet paper or by putting a finger inside the opening. She should note the wetness (presence of mucus), collect mucus, and look at its color and consistency. Findings are recorded on chart each day. Several cycles of mucus changes are recorded to become familiar with the pattern before relying on this method.

Special considerations: Presence and consistency of mucus is altered by vaginal infection, vaginal medications such as creams or suppositories, spermicides, lubricants, douching, sexual arousal, or semen.

When pregnancy is not desired, some advise complete abstinence throughout the *first* cycle, during which a woman charts her mucus changes. This helps her avoid confusing mucus with semen and normal sexual lubrication.

OTHER Additional physical findings that may indicate ovulation include slight vaginal spotting, *mittelschmertz,* increased libido.

Discuss rationale for physical changes. Answer questions.

Evaluation

Teaching has been effective if the nurse discussed BBT and cervical mucus changes associated with ovulation, demonstrated BBT procedure and charting of BBT and cervical mucus changes. The woman feels comfortable with BBT and cervical mucus procedure and completion of charting. The woman is able to describe her body functions, how they change, and how they can be used to identify fertile periods and the time at which ovulation may occur.

(Geerling 1995). As shown in Figure 4–4, the mazelike microscopic mucoid strands align in a parallel manner to allow for easy sperm passage. The mucus is termed inhospitable if these changes do not occur.

Cervical mucus inhospitable to sperm survival can have several causes, some of which are treatable (eg, estrogen secretion may be inadequate for developing of receptive mucus). Therapy with supplemental estrogen for

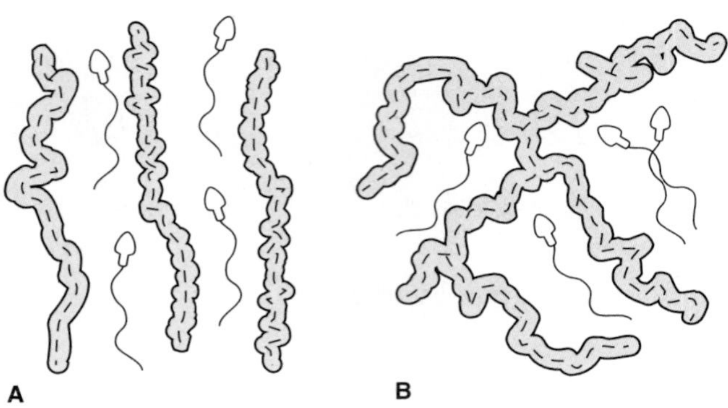

FIGURE 4–4 Sperm passage through cervical mucus. ***A*** Appearance at the time of ovulation with channels favoring efficient sperm penetration and migration upward. ***B*** Unfavorable mazelike configuration found at other times during the menstrual cycle.

Source: Corson S: *Conquering Infertility.* New York: Prentice Hall, 1990, p 16.

approximately 6 days before expected ovulation encourages the formation of suitable spinnbarkeit (Speroff et al 1994). Cervical infection, another cause of mucosal hostility to sperm, can be treated, depending on the type of infection.

Cone biopsy, electrocautery, or cryosurgery of the cervix may remove large numbers of mucus-producing glands, creating a "dry cervix" that decreases sperm survival. Profuse mucus is necessary for a hospitable sperm environment. The cervix can also be the site of secretory immunologic reactions in which antisperm antibodies are produced, causing agglutination or immobilization of sperm. The most widely used serum-sperm bioassay to detect specific classes of antibodies in serum and seminal fluid is immunobead testing by RIA. The treatment for antisperm antibodies may include intrauterine insemination of the male's washed sperm to bypass the cervical factor.

The postcoital examination (**Huhner test** or PCT) is performed 1 or 2 days before the expected date of ovulation by previous BBT charts, the length of prior cycles, or a urinary LH kit. This examination evaluates the cervical mucus, sperm motility, sperm mucus interaction, and the sperm's ability to negotiate the cervical mucus barrier (Tredway 1996).

The couple is asked to have intercourse up to 12 hours before the examination. The optimal time for the exam is 2 to 3 hours after coitus. A small plastic catheter attached to a 10 mL syringe is placed in the cervix. Mucus is aspirated from the internal and external os, measured, and examined microscopically for signs of infection, spinnbarkeit, ferning, and number and motility of active spermatozoa per high-power field (HPF) and number of sperm with poor or no motility. The postcoital exam focuses attention on the timing of intercourse and has the potential for sexual relationship difficulties unless the infertile couple has a satisfying sexual relationship (Oei et al 1996).

Evaluation of Uterine Structures and Tubal Patency

Tubal patency tests are usually done after BBT evaluation, semen analysis, and the other less invasive tests have been done and evaluated. Tubal patency and uterine structure are usually evaluated by hysterosalpingography. Other invasive tests of tubular function are laparoscopy and hysteroscopy. Hysteroscopy may be performed earlier in the evaluation if the woman's history suggests possible tubal damage or uterine abnormalities.

Hysterosalpingography (HSG or hysterogram) involves an instillation of a radiopaque substance into the uterine cavity. As the substance fills the uterus and fallopian tubes and spills into the peritoneal cavity, it is viewed with x-ray techniques. This procedure can reveal tubal patency and any distortions of the uterine cavity. In addition the oil-based dye and injection pressure used in HSG may have a therapeutic effect. This effect may be caused by the flushing of debris, breaking of adhesions, induction of peristalsis by the instillation, or improvement of cervical mucus because the iodine exerts a bacteriostatic effect on the mucous membranes and decreases phagocytosis of sperm (Speroff et al 1994, Karande et al 1995).

The hysterosalpingography should be performed in the proliferative phase of the cycle to avoid interrupting an early pregnancy. This timing also avoids the lush secretory changes in the endometrium that occur after ovulation, which may prevent the passage of the dye through the tubes and present a false picture of cornual obstruction. Hysterosalpingography causes moderate discomfort. The pain is referred from the peritoneum (which is irritated by the subdiaphragmatic collection of gas) to the shoulder. The cramping may be decreased if the radiopaque dye is warmed to body temperature before instillation. Women can take OTC prostaglandin synthesis inhibitor 30 minutes before the procedure to decrease the pain. HSG can also cause recurrence of pelvic inflammatory disease, so prophylactic antibiotics are recommended (Hatcher et al 1994).

Hysteroscopy allows the physician to further evaluate any areas of suspicion within the uterine cavity revealed by the HSG. It is often done in conjunction with a laparoscopy, but it can be done independently and does not require general anesthesia. A fiberoptic instrument is inserted into the uterus for further evaluation of polyps, myomata, or structural variations (Speroff et al 1994).

Laparoscopy enables direct visualization of the pelvic organs and is usually done 6 to 8 months after the HSG unless symptoms suggest the need for earlier evaluation. The woman is usually given a general anesthetic for this procedure. Entry is generally made through an incision in the umbilical area, although it is occasionally done suprapubically. The peritoneal cavity is distended with carbon-dioxide gas so that the pelvic organs can be directly visualized with a fiberoptic instrument. Tubular patency can be assessed by instillation of dye into the uterine cavity through the cervix. The pelvis is evaluated for endometriosis, adhesions, organ fixations, pelvic inflammatory disease, tumors, and cysts. The intraperitoneal gas is usually manually expressed at the end of the procedure. In routine preanesthesia instructions, the woman is told that for 24 to 48 hours after the procedure she may have some discomfort from organ displacement and shoulder and chest pain caused by gas in the abdomen. She should be informed that she can resume normal activities after resting for about 2 days. Using postoperative pain medication and assuming a knee chest position may help relieve any discomfort.

Male Assessment

A semen analysis is the most important initial diagnostic study of the male and should be done early in the couple's evaluation before invasive testing of the woman. Although a postcoital test can provide information about sperm viability, it does not provide sufficient information about normal seminal parameters. To obtain adequate results, the specimen is collected after 2 to 3 days of abstinence and usually by masturbation to avoid contamination or loss of any ejaculate. If the male has difficulty producing sperm by masturbation, special condoms are available to collect the sperm during intercourse. Regular or nonlatex (without nonoxynol-9) condoms should not be used, because they contain spermicidal agents and sperm can be lost in the condom. The man should place the specimen in a sterile container marked with the time of collection and date of previous ejaculation, maintain it at body temperature, and bring it to the laboratory within an hour of collection if possible (2–3 hours maximum). Repeated semen analyses may be required to adequately identify the male's fertility potential. A minimum of two separate analyses are recommended for confirmation. Because the cycle of spermatogenesis is 72 days, semen collections should be repeated at least 74 days apart to allow for new germ cell maturation (Speroff et al 1994).

Sperm analysis provides information about sperm motility and morphology as well as a determination of the absolute number of spermatozoa present (Table 4–4). Debate exists over the absolute number of sperm required for fertility. An infertile specimen is one that has fewer than 20 million sperm per milliliter, less than 50 percent motility at 6 hours, or less than 50 percent normal sperm forms (World Health Organization 1992).

Spermatozoa have been shown to possess intrinsic antigens that can provoke male immunologic infertility. This is especially apparent following vasectomy reversals, where an autoimmunity (the male produces antibodies to his sperm) to sperm develops (Haas 1994). Research now indicates that it is the actual presence of antibodies on the spermatozoal surface (not just the presence of antibodies in the serum) that affects sperm function and thus leads to subfertility. Treatment for the presence of sperm antibodies in the male ejaculate may include immunosuppression and sperm washing or dilution insemination techniques. Donor insemination is a treatment alternative for antibodies in the male and possibly in the female if she reacts only to her partner's sperm (Speroff et al 1994).

TABLE 4–4 Normal Semen Analysis

Factor	Value
Volume	2 to 6 mL
pH	7.0 to 8.0
Total sperm count	20 million
Liquefaction	Complete in 1 hour
Motility	50% or greater
Normal forms	60% or greater

Source: Speroff L, Glass RH, Kase NG: *Clinical Gynecologic Endocrinology and Infertility*, 4th ed. Baltimore: Williams & Wilkins, 1989.

Methods of Infertility Management

Pharmacologic Methods

If an ovulation defect has been detected during the fertility testing, the treatment depends on the specific cause. In the presence of normal ovaries, a normal prolactin level, and intact pituitary gland, *clomiphene citrate* (Clomid, Serophene) is often used. This medication induces ovulation in 80 percent of women by actions at both the hypothalamic and ovarian levels; 40 percent of these women will become pregnant.

Approximately 5 percent of women develop multiple gestation pregnancies, almost exclusively twins (Speroff et al 1994). Clomiphene works by increasing the secretion of LH and FSH, which stimulates follicle growth. The woman takes 50–250 mg per day orally for 5 days starting from day 3 to 5 after last menses (Hammond 1996). The woman usually starts with 50 mg per day and increases the dose by 50 mg per day, if there is no response, to a maximum of 250 mg (Mishell 1991). The clinician may need to give estrogen simultaneously if cervical mucus decreases.

The woman is informed that if ovulation occurs, it is expected to occur 5–10 days after the last dose. The presence of ovulation and evaluation of the response to therapy is assessed by BBT or urinary LH kit for in-home use, ultrasound evaluation, and possibly progesterone assays in conjunction with an endometrial biopsy.

After the first treatment cycle, a pelvic exam should be done to rule out ovarian enlargement, or hyperstimulation syndrome. Ovarian enlargement and abdominal discomfort may result from follicular growth and formation of multiple corpus lutea. Persistence of ovarian cysts is a contraindication for further clomiphene administration. Other side effects include hot flashes, abdominal distention, bloating, breast discomfort, nausea and vomiting, vision problems (such as visual spots), headache, and dryness or loss of hair (Hammond 1996). Supplemental low-dose estrogen may be given to ensure appropriate quality and quantity of cervical mucus.

The nurse determines if the couple has been advised to have sexual intercourse every other day for 1 week beginning 5 days after the last day of medications. The nurse also reminds couples that if the woman doesn't have a period she must be checked for the possibility of pregnancy before another trial of clomiphene is started.

Self-Care Measures

Women can assess the presence of ovulation and possible response to clomiphene therapy by doing BBT and urinary LH tests. The woman should be knowledgeable about side effects and call her health care provider if they occur. When visual disturbances (flashes, blurring, spots) occur, the woman should avoid brightly lit rooms. This side effect disappears within a few days or weeks after discontinuation of therapy (Speroff et al 1994). The occurrence of hot flashes may be due to the antiestrogenic properties of clomiphene. Some relief can be obtained by increasing intake of fluids and using fans.

Human menopausal gonadotropin (hMG), also referred to as *menotropin,* is a combination of FSH and LH obtained from postmenopausal women's urine and administered intramuscularly every day for varying periods of time during the first half of the cycle to stimulate follicular development. The most common commercial preparation is Pergonal. Menotropins require close observation with serum estradiol and ultrasound. Monitoring of follicle development is necessary to minimize the risk of multiple pregnancy and to avoid overstimulation syndrome. When follicle maturation has occurred, *human chorionic gonadotropin (hCG)* may be administered by intramuscular injection to stimulate ovulation. The couple is advised to have intercourse on the day of hCG administration and for the next 2 days. The multiple birth rate is about 20 percent, with less than 1 percent resulting in multiples greater than triplets. Women who elect to have hMG medication usually have passed through all other forms of management without conceiving. Strong emotional support and thorough education are needed because of the numerous office visits and injections. Often the male partner is instructed, with return demonstration, to administer the daily injections.

When hyperprolactinemia accompanies anovulation, the infertility may be treated with *bromocriptine* (Parlodel). This medication acts directly on the prolactin-secreting cells in the anterior pituitary. It inhibits the pituitary's secretion of prolactin—thus preventing suppression of the pulsatile secretion of FSH and LH. This restores normal menstrual cycles and induces ovulation by allowing FSH and LH production. High prolactin levels may impair the glandular production of FSH and LH or block their action on the ovaries. If treatment is successful, the tests of ovulatory function will indicate that ovulation is occurring with a normal luteal phase. Bromocriptine should be discontinued if pregnancy is suspected or at the anticipated time of ovulation because of its possible teratogenic effects. Other side effects include nausea, diarrhea, dizziness, headache, and fatigue.

When endometriosis is determined to be the cause of the infertility, *danazol* (Danocrine) may be given to suppress ovulation and menstruation and to effect atrophy of the ectopic endometrial tissue. Temporary suppression has been shown to result in healing of the endometriosis. The treatment regimen may last for 6–12 months or longer, depending on the severity of the disease.

Other pharmacologic treatments involve use of oral contraceptives, oral medroxyprogesterone acetate, or GnRH agonists (Haney 1994). The management and care of endometriosis is further discussed in Chapter 5.

Gonadotropin-releasing hormone (GnRH) is a therapeutic tool for ovulation stimulation. It is used for women who have insufficient endogenous release of GnRH. Administration is usually by continuous intravenous infusion accomplished by a portable infusion pump with a pulsatile mechanism worn on a belt around the waist. The length of treatment varies from 2 to 4 weeks and hCG is also given to stimulate ovulation. The risk of multiple gestation and hyperstimulation is less than with hMG therapy, and the treatment is also less expensive (Speroff et al 1994). Significant client education and support are necessary for effective use of the pump. Some women find the pump cumbersome. Treatment of luteal phase defects may include the use of progesterone to augment luteal phase progesterone levels or ovulation induction agents, such as clomiphene citrate or menotropins, to augment proliferative phase FSH production of the developing follicle.

Artificial Insemination

Artificial insemination, with either the partner's semen *(AIH)* or that of a donor *(AID),* is the depositing of semen at the cervical os or in the uterus by mechanical means. Some people use the term *therapeutic donor insemination (TDI)* in place of AID (Speroff et al 1994). AIH is used in cases of too small volumes of sperm, decreased motility, and teratospermia (low percentage, abnormal morphology); anatomic defects accompanied by inadequate deposition or penetration of semen; or retrograde ejaculation (Corson 1990).

Donor insemination is considered in cases of azoospermia (absence of sperm), severe oligo- or asthenospermia, inherited male sex-linked disorders, and autosomal dominant disorders. Some states have specified the parental rights of single women and donors, but most are silent on this issue (Speroff et al 1994).

Numerous factors need to be evaluated before AID is performed. Has every possible effort been made to diagnose and treat the cause of the male infertility? Do tests indicate normal fertility and sperm/ovum transport in the woman? Has the couple had an opportunity to discuss this option with an infertility counselor to explore the issues of secrecy, disclosure, and potential feelings of loss the couple (particularly the male partner) may feel about not having a genetic child (Townsend 1992). Are there any religious constraints?

After making the decision, the couple should allow themselves time to further assess their concerns and explore their feelings individually and together to ensure that this option is acceptable to both. Donor insemination now has strict screening and processing procedures to prevent transmission of a genetic defect or sexually transmitted disease to the offspring or recipient. American Fertility Society (1990) guidelines include mandatory medical and infectious disease screening of both donor and recipient, informed consent from all parties, limited number of pregnancies per donor, and accurate means of record keeping (Gutmann and Corson 1994). Because of the risk of infectious disease transmission, donated sperm must be frozen and quarantined for 6 months from the time of acquisition, and the donor must be retested before sperm can be released for use.

Intrauterine insemination (IUI) is an option for many couples with or without ovulation induction therapy before more aggressive treatments such as in vitro fertilization (IVF) and gamete intrafallopian transfer (GIFT) are employed. Success rates vary from 10–25 percent, depending on indications for use and the woman's age.

In Vitro Fertilization

The **in vitro fertilization (IVF)** procedure is selectively used in cases in which infertility has resulted from tubal factors, mucus abnormalities, male infertility, unexplained infertility, male and female immunologic infertility, and cervical factors. In IVF a woman's eggs are collected from her ovaries, fertilized in the laboratory, and placed into her uterus after normal embryo development has begun. If the procedure is successful, the embryo continues to develop in the uterus, and pregnancy proceeds naturally.

The potential for a successful pregnancy with IVF is maximized when three to four embryos are replaced. For this reason ovulation is induced using fertility drugs. Follicular development and oocyte maturity are monitored frequently with ultrasound and hormonal assays.

Women with three to six cycles of IVF have a good chance of achieving pregnancy. Many couples find the emotional, physical, and financial costs of going beyond three to six cycles too difficult (Speroff et al 1994). Clinical delivery rates reported by the Society of Assisted Reproductive Technology (SART) in 1992 were 19 percent per embryo replacement for women under the age of 40 when no male factor was present (SART 1993). It should be noted that some centers show increased maternal and neonatal morbidity associated with IVF because of the multiple gestation rates of 15–30 percent (Tallo et al 1995).

Other Assisted Reproductive Techniques (ART)

Other assisted reproductive technologies being used include **gamete intrafallopian transfer (GIFT)** and **zygote intrafallopian transfer (ZIFT)** (Medical Research International and SART 1992). In GIFT, ovulation is induced as it is in IVF. However, after the eggs are retrieved, they are placed directly into the fallopian tube along with the male's sperm, usually via laparoscopy. Fertilization occurs in the fallopian tube as with normal conception (in vivo), rather than in the laboratory (in vitro), a procedure acceptable to the Catholic church (Mastroyannis 1993). In ZIFT and tubal embryo transfer (TET), eggs are retrieved and incubated with the male's sperm as they are for IVF. However, the eggs are transferred back to the woman's body at a much earlier stage of cell division and, as in GIFT, are placed in the fallopian tube or tubes and not the uterus. In TET this is done at the embryo stage. These procedures allow fertilization to be documented, which is not possible with GIFT, and the pregnancy rate is theoretically increased when the conceptus is placed in the fallopian tube so that normal fertilization and implantation are better mimicked than with IVF, in which replacement is in the uterus.

Other technologies involve oocyte donation (Lessor et al 1993), and cryopreservation of the embryo (Schenker and Ezra 1994). Success rates for these procedures are generally high, and GIFT may be more acceptable by adherents of some religions, since fertilization does not occur outside the woman's body. The success rates are 26.5 percent for GIFT, 28.8 percent for ZIFT (Goode and Hahn 1993, Townsend 1992), 9 percent for frozen embryo transfer, and 22 percent for IVF with donor egg (Medical Research International and SART 1992). Perinatal nurses need to be involved in establishing standards and guidelines for assisted reproductive technologies (Jones 1994).

There are several new reproductive technologies that assist families with genetic problems or infertile women who are unable to carry a pregnancy. The diagnosis of genetic disorders via blastomere analysis before implantation provides couples with the option of foregoing the attempt to establish a pregnancy and thereby avoiding a difficult decision about terminating an affected pregnancy (Pickler and Munro 1994; Guyer and Collins 1993). Use of IVF and gestational carrier allows infertile women who are genetically sound but unable to carry a pregnancy to exercise the option of having their own biologic pregnancy (English 1991; Snowdon 1994; Pergament and Fiddler 1996).

Community-Based Nursing Care

Approximately 8 percent of the childbearing population in the United States (1 out of 12 couples) is unable to conceive or carry a pregnancy to term. The couple may incur tremendous emotional and physical stress, as well as financial expense, for infertility testing. Treatment can cost over $20,000 a year, and insurance coverage may be limited. Years of effort and numerous evaluations and examinations may take place before conception occurs, if it occurs at all. In a society that values children and considers them to be the natural result of marriage, infertile couples face a myriad of tensions and discrimination.

The clinic nurse needs to be constantly aware of the emotional needs of the couple confronting infertility evaluation and treatment. Constant attention to temperature charts and instructions about their sex life from a person outside the relationship naturally affects the spontaneity of a couple's interactions. Tests and treatments may heighten feelings of frustration or anger between the partners. The need to share this intimate area of a relationship may contribute to feelings of guilt or shame, especially when one or the other is identified as "the cause" of infertility. Throughout the evaluation process nurses play a key role in lessening the stress these couples must endure by providing resources and accurate information about what is entailed in treatment and what physical, emotional, and financial demands they can anticipate throughout the process. The nurse's ability to assess and respond to emotional and educational needs is essential to give infertile couples control (Johnson 1996; Jirka et al 1996). It is important to use a nursing framework that recognizes the multidimensional needs of the infertile individual or couple within physical, social, psychospiritual, and environmental contexts (Boxer 1996; Schoener and Krysa 1996).

An assessment tool like the infertility questionnaire in Table 4–5 can assist the nurse in determining the support needs of the couple. Extensive and repeated explanations and written instructions may be necessary to help relieve anxiety.

TABLE 4–5 Infertility Questionnaire

Self-Image

1. I feel bad about my body because of our inability to have a child.
2. Since our infertility, I feel I can do anything as well as I used to.
3. I feel as attractive as before our infertility.
4. I feel less masculine/feminine because of our inability to have a child.
5. Compared with others, I feel I am a worthwhile person.
6. Lately, I feel I am sexually attractive to my wife/husband.
7. I feel I will be incomplete as a man/woman if we cannot have a child.
8. Having an infertility problem makes me feel physically incompetent.

Guilt/Blame

1. I feel guilty about somehow causing our infertility.
2. I wonder if our infertility problem is due to something I did in the past.
3. My spouse makes me feel guilty about our problem.
4. There are times when I blame my spouse for our infertility.
5. I feel I am being punished because of our infertility.

Sexuality

1. Lately I feel I am able to respond to my spouse sexually.
2. I feel sex is a duty, not a pleasure.
3. Since our infertility problem, I enjoy sexual relations with my spouse.
4. We have sexual relations for the purpose of trying to conceive.
5. Sometimes I feel like a "sex machine," programmed to have sex during the fertile period.
6. Impaired fertility has helped our sexual relationship.
7. Our inability to have a child has increased my desire for sexual relations.
8. Our inability to have a child has decreased my desire for sexual relations.

Note: The questionnaire is scored on a Likert scale with responses ranging from "strongly agree" to "strongly disagree." Each question is scored separately, and the mean score is determined for each section (Self-Image, Guilt/Blame, Sexuality). The total mean score is then divided by 3. A final mean score of greater than 3 indicates distress.

Source: Bernstein J: Assessment of psychological dysfunction associated with infertility. *JOGNN* 1985; 14(Suppl):63.

Infertility may be perceived as a loss by one or both partners. The losses experienced have been described as loss of relationship with spouse or family, health, status or prestige, self-esteem, self-confidence, security, and potential child. Often the crisis of infertility touches on all these feelings (Mahlstedt 1985; Schoener and Krysa 1996). Each couple passes through several stages of feelings, not unlike those identified by Kübler-Ross: surprise, denial, anger, isolation, guilt, grief, and resolution (Menning 1988). It is important to remember that partners may progress through the stages at different rates (Sandelowski 1994). Nonjudgmental acceptance and a professional, caring attitude on the nurse's part can go far to dissipate the negative emotions the couple may experience. This is also a time when the nurse may assess the quality of the couple's relationship: Are they able and willing to communicate verbally and share feelings?

Are they mutually supportive? The answers to such questions may help the nurse identify areas of strength and weakness and construct an appropriate plan of care. At times, individual or group counseling with other infertile couples may facilitate the couple's resolution of feelings brought about by their own difficult situation. The community has a wealth of services and education opportunities available for infertile women and couples and the knowledgeable nurse can help them access these services. Couples should be aware of infertility support and education organizations such as RESOLVE, which may help meet some of their needs and validate their feelings. Sawatzky (1981) has identified the essential tasks of the infertile couple (Table 4–6).

TABLE 4–6 Tasks of the Infertile Couple

Tasks	*Nursing Interventions*
Recognize how infertility affects their lives and express feelings (may be negative toward self or mate)	Supportive: help to understand and facilitate free expression of feelings
Grieve the loss of potential offspring	Help to recognize feelings
Evaluate reasons for wanting a child	Help to understand motives
Decide about management	Identify alternatives; facilitate partner communication

Source: Sawatzky M: Tasks of the infertile couple. *JOGNN* 1981; 10:132.

Adoption

Adoption of an infant can be a difficult and frustrating experience for all persons involved (Arms 1990). A waiting period of as long as several years to begin the adoption process is not uncommon. The decrease in number of available infants has occurred because many infants are reared by their single mothers instead of being relinquished for adoption as was customary in the past. In addition, many unwanted pregnancies are terminated by elective abortion. Some couples seek international adoption or consider adopting older children, children with handicaps, or children of mixed parentage, because the adoption process in such cases is quicker and more children are available. Nurses in the community can assist couples considering adoption by providing information on community resources for adoption and support through the adoption process. Some helpful support groups are: Adoptive Families of America, Families for Private Adoption, Concerned United Birthparents Inc, The National Adoption Center, and National Adoption Information Clearinghouse. Couples also need support if they choose to remain childless (Menning 1988).

Pregnancy After Infertility

The feeling of being infertile does not necessarily disappear with pregnancy. Although there may be initial ecstacy, couples may face a whole new arena of fear and anxiety, and they often do not know where they "fit in." Contact with their past "infertile" support system may vanish when peers learn they have resolved their infertility (Braverman and English 1992). The couple may also have concerns about the possible effect of repeated cycles of fertility drugs, IVF technology, or cryopreservation on the fetus. Couples may need reassurance throughout the pregnancy to allay these anxieties.

Genetic Disorders

Even when conception has been achieved, families can have special reproductive concerns. The desired and expected outcome of any pregnancy is the birth of a healthy, "perfect" baby. Parents experience grief, fear, and anger when they discover that their baby has been born with a defect or a genetic disease. Such an abnormality may be evident at birth or may not appear for some time. The baby may have inherited a disease from one parent, creating more guilt and strife within the family (Olsen 1994).

Regardless of the type or scope of the problem, parents will have many questions: "What did I do?" "What caused it?" "Will it happen again?" The nurse must anticipate the couple's questions and concerns and guide, direct, and support the family. To do so, the nurse must have a basic knowledge of genetics and genetic counseling. Many congenital malformations and diseases are genetic or have a strong genetic component. Others are not genetic at all. Professional nurses can help expedite attempts to categorize the problem and answer the family's questions if they already have an understanding of the principles involved and can direct the family to the appropriate resources.

Chromosomes and Chromosomal Analysis

All hereditary material is carried on tightly coiled strands of DNA known as **chromosomes.** The chromosomes carry the genes, the smallest unit of inheritance.

All *somatic (body) cells* contain 46 chromosomes, which is the *diploid number* of chromosomes, while the sperm and egg contain 23 chromosomes, or the *haploid number* (see Chapter 3). There are 23 pairs of homologous chromosomes (a matched pair of chromosomes, one inherited from each parent). Twenty-two of the pairs are known as **autosomes** (nonsex chromosomes),

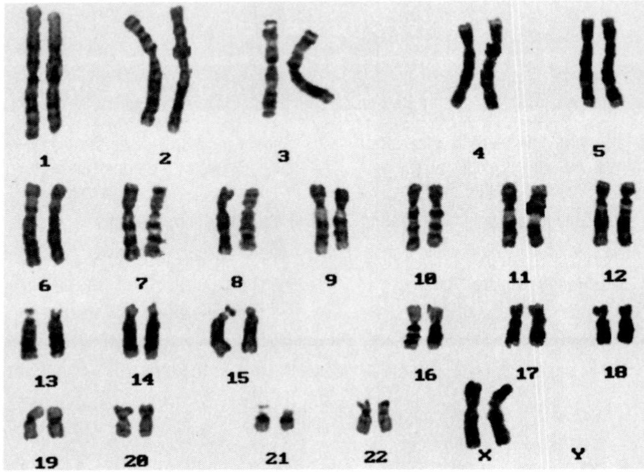

FIGURE 4–5 Normal female karyotype.

Source: Courtesy David Peakman, Reproductive Genetics Center, Denver, CO.

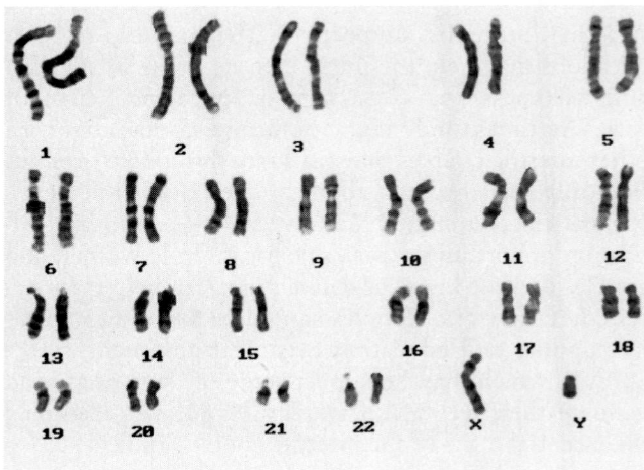

FIGURE 4–6 Normal male karyotype.

Source: Courtesy David Peakman, Reproductive Genetics Center, Denver, CO.

and one pair is the **sex chromosomes,** X and Y. A normal female has a 46,XX chromosome constitution; the normal male a 46,XY (Figures 4–5 and 4–6). The **karyotype,** or pictorial analysis of these chromosomes, is usually obtained from specially treated and stained peripheral blood lymphocytes.

Chromosomal abnormalities can occur in either the autosomes or the sex chromosomes and can be divided into two categories: abnormalities of number and abnormalities of structure. Even small alterations in chromosomes can cause problems, especially those associated with slow growth and development or with mental retardation. The child need not have obvious major congenital malformations to be affected. Some of these abnormalities can be passed on to other offspring. Thus in some cases chromosomal analysis is appropriate even if clinical manifestations are mild. Whatever the case, too much or too little genetic material usually produces adverse effects on normal growth and development.

Autosomal Abnormalities

Abnormalities of chromosome number are most commonly seen as trisomies, monosomies, and mosaicism. In all three cases, the abnormality is most often caused by nondisjunction. Nondisjunction occurs when paired chromosomes fail to separate during cell division. If nondisjunction occurs in either the sperm or the egg before fertilization, the resulting zygote (fertilized egg) will have an abnormal chromosome makeup in all of the cells (trisomy or monosomy). If nondisjunction occurs after fertilization, the developing zygote will have cells with two or more different chromosome makeups, evolving into two or more different cell lines (mosaicism).

Trisomies are the product of the union of a normal gamete (egg or sperm) with a gamete that contains an extra chromosome. The individual will have 47 chromosomes and is trisomic (has three chromosomes the same) for whichever chromosome is extra. Down syndrome (formerly called mongolism) is the most common trisomy abnormality seen in children (see Figure 4–7). The presence of the extra chromosome 21 produces distinctive clinical features (see Table 4–7 on page 80 and Figure 4–8). With the advent of modern surgical techniques and antibiotics, children with Down syndrome are now living into their fifth and sixth decades.

Trisomies can occur among other autosomes, the two most common being trisomy 18 and trisomy 13 (see

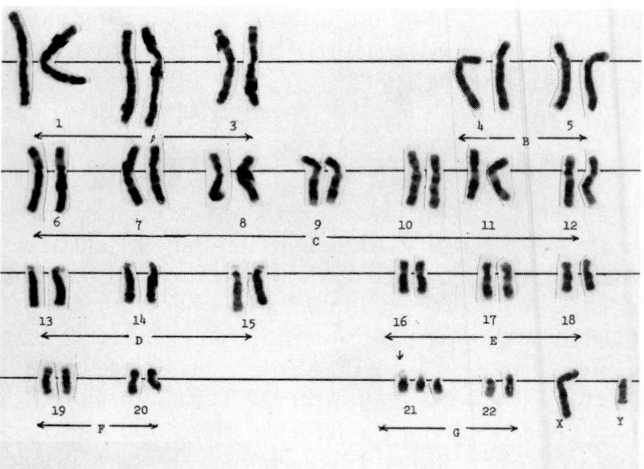

FIGURE 4–7 Karyotype of a male who has trisomy 21, Down syndrome: Note the extra 21 chromosome.

Source: Courtesy Dr Arthur Robinson, National Jewish Hospital and Research Center.

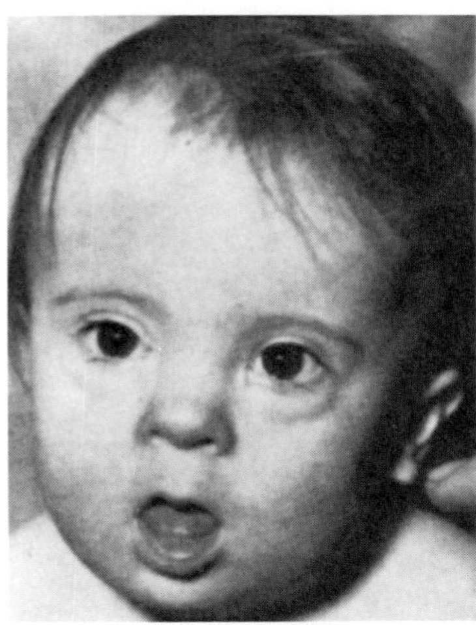

FIGURE 4–8 A child with Down syndrome.
Source: Jones KL: *Smith's Recognizable Patterns of Human Malformations,* 4th ed. Philadelphia: Saunders, 1988.

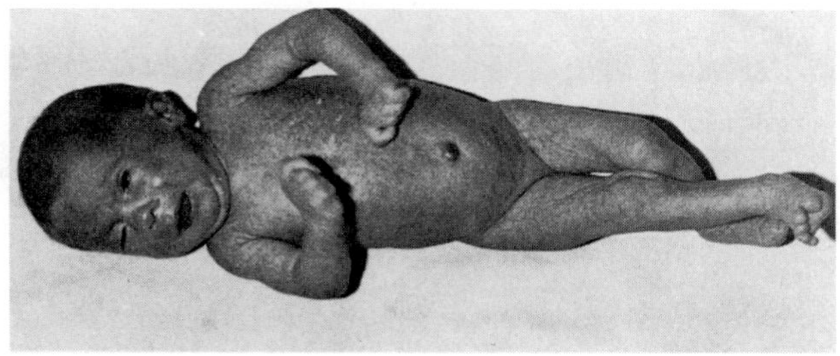

FIGURE 4–9 Infant with trisomy 18.
Source: Smith DW: Autosomal abnormalities. *Am J Obstet Gynecol* December 1964; 90:1055.

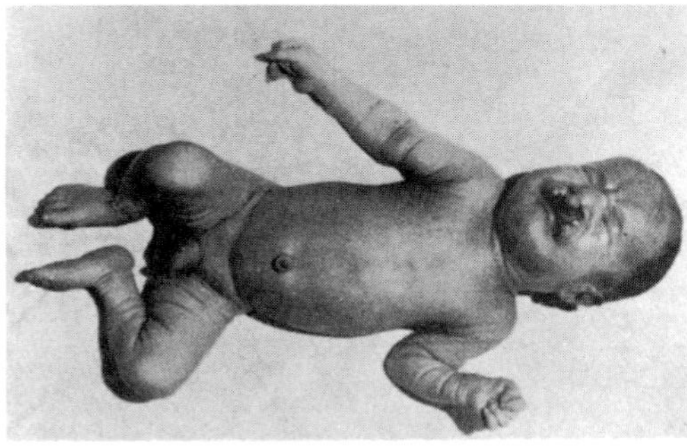

FIGURE 4–10 Infant with trisomy 13.
Source: Smith DW et al: The D_1 trisomy syndrome. *J Pediatr* March 1963; 62:326..

Table 4–7 on page 80 and Figures 4–9 and 4–10). The prognosis for both trisomy 18 and 13 is extremely poor. Most children (70%) die within the first 3 months of life secondary to complications related to respiratory and cardiac abnormalities.

Monosomies occur when a normal gamete unites with a gamete that is missing a chromosome. In this case, the individual has only 45 chromosomes and is said to be monosomic. Monosomy of an entire autosomal chromosome is incompatible with life.

Mosaicism occurs after fertilization and results in an individual who has two different cell lines, each with a different chromosomal number. Mosaicism tends to be more common in the sex chromosomes, but when it does occur in the autosomes it is most common in Down syndrome. An individual with many classic signs of Down syndrome but with normal or near-normal intelligence should be investigated for the possibility of mosaicism.

Abnormalities of chromosome structure involve only parts of the chromosome and occur in two forms: translocation and deletions or additions. Some children born with Down syndrome have an abnormal rearrangement of chromosomal material known as a translocation. Clinically, the two types of Down syndrome are indistinguishable. What is of major importance to the family is that the two different types have significantly different risks of recurrence. The only way to distinguish the two types of Down syndrome is to do a chromosome analysis. Risk of trisomy is 1 in 800 live births, in contrast with 1 in 1500 live births with a balanced translocation (Simpson 1990).

The translocation occurs when the carrier parent has 45 chromosomes, usually with one of the number 21 chromosomes fused to one of the number 14 chromosomes. The parent has one normal 14, one normal 21, and one 14/21 chromosome. Since all the chromosomal material is present and functioning normally, the parent is clinically normal. This individual is known as a *balanced translocation carrier.* When a person who is a balanced translocation carrier has a child with a person who has a structurally normal chromosome constitution, the child can have a normal number of chromosomes, be a carrier, or have an extra chromosome 21. Such a child has an *unbalanced translocation* and has Down syndrome.

The other type of structure abnormality seen is caused by *additions* or *deletions* of chromosomal material. Any portion of a chromosome may be lost or added, generally leading to some adverse effect. Depending on how much chromosomal material is involved, the clinical effects may be mild or severe. Many types of additions and deletions have been described, such as the deletion of the short arm of chromosome 5 (cri du chat, or cat cry, syndrome; see Figure 4–11) or the deletion of the long arm of chromosome 18 (see Table 4–7).

TABLE 4–7 Chromosomal Syndromes	
Altered chromosome: 21 Genetic defect: trisomy 21 (Down syndrome) (secondary nondisjunction or 14/21 unbalanced translocation) Incidence: 1 in 700 live births (Figure 4–8)	**Characteristics:** CNS: mental retardation; hypotonia at birth Head: flattened occiput; depressed nasal bridge; mongoloid slant of eyes; epicanthal folds; white specking of the iris (Brushfield spots); protrusion of the tongue; high, arched palate; low-set ears Hands: broad, short fingers; abnormalities of finger and foot; dermal ridge patterns (dermatoglyphics); transverse palmar crease (simian line) Other: congenital heart disease
Altered chromosome: 18 Genetic defect: trisomy 18 Incidence: 1 in 3000 live births (Figure 4–9)	**Characteristics:** CNS: mental retardation; severe hypotonia Head: prominent occiput; low-set ears; corneal opacities; ptosis (drooping of eyelids) Hands: third and fourth fingers overlapped by second and fifth fingers; abnormal dermatoglyphics; syndactyly (webbing of fingers) Other: congenital heart defects; renal abnormalities; single umbilical artery; gastrointestinal tract abnormalities; rocker-bottom feet; cryptorchidism; various malformations of other organs
Altered chromosome: 18 Genetic defect: deletion of long arm of chromosome 18	**Characteristics:** CNS: severe psychomotor retardation Head: microcephaly; stenotic ear canals with conductive hearing loss Other: various other organ malformations
Altered chromosome: 13 Genetic defect: trisomy 13 Incidence: 1 in 5000 live births (Figure 4–10)	**Characteristics:** CNS: mental retardation; severe hypotonia; seizures Head: microcephaly; microphthalmia and/or coloboma (keyhole-shaped pupil); malformed ears; aplasia of external auditory canal; micrognathia (abnormally small lower jaw); cleft lip and palate Hands: polydactly (extra digits); abnormal posturing of fingers; abnormal dermatoglyphics Other: congenital heart defects; hemangiomas; gastrointestinal tract defects; various malformations of other organs
Altered chromosome: 5p Genetic defect: deletion of short arm of chromosome 5 (cri du chat, or cat cry, syndrome) Incidence: 1 in 20,000 live births (Figure 4–11)	**Characteristics:** CNS: severe mental retardation; a catlike cry in infancy Head: microcephaly; hypertelorism (widely spaced eyes); epicanthal folds; low-set ears Other: failure to thrive; various organ malformations
Altered chromosome: XO (sex chromosome) Genetic defect: only one X chromosome in female (Turner syndrome) Incidence: 1 in 300–7000 live female births (Figure 4–12)	**Characteristics:** CNS: no intellectual impairment; some perceptual difficulties Head: low hairline; webbed neck Trunk: short stature; cubitus valgus (increased carrying angle of arm); excessive nevi (congenital discoloration of skin due to pigmentation); broad shieldlike chest with widely spaced nipples; puffy feet; no toenails Other: fibrous streaks in ovaries; underdeveloped secondary sex characteristics; primary amenorrhea; usually infertile; renal anomalies; coarctation of the aorta
Altered chromosome: XXY (sex chromosome) Genetic defect: extra X chromosome in male (Klinefelter syndrome) Incidence: 1 in 1000 live male births, approximately 1–2% of institutionalized males	**Characteristics:** CNS: mild mental retardation Trunk: occasional gynecomastia (abnormally large male breasts); eunuchoid body proportions (lack of male muscular and sexual development) Other: small, soft testes; underdeveloped secondary sex characteristics; usually sterile

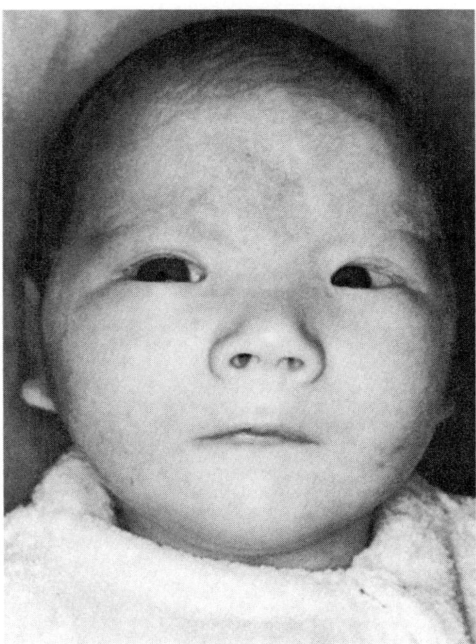

FIGURE 4–11 Infant with cri du chat syndrome resulting from deletion of part of the short arm of chromosome 5. Note characteristic facies with hypertelorism, epicanthus, and retrognathia.

Source: Thompson JS, Thompson MW: *Genetics in Medicine,* 5th ed. Philadelphia: Saunders, 1991.

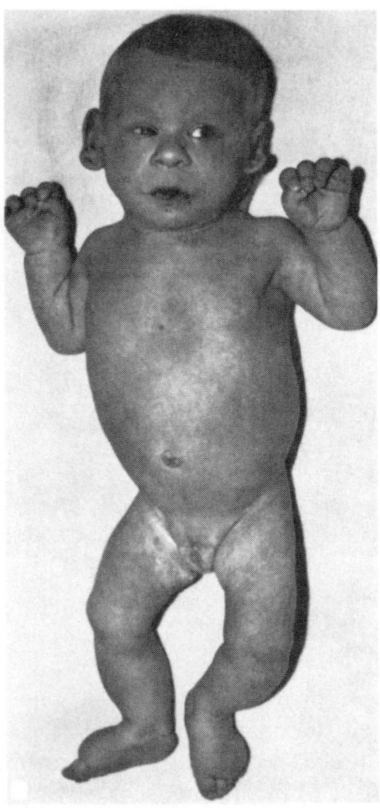

FIGURE 4–12 Infant with Turner syndrome at 1 month of age. Note prominent ears.

Source: Lemli L, Smith DW: The XO syndrome: A study of the differentiated phenotype in 25 patients. *J Pediatr* 1963; 63:577.

Sex Chromosome Abnormalities

To better understand abnormalities of the sex chromosomes, the nurse should know that in females, at an early embryonic stage, one of the two normal X chromosomes becomes inactive. The inactive X chromosome forms a dark staining area known as the *Barr body.* The normal female has one Barr body, since one of her two X chromosomes has been inactivated. The normal male has no Barr bodies, since he has only one X chromosome to begin with.

The most common sex chromosome abnormalities are Turner syndrome in females (45,XO with no Barr bodies present; see Figure 4–12) and Klinefelter syndrome in males (47,XXY with one Barr body present). See Table 4–7 for clinical descriptions of these abnormalities.

Modes of Inheritance

Many inherited diseases are produced by an abnormality in a single gene or pair of genes. In such instances, the chromosomes are grossly normal. The defect is at the gene level. Some of these gene defects can be detected by technologies such as DNA and biochemical assays.

There are two major categories of inheritance: **Mendelian (single-gene) inheritance** and **non-Mendelian (multifactorial) inheritance.** Each single-gene trait is determined by a pair of genes working together. These genes are responsible for the observable expression of the traits (eg, blue eyes, fair skin), referred to as the **phenotype.** The total genetic makeup of an individual is referred to as the **genotype** (pattern of the genes on the chromosomes).

One of the genes for a trait is inherited from the mother, the other from the father. An individual who has two identical genes at a given locus is considered to be *homozygous* for that trait. An individual is considered to be *heterozygous* for a particular trait when he or she has two different *alleles* (alternate forms of the same gene) at a given locus on a pair of homologous chromosomes.

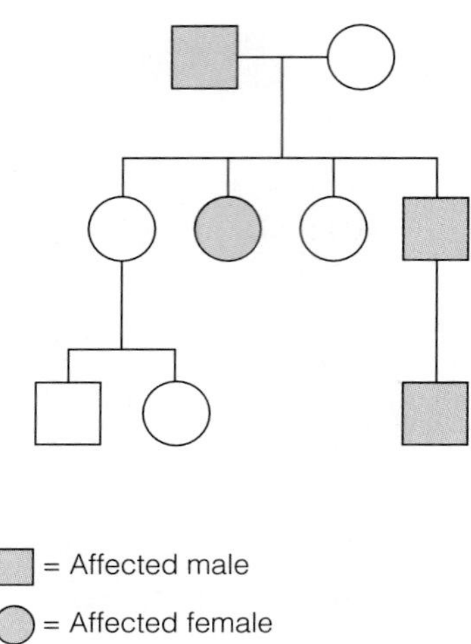

FIGURE 4–13 Autosomal dominant pedigree. One parent is affected. Statistically, 50% of offspring will be affected, regardless of sex.

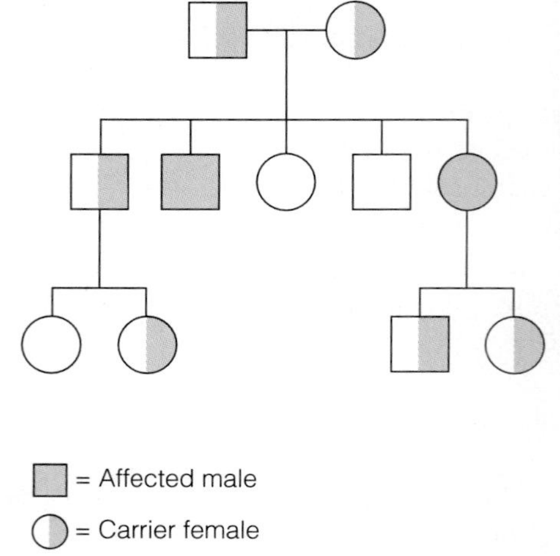

FIGURE 4–14 Autosomal recessive pedigree. Both parents are carriers. Statistically, 25% of offspring are affected, regardless of sex.

The best-known modes of single-gene inheritance are autosomal dominant, autosomal recessive, and X-linked (sex-linked) recessive. There is also an X-linked dominant mode of inheritance that is less common, and a newly identified mode of inheritance, the fragile X syndrome.

Autosomal Dominant Inheritance

An individual is said to have an autosomal dominantly inherited disorder if the disease trait is heterozygous. That is, the abnormal gene overshadows the normal gene of the pair. It is essential to remember that in autosomal dominant inheritance

1. An affected individual generally has an affected parent. Thus the family **pedigree** (graphic representation of a family tree) usually shows multiple generations with the disorder.
2. The affected individual has a 50 percent chance of passing on the abnormal gene to each of his or her children (Figure 4–13).
3. Males and females are equally affected, and a father can pass the abnormal gene on to his son. This is an important principle when distinguishing autosomal dominant disorders from X-linked disorders.
4. Autosomal dominant inherited disorders have varying degrees of presentation. This is an important factor when counseling families concerning autosomal dominant disorders. Although a parent may have a mild form of the disease, the child may have a more severe form.

Some common autosomal dominant inherited disorders are Huntington's disease, polycystic kidney disease, neurofibromatosis (von Recklinghausen disease), and achondroplastic dwarfism.

Autosomal Recessive Inheritance

In an autosomal recessive inherited disorder, the individual must have two abnormal genes to be affected. The notion of a *carrier state* is appropriate here. A carrier is an individual who is heterozygous for the abnormal gene and clinically normal. It is not until two individuals mate and pass on the same abnormal gene that affected children may appear. It is essential to remember that in autosomal recessive inheritance

1. An affected individual may have clinically normal parents, but both parents will be carriers of the abnormal gene (Figure 4–14).
2. There is a 25 percent chance of carrier parents passing the abnormal gene on to any of their offspring.
3. If a child of two carrier parents is clinically normal, there is a 50 percent chance that he or she is a carrier of the gene.
4. Both males and females are equally affected.
5. There is an increased history of consanguineous matings.

Some common autosomal recessive inherited disorders are cystic fibrosis, phenylketonuria (PKU), galactosemia, sickle-cell anemia, Tay-Sachs disease, and most metabolic disorders.

X-Linked Recessive Inheritance

X-linked or sex-linked disorders are those for which the abnormal gene is carried on the X chromosome. Thus an X-linked disorder is manifested in a male who carries the abnormal gene on his X chromosome. His mother is considered to be a carrier when the normal gene on one X chromosome overshadows the abnormal gene on the other X chromosome. It is essential to remember that in X-linked recessive inheritance

1. There is no male-to-male transmission. Affected males are related through the female line (see Figure 4–15).
2. There is a 50 percent chance that a carrier mother will pass the abnormal gene to each of her sons, who will thus be affected. There is a 50 percent chance that a carrier mother will pass the normal gene to each of her sons, who will thus be unaffected. Finally, there is a 50 percent chance that a carrier mother will pass the abnormal gene to each of her daughters, who will become carriers.
3. Fathers affected with an X-linked disorder cannot pass the disorder to their sons, but all their daughters become carriers of the disorder.

Common X-linked recessive disorders are hemophilia, Duchenne muscular dystrophy, and color blindness.

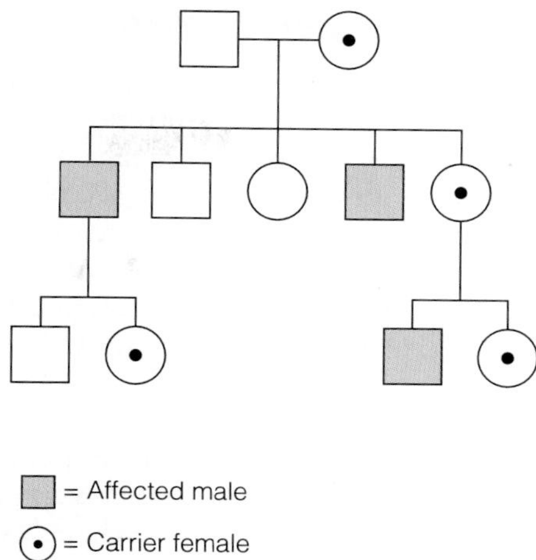

FIGURE 4–15 X-linked recessive pedigree. The mother is the carrier. Statistically, 50% of male offspring are affected, and 50 percent of female offspring are carriers.

X-Linked Dominant Inheritance

X-linked dominant disorders are extremely rare, the most common being vitamin D–resistant rickets. When X-linked dominance does occur, the pattern is similar to X-linked recessive inheritance except that heterozygous females are affected. It is essential to remember that in X-linked dominant inheritance there is no male-to-male transmission. Affected fathers will have affected daughters, but no affected sons.

Fragile X Syndrome

The fragile X syndrome is a common inherited form of mental retardation second only to Down syndrome among all causes of moderate mental retardation in males (Thompson et al 1991). Fragile X syndrome is a CNS disorder linked to a "fragile site" on the X chromosome. Fragile X syndrome is characterized by moderate mental retardation, large protuberant ears, and large testes after puberty. The carrier females are not dysmorphic (having abnormal features), but about one-third are mildly mentally retarded (Thompson et al 1991).

Multifactorial Inheritance

Many common congenital malformations, such as cleft palate, heart defects, spina bifida, dislocated hips, clubfoot, and pyloric stenosis, are caused by an interaction of many genes and environmental factors. They are, therefore, multifactorial in origin. It is essential to remember that in multifactorial inheritance

1. The malformations may vary from mild to severe. For example, spina bifida may range in severity from mild (spina bifida occulta) to more severe (myelomeningocele). It is believed that the more severe the defect, the greater the number of genes present for that defect.
2. There is often a sex bias. Pyloric stenosis is more common in males, whereas cleft palate is more common among females. When a member of the less commonly affected sex shows the condition, a greater number of genes must usually be present to cause the defect.
3. In the presence of environmental influences (such as seasonal changes, altitude, irradiation, chemicals in the environment, or exposure to toxic substances), it may take fewer genes to manifest the disease in the offspring.
4. In contrast to single-gene disorders, there is an additive effect in multifactorial inheritance. The more family members who have the defect, the greater the risk that the next pregnancy will also be affected.

Although most congenital malformations are multifactorial traits, a careful family history should always be taken, since cleft lip and palate, certain congenital heart defects, and other malformations occasionally can be inherited as autosomal dominant or recessive traits. Other disorders thought to be within the multifactorial inheritance group are diabetes, hypertension, some heart diseases, and mental illness.

Prenatal Diagnostic Tests

Parent-child and family planning counseling have become a major responsibility of professional nurses. To be effective counselors, nurses must have the most recent knowledge about prenatal diagnosis. It is essential that the couple be completely informed about the known and potential risks of each of the genetic diagnostic procedures. The nurse must recognize the emotional impact on the family of a decision to have or not to have a genetic diagnostic procedure.

The ability to diagnose certain genetic diseases by various diagnostic tools has enormous implications for the practice of preventive health care. Several methods are available for prenatal diagnosis, although some are still being used on an experimental basis.

Ultrasound may be used to assess the fetus for genetic or congenital problems. With ultrasound, the fetal head can be assessed for abnormalities in size, shape, and structure (for a detailed discussion of ultrasound technology, see Chapter 14). Craniospinal defects (anencephaly, microcephaly, hydrocephalus), thoracic malformations (diaphragmatic hernia), gastrointestinal malformations (omphalocele, gastroschisis), renal malformations (dysplasia or obstruction), and skeletal malformations are only some of the disorders that have been diagnosed in utero by ultrasound (Garmel and D'Alton 1994).

Screening for congenital anomalies is best done at 18 to 20 weeks, when fetal structures have developed completely (Chervenak et al 1993; Simpson and Elias 1993). There is no information documenting harm to the fetus or long-term effects from exposure to ultrasound. However, there is no guarantee of complete safety; therefore, the practitioner and the parents must evaluate the risks against the benefits on an individual basis (Kuller and Laifer 1995).

Genetic Amniocentesis

The major method of prenatal diagnosis is genetic amniocentesis (Figure 4–16). The procedure is described in Chapter 14. The indications for genetic amniocentesis include the following:

1. *Advanced maternal age.* Any woman 35 or older is at greater risk for having children with chromosomal abnormalities. See Chapter 10 for further discussion. Half of the chromosomal abnormalities due to maternal age are trisomy 21, and half are other abnormalities of chromosome number, such as trisomy 13, 18, XXX, XXY, and so on. The risk of having a live born infant with a chromosome problem is 1 in 200 for a 35-year-old woman; the risk for trisomy 21 is 1 in 400 (Hook et al 1988). At age 45, the risks are 1 in 20 and 1 in 40, respectively.
2. *Previous child born with a chromosomal abnormality.* Young couples who have had a child with trisomy 21, 18, or 13 have approximately a 1–2 percent risk of a future child having a chromosomal abnormality.
3. *Parent carrying a chromosomal abnormality (balanced translocation).* For example, a woman who carries a balanced 14/21 translocation has a risk of approximately 10–15 percent that her children will be affected with the unbalanced translocation of Down syndrome; if the father is the carrier, there is a 2–5 percent risk.
4. *Mother carrying an X-linked disease.* In families in which the woman is a known or possible carrier of an X-linked disorder like hemophilia or Duchenne muscular dystrophy, genetic amniocentesis, chorionic villus sampling (CVS), or percutaneous umbilical blood sampling (PUBS) may be appropriate options. For a known female carrier, the risk of an affected male fetus is 50 percent. With new technologies such as DNA testing, it may be possible to identify affected males from the nonaffected males in some disorders. In disorders where female carriers can be distinguished from noncarriers, only the carrier females would be offered prenatal diagnosis.
5. *Parents carrying an inborn error of metabolism that can be diagnosed in utero.* Metabolic disorders detectable in utero include (partial list): argininosuccinicaciduria, cystinosis, Fabry disease, galactosemia, Gaucher disease, homocystinuria, Hunter syndrome, Hurler disease, Krabbe disease, Lesch-Nyhan syndrome, maple syrup urine disease, metachromatic leukodystrophy, methylmalonic aciduria, Niemann-Pick disease, Pompe disease, Sanfilippo syndrome, and Tay-Sachs disease.
6. *Both parents carrying an autosomal recessive disease.* When both parents are carriers of an autosomal recessive disease, there is a 25 percent risk for each pregnancy that the fetus will be affected. Diagnosis is made by testing the cultured amniotic fluid cells (enzyme level, substrate level, product level, or DNA) or the fluid itself. Autosomal recessive diseases identified by amniocentesis are hemoglobinopathies such as sickle-cell anemia and thalassemia. Prenatal diagnosis of these conditions can be accomplished on uncultured amniotic fluid from an amniocentesis using various DNA analyses (D'Alton 1994). With the detection of the deletion that causes 70 percent of the cases of cystic fibrosis, carrier testing and prenatal diagnosis are available for some families. It is theorized that the other 30 percent of cystic fibrosis cases are caused by numerous, varying deletions (Simpson and Elias 1993). For families without a known deletion but with a living affected relative, carrier detection and prena-

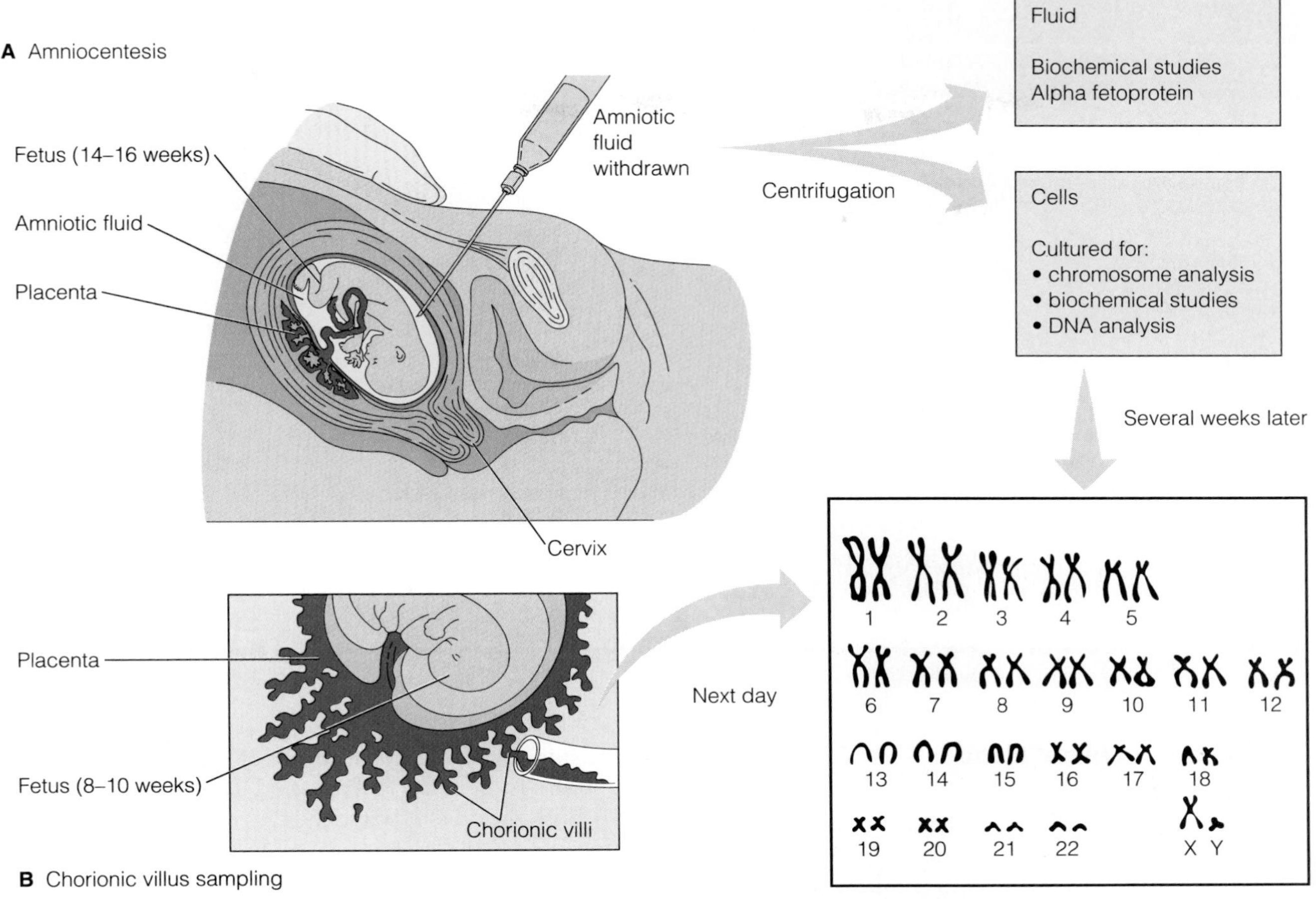

FIGURE 4–16 ***A*** Genetic amniocentesis for prenatal diagnosis is done at 14 to 16 weeks' gestation. ***B*** Chorionic villus sampling is done at 8 to 10 weeks, and the cells are karyotyped within 48 to 72 hours.
Source: adapted from Marieb EN: *Human Anatomy and Physiology*, 3rd ed. Redwood City, CA: Benjamin/Cummings, 1995, p 1037.

tal diagnosis may be possible with DNA testing by restriction endonuclease or biochemical analysis of amniotic fluid with the microvillar enzyme activity (Simpson and Elias 1993).

7. *Family history of neural tube defects.* Neural tube defects (anencephaly, spina bifida, and myelomeningocele) are usually multifactorial traits.

Regardless of the statistical risk for a given family, whether for an isolated neural tube defect or a disorder in which a neural tube defect is a constant feature, recurrence can be detected (possibly as much as 90 percent) through α-fetoprotein (AFP) determination of the amniotic fluid (Simpson and Elias 1993). Alpha fetoprotein is a substance produced in fetal liver, kidney, and gastrointestinal tract. In pregnancies in which the fetus has an open neural tube defect, α-fetoprotein leaks into the amniotic fluid and levels are elevated (Filly et al 1993). Thus genetic amniocentesis allows families for whom the risk of a neural tube defect is increased the opportunity to choose whether to have a child affected with such a disorder. With these babies the preferred birthing method is cesarean section prior to onset of labor (Luthy et al 1992).

Chorionic Villus Sampling (CVS)

Chorionic villus sampling is a new technique that is used in selected regional centers. Its diagnostic capability is similar to amniocentesis. Its advantage is that diagnostic information is available at 8–10 weeks' gestation and that products of conception are tested directly. For further discussion, see Chapter 14.

TABLE 4–8 Genetic Screening Recommendation for Various Ethnic and Age Groups

Background of Population at Risk	*Disorder*	*Screening Test*	*Definitive Test*
Ashkenazic Jewish	Tay-Sachs disease	Decreased serum hexosaminidase-A	CVS* or amniocentesis for hexosaminidase-A assay
African; Hispanic from Caribbean, Central America, South America (*Journal of Black Nurses* 1992)	Sickle-cell anemia	Presence of sickle-cell hemoglobin; confirmatory hemoglobin electrophoresis	CVS or amniocentesis for genotype determination; direct molecular studies
Greek, Italian	β-thalassemia	Mean corpuscular volume <80%; confirmatory hemoglobin electrophoresis	CVS or amniocentesis for genotype determination (direct molecular studies or indirect RFLP† analysis)
Southeast Asian (Vietnamese, Laotian, Cambodian), Philippine	α-thalassemia	Mean corpuscular volume <80%; confirmatory hemoglobin electrophoresis	CVS or amniocentesis for genotype determination (direct molecular studies)
Women over age 35 (EDB) (all ethnic groups)	Chromosomal trisomies	None	CVS or amniocentesis for cytogenetic analysis
Women of any age (all ethnic groups; particularly suggested for women from British Isles, Ireland)	Neural tube defects and selected other anomalies	Maternal serum α-fetoprotein (MSAFP)	Amniocentesis for amniotic fluid, α-fetoprotein, and acetylcholinesterase assays

* Chorionic villus sampling

† Restriction fragment length polymorphism

Percutaneous Umbilical Blood Sampling (PUBS)

Percutaneous umbilical blood sampling is a technique used for obtaining blood that allows for more rapid chromosome diagnosis, for genetic studies, or for transfusion related to Rh isoimmunization or hydrops (Shulman et al 1993). For more discussion, see Chapter 14.

Alpha Fetoprotein (AFP and AFP3)

Alpha fetoprotein tests for AFP in the maternal circulation or amniotic fluid. Maternal serum AFP (MSAFP) is elevated in cases of infants with open neural tube defects, anencephaly, omphalocele, and gastroschisis; fetal death; vaginal bleeding; or multiple gestations (Kuller and Laifer 1995). Women with a family history of neural tube defects should consult their prenatal care provider for recommended folic acid dosages (Centers for Disease Control 1993; King and Schimke 1994). Low MSAFP has been associated with Down syndrome. Testing for AFP3, in addition to hCG and unconjugated estriol (uE3), will detect 60 percent of Down syndrome and about 50 percent of trisomy 18 (D'Alton 1994; ACOG 1994). Maternal serum analyte (MSAFP, hCG, uE3) screening is done at 15 to 20 weeks' gestation (Wright 1994; Kuller and Laifer 1995).

Implications of Prenatal Diagnostic Testing

It is imperative that counseling precede any procedure for prenatal diagnosis. Many questions and points must be considered if the family is to reach a satisfactory decision. See Table 4–8 and Key Facts to Remember: Couples to Be Offered Prenatal Diagnosis.

With the advent of diagnostic techniques such as amniocentesis and chorionic villus sampling, couples at risk, who would not otherwise have additional children,

KEY FACTS TO REMEMBER

Couples to Be Offered Prenatal Diagnosis

- Women 35 or over at time of birth
- Couples having a balanced translocation (chromosomal abnormality)
- Mother carrying X-linked disease (eg, hemophilia)
- Couples having a previous child with chromosomal abnormality
- Couples in which either partner or a previous child is affected with a diagnosable metabolic disorder
- Couples in which both partners are carriers for a diagnosable metabolic or autosomal recessive disorder
- Family or personal history of neural tube defects
- Ethnic groups at increased risk for specific disorders (Table 4–8)
- Couples with history of two or more first trimester spontaneous abortions
- Women with an abnormal maternal serum alpha fetoprotein (MSAFP or AFP3) test

can decide to conceive. Following prenatal diagnosis, a couple can decide not to have a child with a genetic disease. For many couples, prenatal diagnosis is not a solution, however, since the only method of preventing a genetic disease is preventing the birth by aborting the affected fetus. This decision can only be made by the family. Even when termination is not an option, prenatal diagnosis can give parents an opportunity to prepare for the birth of a child with special needs, contact other families with a child with similar problems, or contact support services before the birth.

Every pregnancy has a 3–4 percent risk for an infant to be born with a birth defect, some of which can be diagnosed before birth. When an abnormality is detected or suspected, an attempt is made to determine the diagnosis by assessing the family health history (via the pedigree) and the pregnancy history, and by evaluating the fetal anomaly or anomalies. The parents can then be presented with options. For example, families expecting a baby with a lethal anomaly, such as trisomy 13 or 18, may wish to consider nonaggressive intervention.

Prenatal diagnosis cannot guarantee the birth of a normal child. It can only determine the presence or absence of specific disorders (within the limits of laboratory error). Experts on a specific disorder should be consulted before giving information to couples or discussing options.

Treatment of prenatally diagnosed disorders may begin during the pregnancy, thus possibly preventing irreversible damage. For example, a galactose-free diet may be given to a mother carrying a fetus with galactosemia. In light of the philosophy of preventive health care, information that can be obtained prenatally should be made available to all couples who are expecting a baby or who are contemplating pregnancy.

Postnatal Diagnosis

Questions concerning genetic disorders (cause, treatment, and prognosis) are generally first discussed in the newborn nursery or during the infant's first few months of life. When a child is born with anomalies, has a stormy newborn period, or does not progress as expected, a genetic evaluation may well be warranted. An accurate diagnosis and an optimal treatment plan incorporate the following:

- Complete and detailed histories to determine whether the problem is prenatal (congenital), postnatal, or familial in origin.
- Thorough physical examination, including dermatoglyphics analysis (Figure 4–17).
- Laboratory analysis, which includes chromosome analysis; enzyme assay for inborn errors of metabolism (see Chapter 25 for further discussion on these specific tests); DNA studies; and antibody titers for infectious teratogens, such as toxoplasmosis, rubella, cytomegalovirus, and herpesvirus (**TORCH syndrome**) (see Chapter 13).

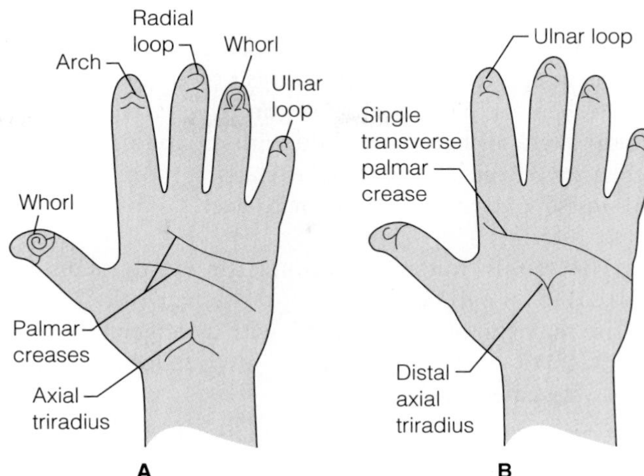

FIGURE 4–17 Dermatoglyphic patterns of the hands in ***A*** a normal individual, and ***B*** a child with Down sydrome. Note the single transverse palmar crease, distally placed axial triradius, and increased number of ulnar loops.

To make an accurate diagnosis, the geneticist consults with other specialists and reviews the current literature. This permits the geneticist to evaluate all the available information before arriving at a diagnosis and plan of action.

Community-Based Nursing Care

Genetic counseling is a communication process in which the family is provided with the most complete and accurate information about the occurrence or the risk of recurrence of a genetic disease in that family (Inati et al 1994).

In retrospective genetic counseling, time is a crucial factor. One cannot expect a couple who has just learned that their child has a birth defect or Down syndrome to take in any information concerning future risks. However, the couple should never be "put off" from counseling for too long a period, only to find that they have borne another affected child. The perinatal nursing team nurse frequently has the first contact with the family who have a newborn with a congenital abnormality. At the birth of an affected child, the nurse can inform the parents that genetic counseling is available before they attempt having another child. Genetic counseling is an appropriate course of action for any family wondering

"Will it happen again?" Asking one or two members of a genetics team to introduce themselves to the family is often enough to bring up the subject of genetic counseling. When the parents have begun to recover from the initial shock of bearing a child with an abnormality, or when they begin to contemplate having more children, the nurse can encourage them to seek counseling and make referrals.

The family nurse practitioner or family-planning nurse is in an excellent position to reach at-risk families before the birth of another baby with a congenital problem. Genetic counseling referral is advised for any of the following categories:

1. *Congenital abnormalities, including mental retardation.* Any couple who has a child or a relative with a congenital malformation may be at increased risk and should be so informed. If mental retardation of unidentified cause has occurred in a family, there may be an increased risk of recurrence.

   In many cases, the genetic counselor will identify the cause of a malformation as a teratogen (see Chapter 9). The family should be aware of teratogenic substances so they can avoid exposure during any subsequent pregnancy.
2. *Familial disorders.* Families should be told that certain diseases may have a genetic component and that the risk of their occurrence in a particular family may be higher than that for the general population. Such disorders as diabetes, heart disease, cancer, and mental illness fall into this category.
3. *Known inherited diseases.* Families may know that a disease is inherited but not know the mechanism or the specific risk for them. An important point to remember is that family members who are not at risk for passing on a disorder should be as well informed as family members who are at risk.
4. *Metabolic disorders.* Any families at risk for having a child with a metabolic disorder or biochemical defect should be referred. Because most inborn errors of metabolism are autosomal recessive inherited ones, a family may not be identified as being at risk until the birth of an affected child. Carriers of the sickle-cell trait can be identified before pregnancy is begun, and the risk of having an affected child can be determined. Prenatal diagnosis of an affected fetus is available on an experimental basis only.
5. *Chromosomal abnormalities.* As discussed previously, any couple who has had a child with a chromosomal abnormality may be at increased risk of having another child similarly affected.

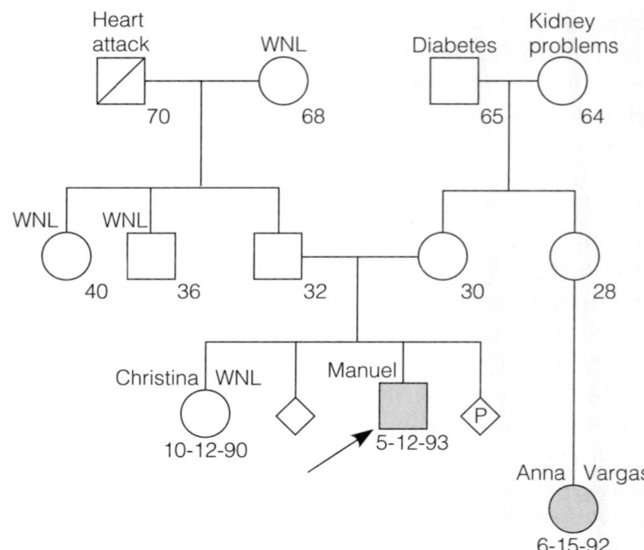

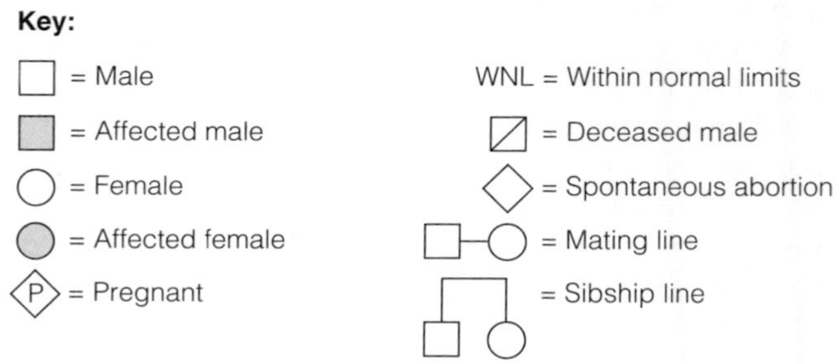

FIGURE 4–18 Screening pedigree. Arrow indicates the nearest family member affected with the disorder being investigated. Basic data have been recorded. Numbers refer to the ages of the family members.

This group includes families in which there is concern about a possible translocation.

After the couple has been referred to the genetics clinic, they are sent a form requesting information on the health status of various family members. At this time, the nurse can help by discussing the form with the family or clarifying the information needed to complete it.

A pedigree and history facilitate identification of other family members who might also be at risk for the same disorder (Figure 4–18). The family being counseled may wish to notify those relatives at risk so that they, too, can be given genetic counseling. When done correctly, the family history and pedigree can be powerful tools for determining a family's risk.

The counselor gathers additional information about the pregnancy, the affected child's growth and development, and the family's understanding of the problem. Generally the child is given a physical examination. Other family members may also be examined. If any laboratory tests, such as chromosomal analysis, metabolic studies, or viral titers, are indicated, they are performed at this time. The genetic counselor may then give the family some preliminary information based on the data at hand.

Finally, information concerning ethnic or religious background and family origin should be elicited. Many genetic disorders are more common among certain ethnic groups or more commonly found in particular geographic areas. For example, families from the British Isles are at higher risk for neural tube defects; Ashkenazic Jews (deriving from eastern Europe) for Tay-Sachs; people of African descent for sickle-cell anemia; and people of Mediterranean heritage for thalassemias.

Follow-Up Counseling

When all the data have been carefully examined and analyzed, the family returns for a follow-up visit. At this time, the parents are given all the information available, including the medical facts, diagnosis, probable course of the disorder, and any available management; the inheritance pattern for this particular family and the risk of recurrence; and the options or alternatives for dealing with the risk of recurrence. The remainder of the counseling session is spent discussing the course of action that seems appropriate to the family in view of their risk and family goals. Among those options or alternatives are prenatal diagnosis and early detection and treatment and, in some cases, adoption, artificial insemination, or delayed childbearing.

The family may consider *artificial insemination by donor (AID),* discussed earlier in this chapter. This alternative is appropriate in several instances; for example, if the male partner is affected with an autosomal dominant disease, AID would decrease to zero the risk of having an affected child, since the child would not inherit any genes from the affected parent. If the man is affected with an X-linked disorder and does not wish to continue the gene in the family (all his daughters will be carriers), AID would be an alternative to terminating all pregnancies with a female fetus. If the man is a carrier for a balanced translocation and if termination of pregnancy is against family ethics, AID is the most appropriate alternative. AID is also appropriate if both parents are carriers of an autosomal recessive disease. AID lowers the risk to a very low level or to zero if a carrier test is available. Finally, AID may be appropriate if the family is at high risk for a multifactorial disorder.

Couples who are young and at risk may decide to delay childbearing for a few years. Medical science and genetics are continually making breakthroughs in early detection and treatment. These couples may find in a few years that prenatal diagnosis is available or that a disease can be detected and treated early to prevent irreversible damage.

The family may return to the genetic counselor a number of times to air their questions and concerns. It is most desirable for the nurse working with the family to attend many or all of these counseling sessions. The nurse, who has already established a rapport with the family, can act as a liaison between the family and the genetic counselor. Hearing directly what the genetic counselor says helps the nurse clarify the issues for the family, which in turn helps them formulate questions.

When the parents have completed the counseling sessions, the counselor sends them and their certified nurse-midwife/physician a letter detailing the contents of the sessions. The family keeps this document for reference. See Key Facts to Remember: Nursing Responsibilities in Genetic Counseling.

Perhaps one of the most important and crucial aspects of genetic counseling in which the nurse is involved is follow-up counseling. The nurse with the appropriate knowledge of genetics is in an ideal position to help families review what has been discussed during the counseling sessions and to answer any additional questions they might have. As the family returns to daily living, the nurse can provide helpful information on the day-to-day aspects of caring for the child, answer questions as they arise, support parents in their decisions, and refer the family to other health and community agencies (Mackta and Weiss 1994).

If the couple is considering having more children, or if siblings want information about their affected brother or sister, the nurse should recommend that the family

KEY FACTS TO REMEMBER

Nursing Responsibilities in Genetic Counseling

Identify families at risk for genetic problems.

Assist families in acquiring accurate information about the specific problem.

Act as liaison between family and genetic counselor.

Assist the family in understanding/dealing with information received.

Provide information on support groups.

Aid families in coping with this crisis.

Provide information about known genetic factors.

Assure continuity of nursing care to the family.

return for another follow-up visit with the genetic counselor. Appropriate options can again be defined and discussed and any new information given to the family. Many genetic centers have found the public health nurse to be the ideal health professional to provide such follow-up care.

Nurses must be careful not to assume a diagnosis, determine carrier status or recurrence risks, or provide genetic counseling without adequate information and training. Inadequate, inappropriate, or inaccurate information may be misleading or harmful. Health care professionals need to learn the appropriate referral systems and options for care in their region.

CHAPTER HIGHLIGHTS

- A couple is considered infertile when they do not conceive after 1 year of unprotected coitus.
- At least 8 percent of couples in the United States are infertile.
- A thorough history and physical of both partners is essential as a basis for infertility investigation.
- General fertility investigations include evaluation of ovarian function, cervical mucus adequacy and receptivity to sperm, sperm number and function, tubal patency, general condition of the pelvic organs, and certain laboratory tests.
- Among cases of infertility, 40 percent involve male factors, 40 percent involve female factors, 10–20 percent have no identifiable cause, and 35 percent have multifactorial etiologies.
- Medications may be prescribed to induce ovulation, facilitate cervical mucus formation, reduce antibody concentration, increase sperm count and motility, and suppress endometriosis.
- The emotional aspects of infertility may be even more difficult for the couple than the testing and therapy.
- The nurse needs to be prepared to dispel myths and provide accurate information about infertility.
- The nurse assesses coping responses and initiates counseling referrals as indicated.
- In autosomal dominant disorders, an affected parent has a 50 percent chance of having an affected child. Such disorders equally affect males and females. The characteristic presentation will vary in each individual with the gene. Some of the common autosomal dominant inherited disorders are Huntington disease, polycystic kidney disease, and neurofibromatosis (von Recklinghausen disease).
- Autosomal recessive disorders are characterized by both parents being carriers; each offspring having a 25 percent chance of having the disease, a 25 percent chance of not being affected, and a 50 percent chance of being a carrier; and males and females being equally affected. Some common autosomal recessive inheritance disorders are cystic fibrosis, phenylketonuria (PKU), galactosemia, sickle-cell anemia, Tay-Sachs disease, and most metabolic disorders.
- X-linked recessive disorders are characterized by no male-to-male transmission; effects limited to males; a 50 percent chance that a carrier mother will pass the abnormal gene to her son; a 50 percent chance that she will not transmit the abnormal gene to her son; a 50 percent chance that her daughter will be a carrier; and a 100 percent chance that daughters of affected fathers will be carriers. Common X-linked recessive disorders are hemophilia, color blindness, and Duchenne muscular dystrophy.
- Multifactorial inheritance disorders include cleft lip and palate, spina bifida, dislocated hips, clubfoot, and pyloric stenosis.
- Some genetic conditions that can currently be diagnosed prenatally are craniospinal defects, renal malformations, hemophilia, fragile X syndrome, thalassemia, cystic fibrosis, many inborn errors of metabolism such as Tay-Sachs disease, and neural tube defects. This list expands daily as new technology allows more conditions to be detected.
- The chief tools of prenatal diagnosis are ultrasound, serum alpha fetoprotein testing, amniocentesis, chorionic villus sampling, and percutaneous umbilical blood sampling.
- Based on sound knowledge about common genetic problems, the nurse should prepare the family for counseling and act as a resource person during and after the counseling sessions.

REFERENCES

American College of Obstetricians and Gynecologists, Committee on Obstetric Practice. *Down Syndrome Screening.* ACOG Committee Opinion No. 141. Washington, DC: Author, 1994.

American Fertility Society: New guidelines for the use of semen donor insemination. *Fertil Steril* 1990; 53(3):1s–3s.

Arms S: *Adoption: A Handful of Hope.* Albany, CA: Celestial Arts, 1990.

Blenner JL: Clomiphene-induced mood swings. *JOGNN* 1991; 20(4):321.

Boxer A: Images of infertility. *Nurse Practitioner Forum* 1996; 7(2):60.

Braverman A, English M: Creating brave new families with advanced reproductive technologies. *Clin Issues Perinat Women Health Nurs* 1992; 3(2):353.

Centers for Disease Control: Recommendations for use of folic acid to reduce number of spina bifida cases and other neural tube defects. *JAMA* 1993; 269(10):1233.

Chervenak FA, Isaacson GC, Campbell S: *Ultrasounds in Obstetrics and Gynecology.* Boston: Little, Brown, 1993.

Corson S: *Conquering Infertility.* New York: Prentice Hall, 1990.

D'Alton ME: Prenatal diagnostic procedures. *Semin Perinatol* 1994; 18(3):140.

English M: Frontiers of reproductive technology: A review of assisted methods of reproduction. In: *Principles of Infertility Nursing.* Garner C (editor). Boston: CRC Press, 1991.

Filly RA, Callen PW, Goldstein RB: Alpha-fetoprotein screening programs: What every obstetric sonologist should know. *Radiology* 1993; 188(1):1.

Garmel SH, D'Alton ME: Diagnostic ultrasound in pregnancy: An overview. *Semin Perinatol* 1994; 18(3):117.

Geerling JH: Natural family planning. *AFP,* 1995; 52(6):1749.

Goode CJ, Hahn SJ: Oocyte donation and in vitro fertilization: The nurse's role with ethical and legal issues. *JOGNN* 1993; 22(2):106.

Gutmann JN, Corson SL: Artificial insemination. In: *Gynecology and Obstetrics, Vol 5.* Sciarra JJ et al (editors). Hagerstown, MD: Harper & Row, 1994.

Guyer MS, Collins FS: The Human Genome Project and the future of medicine. *Am J Disabled Child* 1993; 147:1145.

Haas G: Antisperm antibodies. In: *Progress in Infertility.* Behrman S, Patton G, Holtz G (editors). Boston: Little, Brown, 1994.

Hammond MG: Induction of ovulation with clomiphene citrate. In: *Gynecology and Obstetrics, Vol 5.* Sciarra JJ et al (editors). Hagerstown, MD: Harper & Row, 1996.

Haney A: Treatment of endometriosis. In: *Progress in Infertility.* Behrman S, Patton G, Holtz G (editors). Boston: Little, Brown, 1994.

Hatcher RA et al: *Contraceptive Technology,* 16th ed. New York: Irvington, 1994.

Hill L: Infertility and reproductive assistance. In: *Transvaginal Ultrasound.* Nyberg D et al (editors). St Louis: Mosby, 1992.

Hook EB et al: Maternal age-specific rates of 47,+21 and other cytogenetic abnormalities diagnosed in the first trimester of pregnancy in chorionic villus biopsy specimens: Comparison with rates expected from observations at amniocentesis. *Am J Hum Genet* 1988; 42:797.

Inati MN, Lazar EC, Haskin-Leahy L: The role of the genetic counselor in a perinatal unit. *Semin Perinatol* 1994; 18(3):133.

Jaffe SB, Jewelewicz R: The basic infertility investigation. *Fertil Steril* 1991; 56(4):599.

Jirka J, Schuett S, Foxall MJ: Loneliness and social support in infertile couples. *JOGNN* 1996; 25(1):55.

Johnson CL: Regaining self-esteem: Strategies and interventions for the infertile woman. *JOGNN* 1996; 25(4):291.

Jones SL: Assisted reproductive technologies: Genetic and nursing implications. *JOGNN* 1994; 23(6):492.

Karande VC et al: The limited value of hysterosalpingography in assessing tubal status and fertility potential. *Fertil Steril* 1995; 63(6):1167.

King CR, Schimke RN: Multifactorial inheritance. In: *Gynecology and Obstetrics, Vol 5.* Sciarra JJ et al (editors). Hagerstown, MD: Harper & Row, 1994.

Kuller JA, Laifer SA: Contemporary approaches to prenatal diagnosis. *Am Fam Pract* 1995; 52(8):2277.

Lessor R et al: An analysis of social and psychological characteristics of women volunteering to become oocyte donors. *Fertil Steril* 1993; 59(1):65.

Luthy DA et al: Cesarean section before the onset of labor and subsequent motor function in infants with meningomyolocele diagnosed antenatally. *N Engl J Med* 1992; 324(10):662.

Mackta J, Weiss JO: The role of genetic support groups. *JOGNN* 1994; 23(6):519.

Mahlstedt PP: The psychological components of infertility. *Fertil Steril* 1985; 43:335.

Mastroyannis C: Gamete intrafallopian transfer: Ethical considerations, historical development of the procedure, and comparison with other advanced reproductive technologies. *Fertil Steril* 1993; 60(3):389.

Medical Research International and SART. IVF-ET in the United States during 1990. *Fertil Steril* 1992; 57(1):15.

Menning E: *Infertility: A Guide for the Childless Couple.* 2nd ed. New York: Prentice Hall, 1988.

Mishell DR, Davajan V, Lobo RA: *Infertility, Contraception and Reproductive Endocrinology.* Boston: Blackwell Scientific Publications, 1991.

Mosher WD, Pratt WF: The demography of infertility in the United States. In: *Annual Progress in Reproductive Medicine.* Asch RH, Studd JW (editors). Pearl River, NY: Parthenon Publishing Group, 1993.

Oei SG et al: Effect of the postcoital test on the sexual relationship of infertile couples: A randomized controlled trial. *Fertil Steril* 1996; 65(4):771.

Olsen DG: Parental adjustment to a child with a genetic disease: One parent's reflections. *JOGNN* 1994; 23(6):516.

Pergament E, Fiddler M: Current status of preimplantation diagnosis. In: *Gynecology and Obstetrics, Vol 5.* Sciarri JJ et al (editors). Hagerstown, MD: Harper & Row, 1996.

Pickler RH, Munro CL: Blastomere analysis: Issues for discussion. *JOGNN* 1994; 23(5):379.

Sandelowski M: On infertility. *JOGNN* 1994; 23(9):749.

Sawatzky M: Tasks of the infertile couple. *JOGNN* 1981; 10:132.

Schenler JG, Ezra Y: Complications of assisted reproductive techniques. *Fertil Steril* 1994; 61(3):411.

Schoener CJ, Krysa LW: The comfort and discomfort of infertility. *JOGNN* 1996; 25(2):167.

Shulman LP, Simpson JL, Elias S: Invasive prenatal genetic techniques. In: *Gynecology and Obstetrics, Vol 5.* Sciarra JJ et al (editors). Hagerstown, MD: Harper & Row, 1993.

Simpson JL: Genetic factors in obstetrics and gynecology. In: *Danforth's Obstetrics and Gynecology* 6th ed. Scott JR et al (editors). Philadelphia: Lippincott, 1990.

Simpson JL, Elias S: *Essentials of Prenatal Diagnosis.* New York: Churchill Livingstone, 1993.

Snowdon C: What makes a mother? Interviews with women involved in egg donation and surrogacy. *Birth* 1994; 21(2):77.

Society for Assisted Reproductive Technology (SART): Assisted reproductive technology in the United States and Canada: 1991 results from the Society for Assisted Reproductive Technology generated from the American Fertility Society Registry. *Fertil Steril* 1993; 59(5):956.

Speroff L, Glass RH, Kase NG: *Clinical Gynecologic Endocrinology and Infertility,* 5th ed. Baltimore: Williams & Wilkins, 1994.

Stansberry J: The infertile couple: An overview of pathophysiology and diagnostic evaluation for the primary care clinician. *Nurse Practitioner Forum* 1996; 7(2):76.

Tallo CP et al: Maternal and neonatal morbidity asociated with in vitro fertilization. *J Pediatr* 1995; 127(5):794.

Thompson MW, McInnes RR, Willard HF: *Thompson & Thompson's Genetics in Medicine,* 5th ed. Philadelphia: Saunders, 1991.

Townsend AB: Ethical issues of gamete and embryo donation: Implications for nursing. *J Perinatol* 1992; 12(4):359.

Tredway DR: The postcoital test. In: *Gynecology and Obstetrics, Vol 5.* Sciarri JJ et al (editors). Hagerstown, MD: Harper & Row, 1996.

Wilcox LS, Mosher WD: Use of infertility services in the United States. *Obstet Gynecol* 1993: 82:122.

World Health Organization: *WHO Manual for the Examination of Human Semen and Sperm–Cervical Mucus Interaction.* Cambridge, England: Cambridge Univ Press, 1992.

Wolf GC, Baker CA: Tympanic thermometry for recording basal body temperatures. *Fertil Steril* 1993; 60(5):922.

Wright L: Prenatal diagnosis in the 1990s. *JOGNN* 1994; 23(6):506.

Chapter 5 Women's Health Care

OBJECTIVES

- Summarize information that women may need to implement appropriate self-care measures for dealing with menstruation.
- Compare the advantages, disadvantages, and effectiveness of the various methods of contraception.
- Discuss basic gynecologic screening procedures indicated for well women.
- Discuss the physical and psychologic aspects of menopause.
- Delineate the nurse's role in working with women who are the victims of violence through female partner abuse and rape.
- Contrast the common benign breast disorders.
- Discuss the signs and symptoms, medical therapy, and implications for fertility of endometriosis.
- Compare vulvovaginal candidiasis and bacterial vaginosis.
- Describe the common sexually transmitted infections.
- Summarize the health teaching a nurse should provide to a woman with a sexually transmitted infection.
- Relate the implications of pelvic inflammatory disease (PID) for future fertility to its pathology, signs and symptoms, and treatment.
- Identify the implications of an abnormal finding during a pelvic examination.
- Contrast cystitis and pyelonephritis.

KEY TERMS

Amenorrhea
Breast self-examination (BSE)
Cervical cap
Climacteric
Coitus interruptus
Colposcopy
Condom
Depo-Provera
Diaphragm
Dysmenorrhea
Dyspareunia
Endometriosis
Female partner abuse
Fertility awareness methods
Fibrocystic breast disease
Hormone replacement therapy (HRT)
Intrauterine device (IUD)
Mammogram
Menopause
Oral contraceptives
Osteoporosis
Pap smear
Pelvic inflammatory disease (PID)
Premenstrual syndrome (PMS)
Rape
Sexually Transmitted Infections (STI)
Spermicides
Subdermal implants (Norplant)
Toxic shock syndrome (TSS)
Tubal ligation
Vasectomy

A woman's health care needs change throughout her lifetime. As a young girl she requires health teaching about menstruation, sexuality, and personal responsibility. As a teen she needs information about reproductive choices and safe sexual activity. During this time she should also be introduced to the importance of health care practices such as breast self-examination and regular Pap smears. The mature woman may need to be reminded of these self-care issues and prepared for physical changes that accompany childbirth and aging. By educating women about their bodies, their health care choices, and their right to be knowledgeable consumers, nurses can help women assume responsibility for the health care they receive.

The contemporary woman is likely to encounter various major or minor gynecologic or urinary problems during her lifetime. These problems may provoke a variety of psychologic responses and physical concerns. The nurse can assist a woman in this situation by providing accurate, sensitive, and supportive health education and counseling. To meet the woman's needs, the nurse must have up-to-date information about health care practices and available diagnostic and treatment options.

This chapter provides information about selected aspects of women's health care with an emphasis on conditions typically addressed in a community-based setting.

Community-Based Nursing Care

Women's health refers to a holistic view of women and their health-related needs within the context of their everyday lives. It is based on the awareness that a woman's physical, mental, and social status are interdependent and determine her state of health or illness. The woman's view of her situation, her assessment of her needs, her values, and her beliefs are valid and important factors to be incorporated into any health care intervention.

Nurses can work with women to provide health teaching and information about self-care practices in schools, during routine examinations in a clinic or office, at senior centers, at meetings of volunteer organizations, through classes offered by the local health department or community college, or in the home. This community-based focus is the key to providing effective nursing care to women of all ages.

In reality, the vast majority of women's health care is provided outside of acute care settings. Nurses oriented to community-based care are especially effective in recognizing the autonomy of each individual and in dealing with clients holistically. This is especially important in addressing not only physical problems but also major health issues such as violence against women, which may go undetected unless care providers are alert for signs of it.

The Nurse's Role in Addressing Issues of Sexuality

On occasion most people experience concern and even anxiety about some aspect of sexuality. Societal standards and pressures can cause people to evaluate and compare with others their sexual attractiveness, technical abilities, frequency of sexual interaction, and so on. Appearance and sexual behavior are not the only causes for concern; the reproductive implications of sexual intercourse must also be considered. Some people desire conception; others wish to avoid it. Health factors are another consideration. The increase in the incidence of sexually transmitted infections, especially AIDS and herpes, has caused many people to modify their sexual practices and activities.

Because sexuality and its reproductive implications are such an intrinsic and emotion-laden part of life, people have many concerns, problems, and questions about sex roles, behaviors, education, inhibitions, and morality, and related areas such as family planning. Women frequently voice these concerns to the nurse in a clinic or ambulatory setting. Thus the nurse may need to assume the role of counselor on sexual and reproductive matters.

Nurses who assume this role must be secure about their own sexuality. They must also develop an awareness of their own feelings, values, and attitudes about sexuality so they can be more sensitive and objective when they encounter the values and beliefs of others. Nurses should have accurate, up-to-date information about topics related to sexuality, sexual practices, and common gynecologic problems. They also need to know about the structures and functions of female and male reproductive systems.

Continuing education for the practicing nurse and appropriate courses in undergraduate and graduate nursing education programs can help nurses achieve this sense of security and the requisite knowledge about aspects of sexuality. These courses can teach nurses about sexual values, attitudes, alternative lifestyles, cultural factors, and misconceptions and myths about sex and reproduction.

Taking a Sexual History

Nurses today are often responsible for taking a woman's initial history, including her gynecologic and sexual history. To be effective in this role, the nurse must have good communication skills and should conduct the interview in a quiet, private place free of distractions.

Opening the discussion with a brief explanation of the purpose of such questions is often helpful. For example, the nurse might say, "As your nurse I'm interested in all aspects of your well-being. Often women have concerns or questions about sexual matters, especially when they are pregnant (or starting to be sexually active). I will be asking you some questions about your sexual history as part of your general health history."

It may be helpful to use direct eye contact as much as possible unless the nurse knows it is culturally unacceptable to the woman. The nurse should do little, if any, writing during the interview, especially if the woman seems ill at ease or is discussing very personal issues. Open-ended questions are often useful in eliciting information. For example, "What, if anything, would you change about your sex life?" will elicit more information than "Are you happy with your sex life now?" The nurse should also clarify terminology and proceed from easier topics to those that are more difficult to discuss. Throughout the interview the nurse should be alert to body language and nonverbal cues.

After completing the sexual history, the nurse assesses the information obtained. If there is a problem that requires further medical tests and assessments, the nurse will refer the woman to a nurse practitioner, certified nurse-midwife, physician, or counselor as necessary. In many instances the nurse alone will be able to develop a nursing diagnosis and then plan and implement therapy. For example, if the nurse determines that a woman who is interested in conceiving a child does not have a clear understanding of when she ovulates, the nurse may formulate the nursing diagnosis: *Knowledge deficit related to lack of information about the timing of ovulation.* The nurse can then evaluate the woman's knowledge through discussion and review and work with the woman to provide necessary knowledge. The nurse might also suggest that the woman keep a menstrual calendar and monitor basal body temperatures to identify the time of ovulation.

The nurse must be realistic in making assessments and planning interventions. It requires insight and skill to recognize when a woman's problem requires interventions that are beyond a nurse's preparation and ability. In such situations, the nurse must make appropriate referrals.

Menstruation

Girls today begin to learn about puberty and menstruation at a surprisingly young age. Unfortunately the source of their "education" is sometimes their peers and sometimes the media; thus the information is frequently incomplete, inaccurate, and sensationalized. Nurses who work with young girls and adolescents recognize this and are working hard to provide accurate health teaching and correct misinformation about menarche (the onset of menses) and the menstrual cycle.

Cultural, religious, and personal attitudes about menstruation are part of the menstrual experience and often reflect negative attitudes toward women. In the past, many myths surrounded menstruation. Women were often isolated or restricted to the company of other women during their monthly flow because they were considered "unclean." Today there is a tendency to regard menstruating women as vulnerable or less capable. Current customs include refraining from exercise and showers and hiding the fact of menstruation entirely. Cultural taboos against coitus (sexual intercourse) during menses have long endured, but there are no health reasons for such taboos. Nurses discussing this topic with clients may want to confirm that sexual intercourse during menses is common practice and not contraindicated; however, not all couples desire it. (The physiology of menstruation is discussed in Chapter 2.)

Counseling the Premenstrual Girl About Menarche

Many young women find it embarrassing or stressful to discuss the menstrual experience, both because of the many taboos associated with the subject and because of their immaturity. However, the most critical factor in successful adaptation to menarche is the adolescent's level of preparedness. Information should be given to premenstrual girls over time, rather than all at once. This allows them to absorb information and develop questions.

The following basic information is helpful for young clients:

- *Cycle length.* Cycle length is determined from the first day of one menses to the first day of the next menses. Initially a female's cycle length is about 29 days, but the normal length may vary from 21–35 days. As a woman matures, cycle length often shortens to a median of 25+ days just before menopause. Cycle length often varies by a day or two from one cycle to the next, although greater normal variations may also occur.
- *Amount of flow.* The average flow is approximately 30 mL per period. Usually women characterize the amount of flow in terms of the number of pads or tampons used. Flow often is heavier at first and lighter toward the end of the period.
- *Length of menses.* Menses usually lasts from 2 to 8 days, although this may vary.

The nurse should make it clear that variations in age at menarche, length of cycle, and duration of menses are normal because girls are likely to be concerned if their experience varies from that of their peers. It also is helpful to acknowledge the negative aspects of menstruation (messiness and embarrassment) while stressing its positive role as a symbol of maturity and womanhood.

Educational Topics

The nurse's primary role is to provide accurate information and assist in clarifying misconceptions, so that girls will develop positive self-images and progress smoothly through this phase of maturation.

Pads and Tampons

Since early times women have made pads and tampons from cloth or rags, which required washing but were reusable. Some women made them from gauze or cotton balls. Commercial tampons were introduced in the 1930s.

Today adhesive-stripped minipads and maxipads and flushable tampons have made life easier. However, the deodorants and increased absorbency that manufacturers have added to both sanitary napkins and tampons may prove harmful. The chemical used to deodorize can create a rash on the vulva and damage the tender mucous lining of the vagina. Excessive or inappropriate use of tampons can produce dryness or even small sores or ulcers in the vagina.

Because the use of superabsorbent tampons has been linked to the development of toxic shock syndrome (TSS) (see p 122), women should avoid using them. They should use regular-absorbency tampons only for heavy menstrual flow (during the first 2 or 3 days of the period), not during the whole period, and change them every 3 to 6 hours. Since *Staphylococcus aureus,* the causative organism of TSS, is frequently found on the hands, a woman should wash her hands before inserting a fresh tampon and should avoiding touching the tip of the tampon when unwrapping it or before insertion.

In the absence of a heavy menstrual flow, tampons absorb moisture, leaving the vaginal walls dry and subject to injury. The absorbency of regular tampons varies. If the tampon is hard to pull out or shreds when removed, or if the vagina becomes dry, the tampon is probably too absorbent. If a woman is worried about accidental spotting, she can check the diagrams on the packages of regular tampons. Those that expand in width are better able to prevent leakage without being too absorbent.

A woman may want to use tampons only during the day and switch to napkins at night to avoid vaginal irritation. She should avoid using tampons on the last spotty days of the period and should never use them for midcycle spotting or leukorrhea. If a woman experiences vaginal irritation, itching, or soreness, or notices an unusual odor while using tampons, she should stop using them or change brands or absorbencies to see if that helps.

The choice of sanitary protection must meet the individual's needs and feel comfortable, whether it be napkins or tampons.

Vaginal Sprays and Douching

Vaginal sprays are unnecessary and can cause infections, itching, burning, vaginal discharge, rashes, and other problems. If a woman chooses to use a spray, she needs to know that these sprays are for external use only and should never be applied to irritated or itching skin or used with sanitary napkins.

Although douching is sometimes used to treat vaginal infections, douching as a hygiene practice is unnecessary, since the vagina cleanses itself. Douching washes away the natural mucus and upsets the vaginal ecology, which can make the vagina more susceptible to infection. Douching with one of the perfumed or flavored douches can cause allergic reactions, and too frequent use of an undiluted or strong douche solution can induce severe irritation, even tissue damage. Propelling water up the vagina may also erode the antibacterial cervical plug and force bacteria and germs from the vagina into the uterus. Women should avoid douching during menstruation because the cervix is dilated to permit the downward flow of menstrual fluids from the uterine lining. Douching may force tissue back up into the uterine cavity, which could create endometriosis.

The mucous secretions that continually bathe the vagina are completely odor-free while they are in the vagina; only when they mingle with perspiration and hit the air does odor develop. Keeping one's skin clean and free of bacteria with plain soap and water is the most effective method of controlling odor. A soapy finger or soft washcloth should be used to wash gently between the vulvar folds. Bathing is as important (if not more so) during menses as at any other time. A long leisurely soak in a warm tub will promote menstrual blood flow and relieve cramps by relaxing the muscles.

Keeping the vaginal area fresh throughout the day means keeping it dry and clean. A woman can assure herself of adequate ventilation by wearing cotton panties and clothes loose enough to permit the vaginal area to breathe. After using the toilet, a woman should always wipe herself from front to back and, if necessary, follow up with a moistened paper towel or toilet paper.

The most important thing to remember is that if an unusual odor persists despite these efforts, it may be a sign that something is awry. Certain conditions such as vaginitis produce a foul-smelling discharge.

Relief of Discomfort

Some nutritionists suggest that vitamins B and E help relieve the discomforts associated with menstruation. Vitamin B_6 may help relieve the premenstrual bloating and irritability some women experience. Vitamin E, a mild prostaglandin inhibitor, may help decrease menstrual discomfort. Avoiding salt can decrease discomfort from fluid retention.

Heat is soothing and promotes increased blood flow. Any source of warmth, from sipping herbal tea to soaking in a hot tub or using a heating pad, may be helpful during painful periods. Massage can also soothe aching back muscles and promote relaxation and blood flow.

Daily exercise can ease existing menstrual discomfort and help prevent cramps and other menstrual complaints. Aerobic exercises such as jogging, cycling, aerobic dancing, swimming, and fast-paced walking are especially helpful. Persistent discomfort should be medically evaluated.

Associated Menstrual Conditions

A variety of menstrual irregularities have been identified. An abnormally short duration of menstrual flow is termed *hypomenorrhea;* an abnormally long one is called *hypermenorrhea*. Excessive, profuse flow is called *menorrhagia*, and bleeding between periods is known as *metrorrhagia*. Infrequent and too frequent menses are termed *oligomenorrhea* and *polymenorrhea*, respectively. An anovulatory cycle is one in which ovulation does not occur. Such irregularities should be investigated to rule out any disease process.

Amenorrhea

Amenorrhea, the absence of menses, is classified as primary or secondary. Primary amenorrhea is said to occur if menstruation has not been established by 18 years of age. Secondary amenorrhea is said to occur when an established menses (of longer than 3 months) ceases.

Primary amenorrhea necessitates a thorough assessment of the young woman to determine its cause. Possible causes include congenital obstructions, congenital absence of the uterus, testicular feminization (external genitals appear female but uterus and ovaries are absent and testes are present), or absence or imbalance of hormones. Success of treatment depends on the causative factors. Many causes are not correctable.

Secondary amenorrhea is caused most frequently by pregnancy. Additional causes include lactation, hormonal imbalances, poor nutrition (anorexia nervosa, obesity, fad dieting), ovarian lesions, strenuous exercise (associated with long-distance runners, dancers, and other athletes with low body fat ratios), debilitating systemic diseases, stress of high intensity and/or long duration, stressful life events, a change in season or climate, use of oral contraceptives, the phenothiazine and chlorpromazine group of tranquilizers, and syndromes such as Cushing and Sheehan. Treatment is dictated by the causative factors. The nurse can explain that once the underlying condition has been corrected—for example, when sufficient body weight is gained—menses will resume. Female athletes and women who participate in strenuous exercise routines may be advised to increase their caloric intake or reduce their exercise levels for a month or two to see whether a normal cycle ensues. If it does not, medical referral is indicated.

Dysmenorrhea

Dysmenorrhea, or painful menstruation, occurs at, or a day before, the onset of menstruation and disappears by the end of menses. Dysmenorrhea is classified as primary or secondary. *Primary dysmenorrhea* is defined as cramps without underlying disease. Prostaglandins F_2 and $F_{2\alpha}$, which are produced by the uterus in higher concentrations during menses, are the primary cause. They increase uterine contractility and decrease uterine artery blood flow, causing ischemia. The end result is the painful sensation of cramps. Dysmenorrhea typically disappears after a first pregnancy and does not occur if cycles are anovulatory. Treatment of primary dysmenorrhea incudes oral contraceptives (which block ovulation), prostaglandin inhibitors (such as ibuprofen, aspirin, naproxen), and self-care measures such as regular exercise, rest, heat, and good nutrition. Biofeedback has also been used with some success.

Secondary dysmenorrhea is associated with pathology of the reproductive tract and usually appears after menstruation has been established. Conditions that most frequently cause secondary dysmenorrhea include endometriosis; residual pelvic inflammatory disease (PID); anatomic anomalies such as cervical stenosis, imperforate hymen, uterine displacement; ovarian cysts; or the presence of an IUD. Because primary and secondary dysmenorrhea may coexist, accurate differential diagnosis is essential for appropriate treatment.

Premenstrual Syndrome

Premenstrual syndrome (PMS) refers to a symptom complex associated with the luteal phase of the menstrual cycle. Women over 30 years of age are the most likely to have PMS. The symptoms must, by definition, occur between ovulation and the onset of menses. They repeat at the same stage of each menstrual cycle and include some or all of the following:

- *Psychologic:* irritability, lethargy, depression, low morale, anxiety, sleep disorders, crying spells, and hostility
- *Neurologic:* classic migraine, vertigo, syncope
- *Respiratory:* rhinitis, hoarseness, occasionally asthma
- *Gastrointestinal:* nausea, vomiting, constipation, abdominal bloating, craving for sweets
- *Urinary:* retention and oliguria
- *Dermatologic:* acne
- *Mammary:* swelling and tenderness

Most women experience only some of these symptoms. The symptoms usually are most pronounced 2 or 3 days before the onset of menstruation and subside as menstrual flow begins, with or without treatment.

The exact cause of PMS is unknown, although a variety of theories have been put forth to explain it. These include, for example, hormone imbalance, nutritional deficiency, prostaglandin excess, and endorphin deficiency.

Nursing Care

The nurse can help the woman identify specific symptoms and develop healthy behavior. After assessment, counseling for PMS may include advising the woman to restrict her intake of foods containing methylxanthines such as chocolate, cola, and coffee; restrict her intake of alcohol, nicotine, red meat, and foods containing salt and sugar; increase her intake of complex carbohydrates and protein; and increase the frequency of meals. Supplementation with B complex vitamins, especially B_6, may decrease anxiety and depression. Vitamin E supplements may help reduce breast tenderness, and a program of aerobic exercises such as fast walking, jogging, and aerobic dancing is generally beneficial.

In addition to vitamin supplements, pharmacologic treatments for PMS include progesterone suppositories, diuretics, and prostaglandin inhibitors. All have been effective in some women and not in others.

An empathic relationship with a health care professional to whom the woman feels free to voice concerns is highly beneficial. Encouragement to keep a diary may help the woman identify life events associated with PMS. Self-care groups and self-help literature both help women gain control over their bodies.

Contraception

The decision to use a method of contraception may be made individually by a woman (or, in the case of vasectomy, by a man) or jointly by a couple. The decision may be motivated by a desire to avoid pregnancy, to gain control over the number of children conceived, or to determine the spacing of future children. In choosing a specific method, consistency of use outweighs the absolute reliability of the given method.

Decisions about contraception should be made voluntarily, with full knowledge of advantages, disadvantages, effectiveness, side effects, contraindications, and long-term effects. Many outside factors influence this choice, including cultural practices, religious beliefs, personality, cost, effectiveness, misinformation, practicality of method, and self-esteem. Different methods of contraception may be appropriate at different times in a couple's life.

Fertility Awareness Methods

Fertility awareness methods, also known as *natural family planning,* are based on an understanding of the changes that occur throughout a woman's ovulatory cycle. All these methods require periods of abstinence and recording of certain events throughout the cycle; cooperation of the partners is important.

Fertility awareness methods are free, safe, and acceptable to many whose religious beliefs prohibit other methods; they provide an increased awareness of the body; they involve no artificial substances or devices; they encourage a couple to communicate about sexual activity and family planning; and they are useful in helping a couple plan a pregnancy.

On the other hand, these methods require extensive initial counseling to be used effectively; they may interfere with sexual spontaneity; they require extensive maintenance of records for several cycles before beginning to use them; they may be difficult or impossible for women with irregular cycles to use; and, although theoretically they should be very reliable, in practice they may not be as reliable in preventing pregnancy as other methods.

The *basal body temperature (BBT) method* to detect ovulation requires that a woman take her BBT every morning upon awakening (before any activity) and record the readings on a temperature graph. To do this, she uses a basal body temperature thermometer, which shows tenths of a degree rather than the two tenths shown on standard thermometers. After 3 to 4 months of recording temperatures, a woman with regular cycles should be able to predict when ovulation will occur. The method is based on the fact that the temperature sometimes drops just before ovulation and almost always rises and remains elevated for several days after. The temperature rise occurs in response to the increased progesterone levels that occur in the second half of the cycle. Figure 5–1 shows a sample BBT chart. To avoid conception, the couple abstains from intercourse on the day of the temperature rise and for 3 days after. Because the temperature rise does not occur until after ovulation, a woman who had intercourse just before the rise is at risk of pregnancy. To decrease this risk, some couples abstain from intercourse for several days before the *anticipated* time of ovulation and then for 3 days after.

The *calendar,* or *rhythm, method* is based on the assumptions that ovulation tends to occur 14 days (plus or minus 2 days) before the start of the next menstrual period, sperm are viable for 48–72 hours, and the ovum is viable for 24 hours (Hatcher et al 1994). To use this method, the woman must record her menstrual cycles for 6 to 8 months to identify the shortest and longest cycles. The first day of menstruation is the first day of the cycle. The fertile phase is calculated from 18 days before the end of the shortest recorded cycle through 11 days

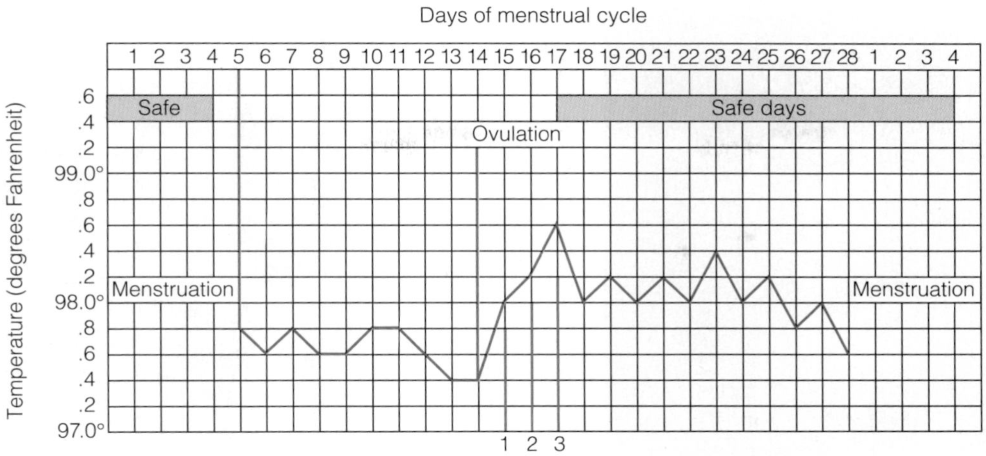

FIGURE 5–1 Sample basal body temperature chart.

Source: Crooks R, Baur K: *Our Sexuality,* 5th ed. Monterey, CA: Brooks Cole, 1993.

from the end of the longest recorded cycle (Hatcher et al 1994). For example, if a woman's cycle lasts from 24–28 days, the fertile phase would be calculated as day 6 through day 17. Once this information is obtained, the woman can identify the fertile and infertile phases of her cycle. For effective use of this method, she must abstain from intercourse during the fertile phase.

The calendar method is the least reliable of the fertility awareness methods and has largely been replaced by other, more scientific approaches.

The *cervical mucus method,* sometimes called the *ovulation method* or the *Billings method,* involves the assessment of cervical mucus changes that occur during the menstrual cycle. The amount and character of cervical mucus change because of the influence of estrogen and progesterone. At the time of ovulation the mucus (estrogen-dominant mucus) is clearer, more stretchable (a quality called spinnbarkeit), and more permeable to sperm. It also shows a characteristic fern pattern when placed on a glass slide and allowed to dry.

During the luteal phase, the cervical mucus is thick and sticky (progesterone-dominant mucus) and forms a network that traps sperm, making their passage more difficult.

To use the cervical mucus method, the woman abstains from intercourse for the first menstrual cycle. Cervical mucus is assessed daily for amount, feeling of slipperiness or wetness, color, clearness, and spinnbarkeit, as the woman becomes familiar with varying characteristics.

The peak day of wetness and clear, stretchable mucus is assumed to be the time of ovulation. To use this method correctly, a woman is advised to abstain from intercourse from the time she first notices that the mucus is becoming clear, more elastic, and slippery until 4 days after the last wet mucus (ovulation) day. Because this method evaluates the effects of hormonal changes, it can be used by women with irregular cycles.

The *symptothermal method* consists of various assessments made and recorded by the couple. These include information regarding cycle days, coitus, cervical mucus changes, and secondary signs such as increased libido, abdominal bloating, mittelschmerz (midcycle abdominal pain), and basal body temperature. Through the various assessments, the couple learns to recognize signs that indicate ovulation. This combined approach tends to improve the effectiveness of fertility awareness as a method of birth control.

Situational Contraceptives

Abstinence can be considered a method of contraception and, partly because of changing values and the increased risk of infection with intercourse, it is gaining increased acceptance.

Coitus interruptus, or withdrawal, is one of the oldest and least reliable methods of contraception. This method requires that the male withdraw from the female's vagina when he feels that ejaculation is impending. He then ejaculates away from the external genitalia of the woman. Failure tends to occur for two reasons:

- This method demands great self-control on the part of the man, who must withdraw just as he feels the urge for deeper penetration with impending orgasm.
- Some preejaculatory fluid, which can contain sperm, may escape from the penis during the excitement phase prior to ejaculation. Because the quantity of sperm in this preejaculatory fluid is increased after a recent ejaculation, this is especially significant for couples who engage in repeated episodes of orgasm within a short period of time.

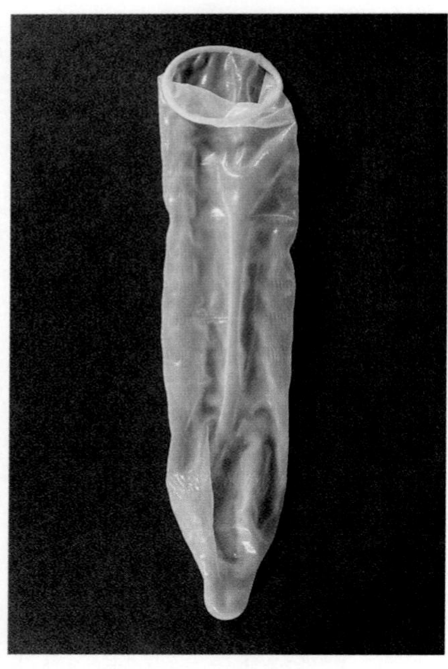

A

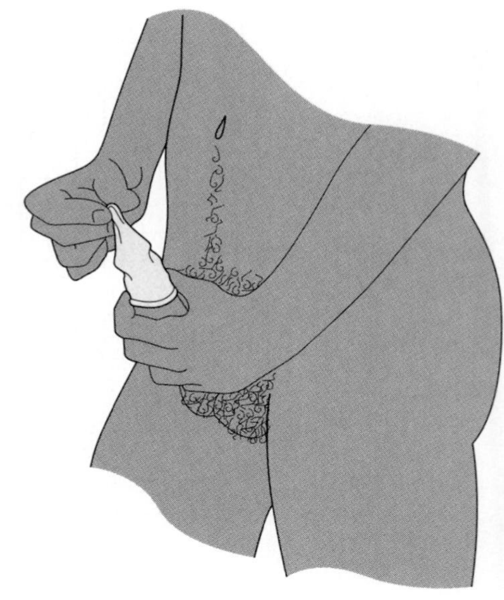

B

FIGURE 5–2 ***A*** Unrolled condom with reservoir tip. ***B*** Correct use of a condom.

Couples who use this method should be aware of postcoital contraceptive options should the man fail to withdraw in time.

Douching after intercourse is an ineffective method of contraception and is not recommended. It may actually facilitate conception by pushing sperm farther up the birth canal.

Mechanical Contraceptives

Mechanical contraceptive methods either prevent the transport of sperm to the ovum or prevent implantation of the ovum/zygote.

The male **condom** offers a viable means of contraception when used consistently and properly (Figure 5–2). Acceptance has been increasing as a growing number of men are assuming responsibility for regulation of fertility. The condom is applied to the erect penis, rolled from the tip to the end of the shaft, before vulvar or vaginal contact. A small space must be left at the end of the condom to allow for collection of the ejaculate, so that the condom will not break at the time of ejaculation. If the condom or vagina is dry, water-soluble lubricants, such as K-Y jelly, should be used to prevent irritation and possible condom breakage. Care must be taken in removing the condom after intercourse. For optimal effectiveness, the man should withdraw his penis from the vagina while it is still erect and hold the condom rim to prevent spillage. If after ejaculation the penis becomes flaccid while still in the vagina, the male should hold onto the edge of the condom while withdrawing to avoid spilling the semen and to prevent the condom from slipping off.

The effectiveness of male condoms is largely determined by their use. The condom is small, lightweight, disposable, and inexpensive; it has no side effects, requires no medical examination or supervision, and offers visual evidence of effectiveness. Latex condoms protect against sexually transmitted infections. Breakage, displacement, perineal or vaginal irritation, and dulled sensation are possible disadvantages.

The male condom is becoming increasingly popular because of the protection latex condoms offer from HIV and other sexually transmitted infections. For women, sexually transmitted infection increases the risk of pelvic inflammatory disease (PID) and resultant infertility. Many women are beginning to insist that their sexual partners use condoms, and many women carry condoms with them.

With their increasing popularity comes increased choice. Condoms are now available with ribbed or smooth sides, tapered or straight-sided, lubricated or unlubricated, with or without spermicide. "Skin condoms" (made from lamb's intestines) are also available and are preferred by some men, especially those who have difficulty tolerating latex. They are not considered effective in preventing the spread of infection, including HIV infection; latex condoms are superior in that regard. Spermicidal condoms or concurrent use of a vaginal spermicide increase the overall effectiveness of skin condoms.

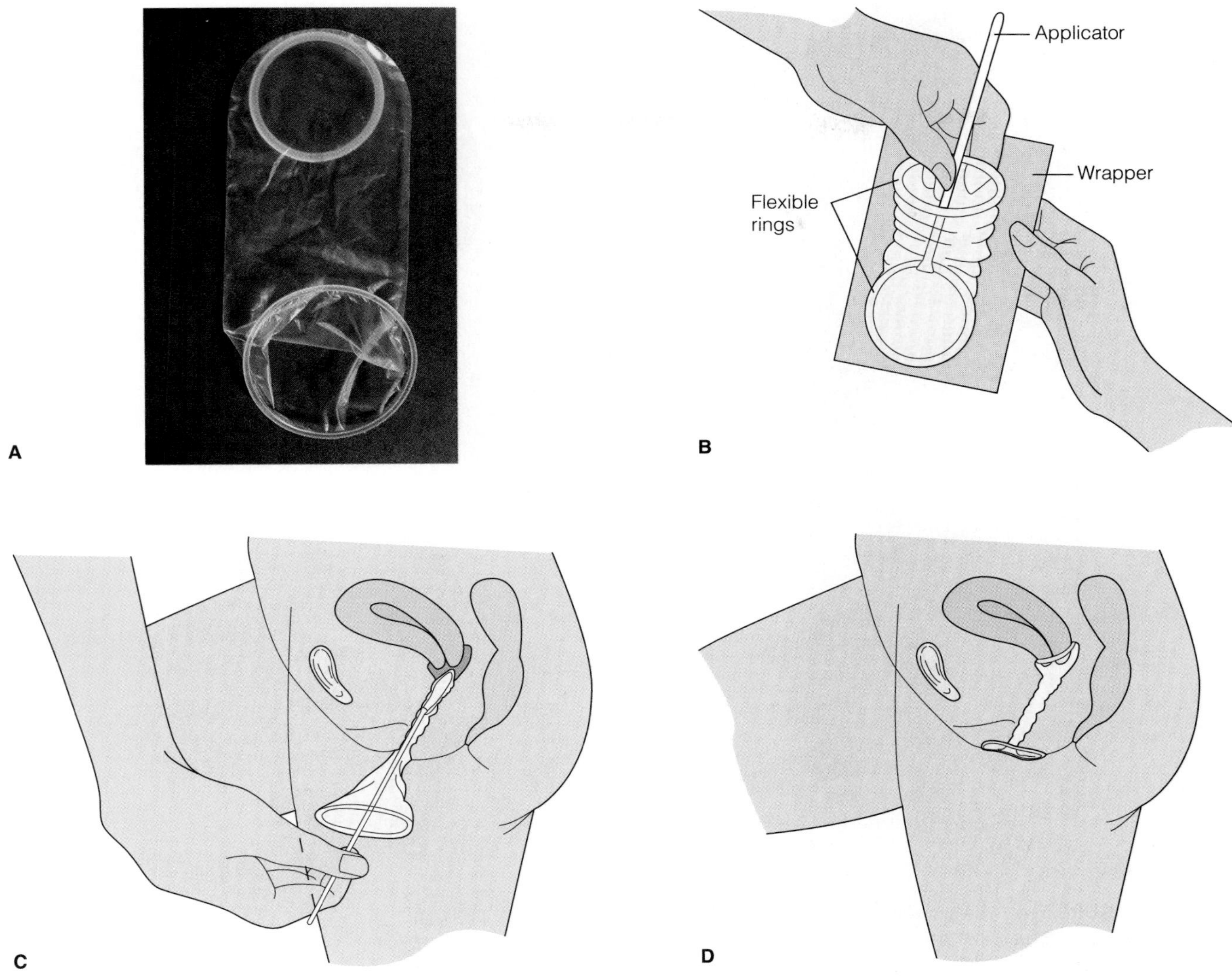

FIGURE 5–3 ***A*** The female condom. To insert the condom: ***B*** Remove condom and applicator from wrapper by pulling up on the ring. ***C*** Insert condom slowly by gently pushing the applicator toward the small of the back. ***D*** When properly inserted, the outer ring should rest on the folds of skin around the vaginal opening, and the inner ring (closed end) should fit loosely against the cervix.

Source: Crooks R, Baur K: *Our Sexuality,* 5th ed. Monterey, CA: Brooks Cole, 1993.

The *Reality female condom* (Figure 5–3) is a thin polyurethane sheath with a flexible ring at each end. The inner ring, at the closed end of the condom, serves as the means of insertion and fits over the cervix like a diaphragm. The second ring remains outside the vagina and covers a portion of the woman's perineum. It also covers the base of the man's penis during intercourse. Available over the counter and designed for one-time use, the condom may be inserted up to eight hours before intercourse. The inner sheath is prelubricated but does not contain spermicide and is not designed to be used with a male condom. Data on its effectiveness against pregnancy are still limited, although the female condom has been compared to other barrier methods. Because it lines the entire vagina, it probably provides better protection against pathogens than other methods. Its cost (about $2.25) may be a factor for some couples. The ultimate acceptance and use of the female condom by women and their partners has not yet been determined (Connell 1994).

The **diaphragm** (Figure 5–4) is used with spermicidal cream or jelly and offers a good level of protection from conception. The woman must be fitted with a diaphragm and instructions given by trained personnel. The diaphragm should be rechecked for correct size after each childbirth and whenever a woman has gained or lost 15 pounds or more.

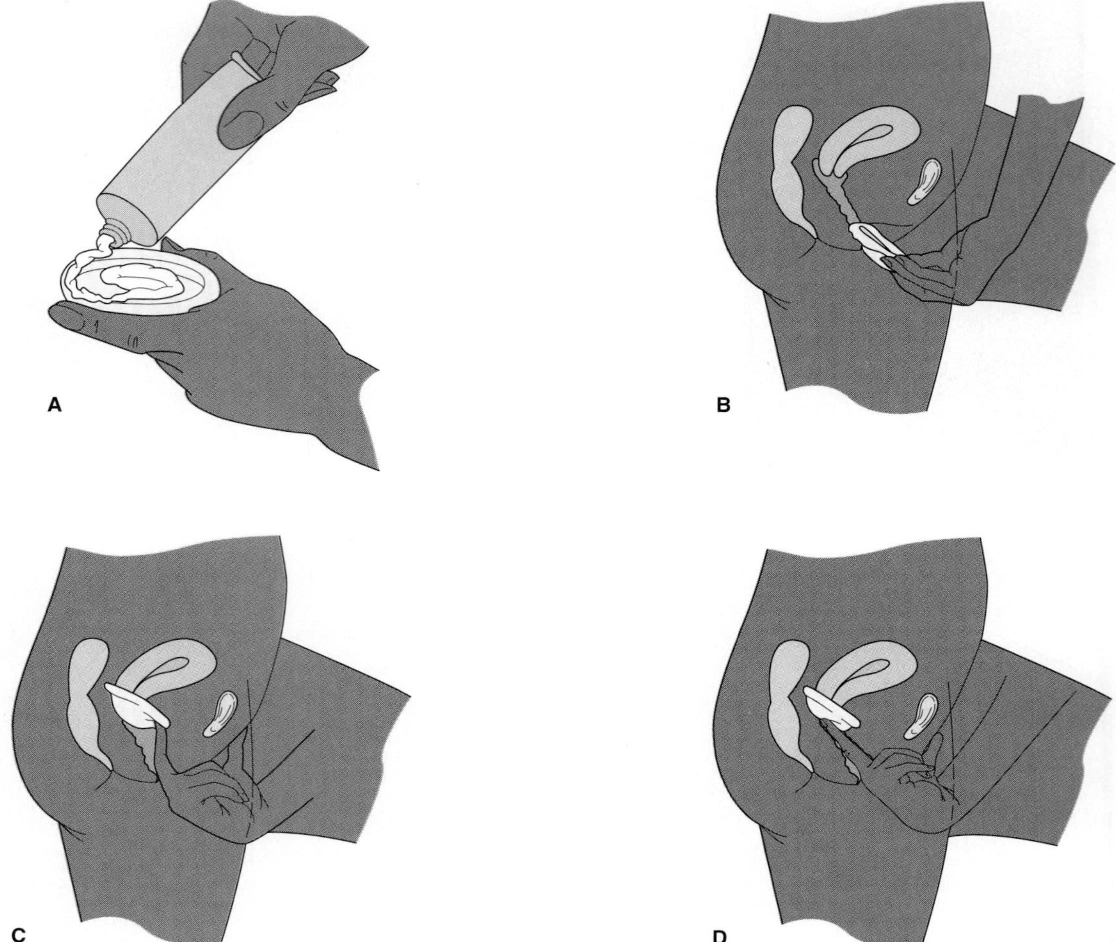

FIGURE 5–4 ***A*** Apply jelly to the rim and center of the diaphragm. ***B*** Insert the diaphragm. ***C*** Push the rim of the diaphragm under the symphysis pubis. ***D*** Check placement of the diaphragm. Cervix should be felt through the diaphragm.

The diaphragm must be inserted before intercourse, with approximately one teaspoonful (or 1.5 inches from the tube) of spermicidal jelly placed around its rim and in the cup. This chemical barrier supplements the mechanical barrier of the diaphragm. The diaphragm is inserted through the vagina and covers the cervix. The last step in insertion is to push the edge of the diaphragm under the symphysis pubis, which may result in a "popping" sensation. When fitted properly and correctly in place, the diaphragm should not cause discomfort to the woman or her partner. Correct placement of the diaphragm can be checked by touching the cervix with a fingertip through the cup. The cervix feels like a small rounded structure and has a consistency similar to that of the tip of the nose. The center of the diaphragm should be over the cervix. If more than 4 hours elapse between insertion of the diaphragm and intercourse, additional spermicidal cream should be used. It is necessary to leave the diaphragm in place for at least 6 hours after coitus. If intercourse is desired again within the 6 hours, another type of contraception must be used or additional spermicidal jelly placed in the vagina with an applicator, taking care not to disturb the placement of the diaphragm. The diaphragm should be periodically held up to the light and inspected for tears or holes.

Some couples feel that the use of a diaphragm interferes with the spontaneity of intercourse. The nurse can suggest that the partner insert the diaphragm as part of foreplay.

Diaphragms are an excellent contraceptive method for women who are lactating, who cannot or do not wish to use the pill (oral contraceptives), or who wish to avoid the increased risk of PID associated with intrauterine devices. They are also a good choice for older women who smoke but don't wish to be sterilized.

Women who object to manipulating their genitals to insert the diaphragm, check its placement, and remove it

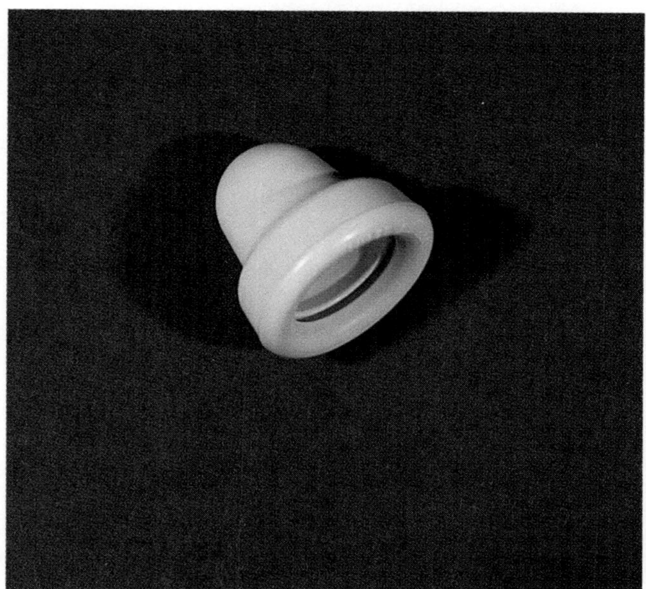

FIGURE 5–5 Cervical cap.

may find this method unsatisfactory. It is not recommended for women with a history of urinary tract infection, because pressure from the diaphragm on the urethra may interfere with complete bladder emptying and lead to recurrent urinary tract infections (UTIs). Women with a history of toxic shock syndrome should not use diaphragms or any of the barrier methods because they are left in place for prolonged periods. For the same reason, the diaphragm should not be used during a menstrual period or if a woman has abnormal vaginal discharge.

The **cervical cap** (Figure 5–5) is a cup-shaped device, used with spermicidal cream or jelly, that fits snugly over the cervix and is held in place by suction. Effectiveness rates and method of insertion are similar to those for the diaphragm. Unlike the diaphragm, however, the cap may be left in place for up to 48 hours, and it does not require additional spermicide for repeated intercourse (Hatcher et al 1994). Advantages, disadvantages, and contraindications are similar to those associated with the diaphragm. The cervical cap may be more difficult to fit because of limited size options. It also tends to be more difficult for women to insert and remove.

The **intrauterine device** (IUD) is designed to be inserted into the uterus by a qualified health care provider and left in place for an extended period, providing continuous contraceptive protection. The exact mechanism of IUD action is not clearly understood. Traditionally the IUD was believed to act by preventing the implantation of a fertilized ovum. Thus the IUD was considered an abortifacient or abortion-causing method. Current evidence on the new generation of IUDs suggests that

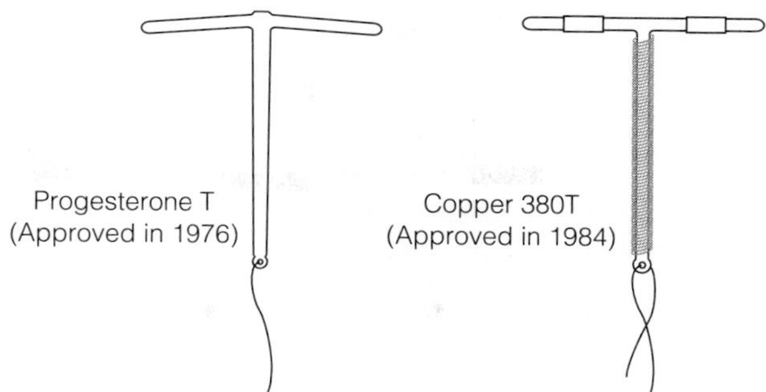

FIGURE 5–6 Two types of IUDs.

they truly are contraceptives; they act by immobilizing sperm in some way and impeding their progress from the cervix through the uterus to the fallopian tubes (Chez and Mishell 1994). Other evidence suggests they may also prevent fertilization by speeding the movement of the ovum through the fallopian tubes to the uterus. The IUD is also known to have local inflammatory effects on the endometrium (Hatcher et al 1994).

Advantages of the IUD include high rate of effectiveness, continuous contraceptive protection, no coitus-related activity, and relative inexpensiveness over time. Possible adverse reactions to the IUD include discomfort to the wearer, increased bleeding during menses, PID, perforation of the uterus, intermenstrual bleeding, dysmenorrhea, expulsion of the device, and ectopic pregnancy.

Two IUDs are currently available (Figure 5–6). The Progesterone T (Progestasert) must be changed annually and should be used only by women with an allergy to copper. The Copper T380A (ParaGard) is highly effective and can be left in place for up to ten years (Nelson 1995). The IUD is recommended only for women who have at least one child and are in a monogamous relationship, because they have the lowest risk of developing a pelvic infection. It is not recommended for women with multiple sexual contacts, because they are at risk for sexually transmitted infections (STIs).

The IUD is inserted into the uterus with its string or tail protruding through the cervix into the vagina. It may be inserted during a menstrual period or during the 4- to 6-week postpartum check. After insertion, the clinician instructs the woman to check for the presence of the string once a week for the first month and then after each menses. She is told that she may have some cramping or bleeding intermittently for 2–6 weeks, and that her first few menses may be irregular. Follow-up examination is suggested 4–8 weeks after insertion.

Women with IUDs should contact their health care providers if they are exposed to a STI or if they develop the following warning signs: late period, abnormal spotting or bleeding, pain with intercourse, abdominal pain, abnormal discharge, signs of infection (fever, chills, malaise), or missing string.

Oral Contraceptives

The use of hormones, specifically the combination of estrogen and progesterone, is a very successful birth control method. **Oral contraceptives** work by inhibiting the release of an ovum and by maintaining cervical mucus that is hostile to sperm. Numerous oral contraceptives are available. The pill is taken daily for 21 days, typically beginning on the Sunday after the first day of the menstrual cycle. In most cases menses will occur 1 to 4 days after the last pill is taken. Seven days after taking her last pill, the woman restarts the pill. Thus the woman always begins the pill on the same day. Some companies offer a 28-day pack with seven "blank" pills so that the woman never stops taking a pill. The pill should be taken at approximately the same time each day—usually upon arising or before retiring in the evening.

Although they are highly effective, oral contraceptives may produce side effects ranging from breakthrough bleeding to thrombus formation. Side effects from oral contraceptives may be either progesterone- or estrogen-related (Table 5–1). The use of low-dose (35 μg or less estrogen) preparations has reduced many of the side effects, but the threat of potential risk is sufficient to deter some women from using oral contraceptives.

Another oral contraceptive is the seldom-used progesterone-only pill, also called the *minipill.* It is used primarily by women who have a contraindication to the estrogen component of the combination preparation, such as history of thrombophlebitis, but are strongly motivated to use this form of contraception. The major problems with this preparation are amenorrhea or irregular spotting and bleeding patterns.

Contraindications to the use of oral contraceptives include pregnancy, previous history of thrombophlebitis or thromboembolic disease, acute or chronic liver disease of cholestatic type with abnormal function, presence of estrogen-dependent carcinomas, undiagnosed uterine bleeding, heavy smoking, hypertension, diabetes, and hyperlipidemia. In addition, women with the following conditions who use oral contraceptives should be examined every 3 months: migraine headaches, epilepsy, depression, oligomenorrhea, and amenorrhea. Women who choose this method of contraception should be fully advised of its potential side effects.

Oral contraceptives also have some important noncontraceptive benefits. Many women experience relief of uncomfortable menstrual symptoms. Cramps are lessened, flow is decreased, and cycle regularity is increased. Mittelschmerz is eliminated and the incidence of functional ovarian cysts is decreased. More importantly, there is a substantial reduction in the incidence of ectopic pregnancy, ovarian cancer, endometrial cancer, iron-deficiency anemia, and benign breast disease. In addition, the FDA recently revised its oral contraceptive labeling to state that for healthy, nonsmoking women over age 40, the benefits of oral contraceptives may outweigh possible risks (Hatcher et al 1994).

TABLE 5–1 Side Effects Associated with Oral Contraceptives

Estrogen Effects	Progestin Effects
Alterations in lipid metabolism	Acne, oily skin
Breast tenderness, engorgement; increased breast size	Breast tenderness; increased breast size
Cerebrovascular accident	Decreased libido
Changes in carbohydrate metabolism	Decreased high-density lipoprotein (HDL) cholesterol levels
Chloasma	Depression
Fluid retention; cyclic weight gain	Fatigue
Headache	Hirsutism
Hepatic adenomas	Increased appetite; weight gain
Hypertension	Increased low-density lipoprotein (LDL) cholesterol levels
Leukorrhea, cervical erosion, ectopia	Oligomenorrhea, amenorrhea
Nausea	Pruritus
Nervousness, irritability	Sebaceous cysts
Telangiectasia	
Thromboembolic complications – thrombophlebitis, pulmonary embolism	

The woman using oral contraceptives should contact her health care provider if she becomes depressed, develops a breast lump, becomes jaundiced, or experiences any of the following warning signs: severe abdominal pain, severe chest pain or shortness of breath, severe headaches, dizziness, changes in vision (vision loss or blurring), speech problems, or severe leg pain.

Spermicides

Spermicides, available as creams, jellies, foams, vaginal film, and suppositories, are inserted into the vagina before intercourse. They destroy sperm or neutralize vaginal secretions and thereby immobilize sperm. Spermicides that effervesce in a moist environment offer more rapid protection, and coitus may take place immediately after they are inserted. Suppositories may require up to 30 minutes to dissolve and will not offer protection until they do so. The nurse instructs the woman to insert these spermicide preparations high in the vagina and maintain a supine position.

Spermicides are minimally effective when used alone, but their effectiveness increases in conjunction with a diaphragm or condom. They provide significant protection from gonorrhea and chlamydia, and some protection against trichomonas and herpes (Hatcher et al 1994).

The major advantages of spermicides are their wide availability and low toxicity. While some studies have suggested that the use of spermicides at the time of conception or early in pregnancy may be associated with an increased risk of congenital anomalies, recent studies show no increased incidence.

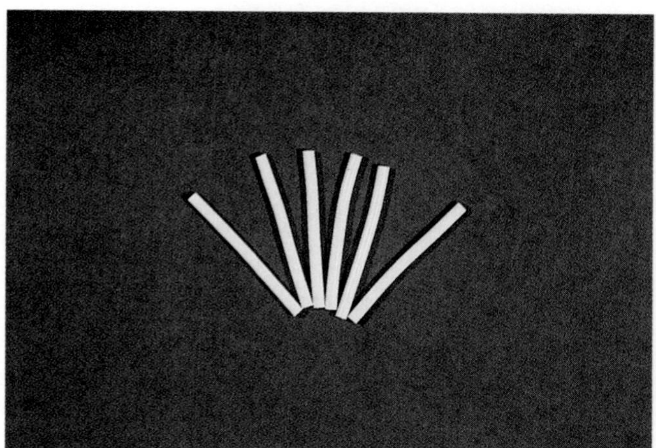

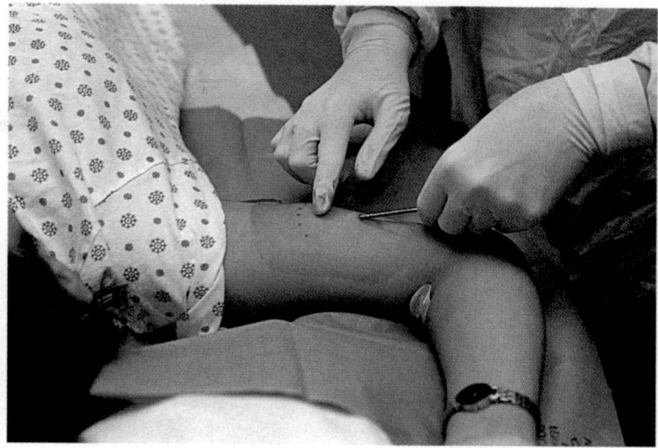

FIGURE 5–7 Norplant, a long-acting progestin contraceptive, is implanted in a woman's upper arm.

Long-Acting Progestin Contraceptives

Subdermal implants (Norplant) consist of six silastic capsules containing levonorgestrel, a progestin, which are implanted in the woman's arm. They are effective for up to five years (Figure 5–7).

Norplant prevents ovulation in most women. It also stimulates the production of thick cervical mucus, which inhibits sperm penetration. Norplant provides effective continuous contraception removed from the act of coitus. Possible side effects include spotting, irregular bleeding or amenorrhea, an increased incidence of ovarian cysts, weight gain, headaches, fluid retention, acne, mood changes, and depression. Women should be advised that the implant may be visible, especially in very slender users, and that it requires a minor surgical procedure to insert and remove the implants. Recent reports of difficulty removing the implants may lead to a decline in their use.

Depot-medroxyprogesterone acetate (DMPA) (**Depo-Provera**), another long-acting progestin, provides highly effective birth control for three months when administered as a single injection of 150 mg. DMPA, which acts primarily by suppressing ovulation, is safe, convenient, private, and relatively inexpensive. It also separates birth control from the act of coitus. It can safely be given to nursing mothers because it contains no estrogen. DMPA provides levels of progesterone high enough to block the LH surge, thereby suppressing ovulation. It also thickens the cervical mucus to block sperm penetration. Side effects include menstrual irregularities, headache, weight gain, breast tenderness, and depression. Return of fertility may be delayed for an average of nine months (Counseling patients 1995).

Emergency Postcoital Contraception

Emergency postcoital contraception is indicated when a woman is worried about pregnancy because of unprotected intercourse or possible contraceptive failure (eg, broken condom, slipped diaphragm, or too long a time between DMPA injections). The most commonly prescribed emergency postcoital contraceptive is norgestrel and ethinyl estradiol (Ovral), a combination oral contraceptive containing 50 μg estrogen. Though sometimes called the "morning-after pill," the phrase is misleading because the woman actually takes two pills as soon after intercourse as possible and two more 12 hours later. Other postcoital regimens involve the use of specific doses of danazol, conjugated estrogens, levonorgestrel alone without an estrogen, and insertion of an IUD (Hanson 1996).

Mifepristone (RU 486), a safe, effective, postcoital contraceptive, blocks progesterone, thereby altering the endometrium and making it unsuitable for implantation. It has excellent results with minimal side effects when given within 72 hours of unprotected intercourse (Hatcher et al 1994). Currently it is being tested in selected US cities although it has already gained widespread recognition as an abortifacient in Europe and China.

Information about postcoital emergency contraception has not been widely disseminated. In 1996, in an effort to increase awareness, an Emergency Contraception Hotline was established and a World Wide Web page was developed (Hanson 1996).

Operative Sterilization

Before sterilization is performed on either partner, the physician provides a thorough explanation of the procedure to both. Each needs to understand that sterilization is not a decision to be taken lightly or entered into when psychologic stresses, such as separation or divorce, exist. Even though both male and female procedures are theoretically reversible, the permanency of the procedure should be stressed and understood.

Male sterilization is achieved through a relatively minor procedure called a **vasectomy.** This involves surgically severing the vas deferens in both sides of the scrotum. It takes about 4 to 6 weeks and 6 to 36 ejaculations to clear the remaining sperm from the vas deferens. During that period, the couple is advised to use another method of birth control and to bring in two or three semen samples for a sperm count. The man is rechecked at 6 and 12 months to ensure that fertility has not been restored by recanalization. Side effects of a vasectomy include pain, infection, hematoma, sperm granulomas, and spontaneous reanastomosis (reconnecting).

Vasectomies can sometimes be reversed by using microsurgery techniques. Restored fertility, as measured by subsequent pregnancy, ranges from 30 to 85 percent (Hatcher et al 1994).

Female sterilization is most frequently accomplished by **tubal ligation.** The tubes are located through a small subumbilical incision or by minilaparotomy techniques and are crushed, ligated, electrocoagulated, or banded or plugged (in the newer, reversible procedures). Tubal ligation may be done at any time. However, the postpartal period is an ideal time to perform a tubal ligation because the tubes are somewhat enlarged and easily located.

Complications of female sterilization procedures include coagulation burns on the bowel, bowel perforation, pain, infection, hemorrhage, and adverse anesthesia effects. Reversal of a tubal ligation depends on many factors, including the portion of the tube excised, the presence or absence of the fimbriae, and the length of the tube remaining. With microsurgical techniques, a pregnancy rate of 40 to 75 percent is possible (Hatcher et al 1994).

Male Contraception

The vasectomy and the condom, discussed previously, are currently the only forms of male contraception available in the United States. Hormonal contraception for men has yet to be developed, although studies are under way.

Nursing Care

In most cases, the nurse who provides information and guidance about contraceptive methods works with the woman partner, because most contraceptive methods are female oriented. Since a man can purchase condoms without seeing a health care provider, only in the case of vasectomy does a man require counseling and interaction with a nurse. The nurse can play an important role in helping a woman choose a method of contraception that is acceptable to her and to her partner.

In addition to completing a history and assessing for any contraindications to specific methods, the nurse can spend time with a woman learning about her lifestyle, personal attitudes about particular contraceptive methods, religious beliefs, personal biases, and plans for future childbearing, before helping the woman select a particular contraceptive method. Once the method is chosen, the nurse can help the woman learn to use it effectively. Table 5–2 summarizes factors to consider in choosing an appropriate method of contraception.

TABLE 5–2 Factors to Consider in Choosing a Method of Contraception

Effectiveness of method in preventing pregnancy

Safety of the method:
- Are there inherent risks?
- Does it offer protection against STIs or other conditions?

Client's age and future childbearing plans

Any contraindications in client's health history

Religious or moral factors influencing choice

Personal preferences, biases

Lifestyle:
- How frequently does client have intercourse?
- Does she have multiple partners?
- Does she have ready access to medical care in the event of complications?
- Is cost a factor?

Partner's support and willingness to cooperate

Personal motivation to use method

The nurse also reviews any possible side effects and warning signs related to the method chosen, and counsels the woman about what action to take if she suspects she is pregnant. In many cases the nurse is involved in telephone counseling of women who call with questions and concerns about contraception. Thus it is vital that the nurse be knowledgeable about this topic and have resources available to find answers to less common questions.

The Teaching Guide: Using a Method of Contraception provides guidelines for helping women use a method of contraception effectively.

Surgical Interruption of Pregnancy

Although abortion was legalized in the United States in 1973, the associated controversy over moral and legal issues continues. This controversy is as readily apparent in the medical and nursing professions as in other groups.

A number of physical and psychosocial factors influence a woman's decision to seek an abortion. The presence of a disease or health state that jeopardizes the

TEACHING GUIDE Using a Method of Contraception

Assessment

The nurse determines the woman's general knowledge about contraceptive methods, identifies the methods the woman has used previously (if any), identifies contraindications or risk factors for any methods, discusses the woman's personal preferences and biases about various methods, and discusses her commitment (and her partner's commitment if appropriate) to a chosen method.

Nursing Diagnosis

Knowledge deficit related to lack of information about the correct use of chosen method of contraception.

Nursing Plan and Implementation

The teaching plan will focus on confirming that a chosen method of contraception is a good choice for the woman. The nurse will then help the woman learn the method so that she can use it effectively.

Client Goals

At the completion of teaching, the woman will be able to:

1. Confirm for herself that the chosen method of contraception is appropriate for her.
2. List the advantages, disadvantages, and risks of the chosen method.
3. Describe (or demonstrate) the correct procedure for using the chosen method.
4. Cite warning signs that should be reported to the caregiver.

Teaching Plan

Content	Teaching Method
Discuss the factors that a woman should consider in choosing a method of contraception (Table 5–2). Stress that the different methods may be appropriate at different times in the woman's life. Review the woman's reasons for selecting a particular method and confirm any contraindications to specific methods.	Contraception is a personal decision, so the discussion should take place in a private area free of interruptions. The nurse should create a supportive, warm, and comfortable atmosphere by her or his attitude and communication style—both verbal and nonverbal. The nurse needs to consciously recognize that her or his personal preferences about contraception may be very different from those of the woman being counseled. The nurse has the responsibility to provide accurate information in an open, nonjudgmental way.
Discuss the advantages, disadvantages, and risks of the chosen method.	Focus on open discussion. It may help to have written information about the method chosen. If a signed permit is required (as with sterilization or IUD insertion), the physician should also discuss the advantages, disadvantages, and risks.
Describe the correct procedure for using a method. Go through step-by-step. Periodically stop and have the woman review the information for you. If a technique is to be learned (as with inserting a diaphragm or charting BBT), demonstrate and then have the woman do a return demonstration as appropriate. (Note: If certain aspects are beyond the nurse's level of expertise, the nurse can review the content and confirm that the woman has the opportunity to do a return demonstration. For example, an office nurse who does not do cervical cap fittings may cover information on its use, have the woman try inserting the cap herself, and then have the placement checked by the nurse practitioner or physician.)	Learning is best accomplished when material is broken down into smaller steps. People learn best when multiple approaches are used, so it is helpful to have a model or chart to enable the woman to visualize what is being described. The nurse can also have a sample of the chosen method available: a package of oral contraceptives, an open IUD, or a symptothermal chart.
Provide information on what the woman should do if unusual circumstances arise (she forgets a pill or misses a morning temperature). Stress warning signs that require immediate action on the part of the woman, and explain why these signs indicate a risk. Carefully delineate the actions the woman should take: Should she contact her caregiver? Stop the method?	Provide a written handout identifying the warning signs and listing the actions a woman should take. The handout should also cover actions the woman should take if an unusual situation develops. For example, what should she do if she vomits or has diarrhea while taking oral contraceptives? What action should she take if she and her partner are using a condom and it breaks?
Arrange to talk with the woman again soon, either on the phone or at a return visit, to determine if she has any questions about the method and to ensure that no problems have arisen.	The woman should know that she is free to call if she has questions or concerns once she starts using the method. This increases her comfort level and enables the nurse to detect potential problems early.

mother's life and serious, life-threatening fetal problems are frequently suggested as indications for abortion. In other instances, the timing or circumstance of the pregnancy creates an inordinate stress on the woman and she chooses an abortion. Some of these situations may involve contraceptive failure, rape, or incest. In all cases, the decision is best made by the woman or couple involved. A woman whose life is threatened by the pregnancy may choose to continue the pregnancy, while one with no obvious threat may choose abortion.

Abortion in the first trimester is technically easier and safer than abortion in the second trimester. It may be performed by dilatation and curettage (D&C), minisuction, or vacuum curettage. The major risks include perforation of the uterus, laceration of the cervix, systemic reaction to the anesthetic agent, hemorrhage, and infection (Stubblefield 1991). Second-trimester abortion may be done using dilatation and extraction (D&E), hypertonic saline, systemic prostaglandins, and intrauterine prostaglandins.

Important aspects of nursing care include providing information about the methods of abortion and associated risks; counseling regarding available alternatives to abortion and their implications; encouraging verbalization by the woman; providing support before, during, and after the procedure; monitoring of vital signs, intake, and output; providing for physical comfort and privacy throughout the procedure; and health teaching about self-care, the importance of the postabortion checkup, and contraception review.

Recommended Gynecologic Screening Procedures

The accepted standard of care for women today involves the regular completion of a variety of screening procedures designed to detect potential problems early to permit the most effective treatment. This section focuses on some of the most commonly used screening procedures: breast self-examination and breast examination by a trained health care provider, mammography, Pap smear, and pelvic examination.

Breast Examination

Like the uterus, the breast undergoes regular cyclical changes in response to hormonal stimulation. Each month, in rhythm with the cycle of ovulation, the breasts become engorged with fluid in anticipation of pregnancy, and the woman may experience sensations of tenderness, lumpiness, or pain. If conception does not occur, the accumulated fluid drains away via the lymphatic network. *Mastodynia* (premenstrual swelling and tenderness of the breasts) is common. It usually lasts for 3–4 days before the onset of menses, but the symptoms may persist throughout the month.

After menopause, adipose breast tissue atrophies and is replaced by connective tissue. Elasticity is lost and the breasts may droop and become pendulous. The recurring breast engorgement associated with ovulation ceases. If estrogen replacement therapy (ERT) is used to counteract other symptoms of menopause, breast engorgement may resume.

Monthly **breast self-examination** (BSE) is the best method for detecting breast masses early. A woman who knows the texture and feel of her own breasts is far more likely to detect changes that develop. Thus it is important for a woman to develop the habit of doing routine BSE as early as possible, preferably as an adolescent. Women at high risk for breast cancer are especially encouraged to be attentive to the importance of early detection through routine BSE.

In the course of a routine physical examination or during an initial visit to the caregiver, the woman should be taught BSE technique and its importance as a monthly practice. The effectiveness of BSE is determined by the woman's ability to perform the procedure correctly.

Breast self-examination should be performed on a regular monthly basis about 1 week after each menstrual period, when the breasts are typically not tender or swollen. After menopause, BSE should be performed on the same day each month (chosen by the woman for ease of remembrance).

Breast self-examination is most effective when it uses a dual approach incorporating both inspection and palpation. See the Teaching Guide: Teaching Breast Self-Examination.

Clinical breast examination (CBE) by a trained health care provider, such as a physician, nurse practitioner, or nurse-midwife, is an essential element of a routine gynecologic examination. Experience in differentiating among benign, suspicious, and worrisome breast changes enables the caregiver to reassure the woman if the findings are normal or move forward with additional diagnostic procedures or referral if the findings are suspicious or worrisome.

Mammography

A **mammogram** is a soft tissue x-ray of the breast without the injection of a contrast medium. It can detect lesions in the breast before they can be felt and has gained wide acceptance as an effective screening tool for breast cancer. Currently the American Cancer Society suggests that all women ages 40 and over have an annual mammogram. The National Cancer Institute (NCI) recommends mammograms every 1–2 years for women ages 40 to 49 and annually for all women ages 50 and older. The National Cancer Advisory Board, which

TEACHING GUIDE Teaching Breast Self-Examination

Assessment
The nurse determines the woman's general knowledge about BSE, identifies previous experience with BSE, identifies risk factors for breast cancer, determines the woman's general knowledge about breast cancer, discusses the woman's feelings about her breasts and BSE, identifies barriers to BSE, and discusses her commitment to practice BSE.

Nursing Diagnosis
Knowledge deficit related to lack of information about breast self-examination

Nursing Plan and Implementation
The teaching plan will focus on assisting the woman to learn BSE so that she can use it effectively.

Client Goals
At completion of teaching, the woman will be able to:

1. Discuss her risk of breast cancer.
2. Describe the use of BSE in breast cancer detection.
3. Demonstrate the correct procedure for BSE.
4. List warning signs of breast cancer to be reported to the caregiver.
5. Incorporate monthly BSE into her personal routine.

Teaching Plan

Content	Teaching Method
Discuss the risk factors associated with breast cancer.	This should be discussed in a private area free of interruptions. The room needs to have a mirror; bed, couch, or examining table; pillows; a patient gown; and a private area for the woman to disrobe.
Stress the unique risk factors associated with the woman's personal history and lifestyle.	The nurse should create a supportive, warm, and comfortable atmosphere by attitude and communication style—both verbal and nonverbal. A discussion of breast cancer may bring forth many emotions in the woman, including grief for previous breast cancer–related losses.
Discuss the use of BSE in breast cancer detection.	Focus on open discussion. A brochure with statistics and illustrations may be useful. Stress the positive outcomes of early detection to counterbalance fears.
Describe and demonstrate the correct procedure for BSE. A. Instruct the woman to inspect her breasts by standing or sitting in front of a mirror. She needs to inspect her breasts in three positions: with both arms relaxed down at her side, both arms stretched straight over her head, and both hands placed on her hips while leaning forward (Figure 5–8).	Learning is best accomplished when material is broken down into smaller steps and presented with multiple approaches. Prior to asking the woman to perform BSE, the nurse should use a model or a chart to demonstrate the procedure. Then the nurse should have the woman perform BSE. The nurse should be very supportive and give a lot of positive feedback because some women may be embarrassed. The nurse needs to demonstrate a nonjudgmental, accepting attitude.

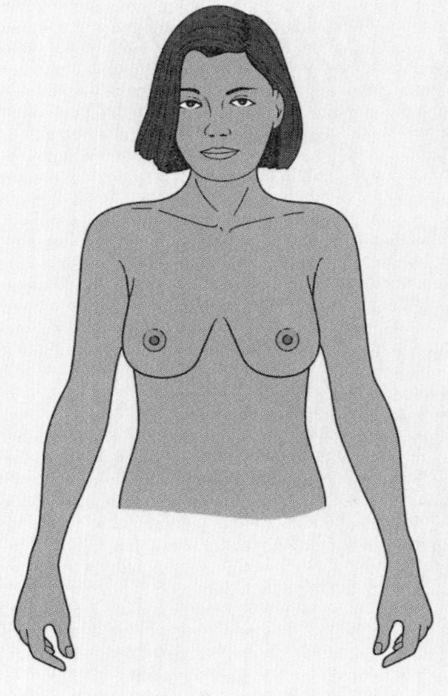
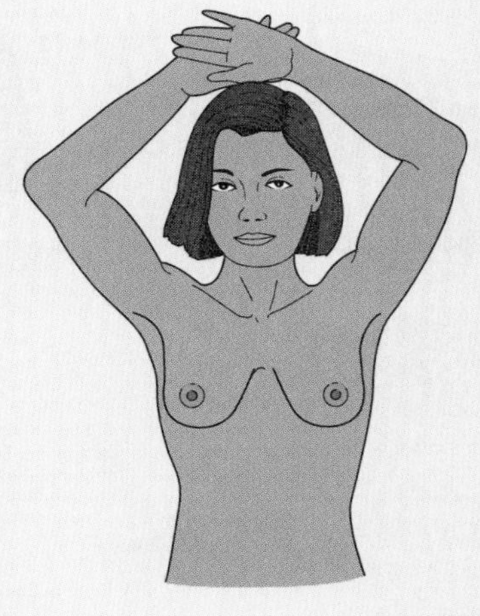
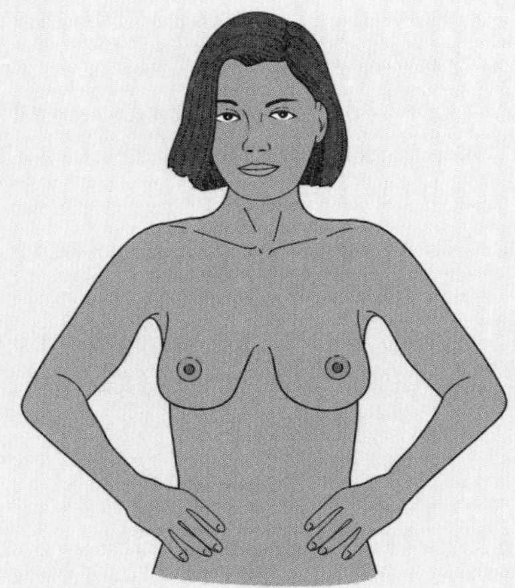

FIGURE 5–8 Positions for inspection of the breasts.

TEACHING GUIDE Teaching Breast Self-Examination continued

B. Advise the woman to look at her breasts individually and in comparison with one another. Note and record the following characteristics for each position:

Size and Symmetry of the Breasts

1. Breasts may vary, but the variations should remain constant during rest or movement—note abnormal contours.
2. Some size difference between the breasts is normal.

Shape and Direction of the Breasts

1. The shape of the breasts can be rounded or pendulous with some variation between breasts.
2. The breasts should be pointing slightly laterally.

Color, Thickening, Edema, and Venous Patterns

1. Check for redness or inflammation.
2. A blue hue with a marked venous pattern that is focal or unilateral may indicate an area of increased blood supply due to tumor. Symmetric venous patterns are normal.
3. Skin edema observed as thickened skin with enlarged pores ("orange peel") may indicate blocked lymphatic drainage due to tumor.

Surface of the Breasts

1. Skin dimpling, puckering, or retraction (pulling) when the woman presses her hands together or against her hips suggests malignancy.
2. Striae (stretch marks) red at onset and whitish with age are normal.

Nipple Size and Shape, Direction, Rashes, Ulcerations, and Discharge

1. Long-standing nipple inversion is normal, but an inverted nipple previously capable of erection is suspicious. Note any deviation, flattening, or broadening of the nipples.
2. Check for rashes, ulcerations, or discharge.

C. Instruct the woman to palpate (feel) her breasts as follows:

1. Lie down. Put one hand behind your head. With the other hand, fingers flattened, gently feel your breast. Press lightly (Figure 5–9*A*). Now examine the breast.
2. Figure 5–9*B* shows you how to check each breast. Begin as you see in B and follow the arrows, feeling gently for a lump or thickening. Remember to feel all parts of each breast.
3. Now repeat the same procedure sitting up, with the hand still behind your head (Figure 5–9*C*).
4. Squeeze the nipple between your thumb and forefinger. Look for any discharge—clear or bloody (Figure 5–9*D*).

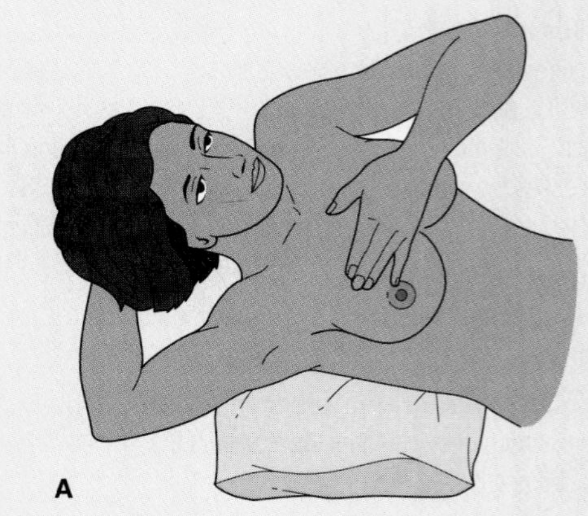

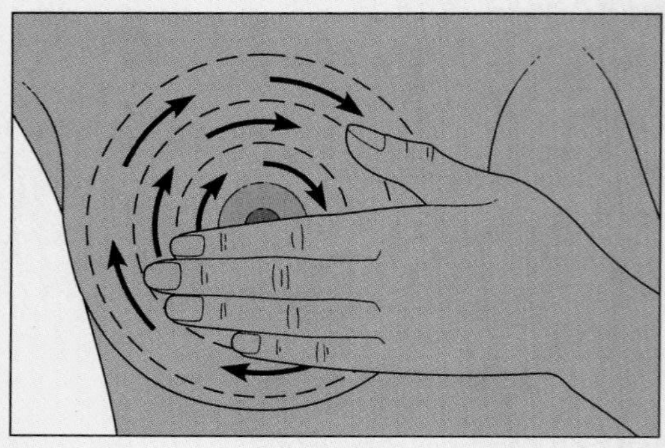

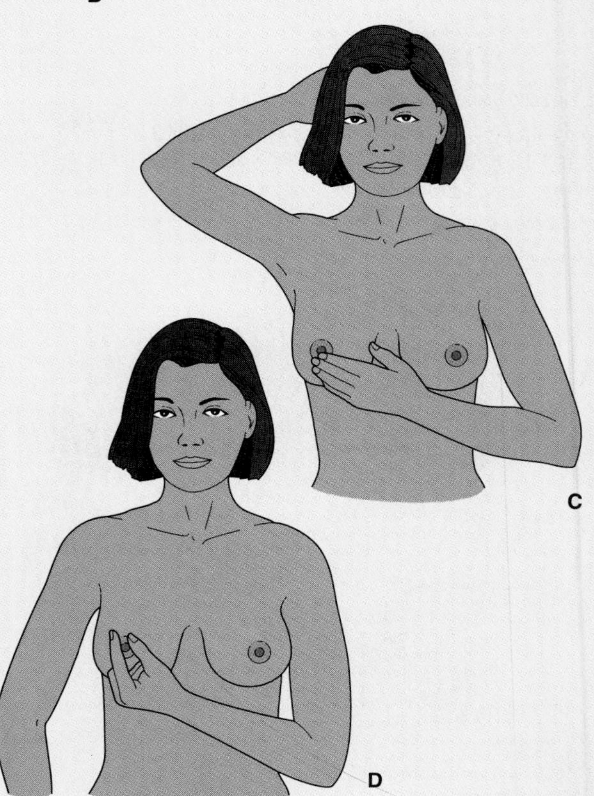

FIGURE 5–9 Breast self-examination (at right).

TEACHING GUIDE continued

D. Take the woman's hand and help her to identify her "normal lumps" (eg, mammary ridge, ribs and nodularity in the upper outer quadrants).	Demonstrate "normal lumps" on the woman herself while guiding her hand and identifying the area.
E. After she examines her breasts and identifies her normal lumps, instruct her to palpate her breasts once more to identify any areas that she may have questions about. If questions arise, the nurse should palpate the area and attempt to identify if it is normal.	Allowing the woman to differentiate normal from abnormal lumps on herself and a model will increase confidence that she will recognize an abnormal finding. Having the nurse check her immediately afterwards will positively reinforce her and diminish the fear associated with BSE.
F. If a breast model is available, instruct the woman to palpate it and identify the lumps.	
G. Provide information on the warning signs of breast cancer and what she should do if she identifies any of these signs during BSE.	Provide a written handout on the warning signs of breast cancer. The handout should also cover actions that she should take if a warning sign is discovered. Stress the positive effects of early detection.
Timing Instruct the woman to perform BSE on a monthly basis. Be specific based on whether she is premenopausal, pregnant, postmenopausal, or postmenopausal receiving hormone replacement therapy.	Provide the woman with a reminder symbol for monthly BSE. The American Cancer Society provides such items to hang in the shower, place on a refrigerator, and so forth. Ask her when she plans to do BSE each month. This will serve as a method of evaluation and reinforcement. Praise her commitment to do monthly BSE. Give the woman a follow-up telephone number (eg, American Cancer Society) to use if she needs additional information or has questions. This will increase her comfort level with BSE and enable her to detect potential problems early.

Source: American Cancer Society: *Breast Self-Examination and the Nurse,* No. 3408 PE. New York, 1973.

offers guidance to NCI, also recommended that women at high risk for breast cancer should ". . . seek medical advice about beginning mammography before age 40 and to determine their mammography schedule in their 40s." (Taubes 1997, p 27).

For women ages 40 to 49, 30 percent are likely to have a false-positive result requiring biopsy. Moreover, mammograms miss about 25 percent of breast cancers for women in this age group (Taubes 1997).

Pap Smear and Pelvic Examination

The purpose of the Papanicolaou test (**Pap smear**) is to detect the presence of cellular abnormalities by obtaining a smear containing cells from the cervix and the endocervical canal. Precancerous and cancerous conditions, as well as atypical findings and inflammatory changes, can be identified by microscopic examination.

Women should be advised to avoid douching, intercourse, female hygiene products, and spermicidal agents immediately before a Pap smear. Pap smears should not be obtained during menstruation or when visible cervicitis exists.

Women who have reached the age of 18 and women, regardless of age, who are or have been sexually active should have a pelvic examination and Pap smear annually. Current guidelines suggest that after the woman has had normal results on three or more consecutive examinations, the Pap test may be performed less frequently at the discretion of her caregiver (DiSaia 1994). The caregiver should consider carefully before making such a recommendation because many changes that occur in a woman's life and lifestyle may alter her risk factors.

The pelvic examination enables the health care provider to assess a variety of factors about the woman's vagina, uterus, ovaries, and lower abdominal area. It is often performed after the Pap smear but may also be performed without a Pap for diagnostic purposes. Women sometimes perceive the pelvic exam as uncomfortable and embarrassing. The negative feelings may cause women to delay having yearly gynecologic examinations, and this avoidance may pose a threat to life and health.

To make the pelvic examination less threatening, and thus improve health-seeking behavior, more health care providers are performing what is called an educational pelvic examination. This includes offering the woman a mirror to watch the procedure, pointing out anatomic parts to her, and positioning and draping her to allow eye-to-eye contact with the practitioner. The woman is encouraged to participate by asking questions and giving feedback.

Nurse practitioners, certified nurse-midwives, and physicians all perform pelvic examinations. Nurses assist the practitioner and the woman during the examination. Procedure 5–1 provides information on assisting with a pelvic examination.

Menopause

Menopause, the time when menses cease, is a time of transition for a woman, marking the end of her reproductive abilities. The current approximate age of menopause in the United States is 51 years. **Climacteric,** or *change of life* (often used synonymously with menopause), refers to the host of psychologic and physical alterations that occur around the time of menopause.

Psychologic Aspects

The old image of menopausal women as socially irrelevant is undergoing revision, as the average woman will live one-third of her life after menopause. A woman's psychologic adaptation to menopause and the climacteric is multifactorial. She is influenced by her own expectations and knowledge, physical well-being, family views, marital stability, and sociocultural expectations. As the number of women reaching menopause increases, the negative emotional connotations society attaches to menopause are diminishing, enabling menopausal women to cope more effectively and even enabling them to view menopause as a time of personal growth.

Physical Aspects

The physical characteristics of menopause are linked to the shift from a cyclic to a noncyclic hormonal pattern. Menopause usually occurs between 45 and 52 years of age. The age of onset may be influenced by nutritional, cultural, or genetic factors. The physiologic mechanisms initiating its onset are not precisely known. The onset of menopause occurs when estrogen levels become so low that menstruation stops.

Generally ovulation ceases 1 to 2 years before menopause, but individual variations exist. Atrophy of the ovaries occurs gradually. FSH levels rise and less estrogen is produced. Menopausal symptoms include atrophic changes in the vagina, vulva, and urethra and in the trigonal area of the bladder.

Many menopausal women experience a vasomotor disturbance commonly known as *hot flashes,* a feeling of heat arising from the chest and spreading to the neck and face. The hot flashes are often accompanied by sweating and sleep disturbances. These episodes may occur as often as 20–30 times a day and generally last 3–5 minutes. Some women also experience dizzy spells, palpitations, and weakness. Many women find their own most effective ways to deal with the hot flashes. Some report that using a fan or drinking a cool liquid helps relieve distress. Still others seek relief through hormone replacement therapy.

The uterine endometrium and myometrium atrophy, as do the cervical glands. The uterine cavity constricts. The fallopian tubes and ovaries atrophy extensively. The vaginal mucosa becomes smooth and thin and the rugae disappear, leading to loss of elasticity. As a result, intercourse can be painful, but this may be overcome by using lubricating gel or saliva. Dryness of the mucus membrane can lead to burning and itching. The vaginal pH level increases as the number of Döderlein's bacilli decreases.

Postmenopausal women can still be multiorgasmic, and sexual interest and activity may even improve as the need for contraception disappears and personal growth and awareness increase.

Vulvar atrophy occurs late, and the pubic hair thins, turns gray or white, and may ultimately disappear. The labia shrivel and lose their heightened pigmentation. Pelvic fascia and muscles atrophy, resulting in decreased pelvic support. The breasts become pendulous and decrease in size and firmness.

Long-range physical changes may include **osteoporosis,** a decrease in the bony skeletal mass. This change is thought to be associated with lowered estrogen and androgen levels, lack of physical exercise, and a chronic low intake of calcium. Moreover, the estrogen deprivation that occurs in menopausal women may significantly increase their risk of coronary heart disease. Loss of protein from the skin and supportive tissues causes wrinkling. Postmenopausal women frequently gain weight, which may be due to excessive caloric intake or to lower caloric need with the same level of intake.

Hormone Replacement Therapy

Hormone replacement therapy (**HRT**), usually involving estrogen with or without a progestin, had been controversial for years, but currently the American College of Obstetricians and Gynecologists recommends HRT in menopause. Estrogen replacement is helpful in stopping hot flashes and night sweats and in reversing atrophic vaginal changes. Perhaps most significantly, HRT may reduce the incidence of coronary artery disease, the leading cause of death in postmenopausal women (Andrews 1995). It also retards bone loss and decreases the fractures associated with osteoporosis.

Osteoporosis puts an individual at risk for nontraumatic fractures. Osteoporosis is more common in

PROCEDURE 5–1 Assisting with a Pelvic Examination

Nursing Action	Rationale
Objective: Provide a warm environment.	
Turn on overhead heat lights, if available, or turn up the thermostat.	
Objective: Assemble and prepare the equipment.	
• Prepare and arrange the following items so that they are easily accessible:	Equipment organization facilitates the examination.
• Various-sized vaginal specula, warmed with water or on a heating pad prior to insertion.	A warmed speculum assists in lubrication and facilitates initial insertion when culture and smears are taken.
• Gloves.	
• Water-soluble lubricant.	
• Materials for Pap smear and cultures.	
• Good light source.	
• Do not use lubricant on the speculum before insertion.	Use of lubricant may alter findings or cultures.
Objective: Prepare the woman.	
• Explain the procedure. If the woman has never had a pelvic examination, show her the equipment and explain the procedure before examination.	Explanation of the procedure decreases anxiety.
• Instruct the woman to empty her bladder and to remove clothing below the waist. She may want to leave her shoes on.	An empty bladder promotes comfort during internal examination. Some women feel more comfortable with shoes on, rather than supporting their weight with bare heels against cold stirrups.
• Give the woman a disposable drape or sheet to place on her lap. Encourage her to sit on the end of the examining table with the drape across her lap.	
• Position the woman in the lithotomy position with her thighs flexed and adducted. Place her feet in stirrups. Her buttocks should extend slightly beyond the end of the examining table.	
• Drape the woman with the sheet, leaving a flap so the perineum can be exposed.	
Objective: Provide support to the woman as the physician or nurse practitioner performs the examination.	
• Explain each part of the examination as it is performed: inspection of external genitals, vagina, and cervix; bimanual examination of internal organs.	Promotes relaxation.
• Instruct the woman to relax and breathe slowly.	
• Advise the woman when the speculum is about to be inserted and ask her to bear down.	When the speculum is inserted, the woman may feel intravaginal pressure. Bearing down helps open vaginal orifice and relaxes perineal muscles.
• Lubricate the examiner's finger prior to bimanual examination.	Lubrication decreases friction and eases insertion.
Objective: Provide for the woman's comfort at the end of the examination.	
• Move to the end of the examination table and face the woman's perineum. Cover the woman with the drape. Apply gentle pressure to the woman's knees and encourage her to move toward the head of the table. Offer your hand to the woman, remove her heels from the stirrups, and assist her to a sitting position. Be sure that she is not dizzy and that she is sitting or standing safely before you leave the room.	The supine position may cause postural hypotension.
• Provide tissues to wipe lubricant from the perineum.	Upon assuming a sitting position, vaginal secretions along with lubricant may be discharged.
• Provide privacy while the woman dresses.	

women who are middle-aged or older. The following risk factors are also associated with osteoporosis:

- White or Asian
- Small-boned and thin
- Family history of osteoporosis
- Lack of regular exercise
- Nulliparous
- Early onset of menopause
- Consistently low intake of calcium
- Cigarette smoking
- Moderate to heavy alcohol intake

Pre- or postmenopausal women with four or more risk factors for osteoporosis should have bone mass measurements done. The woman's height should be measured at each visit, because a loss of height is often an early sign that vertebrae are being compressed because of reduced bone mass (Kase 1993). A variety of conditions, including malabsorption syndrome, cancer, cirrhosis of the liver, chronic use of cortisone, and rheumatoid arthritis, can cause secondary arthritis, which resembles osteoporosis. If these secondary causes have been eliminated, treatment for osteoporosis is instituted.

Prevention of osteoporosis is a primary goal of care. Women are advised to maintain an adequate calcium intake. Approximately 800 mg of elemental calcium is recommended for premenopausal women and 1000 mg for postmenopausal women. Most women require supplements to achieve this level. Women are also advised to participate regularly in exercise, consume only modest quantities of alcohol and caffeine, and to stop smoking. This is especially important because alcohol and smoking have a negative effect on the rate of bone resorption. Women with no contraindications to estrogen who are showing evidence of bone loss are good candidates for HRT.

When estrogen is given alone, it can produce endometrial hyperplasia and increase the risk of endometrial cancer. Thus, in women who still have a uterus, estrogen is opposed by giving a progestin for a portion of the cycle. Currently opinion varies on the number of days that progesterone (Provera) should be included. Typically, estrogen is given the first 25 days of the month with 10 mg Provera added during the last 12 days of the estrogen administration (days 14 to 25). An alternative approach involves the daily administration of 0.625 mg estrogen with 2.5 mg Provera. This regimen is associated with less vaginal bleeding and is sufficient to prevent endometrial hyperplasia and osteoporosis; it also retains most of the cardiovascular beneficial effects of estrogen (Andrews 1995). While most women prefer to take estrogen orally, some choose the transdermal estrogen skin patch. For women experiencing decreased libido, combination estrogen-testosterone preparations are available.

A thorough history, physical examination including Pap smear, and baseline mammogram are indicated before starting HRT. An initial endometrial biopsy is no longer recommended for all women beginning HRT, but is indicated for women with an increased risk of endometrial cancer and if excessive, unexpected, or prolonged vaginal bleeding occurs (McKeon 1994).

Women taking estrogen should be advised to stop immediately if they develop headaches, visual changes, signs of thrombophlebitis, or chest pain.

Alendronate (Fosamax) is a new treatment for osteoporosis that acts by inhibiting bone resorption and increasing bone mass. It is recommended for menopausal women with osteoporosis who cannot take estrogen (Kupecz 1996). Intranasal calcitonin has also been shown to be an effective treatment for osteoporosis and should be more widely accepted than the injectible form, which was used previously. Calcium and vitamin D supplements are generally recommended in addition to the alendronate or calcitonin (Kessenich 1996).

Nursing Care

Menopausal women may need counseling to adjust successfully to this developmental phase of life. Reaction to menopause is determined to a large extent by the kind of life the woman has lived, by the security she has in her feminine identity, and by her feelings of self-worth and self-esteem.

Nurses and other health care professionals can help the menopausal woman achieve high-level functioning at this time in her life. Of paramount importance is the nurse's ability to understand and provide support for the woman's views and feelings. Whether the woman expresses relief and delight or tearfulness and fear, the nurse needs to use an empathic approach in counseling, health teaching, or providing physical care. Touch and caring, as nursing measures, may enhance the self-actualization of both nurse and client.

Nurses should explore the question of the woman's comfort during sexual intercourse. In counseling, the nurse may say, "After menopause many women notice that their vagina seems dryer and intercourse can be uncomfortable. Have you noticed any changes?" This gives the woman information and may open discussion. The nurse can then go on to explain that dryness and shrinking of the vagina can be addressed by use of a water-soluble jelly to help provide relief. Use of estrogen, orally or in vaginal creams, may also be indicated. Increased frequency of intercourse will maintain some elasticity in the vagina. When assessing the menopausal woman, the nurse should address the question of sexual activity openly but tactfully, because the woman may have been socialized to be reticent in discussing sex.

The crucial need of women in the perimenopausal period of life is for adequate information about the changes taking place in their bodies and their lives. Supplying that information provides both a challenge and an opportunity for nurses.

Violence Against Women

Violence against women has reached epidemic proportions in society today. Experts suggest that as many as one in three women will be the victim of abuse at some time in her life. Violence affects women of all ages, races, and ethnic backgrounds, from all socioeconomic levels, all educational levels, and all walks of life. Two of the most common forms of violence are partner abuse and rape. Society not only accepts these forms of violence against women but also shifts the blame for the violence to the woman herself by asking questions such as "What did she do to make him so mad?" "Why does she stay?" "What was she doing out so late?"

Violence against women is a major health concern. It costs the health care system millions of dollars and thousands of lives each year (Campbell 1993). In response to this epidemic a number of health-related organizations have begun to address the issue. Healthy People 2000 (Department of Health and Human Services 1990), a national health promotion and disease prevention project, includes in its summary report objectives to decrease the violence experienced by women. The Joint Commission for the Accreditation of Healthcare Organizations (JCAHO) has mandated that emergency departments have in place protocols for caring for battered women. The American Nurses Association (1991) advocates education for all nurses about identification and prevention of violence against women as well as routine assessment for abuse in all women.

Female Partner Abuse

A variety of terms have been used to describe violence occurring between partners in an ongoing relationship: *domestic violence, partner abuse, spouse abuse, violence between intimates.* These terms suggest a neutrality, a balance of abuse that is totally inaccurate because over 90 percent of the victims of this form of violence are women (Buel 1995). Consequently, this text uses the term **female partner abuse.**

Female partner abuse is the most common form of violence in the United States but the least reported serious crime. Estimates suggest that a battering incident occurs every 15 seconds in the United Sstates. At least two-thirds of the women who lose their lives at the hands of a partner or ex-partner were experiencing physical abuse by the man before the murder (Campbell 1993).

Typically the batterer is male. The woman may or may not be married to her abuser. She may be living with, dating, or divorced from him. Female partner abuse takes many forms, including verbal attacks and insults, intimidation and threats, emotional deprivation and aggravation, social isolation and economic deprivation, intellectual derision and ridicule, sexual demands or deprivation, and physical attacks and injury.

A battered woman is one who has suffered one or more episodes of battery from her male partner or ex-partner (Helton and Snodgrass 1987; Walker 1984). Battering involves coercing a woman with physical, social, or psychologic behaviors. Physical battering includes slapping, kicking, shoving, punching, forms of torture, attacks with objects or weapons, and sexual assault. Women who are physically abused can also suffer psychologic and emotional abuse.

Cycle of Violence

In an effort to explain the experience of battered women, Walker (1984) developed the theory of the cycle of violence. Battering takes place in a cyclic fashion through three phases:

1. The tension-building phase is manifested by the batterer demonstrating power and control. This phase is characterized by anger, arguing, blaming the woman for external problems, and possibly minor battering incidents. The woman may blame herself and believe she can prevent the escalation of the batterer's anger by her own actions.
2. The acute battering incident is typically triggered by some external event or internal state of the batterer. It is an episode of acute violence distinguished by lack of control, lack of predictability, and major destructiveness. The cycle of violence can be interrupted before the acute battering incident if proper interventions take place.
3. The tranquil, loving phase, is sometimes termed the honeymoon period. This phase may be characterized by extremely kind and loving behavior on the part of the batterer as he tries to make up with the woman, or it may simply be manifested as an absence of tension and violence. Without intervention, this phase will end and the cycle of violence will recur. Over time the violence increases in severity and frequency.

Characteristics of Battered Women

Battered women often hold traditional views of sex roles. Most were raised to be submissive, passive, and dependent and to seek approval from male figures. Some battered women were exposed to violence between their parents, while others first experience it from their partners. Many battered women do not work outside the home. They are isolated from family and friends and totally dependent on their partners for their financial and emotional needs.

Battered women typically attribute their beatings to some personal shortcoming or inadequacy. Many believe their partners' insults and accusations of being bad wives or partners and negligent mothers. As these women become more isolated, they find it harder to judge who is right. Eventually they fully believe in their inadequacy, and their low self-esteem reinforces their belief that they deserve to be beaten. Battered women often feel a pervasive sense of guilt, fear, and depression. Their sense of hopelessness and helplessness reduces their problem-solving ability. Some women develop a pattern of behavior termed "learned helplessness," in which the unknown becomes terrifying. Learned helplessness often plays a role in a woman's decision to stay in a known, though abusive, situation rather than leave and face the unknown.

Characteristics of Batterers

Batterers come from all backgrounds, professions, religious groups, and socioeconomic levels. Batterers often have feelings of insecurity, socioeconomic inferiority, powerlessness, and helplessness that conflict with their assumptions of male supremacy. Emotionally immature and aggressive men have a tendency to express these overwhelming feelings of inadequacy through violence. Many batterers feel undeserving of their partners, yet they blame and punish the very person they value.

Battered women often describe their husbands or partners as lacking respect toward women in general, having come from homes where they witnessed abuse of their mothers or were themselves abused as children, and having a hidden rage that erupts occasionally. Batterers accept traditional "macho" values, yet when they are not angry or aggressive, they appear childlike, dependent, seductive, manipulative, and in need of nurturing. They may be well respected in the community. This dual personality of batterers reflects the conflict between their belief that they must live up to their macho image and their feelings of inadequacy in the role of husband or provider. Combined with low frustration tolerance and poor impulse control, their pervasive sense of powerlessness leads them to strike out at life's inequities by abusing women.

Nursing Care

Nurses in many different health care settings often come in contact with abused women but fail to recognize them, especially if their bruises are not visible. Women who are at high risk of battering often have a history of alcohol or drug abuse, child abuse, or abuse in the previous or present relationship. Other possible signs of abuse include expressions of helplessness and powerlessness; low self-esteem revealed by the woman's dress, appearance, and the way she relates to health care providers; signs of depression evidenced by fatigue, hopelessness, and somatic problems such as headache, insomnia, chest, back, or pelvic pain; and possible suicide attempts. In addition, the abused woman may have a history of missed or frequently changed appointments, perhaps because she had signs of abuse that kept her from coming in or her partner prevented it.

Because battering is now so prevalent, it is important to include questions about violence in all primary care encounters. Furniss and associates (1993) recommend asking the following screening questions:

1. Has your partner ever emotionally or physically abused you?
2. During the past year, have you been hurt physically by anyone?
3. (For pregnant women) Since you became pregnant, has anyone hurt you physically?

During the screening the nurse should assure the woman that her privacy will be respected. It is essential that the nurse remain nonjudgmental; create a warm, caring climate conducive to sharing; and demonstrate a willingness to talk about violence. A battered woman often interprets the nurse's willingness to discuss violence as permission for her to discuss it as well (Hoff 1992).

When a woman seeks care for an injury, the nurse should be alert to the following cues of abuse:

- Hesitancy in providing detailed information about the injury and how it occurred.
- Inappropriate affect for the situation.
- Delayed reporting of symptoms.
- Pattern of injury consistent with abuse, including multiple injury sites involving bruises, abrasions, and contusions to the head (eyes and back of the neck), throat, chest, abdomen, or genitals.
- Inappropriate explanation for the injuries.
- Signs of increased anxiety in the presence of the possible batterer.

When a battered woman comes in for treatment, she needs to feel safe physically and safe in talking about her injuries and problems. A battered woman also needs to reestablish a feeling of control over her world. She needs to regain a sense of predictability by knowing what to expect and how she can interact. The nurse should provide sufficient information about what to expect in terms the woman can understand.

In providing care the nurse needs to let the woman work through her story, problems, and situation at her own pace. The nurse should reassure the woman that she is believed and not considered crazy. The nurse should anticipate the woman's ambivalence (due to her love-hate relationship with her batterer) but also respect the woman's capacity to change and grow when she is ready. The woman may require assistance in identifying specific problems and in developing realistic ideas for reducing or eliminating those problems. In all interactions the nurse should stress that no one should be abused and that the abuse is not the woman's fault.

The nurse should inform any woman suspected of being in an abusive situation of the services available in the health care agency and the community. A battered woman may need the following:

- Medical treatment for injuries
- Temporary shelter to provide a safe environment for her and her children
- Counseling to raise her self-esteem and help her understand the dynamics of family violence
- Legal assistance for protection and/or prosecution
- Financial assistance to obtain shelter, food, and clothing
- Job training or employment counseling
- An ongoing support group with counseling about relationships with males and children

If the woman returns to an abusive situation, the nurse should encourage her to develop an exit plan for herself and her children, if any. If possible, the plan should include storing with a friend or relative a change of clothing, an extra set of car keys, money, identification papers, checkbook, other financial information, and information about the children to help her enroll them in school. She should also plan where she will go, regardless of the time of day. The nurse should ensure that the woman has a planned escape route and emergency telephone numbers she can call, including local police, a phone hotline, and a women's shelter if one is available in the community.

Working with battered women is often frustrating, and many health care providers feel impotent when the women repeatedly return to their abusive situations without developing sufficient ego strength or coping abilities. Nurses must realize that they cannot rescue battered women; battered women must decide on their own how to handle their situations. The effective nurse provides battered women with information that empowers them in decision making and supports their decisions, knowing that incremental assistance over the years may be the only alternative until they are ready to explore other options.

Rape

In its broadest sense, **rape** is involuntary sexual contact with another person. The National Crime Victimization Survey defines it as follows: "rape is forced sexual intercourse and includes both psychological coercion as well as physical force. Forced sexual intercourse means vaginal, anal, or oral penetration by the offender(s)" (Bachman and Saltzman 1995).

The person who rapes may be a stranger, acquaintance, spouse, other relative, or employer. Rape is an act of violence expressed sexually—most commonly, a man's aggression and rage acted out against a woman. Rape is one of the most underreported violent crimes in the United States. The National Center for the Prevention and Control of Rape estimates that one out of three women will be raped at some time in her life. The 1994 Criminal Victimization survey indicated that almost two-thirds of victims of completed rapes did not report the assault to the police (Perkins and Klaus 1996). The actual number of rapes occurring in the United States each year is probably about one every 1.2 minutes (Buchwald et al 1993). Even more disturbing, only 1 percent of rapists are arrested and convicted (Herman 1992).

No woman of any age or ethnicity is immune, but statistics indicate that (a) young, unmarried women, (b) women who are unemployed or have a low family income, and (c) students have the highest incidence of rape or attempted rape (Horton 1992).

Like their victims, rapists come from all ethnic backgrounds and walks of life. More than half are under age 25, and three out of five are married and leading "normal" sex lives. Why do men rape? Of the many theories put forth, none provides a completely satisfactory explanation.

So few rapists are actually caught and convicted that a clear characteristic of the assailant has not been developed. Far from being lusty, overly amorous, or perverted, the rapist tends to be emotionally weak and insecure and may have difficulty maintaining interpersonal relationships. Many rapists also have trouble dealing with the stresses of daily life. Such men may become angry and overcome by feelings of powerlessness. They then commit the act of rape as an expression of power or anger (Dupre et al 1993).

Rape has been classified in different ways, which are not mutually exclusive. The classifications categorize the dominant motive in a given rape:

- In *blitz rape* the assailant and the victim are strangers, and the rape is sudden and unexpected.
- In *confidence rape* (also called *acquaintance rape*) the assailant is an individual with whom the victim has had previous, nonviolent interaction.
- In *power rape* the purpose of the assault is control or mastery. The male uses sexual intercourse to place the woman in a powerless situation so he can feel dominant, potent, and strong. He exerts only the amount of force necessary to subdue the victim.
- In *anger rape* the sexual assault is used to express feelings of rage. The attack is often characterized by brutality and degradation.

- In *sadistic rape* the assailant has an antisocial personality and delights in torture and mutilation. Usually the assailant and victim are strangers and the assault is planned. Most rape homicides are sadistic rapes.
- In *gang rape* the assailants are more commonly younger men responding to peer pressure. Typically only one or two of the men has a rapist mentality, but they are able to incite the others to commit acts they would not do individually. Gang rape can escalate to severe violence as the young men seek to outdo each other.

Date rape, a form of acquaintance rape that is an increasing phenomenon on college campuses, occurs between a dating couple. In date rape situations, the male has usually determined to have sex and will do whatever he feels necessary if denied. Thus in date rape the primary motivation is sexual gratification (Crooks and Baur 1993), but it is still expressed as violence against the woman.

Responses to Rape

Rape is a situational crisis. It is a traumatic event that the victim cannot be prepared to handle because it is unforeseen. Following the rape, the victim generally experiences a cluster of symptoms, described by Burgess and Holmstrom (1979) as the rape trauma syndrome, that last far beyond the rape itself. These phases are described in Table 5–3. Although the phases of response are listed individually, they often overlap, as do individual responses and their duration.

Research also suggests that rape survivors may exhibit high levels of posttraumatic stress disorder, the same disorder that developed in many of the veterans of the Vietnam war. Although there are many common characteristics of posttraumatic stress disorder, there is no one set of predictable behaviors; each individual's symptom pattern tends to reflect his or her childhood experiences, adaptive style, and emotional conflicts (Herman 1992). Posttraumatic stress disorder is also marked by varying degrees of intensity. One mitigating factor is individual resiliency. Women who remained calm during a rape attack, used a variety of active strategies, and did their best to thwart the attack tend to fare better and have fewer symptoms of distress afterward than women who were rendered helpless and unable to function because of their terror (Herman 1992).

Posttraumatic stress disorder is difficult to treat. Recovery depends on empowering the woman to seek control of her life within the context of healing relationships.

Care of the Rape Survivor

Rape survivors often enter the health care system by way of the emergency room. Thus the nurse is often the first person to counsel them. Because the values, attitudes, and beliefs of the caregiver will necessarily affect the competence and focus of the care, it is essential that nurses clearly understand their feelings about rape and rape survivors and resolve any conflicts that may exist.

TABLE 5–3 Phases of the Rape Trauma Syndrome

Phase	Response
Acute phase	Fear, shock, disbelief, desire for revenge, anger, denial, anxiety, guilt, embarrassment, humiliation, helplessness, dependency; survivor may seek help or may remain silent.
Outward adjustment phase	Survivor appears outwardly composed, denying and repressing feelings; for example, she returns to work, buys a weapon, adds security measures to her residence, and denies need for counseling.
Reorganizational phase	Survivor experiences sexual dysfunction, phobias, sleep disorders, anxiety, and a strong urge to talk about or resolve feelings; survivor may seek counseling or may remain silent.

The first priority in caring for a rape survivor is to create a safe, secure milieu. Admission information should be gathered in a quiet, private room. The woman should be reassured that she is safe and not alone. The survivor's level of emotional distress must be assessed, both for the purpose of planning care and for possible courtroom evidence. Obtaining a careful, detailed history is essential. A detailed sexual history is usually taken immediately after the woman has received any necessary emergency care. The process of collecting evidence of the rape may, in itself, be traumatic for the woman. It is helpful to have a support person with the woman during these procedures.

The woman's clothing is collected and bagged, swabs of stains and secretions are taken, hair samples and any fingernail scrapings are collected, blood samples are drawn, and photographs are taken. Vaginal and rectal examinations are performed along with a complete physical examination for trauma. The woman is offered prophylactic treatment for sexually transmitted infections. The woman is also questioned about her menstrual cycle and contraceptive practices. If she could become pregnant as a result of the rape, she is offered postcoital contraceptive therapy.

Throughout the experience the nurse acts as the rape survivor's advocate, providing support without usurping decision making. The nurse need not agree with all the survivor's decisions but should respect and defend her right to make them.

The family members and friends on whom the survivor calls will also need nursing care. Like those of the survivor, the reactions of the family will depend on the

COMMUNITY IN FOCUS The SANE Program

In many communities, the treatment of a woman immediately following a rape has been almost as traumatic as the rape itself. Often the woman is taken to the local emergency room accompanied by a police officer, and sits in the waiting room while others speculate as to why she requires a police escort. She may have to wait 4–8 hours or more to be seen by the physician, who first has to treat life-threatening emergencies. During this period, she is not allowed to urinate, shower, eat or drink anything, or change her clothes, because these activities might destroy or alter physical evidence. The police officer who accompanies the rape victim is also detained, unable to leave the victim until the examination is completed and specimens obtained, thus preserving the chain of evidence.

In Tulsa, Oklahoma, the Sexual Assault Nurse Examiner (SANE) Program is designed to address this problem. SANE is coordinated by the police department and provides a seamless program of post-rape health care, personal counseling, and prosecution by combining the resources of seven community organizations: the police department, the District Attorney's office, Call Rape (rape crisis center), the Victim/Witness Center, the Tulsa City/County Health Department, the University of Oklahoma College of Medicine, and Hillcrest Medical Center (Kauffold 1996).

Following the report of a rape, provided the woman's physical injuries are not severe, a police officer brings the rape victim to a special examination suite, away from the busy emergency room. They are met there by a specially trained female sexual assault nurse examiner and a rape crisis counselor. The victim is examined immediately by the SANE nurse, who completes the lengthy examination and gathers all necessary forensic evidence. The hospital ob/gyn resident is available to the nurse if there is a need for further examination and treatment.

Because the evidence collected by the SANE nurses has been of such high quality, the Tulsa District Attorney has designated SANE nurses as expert witnesses in rape trials. Each SANE nurse participates in an extensive training program, agrees to serve as an expert witness if necessary, and takes calls so that nurses are always available to respond when a rape occurs.

Similar programs exist elsewhere. The Sexual Assault Response Team (SART), which started in San Diego, is a multidisciplinary approach that also makes use of SANE nurses. The SART Program is designed to ensure that victims receive necessary health care, emotional support, evidentiary examinations, and referral information. The International Association of Forensic Nurses (the terms *sexual assault nurse examiner* and *forensic nurse* are comparable) estimates that 30–40 new SART programs have started in the United States in the past year (Voelker 1996).

These programs are highly effective in addressing a real community need. In Tulsa, for example, successful convictions of accused rapists are up significantly (Kauffold 1996). Equally important, however, the victim of a rape is treated with care and compassion and not victimized a second time.

values to which they ascribe. Many families or mates blame the survivor for the assault and feel angry with her for not having been more careful. They may also incorrectly view the rape as a sexual act rather than an act of violence. They may feel personally wronged and see the survivor as devalued or unclean. Their reactions may compound the survivor's crisis.

By spending some time with family members before their first interaction with the rape survivor, the nurse can reduce their anxiety and absorb some of their frustrations, sparing the woman further trauma.

Rape counseling, provided by qualified nurses or other counselors, is a valuable tool in helping the rape survivor come to terms with her assault and its impact on her life. In counseling the woman is encouraged to explore and identify her feelings and determine appropriate actions to resolve her problems and concerns. It is important for the counselor to avoid reinforcing the prevalent myth that the rape was somehow the woman's fault. The fault lies with the rapist. The counselor also plays an important role in emphasizing that the loss of control the woman experienced during the rape was temporary and that the woman does have control over other aspects of her life.

Prosecution of the Rapist

Legally, rape is considered a crime against the state and prosecution of the assailant is a community responsibility. The survivor, however, must begin the process by reporting the assault and pressing charges against her assailant. In the past, the police and the judicial system have been notoriously insensitive in dealing with rape survivors. Many communities, however, now have classes designed to help officers work effectively with rape survivors or have special teams to carry out this important task.

Many women who have sought to use the judicial process have had such a traumatic experience that they refer to it as a second rape. The woman may be asked repeatedly to describe the experience in intimate detail and her reputation and testimony will be attacked by the defense attorney. In addition, publicity may intensify her feelings of humiliation and, if the assailant is released on bail, she may fear retaliation.

The nurse acting as a counselor needs to be aware of the judicial sequence to anticipate rising tension and frustration in the survivor and her support system. She will need consistent, effective support at this crucial time.

Care of the Woman with a Disorder of the Breast

Throughout her lifetime a woman may experience a variety of breast disorders. Some, like mastitis, are acute disorders, while others, such as fibrocystic breast disease, are chronic. This section deals with some of the common breast disorders a woman may encounter. For information on breast cancer, readers are referred to a medical-surgical nursing text.

Fibrocystic breast disease, the most common of the benign breast disorders, is most prevalent in women 30 to 50 years of age (Mansel 1992). Only women with fibrocystic breast disease who show certain histologic changes (usually found incidentally when a biopsy is done) have an increased risk of developing cancer (Simpson 1992). Fibrosis is a thickening of the normal breast tissue. Cyst formation that may accompany fibrosis is considered a later change in the condition. Fibrocystic breast disease is probably caused by an imbalance in estrogen and progesterone that distorts the normal changes of the menstrual cycle. The symptoms often increase as the woman approaches menopause, while the condition generally improves following menopause. However, if a postmenopausal woman is treated with hormone replacement therapy, the cyclic breast changes may resume.

The woman often reports pain, tenderness, and swelling that occurs cyclically and is most pronounced just before menses. Physical examination may reveal only mild signs of irregularity, or the breasts may feel dense, with areas of irregularity and nodularity. Women often refer to this as "lumpiness." Some women may also have expressible nipple discharge. Although unilateral discharge and serosanguinous discharge are the most worrisome findings, all breast discharge should be investigated further (Edge and Segatore 1993).

If the woman has a large, fluid-filled cyst, she may experience a localized painful area as the capsule containing the accumulated fluid distends coincident with her cycle. However, if small cysts form, the woman may experience not a solitary tender lump but a diffuse tenderness. A cyst may often be differentiated from a malignancy because a cyst is more mobile and tender and is not associated with skin retraction (pulling) in the surrounding tissue.

Mammography, sonography, palpation, and fine-needle aspiration are used to confirm fibrocystic breast disease. Often, fine-needle aspiration is the treatment as well, affording relief from the tenderness or pain. Treatment of palpable cysts is conservative; invasive procedures such as biopsy are used only if the diagnosis is questionable.

Women with mild symptoms may benefit from restricting sodium intake and taking a mild diuretic during the week before the onset of menses. This counteracts fluid retention, relieves pressure in the breast, and helps decrease the pain. In other cases, a mild analgesic is necessary. Other treatment approaches include the use of thiamine and vitamin E. In severe cases, the hormone inhibitor danazol is the drug of choice.

Some researchers suggest that methylxanthines (found in caffeine products, such as coffee, tea, colas, and chocolate, and some medications) may contribute to the development of fibrocystic breast changes and that limiting intake of these substances will help decrease fibrocystic changes (Bullough et al 1990). Other research fails to demonstrate a clear association between methylxanthines and fibrocystic breast changes (Norwood 1990). Additional medical therapies that are helpful in varying degrees include oral contraceptives, progestins, and bromocriptine. All work on the principle of estrogen suppression and progesterone stimulation or augmentation.

Fibroadenoma is a common benign tumor seen in women in their teens and early twenties. It has not been significantly associated with breast cancer. Fibroadenomas are freely movable, solid tumors that are well defined, sharply delineated, and rounded, with a rubbery texture. They are asymptomatic and nontender.

If there are any disquieting features to the appearance of a lump, fine-needle biopsy or excision of the mass may be indicated. Caution is exercised when deciding upon biopsy because excision of the mass in a young girl may interfere with normal breast development. Watchful observation and possible surgical excision are the only treatments for fibroadenomas. Surgery is often deferred. When advisable, surgical removal of the fibroadenoma concludes its treatment.

Intraductal papillomas, most often occurring during the menopausal years, are tumors growing in the terminal portion of a duct or, sometimes, throughout the duct system within a section of the breast. They are typically benign but have the potential to become malignant (Morrow 1992). Although relatively uncommon, they are the most common cause of nipple discharge in women who are not pregnant or lactating.

The majority of papillomas present as solitary nodules. These small ball-like lesions may be detected on mammography but often are nonpalpable. The presence of a papilloma is often frightening to the woman, because her primary symptom is a discharge from the nipple that may be serosanguineous or brownish-green due to old blood. The location of the papilloma within the duct system and its pattern of growth determine whether nipple discharge will be present.

If the woman reports a nipple discharge, the breast should be milked to obtain fluid. The fluid obtained is sent for a Pap smear. The diagnosis is confirmed if papilloma cells are present. The lesion must be excised and histologically examined because of the difficulty in differentiating between a benign papilloma and a papillary carcinoma. Treatment for benign intraductal papilloma is excision with follow-up care.

Duct ectasis (comedomastitis), an inflammation of the ducts behind the nipple, commonly occurs during or near the onset of menopause and is not associated with malignancy. The condition typically occurs in women who have borne and nursed children. It is characterized by a thick, sticky nipple discharge and by burning pain, pruritus, and inflammation. Nipple retraction may also be noted, especially in postmenopausal women. Treatment is conservative, with drug therapy aimed at symptomatic relief. The major central ducts of the breast occasionally have to be excised.

APPLYING THE NURSING PROCESS

Nursing Assessment

During the period of diagnosis, the woman may be anxious about a possible change in body image or a diagnosis of cancer. The nurse can use therapeutic communication to assess the significance the woman places on her breasts; her current emotional status, coping mechanisms used during periods of stress, and knowledge and beliefs about cancer; and other variables that may influence her coping and adjustment.

Nursing Diagnosis

Nursing diagnoses that may apply to a woman with a benign disorder of the breast include the following:

- Knowledge deficit related to a lack of information about the diagnostic procedures.
- Anxiety related to threat to body image.

Nursing Plan and Implementation

During the prediagnosis period the nurse should clarify misconceptions and encourage the woman to express her anxiety. Once a diagnosis has been made, the nurse should ensure that the woman clearly understands her condition, its association to breast malignancy, and treatment options.

The nurse can also point out that frequent professional breast examinations and regular mammograms are tools that help detect any abnormalities and that the woman who practices monthly BSE, follows her caregiver's advice, and is examined regularly has taken positive action to protect her health.

Evaluation

Anticipated outcomes of nursing care include

- The woman is able to discuss her fears, concerns, and questions during the period of diagnosis.
- The diagnosis is made quickly and accurately.

Care of the Woman with Endometriosis

Endometriosis is a condition characterized by the presence of endometrial tissue outside the endometrial cavity. Endometriosis has been found almost everywhere in the body, including the vagina, lungs, cervix, central nervous system, and gastrointestinal tract. The most common location, however, is the pelvis (Nachtigall et al 1994). This tissue responds to the hormonal changes of the menstrual cycle and bleeds in a cyclic fashion. The bleeding results in inflammation, scarring of the peritoneum, and formation of adhesions.

Endometriosis may occur at any age after puberty, although it is most common in women between ages 30 and 40 and is rare in postmenopausal women. The exact cause of endometriosis is unknown. Proposed causative factors include retrograde menstrual flow and inflammation of the endometrium, hereditary tendency, and a possible immunologic defect (Kauppila 1993).

The most common symptom of endometriosis is pelvic pain, which is often dull or cramping. Usually the pain is related to menstruation and is thought to be dysmenorrhea by the affected woman. **Dyspareunia** (painful intercourse) and abnormal uterine bleeding are other common signs. The condition is often diagnosed when the woman seeks evaluation for infertility. Bimanual examination may reveal a fixed, tender, retroverted uterus and palpable nodules in the cul-de-sac. Diagnosis is confirmed by laparoscopy.

Treatment may be medical, surgical, or a combination of the two. During the laparoscopic examination, the physician may surgically resect any visible implants of endometrial tissue, taking care to avoid damaging any organs. Laser vaporization can be used for all but the deepest implants (Younger 1993). This allows for more exact removal of tissue, less adjacent tissue damage, and decreased bleeding. If the woman does not desire pregnancy at the present time, she may be started on oral contraceptives. In women with minimal disease and symptoms, treatment includes observation, analgesics, and nonsteroidal anti-inflammatory drugs (NSAIDs). The woman who desires pregnancy and has been unsuccessful in her attempts to conceive is often treated with a 6-month course of danazol. Danazol is a testosterone derivative with a mild androgenic effect. It suppresses both follicle-stimulating hormone (FSH) and luteinizing hormone (LH). This suppresses ovulation and causes amenorrhea. Danazol does have some significant side effects including hirsutism, vaginal bleeding, acne, oily skin, weight gain, reduced libido, voice changes and hoarseness, clitoral enlargement, and decreased breast size.

Gonadotropin-releasing hormone (GnRH) agonists such as nafarelin acetate (given as a metered nasal spray twice daily), and leuprolide acetate (Lupron) (given once a month as an intramuscular injection) are gaining popularity because many women tolerate them better than danazol and their results in treating endometriosis are comparable. GnRH agonists suppress the menstrual cycle through estrogen antagonism. This may result in the hypoestrogen side effects of hot flashes, vaginal dryness, and loss of bone density, but these side effects can be modified by combining GnRH agonists with a progestin (Kauppila 1993).

In more advanced cases, surgery may be done to remove implants and break up adhesions. If severe dyspareunia or dysmenorrhea are symptoms, the surgeon may perform a presacral neurectomy. In advanced cases in which childbearing is not an issue, treatment may be a hysterectomy with bilateral salpingo-oophorectomy.

APPLYING THE NURSING PROCESS

Nursing Assessment

The nurse should be aware of the common symptoms of endometriosis and elicit an accurate history if a woman mentions these symptoms. If a woman is being treated for endometriosis, the nurse should assess the woman's understanding of the condition, its implications, and the treatment alternatives.

Nursing Diagnosis

Nursing diagnoses that may apply to a woman with endometriosis include the following:

- Pain related to peritoneal irritation secondary to endometriosis.
- Ineffective individual coping related to depression secondary to infertility.

Nursing Plan and Implementation

The nurse can be available to explain the condition, its symptoms, treatment alternatives, and prognosis. The nurse can help the woman evaluate treatment options and make appropriate choices. If medication is begun, the nurse can review the dosage, schedule, possible side effects, and any warning signs. Women are often advised to avoid delaying pregnancy because of the risk of infertility. The woman may wish to discuss the implications of this decision on her life choices, relationship with her partner, and personal preferences. The nurse can be a nonjudgmental listener and help the woman consider her options.

Evaluation

Anticipated outcomes of nursing care include

- The woman is able to discuss her condition, its implications for fertility, and her treatment options.
- After considering the alternatives, the woman chooses appropriate treatment options.

Care of the Woman with Toxic Shock Syndrome (TSS)

Although **toxic shock syndrome** (TSS) has been reported in children, postmenopausal women, and men, it is primarily a disease of women in their reproductive years, especially women at or near menses or during the postpartum period. The causative organism is a strain of *Staphylococcus aureus*. As discussed earlier, the use of superabsorbent tampons has been widely related to an increased incidence of TSS. However, occluding the cervical os with a contraceptive device such as a diaphragm or cervical cap, especially if it is left in place for more than 24 hours, may also increase the risk of TSS.

Early diagnosis and treatment are important in preventing a fatal outcome. The most common signs of TSS include fever (often greater than 38.9C, or 102F); desquamation of the skin, especially the palms and soles, which usually occurs 1–2 weeks after the onset of symptoms; rash; hypotension; and dizziness. Systemic symptoms often include vomiting, diarrhea, severe myalgia, and inflamed mucous membranes (oropharyngeal, conjunctival, or vaginal). Disorders of the central nervous system, including alterations in consciousness, disorientation, and coma, may also occur.

Laboratory findings reveal elevated blood urea nitrogen (BUN), creatinine, SGOT, SGPT, and total bilirubin, while platelets are often less than 100,000/mm^3.

Women with TSS are generally hospitalized and given supportive therapy, including intravenous fluids to maintain blood pressure. Severe cases may require renal dialysis, administration of vasopressors, and intubation. Penicillinase-resistant antibiotics, while of limited value during the acute phase, do help reduce the risk of recurrence (Eschenbach 1994).

Nursing Care

Nurses play a major role in helping educate women about ways to prevent the development of TSS. Women should understand the importance of avoiding prolonged use of tampons. They should change tampons every 3 to 6 hours, and avoid using superabsorbent tampons. Some women may choose to use other products, such as sanitary napkins or minipads. The woman who chooses to continue using tampons may reduce her risk by alternating them with napkins and avoiding overnight use of tampons.

Postpartal women should avoid the use of tampons for 6–8 weeks after childbirth. Women with a history of TSS should never use tampons.

Women who use diaphragms or cervical caps should not leave them in place for prolonged periods and should not use them during the postpartum period or when they are menstruating.

Nurses can also help make women aware of the signs and symptoms of TSS so that they can seek treatment promptly if symptoms occur.

Care of the Woman with a Vaginal Infection

Vulvovaginal Candidiasis

Vulvovaginal candidiasis (VVC), also called moniliasis or yeast infection, is the most common form of vaginitis affecting the vagina and vulva. Recurrences are frequent for some women. Factors that contribute to the occurrence of this infection are use of oral contraceptives, use of antibiotics, frequent douching, pregnancy, diabetes mellitus, and premenstrual factors that are unclear. A gram-positive fungus *(Candida albicans)* is the causative organism.

The woman often complains of thick, curdy vaginal discharge; severe itching; dysuria; and dyspareunia. A male sexual partner may experience a rash or excoriation of the skin of the penis, and possibly pruritus. The male may be symptomatic and the female asymptomatic.

On physical examination, the woman's labia may be swollen and excoriated if pruritus has been severe. A speculum examination reveals thick, white, tenacious cheeselike patches adhering to the vaginal mucosa. Diagnosis is confirmed by microscopic examination of the vaginal discharge; hyphae and spores are usually seen on a wet mount preparation (Figure 5–10).

Medical treatment of monilial vaginitis includes intravaginal insertion of miconazole, tioconazole, butoconazole, terconazole, or clotrimazole suppositories or

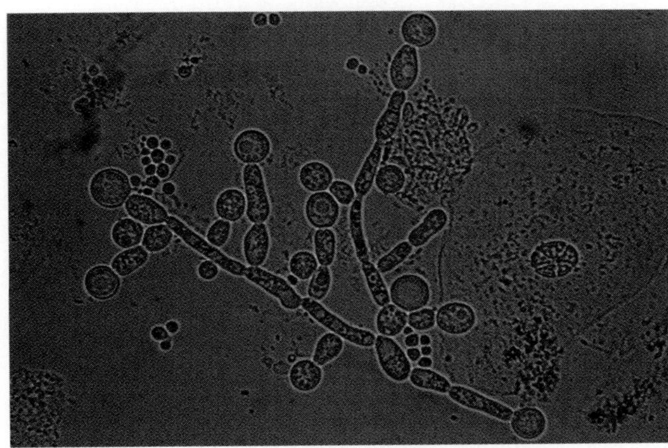

FIGURE 5–10 The hyphae and spores of *Candida albicans.*
Source: Courtesy Centers for Disease Control and Prevention.

cream at bedtime for 3 days to 1 week. If the vulva is also infected, the cream is prescribed and may be applied topically. Some of these medications are available over the counter. They are indicated for women with a history of yeast infections who clearly recognize the symptoms.

Topical miconazole usually eliminates the yeast infection from the male. However, the CDC states that treatment of the male partner is not necessary unless candidal balanitis (inflammation of the glans penis) is present or chronicity is a problem (CDC 1993).

If a woman experiences frequent recurrences of monilial vaginitis, she should be tested for an elevated blood glucose level to determine whether a diabetic or prediabetic condition is present. Women at high risk for HIV disease should also be tested for HIV infection. Pregnant women are treated the same as nonpregnant women (CDC 1993). Infection at the time of birth may cause thrush (a mouth infection) in the newborn.

APPLYING THE NURSING PROCESS

Nursing Assessment

The nurse caring for the woman should suspect VVC if the woman complains of intense vulvar itching and a curdy, white discharge. Because pregnant women with diabetes mellitus are especially susceptible to this infection, the nurse should be alert for symptoms in these women. In some areas nurses are trained to do speculum examinations and wet-mount preparations and can confirm the diagnosis themselves. In most cases, however, the nurse who suspects a vaginal infection reports it to the woman's health care provider. See Key Facts to Remember: Vaginitis.

KEY FACTS TO REMEMBER

Vaginitis

To distinguish among the common types of vaginitis and their treatments, it is useful to remember the following:

Vulvovaginal candidiasis (moniliasis)

Cause: *Candida albicans.*

Appearance of discharge: Thick, curdy, like cottage cheese.

Diagnostic test: Slide of vaginal discharge (treated with potassium hydroxide [KOH]) shows characteristic hyphae and spores.

Treatment: Clotrimazole vaginal cream or suppositories.

Bacterial vaginosis* (Gardnerella vaginalis *vaginitis)

Cause: *Gardnerella vaginalis.*

Appearance of discharge: Gray, milky.

Diagnostic test: Slide of vaginal discharge shows characteristic "clue" cells.

Treatment: Metronidazole.

Trichomoniasis

Cause: *Trichomonas vaginalis.*

Appearance of discharge: Greenish-white and frothy.

Diagnostic test: Saline slide of vaginal discharge shows motile flagellated organisms.

Treatment: Metronidazole.

Nursing Diagnosis

Nursing diagnoses that might apply to the woman with VVC include the following:

- Risk for impaired skin integrity related to scratching secondary to discomfort of the infection.
- Knowledge deficit related to lack of information about ways of preventing the development of VVC.

Nursing Plan and Implementation

If the woman is experiencing discomfort because of pruritus, the nurse can recommend gentle bathing of the vulva with a weak sodium bicarbonate solution. If a topical treatment is being used, the woman will need to bathe the area before applying the medication.

The nurse also discusses with the woman the factors that contribute to the development of VVC and suggests ways to prevent recurrences, such as wearing cotton underwear and avoiding vaginal powders or sprays that may irritate the vulva. Some women report that the addition of yogurt to the diet or the use of activated culture of plain yogurt as a vaginal douche helps prevent recurrence by maintaining high levels of lactobacillus.

Evaluation

Anticipated outcomes of nursing care include

- The woman's symptoms are relieved, and the infection is cured.
- The woman is able to identify self-care measures to prevent further episodes of VVC.

Bacterial Vaginosis (BV) (*Gardnerella vaginalis vaginitis*)

Many flora normally inhabit the vagina of the healthy woman. Some of these organisms are potentially pathogenic. In some women these bacteria begin to "overgrow," causing a vaginitis. The cause of this overgrowth is not clear, although tissue trauma and sexual intercourse are sometimes identified as contributing factors. The *Gardnerella vaginalis* organism (formerly referred to as *Hemophilus vaginalis*) has been found in the vast majority of cases, along with an increased concentration of anaerobic bacteria. The infected woman often notices an excessive amount of thin, watery, yellow-gray vaginal discharge with a foul odor described as "fishy." The characteristic "clue" cell is seen on a wet mount preparation (Figure 5–11).

The nonpregnant woman is generally treated with metronidazole (Flagyl) (see Key Facts to Remember: Vaginitis). Because of its potential teratogenic effects,

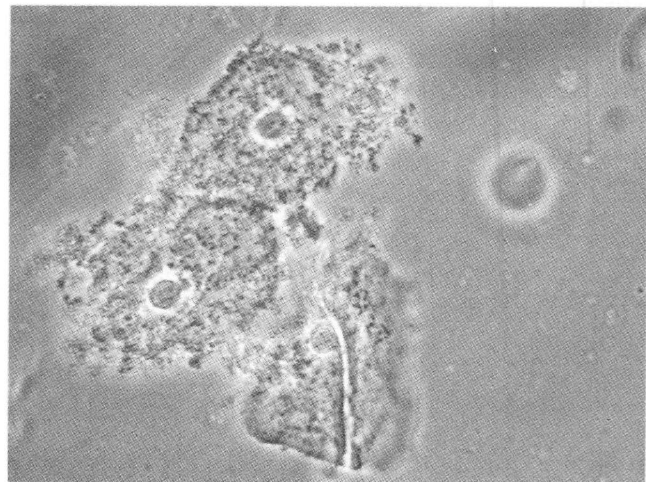

FIGURE 5–11 Depiction of the clue cells characteristically seen in bacterial vaginosis *(Gardnerella vaginalis).*

metronidazole is avoided during the first trimester of pregnancy; one full applicator of clindamycin is inserted intravaginally at bedtime instead (CDC 1993). During the second and third trimesters, oral metronidazole can be used, although vaginal metronidazole or clindamycin cream may be preferable. BV during pregnancy may be a factor in premature rupture of the membranes and preterm birth (CDC 1993).

Care of the Woman with a Sexually Transmitted Infection

The occurrence of **sexually transmitted infections** (STI), also called a *sexually transmitted disease (STD),* has increased over the past few decades. In fact, vaginitis and sexually transmitted infections are the most common reasons for outpatient, community-based treatment of women.

Trichomoniasis

Trichomonas vaginalis is a microscopic motile protozoan that thrives in an alkaline environment. Most infections are acquired through sexual intimacy. Transmission by shared bath facilities, wet towels, or wet swimsuits may also be possible (CDC 1993).

Symptoms of trichomoniasis include a yellow-green, frothy, odorous discharge frequently accompanied by inflammation of the vagina and cervix, dysuria, and dyspareunia. Visualization of *T vaginalis* under the microscope on a wet-mount preparation of vaginal discharge confirms the diagnosis (Figure 5–12).

Treatment for trichomoniasis is metronidazole (Flagyl) administered over 7 days or in a single 2 g dose for both male and female sexual partners. Partners should avoid intercourse until both are cured (see Key Facts to Remember: Vaginitis).

The woman should be informed that metronidazole is contraindicated in the first trimester of pregnancy because of possible teratogenic effects on the fetus. However, no other adequate treatment exists. For women with severe symptoms after the first trimester, treatment with 2 g metronidazole in a single dose may be considered (CDC 1993). The woman and her partner should be cautioned to avoid alcohol while taking metronidazole; the combination has an effect similar to that of alcohol and Antabuse—abdominal pain, flushing, or tremors (CDC 1993).

Chlamydial Infection

Chlamydial infection, caused by *Chlamydia trachomatis,* is the most common STI in the United States. The

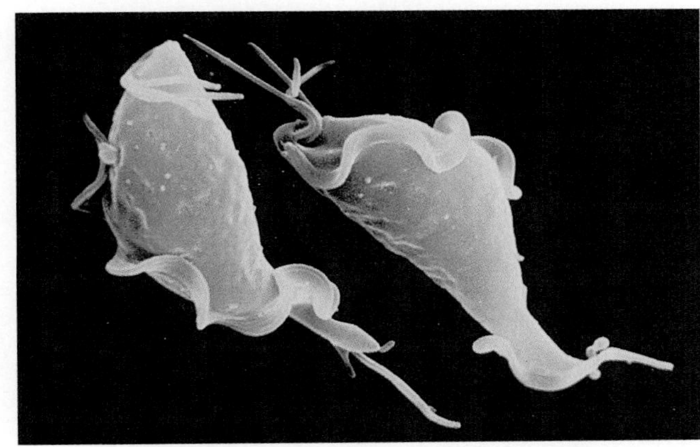

FIGURE 5–12 Microscopic appearance of *Trichomonas vaginalis.*

organism is an intracellular bacterium with several different immunotypes. Immunotypes of chlamydia are responsible for lymphogranuloma venereum and trachoma, which is the world's leading cause of preventable blindness.

Chlamydia is a major cause of nongonococcal urethritis (NGU) in men. In women it can cause infections similar to those that occur with gonorrhea. It can infect the fallopian tubes, cervix, urethra, and Bartholin's glands. Pelvic inflammatory disease, infertility, and ectopic pregnancy are associated with chlamydia. The infant of a woman with untreated chlamydia is at risk of developing ophthalmia neonatorum, which responds to erythromycin ophthalmic ointment but not to silver nitrate prophylaxis. The newborn may also develop chlamydia pneumonia.

Symptoms of chlamydia include a thin or purulent discharge, burning and frequency of urination, and lower abdominal pain. Women, however, are often asymptomatic. Diagnosis is frequently made after treatment of a male partner for NGU or in a symptomatic woman with a negative gonorrhea culture. Laboratory detection is now simpler, due to the availability of a test to detect monoclonal antibodies specific for Chlamydia.

The usual prescribed treatment is azithromycin or doxycycline. Pregnant women should be treated with erythromycin ethylsuccinate because doxycycline taken during the time of fetal tooth development can cause permanent staining of teeth in the infant (CDC 1993).

Herpes Genitalis

Herpes infections are caused by the herpes simplex virus. Estimates suggest that 30 million people in the United States have genital herpes and that 500,000 new cases occur each year (CDC 1993). Two types of herpes infections can occur: Type I (the "cold sore") typically occurs above the waist and is not sexually transmitted; type II is usually associated with genital infections. However, as a result of oral-genital contact, type I lesions can occur in the genital area and type II lesions can occur around the mouth. The clinical symptoms and treatment of both types are the same.

The primary episode of herpes genitalis is characterized by the development of single or multiple blisterlike vesicles, which usually occur in the genital area and sometimes affect the vaginal walls, cervix, urethra, and anus. The vesicles may appear within a few hours to 20 days after exposure and rupture spontaneously to form very painful, open, ulcerated lesions. Inflammation and pain secondary to the presence of herpes lesions can cause difficult urination and urinary retention. Inguinal lymph node enlargement may be present. Flulike symptoms and genital pruritus or tingling also may be noticed. Primary episodes usually last the longest and are the most severe. Lesions heal spontaneously in 2–4 weeks.

After the lesions heal, the virus enters a dormant phase, residing in the nerve ganglia of the affected area. Some individuals never have a recurrence, whereas others have regular recurrences. Recurrences are usually less severe than the initial episode and seem to be triggered by emotional stress, menstruation, ovulation, pregnancy, frequent or vigorous intercourse, poor health status or a generally run-down physical condition, tight clothing, or overheating. Diagnosis is made on the basis of the clinical appearance of the lesions, Pap smear or culture of the lesions, and sometimes blood testing for antibodies.

No known cure for herpes exists. Prescriptive treatment is available to provide relief from pain and prevent complications from secondary infection. The recommended treatment of the first clinical episode of genital herpes is oral acyclovir (200 mg five times a day for 7–10 days or until clinical resolution). Oral acyclovir may also be used to treat recurrences. Therapy should be started during the prodromal period for the greatest benefit. Acyclovir should not be used during pregnancy because its safety has not been established (CDC 1993).

Self-help suggestions include cleansing with povidone-iodine (Betadine) solution to prevent secondary infection and with Burow's solution to relieve discomfort. Use of vitamin C or lysine is frequently suggested to prevent recurrence, although studies have not documented the effectiveness of these supplements. Keeping the genital area clean and dry, wearing loose clothing, and wearing cotton underwear or none at all will promote healing. Primary or recurrent lesions will heal without prescriptive therapies.

If herpes is present in the genital tract of a woman during childbirth, it can have a devastating, even fatal, effect on the newborn. For further discussion, see Chapter 13.

Syphilis

Syphilis is a chronic infection caused by the spirochete *Treponema pallidum.* Syphilis can be acquired congenitally through transplacental inoculation and can result from maternal exposure to infected exudate during sexual contact or from contact with open wounds or infected blood. The incubation period varies from 10 to 90 days, and even though no symptoms or lesions are noted during this time, the woman's blood contains spirochetes and is infectious.

Syphilis is divided into early and late stages. During the early stage (primary), a chancre appears at the site where the *Treponema pallidum* organism entered the body. Symptoms include slight fever, loss of weight, and malaise. The chancre persists for about 4 weeks and then disappears. In 6 weeks to 6 months, secondary symptoms appear. Skin eruptions called condylomata lata, which resemble wartlike plaques and are highly infectious, may appear on the vulva. Other secondary symptoms are acute arthritis, enlargement of the liver and spleen, nontender enlarged lymph nodes, iritis, and a chronic sore throat with hoarseness. When infected in utero, the newborn will exhibit secondary stage symptoms of syphilis. Transplacentally transmitted syphilis may cause preterm birth, stillbirth, and neonatal death (CDC 1993).

As a result of the disease's impact on the fetus in utero, serologic testing of every pregnant woman is recommended; some state laws require it. Testing is done at the initial prenatal screening and repeated in the third trimester. Blood studies may be negative if blood is drawn too early in the pregnancy.

Diagnosis is made by dark-field examination for spirochetes. Blood tests such as VDRL (Venereal Disease Research Laboratories), RPR (Rapid Plasma Reagin), or the more specific FTA-ABS (fluorescent treponemal antibody absorption test) are commonly done.

For pregnant and nonpregnant women with syphilis of less than a year's duration, the CDC recommends 2.4 million units of benzathine penicillin G intramuscularly. If syphilis is of long (more than a year) duration, 2.4 million units of benzathine penicillin G is given intramuscularly once a week for 3 weeks. If a woman is allergic to penicillin, doxycycline can be given. Maternal serologic testing may remain positive for 8 months, and the newborn may have a positive test for 3 months.

Gonorrhea

Gonorrhea is an infection caused by the bacteria *Neisseria gonorrhoeae.* If a nonpregnant woman contracts the disease, she is at risk to develop pelvic inflammatory disease. If a woman becomes infected after the third month of pregnancy, the mucous plug in the cervix will prevent the infection from ascending, and it will remain localized in the urethra, cervix, and Bartholin's glands until the membranes rupture. Then it can spread upward.

The majority of women with gonorrhea are asymptomatic. Thus it is accepted practice to screen for this infection by doing a cervical culture during the initial prenatal examination. For women at high risk, the culture may be repeated during the last month of pregnancy. Cultures of the urethra, throat, and rectum may also be required for diagnosis, depending on the body orifices used for intercourse.

The most common symptoms of gonorrheal infection include a purulent, greenish-yellow vaginal discharge; dysuria; and urinary frequency. Some women also develop inflammation and swelling of the vulva. The cervix may appear swollen and eroded and may secrete a foul-smelling discharge in which gonococci are present.

Treatment consists of antibiotic therapy with 125 mg ceftriaxone intramuscularly once plus 100 mg doxycycline by mouth twice a day for 7 days. If the woman is allergic to ceftriaxone, spectinomycin is given followed by the doxycycline. Additional treatment may be required if the cultures remain positive 7–14 days after completion of treatment. All sexual partners must also be treated or the woman may become reinfected. Pregnant women should be treated with 250 mg ceftriaxone intramuscularly once plus 500 mg erythromycin by mouth twice a day for 7 days (CDC 1993).

Women should be informed of the need for reculture to verify cure and the need for abstinence or condom use until cure is confirmed. Both sexual partners should be treated if either has a positive test for gonorrhea.

Condyloma Acuminata (Venereal Warts)

Condylomata acuminata, also called venereal warts, is a relatively common, sexually transmitted infection caused by the human papilloma virus (HPV). Because of the increasing evidence of a link between HPV and cervical cancer, the condition is receiving increasing attention.

Often a woman seeks medical care after noticing single or multiple soft, grayish-pink, cauliflowerlike lesions in her genital area (Figure 5–13). The moist, warm environment of the genital area is conducive to the growth of the warts, which may be present on the vulva, vagina, cervix, and anus. The incubation period following exposure is 3 weeks to 3 years.

Because condylomata sometimes resemble other lesions and malignant transformation is possible, all atypical, pigmented, and persistent warts should be biopsied and treatment should be instituted promptly. The treatment of choice for pregnant and nonpregnant women is cryothrapy with liquid nitrogen to destroy the lesions (CDC 1993). An alternative therapy is topical podophyllin, which is applied by health care providers who instruct the woman to wash it off four hours after application. Podofilox, also applied topically and washed off after four hours, is used for self-treatment. These drugs are not used during pregnancy because they are thought to be teratogenic and in large doses have been associated with fetal death. If the woman is pregnant or if the lesions do not respond to podophyllin, trichloroacetic acid (TCA) may be used; 5-Fluorouracil (5-FU), another topical agent, is used for multiple small vaginal or vulvar lesions. Carbon dioxide laser therapy, performed under colposcopy, has a good success rate, probably because use of the colposcope aids in detecting tiny satellite lesions.

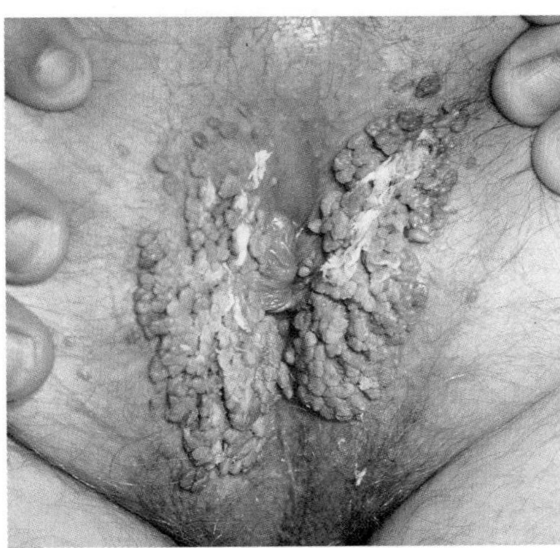

FIGURE 5–13 Condylomata acuminata on the vulva.

Loop electrosurgical excision procedure (LEEP), long popular in Europe for the excision of HPV lesions of the cervix, is becoming more common in the United States. The procedure involves using a loop attached to an electrode handle to excise a lesion. Because the specimen is removed intact (rather than vaporized, as with laser) it can be examined by the pathologist. LEEP is also less expensive than laser therapy and can be done as an office procedure. Opinions vary about the use of LEEP for large areas of condylomata on the vulva because the hand-held device is less precise than the laser (Symposium 1992).

Acquired Immunodeficiency Syndrome (AIDS)

Acquired immunodeficiency syndrome (AIDS) is a fatal disorder caused by the human immunodeficiency virus (HIV), which may be transmitted sexually. The care of a person with AIDS is primarily supportive, although some medications are being developed that seem to prolong life. A medical-surgical text will more fully describe this care. However, because the diagnosis of HIV/AIDS or the presence of the HIV antibody has profound implications for a fetus if the woman is pregnant, AIDS is discussed in greater detail in Chapter 12.

APPLYING THE NURSING PROCESS

Nursing Assessment

The nurse working with women must become adept at taking a thorough history and identifying women at risk for sexually transmitted infections. Risk factors include multiple sexual partners, a partner's involvement with other partners, high-risk sexual behaviors such as intercourse without barrier contraception or anal intercourse, partners with high-risk behaviors, treatment with antibiotics while taking oral contraceptives, and young age at onset of sexual activity. The nurse should be alert for signs and symptoms of sexually transmitted infections and be familiar with diagnostic procedures if STI is suspected.

While each STI has certain distinctive characteristics, the following complaints suggest the possibility of infection and warrant further investigation:

- Presence of a "sore" or lesion on the vulva
- Increased vaginal discharge or malodorous vaginal discharge
- Burning with urination
- Dyspareunia
- Bleeding after intercourse
- Pelvic pain

In many instances the woman is asymptomatic, but may report symptoms in her partner, especially painful urination or urethral discharge. It is often helpful to ask the woman whether her partner is experiencing any symptoms.

Nursing Diagnosis

Nursing diagnoses that may apply when a woman has a sexually transmitted infection include the following:

- Altered family processes related to the effects of a diagnosis of sexually transmited infection on the couple's relationship.
- Knowledge deficit related to lack of information about the long-term effects of the diagnosis on childbearing status.

Nursing Plan and Implementation

In a supportive, nonjudgmental way the nurse provides the woman who has a sexually transmitted infection with information about the infection, methods of transmission, implications for pregnancy or future fertility, and importance of thorough treatment. If treatment of her partner is indicated, the woman must understand that it is necessary to prevent a cycle of reinfection. She should also understand the need to abstain from sexual activity, if necessary, during treatment.

Some sexually transmitted infections such as trichomoniasis or chlamydia may cause a woman concern but, once diagnosed, are rather simply treated. Other STIs may also be fairly simple to treat medically but may carry a stigma and be emotionally devastating for the woman. Thus the nurse should stress prevention with all women and encourage them to require partners, especially new partners, to use a condom.

The sensitive nurse can be especially helpful in encouraging the woman to explore her feelings about the diagnosis. She may experience anger or feel "betrayed" by a partner; she may feel guilt or see her diagnosis as a form of "punishment"; or she may feel concern about the long-term implications for future childbearing or ongoing intimate relationships. She may experience a myriad of emotions that she never expected. Opportunities to discuss her feelings in a nonjudgmental environment can be especially helpful. The nurse can offer suggestions about support groups, if indicated, and assist the woman in planning for her future with regard to sexual activity.

More subtly, the nurse's attitude of acceptance and matter-of-factness conveys to the woman that she is still an acceptable person who happens to have an infection. See Key Facts to Remember: Information About Sexually Transmitted Infections.

Evaluation

Anticipated outcomes of nursing care include

- The infection is identified and cured, if possible. If not, supportive therapy is provided.
- The woman and her partner can describe the infection, its method of transmission, its implications, and the therapy.
- The woman copes successfully with the impact of the diagnosis on her self-concept.

KEY FACTS TO REMEMBER

Information About Sexually Transmitted Infections

- The risk of contracting a sexually transmitted infection increases with the number of sexual partners. Because of the extended periods of time between infection with the HIV virus and evidence of infection, intercourse with an individual exposes a woman or man to all the other sex partners of that individual for the past 5 or more years.
- The condom is the best contraceptive method currently available (other than abstinence) for protection from sexually transmitted infections.
- Other contraceptive methods such as the diaphragm, cervical cap, and spermicides also offer some protection against sexually transmitted infections.
- A person diagnosed with a sexually transmitted infection has a responsibility to notify any sexual partners so they can obtain treatment.
- Absence of symptoms or disappearance of symptoms does not mean that treatment is unnecessary if a person suspects a sexually transmitted infection. She or he should be seen for evaluation and treatment. All prescribed medications should be taken completely.
- The presence of a genital infection may lead to an abnormal Pap smear. Women with certain infections should have more frequent Pap tests according to a schedule recommended by their caregiver.

Care of the Woman with Pelvic Inflammatory Disease

Pelvic inflammatory disease (PID) occurs in approximately 1 percent of women between ages 15 and 39, although sexually active young women between 15 and 24 have the highest infection rate. The disease is more common in women who have had multiple sexual partners, a history of PID, early onset of sexual activity, a recent gynecologic procedure, or an intrauterine device. It usually produces a tubal infection (salpingitis) that may or may not be accompanied by a pelvic abscess. However, perhaps the greatest problem of PID is postinfection tubal damage, which is closely associated with infertility.

The organisms most frequently identified with PID include *Chlamydia trachomatis* and *Neisseria gonorrhoeae,* although other aerobic and anaerobic organisms that are often part of the normal vaginal flora have also been found in women with PID (CDC 1993).

Symptoms of PID include bilateral sharp, cramping pain in the lower quadrants, fever, chills, purulent vaginal discharge, irregular bleeding, malaise, nausea, and vomiting. However, it is also possible to be asymptomatic and have normal laboratory values.

Diagnosis consists of a clinical examination to define symptoms, plus blood tests and a gonorrhea culture and test for chlamydia. Physical examination usually reveals direct abdominal tenderness with palpation, adnexal tenderness, and cervical and uterine tenderness with movement (Chandelier sign). A palpable mass is evaluated with ultrasound. Laparoscopy may be used to confirm the diagnosis and to enable the examiner to obtain cultures from the fimbriated ends of the fallopian tubes.

Except in mild cases, the woman is hospitalized and treated with intravenous administration of cefoxitan sodium, cefotetan disodium, or clindamycin plus gentamicin. Outpatient therapy usually includes antibiotics such as cefoxitan, ceftriaxone, doxycycline, and clindamycin used singly or in combination. A new antibiotic, ofloxacin (Floxin), is now available for women with PID caused by chlamydia or gonorrhea. Ofloxacin, taken twice daily for 10–14 days, has a 98 percent cure rate (A simpler cure 1997). In addition, supportive therapy is often indicated for severe symptoms. The sexual partner should also be treated. If the woman has an IUD, it is generally removed 24 to 48 hours after antibiotic therapy is started.

After the infection is treated, microsurgical techniques are sometimes used to release any adhesions and repair tubal damage if the woman wishes to bear children (Ault and Faro 1993).

APPLYING THE NURSING PROCESS

Nursing Assessment

The nurse is alert to factors in a woman's history that put her at risk for PID. Even though fewer types of IUDs are available, many women still have them, and the nurse should question the woman about possible symptoms, such as aching pain in the lower abdomen, foul-smelling discharge, malaise, and the like. The woman who is acutely ill will have obvious symptoms, but a low-grade infection is more difficult to detect.

Nursing Diagnosis

Nursing diagnoses that may apply to a woman with PID include the following:

- Pain related to peritoneal irritation.
- Knowledge deficit related to a lack of information about the possible effects of PID on fertility.

Nursing Plan and Implementation

The nurse plays a vital role in helping to prevent or detect PID. Accordingly, the nurse spends time discussing risk factors related to this infection. The woman who uses an IUD for contraception and has multiple sexual partners needs to understand clearly the risk she faces. The nurse discusses signs and symptoms of PID and stresses the importance of early detection.

The woman who develops PID needs to understand the importance of completing her antibiotic treatment and of returning for follow-up evaluation. She should also understand the possibility of decreased fertility following the infection.

Evaluation

Anticipated outcomes of nursing care include

- The woman describes her condition, her therapy, and the possible long-term implications of PID on her fertility.
- The woman completes her course of therapy and the PID is cured.

Care of the Woman with an Abnormal Finding During Pelvic Examination

Abnormal Pap Smear Results

The Bethesda System (TBS) (Table 5–4) has become the most widely used system in the United States for reporting Pap smear results. The new system was established to provide a uniform format and classification of terminiology based on current understanding of cervical disease (Isacson and Kurman 1995). Early detection of abnormalities allows early changes to be treated before cells reach the precancerous or cancerous stage.

Notification of an abnormal Pap smear may cause anxiety for the woman, so it is important that she be told in a caring way and then given accurate and complete information about the meaning of the results and the next steps to be taken. She should also be given time to ask questions and express her concerns.

Diagnostic or therapeutic procedures employed in cases of cellular abnormalities include repetition of Pap smears at shorter intervals, colposcopy and endocervical biopsy, cryotherapy, laser conization, or LEEP. Decisions for management are based on the specific report.

Colposcopy has evolved as an appropriate "second step" in many cases when a Pap smear is abnormal. The examination, typically done in an office or clinic, permits more detailed visualization of the cervix in bright light, using a microscope with 6 to 40 times magnification. The cervix can be visualized directly and again following application of 3 percent acetic acid. The acetic acid causes abnormal epithelium to assume a characteristic white appearance. The colposcope can be used to localize and obtain a "directed biopsy."

Women who had first coitus at an early age or have a history of, or a sex partner with a history of, multiple sexual partners, exposure to sexually transmitted infections, immunosuppressive therapy, or antenatal exposure to diethylstilbestrol (DES) have an increased risk of abnormal cell changes and cervical cancer.

Ovarian Masses

Between 70 and 80 percent of ovarian masses are benign. More than 50 percent are functional cysts, occurring most commonly in women 20 to 40 years of age. Functional cysts are rare in women who take oral contraceptives.

Ovarian cysts usually represent physiologic variations in the menstrual cycle. Dermoid cysts (cystic teratomas) comprise 10 percent of all benign ovarian masses. Cartilage, bone, teeth, skin, or hair can be observed in these cysts. Endometriomas, or "chocolate cysts," are another common type of ovarian mass.

No relationship exists between ovarian masses and ovarian cancer. However, ovarian cancer is the most fatal of all cancers in women because it is difficult to diagnose and often has spread throughout the pelvis before it is detected.

A woman with an ovarian mass may be asymptomatic; the mass may be noted on a routine pelvic examination. She may experience a sensation of fullness or cramping in the lower abdomen (often unilateral), dyspareunia, irregular bleeding, or delayed menstruation.

Diagnosis is made on the basis of a palpable mass with or without tenderness and other related symptoms. Radiography or ultrasonography may be used to assist or confirm the diagnosis.

The woman is frequently kept under observation for a month or two because most cysts will resolve on their own and are harmless. Oral contraceptives may be prescribed for 1 to 2 months to suppress ovarian function. If this regimen is effective, a repeat pelvic examination should be normal. If the mass is still present after 60 days of observation and oral contraceptive therapy, a diagnostic laparoscopy or laparotomy may be considered. Tubal or ovarian lesions, ectopic pregnancy, cancer, infection, or appendicitis also must be ruled out before a diagnosis can be confirmed.

Surgery is not always necessary, but will be considered if the mass is larger than 6–7 cm in circumference; if the woman is over 40 years of age with an adnexal mass, a persistent mass, or continuous pain; or if the woman is taking oral contraceptives. Surgical explo-

TABLE 5–4 The Bethesda System (TBS) for Classifying Pap Smears

Adequacy of the Specimen

Satisfactory for evaluation

Satisfactory for evaluation but limited by . . . (specify reason)

Unsatisfactory for evaluation

General Categorization (optional)

Within normal limits

Benign cellular changes (See descriptive diagnoses.)

Epithelial cell abnormality (See descriptive diagnoses.)

Descriptive Diagnoses

Benign cellular changes
- Infection
  - *Trichomonas vaginalis*
  - Fungal organisms morphologically consistent with *Candida* spp
  - Predominance of coccobacilli consistent with shift in vaginal flora
  - Bacteria morphologically consistent with *Actinomyces* spp
  - Cellular changes associated with herpes simplex virus
  - Other

Reactive changes
- Reactive cellular changes associated with:
  - Inflammation (includes typical repair)
  - Atrophy with inflammation ("atrophic vaginitis")
  - Radiation
  - Intrauterine contraceptive device (IUD)
  - Other

Reactive changes *continued*
- Epithelial cell abnormalities
  - Squamous cell
    - Atypical squamous cells of undetermined significance (ASCUS): Qualify*
    - Low-grade squamous intraepithelial lesion (SIL) encompassing HPV† mild dysplasia/CIN 1
    - High-grade squamous intraepithelial lesion encompassing: Moderate and severe dysplasia, CIS/CIN 2 and CIN 3
    - Squamous cell carcinoma
  - Glandular cell
    - Endometrial cells, cytologically benign, in a postmenopausal woman
    - Atypical glandular cells of undetermined significance: Qualify*
    - Endocervical adenocarcinoma
    - Endometrial adenocarcinoma
    - Extrauterine adenocarcinoma
    - Adenocarcinoma, not otherwise specified
  - Other malignant neoplasms: Specify
    - Hormonal evaluation (applies to vaginal smears only)
    - Hormonal pattern compatible with age and history
    - Hormonal pattern incompatible with age and history: Specify
    - Hormonal evaluation not possible due to: Specify

*Atypical squamous or glandular cells of undetermined significance should be further qualified as to whether a reactive or a premalignant/malignant process is favored.

†Cellular changes of human papillomavirus (HPV)—previously termed koilocytosis, koilocytotic atypia, or condylomatous atypia—are included in the category of low-grade squamous intraepithelial lesion.

ration is also indicated when a palpable mass is found in an infant, a young girl, or a postmenopausal woman.

Women who are taking oral contraceptives should be informed of their preventive effect against ovarian masses. Women may need clear explanations about why the initial therapy is observation. A discussion of the origin and resolution of ovarian cysts may clarify this treatment plan. If a surgical treatment removes or impairs the function of one ovary, the woman needs to be assured that the remaining ovary can be expected to take over ovarian functioning and that pregnancy is still possible.

Uterine Masses

Fibroid tumors, or leiomyomas, are among the most common benign disease entities in women and are the most common reason for gynecologic surgery. Between 20 and 50 percent of women develop leiomyomas by 40 years of age. The potential for cancer is minimal. Leiomyomas are more common in women of African heritage.

Fibroid tumors develop when smooth muscle cells are present in whorls and arise from uterine muscles and connective tissue. The size varies from 1–2 cm to the size of a 10-week fetus. Frequently the woman is asymptomatic. Lower abdominal pain, fullness or pressure, menorrhagia, metrorrhagia, or increased dysmenorrhea may occur, particularly with large leiomyomas. Ultrasonography revealing masses or nodules can assist and confirm the diagnosis. Leiomyoma is also considered a possible diagnosis when masses or nodules involving the uterus are palpated on a pelvic examination.

The majority of these masses require no treatment and will shrink after menopause. Close observation for symptoms or an increase in size of the uterus or the masses may be the only management most women will require. Routine pelvic examinations every 3–6 months are recommended unless new symptoms appear.

If a woman notices symptoms, or pelvic examination reveals that the mass is increasing in size, surgery (myomectomy, D&C, or hysterectomy) will be recommended. The choice of surgery depends on the age and reproductive status of the woman and the significance of the noted changes. There are no medications or therapies to prevent fibroids.

Endometrial cancer, most commonly a disease of postmenopausal women, has a high rate of cure if detected early. The hallmark sign is vaginal bleeding in postmenopausal women not treated with hormone replacement therapy. Diagnosis is made by endometrial biopsy or posthysterectomy pathology examination of the uterus. The treatment is total abdominal hysterectomy (TAH) and bilateral salpingo-oophorectomy. Radiation therapy may also be indicated, depending on the staging of the cancer.

Role of the Nurse

Except for nurses with special training, pelvic examinations and Pap smears are not done by nurses. In most cases, nursing assessment is directed toward an evaluation of the woman's understanding of the findings and their implications and her psychosocial response.

The woman needs accurate information on etiology, symptomatology, and treatment options. She should be encouraged to report symptoms and keep appointments for follow-up examination and evaluation. The woman needs realistic reassurance if her condition is benign; she may require counseling and effective emotional support if a malignancy is likely. If the management plan includes surgery, she may need the nurse's support in obtaining a second opinion and making her decision.

Care of the Woman with a Urinary Tract Infection

A urinary tract infection (UTI) may be life-threatening or a mere inconvenience. Bacteria usually enter the urinary tract by way of the urethra. The organisms are capable of migrating against the downward flow of urine. The shortness of the female urethra facilitates the passage of bacteria into the bladder. Other conditions that are associated with bacterial entry are relative incompetence of the urinary sphincter, frequent enuresis (bedwetting) before adolescence, and urinary catheterization. Wiping from back to front after urination may transfer bacteria from the anorectal area to the urethra.

Voluntarily suppressing the desire to urinate is a predisposing factor. Retention overdistends the bladder and can lead to an infection. There also seems to be a relationship between recurring UTI and sexual intercourse. General poor health or lowered resistance to infection can increase a woman's susceptibility to UTI.

Asymptomatic bacteriuria (ASB) (bacteria in the urine actively multiplying without accompanying clinical symptoms) constitutes about 6 to 8 percent of UTI. This becomes especially significant if the woman is pregnant. Between 20 and 30 percent of pregnant women with untreated ASB will go on to develop cystitis or pyelonephritis (Kiningham 1993). Asymptomatic bacteriuria is almost always caused by a single organism. If more than one type of bacteria is cultured, the possibility of urine-culture contamination must be considered. The most common cause of ASB is *Escherichia coli*. Other commonly found causative organisms include *Klebsiella* and *Proteus*.

A woman who has had a UTI is susceptible to recurrent infection. If a pregnant woman develops an acute UTI, especially with a high temperature, amniotic fluid infection may develop and retard the growth of the placenta.

Lower Urinary Tract Infection (Cystitis)

Because urinary tract infections are ascending, it is important to recognize and diagnose a lower UTI early to avoid the sequelae associated with upper UTI.

Symptoms of frequency, pyuria, and dysuria without bacteriuria may indicate urethritis caused by *Chlamydia trachomatis;* it has become a common pathogen in the genitourinary system.

When cystitis develops, the initial symptom is often dysuria, specifically at the end of urination. Urgency and frequency also occur. Cystitis is usually accompanied by a low-grade fever (38.3C, or 101F, or lower), and hematuria is occasionally seen. Urine specimens usually contain an abnormal number of leukocytes and bacteria.

Oral sulfonamides, particularly sulfisoxazole, are generally effective against lower UTI. If the woman is pregnant, these should be used only in early pregnancy because they interfere with protein binding of bilirubin in the fetus; use in the last few weeks of pregnancy can lead to neonatal hyperbilirubinemia and kernicterus. Other drugs that are usually effective (and apparently safe for a fetus) are ampicillin and nitrofurantoin (Furadantin). Nitrofurantoin crosses the placenta, but no harm to the fetus has been demonstrated (Tan and File 1992). Phenazopyridine (Pyridium), a bladder analgesic, may also be prescribed to treat the dysuria.

APPLYING THE NURSING PROCESS

Nursing Assessment

During each visit the nurse notes any complaints from the woman of pain on urination or other urinary difficulties. If any concerns arise, the nurse obtains a clean-catch urine specimen from the woman.

Nursing Diagnosis

Nursing diagnoses that may apply to a woman with a lower UTI include the following:

- Pain related to dysuria secondary to the urinary tract infection.
- Knowledge deficit related to a lack of information about self-care measures to help prevent recurrence of UTI.

Nursing Plan and Implementation

The nurse should make sure the woman is aware of good hygiene practices, since most bacteria enter through the urethra after having spread from the anal area. See Key Facts to Remember: Information for Women About Ways to Avoid Cystitis. The nurse should also reinforce instructions or answer questions regarding the prescribed antibiotic, the amount of liquids to take, and the reasons for these treatments. Cystitis usually responds rapidly to treatment, but follow-up urinary cultures are important.

Evaluation

Anticipated outcomes of nursing care include

- The woman implements self-care measures to help prevent cystitis as part of her personal routine.
- The woman can identify the signs, symptoms, therapy, and possible complications of cystitis.
- The woman's infection is cured.

KEY FACTS TO REMEMBER

Information for Women About Ways to Avoid Cystitis

- If you use a diaphragm for contraception, try changing methods or using another size of diaphragm.
- Avoid bladder irritants such as alcohol, caffeine products, and carbonated beverages.
- Increase fluid intake, especially water, to a minimum of 6 to 8 glasses per day.
- Make regular urination a habit; avoid long waits.
- Practice good genital hygiene, including wiping from front to back after urination and bowel movements.
- Be aware that vigorous or frequent sexual activity may contribute to urinary tract infection.
- Urinate before and after intercourse to empty the bladder and cleanse the urethra.
- Complete medication regimens even if symptoms decrease.
- Do not use medication left over from previous infections.
- Drink cranberry juice to acidify the urine. This has been found to relieve symptoms in some cases.

Upper Urinary Tract Infection (Pyelonephritis)

Pyelonephritis (inflammatory disease of the kidneys) is less common but more serious than cystitis and is often preceded by lower UTI. It is more common during the latter part of pregnancy or early postpartum and poses a serious threat to maternal and fetal well-being. Women with symptoms of pyelonephritis during pregnancy have an increased risk of preterm birth, as well as intrauterine growth retardation.

Acute pyelonephritis has a sudden onset with chills, high temperature of 39.6–40.6C (103–105F), and flank pain (either unilateral or bilateral). The right side is almost always involved if the woman is pregnant because the large bulk of intestines to the left pushes the uterus to the right, putting pressure on the right ureter and kidney. Nausea, vomiting, and general malaise may ensue. With accompanying cystitis, the woman may experience frequency, urgency, and burning with urination.

Edema of the renal parenchyma or ureteritis with blockage and swelling of the ureter may lead to temporary suppression of urinary output. This is accompanied by severe colicky (spastic, intense) pain, vomiting, dehydration, and ileus of the large bowel. The woman with acute pyelonephritis will generally have increased diastolic blood pressure, positive fluorescent antibody titer (FA-test), low creatinine clearance, significant bacteremia in urine culture, pyuria, and presence of white blood cell casts.

Often the woman is hospitalized and started on intravenous antibiotics. In the case of obstructive pyelonephritis, a blood culture is necessary. The woman is kept on bed rest. After the sensitivity report is received, the antibiotic is changed as necessary. If signs of urinary obstruction occur or continue, the ureter may be catheterized to establish adequate drainage.

With appropriate drug therapy, the woman's temperature should return to normal. The pain subsides and the urine shows no bacteria within 2 to 3 days. Follow-up urinary cultures are needed to determine that the infection has been eliminated completely.

APPLYING THE NURSING PROCESS

Nursing Assessment

During the woman's visit, the nurse obtains a sexual and medical history to identify whether she is at risk for UTI. A clean-catch urine specimen is evaluated for evidence of ASB.

Nursing Diagnosis

Nursing diagnoses that may apply to a woman with an upper urinary tract infection include the following:

- Knowledge deficit related to lack of information about the disease and its treatment.
- Fear related to the possible long-term effects of the disease.

Nursing Plan and Implementation

The nurse provides the woman with information to help her recognize the signs of UTI, so she can contact her caregiver as soon as possible. The nurse also discusses hygiene practices, the advantages of wearing cotton underwear, and the need to void frequently to prevent urinary stasis.

The nurse stresses the importance of maintaining a good fluid intake. Drinking cranberry juice daily and taking 500 mg vitamin C help acidify the urine and may help prevent recurrence of infection. Women with a history of UTI find it helpful to drink a glass of fluid before sexual intercourse and to void afterward.

Evaluation

Anticipated outcomes of nursing care include

- The woman completes her prescribed course of antibiotic therapy.
- The woman's infection is cured.
- The woman incorporates preventive self-care measures into her daily regimen.

Cystocele and Pelvic Relaxation

A cystocele is the downward displacement of the bladder, which appears as a bulge in the anterior vaginal wall. Arbitrary classifications of mild to severe are frequently given. Genetic predisposition, childbearing, obesity, and increased age are factors that may contribute to cystocele.

Symptoms of stress incontinence are most common, including loss of urine with coughing, sneezing, laughing, or sudden exertion. Vaginal fullness, a bulging out of the vaginal wall, or a dragging sensation may also be noticeable.

If pelvic relaxation is mild, Kegel exercises are helpful in restoring tone. The exercises involve contraction and relaxation of the pubococcygeal muscle. (See Chapter 9). Women have found these exercises helpful before and after childbirth in maintaining vaginal muscle tone. Estrogen may improve the condition of vaginal mucous membranes—especially in menopausal women. Vaginal pessaries or rings may be used if surgery is undesirable or impossible, or until surgery can be scheduled. Surgery may be considered for cystoceles considered moderate to severe.

The nurse may instruct the woman in the use of Kegel exercises. Information on causes and contributing factors and discussion of possible alternative therapies will greatly assist the woman.

CHAPTER HIGHLIGHTS

- Girls and women should be provided with clear information about menstrual issues, such as use of tampons (deodorant and absorbency); vaginal spray and douching practices; and self-care comfort measures during menstruation, such as nutrition, exercise, and use of heat and massage.
- Dysmenorrhea usually begins at, or a day before, onset of menses and disappears by the end of menstruation. Therapy with hormones such as oral contraceptives, or the use of nonsteroidal anti-inflammatory drugs or prostaglandin inhibitors is useful. Self-care measures include improved nutrition, exercise, applications of heat, and extra rest.
- Premenstrual syndrome occurs most often in women over 30, and symptoms occur 2 to 3 days before onset of menstruation and subside as menstruation starts, with or without treatment. Medical management usually includes progesterone agonists and prostaglandin inhibitors. Self-care measures include improved nutrition (vitamin B complex and E supplementation and avoidance of methylxanthines found in chocolate and caffeine), a program of aerobic exercise, and participation in self-care support groups.
- Fertility awareness methods are "natural," noninvasive methods of contraception often used by people whose religious beliefs prevent their using other methods.

- Mechanical contraceptives such as the diaphragm, cervical cap, and condom act as barriers to prevent the transport of sperm. These methods are used in conjunction with a spermicide.
- The IUD is a mechanical contraceptive. Although its exact method of action is not clearly understood, research suggests it acts by immobilizing sperm or by impeding the progress of sperm from the cervix to the fallopian tubes. The IUD may also act by speeding the movement of the ovum through the fallopian tube. In addition, the IUD does have a local inflammatory effect.
- Oral contraceptives (the pill) are combinations of estrogen and progesterone. When taken correctly, they are the most effective of the reversible methods of fertility control.
- Spermicides are far less effective in preventing pregnancy when they are not used with a barrier method.
- Permanent sterilization is accomplished by tubal ligation for women and vasectomy for men. Although theoretically reversible, clients are advised that the method should be considered irreversible.
- The breasts function in a cyclic process that is regulated by nervous and hormonal systems. Thus many women experience breast tenderness and swelling premenstrually.
- Recommendations about the frequency of screening mammograms vary somewhat.
    - The American Cancer Society recommends screening mammograms annually from age 40.
    - The National Cancer Institute recommends mammograms every 1–2 years between ages 40 and 49, and annually for all women ages 50 and older.
- Menopause is a physiologic, maturational change in a woman's life. Physiologic changes include the cessation of menses and decrease in circulating hormones. Hormonal changes sometimes bring unsettling emotional responses. The more common physiologic symptoms are "hot flashes," palpitations, dizziness, and increased perspiration at night. The woman's anatomy also undergoes changes, such as atrophy of the vagina, reduction in size and pigmentation of the labia, and myometrial atrophy. Osteoporosis becomes an increasing concern.
- Current management of menopause centers around hormone replacement therapy and client health care education.
- Battering occurs in a cyclic pattern called the "cycle of violence" and increases in frequency and severity over time.
- Nurses are in an excellent position to intervene and assist battered women by recognizing their cues, diagnosing their problems appropriately, and understanding the complex dynamics of the battering family. The nurse provides information about available community resources, medical attention, and community support.
- Rape is an act of violence acted out sexually. Most rapes are expressions of anger or power.
- Following rape the survivor will usually experience an assortment of symptoms known as the rape trauma syndrome. Research also links the effects of rape to the posttraumatic stress disorder experienced by many veterans following the Vietnam War.
- In fibrocystic breast disease the cysts tend to be round, mobile, and well delineated. The woman generally experiences increased discomfort premenstrually. Because of the increased risk of breast cancer, women with FBD should understand the importance of monthly BSE.
- Endometriosis is a condition in which endometrial tissue occurs outside the endometrial cavity. This tissue bleeds in a cyclic fashion in response to the menstrual cycle. The bleeding leads to inflammation, scarring, and adhesions. The prime symptoms include dysmenorrhea, dyspareunia, and infertility.
- Treatment of endometriosis may be medical, surgical, or a combination. For the woman not desiring pregnancy at present, oral contraceptives are used. Women desiring pregnancy are treated with danazol.
- Toxic shock syndrome, caused by a toxin of *Staphylococcus aureus,* is most common in women of childbearing age. There is an increased incidence in women who use tampons or barrier methods of contraception, such as the diaphragm and cervical cap.
- Vulvovaginal candidiasis (moniliasis), a vaginal infection caused by *Candida albicans,* is most common in women who use oral contraceptives, are on antibiotics, are currently pregnant, or have diabetes mellitus. It is generally treated with intravaginal miconazole or clotrimazole suppositories.
- Bacterial vaginosis (*Gardnerella vaginalis* vaginitis), a common vaginal infection, is diagnosed by its characteristic fishy odor and by the presence of "clue" cells on a vaginal smear. It is treated with metronidazole unless the woman is in the first trimester of pregnancy.
- Chlamydial infection is difficult to detect in a woman, but may result in PID and infertility. It is treated with antibiotic therapy.
- Herpes genitalis, caused by the herpes simplex virus, is a recurrent infection with no known cure. Acyclovir (Zovirax) may reduce the symptoms.

- Syphilis, caused by *Treponema pallidum,* is a sexually transmitted infection that is treatable if diagnosed. The characteristic lesion is the chancre. Syphilis can also be transmitted in utero to the fetus of an infected woman. The treatment of choice is penicillin.
- Gonorrhea, a common sexually transmitted infection, may be asymptomatic in women initially but may cause PID if not diagnosed early. The treatment of choice is penicillin.
- Condyloma accuminata (venereal warts) is transmitted by the human papilloma virus (HPV). Treatment is indicated, because research suggests a possible link with abnormal cervical changes. The treatment chosen depends on the size and location of the warts.
- Pelvic inflammatory disease may be life threatening and may lead to infertility.
- Women with an abnormal finding on a pelvic examination will need careful explanation of the finding and techniques of diagnosis and emotional support during the diagnostic period.
- The classic symptoms of a lower UTI are dysuria, urgency, frequency, and sometimes hematuria. Oral sulfonamides are the treatment of choice except in mid- to late pregnancy.
- An upper UTI is a serious infection that can permanently damage the kidneys if untreated. Generally the woman is acutely ill and may require supportive therapy as well as antibiotics.
- A cystocele is a downward displacement of the bladder into the vagina. Often it is accompanied by stress incontinence. Kegel exercises may help restore tone in mild cases.

REFERENCES

A simpler cure for pelvic infections. *Health* April 1997, p18.

American Nurses Association: *Position Statement on Physical Violence Against Women.* Washington, DC: ANA, 1991.

Andrews WC: Continuous combined estrogen/progestin hormone replacement therapy. *Nurse Pract* 1995; Suppl 2:1.

Ault KA, Faro S: Pelvic inflammatory disease: Current diagnostic criteria and treatment guidelines. *Postgrad Med* February 1993; 93(2):85.

Bachman R, Saltzman LE: *Violence Against Women: Estimates from the Redesigned Survey.* Bureau of Justice Statistics Special Report, August 1995; Washington, DC: US Department of Justice, NCJ-154348.

Buchwald E et al: *Transforming a Rape Culture.* Minneapolis, MN: Milkweed Editions, 1993.

Buel SM: Family violence: Practical recommendations for physicians and the medical community. *Women Health Issues* 1995; 5(4):158.

Bullough B et al: Methylxanthines and fibrocystic breast disease: A study of correlations. *Nurse Pract* 1990; 15(3):36.

Burgess AW, Holmstrom LL: *Rape: Crisis and Recovery.* Englewood Cliffs, NJ: Prentice Hall, 1979.

Campbell JC: Woman abuse and public policy: Potential for nursing action. *Clin Issues Perinatal Women Health Nurs* 1993; 4(3):503.

Centers for Disease Control and Prevention: 1993 Sexually transmitted disease treatment guidelines. *MMWR* 1993; 42(RR-14):4.

Chez RA, Mishell DR: Control of human reproduction: Contraception, sterilization, and pregnancy termination. In: *Danforth's Obstetrics and Gynecology,* 7th ed. Scott JR et al (editors). Philadelphia: Lippincott, 1994.

Connell EB: The female condom: A new contraception option. *Contemp OB/GYN* 1994; 39(1):66.

Counseling patients about injectible contraception. *Contraception Rep* 1995; 6(5):4.

Crooks R, Baur K: *Our Sexuality,* 5th ed. Redwood City, CA: Benjamin/Cummings, 1993.

Department of Health & Human Services, Public Health Services: *Healthy People 2000.* Washington, DC: Author. Publication No. PHS 91-50213, 1990.

DiSaia PJ: Disorders of the uterine cervix. In: *Danforth's Obstetrics and Gynecology,* 7th ed. Scott JR et al (editors). Philadelphia: Lippincott, 1994.

Dupre AR et al: Sexual assault. *Obstet Gynecol Survey* 1993; 48(9):640.

Edge DS, Segatore M: Assessment and management of galactorrhea. *Nurse Pract* 1993; 18(6):35.

Eschenbach DA: Pelvic infections and sexually transmitted diseases. In: *Danforth's Obstetrics and Gynecology,* 7th ed. Scott JR et al (editors). Philadelphia: Lippincott, 1994.

Furniss K et al: What you can do to stop domestic violence. *Contemp OB/GYN* November 1993; 1(4):5.

Hanson V: Facing facts on emergency postcoital contraception. *Contemp OB/GYN* 1996; 41(6):31.

Hatcher RA et al: *Contraceptive Technology,* 15th revised ed. New York: Irvington, 1994.

Helton AS, Snodgrass FG: Battering during pregnancy: Intervention strategies. *Birth* 1987; 14(3):142.

Herman JL: *Trauma and Recovery.* New York: Basic Books, 1992.

Hoff LA: Battered women: Understanding, identification, and assessment. *J Am Acad Nurs Pract* October/December 1992; 4(4):148.

Horton JA: *The Women's Health Data Book.* Washington, DC: Elsevier, 1992.

Isacson C, Kurman RJ: The Bethesda System: A new classification for managing Pap smears. *Contemp OB/GYN* 1995; 40(6):67.

Kase NG et al: *Principles and Practices of Clinical Gynecology.* New York: Wiley, 1993.

Kauffold MP: The SANE solution: Easing the trauma of rape. *Trustee* September 1996; 49(8):6.

Kaunitz AM: DMPA: A new contraceptive option. *Contemp OB/GYN-NP* April 1993; 1(1):5.

Kauppila A: Changing concepts of medical treatment of endometriosis. *Acta Obstet Gynecol Scand* July 1993; 72(5):324.

Kessenich CR: Update on pharmacologic therapies for osteoporosis. *Nurse Pract* 1996; 21(8):19.

Kiningham RB: Asymptomatic bacteriuria in pregnancy. *Am Fam Phys* April 1993; 47(5):1232.

Kupecz D: Alendronate for the treatment of osteoporosis. *Nurse Pract* 1996; 21(1):86.

Mansel R: Benign breast disease. *Practitioner* September 1992; 236(1518):830.

McKeon VA: Hormone replacement therapy: Evaluating the risks and benefits. *JOGNN* October 1994; 23(8):647.

Morrow M: Pre-cancerous breast lesions: Implications for breast cancer prevention trials. *Internat J Radiol Oncol Biol Physiol* 1992; 23(5):1071.

Nachtigall MJ et al: Endometriosis. In: *Danforth's Obstetrics and Gynecology,* 7th ed. Scott JR et al (editors). Philadelphia: Lippincott, 1994.

Nelson A: Patient selection key to IUD success. *Contemp OB/GYN* 1995; 40(10):49.

Norwood SL: Fibrocystic breast disease: An update and review. *JOGNN* 1990; 19(2):116.

Perkins C, Klaus P: *Criminal Victimization 1994. Bureau of Justice Statistics Bulletin, April 1996.* Washington, DC: US Department of Justice, NCJ-158022.

Schnorr TM: NIOSH epidemiologic studies of pregnancy outcomes. *Reprod Toxicology* 1988; 2:247.

Simpson JF: Benign conditions affecting the breast. *Contemp OB/GYN* 15, 1992; 37S:11.

Stubblefield PG: Pregnancy termination. In: *Obstetrics: Normal and Problem Pregnancies,* 2nd ed. Gabbe SG et al (editors). New York: Churchill-Livingstone, 1991.

Symposium: Ways of using LEEP for external lesions. *Contemp OB/GYN* 1992; 37(5):138.

Tan JS, File TM Jr: Treatment of bacteriuria in pregnancy. *Drugs* 1992; 44(6):972.

Taubes G: NCI reverses on expert panel, sides with another. *Science* April 4, 1997; 276:27.

Voelker R: Experts hope team approach will improve the quality of rape exams. *JAMA* April 3, 1996; 275(13):973.

Younger JB: Endometriosis. *Curr Op Obstet Gynecol* June 1993; 5(3):333.

Walker L: *The Battered Woman Syndrome.* New York: Springer, 1984.

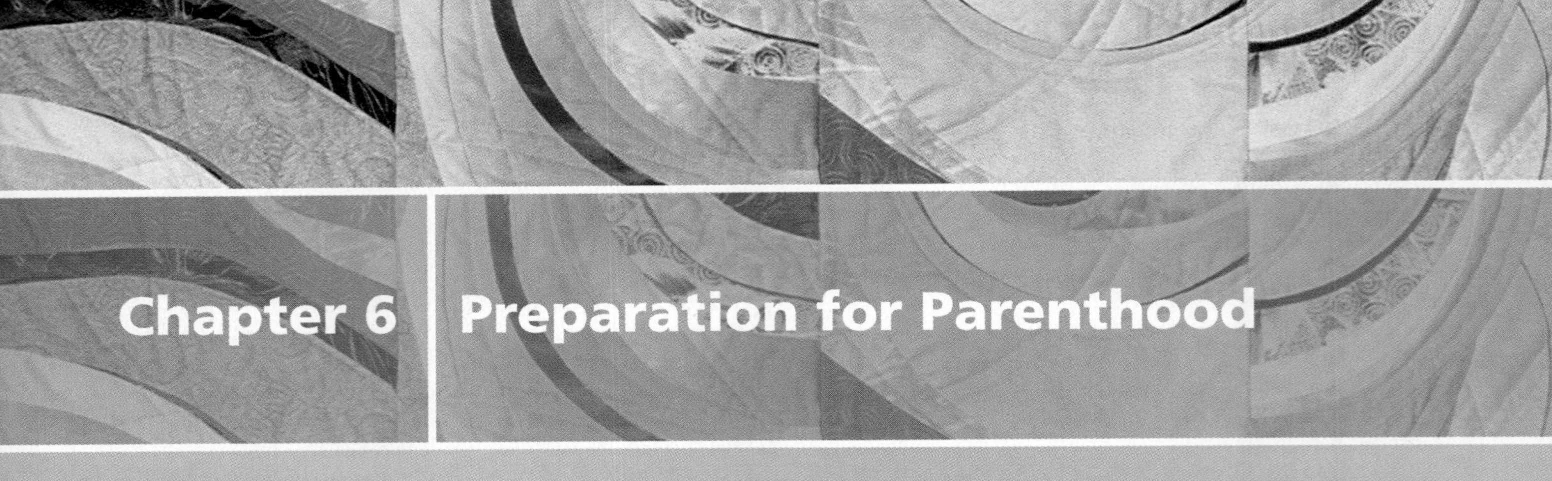

Chapter 6 Preparation for Parenthood

OBJECTIVES

- Apply the nursing process to help couples prepare for parenthood.
- Identify the various issues related to pregnancy, labor, and birth that require decision making by the parents.
- Discuss the basic goals of childbirth education.
- Describe the types of antepartal education programs available to expectant couples and their families.
- Describe the childbirth educator's role in decreasing pregnant women's anxiety.
- Compare methods of childbirth preparation.

KEY TERMS

Abdominal effleurage
Antepartal education
Birth plan
La Leche League
Psychoprophylactic method

As pregnancy progresses, expectant parents begin to look forward to their birth experience and the challenges of parenthood. In addition to gathering information about the pregnancy, there are many decisions and plans to be made. Where will the birth be? Who do they wish to be present? What steps can they take to prepare themselves for this wonderful occasion? How do they approach their new roles as parents?

Today's professional nurse has many opportunities to assist expectant parents in making the decisions that are part of pregnancy and birth. The nurse can help them select a health care provider, find prenatal classes that meet their needs, and make informed choices based on adequate information. Even more important, as the parents work through these decisions, the nurse is able to affirm their decision-making abilities and the taking on of the parenting role. For first-time parents, the decisions may seem numerous and complicated, and the nurse has a unique opportunity to help them establish a pattern of decision making that will serve them well in their years as parents (Figure 6–1).

Preconception Counseling

One of the first questions a couple should ask before conception is whether they wish to have children. This involves consideration of each person's goals, expectations of the relationship, and desire to be a parent. Often one individual wishes to have a child, while the other does not. In such situations, an open discussion is essential to reach a mutually acceptable decision. In some cases this may require counseling.

Couples who wish to have children face a decision about the timing of pregnancy. At what point in their lives do they believe it would be best to become parents? Pregnancy comes as a surprise even when the decision about timing is made, but at least the couple can have some control over it.

For couples who have religious beliefs that do not support contraception or who feel that fertility planning is unnatural, planning the timing of the pregnancy is unacceptable and irrelevant. These couples can still take steps to ensure that they are in the best possible physical and mental health when pregnancy occurs.

Preconception Health Measures

The couple is taught about known or suspected health risks. The nurse advises the woman to cease smoking if possible, or to limit her cigarette intake to less than half a pack per day (Tirosh et al 1997). Because of the hazards of second-hand smoke, it is helpful if her partner refrains from smoking around her. Since the effects of caffeine are less clearly understood, the woman is advised to avoid caffeine or limit her intake. Alcohol, social drugs, and street drugs pose a real threat to the fetus. A woman who uses any prescription or over-the-counter medications needs to discuss the implications of their use with her health care provider. It is best to avoid using any medication if possible. Because of the possible teratogenic effects of environmental hazards in the workplace, the nurse urges the couple contemplating pregnancy to determine whether they are exposed to any environmental hazards at work or in their community.

Physical Examination

It is advisable for both partners to have a physical examination to identify any health problems so that they can be corrected if possible. These might include medical conditions such as high blood pressure or obesity; problems that pose a threat to fertility, such as certain sexually transmitted diseases; or conditions that keep the individual from achieving optimal health, such as anemia or colitis. If the family history indicates previous genetic disorders, or if the couple is planning pregnancy when the woman is over age 35, the health care provider may suggest that the couple consider genetic counseling. In addition to the history and physical exam, the woman may have the following laboratory tests: urinalysis, complete blood count, Rh factor, Venereal Disease Research Laboratory (VDRL) test, Pap smear, gonorrhea culture, and rubella and hepatitis screens (Olds 1997). Prior to conception the woman is also advised to have a dental examination and any necessary dental work to avoid exposure to x-rays and the risk of infection.

Nutrition

Prior to conception it is advisable for the woman to be at an average weight for her body build and height. The woman is advised to follow a nutritious diet that contains ample quantities of all the essential nutrients. Some nutritionists advocate emphasizing the following nutrients: calcium, protein, iron, B complex vitamins, vitamin C, folic acid, and magnesium. Excessive vitamin intake can cause severe fetal problems and should be avoided.

Exercise

A woman is advised to establish a regular exercise plan beginning at least 3 months before she plans to attempt to become pregnant. The exercise should be one she enjoys and will continue. It needs to provide some aerobic

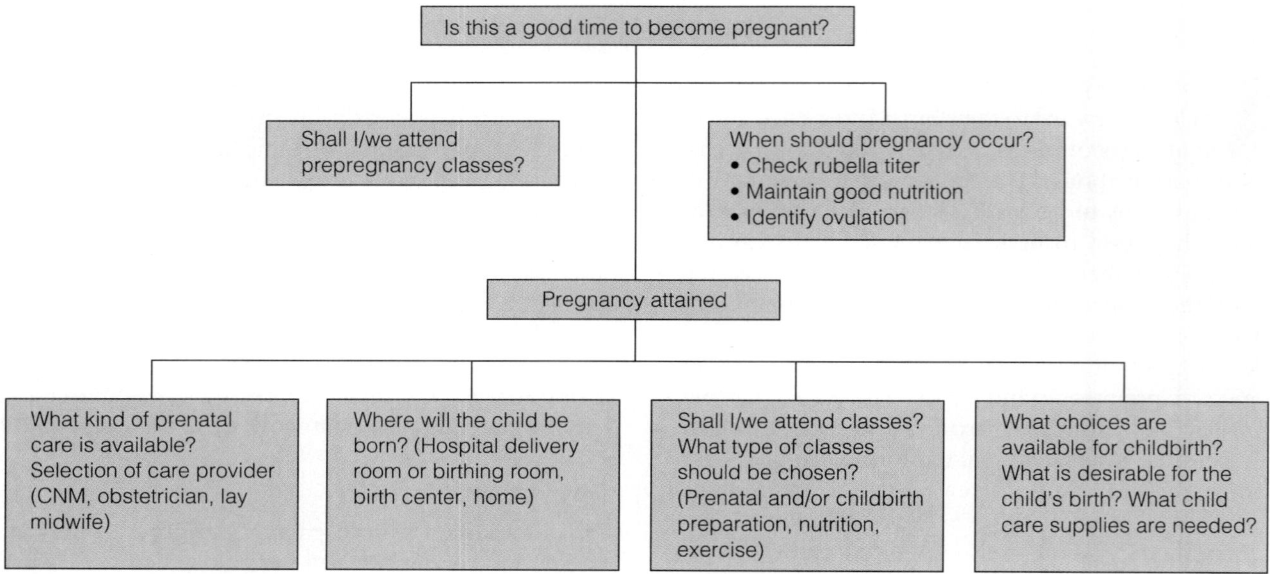

FIGURE 6–1 Pregnancy decision tree.

conditioning and some general toning. Exercise improves the woman's circulation and general health and tones her muscles. Once an exercise program is well established, the woman is generally encouraged to continue it during pregnancy.

Contraception

A woman who takes birth control pills is advised to stop the pill and have two or three normal menses before attempting to conceive. This allows the natural hormonal cycle to return and facilitates dating the subsequent pregnancy. A woman using an intrauterine device is advised to have it removed and wait 1 month before attempting to conceive. This allows the endometrium to be resterilized. During the waiting period, she can use barrier methods of contraception (condoms, diaphragm, cervical cap, or spermicides).

Conception

Most preconception recommendations focus on helping the couple attain their best possible health state so that they do not enter pregnancy with unnecessary risks. Conception is a personal and emotional experience, and even if a couple is prepared, they may feel some ambivalence. This is a normal response, but they may require reassurance that the ambivalence will pass. A couple may get so caught up in preparation and in their efforts to "do things right" that they lose sight of the pleasure they derive from each other and their lives together and cease to value the joy of spontaneity in their relationship. It is often helpful for the health care provider to remind an overly zealous couple that moderation is always appropriate and that there is value in "taking time to smell the roses."

Childbearing Decisions

Care Provider

One of the first decisions facing expectant parents is the selection of a health care provider. The nurse assists them by explaining the various options and outlining what can be expected from each. A thorough understanding of the differences of education preparation, skill level, and general philosophy and characteristics of practice of certified nurse-midwives, obstetricians, family practice physicians, and lay midwives is essential (Harvey et al 1997). The nurse can encourage expectant parents to investigate the care provider's credentials, basic and special education and training, fee schedule, and availability to new clients; this is often accomplished by telephoning the provider's office. The nurse can also help them develop a list of interview questions for their first visit to a care provider. These could include

- Who is in practice with you, or who covers for you when you are unavailable?
- How do your partners' philosophies compare to yours?
- How do you feel about my partner, other support person, or other children coming to the prenatal visits?
- What weight gain do you recommend and why?

Choice	I would like to have: Yes	I would like to have: No	Available: Yes	Available: No
Care provider:				
Certified nurse-midwife	____	____	____	____
Obstetrician	____	____	____	____
Lay midwife	____	____	____	____
Birth setting	____	____	____	____
Hospital:				
Birthing room	____	____	____	____
Delivery room	____	____	____	____
Birth center	____	____	____	____
Home	____	____	____	____
Partner present	____	____	____	____
During labor	____	____	____	____
During birth	____	____	____	____
During cesarean	____	____	____	____
During whole postpartum period	____	____	____	____
During labor:				
Ambulate as desired	____	____	____	____
Shower if desired	____	____	____	____
Wear own clothes	____	____	____	____
Use hot tub	____	____	____	____
Use own rocking chair	____	____	____	____
Have perineal prep	____	____	____	____
Have enema	____	____	____	____
Water birth	____	____	____	____
Electronic fetal monitor	____	____	____	____
Membranes:				
Rupture naturally	____	____	____	____
Amniotomy if needed	____	____	____	____
Labor stimulation if needed	____	____	____	____
Medication:				
Identify type desired	____	____	____	____
Fluids or ice as desired	____	____	____	____
Music during labor and birth	____	____	____	____
Position during birth:				
On side	____	____	____	____
Hands and knees	____	____	____	____
Kneeling	____	____	____	____
Squatting	____	____	____	____
Birthing chair	____	____	____	____
Birthing bed	____	____	____	____
Other:	____	____	____	____
Family present (sibs)	____	____	____	____
Filming of birth	____	____	____	____
Leboyer	____	____	____	____
Episiotomy	____	____	____	____
No sterile drapes	____	____	____	____
Partner to cut umbilical cord	____	____	____	____
Hold baby immediately after birth	____	____	____	____
Breastfeed immediately after birth	____	____	____	____
No separation after birth	____	____	____	____
Save the placenta	____	____	____	____
Newborn care:				
Eye treatment for the baby	____	____	____	____
Vitamin K injection	____	____	____	____
Breastfeeding	____	____	____	____
Formula feeding	____	____	____	____
Glucose water	____	____	____	____
Circumcision	____	____	____	____
Postpartum care:				
Rooming-in	____	____	____	____
Short stay	____	____	____	____
Sibling visitation	____	____	____	____
Infant care classes	____	____	____	____
Self-care classes	____	____	____	____
Other:	____	____	____	____

FIGURE 6–2 Birth plan for childbirth choices. The column on the left lists various choices that the couple may consider during their childbirth experience. Once the couple has considered each of the choices, they may mark the "yes" or "no" space in the middle columns. The right columns are used to note the availability of some of the choices. For instance, the couple may want to use a hot tub during labor, but the birthing settings in their community do not have hot tubs available. All choices need to be made in the context of what is available in the couple's community.

- What are your feelings about (fill in special desires for the birth event, such as different positions assumed during labor, episiotomy, induction of labor, other people present during the birth, breastfeeding immediately after the birth, no separation of infant and parents following birth, and so on)?
- If a cesarean is necessary could my partner be present?

Choosing a care provider is just one of the decisions pregnant women and couples will make. A method that has assisted many couples in making these choices is called a **birth plan.** In the birth plan, prospective parents identify aspects of the childbearing experience that are most important to them. (A sample birth plan is presented in Figure 6–2.) The birth plan helps identify available options and becomes a tool for communication among the expectant parents, the health care providers, and the health care professionals at the birth setting (Kitzinger 1992).

The plan also helps pregnant women and couples set priorities. Using the plan, they identify areas that they want to incorporate in their own birth experience. Then they can take the birth plan to a visit with their certified nurse-midwife or other care provider and use it in discussing and comparing their wishes with the philosophy and beliefs of the provider. They can also take the birth plan to the birth setting and use it as a basis for communicating their wishes during the childbirth experience.

Expectant parents also need to discuss the qualities they want in a care provider for the newborn, and they may want to visit several before the birth to assure a selection of someone who will meet their needs and those of their child.

There are many more choices that pregnant women and couples will make. Some of these are explored in Table 6–1. Although most birth experiences are very close to the desired experience, at times expectations cannot be met. This may be due to unavailability of some choices in the community or in the presence of unexpected problems during pregnancy or birth. It is important for nurses to help expectant parents keep sight of what is realistic for their situation.

Choosing the Birth Setting

The nurse can help expectant parents choose a birth setting by suggesting they tour facilities and talk with

TABLE 6–1 Benefits and Risks of Some Consumer Decisions During Pregnancy, Labor, and Birth

Issue	Benefits	Risks
Breastfeeding	No additional expense. Contains maternal antibodies. Decreases incidence of infant otitis media, vomiting, and diarrhea. Easier to digest than formula. Immediately after birth, promotes uterine contractions and decreases incidence of postpartum hemorrhage.	Transmission of pollutants to newborn. Irregular ovulation and menses can cause false sense of security and nonuse of contraceptives. Increased nutritional requirement in mother.
Perineal prep	May decrease risk of infection. Facilitates episiotomy repair.	Nicks can be portal for bacteria. Discomfort as hair grows back.
Enema	May facilitate labor. Increases space for infant in pelvis. May increase strength of contractions. May prevent contamination of sterile field.	Increases discomfort and anxiety.
Ambulation during labor	Comfort for laboring woman. May assist in labor progression by a. Stimulating contractions. b. Allowing gravity to help descent of fetus. c. Giving sense of independence and control.	Cord prolapse with rupture membranes unless engagement has occurred. Birth of infant in undesirable situations.
Electronic fetal monitoring	Helps evaluate fetal well-being. Helps identify fetal stress. Useful in diagnostic testing. Helps evaluate labor progress.	Supine postural hypotension. Intrauterine perforation (with internal uterine pressure device). Infection (with internal monitoring). Decreases personal interaction with mother because of attention paid to the machine. Mother is unable to ambulate or change her position freely.
Whirlpool (jet hydrotherapy)	Increased relaxation. Decreased anxiety. Stimulation of labor. Nonmedicated pain relief. Slight decrease in B/P. Increased diuresis.	May slow contractions if used before active labor is established. Possible risk of infection if membranes are ruptured. Slight increase in maternal temperature and heart rate and fetal heart rate during whirlpool and/or in first 30 min after being in tub (Rogers and Davis 1995).
Analgesia	Maternal relaxation facilitates labor.	All drugs reach the fetus in varying degrees and with varying effects.
Episiotomy	Decreases irregular tearing of perineum.	Increased pain after birth and for 3 months following birth. Infection. Increased frequency of 3rd- and 4th-degree lacerations (Woolley 1995).

Note: For additional information regarding these issues, refer to Chapter 17.

nurses there, and by talking with friends or acquaintances who are recent parents. Questions that may be asked of new parents include

- What kind of support did you receive during labor? Was it what you wanted?
- If the setting has both labor and delivery rooms and birthing rooms, was a birthing room available when you wanted it?
- Were you encouraged to be mobile during labor or to do what you wanted to do (walking, sitting in a rocking chair, remaining in bed, sitting in a hot tub, standing in a shower, and so on)?
- Was your labor partner or coach treated well?
- Was your birth plan respected? Did you share it with the facility before the birth? If something didn't work, why do you think there were problems?
- How were medications handled during labor? Were you comfortable with this?
- Were siblings welcomed in the birth setting? After the birth?
- Was the nursing staff helpful after the baby was born? Did you receive self-care and infant-care information? Was it in a usable form? Did you have a choice about what information you got? Did they let you decide what information you needed?

The nurse helps expectant parents understand the array of choices available to them. The nurse can encourage them to consider options early in the pregnancy to allow time for talking with other parents and touring facilities.

Sibling Preparation for Birth

Some expectant parents may wish to have their other children present at the birth. Children who will attend a birth can be prepared through books, audiovisual materials, models, discussion, and sibling classes. Nurses can assist parents with sibling preparation by helping them understand the stresses a child may experience. For example, the child may feel left out when there is a new child to love or disappointed if a brother is born when a sister is expected.

It is highly recommended that the child have his or her own support person or coach whose sole responsibility is tending to the needs of the child. The support person should be well known to the child; warm, sensitive, and flexible; knowledgeable about the birth process; and comfortable with sexuality and birth. This person must be prepared to interpret what is happening to the child and to intervene when necessary. For example, the support person should not be one who would hesitate to leave the birthing room (such as a maternal grandmother) but should be amenable to the child's desire to leave.

The child should be given the option of relating to the birth in whatever manner she or he chooses as long as it is not disruptive. Children should understand that it is their own choice to be there and that they may stay or leave the room as they choose. To help the child meet her or his goal, the nurse may wish to elicit from the child exactly what she or he expects from the experience. The child needs to feel free to ask questions and express feelings.

In general, the presence of siblings at birth engenders feelings of interest and the desire to nurture "our" baby, as opposed to jealousy and rivalry directed at "Mom's" baby. The mother does not disappear mysteriously into the hospital and return with a demanding outsider. Instead, the family attending the birth together finds a new opportunity for closeness and growth by sharing in the birth of a new member.

Classes for Family Members During Pregnancy

Antepartal education programs provide important opportunities to share information about pregnancy and childbirth and to enhance the parents' decision-making skills (Humenick 1996; Monto 1996). The content of each class is generally directed by the overall goals of the program. For example, in classes that aim to provide preconceptual information, preparations for becoming pregnant would be the major topics. Other classes may be directed toward childbirth choices available today, preparation of the mother for pregnancy and birth, preparation for cesarean birth, and preparation of specific people such as grandparents or siblings for the birth. The nurse who knows the types of prenatal programs available in the community can direct expectant parents to programs that meet their special needs and learning goals (Walden et al 1996).

Class Content

Childbirth preparation classes usually contain information about changes in the woman and the developing baby. See Key Facts to Remember: Possible Content of Preparation for Childbirth Classes.

From the expectant parents' point of view, class content is best presented in chronology with the pregnancy.

KEY FACTS TO REMEMBER

Possible Content of Preparation for Childbirth Classes

Early Classes (first trimester)

- Early gestational changes
- Self-care during pregnancy
- Fetal development, environmental dangers for the fetus
- Sexuality in pregnancy
- Birth settings and types of care providers
- Nutrition, rest, and exercise suggestions
- Relief measures for common discomforts of pregnancy
- Psychologic changes in pregnancy
- Information for getting pregnancy off to a good start

Later classes (second and third trimesters)

- Preparation for birth process
- Postpartum self-care
- Birth choices (episiotomy, medications, fetal monitoring, perineal prep, enema, etc.)
- Relaxation techniques
- Breathing techniques
- Infant stimulation
- Newborn safety issues, such as car seats

Adolescent preparation classes

- How to be a good parent
- Newborn care
- Health dangers for the baby
- Healthy diet during pregnancy
- How to recognize when baby is ill
- Baby care: physical and emotional

Breastfeeding programs

- Advantages and disadvantages
- Techniques of breastfeeding
- Methods of breast preparation
- Involvement of fathers in feeding process

While both parents expect to learn breathing and relaxation techniques and infant care, fathers usually expect facts and mothers expect coping strategies. It is important that the classes begin by finding out what each parent wants to learn and birth alternatives (Humenick 1996). At times prenatal classes are divided into early and late classes.

Early Classes: First Trimester

Early prenatal classes should include prepregnant women and couples as well as those in early pregnancy. The classes cover early gestational changes; self-care during pregnancy; fetal development and environmental dangers for the fetus; sexuality in pregnancy; birth settings and types of care providers; nutrition, rest, and exercise suggestions; common discomforts of pregnancy and relief measures; psychologic changes in pregnancy for the woman and man; and getting the pregnancy off to a good start by following a healthful lifestyle, learning methods of coping with stress, and avoiding alcohol and smoking. Early classes should provide information about factors that place the woman at risk for preterm labor and about how to recognize symptoms of preterm labor. Early classes should also present the advantages and disadvantages of breast- and bottle-feeding. The majority of women (50–80%) have made their infant feeding decision before the sixth month of pregnancy.

Later Classes: Second and Third Trimesters

The later classes focus on preparation for the birth, infant care and feeding, postpartum self-care, birth choices (episiotomy, medications, fetal monitoring, perineal prep, enema, and so forth), and newborn safety issues. Since many parents purchase a car seat before birth, later classes should also include information about the importance of car seats, how they work, and how to select an approved car seat (Baer 1992).

Broussard and Rich (1990) suggest that infant stimulation concepts be incorporated into childbirth preparation classes. This will aid in the development of parenting skills and enhance prenatal and neonatal bonding. Methods that can be used include tactile, vestibular, auditory, and visual stimulation. Information regarding tactile stimulation can be presented while discussing maternal anatomy and physiology. As the uterine wall thins during the pregnancy, the mother and father are better able to feel the baby, and the fetus can sense the parents' stroking and patting through the abdominal wall. **Abdominal effleurage** (a light stroking movement made over the abdominal wall with the fingertips) can also be used to provide tactile stimulation to the fetus.

Vestibular stimulation through movement of the fetus is provided while the expectant woman does the pelvic-tilt exercise. Rocking in a rocking chair is also a comfortable way to provide relaxation for the expectant woman and vestibular stimulation for the fetus. Auditory stimulation can be provided by playing music. Classical music (such as Vivaldi, Mozart, Beethoven, and Bach) is found to be pleasing to the fetus. In the prenatal period, actual visual stimulation for the fetus is not possible. However, the parents can be encouraged to visualize the fetus "as lying calmly inside, all flexed, sucking its thumb, swallowing amniotic fluid, and opening its eyes to look toward the sunlight filtering through the abdominal wall" (Broussard and Rich 1990, p 384).

Adolescent Parenting Classes

Adolescents have special learning needs during pregnancy. In a study by Roye and Balk (1996) teens identified informational needs during pregnancy. Areas of concern were how to be a good parent, how to care for the new baby, health dangers to the baby, and healthy foods to eat during pregnancy. Teens also identified information needs about how to recognize when the baby is sick, take care of the baby, protect the baby from accidents, and make the baby feel happy and loved. They were also eager to hear more about the birth process (especially pain during the birth process), the personal health of the mother, the discomforts of pregnancy, changes in life with pregnancy, and sexuality.

Breastfeeding Programs

Programs offering information on breastfeeding are increasing. For many years, a primary source of information has been **La Leche League.** Information can also be obtained from lactation consultants, birthing centers, hospitals, and health clinics. Content includes advantages and disadvantages, techniques of breastfeeding, and methods of breast preparation. The father's support and encouragement of the mother is vital so it is important to include him in the educational programs decision making. Some fathers may feel negative and resentful about breastfeeding and need opportunities in the prenatal period for discussion and sharing of information.

Sibling Preparation: Adjustment to a Newborn

The birth of a new sibling is a significant event in a child's life. Positive adjustment can be enhanced by attendance at formal sibling preparation classes (see Figure 6–3). The classes are usually focused on reducing anxiety in the child, providing opportunities for the child to express feelings and concerns, and encouraging realistic expectations of the newborn. Parents learn strategies to help prepare the child for the birth and to assist the child in coping with a newcomer (Fortier et al 1991).

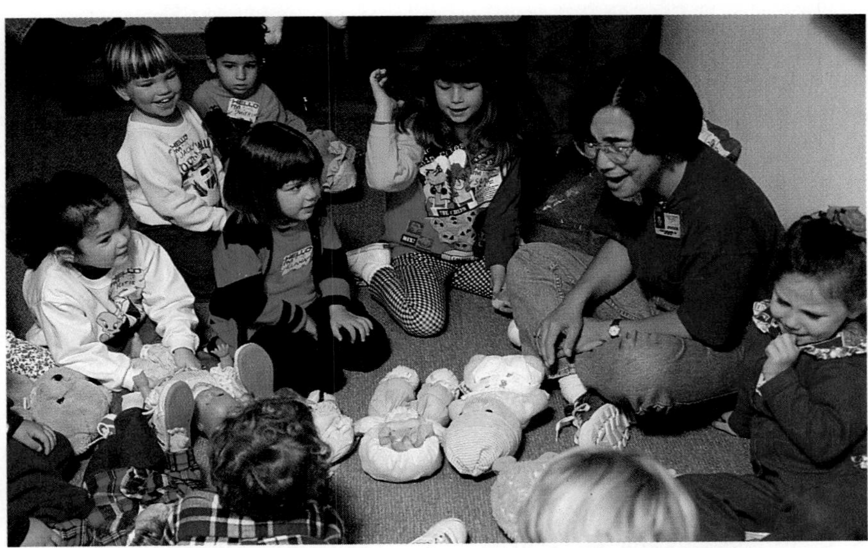

FIGURE 6–3 It is especially important that siblings be well prepared when they are going to be present for the birth. However, all siblings can benefit from information about birth and the new baby ahead of time.

Fortier and associates (1991) found that a sibling preparation class made a significant difference in the adjustment of the child to the birth. The child demonstrated fewer behaviors associated with sibling rivalry (crying, whining, clinging, and eating problems). The mothers also felt that they were able to cope more effectively.

The classes in the study were entitled "Siblings Are Special." Parents and their children attended the class together. Many activities were devised to help each child feel special: Children were greeted with badges saying "I'm a big sister" or "I'm a big brother" and "I'm special"; an instant photo was taken of the child so that the picture could be placed in the newborn's hospital crib; and the child decorated a bib for the new baby. Time was allotted at the end of the class for talking with parents about coping skills and providing hints about dealing with sibling jealousy.

Sibling preparation can be addressed through a formal class such as the one just described, or in a less formal way by preparing a booklet for parents that addresses issues affecting both parents and children.

Classes for Grandparents

Grandparents are an important source of support and information for prospective and new parents. They are now being included in the birthing process more frequently. Prenatal programs for grandparents can be an important source of information about current beliefs and practices in childbearing (Roye and Balk 1997). The most useful content may include changes in birthing and parenting practices and helpful tips for being a supportive grandparent. Grandparents who will be integral members of the labor and birth team need information about being coaches.

Education of the Family Having Cesarean Birth

Preparation for Cesarean Birth

Cesarean birth is an alternative method of birth. Since one out of every four or five births is a cesarean, preparation for this possibility should be an integral part of every childbirth education curriculum. The instructor should treat cesarean birth as a normal event and present factual information that will allow expectant parents to make choices and be full participants in their birth experience. The instructor can emphasize the similarities between cesarean and vaginal births to minimize undertones of "normal" versus "abnormal" birth. This will diminish the feelings of anger, loss, and grief that often accompany cesarean births.

Cesarean birth classes should cover what the parents can expect to happen during a cesarean birth, what they will feel, and what they can do. All pregnant women and couples should be encouraged to discuss with their certified nurse-midwife/physician what the approach would be in the event of a cesarean. They can also discuss their needs and preferences regarding

- Participating in the choice of anesthetic
- Father (or significant other) being present during the birth
- Planning initial contact with their newborn

TABLE 6–2 Summary of Selected Childbirth Preparation Methods

Method	Characteristics	Breathing Technique
Lamaze	See narrative discussion.	
Bradley	Frequently referred to as partner- or husband-coached natural childbirth. Uses various exercises and slow controlled abdominal breathing to accomplish relaxation.	Primarily abdominal.
Kitzinger	Uses sensory memory to help the woman understand and work with her body in preparation for birth. Incorporates the Stanislavsky method of acting as a way to teach relaxation.	Uses chest breathing in conjunction with abdominal relaxation.

Preparation for Repeat Cesarean Birth

When expectant parents are anticipating a repeat cesarean birth, they have time to plan and prepare. Many hospitals or local groups (such as C-Sec, Inc.) provide preparation classes for cesarean birth. Parents who have had previous negative experiences need an opportunity to describe what contributed to their feelings. They should be encouraged to identify what they would like to change and to list interventions that would make the experience more positive. Those who have had positive experiences need reassurance that their needs and desires will be met in the same manner. In addition, all parents are encouraged to air any fears or anxieties.

A specific concern of the woman facing a repeat cesarean is anticipation of pain. She needs reassurance that subsequent cesareans are often less painful than the first. If her first cesarean was preceded by a long or strenuous labor, she will not experience the same fatigue. Giving this information will help her cope more effectively with all stressful stimuli, including pain. The nurse can remind the client that she has already had experience with how to prevent, cope with, and alleviate painful stimuli.

Preparation for Parents Desiring Vaginal Birth after Cesarean Birth (VBAC)

Parents who have had a cesarean birth and are now anticipating a vaginal birth have unique needs. Because they may have unresolved questions and concerns about the last birth, it is helpful to begin the series of classes with an informational session. During this session, they can ask questions, share experiences, and begin to form bonds with each other. The nurse can supply information regarding the criteria necessary to attempt a trial of labor and identify decisions regarding the birth experience. Some childbirth educators find it is helpful to have the parents prepare two birth plans: one for vaginal birth and one for cesarean birth. The preparation of the birth plans seems to help parents take more control of the birth experience and tends to increase the positive aspects of the experience.

After an informational session, the classes may be divided according to the needs of the expectant parents. Those with recent coached childbirth experiences may need only refresher classes, while others may need complete training. Some parents may choose to attend regular classes after participating in the informational session.

Methods of Childbirth Preparation

Overview of Selected Methods

Various methods of childbirth preparation are taught in North America. Some antepartal classes are specifically oriented to preparation for labor and birth, have a name associated with a theory of pain reduction in childbirth, and teach specific exercises to reduce pain. The most common methods of this type are the Lamaze (psychoprophylactic), Kitzinger (sensory-memory), and Bradley (partner-coached childbirth). Each of these methods is designed to provide the woman or couple with self-help measures so that the pregnancy and birth are healthy and happy events. See Table 6–2 for differentiating characteristics of each method.

The programs in prepared childbirth have some similarities. All have an educational component to help eliminate fear. The classes vary in coverage of subjects related to the maternity cycle, but all teach relaxation techniques and all prepare the participants for what to expect during labor and birth. Except for hypnosis, these methods also feature exercises to condition muscles and breathing patterns used in labor. The greatest differences among the methods lie in the theories of why they work and in the relaxation techniques and breathing patterns they teach (see Table 6–2).

There are several advantages to these methods of childbirth preparation. Most important is that the baby may be healthier because of the reduced need for analgesics and anesthetics. Another is the satisfaction of the parents, for whom childbirth becomes a shared and profound emotional experience. In addition, each method has been shown to shorten labor. All nurses must know how these methods differ, so that they can support each birth experience effectively.

Psychoprophylactic (Lamaze) Method

The **psychoprophylactic method** is the childbirth preparation method generally called "Lamaze classes." *Psychoprophylactic* means "mind prevention." Dr. Fernand Lamaze, a French obstetrician, was the first person to introduce this method of childbirth preparation to the Western world. Proponents of the method formed a nonprofit group called the American Society for Psychoprophylaxis in Obstetrics (ASPO). This organization helped establish many programs throughout the country, and Lamaze has become one of the most popular methods of childbirth education.

The major components of Lamaze classes are education and training. In Lamaze classes, the woman learns about the developing fetus and the changes that occur in the pregnant woman. The woman also learns body-conditioning exercises that can be used during the pregnancy and specific relaxation and breathing techniques for labor (Monto 1996).

Body-Conditioning Exercises

Some body-conditioning exercises, such as the pelvic tilt, pelvic rock, and Kegel exercises, are taught in childbirth preparation classes. Other exercises strengthen the abdominal muscles for the expulsive phase of labor. (See Chapter 8 for a description of recommended exercises.)

Relaxation Exercises

Relaxation during labor allows the woman to conserve energy and the uterine muscles to work more efficiently. Without practice it is very difficult to relax the whole body in the midst of intense uterine contractions. However, many people are familiar with progressive relaxation exercises such as those taught to induce sleep. One example follows:

> Lie down on your back or side. (The left side position is best for pregnant women.)
>
> Tighten your muscles in both feet. Hold the tightness for a few seconds and then relax the muscles completely, letting all the tension drain out.
>
> Tighten your lower legs, hold for a few seconds, and then relax the muscles, letting all the tension drain out.
>
> Continue tensing and relaxing parts of your body, moving up the body as you do so.

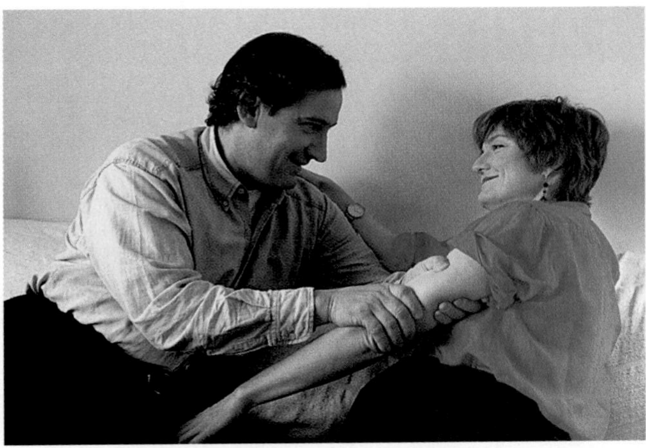

FIGURE 6–4 To help the woman practice relaxing in the presence of discomfort, the coach can induce discomfort by "twisting" the skin of her upper arm or by pinching her inner thigh.

Another type of relaxation exercise, called touch relaxation, requires cooperation between the woman and her coach. It is particularly useful in working together during labor (see Table 6–3 on page 148).

An additional exercise specific to Lamaze is disassociation relaxation. This pattern of active relaxation is in contrast to the Read method of passive relaxation (where the woman is taught progressive contraction and relaxation of muscle groups moving from head to toe to promote sleep). The woman is taught to become familiar with the sensation of contracting and relaxing the voluntary muscle groups throughout her body. She then learns to contract a specific muscle group and relax the rest of her body. This process of isolating the action of one group of voluntary muscles from the rest of the body is called neuromuscular disassociation and is basic to the psychoprophylaxis method of prepared childbirth. The exercise conditions the woman to relax uninvolved muscles while the uterus contracts, creating an active relaxation pattern (see Table 6–4 on page 149).

In order to practice the relaxation exercises in a more realistic setting the coach may use two methods to induce some discomfort:

1. The coach places both hands in a grasping position firmly on the upper arm and turns them in opposite directions to create a burning sensation. This is begun slowly and gently and increased at the direction of the woman as she continues to practice relaxation breathing techniques (Figure 6–4).
2. The coach places a hand on the woman's inner thigh just above the knee and pinches the area.

While practicing, the coach checks the woman's neck, shoulders, arms, and legs for relaxation. As tense areas are found, the coach encourages the woman to relax those particular body parts. The woman learns to

TABLE 6–3 Touch Relaxation

Practice is vital to the following exercises, which require that the pregnant woman and her partner work very closely together. Tell the woman, "With practice you will train yourself to release not only in response to your partner's touch but also to the touch of doctors or nurses as they examine you. This technique will also help you to be more comfortable with your own body."

Goals:

(For her) To recognize and release tension in response to partner's touch; to be able to do this automatically and spontaneously.
(For partner) To recognize her tension in its very early stages; to learn how to touch in a firm yet sensitive way; to concentrate on her problem areas.

Tools:

(For her) Conscious relaxation, comfortable positioning, and trust.
(For partner) Sensitivity, patience, and warm hands!

Procedure:

She tenses.
Partner touches.
She immediately releases towards touch.
Partner strokes, "drawing" tension from her.
She releases all residual tension.

Sequence:

- Contract muscles of the scalp and raise eyebrows. Partner cups hands on either side of the scalp. Immediately release tension in response to the pressure of your partner's touch. Then release any residual tension as your partner strokes your head.
- Frown, wrinkle nose, and squeeze eyes shut. Partner rests hands on brow and then strokes down over temples. Release.
- Grit teeth and clench jaw. Partner rests hands on either side of jaw. Release.
- Press shoulder blades back. Partner rests hands on front of shoulders. Release.
- Pull abdominal wall towards spine. Partner rests hands on sides of abdomen and then strokes down over her hips. Partner might also stroke the lower curve of abdomen across pubic symphysis. Release.
- Press thighs together. Partner touches outside of each leg. Relax and let legs move apart. Partner strokes firmly down outside of leg with light strokes up on inner thigh.
- Press legs outward, still flexed but forcing thighs apart. Partner rests hands with fingers pointing downward, on inner thighs. Firmly strokes down to knees, then lightly strokes upward on outside of leg. Release.
- Tense arm muscles. Partner places hands on the upper arm and shoulder area, one on the inside and one on the outside of the arm. Strokes down to the elbow and then down forearm to wrist, and over fingertips. Release. Repeat with other arm.
- Tighten leg muscles, being careful not to cramp them. Partner touches foot around the instep, firmly without tickling. Release whole leg. Partner moves hands up, placing one on either side of the thigh, stroking down to the knee then down the calf to the foot and over the toes. Release. Repat with other leg.
- Change to the Sims lateral or side-lying position. Raise chin, contracting the muscles at the back of the neck. Partner rests hand on nape of neck and massages. Release.
- Curl into fetal position, crawing shoulders forward. Partner applies pressure to back of shoulders. Strokes upper back. Release.
- Hollow the small of back by arching back. Partner rests hands against either side of spine and follows with stroking down over buttocks. Release.
- Press buttocks together. Partner rests one hand on each buttock. After initial release, strokes down toward thighs.

Source: O'Halloran, S. (1984). *Pregnant and Prepared: A Guide to Preparing for Childbirth.* Wayne, NJ: Avery Publishing Group, p. 45.

respond to her own perceptions of tense muscles and also to the suggestion from others. The suggestion can come verbally or from touch. The exercises are usually practiced each day so that they become comfortable and easy to do.

A specific type of cutaneous stimulation used prior to the transitional phase of labor is known as abdominal effleurage (Figure 6–5). This light abdominal stroking is used in the Lamaze method of childbirth preparation. It effectively relieves mild to moderate pain, but not intense pain. Deep pressure over the sacrum is more effective for relieving back pain. In addition to the measures just described, the nurse can promote relaxation by encouraging and supporting the client's controlled breathing.

Breathing Techniques

Breathing techniques are a key element of most childbirth preparation programs. They help keep the mother and her unborn baby adequately oxygenated and help the mother relax and focus her attention appropriately. Breathing techniques are best taught during the final trimester of pregnancy when the expectant mother's attention is focused on the birth experience. The nurse then supports the mother's use of breathing techniques during labor. See Key Facts to Remember: Goals of Breathing Techniques. Breathing techniques are described in detail in Chapter 17.

KEY FACTS TO REMEMBER

Goals of Breathing Techniques

- Provide adequate oxygenation of mother and baby, open maternal airways, and avoid inefficient use of muscles.
- Increase physical and mental relaxation.
- Decrease pain and anxiety.
- Provide a means of focusing attention.
- Control inadequate ventilation patterns that are related to pain and stress.

TABLE 6–4 Disassociation Relaxation

The uterus, an involuntary muscle over which you have no control, will work most efficiently and effectively when the rest of your body is free from tension. The following exercises will give you further practice in conscious release. They will also give you and your partner a way to evaluate your progress.

Goals:

During pregnancy, disassociation relaxation will teach you consciously to release certain sets of muscles, while contracting others, and to disassociate yourself from voluntary tension. During labor, this technique will release all voluntary muscles of your body at will, while the uterus contracts. This conserves energy and fights fatigue.

Tools:

Body awareness, touch release, and concentration.

Procedure:

Partner gives consistent suggestions.

Partner checks relaxation using touching.

Example:

Partner: "Contraction begins."

Mother: Relaxation breath (following with a comfortable rate of breathing).

Partner: [See suggested patterns below.]

Mother: Relaxation breath.

Sequence:

"Contract right arm. Hold. Release."

"Contract left arm. Hold. Release."

"Contract right leg. Hold. Release."

"Contract left leg. Hold. Release."

"Contract both arms. Hold. Release."

"Contract both legs. Hold. Release."

"Contract right side (arm and leg). Hold. Release."

"Contract left side (arm and leg). Hold. Release."

"Contract right arm and left leg. Hold. Release."

"Contract left arm and right leg. Hold. Release."

For Variety:

- Contract right arm and left leg.
- Release left leg. Contract right leg. Release right arm. Contract left arm.
- Release

Source: O'Halloran S. (1984). *Pregnant and Prepared: A Guide to Preparing for Childbirth.* Wayne, NJ: Avery Publishing Group, pp. 45–46.

Client Education

Nurses involved in childbirth education need to include the concept of individuality when providing information to expectant parents about the process of childbirth and their own pattern of coping. Controversy exists over the use of ritualistic breathing techniques in childbirth. The wave of the future in childbirth education is to encourage women to incorporate their natural responses into coping with the pain of labor and birth. Self-care activities that may be used include

Vocalization or "sounding" to relieve tension in pregnancy and labor.

Massage (light touch) to facilitate relaxation.

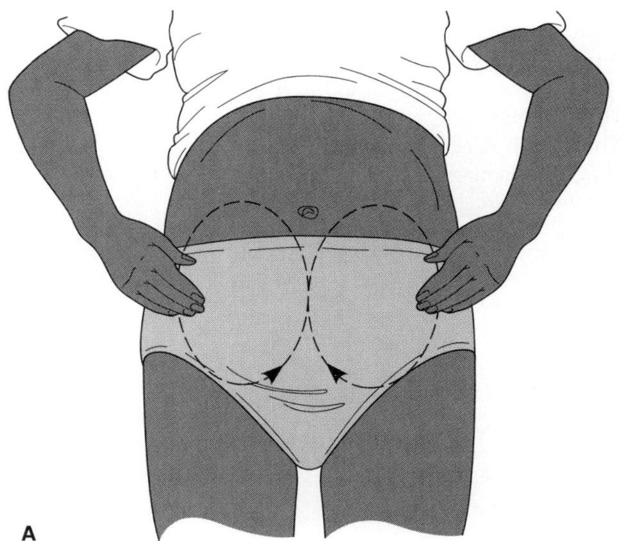

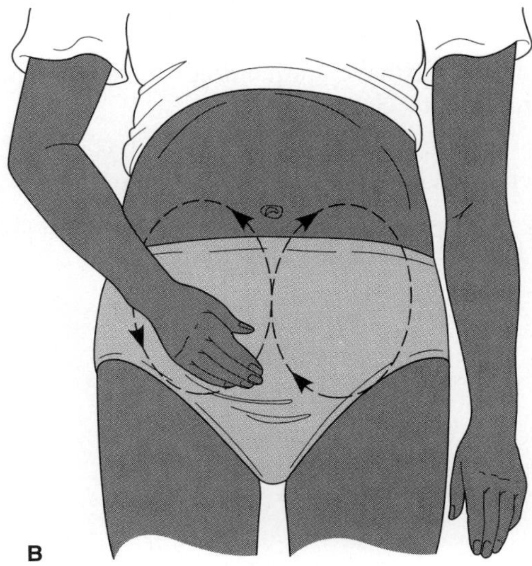

FIGURE 6–5 Effleurage is light stroking of the abdomen with the fingertips. ***A*** Starting at the symphysis, the woman lightly moves her fingertips up and around in a circular pattern. ***B*** An alternative approach involves using one hand in a figure eight pattern. This light stroking can also be done by the support person.

Use of warm water for showers or bathing during labor.

Visualization (imagery).

Relaxing music and subdued lighting.

Nurses should encourage expectant women and couples to make the birth a personal experience. The woman might plan, for example, to bring items from home to enhance relaxation and comfort, such as warm socks, slippers, bath powder, lotion, or a favorite blanket. She may wish to bring photographs of parents or friends who cannot be with them in person to share the birth experience. Many expectant parents enjoy listening to tapes of favorite music or watching home videotapes or favorite films. Such personalization of the birth experience may give expectant parents feelings of increased serenity and empowerment.

CHAPTER HIGHLIGHTS

- Prenatal education programs vary in their goals, content, leadership techniques, and method of teaching.
- Prenatal classes may be offered early and/or late in the pregnancy. The class content varies depending on the type of class and the individual offering it. Expectant parents tend to want information in chronological sequence with the pregnancy. Adolescents have special learning needs.
- Breastfeeding programs are offered in the prenatal period.
- Siblings are included in the whole birthing process, and classes for them are available from many sources.
- Grandparents have unique needs for information in grandparents' classes.
- Information regarding cesarean birth is included in antepartal classes to help prepare parents.
- The major types of childbirth preparation methods are Lamaze, Kitzinger, and Bradley.
- Lamaze is a type of psychoprophylactic method. The classes include information on toning exercises, relaxation exercises and techniques, and breathing methods for labor.

REFERENCES

Baer D: Buckle Up! *Lamaze Parent's Magazine,* 1992, p 95.

Broussard AB, Rich SK: Incorporating infant stimulation concepts into prenatal classes. *JOGNN* September/October 1990; 19(5): 381.

Fortier JC et al: Adjustment to a newborn: Sibling preparation makes a difference. *JOGNN* January/February 1991; 20(1): 73.

Harvey S et al: A randomized, controlled trial of nurse-midwifery care. *Birth* September 1996; 23:128.

Kitzinger S: Sheila Kitzinger's letter from England: Birth plans. *Birth* 1992; 19(1): 36.

Monto M: Lamaze and Bradley childbirth classes: Contrasting perspectives toward the medical model of birth. *Birth* December 1996; 23:193.

Mynaugh PA: A randomized study of two methods of teaching perineal massage: Effects of practice rates, episiotomy rates, and lacerations. *Birth* September 1991; 18(3): 153.

Nichols FH, Humenick SS: *Childbirth Education: Practice, Research and Theory.* Philadelphia: Saunders, 1988.

Olds SB: Care of the childbearing family. In: *Saunders Manual of Nursing Care.* Luckman J (editor). Philadelphia: Saunders, 1997.

Rogers J, Davis BA: How risky are hot tubs and saunas for pregnant women? *MCN* May/June 1995; 20:137.

Roye C, Balk SJ: Evaluation of an intergenerational program for pregnant and parenting adolescents. *MCN* January/March 1996; 21:32.

Tirosh E, Libon D, Bader D: The effect of maternal smoking during pregnancy on sleep respiratory and arousal patterns in neonates. *J Perinatol* November/December 1996; 16:435.

Walden C et al: Perinatal effects of a pregnancy wellness program in the workplace. *MCN* November/December 1996; 21:288.

Woolley RJ: Benefits and risks of episiotomy: A review of the English-language literature since 1980. Part II. *Obstet Gynecol Surv* 1995; 50(11):821.

Part Two | Pregnancy

Choices are important. They determine how you experience giving birth and how your baby enters the world. They must be made in the present and lived with in the future.

—Pregnant Feelings

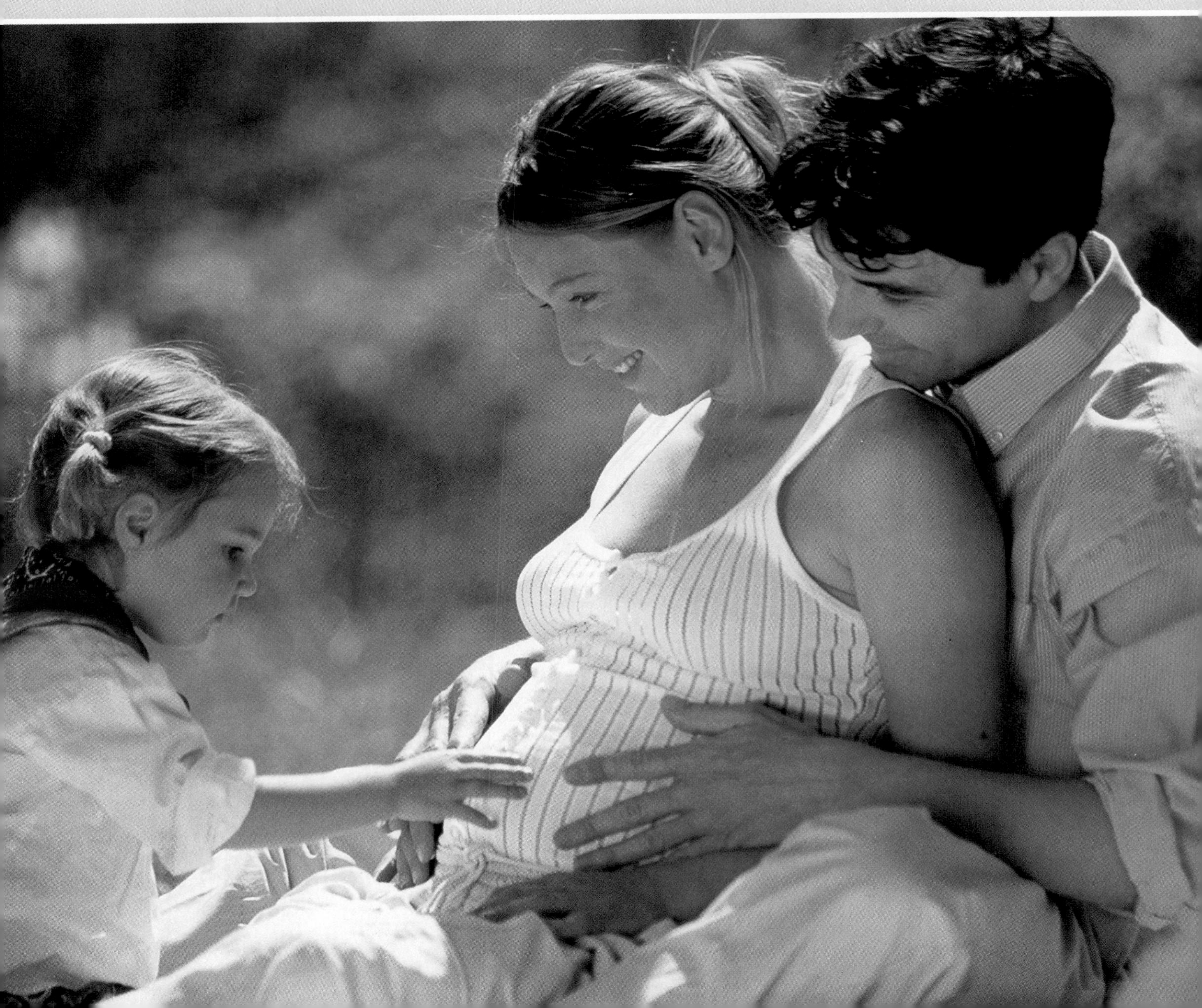

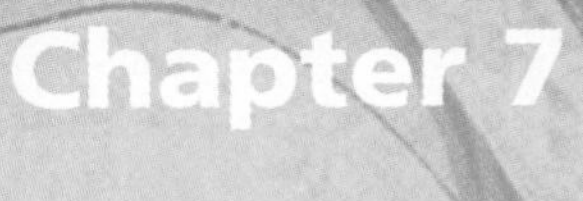

Chapter 7 Physical and Psychologic Changes of Pregnancy

OBJECTIVES

- Identify the anatomic and physiologic changes that occur during pregnancy.
- Relate the physiologic and anatomic changes that occur in the body systems during pregnancy to the signs and symptoms that develop in the woman.
- Compare subjective (presumptive), objective (probable), and diagnostic (positive) changes of pregnancy.
- Contrast the various types of pregnancy tests.
- Discuss the emotional and psychologic changes that commonly occur in a woman, her partner, and her family during pregnancy.
- Summarize cultural factors that may influence a family's response to pregnancy.

KEY TERMS

Braxton Hicks contractions
Chadwick's sign
Chloasma
Couvade
Diastasis recti
Ethnocentrism
Goodell's sign
Hegar's sign
Last menstrual period (LMP)
Linea nigra
McDonald's sign
Striae
Vena caval syndrome

No matter how much we learn about pregnancy and the changes that occur in the woman and the developing fetus, we never cease to be amazed! First, it is nothing short of a miracle that the union of two microscopic entities—an ovum and a sperm—can produce a living being. Second, the woman's body must undergo extraordinary physical changes to maintain a pregnancy.

Pregnancy is divided into three trimesters, each a 3-month period. Each trimester brings predictable changes for both the mother and fetus. This chapter describes the physical and psychologic changes caused by pregnancy. It also presents the various cultural factors that can affect a pregnant woman's well-being. Subsequent chapters build on this information in describing effective approaches to planning and providing care.

Anatomy and Physiology of Pregnancy

Reproductive System

Uterus

The changes in the uterus during pregnancy are phenomenal. Before pregnancy, the uterus is a small, semisolid, pear-shaped organ measuring approximately 7.5 by 5 by 2.5 cm and weighing about 60 g (2 oz). At the end of pregnancy it measures about 28 by 24 by 21 cm and weighs approximately 1000 g; its capacity has also increased from about 10 mL to 5 L or more.

The enlargement of the uterus is primarily due to the enlargement (hypertrophy) of the preexisting myometrial cells as a result of the stimulating influence of estrogen and the distention caused by the growing fetus. Only a limited increase in cell number (hyperplasia) occurs. The fibrous tissue between the muscle bands increases markedly, which adds to the strength and elasticity of the muscle wall. The enlarging uterus, developing placenta, and growing fetus require additional blood flow to the uterus. By the end of pregnancy, one-sixth of the total maternal blood volume is contained within the vascular system of the uterus.

Braxton Hicks contractions, which are irregular, generally painless contractions of the uterus, occur intermittently throughout pregnancy. They may be felt through the abdominal wall beginning about the fourth month of pregnancy. In later pregnancy, these contractions become uncomfortable and may be confused with true labor contractions.

Cervix

Estrogen stimulates the glandular tissue of the cervix, which increases in cell number and becomes hyperactive. The endocervical glands secrete a thick, sticky mucus that accumulates and forms a plug, which seals the endocervical canal and prevents the ascent of organisms into the uterus. This mucous plug is expelled when cervical dilatation begins. The hyperactivity of the glandular tissue also increases the normal physiologic mucorrhea, at times resulting in profuse discharge. Increased cervical vascularity also causes both the softening of the cervix (Goodell's sign) and its bluish discoloration (Chadwick's sign).

Ovaries

The ovaries stop producing ova during pregnancy, but the corpus luteum continues to produce hormones until about weeks 10 to 12. The progesterone it secretes maintains the endometrium until the placenta assumes the task. The corpus luteum begins to regress and is almost completely obliterated by the middle of pregnancy.

Vagina

Estrogen causes a thickening of the vaginal mucosa, a loosening of the connective tissue, and an increase in vaginal secretions. These secretions are thick, white, and acidic (pH 3.5–6.0). The acid pH helps prevent bacterial infection but favors the growth of yeast organisms. Thus the pregnant woman is more susceptible to monilial infection than usual.

The supportive connective tissue of the vagina loosens throughout pregnancy. By the end of pregnancy, the vagina and perineal body are sufficiently relaxed to permit passage of the infant. Because blood flow to the vagina is increased, the vagina may show the same blue-purple color (Chadwick's sign) as the cervix.

Breasts

Estrogen and progesterone cause many changes in the mammary glands. The breasts enlarge and become more nodular as the glands increase in size and number in preparation for lactation. Superficial veins become more prominent, the nipples become more erectile, and the areolas darken. Montgomery's follicles (sebaceous glands) enlarge, and striae (stretch marks) may develop.

Colostrum, an antibody-rich yellow secretion, may leak or be expressed from the breasts during the last trimester. Colostrum gradually converts to mature milk during the first few days after childbirth.

Respiratory System

Many respiratory changes occur to meet the increased oxygen requirements of a pregnant woman. Progesterone decreases airway resistance, permitting a 15 to 20 percent increase in oxygen consumption and a 30 to 40 percent increase in the volume of air breathed each minute. These changes permit increases in oxygen consumption, carbon dioxide production, and respiratory functional reserve.

As the uterus enlarges, it presses upward and elevates the diaphragm. The substernal angle increases so that the rib cage flares. The anteroposterior diameter increases, and the chest circumference expands by as much as 6 cm; for this reason, there is no significant loss of intrathoracic volume. Breathing changes from abdominal to thoracic as pregnancy progresses, and descent of the diaphragm on inspiration becomes less possible. The respiratory rate may increase slightly, and some hyperventilation and difficulty in breathing may occur.

Nasal stuffiness and epistaxis (nose bleeds) may also occur because of estrogen-induced edema and vascular congestion of the nasal mucosa.

Cardiovascular System

During pregnancy, blood flow increases to those organ systems with an increased workload. Thus blood flow increases to the uterus and kidneys, while hepatic and cerebral flow remains unchanged. Cardiac output begins to increase early in pregnancy and remains elevated for the remainder of the pregnancy.

The pulse may increase by as many as 10–15 beats per minute at term. The blood pressure decreases slightly and reaches its lowest point during the second trimester. It gradually increases to near prepregnant levels during the third trimester.

The enlarging uterus may press on pelvic and femoral vessels, interfering with returning blood flow and causing stasis of blood in the lower extremities. This condition may lead to dependent edema and varicosity of the veins in the legs, vulva, and rectum (hemorrhoids) in late pregnancy. This increased blood volume in the lower legs may also make the pregnant woman more prone to postural hypotension.

The enlarging uterus may press on the vena cava when the pregnant woman lies supine, thus reducing blood flow to the right atrium, lowering blood pressure and causing dizziness, pallor, and clamminess. This is called the *supine hypotensive syndrome* or **vena caval syndrome** (Figure 7–1). It can be corrected by having the woman lie on her left side or by placing a pillow or wedge under her right hip. Because the enlarging uterus may also press on the aorta and its collateral circulation, some researchers suggest that the term *aortocaval compression* is more accurate (Blackburn and Loper 1992).

Blood volume progressively increases beginning in the first trimester, increasing rapidly in the second trimester, and slowing in the third. It peaks in the middle of the third trimester at about 45 percent above nonpregnant levels.

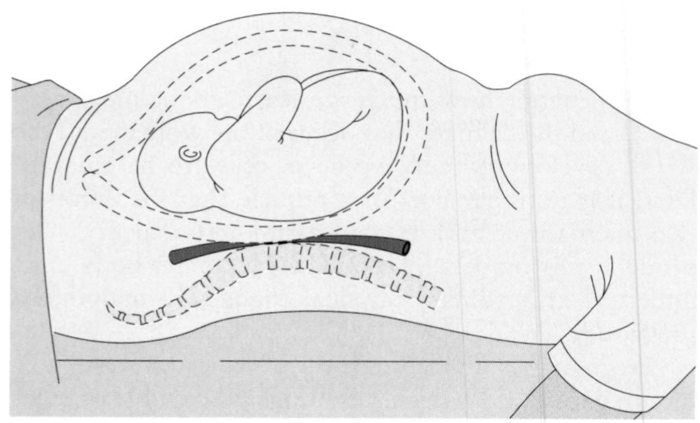

FIGURE 7–1 Vena caval syndrome. The gravid uterus compresses the vena cava when the woman is supine. This reduces the blood flow returning to the heart and may cause maternal hypotension.

The total erythrocyte (red blood cell) volume increases by about 30 percent in women who receive iron supplementation (but only about 18 percent without iron supplementation) (Cruikshank et al 1996). This increase in erythrocytes is necessary to transport the additional oxygen required during pregnancy. However, the increase in plasma volume during pregnancy averages about 50 percent. Because the plasma volume increase (50%) is greater than the erythrocyte increase (30%), the hematocrit, which measures the concentration of red blood cells in the plasma, decreases by an average of about 7 percent. This decrease is referred to as the *physiologic anemia of pregnancy (pseudoanemia)*.

Iron is necessary for hemoglobin formation, and hemoglobin is the oxygen-carrying component of erythrocytes. Thus the increase in erythrocyte levels results in an increased need for iron by the pregnant woman. Even though the gastrointestinal absorption of iron is moderately increased during pregnancy, it is usually necessary to add supplemental iron to the diet to meet the expanded red blood cell and fetal needs.

Leukocyte production increases slightly to an average of 5,000–12,000 per mm^3; a few women develop levels as high as 15,000 per mm^3. During labor and the early postpartum period, these levels may reach 25,000 per mm^3.

Both the fibrin and plasma fibrinogen levels increase during pregnancy. Although the blood-clotting time of the pregnant woman does not differ significantly from that of the nonpregnant woman, clotting factors VII, VIII, IX, and X increase; thus pregnancy is a somewhat hypercoagulable state. These changes, coupled with venous stasis in late pregnancy, increase the pregnant woman's risk of developing venous thrombosis.

Gastrointestinal System

Nausea and vomiting are common during the first trimester because of elevated human chorionic gonadotropin (hCG) levels and changed carbohydrate metabolism. Gum tissue may soften and bleed easily. The secretion of saliva may increase and even become excessive *(ptyalism)*.

Elevated progesterone levels cause smooth muscle relaxation, resulting in delayed gastric emptying and decreased peristalsis. As a result, the pregnant woman may complain of bloating and constipation. These symptoms are aggravated as the enlarging uterus displaces the stomach upward and the intestines laterally and posteriorly. The cardiac sphincter also relaxes, and heartburn *(pyrosis)* may occur due to reflux of acidic secretions into the lower esophagus.

Hemorrhoids frequently develop in late pregnancy from constipation and from pressure on vessels below the level of the uterus.

Only minor liver changes occur with pregnancy. Plasma albumin concentrations and serum cholinesterase activity decrease with normal pregnancy, as with certain liver diseases.

The emptying time of the gallbladder is prolonged during pregnancy as a result of smooth muscle relaxation from progesterone. This, coupled with the elevated levels of cholesterol in the bile, can predispose the woman to gallstone formation.

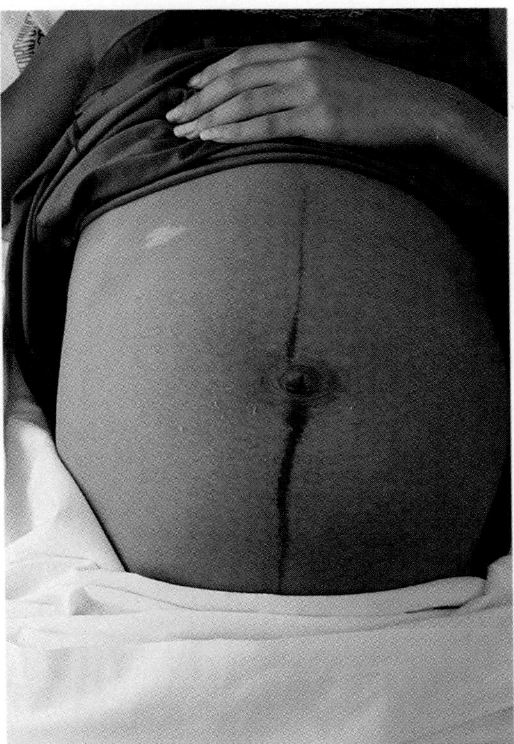

FIGURE 7–2 Linea nigra.

Urinary Tract

During the first trimester, the enlarging uterus is still a pelvic organ and presses against the bladder, producing urinary frequency. This symptom decreases during the second trimester when the uterus becomes an abdominal organ and pressure against the bladder lessens. Frequency reappears during the third trimester, when the presenting part descends into the pelvis and again presses on the bladder, reducing bladder capacity, contributing to hyperemia, and irritating the bladder.

The ureters (especially the right ureter) elongate and dilate above the pelvic brim. The glomerular filtration rate (GFR) rises by as much as 50 percent beginning in the second trimester and remains elevated until birth. To compensate for this, renal tubular reabsorption also increases. However, glycosuria is sometimes seen during pregnancy because of the kidneys' inability to reabsorb all the glucose filtered by the glomeruli. This may be normal or may indicate gestational diabetes, so glycosuria always warrants further testing.

Skin

Changes in skin pigmentation commonly occur during pregnancy. They are thought to be stimulated by increased estrogen and, perhaps, by increased progesterone, because these hormones are melanogenic stimulants (Blackburn and Loper 1992). Pigmentation of the skin increases primarily in areas that are already hyperpigmented: the areola, the nipples, the vulva, and the perianal area. The skin in the middle of the abdomen may develop a pigmented line, the **linea nigra,** which usually extends from the umbilicus or above to the pubic area (Figure 7–2). Facial **chloasma** (also known as the mask of pregnancy), a darkening of the skin over the forehead and around the eyes, may develop. Chloasma is more prominent in dark-haired women and is aggravated by exposure to the sun. Fortunately, chloasma fades or becomes less prominent soon after childbirth when the hormonal influence of pregnancy subsides.

Striae (reddish, irregular streaks) may appear on the abdomen, thighs, buttocks, and breasts. Commonly called stretch marks, they result from reduced connective tissue strength due to elevated adrenal steroid levels. Vascular spider nevi, small, bright-red elevations of the skin radiating from a central body, may develop on the chest, neck, face, arms, and legs. They may be caused by increased subcutaneous blood flow in response to elevated estrogen levels.

The sweat and sebaceous glands are often hyperactive during pregnancy.

The rate of hair growth may decrease during pregnancy; the number of hair follicles in the resting or dormant phase also decreases. After birth, the number of hair follicles in the resting phase increases sharply and the woman may notice increased hair shedding for 1–4 months. Practically all hair is replaced within 6–12 months, however (Cunningham et al 1997).

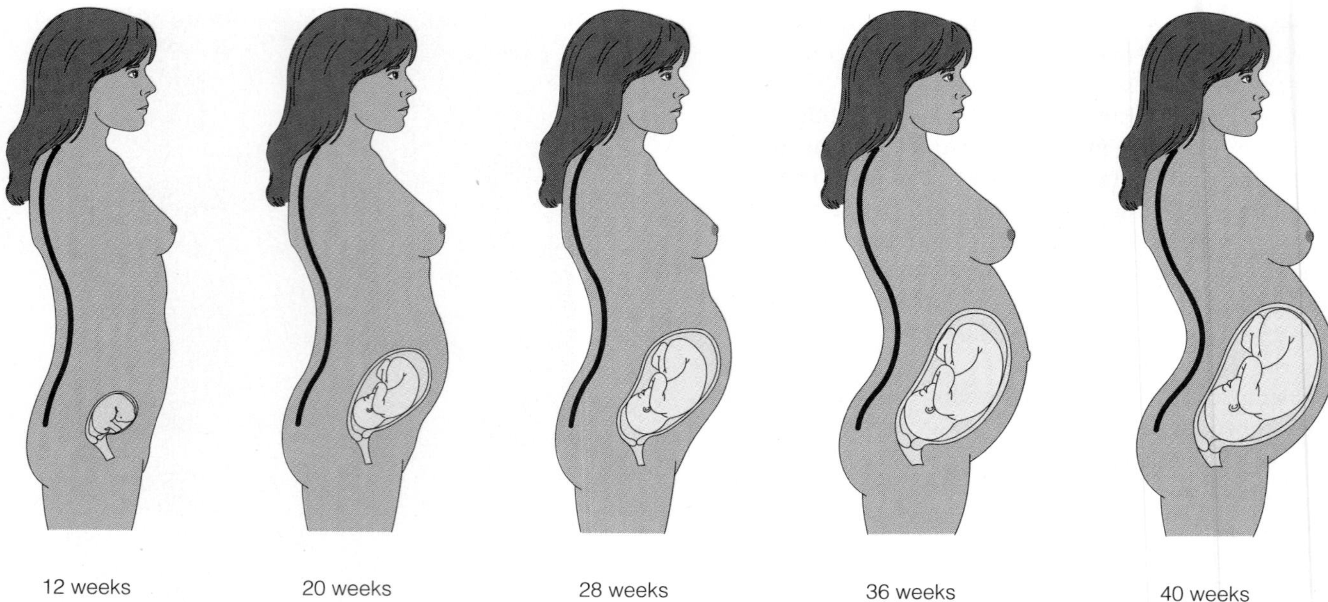

FIGURE 7–3 Postural changes during pregnancy. Note the increasing lordosis of the lumbosacral spine and the increasing curvature of the thoracic area.

Musculoskeletal System

No demonstrable changes occur in the teeth of pregnant women. The dental caries that sometimes accompany pregnancy are probably caused by the slightly more acidic saliva during pregnancy and by inadequate oral hygiene, especially if the woman has problems with bleeding gums.

The joints of the pelvis relax somewhat because of hormonal influences. The result is often a waddling gait. As the pregnant woman's center of gravity gradually changes, the lumbar spinal curve becomes accentuated, and her posture changes (Figure 7–3). This posture change compensates for the increased weight of the uterus anteriorly and frequently results in low backache.

Pressure of the enlarging uterus on the abdominal muscles may cause the rectus abdominis muscle to separate, producing **diastasis recti.** If the separation is severe and muscle tone is not regained postpartally, subsequent pregnancies will not have adequate support and the woman's abdomen may appear pendulous.

Metabolism

Most metabolic functions increase during pregnancy because of the increased demands of the growing fetus and its support system. The expectant mother must meet both her own tissue replacement needs and those of her unborn child. Her body must also anticipate the needs of labor and lactation.

For a detailed discussion of nutrient, vitamin, and mineral metabolism, see Chapter 11.

Weight Gain

The recommended weight gain for women of normal weight before pregnancy is 25–35 lb (11.5–16 kg); for women who were overweight, the recommended gain is 15–25 lb (7–11.5 kg); and for underweight women, 28–40 lb (12.5–18 kg) (Institute of Medicine 1990). The average pattern of weight gain is 3–5 lb (1.4–2.3 kg) during the first trimester, and 12–15 lb (5.5–6.8 kg) during each of the last two trimesters. Adequate nutrition and weight gain are important during pregnancy (see discussion in Chapter 11).

Water Metabolism

Increased water retention is a basic alteration of pregnancy. Several interrelated factors cause this phenomenon. The increased level of steroid sex hormones affects sodium and fluid retention. The lowered serum protein also influences the fluid balance, as do increased intracapillary pressure and permeability. The extra water is due to the products of conception—the fetus, placenta, and amniotic fluid—and the mother's increased blood volume, interstitial fluids, and enlarged organs.

Nutrient Metabolism

The fetus makes its greatest protein and fat demands during the second half of pregnancy, and doubles in weight during the last 6 to 8 weeks. Protein (contributing nitrogen) must be stored during pregnancy to maintain a constant level within the breast milk and to avoid depletion of maternal tissues. Carbohydrate needs also increase, especially during the second and third trimesters.

Fats are more completely absorbed during pregnancy, and the level of free fatty acids increases in response to human placental lactogen (hPL). The levels of lipoproteins and cholesterol also increase. Because of these changes, increased levels of dietary fat or reduced carbohydrate production may lead to ketonuria in the pregnant woman.

Endocrine System

Thyroid

The thyroid gland often enlarges slightly during pregnancy because of increased vascularity and hyperplasia of glandular tissue. Its capacity to bind thyroxine is greater, resulting in an increase in serum protein-bound iodine (PBI). These changes are due to higher blood levels of estrogen.

The basal metabolic rate increases by 25 percent during pregnancy. However, within a few weeks after birth all thyroid function returns to normal limits.

Pituitary

Pregnancy is made possible by the hypothalamic stimulation of the anterior pituitary gland, which in turn produces the hormones follicle-stimulating hormone (FSH), which stimulates ovum growth, and luteinizing hormone (LH), which brings about ovulation. Stimulation of the pituitary also prolongs the ovary's corpus luteal phase, which maintains the endometrium for development of the pregnancy. Prolactin, another anterior pituitary hormone, is responsible for initial lactation.

The posterior portion of the pituitary secretes vasopressin (antidiuretic hormone) and oxytocin. Vasopressin causes vasoconstriction, which results in increased blood pressure; it also helps regulate water balance. Oxytocin promotes uterine contractility and stimulates ejection of milk from the breasts (the *let-down reflex*) in the postpartum period.

Adrenals

No significant increase in the weight of the adrenal glands occurs during pregnancy. Circulating cortisol, which regulates carbohydrate and protein metabolism, increases in response to increased estrogen levels. Cortisol blood levels return to normal within 1 to 6 weeks postpartum.

The adrenals secrete increased levels of aldosterone by the early part of the second trimester. This increase in aldosterone in a normal pregnancy may be the body's protective response to the increased sodium excretion associated with progesterone (Cunningham et al 1997).

Pancreas

The pregnant woman has increased insulin needs and the pancreatic islets of Langerhans, which secrete insulin, are stressed to meet this increased demand. Any marginal pancreatic function quickly becomes apparent, and the woman may show signs of gestational diabetes.

Hormones in Pregnancy

Human Chorionic Gonadotropin (hCG)

The trophoblast secretes hCG in early pregnancy. This hormone stimulates progesterone and estrogen production by the corpus luteum to maintain the pregnancy until the placenta is developed sufficiently to assume that function.

Human Placental Lactogen (hPL)

Also called human chorionic somatomammotropin, hPL is produced by the syncytiotrophoblast. Human placental lactogen is an antagonist of insulin; it increases the amount of circulating free fatty acids for maternal metabolic needs and decreases maternal metabolism of glucose to favor fetal growth.

Estrogen

Estrogen, secreted originally by the corpus luteum, is produced primarily by the placenta as early as week 7. Estrogen stimulates uterine development to provide a suitable environment for the fetus. It also helps develop the ductal system of the breasts in preparation for lactation.

Progesterone

Progesterone, also produced initially by the corpus luteum and then by the placenta, plays the greatest role in maintaining pregnancy. It maintains the endometrium and inhibits spontaneous uterine contractility, thus preventing early spontaneous abortion. Progesterone also helps develop the acini and lobules of the breasts in preparation for lactation.

Relaxin

Relaxin is detectable in the serum of a pregnant woman by the time of the first missed menstrual period. Relaxin inhibits uterine activity, diminishes the strength of uterine contractions, aids in the softening of the cervix, and has the long-term effect of remodeling collagen. Its primary source is the corpus luteum, but small amounts are believed to be produced by the placenta and uterine decidua (Buster and Carson 1996).

Prostaglandins in Pregnancy

Prostaglandins (PGs) are lipid substances that can arise from most body tissues but occur in high concentrations in the female reproductive tract and are present in the decidua during pregnancy. The exact functions of PGs during pregnancy are still unknown, although it has

KEY FACTS TO REMEMBER

Differentiating the Signs of Pregnancy

These guidelines help differentiate among the presumptive, probable, and positive changes of pregnancy.

Subjective (Presumptive) Changes

- Symptoms the woman experiences and reports
- May have causes other than pregnancy

Objective (Probable) Changes

- Signs perceived by the examiner
- May have causes other than pregnancy

Diagnostic (Positive) Changes

- Signs perceived by the examiner
- Can be caused only by pregnancy

been proposed that they are responsible for maintaining reduced placental vascular resistance. Decreased prostaglandin levels may contribute to pregnancy-induced hypertension (PIH). Prostaglandins are also believed to play a role in the complex biochemistry that initiates labor (Blackburn and Loper 1992).

TABLE 7–1 Differential Diagnosis of Pregnancy—Subjective Changes

Subjective Changes	*Possible Causes*
Amenorrhea	Endocrine factors: early menopause; lactation; thyroid, pituitary, adrenal, ovarian dysfunction Metabolic factors: malnutrition, anemia, climatic changes, diabetes mellitus, degenerative disorders, long-distance running Psychologic factors: emotional shock, fear of pregnancy or sexually transmitted infection, intense desire for pregnancy (pseudocyesis), stress Obliteration of endometrial cavity by infection or curettage Systemic disease (acute or chronic), such as tuberculosis or malignancy
Nausea and vomiting	Gastrointestinal disorders Acute infections such as encephalitis Emotional disorders such as pseudocyesis or anorexia nervosa
Urinary frequency	Urinary tract infection Cystocele Pelvic tumors Urethral diverticula Emotional tension
Breast tenderness	Premenstrual tension Chronic cystic mastitis Pseudocyesis Hyperestrinism
Quickening	Increased peristalsis Flatus ("gas") Abdominal muscle contractions Shifting of abdominal contents

Signs of Pregnancy

Many of the changes women experience during pregnancy are used to diagnose the pregnancy itself. They are called the *subjective* or *presumptive* changes, the *objective* or *probable* changes, and the *diagnostic* or *positive* changes of pregnancy. The guidelines for differentiating among these three are identified in Key Facts to Remember: Differentiating the Signs of Pregnancy.

Subjective (Presumptive) Changes

The subjective changes of pregnancy are the symptoms the woman experiences and reports. Because they can be caused by other conditions, they cannot be considered proof of pregnancy (Table 7–1). The following subjective signs can be diagnostic clues when other signs and symptoms of pregnancy are also present.

Amenorrhea, or the absence of menses, is the earliest symptom of pregnancy. The missing of more than one menstrual period, especially in a woman whose cycle is ordinarily regular, is an especially useful diagnostic clue.

Nausea and vomiting in pregnancy (NVP) occur frequently during the first trimester. Because these symptoms often occur in the early part of the day, they are commonly referred to as *morning sickness.* In reality, the symptoms may occur at any time and can range from merely a distaste for food to severe vomiting. Research suggests that women who experience NVP have a decreased incidence of spontaneous abortion and perinatal mortality (Blackburn and Loper 1992).

Excessive fatigue may be noted within a few weeks after the first missed menstrual period and may persist throughout the first trimester.

Urinary frequency is experienced during the first trimester as the enlarging uterus presses on the bladder.

Changes in the breasts are frequently noted in early pregnancy. These changes include tenderness and tingling sensations, increased pigmentation of the areola and nipple, and changes in Montgomery's glands. The veins also become more visible and form a bluish pattern beneath the skin.

Quickening, or the mother's perception of fetal movement, occurs about 18 to 20 weeks after the **last menstrual period (LMP)** in a woman pregnant for the first time but may occur as early as 16 weeks in a woman who has been pregnant before. Quickening is a fluttering sensation in the abdomen that gradually increases in intensity and frequency.

TABLE 7–2 Differential Diagnosis of Pregnancy—Objective Changes

Objective Changes	Possible Causes
Changes in pelvic organs	Increased vascular congestion
Goodell's sign	Estrogen-progestin oral contraceptives
Chadwick's sign	Vulvar, vaginal, cervical hyperemia
Hegar's sign	Excessively soft walls of nonpregnant uterus
Uterine enlargement	Uterine tumors
Braun von Fernwald's sign	Uterine tumors
Piskacek's sign	Uterine tumors
Enlargement of abdomen	Obesity, ascites, pelvic tumors
Braxton Hicks contractions	Hematometra, pedunculated, submucous, and soft myomas
Uterine souffle	Large uterine myomas, large ovarian tumors, or any condition with greatly increased uterine blood flow
Pigmentation of skin	Estrogen-progestin oral contraceptives
Choasma	Melanocyte hormonal stimulation
Linea nigra	
Nipples/areola	
Abdominal striae	Obesity, pelvic tumor
Ballottement	Uterine tumors/polyps, ascites
Pregnancy tests	Increased pituitary gonadotropins at menopause, choriocarcinoma, hydatidiform mole
Palpation for fetal outline	Uterine myomas

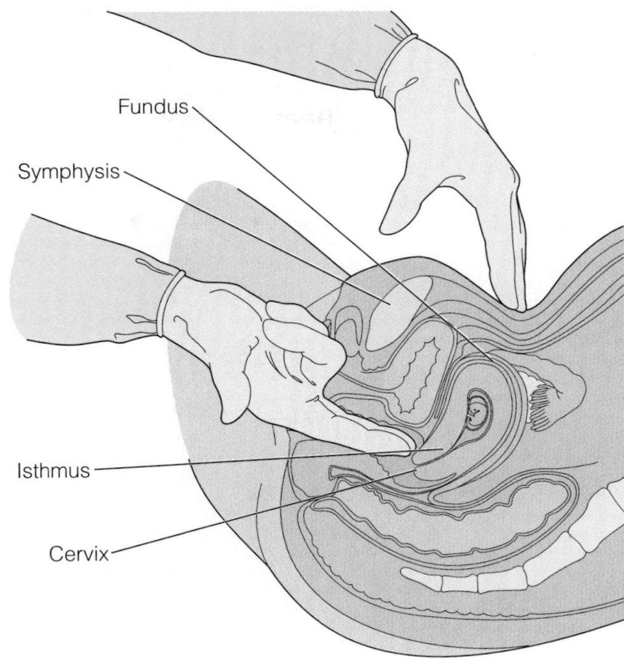

FIGURE 7–4 Hegar's sign, a softening of the isthmus of the uterus, can be determined by the examiner during a vaginal examination.

Objective (Probable) Changes

An examiner can perceive the objective changes that occur in pregnancy. Since these changes can also have other causes, they do not confirm pregnancy (Table 7–2).

Changes in the pelvic organs—the only physical changes detectable during the first 3 months of pregnancy—are caused by increased vascular congestion. These changes are noted on pelvic examination. There is a softening of the cervix called **Goodell's sign. Chadwick's sign** is a bluish, purple, or deep red discoloration of the mucous membranes of the cervix, vagina, and vulva (some sources consider this a presumptive sign). **Hegar's sign** is a softening of the isthmus of the uterus, the area between the cervix and the body of the uterus (Figure 7–4). **McDonald's sign** is an ease in flexing the body of the uterus against the cervix.

General enlargement and softening of the body of the uterus can be noted after the eighth week of pregnancy. The fundus of the uterus is palpable just above the symphysis pubis at about 10 to 12 weeks' gestation and at the level of the umbilicus at 20 to 22 weeks' gestation (Figure 7–5).

Enlargement of the abdomen during the childbearing years is usually regarded as evidence of pregnancy, especially if it is continuous and accompanied by amenorrhea.

Braxton Hicks contractions are ordinarily painless uterine contractions that occur at irregular intervals throughout pregnancy but can be felt most commonly after the 28th week. As the woman approaches the end of pregnancy, these contractions may become more uncomfortable. They are then often called "false labor."

Uterine souffle may be heard when the examiner auscultates the abdomen over the uterus. This is a soft, blowing sound that occurs at the same rate as the maternal pulse and is caused by the increased uterine blood flow and blood pulsating through the placenta. It is sometimes confused with the *funic souffle,* a soft blowing sound of blood pulsating through the umbilical cord. The funic souffle occurs at the same rate as the fetal heart rate.

Changes in pigmentation of the skin are common in pregnancy. The nipples and areola may darken, and the linea nigra may develop. Facial chloasma may become noticeable and striae may appear.

The *fetal outline* may be identified by palpation in many pregnant women after 24 weeks' gestation.

Ballottement is the passive fetal movement elicited by pushing up against the cervix with two fingers. This pushes the fetal body up, and a rebound is felt as it falls back.

Pregnancy tests detect the presence of hCG in the maternal blood or urine. These are not considered a positive sign of pregnancy because other conditions can cause elevated hCG levels.

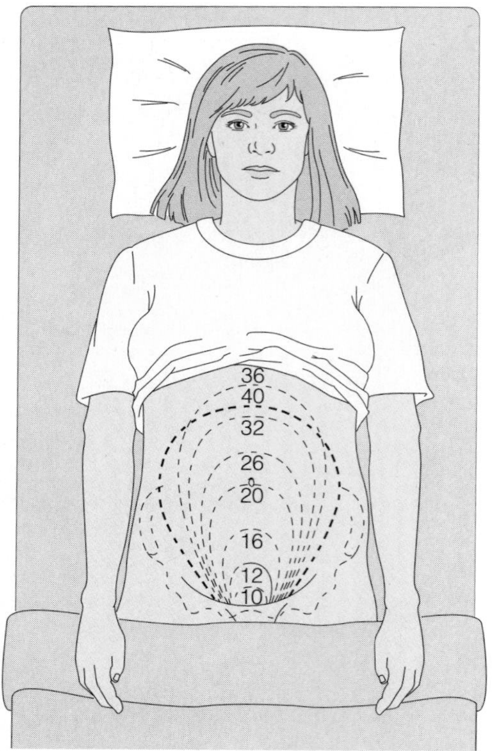

FIGURE 7–5 Approximate height of the fundus at various weeks of pregnancy.

Pregnancy Tests

Today's pregnancy tests are immunoassays and radioreceptor assays.

Immunoassay tests are based on the antigenic properties of hCG. In the *hemagglutination-inhibition test (Pregnosticon R),* no clumping of cells occurs when the urine of a pregnant woman is added to the hCG-sensitized red blood cells of sheep. In the *latex agglutination tests (Gravindex and Pregnosticon Slide tests),* latex particle agglutination is inhibited in the presence of urine containing hCG. Both these tests are done on the first early morning urine specimen of the woman because it is adequately concentrated. The tests become positive within 10–14 days after the first missed period.

The *β subunit radioimmunoassay,* or RIA, uses an antiserum with specificity for the β subunit of hCG in maternal blood. This is a very accurate pregnancy test that becomes positive a few days after presumed implantation, thereby permitting earlier diagnosis of pregnancy. This test is also used in the diagnosis of ectopic pregnancy or trophoblastic disease. However, because it requires several hours to perform and has only limited sensitivity, it is being replaced by other, technically simpler tests such as the *immunoradiometric assay (IRMA)* (Buster and Carson 1996). IRMA (Neocept, Pregnosis), an assay that uses a radioactive antibody to identify the presence of hCG in the serum, can detect very low concentrations of hCG. It requires only about 30 minutes to perform. The *enzyme-linked immunosorbent assay (ELISA)* (Model Sensichrome, Quest Confidot) does not use radioisotopes but a substance that results in a color change after binding. The test is sensitive and quick, and can detect hCG levels as early as 7–9 days after ovulation and conception, which is 5 days before the first missed period (Buster and Carson 1996).

Radioreceptor assay (Biocept-G) uses the principle of high-affinity receptors to detect pregnancy. It is a sensitive test and can be performed in 1 hour, but because it fails to distinguish between hCG and LH, cross-reactions may occur.

Over-the-Counter Pregnancy Tests

Home pregnancy tests are available over the counter at a reasonable cost. These enzyme immunoassay tests, performed on urine, are quite sensitive and detect even low levels of hCG.

Home pregnancy test instructions are quite explicit and should be followed carefully for optimal results. Best results are obtained with a first morning urine specimen, although some of the tests can be used on any voided specimen. Furthermore, because the newer kits require only a short wait (usually 3–5 minutes), the margin for error is very small. Most of the current kits can detect a pregnancy as early as the day of the missed period, but to avoid false-negative results, women should be encouraged to wait 6–9 days after a missed period before using the test.

Diagnostic (Positive) Changes

A sign of pregnancy is positive if it proves conclusively that a woman is pregnant, but such signs are usually not present until after the fourth month of gestation.

The *fetal heartbeat* can be detected with a fetoscope by weeks 17 to 20 of pregnancy. The electronic Doppler device allows the examiner to detect the fetal heartbeat as early as weeks 10 to 12.

Fetal movement is actively palpable by a trained examiner after about the 20th week of pregnancy.

Visualization of the fetus by ultrasound examination confirms a pregnancy. The gestational sac can be observed by 4 to 5 weeks' gestation (2 to 3 weeks after conception). Fetal parts and fetal movement can be seen as early as 8 weeks. More recently ultrasound using a vaginal probe has been used to detect a gestational sac as early as 10 days after implantation (Cunningham et al 1997).

Psychologic Response of the Expectant Family to Pregnancy

Pregnancy is a developmental challenge, a turning point in a family's life, and thus it is accompanied by stress and anxiety whether the pregnancy is desired or not. Pregnancy confirms the biologic capability to reproduce. It is evidence of participation in sexual activity and an affirmation of sexuality. For beginning families, pregnancy is the transition period from childlessness to parenthood. If the pregnancy results in the birth of a child, the couple enters a new stage of their life together, one that is irreversible and characterized by awesome responsibilities.

The expectant couple may be unaware of the physical, emotional, and cognitive changes of pregnancy and may anticipate no problems from such a normal event. Thus they may be confused and distressed by new feelings and behaviors that are essentially normal.

Parenthood brings significant role changes for the couple. Career goals and mobility may be affected, and the couple's relationship takes on a different meaning to them and their families and community. Routines and family dynamics are altered with each pregnancy, requiring readjustment and realignment.

The couple must make decisions about financial matters, such as whether the woman will work during her pregnancy and return to work after her child is born. They may also need to decide about the division of domestic tasks. Any differences of opinion must be discussed openly and resolved so that the family can meet the needs of its members.

The couple must face the anxieties of labor and birth and must also deal with fears that the baby may be ill or disfigured. Classes in prepared childbirth can help the couple overcome concerns based on misinformation or lack of information.

If the pregnant woman has no stable partner, she must deal alone with the role changes, fears, and adjustments of pregnancy or seek support from family or friends. She also faces the reality of planning for the future as a single parent.

Even if the pregnant woman plans to relinquish her infant, she must still deal with the adjustments of pregnancy. She is no longer a separate individual; she must consider the needs of another being who depends on her totally, at least during pregnancy. This adjustment can be especially difficult without a good support system.

In most pregnancies, whether of a woman with a supportive partner, a single mother, or a relinquishing mother, finances are an important consideration. Traditional lore relegates to the father the role of primary breadwinner, and indeed finances are often a very real concern for fathers. However, in today's society even pregnant women with stable partners recognize the financial impact of a child and may feel concern about financial issues. For the single mother, finances may be a major source of concern.

Pregnancy can be viewed as a developmental stage with its own distinct developmental tasks. It can be a time of support or conflict for a couple, depending on the amount of adjustment each is willing to make to maintain the family's equilibrium.

During a first pregnancy, the couple plans together for the child's arrival, collecting information on how to be parents. At the same time, each continues to participate in some separate activities with friends or family members. The availability of social support is an important factor in psychosocial well-being during pregnancy. The social network is often a major source of advice for the pregnant woman. However, evidence indicates that both sound and unsound information is given.

Although individual activities are important, some conflict may arise if the couple's activities become too divergent. Thus they may find it necessary to limit their outside associations.

During pregnancy, the expectant mother and father both face significant changes and must deal with major psychosocial adjustments (Table 7–3). Other family members, especially the couple's other children and the grandparents-to-be, must also adjust to the pregnancy.

For some couples, pregnancy is more than a developmental stage; it is a crisis. *Crisis* can be defined as a disturbance or conflict in which the individual cannot maintain a state of equilibrium. Pregnancy can be considered a *maturational crisis,* since it is a common event in the normal growth and development of the family. During such a crisis, the individual or family is in disequilibrium. Egos weaken, usual defense mechanisms are not effective, unresolved material from the past reappears, and relationships shift. The period of disequilibrium and disorganization is marked by unsuccessful attempts to solve the perceived problems. If the crisis is not resolved, it will result in maladaptive behaviors in one or more family members, and possible disintegration of the family. Families who are able to resolve a maturational crisis successfully will return to normal functioning and can even strengthen the bonds in the family relationship.

The Mother

Pregnancy is a condition that alters body image and also necessitates a reordering of social relationships and changes in roles of family members. The way a particular woman meets the stresses of pregnancy is influenced by her emotional makeup, her sociologic and cultural background, and her acceptance or rejection of the pregnancy. Many women manifest similar psychologic and

TABLE 7–3 Parental Reactions to Pregnancy

First Trimester	Second Trimester	Third Trimester
Mother's reactions	**Mother's reactions**	**Mother's reactions**
Informs father secretively or openly Feels ambivalent toward pregnancy, anxious about labor and responsibility of child Is aware of physical changes, daydreams of possible miscarriage Develops special feelings for, renewed interest in her own mother, with formation of a personal identity	Remains regressive and introspective, projects all problems with authority figures onto partner, may become angry as if lack of interest is sign of weakness in him Continues to deal with feelings as a mother and looks for furniture as something concrete May have other extreme of anxiety and wait until ninth month to look for furniture and clothes for baby Feels movement and is aware of fetus and incorporates it into herself Dreams that partner will be killed, telephones him often for reassurance Experiences more distinct physical changes, sexual desires may increase or decrease	Experiences more anxiety and tension, with physical awkwardness Feels much discomfort and insomnia from physical condition Prepares for birth, assembles layette, picks out names Dreams often about misplacing baby or not being able to give birth, fears birth of deformed baby Feels ecstasy and excitement, has spurt of energy during last month
Father's reactions	**Father's reactions**	**Father's reactions**
Differ according to age, parity, desire for child, economic stability Acceptance of pregnant woman's attitude, or complete rejection and lack of communication Is aware of his own sexual feelings, may develop more or less sexual arousal Accepts, rejects, or resents mother-in-law May develop new hobby outside of family as sign of stress	If he can cope, will give her extra attention she needs; if he cannot cope, will develop a new time-consuming interest outside of home May develop a creative feeling and a "closeness to nature" May become involved in pregnancy and buy or make furniture Feels for movement of baby, listens to heartbeat, or remains aloof, with no physical contact May have fears and fantasies about himself being pregnant, may become uneasy with this feminine aspect in himself May react negatively if partner is too demanding, may become jealous of physician and of his/her importance to partner and her pregnancy	Adapts to alternative methods of sexual contact Becomes concerned over financial responsibility May show new sense of tenderness and concern, treat partner like doll Daydreams about child as if older and not newborn, dreams of losing partner Renewed sexual attraction to partner Feels he is ultimately responsible for whatever happens

emotional responses during pregnancy, including ambivalence, acceptance, introversion, mood swings, and changes in body image.

Even if the pregnancy is planned, there is an element of surprise at first. Many women commonly experience feelings of ambivalence during early pregnancy. This may be related to feelings that the timing is somehow wrong; worries about the need to modify existing relationships or career plans; fears about assuming a new role; unresolved emotional conflicts with the woman's own mother; and fears about pregnancy, labor, and birth. These feelings may be more pronounced if the pregnancy is unplanned or unwanted. Indirect expressions of ambivalence include complaints about considerable physical discomfort, prolonged or frequent depression, significant dissatisfaction with changing body shape, excessive mood swings, and difficulty in accepting the life changes resulting from the pregnancy (Lederman 1996).

Pregnancy produces marked changes in a woman's body within a relatively short period of time. Women perceive that they require more body space as pregnancy progresses (Mercer 1995). They also experience changes in body image. The degree of this change is related to a certain extent to personality factors, social network responses, and attitudes toward pregnancy. Although changes in body image are normal, they can be very stressful for the woman. Explanation and discussion of the changes may help both the woman and her partner deal with the stress associated with this aspect of pregnancy.

First Trimester

During the first trimester, feelings of disbelief and ambivalence are paramount. The woman's baby does not seem real to her, and she focuses on herself and her pregnancy (Rubin 1984). She may experience one or more of the early symptoms of pregnancy, such as breast tenderness or morning sickness, which are unsettling and at times unpleasant.

During the first trimester, the expectant mother begins to exhibit some characteristic behavioral changes. She may become increasingly introspective and passive. She may be emotionally labile, with characteristic mood swings from joy to despair. She may fantasize about a miscarriage and feel guilt because of these fantasies. She may worry that these thoughts will harm the baby in some way (Robinson and Stewart 1990).

Second Trimester

During the second trimester, quickening occurs. This perception of fetal movement helps the woman think of her baby as a separate person, and she generally becomes excited about the pregnancy even if earlier she was not.

The woman becomes increasingly introspective as she evaluates her life, her plans, and her child's future. This introspection helps the woman prepare for her new mothering role. Emotional lability, which may be unsettling to her partner, persists. In some instances, he may react by withdrawing. This is especially distressing to the woman, because she needs increased love and affection. Once the couple understands that these behaviors are characteristic of pregnancy, it is easier for the couple to deal with them effectively, although they will be sources of stress to some extent throughout pregnancy.

As pregnancy becomes more noticeable, the woman's body image changes. She may feel great pride, embarrassment, or concern. Generally women feel best during the second trimester, which is a relatively tranquil time.

Third Trimester

In the third trimester, the woman feels both pride about her pregnancy and anxiety about labor and birth. Physical discomforts increase, and the woman is eager for the pregnancy to end. She experiences increased fatigue, her body movements are more awkward, and her interest in sexual activity may decrease. During this time, the woman tends to be concerned about the health and safety of her unborn child and may worry that she will not behave well during childbirth (Robinson and Stewart 1990). Toward the end of this period, there is often a surge of energy as the woman prepares a "nest" for the infant. Many women report bursts of energy, during which they vigorously clean and organize their homes.

Psychologic Tasks of the Mother

Rubin (1984) has identified four major tasks that the pregnant woman undertakes to maintain her intactness and that of her family and at the same time incorporate her new child into the family system. These tasks form the foundation for a mutually gratifying relationship with her infant.

1. *Ensuring safe passage through pregnancy, labor, and birth.* The pregnant woman feels concern for both her unborn child and herself. She seeks competent maternity care to provide a sense of control. She may also seek information from literature, observation of other pregnant women and new mothers, and discussion with others. She also seeks to ensure safe passage by engaging in self-care activities related to diet, exercise, alcohol consumption, and so forth (Patterson et al 1990). In the third trimester she becomes more aware of external threats in the environment—a toy on the stairs, the awkwardness of an escalator—that pose a threat to her well-being. She may worry if her partner is late or if she is home alone. Sleep becomes more difficult and she longs for birth even though it, too, is frightening.
2. *Seeking acceptance of this child by others.* The birth of a child alters a woman's primary support group (her family) and her secondary affiliative groups. The woman slowly and subtly alters her network to meet the needs of her pregnancy. In this adjustment the woman's partner is the most important figure. The partner's support and acceptance help form a maternal identity. If there are other children in the home, the mother also works to ensure their acceptance of the coming child. Acceptance of the anticipated change is sometimes stressful, and the woman may work to maintain some special time with her partner or older child. The woman without a partner looks to others such as a family member or friend for this support.
3. *Seeking commitment and acceptance of herself as mother to the infant (binding-in).* During the first trimester the child remains a rather abstract concept. With quickening, however, the child begins to become a real person, and the mother begins to develop bonds of attachment. The mother experiences the movement of the child within her in an intimate, exclusive way and, out of this experience, bonds of love form. The mother develops a fantasy image of her ideal child. This binding-in process, characterized by its strong emotional component, motivates the pregnant woman to become competent in her role and provides satisfaction for her in the role of mother (Mercer 1995). This possessive love increases her maternal commitment to protect her fetus now and her child after he or she is born.
4. *Learning to give of oneself on behalf of one's child.* Childbirth involves many acts of giving. The man "gives" a child to the woman; she in turn "gives" a child to the man. Life is given to an infant; a sibling is given to older children of the family. The woman begins to develop a capacity for self-denial and learns to delay immediate personal gratification to meet the needs of another. Baby showers and baby

gifts are acts of giving that increase the mother's self-esteem and help her acknowledge the separateness and needs of the coming baby.

Accomplishment of these tasks helps the expectant woman develop her self-concept as mother. The expectant woman who was well nurtured by her own mother may view her mother as a role model and emulate her; the woman who views her own mother as a "poor mother" may worry that she will make similar mistakes (Lederman 1996). A woman's self-concept as a mother expands with actual experience and continues to grow through subsequent childbearing and childrearing. Occasionally a woman fails to accept the mother role, instead playing the role of babysitter or older sister.

The Father

For the expectant father, pregnancy is a psychologically stressful time because he, too, must adjust to a new child. Initially, expectant fathers may feel pride in their virility, which pregnancy confirms, but also have many of the same ambivalent feelings expectant mothers have. The extent of ambivalence depends on many factors, including the father's relationship with his partner, previous experience with pregnancy, and age and economic stability. Another important factor is whether the pregnancy was planned.

In adjusting to his role, the expectant father must first deal with the reality of the pregnancy and then struggle to gain recognition as a parent from his partner, family, friends, coworkers, society—and from his baby as well. The expectant mother can help her partner be a participant and not merely a helpmate to her if she has a definite sense of the experience as *their* pregnancy and *their* infant and not *her* pregnancy and *her* infant (Jordan 1990).

The expectant father must establish a fatherhood role, just as the woman develops a motherhood role. Fathers who are most successful at this generally like children, are excited about the prospect of fatherhood, are eager to nurture a child, and have confidence in their ability to be a parent. They also share the experiences of pregnancy and birth with their partners (Lederman 1996). See Table 7–3 on p 162.

First Trimester

After the initial excitement attending the announcement of the pregnancy, an expectant father may begin to feel left out. He may be confused by his partner's mood changes. He might resent the attention she receives and her need to modify their relationship as she experiences fatigue and possibly a decreased interest in sex. In addition, he might be concerned about what kind of father he will be.

During this time his child is a "potential" baby. Fathers often picture interacting with a child of 5 or 6 years, not a newborn. The pregnancy itself may seem unreal until the woman shows more physical signs (Jordan 1990).

Second Trimester

The father's role in the pregnancy is still vague in the second trimester, but his involvement may increase as he watches and feels fetal movement and listens to the fetal heartbeat during a visit to the certified nurse-midwife or physician. Like expectant mothers, expectant fathers need to confront and resolve some of their conflicts about the fathering they received. A father needs to sort out which behaviors of his own father he wants to imitate and which he wants to avoid.

Evidence suggests that the father-to-be's anxiety is lessened if both parents agree on the paternal role the man is to assume. For example, if both see his role as that of breadwinner, the man's stress is low. However, if the man views his role as that of breadwinners and the woman expects him to be actively involved in child care, his stress increases. Agreement between partners tends to increase with age and combined family income (Fishbein 1984).

As the woman's appearance begins to change, her partner may have several reactions. Her changed appearance may decrease his sexual interest, or it may have the opposite effect. Because of the variety of emotions both partners may feel, continued communication and acceptance are important.

Third Trimester

If the couple's relationship has grown through effective communication of their concerns and feelings, the third trimester is a special and rewarding time. They may attend childbirth classes and make concrete preparations for the arrival of the baby. If the father has developed a detached attitude about the pregnancy, however, it is unlikely he will become a willing participant, even though his role becomes more obvious.

Concerns and fears may recur. The father may worry about hurting the unborn baby during intercourse or become concerned about labor and birth. Also, he may wonder what kind of parents he and his partner will be.

Couvade

Couvade has traditionally referred to the observance of certain rituals and taboos by the male to signify the transition to fatherhood. This affirms his psychosocial and biophysical relationship to the woman and child. Some taboos restrict his actions. For example, in some cultures the man may be forbidden to eat certain foods or carry certain weapons before and immediately after the birth.

More recently, the term has been used to describe the unintentional development of physical symptoms such as fatigue, increased appetite, difficulty sleeping, depression, headache, or backache by the partner of the pregnant woman. Research suggests that men who demonstrate couvade syndrome tend to have a higher degree of paternal role preparation and are involved in more activities related to this preparation (Longobucco and Freston 1989).

Siblings

Bringing a new baby home usually marks the beginning of sibling rivalry. The siblings view the baby as a threat to the security of their relationships with their parents. Parents who recognize this potential problem early in pregnancy and begin constructive actions can minimize the problem of sibling rivalry.

Preparation of the young child begins several weeks before the anticipated birth. Because they do not have a clear concept of time, young children should not be told too early about the pregnancy. From the toddler's point of view "several weeks" is an extremely long time. The mother may let the child feel the baby moving in her uterus, explaining that the uterus is "a special place where babies grow." The child can help the parents put the baby clothes in drawers or prepare the nursery.

The concept of consistency is important in dealing with young children. They need reassurance that certain people, special things, and familiar places will continue to exist after the new baby arrives. The crib is an important though transient object in a child's life. If it is to be given to the new baby, the parents should thoughtfully help the child adjust to this change. Any move from crib to bed or from one room to another should precede the baby's birth by at least several weeks. If the new baby must share a room with siblings, the parents must also discuss this with siblings.

If the child is ready, toilet training is most effective several months before or after the baby's arrival. It is not unusual for the older, toilet-trained child to regress to wetting or soiling due to the attention the newborn gets for such behavior. The older, weaned child may want to nurse or drink from the bottle again after the baby comes. If the new mother anticipates these behaviors, they will be less frustrating during her early postpartum days.

Pregnant women may find it helpful to bring their children on a prenatal visit to the certified nurse-midwife or physician to give them an opportunity to listen to the fetal heartbeat. This helps make the baby more real to the children; they may also become involved in the prenatal care.

If siblings are school-age children, pregnancy should be viewed as a family affair. Teaching should be suitable to the child's level of understanding and may be supplemented with appropriate books. Taking part in family discussions, attending sibling preparation classes, feeling fetal movement, and listening to the fetal heartbeat help the school-age child take part in the experience of pregnancy and not feel like an outsider.

Older children or adolescents may appear to have sophisticated knowledge, but may have many misconceptions about pregnancy and birth. The parents should make opportunities to discuss their concerns and involve the children in preparations for the new baby.

Even after birth, siblings need to feel that they are taking part. Permitting siblings to visit their mother and the new baby at the hospital or birthing center will help. After the baby comes home, siblings can share in "showing off" the new baby.

Sibling preparation is essential, but other factors are equally important. These include how much parental attention the new arrival receives, how much attention the older child receives after the baby comes home, and how well the parents handle regressive or aggressive behavior.

For further information about sibling preparation, see Chapter 9.

Grandparents

The first relatives told about a pregnancy are usually the grandparents. Often, the expectant grandparents become increasingly supportive of the couple, even if conflicts previously existed. But it can be difficult for even sensitive grandparents to know how deeply to become involved in the childrearing process.

Younger grandparents leading active lives may not demonstrate as much interest as the young couple would like. In other cases, expectant grandparents may give advice and gifts unsparingly. For grandparents, conflict may be related to the expectant couple's need to feel in control of their own lives, or it may stem from events signalling changing roles in their own lives (for example, retirement, financial concerns, menopause, death of a friend). Some parents of expectant couples may already be grandparents with a developed style of grandparenting. This influences their response to the pregnancy.

Because childbearing and childrearing practices have changed, family cohesiveness is promoted by frank discussion between young couples and interested grandparents about the changes and the reasons for them. Effective communication between new parents and grandparents is important. Clarifying the role of the helping grandparent ensures a comfortable situation for all.

In some areas, classes for grandparents provide information about changes in birth and parenting practices. These classes help familiarize grandparents with new parents' needs and may offer suggestions for ways in which the grandparents can support the childbearing couple.

Cultural Values and Reproductive Behavior

A universal tendency exists to create ceremonial rituals and rites around important life events. Thus pregnancy, childbirth, marriage, and death are often tied to ritual.

The rituals, customs, and practices of a group are a reflection of the group's values. Thus the identification of cultural values is useful in predicting reactions to pregnancy. An understanding of male and female roles, family lifestyles, religious values, or the meaning of children in a culture may explain reactions of joy or shame. Pregnancy is a joyful event in a culture that values children. In some cultures, however, pregnancy is a shameful event if it occurs outside of marriage.

Health values and beliefs are also important in understanding reactions and behavior. Certain behaviors can be expected if a culture views pregnancy as a sickness, whereas other behaviors can be expected if the culture views pregnancy as a natural occurrence. Prenatal care may not be a priority for women who view pregnancy as a natural phenomenon or for women challenged by financial constraints.

Generalization about cultural characteristics or values is difficult because not every individual in a culture may display these characteristics. Just as variations are seen between cultures, variations are also seen within cultures. For example, because of their exposure to the American culture, a third-generation Chinese-American family might have very different values and beliefs from those of a Chinese family who has recently immigrated to America. For this reason, the nurse needs to supplement a general knowledge of cultural values and practices with a complete assessment of the individual's values and practices.

The meaning assigned to childbearing may vary from culture to culture. For example, children can improve the social standing of the traditional Chinese family; a woman who gives birth, especially to a son, achieves higher status. Similarly, in the western United States, people of the Mormon faith view motherhood as the most important aspect of a woman's life, comparable to the male role of priesthood (Conley 1990). In traditional Mexican-American families, having children may be seen as proving the male's manliness, or *machismo,* a desired trait among many Mexican-American men.

Health Beliefs

Although many cultures view pregnancy as a natural occurrence, it may also be seen as a time of increased vulnerability. Individuals with European/Western ideas might expect the woman to be away from work before and right after childbirth. Individuals of many cultures take certain protective precautions based on their beliefs. For example, many Southeast Asian women fear that they will have a complicated labor and birth if they sit in a doorway or on a step. Thus they tend to avoid areas near doors in waiting rooms and examining rooms. Similarly, many Hmong women fear that sharp instruments may cause cleft lip or abortion. Consequently they avoid contact with knives or scissors during pregnancy (Mattson 1995). Many Vietnamese and Laotian women believe that overeating or inactivity during pregnancy leads to a difficult labor (Lee 1989). In the Mexican-American culture, the concept of *mal aire,* or bad air, is sometimes related to evil spirits. It is thought that air, especially night air, may enter the body and cause harm. For many Southeast Asians, "wind" represents a bad external influence that may enter a person when the body is vulnerable, such as during and after childbirth (Mattson 1995).

Most of the taboos stemming from the belief in evil spirits are grounded in fear of injuring the unborn child. Taboos also arise from the belief that a pregnant woman has evil powers. For this reason, pregnant women are sometimes prohibited from taking part in certain activities with other people.

The equilibrium model of health is based on the concept of balance between light and dark, heat and cold. Eastern philosophical belief focuses on the notion of yin and yang. Yin represents the female, passive principle—darkness, cold, wetness—while yang is the masculine, active principle—light, heat, and dryness. When the two are combined, they are all that can be. The hot-cold classification is seen in cultures in Latin America, the Near East, and Asia.

Mexican-Americans may consider illness to be an excess of either hot or cold. To restore health, imbalances are often corrected by the proper use of foods, medications, or herbs. These substances are also classified as hot or cold. For example, an illness attributed to an excess of cold will be treated only with hot foods or medications. Similarly, women of Hispanic background may consider the third trimester of pregnancy as hot, and they may prefer to avoid hot foods during this time (Andrews 1989). The classification of foods is not always consistent but it does conform to a general structure of traditional knowledge. Certain foods, spices, herbs, and medications are perceived to cool or heat the body. These perceptions do not necessarily correspond to the actual temperature; some hot dishes are said to have a cooling quality.

Southeast Asians believe it is important to keep the woman "warm" after birth, because blood, which is considered "hot," has been lost, and the woman is at risk of becoming "cold." Therefore they avoid cold drinks and food following birth (Mattson and Lew 1992). Some Hindu women, on the other hand, consider pregnancy a hot period and eat "cool" foods to balance the hot state (Wollett and Dosanjh-Matwala 1990).

The concepts of hot and cold are not as important in Native-American or African-American beliefs. There are some similarities, however, in all of these groups because of their emphasis on a balance in nature.

Health Practices

Health care practices during pregnancy are influenced by numerous factors, such as the prevalence of traditional home remedies and folk beliefs, the importance of indigenous healers, and the influence of professional health care workers. In an urban setting, the age, length of time in the city, marital status, and strength of the family may affect these patterns. Socioeconomic status is also important, since modern medical services are more accessible to those who can afford them.

An awareness of alternative health sources is crucial for health professionals, since these practices affect health outcomes. Often, for example, in the traditional Mexican-American culture, mothers are influenced by familism and will seek and follow the advice of their mothers or older women in the childbearing period.

Indigenous healers are also important to specific cultures. In the Mexican-American culture, the healer is called a *curandero* or *curandera.* In some Native American tribes, the medicine man or woman may fulfill the healing role. Herbalists are often found in Asian cultures, and faith healers, root doctors, and spiritualists are sometimes consulted by members of some African cultures.

Cultural Factors and Nursing Care

Health care providers are often unaware of the cultural characteristics they themselves demonstrate. Without cultural awareness, caregivers tend to project their own cultural responses onto foreign-born clients; clients from different socioeconomic, religious, or educational groups; or clients from different regions of the country. This leads the caregiver to assume that the clients are demonstrating a specific behavior for the same reason that they themselves would. For example, health care providers sometimes label a pregnant or postpartum Filipina as "lazy" because of her rather sedentary lifestyle. In reality, this results from the cultural belief that inactivity is necessary to protect the mother and child (Stern et al 1985). If health care providers fail to understand the reasons for a person's behavior, it is impossible for them to intervene appropriately and ensure cooperation.

To a certain extent, all of us are guilty of ethnocentrism at least some of the time. **Ethnocentrism** is the conviction that the values and beliefs of one's own cultural group are the best or only acceptable ones. It is characterized by an inability to understand the beliefs and world view of another culture (Eliason 1993). Thus the nurse who values stoicism during labor may be uncomfortable with the more vocal response of some Latin American women. Another nurse may be disconcerted by a Southeast Asian woman who believes that pain is something to be endured rather than alleviated and is intent on maintaining self-control in labor (Mattson and Lew 1992).

Cultural assessment is an important aspect of prenatal care. Health care professionals are becoming increasingly aware that they must address cultural needs in the prenatal assessment to provide culturally sensitive health care during pregnancy. The nurse needs to identify the prospective parents' main beliefs, values, and behaviors related to pregnancy and childbearing. This includes information about ethnic background, amount of affiliation with the ethnic group, patterns of decision making, religious preference, language, communication style, and common etiquette practices (Tripp-Reimer et al 1984). The nurse can also explore the woman's (or family's) expectations of the health care system.

In planning care, the nurse considers the extent to which the woman's personal values, beliefs, and customs are in accord with the values, beliefs, and customs of the woman's identified cultural group, the nurse providing care, and the health care agency. If discrepancies exist, the nurse then considers whether the woman's system is supportive, neutral, or harmful in relation to possible interventions (Tripp-Reimer et al 1984). If the woman's system is supportive or neutral, it can be incorporated into the plan. For example, individual food practices or methods of pain expression may differ from those of the nurse or agency but would not necessarily interfere with the nursing plan. On the other hand, certain cultural practices might pose a threat to the health of the childbearing woman. For example, some Filipinas will not take any medication during pregnancy. The health care provider may consider a certain medication essential to the woman's well-being. In this case, the woman's cultural belief may be detrimental to her own health. The nurse and client must carefully discuss the reasons for her refusal. After discussing and understanding the reasons, the nurse faces three possible outcomes: (a) identifying ways to persuade the woman to accept the proposed medication; (b) accepting the woman's decision to refuse the medication; or (c) explaining alternate therapies that might be acceptable to the woman in light of her cultural beliefs.

Key Facts to Remember: Providing Effective Prenatal Care to Families of Different Cultures (on the next page) summarizes the key actions a nurse can take to become more culturally aware.

KEY FACTS TO REMEMBER

Providing Effective Prenatal Care to Families of Different Cultures

Nurses who are interacting with expectant families from a different culture or ethnic group can provide more effective, culturally sensitive nursing care by:

- Critically examining their own cultural beliefs
- Identifying personal biases, attitudes, stereotypes, and prejudices
- Making a conscious commitment to respect the values and beliefs of others
- Using sensitive, current language when describing their culture
- Learning the rituals, customs, and practices of the major cultural and ethnic groups with whom they have contact
- Including cultural assessment and assessment of the family's expectations of the health care system as a routine part of prenatal nursing care
- Incorporating the family's cultural practices into prenatal care as much as possible
- Fostering an attitude of respect for and cooperation with alternative healers and caregivers whenever possible
- Providing for the services of an interpreter if language barriers exist
- Learning the language (or at least several key phrases) of at least one of the cultural groups with whom they interact
- Recognizing that ultimately it is the woman's right to make her own health care choices
- Evaluating whether the client's health care beliefs have any potential negative consequences for her health

CHAPTER HIGHLIGHTS

- Virtually all systems of a woman's body are altered in some way during pregnancy.
- Blood pressure decreases slightly during pregnancy. It reaches its lowest point in the second trimester and gradually increases to near normal levels in the third trimester.
- The enlarging uterus may cause pressure on the vena cava when the woman lies supine. This is called the vena caval syndrome.
- A physiologic anemia may occur during pregnancy because the total plasma volume increases more than the total number of erythrocytes. This produces a drop in the hematocrit.
- The glomerular filtration rate increases somewhat during pregnancy. Glycosuria may be caused by the body's inability to reabsorb all the glucose filtered by the glomeruli.
- Changes in the skin include the development of chloasma; linea nigra; darkened nipples, areola, and vulva; striae; and spider nevi.
- Insulin needs increase during pregnancy. A woman with a latent deficiency state may respond to the increased stress on the islets of Langerhans by developing gestational diabetes.
- The subjective (presumptive) signs of pregnancy are symptoms experienced and reported by the woman, such as amenorrhea, nausea and vomiting, fatigue, urinary frequency, breast changes, and quickening.
- The objective (probable) signs of pregnancy can be perceived by the examiner but may be caused by conditions other than pregnancy.
- The diagnostic (positive) signs of pregnancy can be perceived by the examiner and can be caused only by pregnancy.
- During pregnancy, the expectant woman may experience ambivalence, acceptance, introversion, emotional lability, and changes in body image.
- Rubin (1984) has identified four developmental tasks for the pregnant woman: (1) ensuring safe passage through pregnancy, labor, and birth; (2) seeking acceptance of this child by others; (3) seeking commitment and acceptance of herself as mother to the infant; and (4) learning to give of oneself on behalf of one's child.
- The father faces a series of adjustments as he accepts his new role. The father must deal with the reality of pregnancy, gain recognition as a parent, and confront and resolve any personal conflicts about the fathering he himself received.
- Siblings of all ages require assistance in dealing with the birth of a new baby.
- Cultural values, beliefs, and behaviors influence a family's response to childbearing and the health care system.
- Ethnocentrism is the belief that one's own cultural beliefs, values, and practices are the best ones, indeed the only ones worth considering.
- A cultural assessment does not have to be exhaustive, but it should focus on factors that will influence the practices of the childbearing family with regard to their health needs.

REFERENCES

Andrews MA: Culture and nutrition. In: *Transcultural Concepts in Nursing Care.* Boyle JS, Andrews MM (editors). Glenview, IL: Scott, Foresman, 1989.

Blackburn ST, Loper DL: *Maternal, Fetal, and Neonatal Physiology: A Clinical Perspective.* Philadelphia: Saunders, 1992.

Buster JE, Carson SA: Endocrinology and diagnosis of pregnancy. In: *Obstetrics: Normal and Problem Pregnancies,* 3rd ed. Gabbe SG et al (editors). New York: Churchill-Livingstone, 1996.

Conley LJ: Childbearing and childrearing practices in Mormonism. *Neonatal Network* October 1990; 9(3):41.

Cruikshank DP, Wigton TR, Hays PM: Maternal physiology in pregnancy. In: *Obstetrics: Normal and Problem Pregnancies,* 3rd ed. Gabbe SG et al (editors). New York: Churchill-Livingstone, 1996.

Cunningham FG et al: *Williams Obstetrics,* 20th ed. Stamford, CT: Appleton & Lange, 1997.

Eliason MJ: Ethics and transcultural nursing care. *Nurs Outlook* September/October 1993; 41(5):225.

Fishbein EG: Expectant father's stress—Due to mother's expectations? *JOGNN* September/October 1984; 13:325.

Institute of Medicine, National Academy of Sciences, Food and Nutrition Board: *Nutrition During Pregnancy: Part 1. Weight Gain.* Washington, DC: National Academy Press, 1990.

Jordan PL: Laboring for relevance: Expectant and new fatherhood. *Nurs Res* January/February 1990; 39:11.

Lederman RP: *Psychosocial Adaptation in Pregnancy,* 2nd ed. New York: Springer, 1996.

Lee RV: Understanding Southeast Asian mothers-to-be. *Childbirth Educator* Spring 1989; p. 32.

Longobucco DC, Freston MS: Relation of somatic symptoms to degree of paternal-role preparation of first-time expectant fathers. *JOGNN* November/December 1989; 18:482.

Mattson S: Culturally sensitive perinatal care for Southeast Asians. *JOGNN* May 1995; 24(4):335.

Mattson S, Lew L: Culturally sensitive prenatal care for Southeast Asians. *JOGNN* 1992; 21(1):48.

Mercer RT: *Becoming a Mother.* New York: Springer, 1995.

Patterson ET et al: Seeking safe passage: Utilizing health care during pregnancy. *Image* Spring 1990; 22(1):27.

Robinson GE, Stewart DE: Motivation for motherhood and the experience of pregnancy. *Can J Psychiatry* December 1990; 34:861.

Rubin R: *Maternal Identity and the Maternal Experience.* New York: Springer, 1984.

Stern PN et al: Culturally induced stress during childbearing: The Philippine-American experience. *Health Care Women Int* 1985; 6:105.

Tripp-Reimer T et al: Cultural assessment: Content and process. *Nurs Outlook* March/April 1984; 32:78.

Wollett A, Dosanjh-Matwala N: Pregnancy and antenatal care: The attitudes and experiences of Asian women. *Child Care Health Dev* 1990; 16:63.

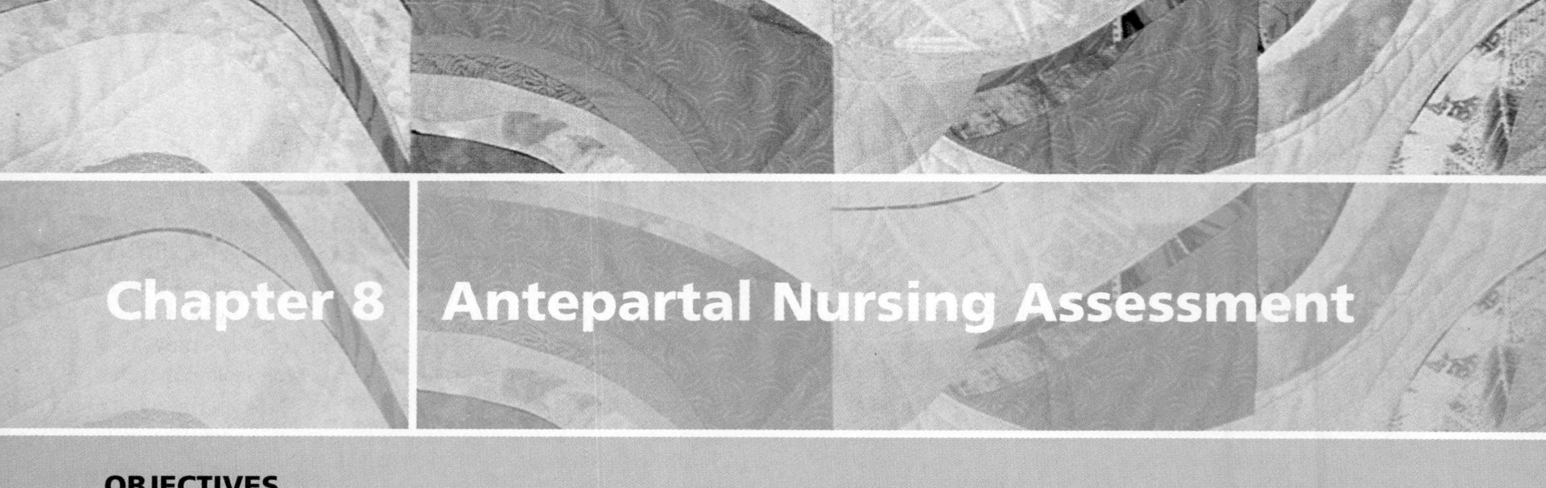

Chapter 8 Antepartal Nursing Assessment

OBJECTIVES

- Summarize the essential components of a prenatal history.
- Define the common obstetric terminology found in the history of a maternity client.
- Identify factors related to the father's health that should be recorded on the prenatal record.
- Describe areas that should be evaluated as part of the initial assessment of psychosocial and cultural factors related to a woman's pregnancy.
- Describe the normal physiologic changes one would expect to find when performing a physical assessment of a pregnant woman.
- Compare the methods most commonly used to determine the estimated date of birth.
- Develop an outline of the essential measurements that can be determined by clinical pelvimetry.
- Delineate the possible causes of the danger signs of pregnancy.
- Relate the components of the subsequent prenatal history and assessment to the progress of pregnancy.

KEY TERMS

Abortion
Antepartum
Diagonal conjugate
Estimated date of birth (EDB)
Gestation
Gravida
Intrapartum
Multigravida
Multipara
Nägele's rule
Nulligravida
Nullipara
Obstetric conjugate
Para
Postpartum
Postterm labor
Preterm or premature labor
Primigravida
Primipara
Risk factors
Stillbirth
Term

Today nurses are assuming a more important role in prenatal care, particularly in the area of assessment. The certified nurse-midwife has the education and skill to perform full and complete prenatal assessments. The nurse practitioner may share the assessment responsibilities with a physician. An office nurse, whose primary role may be to counsel and meet the psychologic needs of the expectant family, performs assessments in those areas.

An environment of comfort and open communication should be established with each antepartal visit. The nurse conveys concern for the woman as an individual and is available to listen and discuss the woman's concerns and desires. A supportive atmosphere, coupled with the information found in the physical and psychosocial assessment guides in this chapter, will help the nurse identify needed areas of education and counseling.

Initial Client History

The course of a pregnancy depends on a number of factors, including the prepregnancy health of the woman, presence of disease states, emotional status, and past health care. Ideally, health care before the advent of pregnancy has been adequate, and antenatal care will be a continuation of that established care. One important method of determining the adequacy of a woman's prepregnancy care is a thorough history.

Definition of Terms

The following terms are used in recording the history of maternity clients:

Gestation: the number of weeks since the first day of the last menstrual period (LMP).

Abortion: birth that occurs before the end of 20 weeks' gestation.

Term: the normal duration of pregnancy (38 to 42 weeks' gestation).

Preterm or premature labor: labor that occurs after 20 weeks but before completion of 37 weeks' gestation.

Postterm labor: labor that occurs after 42 weeks' gestation.

Antepartum: time between conception and the onset of labor; usually used to describe the period during which a woman is pregnant; used interchangeably with *prenatal.*

Intrapartum: time from the onset of true labor until the birth of the infant and placenta.

Postpartum: time from birth until the woman's body returns to an essentially prepregnant condition.

Gravida: any pregnancy, regardless of duration, including present pregnancy.

Nulligravida: a woman who has never been pregnant.

Primigravida: a woman who is pregnant for the first time.

Multigravida: a woman who is in her second or any subsequent pregnancy.

Para: birth after 20 weeks' gestation regardless of whether the infant is born alive or dead.

Nullipara: a woman who has not given birth at more than 20 weeks' gestation.

Primipara: a woman who has had one birth at more than 20 weeks' gestation, regardless of whether the infant was born alive or dead.

Multipara: a woman who has had two or more births at more than 20 weeks' gestation.

Stillbirth: an infant born dead after 20 weeks' gestation.

The terms *gravida* and *para* are used in relation to pregnancies, not to the number of fetuses. Thus twins, triplets, and so forth count as one pregnancy and one birth.

The following examples illustrate how these terms are applied in clinical situations:

1. Jean Smith has one child born at 38 weeks and is pregnant for the second time. At her initial prenatal visit, the nurse indicates her obstetric history as "gravida 2 para 1 ab 0." Jean Smith's present pregnancy terminates at 16 weeks' gestation. She is now "gravida 2 para 1 ab 1."
2. Sue Sanchez is pregnant for the fourth time. She has a child born at 35 weeks at home. One pregnancy ended at 10 weeks' gestation, and she gave birth to another infant stillborn at term. At her prenatal assessment the nurse records her obstetric history as "gravida 4 para 2 ab 1."

To provide more comprehensive data, a more detailed approach is used in some settings. Using the detailed system, *gravida* keeps the same meaning, while *para* changes to mean the number of infants born rather than the number of deliveries. A useful acronym for remembering the system is TPAL:

T: number of *term* infants born; that is, the number of infants born after 37 weeks' gestation or more.

P: number of *preterm* infants born; that is, the number of infants born after 20 weeks' but before the completion of 37 weeks' gestation.

A: number of pregnancies ending in either spontaneous or therapeutic *abortion.*

L: number of currently *living* children.

Name	Gravida	Term	Preterm	Abort	Living Child
Jean Smith	2	1	0	0	1
Sue Sanchez	4	1	1	1	1

FIGURE 8–1 The TPAL approach provides more detailed information about the woman's pregnancy history.

Using this approach, the nurse would have described Jean Smith (see the first example above) initially as "gravida 2 para 1001." Following her spontaneous abortion she would be "gravida 2 para 1011." Sue Sanchez would be described as "gravida 4 para 1111." (Figure 8–1 illustrates this method.)

Client Profile

The history is essentially a screening tool that identifies factors that may negatively affect the course of a pregnancy. The following information should be obtained for each maternity client at the first prenatal assessment:

1. Current pregnancy
   - First day of last normal menstrual period (LMP)
   - Presence of cramping, bleeding, or spotting since LMP
   - Woman's opinion about when conception occurred and when infant is due
   - Woman's attitude toward pregnancy (Is this pregnancy planned? Wanted?)
   - Results of pregnancy tests, if completed
   - Any discomforts since LMP such as nausea, vomiting, and frequency of these
2. Past pregnancies
   - Number of pregnancies
   - Number of abortions, spontaneous or induced
   - Number of living children
   - History of previous pregnancies; length of pregnancy; length of labor and birth; type of birth (vaginal, forceps or silastic cup, cesarean, etc); type of anesthesia used, if any; woman's perception of the experience; complications (antepartal, intrapartal, postpartal)
   - Perinatal status of previous children: Apgar scores, birth weights, general development, complications, feeding patterns
   - Blood type and Rh factor (if negative, medication after birth to prevent sensitization)
   - Prenatal education classes, resources (books)
3. Gynecologic history
   - Date of last Pap smear; any history of abnormal Pap smear
   - Previous infections: vaginal, cervical, sexually transmitted
   - Previous surgery
   - Age at menarche
   - Regularity, frequency, and duration of menstrual flow
   - History of dysmenorrhea
   - Contraceptive history (If birth control pills were used, did pregnancy occur immediately following cessation of pills? If not, how long after?)
   - Sexual history
4. Current medical history
   - Weight
   - Blood type and Rh factor, if known
   - General health including nutrition, normal dietary practices, regular exercise program (type, frequency, duration)
   - Any medications presently being taken (including nonprescription medications) or taken since the onset of pregnancy
   - Previous or present use of alcohol, tobacco, or caffeine (Ask specifically about the amounts of alcohol, cigarettes, and caffeine consumed each day)
   - Illicit drug use or abuse (Ask about specific drugs such as cocaine, crack, marijuana)
   - Drug allergies and other allergies
   - Potential teratogenic insults to this pregnancy (such as viral infections; medications; x-ray examinations; surgery; or cats in the home, which may be a source of toxoplasmosis)
   - Presence of disease conditions such as diabetes, hypertension, cardiovascular disease, renal problems, thyroid disorders
   - Record of immunizations (especially rubella)
   - Presence of any abnormal symptoms
5. Past medical history
   - Childhood diseases
   - Past treatment for any disease condition: Any hospitalizations? History of hepatitis? Rheumatic fever? Pyelonephritis?

- Surgical procedures
- Presence of bleeding disorders or tendencies (Has she received blood transfusions?)

6. Family medical history
   - Presence of diabetes, cardiovascular disease, hypertension, hematologic disorders, tuberculosis, preeclampsia-eclampsia (pregnancy-induced hypertension)
   - Occurrence of multiple births
   - History of congenital diseases or deformities
   - Occurrence of cesarean births
7. Religious/cultural history
   - Does the woman wish to specify a religious preference on her chart? Does she have any religious beliefs or practices that might influence her health care or that of her child, such as prohibition against receiving blood products, dietary considerations, circumcision rites?
   - Are there practices in her culture or that of her partner that might influence her care or that of her child?
8. Occupational history
   - Occupation
   - Does she stand all day, or are there opportunities to sit and elevate her legs? Any heavy lifting?
   - Exposure to harmful substances
   - Opportunity for regular lunch, breaks for nutritious snacks
   - Provision for maternity leave
9. Partner's history
   - Presence of genetic conditions or diseases
   - Age
   - Significant health problems
   - Previous or present alcohol intake, drug or tobacco use
   - Blood type and Rh factor
   - Occupation
   - Educational level
   - Attitude toward the pregnancy
10. Personal information
    - Age
    - Educational level
    - Acceptance of pregnancy
    - Race or ethnic group (to identify need for prenatal genetic screening or counseling)
    - Stability of living conditions
    - Economic level
    - Housing
    - Any history of emotional or physical deprivation (herself or children)
    - History of emotional problems
    - Support systems
    - Personal preferences about the birth (expectations of both the woman and her partner, presence of others, and so on)
    - Plans for care of child following birth
    - Overuse or underuse of health care system

Obtaining Data

A questionnaire is used in many instances to obtain information. The woman should complete the questionnaire in a quiet place with a minimum of distractions.

The nurse can obtain further information in a direct interview, which allows the pregnant woman to expand or clarify her responses to questions, and gives the nurse and client the opportunity to begin developing a good relationship.

The expectant father should be encouraged to attend the prenatal examinations. He is often able to contribute information to the history and may use the opportunity to ask questions or express concerns that are of particular importance to him.

Prenatal High-Risk Screening

Risk factors are any findings that suggest the pregnancy may have a negative outcome, either for the woman or her unborn child. Screening for risk factors is an important part of the prenatal assessment.

Many risk factors can be identified during the initial prenatal assessment; others may be detected during subsequent prenatal visits. It is important to identify high-risk pregnancies early so that appropriate interventions can be started immediately. Not all high-risk factors threaten the pregnancy equally; thus many agencies use a risk scoring sheet to determine the degree of risk. Information must be updated throughout pregnancy as necessary. It is always possible that a pregnancy may begin as low-risk and change to high-risk because of complications.

Table 8–1 identifies the major risk factors currently recognized. The table also identifies maternal and fetal/newborn implications if the risk is present in the pregnancy.

Text continues on page 176

TABLE 8–1 Prenatal High-Risk Factors

Factor	Maternal Implications	Fetal/Neonatal Implications
Social-Personal		
Low income level and/or low educational level	Poor antenatal care Poor nutrition ↑ risk of preeclampsia	Low birth weight Intrauterine growth retardation (IUGR)
Poor diet	Inadequate nutrition ↑ risk anemia ↑ risk preeclampsia	Fetal malnutrition Prematurity
Living at high altitude	↑ hemoglobin	Prematurity IUGR
Multiparity > 3	↑ risk antepartum/postpartum hemorrhage	Anemia Fetal death
Weight < 45.5 kg (100 lb)	Poor nutrition Cephalopelvic disproportion Prolonged labor	IUGR Hypoxia associated with difficult labor and birth
Weight > 91 kg (200 lb)	↑ risk hypertension ↑ risk cephalopelvic disproportion	↓ fetal nutrition
Age < 16	Poor nutrition Poor antenatal care ↑ risk preeclampsia ↑ risk cephalopelvic disproportion	Low birth weight ↑ fetal demise
Age > 35	↑ risk preeclampsia ↑ risk cesarean birth	↑ risk congenital anomalies ↑ chromosomal aberrations
Smoking one pack/day or more	↑ risk hypertension ↑ risk cancer	↓ placental perfusion → ↓ 0_2 and nutrients available Low birth weight IUGR Preterm birth
Use of addicting drugs	↑ risk poor nutrition ↑ risk of infection with IV drugs	↑ risk congenital anomalies ↑ risk low birth weight Neonatal withdrawal Lower serum bilirubin
Excessive alcohol consumption	↑ risk poor nutrition Possible hepatic effects with long-term consumption	↑ risk fetal alcohol syndrome
Preexisting Medical Disorders		
Diabetes mellitus	↑ risk preeclampsia, hypertension Episodes of hypoglycemia and hyperglycemia ↑ risk cesarean birth	Low birth weight Macrosomia Neonatal hypoglycemia ↑ risk congenital anomalies ↑ risk respiratory distress syndrome
Cardiac disease	Cardiac decompensation Further strain on mother's body ↑ maternal death rate	↑ risk fetal demise ↑ perinatal mortality
Anemia: hemoglobin < 9 g/dL (White) < 29% hematocrit (White) < 8.2 g/dL hemoglobin (Black) < 26% hematocrit (Black)	Iron deficiency anemia Low energy level Decreased oxygen-carrying capacity	Fetal death Prematurity Low birth weight
Hypertension	↑ vasospasm ↑ risk CNS irritability → convulsions ↑ risk CVA ↑ risk renal damage	↓ placental perfusion → low birth weight Preterm birth
Thyroid disorder Hypothyroidism	↑ infertility ↓ BMR, goiter, myxedema	↑ spontaneous abortion ↑ risk congenital goiter Mental retardation → cretinism ↑ incidence congenital anomalies

TABLE 8–1 continued

Factor	Maternal Implications	Fetal/Neonatal Implications
Preexisting Medical Disorders *continued*		
Thyroid disorder *continued*		
Hyperthyroidism	↑ risk postpartum hemorrhage ↑ risk preeclampsia Danger of thyroid storm	↑ incidence preterm birth ↑ tendency to thyrotoxicosis
Renal disease (moderate to severe)	↑ risk renal failure	↑ risk IUGR ↑ risk preterm birth
DES exposure	↑ infertility, spontaneous abortion ↑ cervical incompetence	↑ spontaneous abortion ↑ risk preterm birth
Obstetric Considerations		
Previous Pregnancy		
Stillborn	↑ emotional/psychologic distress	↑ risk IUGR ↑ risk preterm birth
Habitual abortion	↑ emotional/psychologic distress ↑ possibility diagnostic workup	↑ risk abortion
Cesarean birth	↑ possibility repeat cesarean birth	↑ risk preterm birth ↑ risk respiratory distress
Rh or blood group sensitization	↑ financial expenditure for testing	Hydrops fetalis Icterus gravis Neonatal anemia Kernicterus Hypoglycemia
Large baby	↑ risk cesarean birth ↑ risk gestational diabetes	Birth injury Hypoglycemia
Current Pregnancy		
Rubella (first trimester)		Congenital heart disease Cataracts Nerve deafness Bone lesions Prolonged virus shedding
Rubella (second trimester)		Hepatitis Thrombocytopenia
Cytomegalovirus		IUGR Encephalopathy
Herpesvirus type 2	Severe discomfort Concern about possibility of cesarean birth, fetal infection	Neonatal herpesvirus type 2 2° hepatitis with jaundice Neurologic abnormalities
Syphilis	↑ incidence abortion	↑ fetal demise Congenital syphilis
Abruptio placenta and placenta previa	↑ risk hemorrhage Bed rest Extended hospitalization	Fetal/neonatal anemia Intrauterine hemorrhage ↑ fetal demise
Preeclampsia/eclampsia (PIH)	See hypertension	↓ placental perfusion → low birth weight
Multiple gestation	↑ risk postpartum hemorrhage	↑ risk preterm birth ↑ risk fetal demise
Elevated hematocrit > 41% (White) > 38% (Black)	Increased viscosity of blood	Fetal death rate 5 times normal rate
Spontaneous premature rupture of membranes	↑ uterine infection	↑ risk preterm birth ↑ fetal demise

COMMUNITY IN FOCUS Baby Network

The Baby Network in Clarement, New Hampshire, is an example of the success that can result when a multidisciplinary group of health care and human service professionals works together to address a community need. Although Clarement is a small community, it has many resources available to address the health needs of pregnant women and their families. However, before Baby Network began, there was no established method for coordinating services for all women.

In 1994, representatives from Valley Regional Hospital, Planned Parenthood, several Physician offices, Connecticut Valley Home Care, University of New Hampshire Cooperative Extension, WIC, and support programs such as Early Interventions and Good Beginnings met to plan an approach that would provide comprehensive, fully integrated care for the childbearing family including prenatal care and education, inpatient services, post-birth care, and parenting support. The outcomes included a common mission and goal setting among the various providers and a commitment to monthly meetings for ongoing collaboration. The Baby Network supports a case management model of care delivery to coordinate all resources.

When a pregnancy is diagnosed, either in a physician's office or the prenatal clinic, a care manager from Valley Regional Hospital or Planned Parenthood's Prenatal Program is assigned to the woman. The care manager, an experienced, specially trained maternal-child health nurse, conducts an initial assessment interview, usually at the woman's second prenatal visit, and assigns the woman to one of four categories:

1. No need for further care management because of very low risk, adequate support and knowledge
2. 4–8 visit plan will be started
3. Multiple high-risk parameters warrant an extended visit plan as the need presents
4. Future consultations are refused by the woman

The majority of primigravidas fall into category 2.

The care manager follows a standard protocol of nutritional guidance, general health maintenance, education, psychosocial interventions, and community referrals throughout the pregnancy, tailoring the care plan as necessary when unique concerns or problems arise. The care manager works closely with the woman and her family as well as the physicians and clinic staff to address needs. Community referrals and connections to parent support agencies such as Good Beginnings or WIC are part of the philosophy of continuity of care and "wrapping" of services around the family.

Because of the integration of Connecticut Valley Home Care, the care managers can offer skilled nursing home visits as part of the service they provide, thereby decreasing the need for more expensive inpatient care for needs such as mild pregnancy-induced hypertension monitoring, glucose control for diabetics, and IV hydration therapy. The care managers make daily rounds in the LDRP unit, have case conferences as needed, and complete a summary for the acute care team so that they are also familiar with the woman and her family prior to admission. When the woman is admitted for labor, the acute care team notifies the care manager so that postpartum plans can be finalized. The care manager completes maternal-newborn home assessments and provides skilled, in-home nursing care if necessary. In addition, for the three months following birth, a Good Beginnings volunteer is available to provide additional family support.

Baby Network continues to develop as the members explore new, creative ways of enhancing the provision of health services to improve pregnancy outcomes and ensure a consistent high quality of care for childbearing families. The program is making a difference to the people it serves and to the care providers working within it.

Source: Personal communication with Becky Gentes, RN, Maternal/Child Services Director for Valley Regional Healthcare, and printed materials.

Initial Antepartal Assessment

The antepartal assessment focuses on the woman holistically by considering physical, cultural, and psychosocial factors that influence her health. At the initial visit the woman may be concerned primarily with the diagnosis of pregnancy. However, during this visit she and her primary support person are also evaluating the health team she has chosen. The establishment of the nurse-client relationship will help the woman evaluate the health team and also provide the nurse with a basis for developing an atmosphere that is conducive to interviewing, support, and education. Because many women are excited and anxious at the first antepartal visit, the initial psychosocial-cultural assessment is general.

As part of the initial psychosocial-cultural assessment, the nurse discusses with the woman any religious, cultural, or socioeconomic factors that influence the woman's expectations of the childbearing experience. It is especially helpful if the nurse is familiar with common practices of various religious and cultural groups who reside in the community. If the nurse gathers this data in a tactful, caring way, it can help make the childbearing woman's experience a positive one.

After obtaining the history, the nurse prepares the woman for the physical examination. The physical examination begins with assessment of vital signs, then the woman's body is examined. The pelvic examination is performed last.

Before the examination, the woman should provide a clean urine specimen. When her bladder is empty, the woman is more comfortable during the pelvic examination and the examiner can palpate the pelvic organs more easily. After emptying her bladder, the nurse asks the woman to disrobe and gives her a sheet or some other protective covering.

In a clinic or office setting, gowns and goggles are usually not necessary because splashing of body fluids is unlikely. Gloves should be worn for procedures that involve contact with body fluids such as drawing blood for lab work, handling urine specimens, or pelvic examinations (sterile gloves).

Increasing numbers of nurses, such as certified nurse-midwives and other nurses in advanced practice, are prepared to perform physical examinations. The nurse who has not yet fully developed specific assessment skills assesses the woman's vital signs, explains the procedures to allay apprehension, positions her for examination, and assists the examiner as necessary.

Each nurse is responsible for operating at the expected standard for someone with that individual nurse's skill and knowledge base.

Thoroughness and a systematic procedure are the most important considerations when performing the physical portion of an antepartal examination (see the Initial Prenatal Assessment Guide starting on p 178). To promote completeness, the Initial Prenatal Assessment Guide is organized in three columns that address the areas to be assessed (and normal findings), the variations or alterations that may be observed, and nursing responses to the data. The nurse should be aware that certain organs and systems are assessed concurrently with others during the physical portion of the examination.

Nursing interventions based on assessment of the normal physical and psychosocial changes, as well as the cultural influences associated with pregnancy and client teaching and counseling needs that have been mutually defined, are discussed further in Chapter 9.

Determination of Due Date

Childbearing families generally want to know the "due date," or the date around which childbirth will occur. Historically the due date has been called the estimated date of confinement (EDC). The concept of confinement is, however, rather negative, and there is a trend in the literature to avoid it by referring to the delivery date as the *EDD* or *estimated date of delivery.* Childbirth educators often stress that babies are not "delivered" like a package; they are *born.* In keeping with a view that emphasizes the normalcy of the process, this text refers to the due date as the **estimated date of birth (EDB).**

To calculate the EDB it is helpful to know the LMP. However, some women have episodes of irregular bleeding or fail to keep track of menstrual cycles. Thus other techniques also help to determine how far along a woman is in her pregnancy, that is, at how many weeks' gestation she is. Other techniques that can be used include evaluating uterine size, determining when quickening occurs, and auscultating fetal heart rate with a Doppler device and later a fetoscope.

Nägele's Rule

The most common method of determining the EDB is **Nägele's rule.** To use this method, one begins with the first day of the last menstrual period, subtracts 3 months, and adds 7 days. For example,

First day of LMP		November 21
Subtract 3 months	−	3 months
		August 21
Add 7 days	+	7 days
EDB		August 28

It is simpler to change the months to numeric terms:

November 21 becomes		11–21
Subtract 3 months	−	3
		8–21
Add 7 days	+	7
EDB		August 28

If a woman with a history of menses every 28 days remembers her LMP and was not taking oral contraceptives before becoming pregnant, Nägele's rule may be a fairly accurate determiner of her predicted birth date. However, if her cycle is irregular, or 35–40 days long, the time of ovulation may be delayed by several days. If she has been using oral contraceptives, ovulation may be delayed several weeks following her last menses. *Ovulation usually occurs 14 days before the onset of the next menses,* not 14 days after the previous menses. Thus the Nägele method, while helpful, is not foolproof. One study (Mittendorf et al 1990) found that the average length of gestation in uncomplicated pregnancies is longer than Nägele's rule suggests, especially for white primigravidas (+7 days). A gestation calculator or "wheel" permits the caregiver to calculate the EDB even more quickly (Figure 8–2).

Text continues on page 186

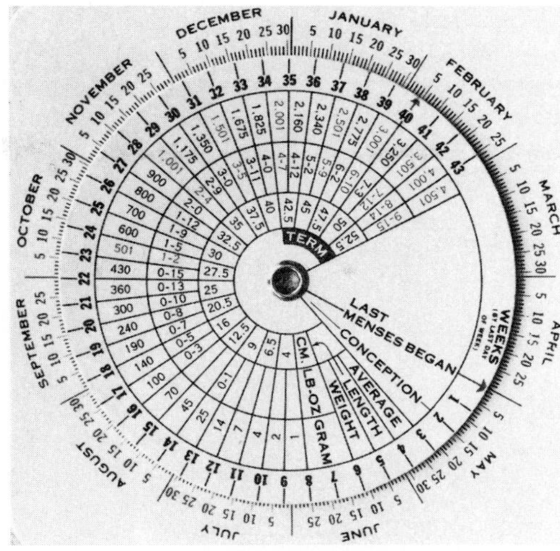

FIGURE 8–2 The EDB wheel can be used to calculate the due date. To use it, place the *last menses began* arrow on the date of the woman's LMP. Then read the EDB at the arrow labeled *40.* In this case the LMP is April 30 and the EDB is February 4.

INITIAL PRENATAL ASSESSMENT GUIDE

Physical Assessment/ Normal Findings	Alterations and Possible Causes*	Nursing Responses to Data[†]
Vital Signs		
Blood pressure (BP): 90–140/60–90	High BP (essential hypertension; renal disease; pregestational hypertension; apprehension or anxiety associated with pregnancy diagnosis, exam, or other crises; PIH if initial assessment not done until after 20 weeks' gestation)	BP > 140/90 requires immediate consideration; establish woman's BP; refer to physician if necessary. Assess woman's knowledge about high BP; counsel on self-care and medical management.
Pulse: 60–90 beats/min. Rate may increase 10 beats/min during pregnancy	Increased pulse rate (excitement or anxiety, cardiac disorders)	Count for 1 full minute; note irregularities.
Respiration: 16–24 breaths/min (or pulse rate divided by four). Pregnancy may induce a degree of hyperventilation; thoracic breathing predominant	Marked tachypnea or abnormal patterns	Assess for respiratory disease.
Temperature: 36.2–37.6C (98–99.6F)	Elevated temperature (infection)	Assess for infection process or disease state if temperature is elevated; refer to physician/CNM.
Weight		
Depends on body build	Weight < 45 kg (100 lb) or > 91 kg (200 lb); rapid, sudden weight gain (PIH)	Evaluate need for nutritional counseling; obtain information on eating habits, cooking practices, foods regularly eaten, income limitations, need for food supplements, pica and other abnormal food habits. Note initial weight to establish baseline for weight gain throughout pregnancy.
Skin		
Color: Consistent with racial background; pink nail beds	Pallor (anemia); bronze, yellow (hepatic disease, other causes of jaundice)	The following tests should be performed: complete blood count (CBC), bilirubin level, urinalysis, and blood urea nitrogen (BUN).
	Bluish, reddish, mottled; dusky appearance or pallor of palms and nail beds in dark-skinned women (anemia)	If abnormal, refer to physician.
Condition: Absence of edema (slight edema of lower extremities is normal during pregnancy)	Edema (PIH); rashes, dermatitis (allergic response)	Counsel on relief measures for slight edema. Initiate PIH assessment; refer to physician.
Lesions: Absence of lesions	Ulceration (varicose veins, decreased circulation)	Further assess circulatory status; refer to physician if lesion severe.
Spider nevi common in pregnancy	Petechiae, multiple bruises, ecchymosis (hemorrhagic disorders; abuse)	Evaluate for bleeding or clotting disorder. Provide oportunities to discuss abuse if suspected.
Moles	Change in size or color (carcinoma)	Refer to physician.

*Possible causes of alterations are placed in parentheses.

[†]This column provides guidelines for further assessment and initial nursing intervention.

INITIAL PRENATAL ASSESSMENT GUIDE continued

Physical Assessment/ Normal Findings	Alterations and Possible Causes*	Nursing Responses to Data†
Pigmentation: Pigmentation changes of pregnancy include linea nigra, striae gravidarum, chloasma		Assure woman that these are normal manifestations of pregnancy and explain the physiologic basis for the changes.
Café-au-lait spots	Six or more (Albright's syndrome or neurofibromatosis)	Consult with physician.
Nose		
Character of mucosa: Redder than oral mucosa; in pregnancy nasal mucosa is edematous in response to increased estrogen, resulting in nasal stuffiness and nosebleeds	Olfactory loss (first cranial nerve deficit)	Counsel woman about possible relief measures for nasal stuffiness and nosebleeds (epistaxis); refer to physician for olfactory loss.
Mouth		
May note hypertrophy of gingival tissue because of estrogen	Edema, inflammation (infection); pale in color (anemia)	Assess hematocrit for anemia; counsel regarding dental hygiene habits. Refer to physician or dentist if necessary. Routine dental care appropriate during pregnancy (no x-rays, no gas).
Neck		
Nodes: Small, mobile, nontender nodes	Tender, hard, fixed or prominent nodes (infection, carcinoma)	Examine for local infection; refer to physician.
Thyroid: Small, smooth, lateral lobes palpable on either side of trachea; slight hyperplasia by third month of pregnancy	Enlargement or nodule tenderness (hyperthyroidism)	Listen over thyroid for bruits, which may indicate hyperthyroidism. Question woman about dietary habits (iodine intake). Ascertain history of thyroid problems; refer to physician.
Chest and Lungs		
Chest: Symmetric, elliptical, smaller anteroposterior (A-P) than transverse diameter	Increased A-P diameter, funnel chest, pigeon chest (emphysema, asthma, chronic obstructive pulmonary disease [COPD])	Evaluate for emphysema, asthma, pulmonary disease (COPD).
Ribs: Slope downward from nipple line	More horizontal (COPD) Angular bumps Rachitic rosary (vitamin C deficiency)	Evaluate for COPD. Evaluate for fractures. Consult physician. Consult nutritionist.
Inspection and palpation: No retraction or bulging of intercostal spaces (ICS) during inspiration or expiration; symmetrical expansion	ICS retractions with inspiration, bulging with expiration; unequal expansion (respiratory disease)	Do thorough initial assessment. Refer to physician.
Tactile fremitus	Tachypnea, hyperpnea, Cheyne-Stokes respirations (respiratory disease)	Refer to physician.
Percussion: Bilateral symmetry in tone	Flatness of percussion, which may be affected by chest wall thickness	Evaluate for pleural effusions, consolidations, or tumor.

*Possible causes of alterations are placed in parentheses.

†This column provides guidelines for further assessment and initial nursing intervention.

INITIAL PRENATAL ASSESSMENT GUIDE continued

Physical Assessment/ Normal Findings	Alterations and Possible Causes*	Nursing Responses to Data†
Low-pitched resonance of moderate intensity	High diaphragm (atelectasis or paralysis), pleural effusion	Refer to physician.
Auscultation: Upper lobes: bronchovesicular sounds above sternum and scapulas; equal expiratory and inspiratory phases	Abnormal if heard over any other area of chest	Refer to physician.
Remainder of chest: vesicular breath sounds heard; inspiratory phase longer (3:1)	Rales, rhonchi, wheezes; pleural friction rub; absence of breath sounds; bronchophony, egophony, whispered pectoriloquy	Refer to physician.
Breasts		
Supple; symmetric in size and contour; darker pigmentation of nipple and areola; may have supernumerary nipples, usually 5–6 cm below normal nipple line	"Pigskin" or orange-peel appearance, nipple retractions, swelling, hardness (carcinoma); redness, heat, tenderness, cracked or fissured nipple (infection)	Encourage monthly self-breast checks; instruct woman how to examine own breasts.
Axillary nodes unpalpable or pellet sized	Tenderness, enlargement, hard node (carcinoma); may be visible bump (infection)	Refer to physician if evidence of inflammation.
Pregnancy changes: 1. Size increase noted primarily in first 20 weeks. 2. Become nodular. 3. Tingling sensation may be felt during first and third trimester; woman may report feeling of heaviness. 4. Pigmentation of nipples and areolas darkens. 5. Superficial veins dilate and become more prominent. 6. Striae seen in multiparas. 7. Tubercles of Montgomery enlarge. 8. Colostrum may be present after 12th week. 9. Secondary areola appears at 20 weeks, characterized by series of washed-out spots surrounding primary areola. 10. Breasts less firm, old striae may be present in multiparas.		Discuss normalcy of changes and their meaning with the woman. Teach and/or institute appropriate relief measures. Encourage use of supportive, well-fitting brassiere.
Heart		
Normal rate, rhythm, and heart sounds *Pregnancy changes:* 1. Palpitations may occur due to sympathetic nervous system disturbance.	Enlargement, thrills, thrusts, gross irregularity or skipped beats, gallop rhythm or extra sounds (cardiac disease)	Complete an initial assessment. Explain normalcy of pregnancy-induced changes. Refer to physician if indicated.

*Possible causes of alterations are placed in parentheses.

†This column provides guidelines for further assessment and initial nursing intervention.

INITIAL PRENATAL ASSESSMENT GUIDE continued

Physical Assessment/ Normal Findings	Alterations and Possible Causes*	Nursing Responses to Data†
2. Short systolic murmurs that ↑ in held expiration are normal due to increased volume.		
Abdomen		
Normal appearance, skin texture, and hair distribution; liver nonpalpable; abdomen nontender *Pregnancy changes:* 1. Purple striae may be present (or silver striae on a multipara) as well as linea nigra. 2. Diastasis of the rectus muscles late in pregnancy.	Muscle guarding (anxiety, acute tenderness); tenderness, mass (ectopic pregnancy, inflammation, carcinoma)	Assure client of normalcy of diastasis. Provide initial information about appropriate postpartum exercises. Evaluate client anxiety level. Refer to physician if indicated.
3. Size: Flat or rotund abdomen; progressive enlargement of uterus due to pregnancy. 10–12 weeks: Fundus slightly above symphysis pubis. 16 weeks: Fundus halfway between symphysis and umbilicus. *20–22 weeks:* Fundus at umbilicus. *28 weeks:* Fundus three finger breadths above umbilicus. *36 weeks:* Fundus just below ensiform cartilage.	Size of uterus inconsistent with length of gestation (intrauterine growth retardation [IUGR], multiple pregnancy, fetal demise, hydatidiform mole)	Reassess menstrual history regarding pregnancy dating. Evaluate increase in size using McDonald's method. Use ultrasound to establish diagnosis.
4. Fetal heartbeats: 120–160 beats/min may be heard with Doppler at 10–12 weeks' gestation; may be heard with fetoscope at 17–20 weeks.	Failure to hear fetal heartbeat with stethoscope after 17–20 weeks (fetal demise, hydatidiform mole)	Refer to physician. Administer pregnancy tests. Use ultrasound to establish diagnosis.
5. Fetal movement palpable by a trained examiner after the 18th week.	Failure to feel fetal movements after 20 weeks' gestation (fetal demise, hydatidiform mole)	Refer to physician for evaluation of fetal status.
6. Ballottement: During fourth to fifth month fetus rises and then rebounds to original position when uterus is tapped sharply.	No ballottement (oligohydramnios)	Refer to physician for evaluation of fetal status.
Extremities		
Skin warm, pulses palpable, full range of motion; may be some edema of hands and ankles in late pregnancy; varicose veins may become more pronounced; palmar erythema may be present.	Unpalpable or diminished pulses (arterial insufficiency); marked edema (PIH)	Evaluate for other symptoms of heart disease; initiate follow-up if woman mentions that her rings feel tight. Discuss prevention and self-treatment measures for varicose veins; refer to physician if indicated.

*Possible causes of alterations are placed in parentheses.

†This column provides guidelines for further assessment and initial nursing intervention.

INITIAL PRENATAL ASSESSMENT GUIDE continued

Physical Assessment/ Normal Findings	Alterations and Possible Causes*	Nursing Responses to Data†
Spine		
Normal spinal curves: Concave cervical, convex thoracic, concave lumbar	Abnormal spinal curves: flatness, kyphosis, lordosis	Refer to physician for assessment of cephalopelvic disproportion (CPD).
In pregnancy lumbar spinal curve may be accentuated	Backache	May have implications for administration of spinal anesthetics; see Chapter 9 for relief measures.
Shoulders and iliac crests should be even	Uneven shoulders and iliac crests (scoliosis)	Refer very young women to a physician; discuss back-stretching exercises with older women.
Reflexes		
Normal and symmetrical	Hyperactivity, clonus (PIH)	Evaluate for other symptoms of PIH.
Pelvic Area		
External female genitals: Normally formed with female hair distribution; in multiparas, labia majora loose and pigmented; urinary and vaginal orifices visible and appropriately located	Lesions, hematomas, varicosities, inflammation of Bartholin's glands; clitoral hypertrophy (masculinization)	Explain pelvic examination procedure (Procedure 5–1). Encourage woman to minimize her discomfort by relaxing her hips. Provide privacy.
Vagina: Pink or dark pink; vaginal discharge odorless, nonirritating; in multiparas, vaginal folds smooth and flattened; may have episiotomy scar	Abnormal discharge associated with vaginal infections	Obtain vaginal smear. Provide understandable verbal and written instructions about treatment for woman and partner, if indicated.
Cervix: Pink color; os closed except in multiparas, in whom os admits fingertip	Eversion, reddish erosion, Nabothian or retention cysts, cervical polyp; granular area that bleeds (carcinoma of cervix); lesions (herpes, human papilloma virus [HPV]) Presence of string or plastic tip from cervix (intrauterine device [IUD] in uterus)	Provide woman with a hand mirror and identify genital structures for her; encourage her to view her cervix if she wishes. Refer to physician if indicated. Advise woman of potential serious risks of leaving an IUD in place during pregnancy; refer to physician for removal.
Pregnancy changes:		
1–4 weeks' gestation: Enlargement in anteroposterior diameter	Absence of Goodell's sign (inflammatory conditions, carcinoma)	Refer to physician.
4–6 weeks' gestation: Softening of cervix (Goodell's sign), softening of isthmus of uterus (Hegar's sign); cervix takes on bluish coloring (Chadwick's sign)		
8–12 weeks' gestation: Vagina and cervix appear bluish-violet in color (Chadwick's sign)		
Uterus: Pear-shaped, mobile; smooth surface	Fixed (pelvic inflammatory disease [PID]); nodular surface (fibromas)	Refer to physician.
Ovaries: Small, walnut-shaped, nontender (ovaries and fallopian tubes are located in the adnexal areas)	Pain on movement of cervix (PID); enlarged or nodular ovaries (cyst, tumor, tubal pregnancy, corpus luteum of pregnancy)	Evaluate adnexal areas; refer to physician.

*Possible causes of alterations are placed in parentheses.

†This column provides guidelines for further assessment and initial nursing intervention.

INITIAL PRENATAL ASSESSMENT GUIDE continued

Physical Assessment/ Normal Findings	Alterations and Possible Causes*	Nursing Responses to Data†
Pelvic Measurements		
Internal measurements:	Measurement below normal	Vaginal birth may not be possible if deviations are present.
1. Diagonal conjugate at least 11.5 cm (Figure 8–5)		
2. Obstetric conjugate estimated by subtracting 1.5–2 cm from diagonal conjugate	Disproportion of pubic arch	
3. Inclination of sacrum	Abnormal curvature of sacrum	
4. Motility of coccyx; external intertuberosity diameter > 8 cm	Fixed or malposition of coccyx	
Anus and Rectum		
No lumps, rashes, excoriation, tenderness; cervix may be felt through rectal wall	Hemorrhoids, rectal prolapse; nodular lesion (carcinoma)	Counsel about appropriate prevention and relief measures; refer to physician for further evaluation.
Laboratory Evaluation		
Hemoglobin: 12–16 g/dL; women residing in high altitudes may have higher levels of hemoglobin	< 12 g/dL (anemia)	Note: Wear gloves when drawing blood. Hemoglobin < 12 g/dL requires nutritional counseling. < 11 g/dL requires iron supplementation.
ABO and Rh typing: Normal distribution of blood types	Rh negative	If Rh negative, check for presence of anti-Rh antibodies. Check partner's blood type; if partner is Rh positive, discuss with woman the need for antibody titers during pregnancy, management during the intrapartal period, and possible candidacy for RhIgG.
Complete blood count (CBC)		
Hematocrit: 38%–47%; physiologic anemia (pseudoanemia) may occur	Marked anemia or blood dyscrasias	Perform CBC and Schilling differential cell count.
Red blood cells (RBC): 4.2–5.4 million/μL		
White blood cells (WBC): 4500–11,000/μL	Presence of infection; may be elevated in pregnancy and with labor	Evaluate for other signs of infection.
Differential		
Neutrophils: 40%–60%		
Bands: up to 5%		
Eosinophils: 1%–3%		
Basophils: up to 1%		
Lymphocytes: 20%–40%		
Monocytes: 4%–8%		

*Possible causes of alterations are placed in parentheses.

†This column provides guidelines for further assessment and initial nursing intervention.

INITIAL PRENATAL ASSESSMENT GUIDE continued

Physical Assessment/ Normal Findings	Alterations and Possible Causes*	Nursing Responses to Data†
Syphilis tests—serologic test for syphilis (STS), complement fixation test, Venereal Disease Research Laboratory (VDRL) test—nonreactive	Positive reaction STS—tests may have 25%–45% incidence of biologic false-positive results; false results may occur in individuals who have acute viral or bacterial infections, hypersensitivity reactions, recent vaccinations, collagen disease, malaria, or tuberculosis.	Positive results may be confirmed with the fluorescent treponemal antibody absorption (FTA-ABS) tests; all tests for syphilis give positive results in the secondary stage of the disease; antibiotic tests may cause negative test results.
Gonorrhea culture: Negative	Positive	Refer for treatment.
Urinalysis (u/a): Normal color, specific gravity; pH 4.6–8.0	Abnormal color (porphyria, hemoglobinuria, bilirubinemia); alkaline urine (metabolic alkalemia, *Proteus* infection, old specimen)	Repeat u/a; refer to physician.
Negative for protein, red blood cells, white blood cells, casts	Positive findings (contaminated specimen, kidney disease)	Repeat u/a; refer to physician.
Glucose: Negative (small degree of glycosuria may occur in pregnancy)	Glycosuria (low renal threshold for glucose, diabetes mellitus)	Assess blood glucose; test urine for ketones.
Rubella titer: Hemagglutination-inhibition test (HAI) $>$ 1:10 indicates woman is immune	HAI titer $<$ 1:10	Immunization will be given postpartally or within 6 weeks after childbirth. Instruct woman whose titers are $<$ 1:10 to avoid children who have rubella.
HIV screen: Offered to all women; encouraged for those at risk; negative	Positive	Refer to physician.
Illicit drug screen: Offered to all women; negative	Positive	Refer to physician.
Sickle cell screen for clients of African descent: Negative	Positive; test results would include a description of cells	Refer to physician.
Pap test: Negative	Test results that show atypical cells	Refer to physician. Discuss the meaning of the findings with the woman and importance of follow-up.

Cultural Assessment	Variations to Consider	Nursing Responses to Data†
Determine the woman's fluency in English.	Woman may be fluent in a language other than English.	Work with a knowledgeable translator to provide information and answer questions.
Ask the woman how she prefers to be addressed.	Some women prefer informality; others prefer to use titles.	Address the woman according to her preference. Maintain formality in introducing oneself if that seems preferred.
Determine customs and practices regarding prenatal care:	Practices are influenced by individual preference, cultural expectations, or religious beliefs.	Honor a woman's practices and provide for specific preferences unless they are contraindicated because of safety.

*Possible causes of alterations are placed in parentheses.

†This column provides guidelines for further assessment and initial nursing intervention.

INITIAL PRENATAL ASSESSMENT GUIDE continued

Cultural Assessment	Variations to Consider	Nursing Responses to Data†
• Ask the woman if there are certain practices she expects to follow when she is pregnant.	Some women believe that they should perform certain acts related to sleep, activity, or clothing.	Have information printed in the language of different cultural groups that live in the area.
• Ask the woman if there are any activities she cannot do while she is pregnant.	Some women have restrictions or taboos they follow related to work; activity; or sexual, environmental, or emotional factors (Boyle and Andrews 1989).	
• Ask the woman whether there are certain foods she is expected to eat or avoid while she is pregnant. Determine whether she has lactose intolerance.	Foods are an important cultural factor. Some women may have certain foods they must eat or avoid; many women have lactose intolerance and have difficulty consuming sufficient calcium.	Respect the woman's food preferences, help her plan an adequate prenatal diet within the framework of her preferences, and refer to a dietician if necessary.
• Ask the woman whether the gender of her caregiver is of concern.	Some women are comfortable only with a female caregiver.	Arrange for a female caregiver if it is the woman's preference.
• Ask the woman about the degree of involvement in her pregnancy that she expects or wants from her support person, mother, and other significant people.	If the woman does have a partner, she may not want this person involved in the pregnancy. For some the role falls to the woman's mother or a female relative or friend.	Respect the woman's preferences about her partner/husband's involvement; avoid imposing personal values or expectations.
• Ask the woman about her sources of support/counseling during pregnancy.	Some women seek advice from a family member, *curandera,* tribal healer, and so forth.	Respect and honor the woman's sources of support.

Psychosocial Assessment	Variations to Consider*	Nursing Responses to Data†
Psychologic Status		
Excitement and/or apprehension; ambivalence	Marked anxiety (fear of pregnancy diagnosis, fear of medical facility)	Establish lines of communication. Active listening is useful. Establish trusting relationship. Encourage woman to take active part in her care.
	Apathy Display of anger with pregnancy diagnosis	Establish communication and begin counseling. Use active listening techniques.
Educational Needs		
May have questions about pregnancy or may need time to adjust to reality of pregnancy		Establish educational, supporting environment that can be expanded throughout pregnancy.
Support Systems		
Can identify at least two or three individuals with whom woman is emotionally intimate (partner, parent, sibling, friend)	Isolated (no telephone, unlisted number); cannot name a neighbor or friend whom she can call on in an emergency; does not perceive parents as part of her support system	Institute support system through community groups. Help woman to develop trusting relationship with health care professionals.

*Possible causes of alterations are placed in parentheses.

†This column provides guidelines for further assessment and initial nursing intervention.

INITIAL PRENATAL ASSESSMENT GUIDE continued

Psychosocial Assessment	Variations to Consider*	Nursing Responses to Data†
Family Functioning		
Emotionally supportive Communications adequate Mutually satisfying Cohesiveness in times of trouble No evidence of physical or psychologic abuse	Long-term problems or specific problems related to this pregnancy, potential stressors within the family, pessimistic attitudes, unilateral decision making, unrealistic expectations of this pregnancy and/or child; signs of female partner abuse (see Chapter 5)	Help identify the problems and stressors, encourage communication, discuss role changes and adaptations. Refer as appropriate.
Economic Status		
Stable and sufficient income to meet basic needs of daily living and medical needs	Limited prenatal care Poor physical health Limited use of health care system Unstable economic status	Discuss available resources for health maintenance and the birth. Institute appropriate referral for meeting expanding family's needs—food stamps and so forth.
Stability of Living Conditions		
Adequate, stable housing for expanding family's needs	Crowded living conditions Questionable supportive environment for newborn	Refer to appropriate community agency. Work with family on self-help ways to improve situation.

*Possible causes of alterations are placed in parentheses.

†This column provides guidelines for further assessment and initial nursing intervention.

Uterine Assessment

Physical Examination

When a woman is examined in the first 10 to 12 weeks of her pregnancy and her uterine size is compatible with her menstrual history, uterine size may be the single most important clinical method for dating her pregnancy. In many cases, however, women do not seek obstetric care until well into their second trimester, when it becomes much more difficult to evaluate specific uterine size. In the obese woman, it is difficult to determine uterine size early in a pregnancy.

Fundal Height

Fundal height may be used as an indicator of uterine size, although this method cannot be used late in pregnancy. A centimeter tape measure is used to measure the distance abdominally from the top of the symphysis pubis to the top of the uterine fundus (McDonald's method) (Figure 8–3). Fundal height in centimeters usually correlates well with weeks of gestation between 22–24 weeks and 34 weeks. Thus, at 26 weeks' gestation, fundal height is probably about 26 cm. If the woman is very tall or very short, fundal height will differ. To be most accurate, fundal height should be measured by the same examiner each time. The woman should have voided within one-half hour of the exam, and should lie in the same position each time (Engstrom et al 1993). In the third trimester, variations in fetal weight decrease the accuracy of fundal height measurements.

Measurements of fundal height from month to month and week to week may signal intrauterine growth retardation (IUGR) if there is a lag in progression. A sudden increase in fundal height may indicate twins or hydramnios (excessive amount of amniotic fluid).

Fetal Development

Quickening

Fetal movements felt by the mother, called quickening, may indicate that the fetus is nearing 20 weeks' gestation. However, quickening may be experienced between 16 and 22 weeks' gestation, so this method is not completely accurate.

Fetal Heartbeat

The fetal heartbeat can be detected with a fetoscope as early as week 16 and almost always by 19 or 20 weeks'

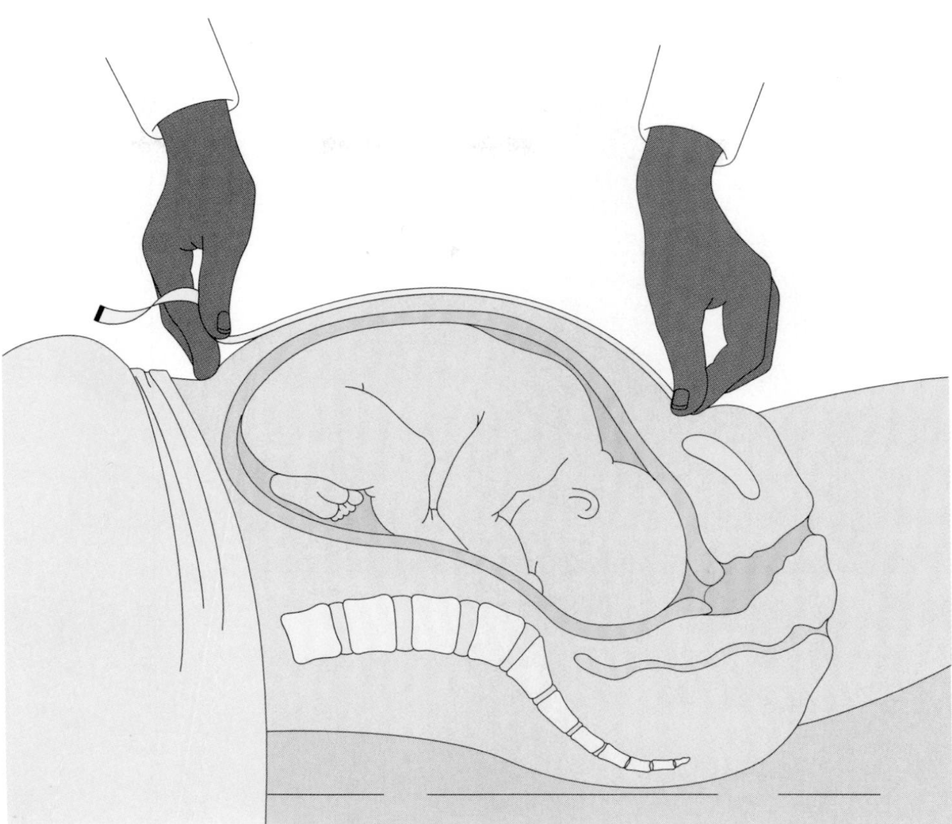

FIGURE 8–3 A cross-sectional view of fetal position when McDonald's method is used to assess fundal height.

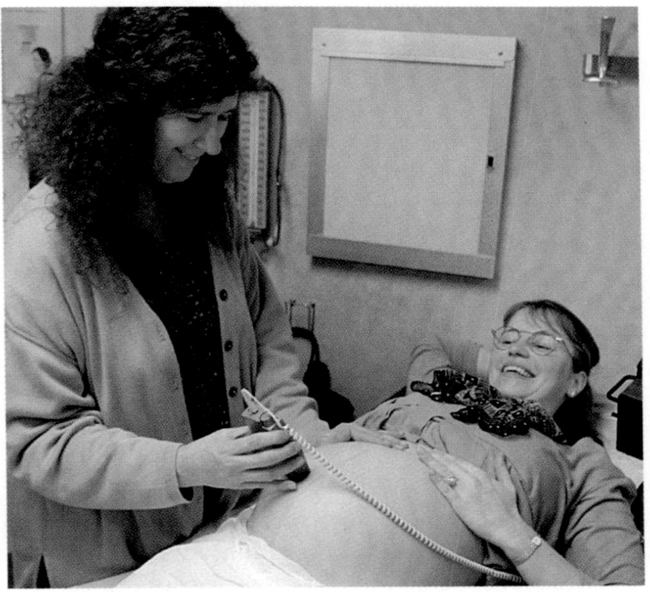

FIGURE 8–4 Listening to the fetal heartbeat with a Doppler device.

gestation. Fetal heartbeat may be detected with the ultrasonic Doppler device (Figure 8–4) as early as 8 weeks, but it is first heard, on average, at 10 to 12 weeks' gestation.

Ultrasound Findings

In the first trimester, ultrasound scanning can detect a gestational sac as early as 5–6 weeks after the LMP, fetal heart activity by 9–10 weeks, and fetal breathing movement by 11 weeks of pregnancy. Crown-to-rump (C–R) measurements can be used to assess fetal age until the fetal head can be visualized clearly. Biparietal diameter (BPD) can then be used. BPD measurements can be made by approximately 12–13 weeks and are most accurate between 20 and 30 weeks, when rapid growth in the biparietal diameter occurs. (See Chapter 14 for an in-depth discussion of ultrasound scanning of the fetus.)

Assessment of Pelvic Adequacy (Clinical Pelvimetry)

The pelvis can be assessed vaginally to determine whether its size is adequate for a vaginal birth. This procedure, referred to as *clinical pelvimetry,* is performed by physicians or by advanced practice nurses such as certified nurse-midwives or nurse practitioners. Some caregivers assess pelvic adequacy as part of the initial physical examination. Others wait until later in the pregnancy, when hormonal effects are greatest and it is possible to make some determination of fetal size.

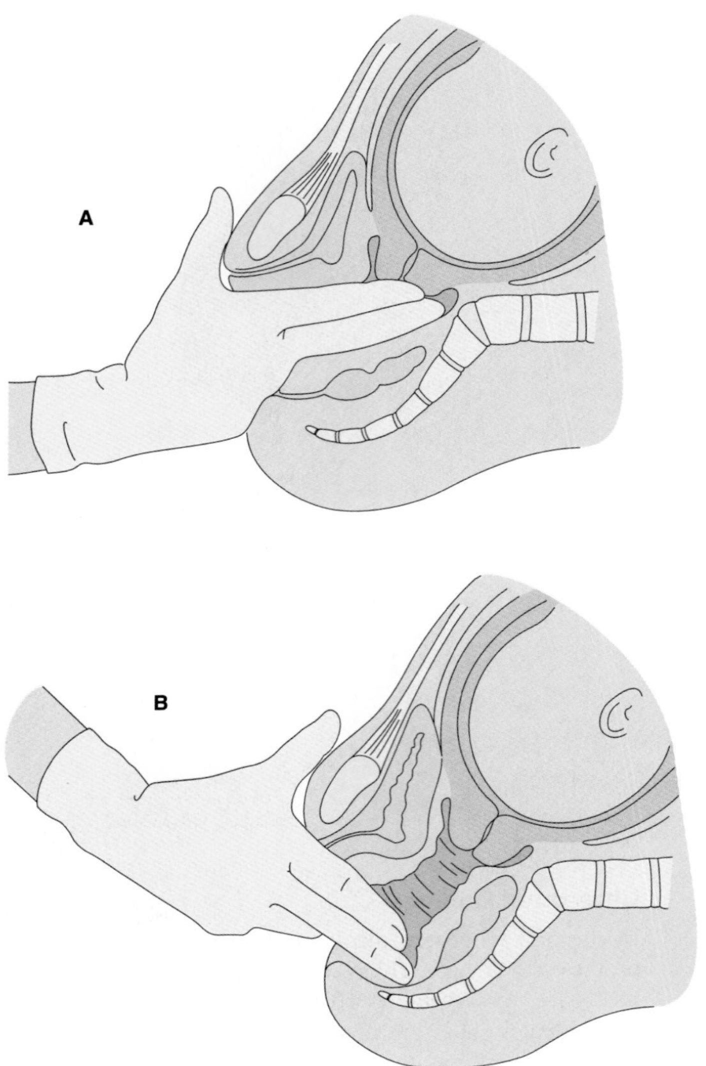

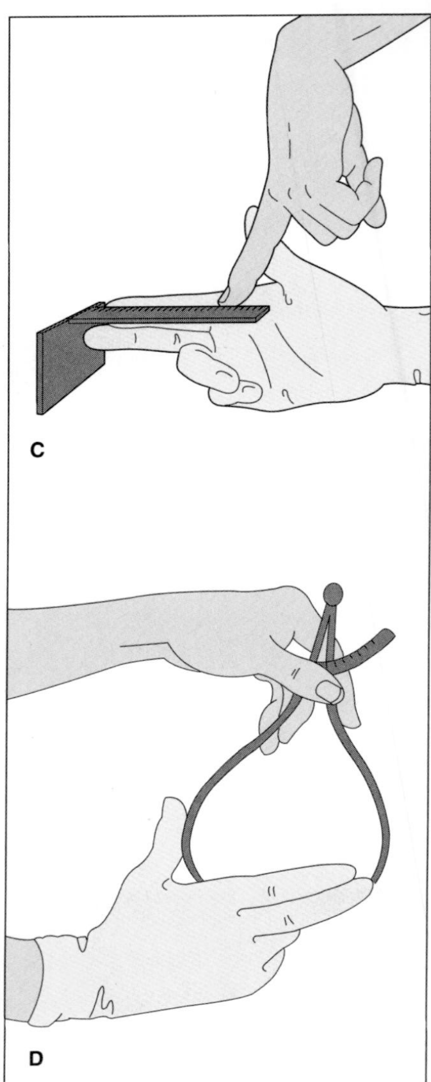

FIGURE 8–5 Manual measurement of inlet and outlet. ***A*** Estimation of the diagonal conjugate, which extends from the lower border of the symphysis pubis to the sacral promontory. ***B*** Estimation of the anteroposterior diameter of the outlet, which extends from the lower border of the symphysis pubis to the tip of the sacrum. ***C** and **D*** Methods that may be used to check the manual estimation of anteroposterior measurements.

The method of measurement is depicted in Figures 8–5, 8–6, and 8–7. The parts of the pelvis that are evaluated and their normal measurements include the following:

1. Pelvic inlet (Figure 8–5)
   - **Diagonal conjugate** (the distance from the lower posterior border of the symphysis pubis to the sacral promontory) at least 11.5 cm
   - **Obstetric conjugate** (a measurement approximately 1.5 cm smaller than the diagonal conjugate) 10 cm or more
2. Pelvic cavity (midpelvis)
   - Plane of least dimension (midplane), 11.5–12 cm
   - Posterior sagittal diameter, 4.5–5 cm
   - Transverse diameter (interspinous), 10 cm

   The planes of the midpelvis cannot be accurately measured by clinical examination. An evaluation of adequacy is based on the prominence of the ischial spines and the degree of convergence of the side walls of the pelvis.
3. Pelvic outlet (Figures 8–5, 8–6, 8–7)
   - Anteroposterior diameter, 9.5–11.5 cm
   - Transverse diameter, 8–10 cm

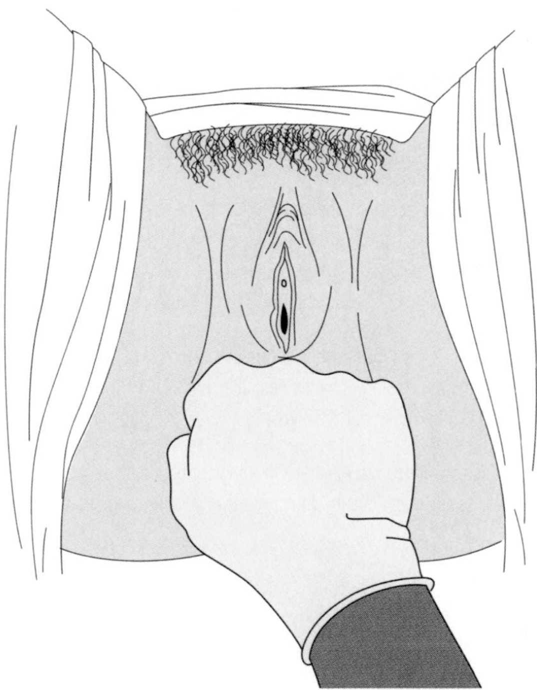

FIGURE 8–6 Use of a closed fist to measure the outlet. Most examiners know the distance between their first and last proximal knuckles. If they don't, they can use a measuring device.

Subsequent Client History

At subsequent prenatal visits the nurse continues to gather data about the course of the pregnancy to date and the woman's responses to it. The nurse asks specifically whether the woman has experienced any discomfort, especially the kinds of discomfort that are often seen at specific times during a pregnancy. The nurse inquires about physical changes that relate directly to the pregnancy, such as fetal movement. The nurse also asks about the danger signs of pregnancy (see Key Facts to Remember: Danger Signs in Pregnancy on p 192).

Other pertinent information includes any exposure to contagious illnesses, medical treatment and therapy prescribed for nonpregnancy problems since the last visit, and any prescription or over-the-counter medications that were not prescribed as part of the woman's prenatal care.

Periodic prenatal examinations offer the nurse an opportunity to assess the childbearing woman's psychologic needs and emotional status. If the woman's partner attends the prenatal visits, the nurse can also identify his needs and concerns.

Text continues on page 192

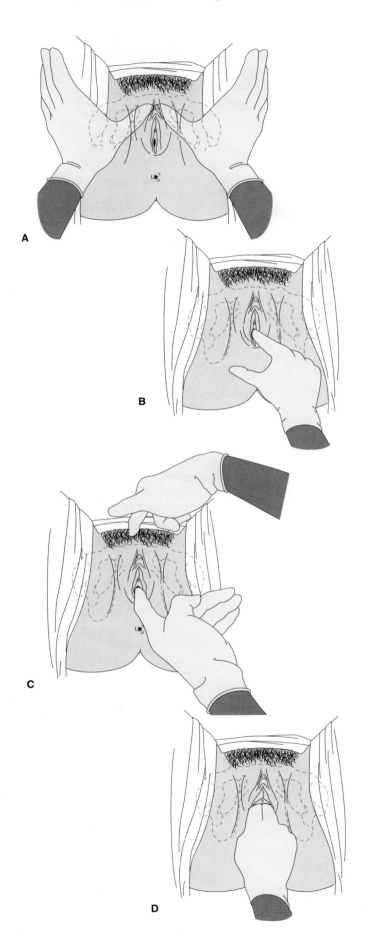

FIGURE 8–7 Evaluation of the outlet. ***A*** Estimation of the subpubic angle. ***B*** Estimation of the length of the pubic ramus. ***C*** Estimation of the depth and inclination of the pubis. ***D*** Estimation of the contour of the subpubic angle.

TABLE 8–2 Prenatal Assessment of Parenting Guide

Areas Assessed	Sample Questions
I. Perception of complexities of mothering	
A. Desires baby for itself Positive: 1. Feels positive about pregnancy Negative: 1. Wants baby to meet own needs such as someone to love her, someone to get her out of unhappy home	1. Did you plan on getting pregnant? 2. How do you feel about being pregnant? 3. Why do you want this baby?
B. Expresses concern about impact of mothering role on other roles (wife, career, school) Positive: 1. Realistic expectations of how baby will affect job, career, school, and personal goals 2. Interested in learning about child care Negative: 1. Feels pregnancy and baby will make no emotional, physical, or social demands on self 2. Has no insight that mothering role will affect other roles or lifestyle	1. What do you think it will be like to take care of a baby? 2. How do you think your life will be different after you have your baby? 3. How do you feel this baby will affect your job, career, school, and personal goals? 4. How will the baby affect your relationship with your boyfriend or husband? 5. Have you done any reading, babysitting, or made any things for a baby?
C. Gives up routine habits because "not good for baby" (eg, quits smoking, adjusts time schedule) Positive: 1. Gives up routines not good for baby (quits smoking, adjusts eating habits)	
II. Attachment	
A. Strong feelings regarding sex of baby. Why? Positive: 1. Verbalizes positive thoughts about the baby Negative: 1. Baby will be like negative aspects of self and partner	1. Why do you prefer a certain sex? (Is reason inappropriate for a baby?) 2. Note comments client makes about baby not being normal and why client feels this way.
B. Interested in data regarding fetus (eg, growth and development, heart tones) Positive: 1. As above Negative: 1. Shows no interest in fetal growth and development, quickening, and fetal heart tones 2. Expresses negative feelings about fetus by rejecting counseling regarding nutrition, rest, hygiene	
C. Fantasies about baby Positive: 1. Follows cultural norms regarding preparation 2. Time of attachment behaviors appropriate to her history of pregnancy loss Negative: 1. Bonding conditional depending on sex, age of baby, and/or labor and birth experience 2. Woman considers only own needs when making plans for baby 3. Exhibits no attachment behaviors after critical period of previous pregnancy 4. Failure to follow cultural norms regarding preparation	1. What did you think or feel when you first felt the baby move? 2. Have you started preparing for the baby? 3. What do you think your baby will look like—what age do you see your baby at? 4. How would you like your new baby to look?

TABLE 8–2 continued

Areas Assessed	Sample Questions
III. Acceptance of child by significant others	
A. Acknowledges acceptance by significant other of the new responsibility inherent in child Positive: 1. Acknowledges unconditional acceptance of pregnancy and baby by significant others 2. Partner accepts new responsibility inherent with child 3. Timely sharing of experience of pregnancy with significant others Negative: 1. Significant others not supportively involved with pregnancy 2. Conditional acceptance of pregnancy depending on sex, race, age of baby 3. Decision making does not take in needs of fetus (eg, spends food money on new car) 4. Takes no/little responsibility for needs of pregnancy, woman/fetus	1. How does your partner feel about this pregnancy? 2. How do your parents feel? 3. What do your friends think? 4. Does your partner have a preference regarding the baby's sex? Why? 5. How does your partner feel about being a father? 6. What do you think he'll be like as a father? 7. What do you think he'll do to help you with child care? 8. Have you and your partner talked about how the baby might change your lives? 9. Who have you told about your pregnancy?
B. Concrete demonstration of acceptance of pregnancy/baby by significant others (eg, baby shower, significant other involved in prenatal education) Positive: 1. Baby shower 2. Significant other attends prenatal class with client	1. Note if partner attends clinic with client (degree of interest; eg, listens to heart tones). Significant other plans to be with client during labor and birth. 2. Is your partner contributing financially?
IV. Ensures physical well-being	
A. Concerns about having normal pregnancy, labor and birth, and baby Positive: 1. Preparing for labor and birth, attends prenatal classes, interested in labor and birth 2. Aware of danger signs of pregnancy 3. Seeks and uses appropriate health care (eg, time of initial visit, keeps appointments, follows through on recommendations) Negative: 1. Denies signs and symptoms that might suggest complications of pregnancy 2. Verbalizes extreme fear of labor and birth—refuses to talk about labor and birth 3. Fails appointments, fails to follow instructions, refuses to attend prenatal classes	1. What have you heard about labor and birth? 2. Note data about client's reaction to prenatal class.
B. Family/client decisions reflect concern for health of mother and baby (eg, use of finances, time) Positive: 1. As above	

Note: When "Negative" is not listed in a section, the reader may assume that negative is the absence of positive responses.

Source: Modified and used with permission of the Minneapolis Health Dept, Minneapolis, MN.

KEY FACTS TO REMEMBER

Danger Signs in Pregnancy

The woman should report the following danger signs in pregnancy immediately:

Danger Sign	*Possible Cause*
Sudden gush of fluid from vagina	Premature rupture of membranes
Vaginal bleeding	Abruptio placentae, placenta previa Lesions of cervix or vagina "Bloody show"
Abdominal pain	Premature labor, abruptio placentae
Temperature above 38.3C (101F) and chills	Infection
Dizziness, blurring of vision, double vision, spots before eyes	Hypertension, preeclampsia
Persistent vomiting	Hyperemesis gravidarum
Severe headache	Hypertension, preeclampsia
Edema of hands, face, legs, and feet	Preeclampsia
Muscular irritability, convulsions	Preeclampsia, eclampsia
Epigastric pain	Preeclampsia–ischemia in major abdominal vessel
Oliguria	Renal impairment, decreased fluid intake
Dysuria	Urinary tract infection
Absence of fetal movement	Maternal medication, obesity, fetal death

The interchange between the nurse and the woman or her partner will be facilitated if it takes place in a friendly, trusting environment. The woman should have sufficient time to ask questions and air concerns. If the nurse provides the time and demonstrates genuine interest, the woman will be more at ease bringing up questions that she may believe are silly or has been afraid to verbalize. The nurse who has an accurate understanding of all the changes of pregnancy is most able to answer questions and provide information.

CRITICAL THINKING IN ACTION

At 33 weeks' gestation, Elena Martinez, gr 2 p1, who is 5 feet 4 inches tall and who weighs 144 lb (prepregnancy weight = 120), is examined by her certified nurse-midwife. At that time her fundal height is measured as 33 cm. Because of a vacation trip she is not seen again by her midwife until 36 weeks' gestation. At that time her fundus measures 35 cm. and she weighs 147 lb. Elena asks you if there is something wrong with her baby's growth. What is your assessment?

Answer may be found in Appendix H.

The nurse should also be sensitive to religious, cultural, and socioeconomic factors that may influence a family's response to pregnancy, as well as to the woman's expectations of the health care system. The nurse can avoid stereotyping clients simply by asking each woman about her expectations for the antepartal period. While the responses of many women may reflect traditional norms, other women will have decidedly different views or expectations that represent a blending of beliefs or cultures.

During the prenatal period, it is essential to begin assessing the ability of the woman and her partner (if possible) to assume their responsibilities as parents successfully. Table 8–2 on pp 190–191 identifies areas for assessment of parenting ability.

Subsequent Antepartal Assessment

The Subsequent Prenatal Assessment Guide (starting on p 193) provides a systematic approach to the regular physical examinations the pregnant woman should undergo for optimal prenatal care, and also provides a model for evaluating both the pregnant woman and the expectant father, if he is involved in the pregnancy.

The recommended frequency of prenatal visits in an uncomplicated pregnancy is as follows:

- Every 4 weeks for the first 28 weeks of gestation
- Every 2 weeks until 36 weeks' gestation
- After week 36, every week until childbirth

During the subsequent psychosocial and cultural portions of the antepartal assessments, a woman may exhibit psychologic problems such as the following:

- Increasing anxiety
- Inability to establish communication

SUBSEQUENT PRENATAL ASSESSMENT GUIDE

Physical Assessment/ Normal Findings	Alterations and Possible Causes*	Nursing Responses to Data[†]
Vital Signs		
Temperature: 36.2–37.6C (98–99.6F)	Elevated temperature (infection)	Evaluate for signs of infection. Refer to physician.
Pulse: 60–90/min Rate may increase 10 beats/min during pregnancy	Increased pulse rate (anxiety, cardiac disorders)	Note irregularities. Assess for anxiety and stress.
Respiration: 16–24/min	Marked tachypnea or abnormal patterns (respiratory disease)	Refer to physician.
Blood pressure: 90–140/60–90 (falls in second trimester)	> 140/90 or increase of 30 mm systolic and 15 mm diastolic (PIH)	Assess for edema, proteinuria, hyperreflexia. Refer to physician. Schedule appointments more frequently.
Weight Gain		
First trimester: 1.4–2.3 kg (3–5 lb) *Second trimester:* 5.5–6.8 kg (12–15 lb) *Third trimester:* 5.5–6.8 kg (12–15 lb)	Inadequate weight gain (poor nutrition, nausea, IUGR) Excessive weight gain (excessive caloric intake, edema, PIH)	Discuss appropriate weight gain. Provide nutritional counseling. Assess for presence of edema or anemia.
Edema		
Small amount of dependent edema, especially in last weeks of pregnancy	Edema in hands, face, legs, feet (PIH)	Identify any correlation between edema and activities, blood pressure, or proteinuria. Refer to physician if indicated.
Uterine Size		
See Initial Prenatal Assessment Guide for normal changes during pregnancy	Unusually rapid growth (multiple gestation, hydatidiform mole, hydramnios, miscalculation of EDB)	Evaluate fetal status. Determine height of fundus (p 186). Use diagnostic ultrasound.
Fetal Heartbeat		
120–160/min Funic souffle	Absence of fetal heartbeat after 20 weeks' gestation (maternal obesity, fetal demise)	Evaluate fetal status.
Laboratory Evaluation		
Hemoglobin: 12–16 g/dL Pseudoanemia of pregnancy	< 12 g/dL (anemia)	Provide nutritional counseling. Hemoglobin is repeated at 7 months' gestation. Women of Mediterranean heritage need a close check on hemoglobin because of possibility of thalassemia.
Maternal serum α-fetoprotein (MSAFP): normal levels (done at 16–18 weeks' gestation)	Elevated (neural tube defect, underestimated gestational age, multiple gestation, fetal demise, Rh disease)	Refer to physician.

*Possible causes of alterations are placed in parentheses.

[†]This column provides guidelines for further assessment and initial nursing intervention.

SUBSEQUENT PRENATAL ASSESSMENT GUIDE continued

Physical Assessment/ Normal Findings	Alterations and Possible Causes*	Nursing Responses to Data[†]
50 g, 1-hour glucose screen (done between 24 and 28 weeks' gestation)	Plasma glucose level > 140 mg/dL (gestational diabetes mellitus [GDM])	Discuss implications of GDM. Refer for a diagnostic glucose tolerance test.
Urinalysis: See Initial Prenatal Assessment Guide for normal findings	See Initial Prenatal Assessment Guide for deviations	Repeat urinalysis at 7 months' gestation. Dipstick test at each visit.
Protein: Negative	Proteinuria, albuminuria (contamination by vaginal discharge, urinary tract infection, PIH)	Obtain dipstick urine sample. Refer to physician if deviations are present.
Glucose: Negative *Note:* Glycosuria may be present due to physiologic alterations in glomerular filtration rate and renal threshold	Persistent glycosuria (diabetes mellitus)	Refer to physician.

Cultural Assessment	Variations to Consider	Nursing Responses to Data[†]
Determine the mother's (and family's) attitudes about the sex of the unborn child.	Some women have no preference about the sex of the child; others do. In many cultures boys are especially valued as firstborn children.	Provide opportunities to discuss preferences and expectations; avoid a judgmental attitude to the response.
Ask about the woman's expectations of childbirth. Will she want someone with her for the birth? Whom does she choose? What is the role of her partner?	Some women want their partner present for labor and birth; others prefer a female relative or friend. Some women expect to be separated from their partner once cervical dilatation has occurred (Boyle and Andrews 1989).	Provide information on birth options, but accept the woman's decision about who will attend.
Ask about preparations for the baby. Determine what is customary for the woman.	Some women may have a fully prepared nursery; others may not have a separate room for the baby.	Explore reasons for not preparing for the baby. Support the mother's preferences, and provide information about possible sources of assistance if the decision is related to a lack of resources.

Psychosocial Assessment	Variations to Consider*	Nursing Responses to Data[†]
Expectant Mother *Psychologic status:* *First trimester:* Incorporates idea of pregnancy; may feel ambivalent, especially if she must give up desired role; usually looks for signs of verification of pregnancy, such as increase in abdominal size or fetal movement *Second trimester:* Baby becomes more real to woman as abdominal size increases and she feels movement; she begins to turn inward, becoming more introspective	Increasing stress and anxiety Inability to establish communication; inability to accept pregnancy; inappropriate response or actions; denial of pregnancy; inability to cope	Encourage woman to take an active part in her care. Establish lines of communication. Establish a trusting relationship. Counsel as necessary. Refer to appropriate professional as needed.

*Possible causes of alterations are placed in parentheses.

[†]This column provides guidelines for further assessment and initial nursing intervention.

SUBSEQUENT PRENATAL ASSESSMENT GUIDE continued

Psychosocial Assessment	Variations to Consider*	Nursing Responses to Data†
Third trimester: Begins to think of baby as separate being; may feel restless and may feel that time of labor will never come; remains self-centered and concentrates on preparing place for baby		
Educational needs: *Self-care measures and knowledge about following:* Health promotion Breast care Hygiene Rest Exercise Nutrition Relief measures for common discomforts of pregnancy Danger signs in pregnancy (See Key Facts to Remember, p 192)	Inadequate information	Teach and/or institute appropriate relief measures (Chapter 9).
Sexual activity: Woman knows how pregnancy affects sexual activity	Lack of information about effects of pregnancy and/or alternative positions during sexual intercourse	Provide counseling.
Preparation for parenting: Appropriate preparation (Table 8–2)	Lack of preparation (denial, failure to adjust to baby, unwanted child) See Table 8–2	Counsel. If lack of preparation is due to inadequacy of information, provide information (Chapter 9).
Preparation for childbirth: *Client aware of following:* 1. Prepared childbirth techniques 2. Normal processes and changes during childbirth		If couple chooses particular technique, refer to classes (see Chapter 6 for description of childbirth preparation techniques). Encourage prenatal class attendance. Educate woman during visits based on current physical status. Provide reading list for more specific information.
3. Problems that may occur as a result of drug and alcohol use and of smoking	Continued abuse of drugs and alcohol; denial of possible effect on self and baby	Review danger signs that were presented on initial visit.
Woman has met other physician and/or nurse-midwife who may be attending her birth in the absence of primary caregiver	Introduction of new individual at birth may increase stress and anxiety for woman and partner	Introduce woman to all members of group practice.
Impending labor: *Client knows signs of impending labor:* 1. Uterine contractions that increase in frequency, duration, intensity 2. Bloody show 3. Expulsion of mucus plug 4. Rupture of membranes	Lack of information	Provide appropriate teaching, stressing importance of seeking appropriate medical assistance.

*Possible causes of alterations are placed in parentheses.

†This column provides guidelines for further assessment and initial nursing intervention.

SUBSEQUENT PRENATAL ASSESSMENT GUIDE continued

Psychosocial Assessment	Variations to Consider*	Nursing Responses to Data†
Expectant Father		
Psychologic status:		
First trimester: May express excitement over confirmation of pregnancy and of his virility; concerns move toward providing for financial needs; energetic; may identify with some discomforts of pregnancy and may even exhibit symptoms	Increasing stress and anxiety Inability to establish communication Inability to accept pregnancy diagnosis Withdrawal of support Abandonment of the mother	Encourage expectant father to come to prenatal visits. Establish lines of communication. Establish trusting relationship.
Second trimester: May feel more confident and be less concerned with financial matters; may have concerns about wife's changing size and shape, her increasing introspection		Counsel. Let expectant father know that it is normal for him to experience these feelings.
Third trimester: May have feelings of rivalry with fetus, especially during sexual activity; may make changes in his physical appearance and exhibit more interest in himself; may become more energetic; fantasizes about child but usually imagines older child; fears of mutilation and death of woman and child		Include expectant father in pregnancy activities as he desires. Provide education, information, and support. Increasing numbers of expectant fathers are demonstrating desire to be involved in many or all aspects of prenatal care, education, and preparation.

*Possible causes of alterations are placed in parentheses.

†This column provides guidelines for further assessment and initial nursing intervention.

- Inappropriate responses or actions
- Denial of pregnancy
- Inability to cope with stress
- Failure to acknowledge quickening
- Failure to plan and prepare for the baby (for example, living arrangements, clothing, feeding methods)
- Indications of substance abuse

If the woman appears to have these or other critical problems, the nurse should provide ongoing support and counseling and refer her to appropriate professionals.

CHAPTER HIGHLIGHTS

- A complete history forms the basis of prenatal care and is reevaluated and updated as necessary throughout the pregnancy.
- The initial prenatal physical assessment is a careful and thorough physical examination designed to identify physical variations and potential risk factors.
- Laboratory tests completed at the initial visit, such as a complete blood count, ABO and Rh typing, urinalysis, Pap smear, gonorrhea culture, rubella titer, and various blood screens, provide information about the woman's health during early pregnancy and also help detect potential problems.
- The estimated date of birth (EDB) can be calculated by using Nägele's rule. Using this approach, one begins with the first day of the last menstrual period, subtracts 3 months, and adds 7 days. A "wheel" may also be used to calculate the EDB.
- Accuracy of the EDB may be evaluated by physical examination to assess uterine size, measurement of fundal height, and ultrasound. Perception of quickening and auscultation of fetal heartbeat are also useful tools in confirming the gestation of a pregnancy.
- The diagonal conjugate is the distance from the lower posterior border of the symphysis pubis to the sacral promontory. The obstetric conjugate is estimated by subtracting 1.5 cm from the length of the diagonal conjugate.

- The nurse begins evaluating the woman psychosocially during the initial prenatal assessment. This assessment continues and is modified throughout the pregnancy.
- Religious, cultural, and ethnic beliefs may strongly influence the woman's attitudes and apparent cooperation with care during pregnancy.

REFERENCES

Boyle JS, Andrews MM: *Transcultural Concepts in Nursing Care*. Glenview, IL: Scott, Foresman/Little, Brown, 1989.

Engstrom JL et al: Fundal height measurements. *J Nurse-Midwifery* January/February 1993; 38:26.

Mittendorf R et al: The length of uncomplicated human gestation. *Obstet Gynecol* June 1990; 75:929.

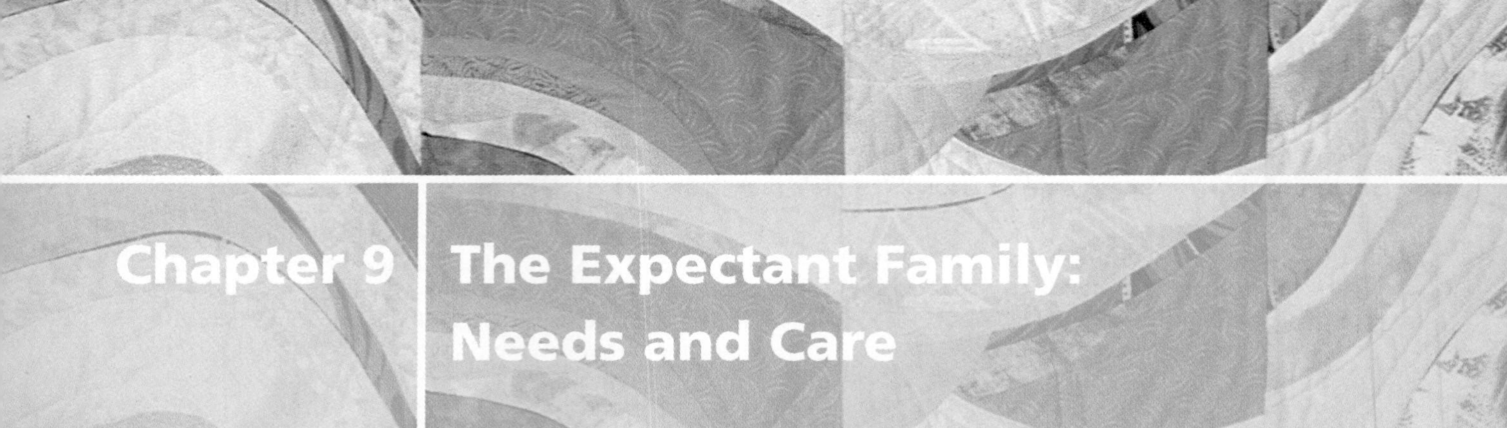

Chapter 9 The Expectant Family: Needs and Care

OBJECTIVES

- Develop sample nursing diagnoses that may apply to a woman experiencing an uncomplicated pregnancy.
- Explain the causes of the common discomforts of pregnancy and appropriate measures to alleviate these discomforts.
- Discuss the basic information that the nurse should provide to the expectant family to allow them to carry out appropriate self-care.
- Identify some of the concerns that the expectant couple may have about sexual activity.
- Relate the significance of cultural considerations to the provision of effective prenatal care.

KEY TERMS

Fetal activity diary (FAD)
Fetal alcohol syndrome (FAS)
Fetal movement records (FMR)
Kegel's exercises
Leukorrhea
Lightening
Nipple preparation
Pelvic tilt
Ptyalism
Teratogens

From the moment a woman finds out she is pregnant, she faces a future marked by dramatic changes. Her appearance will alter. Her relationships will change. She will experience a variety of bodily changes throughout the pregnancy. Even her psychologic state will be affected. To cope with these changes, she will need to make numerous adjustments.

The pregnant woman's family, too, must adjust to the pregnancy. Roles and responsibilities of family members will be altered as the woman's ability to perform certain activities changes. They too must adapt psychologically to the expected arrival of a new family member.

The expectant woman and her family will probably have many questions about the pregnancy and its impact on all of them. The daily activities and health care practices of the woman are important for her well-being and the well-being of the unborn child.

Nurses caring for pregnant women need an up-to-date understanding of pregnancy if they are to be effective in implementing the nursing process as they plan and provide care. With this in mind, Chapter 7 provided a database for the nurse by presenting material related to the normal physical, social, cultural, and psychologic changes of pregnancy. Chapter 8 then used that database to begin the nursing process by focusing on client assessment. This chapter continues the application of the nursing process to the expectant woman by discussing analysis and nursing diagnosis, planning, implementation, and evaluation. Planning and implementation are combined here to avoid redundancy.

Nursing Diagnosis During Pregnancy

The nurse may see a pregnant woman only once every 3 to 4 weeks during the first several months of her pregnancy. Therefore a written care plan that incorporates the database, nursing diagnoses, and client goals is essential to ensure continuity of care.

The nurse can anticipate that, for many women with a low-risk pregnancy, certain nursing diagnoses will be made more frequently than others. This will, of course, vary from woman to woman and according to the time in the pregnancy. Common nursing diagnoses include

- Constipation related to the physiologic effects of pregnancy
- Altered sexuality patterns related to discomfort during late pregnancy

After formulating an appropriate diagnosis, the nurse establishes related goals to guide the nursing plan and interventions.

Nursing Plan and Implementation During Pregnancy

Once nursing diagnoses have been identified, the next step is to establish priorities of nursing care. Sometimes priorities of care are based on the most immediate needs or concerns expressed by the woman. For example, during the first trimester, when she is experiencing nausea or is concerned about sexual intimacy with her partner, the woman is not likely to want to hear about labor and birth.

The woman's priorities may not always be the same as the nurse's. If the safety of the woman or her fetus is at issue, that takes priority over other concerns of the woman or her family. It is the responsibility of medical and nursing professionals to help the woman and her family understand the significance of a problem and to plan appropriate interventions to deal with it.

The intervention methods most used by nurses in caring for the expectant woman and her family are communication techniques and teaching-learning strategies. These intervention methods are often used in groups such as early pregnancy classes and childbirth education classes (see Chapter 6), but the nurse in the prenatal setting also applies these techniques with individuals.

Community-Based Nursing Care

Prenatal care, especially for women with low-risk pregnancies, is community based, typically in a clinic or a private office. The value of providing a primary care nurse in these settings to coordinate holistic care for each childbearing family is recognized. The nurse in a clinic or health maintenance organization (HMO) may be the only source of continuity for the woman, who may see a different physician or certified nurse-midwife at each visit. The nurse can be extremely effective in working with the expectant family by providing complete information about pregnancy, prenatal health care activities, and community resources. Communities often have a wealth of services and educational opportunities available for pregnant women and their families and the knowledgeable nurse can help the woman access these services. This allows the family to assume equal responsibility with health care providers in working toward their common goal of a positive birth experience. See Key Facts to Remember: Key Antepartal Nursing Interventions.

KEY FACTS TO REMEMBER

Key Antepartal Nursing Interventions

Antepartal nursing interventions focus on the following:

- Explaining the normal changes of pregnancy to the childbearing family.
- Specifying those signs or symptoms that indicate a problem may be developing.
- Providing appropriate information about self-care measures the pregnant woman may employ to relieve the common discomforts of pregnancy.
- Answering questions about the common concerns that arise during pregnancy.
- Referring the woman for additional or more specialized assistance when necessary.

Throughout the prenatal period, the nurse provides both informal and formal education to the childbearing family. This prenatal education is designed to help the family carry out self-care when appropriate and to report changes that may indicate a health problem. The nurse also provides anticipatory guidance to help the family plan for changes that will occur after childbirth. The expectant couple needs to discuss issues that could be sources of postpartal stress. Issues to be resolved beforehand may include the sharing of infant and household chores, help in the first few days, options for babysitting to allow the mother (and couple) some free time, the mother's return to work after the baby's birth, and sibling rivalry. Couples resolve these issues in different ways, but postpartal adjustment is easier for couples who agree on the issues beforehand than for couples who do not confront and resolve these issues.

The problems and concerns of the pregnant woman, the relief of her discomforts, and the maintenance of her physical health receive much attention. However, her well-being also depends on the well-being of those to whom she is closest. Thus the nurse must help meet the needs of the woman's family to maintain the integrity of the family unit. Although the father of the baby is present in most cases, his presence cannot be assumed. If he is not part of the family structure, it is important to assess the woman's support system to determine which significant persons in her life will play a major role during this childbearing experience.

Anticipatory guidance of the expectant father, if he is involved in the pregnancy, is a necessary part of any plan of care. He may need information about the anatomic, physiologic, and emotional changes that occur during and after pregnancy, the couple's sexuality and sexual response, and the reactions that he is experiencing. He may wish to express his feelings about breast- versus bottle-feeding, the sex of the child, and other topics. If it is culturally acceptable to the couple and personally acceptable to him, the nurse refers the couple to expectant parents' classes for information and support from other couples.

The nurse assesses the father's intended degree of participation during labor and birth and his knowledge of what to expect. If the couple prefers that his participation be minimal or restricted, the nurse supports the decision. With this type of consideration and collaboration, the father is less apt to develop feelings of alienation, helplessness, and guilt during the pregnancy. As the couple's relationship is strengthened and the father's self-esteem raised, he is better able to provide physical and emotional support to his partner during labor and birth.

In the plan for prenatal care, the nurse also incorporates a discussion about the negative feelings older children may develop. Parents may be distressed to see an older child become aggressive toward the newborn. Parents who are unprepared for the older child's feelings of anger, jealousy, and rejection may respond inappropriately in their confusion and surprise. The nurse emphasizes that open communication between parents and children (or acting out feelings with a doll if the child is too young to verbalize) helps children master their feelings and may prevent their hurting the baby when they are unsupervised. Children may feel less neglected and more secure if they know that their parents are willing to help with their anger and aggressiveness.

Parents may be encouraged to bring their children to antepartal visits. For siblings, seeing what is involved and listening to the fetal heartbeat may make the pregnancy more real. Many agencies also provide sibling classes geared to different ages and levels of understanding.

HOME CARE

Home care can be of benefit to any pregnant woman, but it is especially effective in removing barriers for women who have difficulty accessing health care. These barriers may include lack of locally available health care facilities, problems with transportation to the facility, or schedule conflicts with available appointment times be-

TABLE 9–1 Cultural Beliefs and Activity During Pregnancy

Here are a few examples of cultural beliefs and activities related to pregnancy. It is important not to make assumptions about a client's beliefs since cultural norms vary greatly within a culture and from generation to generation. The nurse should observe the client carefully and take the time to ask questions. The client will benefit greatly from this awareness of differences.

Belief or Activity	*Nursing Considerations*
Home Remedies	
People of European background may use nonprescription medications to relieve discomfort or ensure better health. People of Mexican background may use spearmint or sassafras tea to ease morning sickness and cathartics during the last month of pregnancy to ensure a healthy birth (Brown 1976). Clients of Chinese descent may drink ginseng tea for faintness after childbirth or as a sedative when mixed with bamboo leaves (Spector 1991).	Find out what medications and home remedies your client is using, and counsel your client regarding overall effects. It is common for individuals to avoid telling health care workers about home remedies—the client may feel this will be judged unfavorably. Phrase your questions in a sensitive, accepting way.
Some people of African heritage may use self-medication for pregnancy discomforts—for example, castor oil for constipation, herbs for nausea and vomiting, and vinegar and baking soda for heartburn (Carrington 1978).	In some cases you might want to suggest remedies that may be more effective—for example, eating high-fiber foods to reduce constipation. If the home remedy is not harmful, there is no reason to ask a client to discontinue this practice.
Clothing	
Women of Mexican background may wear certain clothing—for example, a munecocord worn beneath the breasts and knotted over the umbilicus to ensure a safe birth (Brown 1976).	Ask your client how she feels about hospital clothing. You may want to find out if certain styles of clothing or jewelry have special meaning for her. Respect these clothing choices, intervening only if the clothing could be harmful in any way.
Some women of European heritage may be concerned that they look fat while pregnant and may choose clothing based on self-image.	Discuss these concerns about self-image with your client.
Exercise	
Some people of African, European, and Mexican cultural heritage feel that reaching over the head can harm the baby. Some people of European background may fear that lifting heavy objects will cause the placenta to separate.	Ask your client if there are any activities she is afraid to do because of the pregnancy. Assure her that reaching over her head will not harm the baby, and evaluate other activities related to their effect on the pregnancy.
Spirituality	
Navajo Indians may meet with the medicine man 2 months before birth, feeling that the prayers will ensure a safe birth and healthy baby. Some people of European background may tend to pay more attention to spirituality in their life to alleviate fears and assure a safe birth.	Encourage the use of support systems and spiritual aids that provide comfort for the mother.

cause of employment hours or family responsibilities (Stringer et al 1994).

In-home nursing assessments vary according to the scope of practice of the nurse and include current history and those screening procedures typically completed in an office or clinic: vital signs, weight, urine screen, physical activity, dietary intake. Advanced practice nurses can also assess reflexes, perform tests of fetal well-being, and even do cervical examinations. Once the assessments are completed the level of follow-up home care or telephone contact can be determined (Stringer et al 1994).

A prenatal home care visit or phone contact can also be useful for women who anticipate a short inpatient stay (24 hours or less) after childbirth. At the prenatal contact, the nurse explains the postpartum program and answers any questions the woman or her family have.

Although the use of home care for women with uncomplicated pregnancies is growing, it is most often used for women with prenatal complications that can be managed without hospitalization if effective nursing assessment and care are provided in the home (see Chapters 12 and 13).

Cultural Considerations in Pregnancy

As discussed in Chapter 8, actions during pregnancy are often determined by cultural beliefs. Table 9–1 presents activities encouraged or forbidden by some specific cultures. The table is not inclusive, and it is not meant to imply that all members of a given culture hold these beliefs. Nevertheless, it offers a few examples of cultural activities that may be important to some clients during the prenatal period.

In working with clients of another culture, the health professional is as open as possible to other beliefs. If activities are not harmful, there is no need to ask the client to change them. If the activities are harmful, the nurse can consult, or work with, someone within the culture or someone aware of cultural beliefs and values to help modify a client's behavior or to determine alternatives.

Language barriers often pose a special challenge in providing effective prenatal nursing care. Whenever possible it is important to have an interpreter—family member, friend, or staff person—present at prenatal visits so the nurse can provide basic information about

TABLE 9–2 Self-Care Measures for Common Discomforts of Pregnancy

Discomfort	Influencing Factors	Self-Care Measures
First Trimester		
Nausea and vomiting	Increased levels of hCG Changes in carbohydrate metabolism Emotional factors Fatigue	Avoid odors or causative factors. Eat dry crackers or toast before arising in morning. Have small but frequent meals. Avoid greasy or highly seasoned foods. Take dry meals with fluids between meals. Drink carbonated beverages.
Urinary frequency	Pressure of uterus on bladder in both first and third trimesters	Void when urge is felt. Increase fluid intake during the day. Decrease fluid intake *only* in the evening to decrease nocturia.
Fatigue	Specific causative factors unknown May be aggravated by nocturia due to urinary frequency	Plan time for a nap or rest period daily. Go to bed earlier. Seek family support and assistance with responsibilities so that more time is available to rest.
Breast tenderness	Increased levels of estrogen and progesterone	Wear well-fitting, supportive bra.
Increased vaginal discharge	Hyperplasia of vaginal mucosa and increased production of mucus by the endocervical glands due to the increase in estrogen levels	Promote cleanliness by daily bathing. Avoid douching, nylon underpants, and pantyhose; cotton underpants are more absorbent; powder can be used to maintain dryness if not allowed to cake.
Nasal stuffiness and nosebleed (epistaxis)	Elevated estrogen levels	May be unresponsive, but cool air vaporizer may help; avoid use of nasal sprays and decongestants.
Ptyalism (excessive, often bitter salivation)	Specific causative factors unknown	Use astringent mouthwashes, chew gum, or suck hard candy.
Second and Third Trimesters		
Heartburn (pyrosis)	Increased production of progesterone, decreasing gastrointestinal motility and increasing relaxation of cardiac sphincter, displacement of stomach by enlarging uterus, thus regurgitation of acidic gastric contents into esophagus	Eat small and more frequent meals. Use low-sodium antacids. Avoid overeating, fatty and fried foods, lying down after eating, and sodium bicarbonate.
Ankle edema	Prolonged standing or sitting Increased levels of sodium due to hormonal influences Circulatory congestion of lower extremities Increased capillary permeability Varicose veins	Practice frequent dorsiflexion of feet when prolonged sitting or standing is necessary. Elevate legs when sitting or resting. Avoid tight garters or restrictive bands around legs.
Varicose veins	Venous congestion in the lower veins that increases with pregnancy Hereditary factors (weakening of walls of veins, faulty valves) Increased age and weight gain	Elevate legs frequently. Wear supportive hose. Avoid crossing legs at the knees, standing for long periods, garters, and hosiery with constrictive bands.

pregnancy and prenatal care. The nurse should also provide opportunities for the woman to ask questions or express concerns. It is especially useful to have printed material available in the woman's language.

Relief of the Common Discomforts of Pregnancy

The common discomforts of pregnancy result from physiologic and anatomic changes and are fairly specific to each of the three trimesters. Health professionals often refer to these discomforts as minor, but they are not minor to the pregnant woman. They can make her quite uncomfortable and, if they are unexpected, anxious. Table 9–2 identifies the common discomforts of pregnancy, their possible causes, and the self-care measures that may relieve the discomfort.

First Trimester

Nausea and Vomiting

Nausea and vomiting are early symptoms in pregnancy. These symptoms appear sometime after the first missed menstrual period and usually cease by the fourth missed menstrual period. Approximately 50 to 88 percent of pregnant women in Western cultures experience some degree of nausea (Blackburn and Loper 1992). Some women develop an aversion to specific foods, some develop nausea related to specific odors, many experience nausea upon arising in the morning, and others experience nausea throughout the day. Vomiting does not occur in the majority of these women.

Nausea and vomiting in early pregnancy are believed to be caused by elevated human chorionic gonadotropin (hCG) levels and changes in carbohydrate metabolism, but fatigue and emotional factors may also play a part.

TABLE 9–2 Self-Care Measures for Common Discomforts of Pregnancy continued

Discomfort	Influencing Factors	Self-Care Measures
Second and Third Trimesters continued		
Hemorrhoids	Constipation (see following discussion) Increased pressure from gravid uterus on hemorrhoidal veins	Avoid constipation. Apply ice packs, topical ointments, anesthetic agents, warm soaks, or sitz baths; gently reinsert into rectum as necessary.
Constipation	Increased levels of progesterone, which cause general bowel sluggishness Pressure of enlarging uterus on intestine Iron supplements Diet, lack of exercise, and decreased fluids	Increase fluid intake, fiber in the diet, and exercise. Develop regular bowel habits. Use stool softeners as recommended by physician.
Backache	Increased curvature of the lumbosacral vertebrae as the uterus enlarges Increased levels of hormones, which cause softening of cartilage in body joints Fatigue Poor body mechanics	Use proper body mechanics. Practice the pelvic tilt exercise. Avoid uncomfortable working heights, high-heeled shoes, lifting heavy loads, and fatigue.
Leg cramps	Imbalance of calcium/phosphorus ratio Increased pressure of uterus on nerves Fatigue Poor circulation to lower extremities Pointing the toes	Practice dorsiflexion of feet in order to stretch affected muscle. Evaluate diet. Apply heat to affected muscles.
Faintness	Postural hypotension Sudden change of position causing venous pooling in dependent veins Standing for long periods in warm area Anemia	Arise slowly from resting position. Avoid prolonged standing in warm or stuffy environments.
Dyspnea	Decreased vital capacity from pressure of enlarging uterus on the diaphragm	Use proper posture when sitting and standing. Sleep propped up with pillows for relief if problem occurs at night.
Flatulence	Decreased gastrointestinal motility leading to delayed emptying time Pressure of growing uterus on large intestine Air swallowing	Avoid gas-forming foods. Chew food thoroughly. Get regular daily exercise. Maintain normal bowel habits.
Round ligament pain	Stretching and hypertrophy of round ligaments	Apply heating pad to the abdomen. Draw knees up to abdomen.
Carpal tunnel syndrome	Compression of median nerve in carpal tunnel of wrist Aggravated by repetitive hand movements	Avoid aggravating hand movements. Use splint as prescribed. Elevate affected arm.

A woman should be advised to contact her health care provider if she vomits more than once a day or shows signs of dehydration such as dry mouth and concentrated urine. In such cases, the physician/certified nurse-midwife might order antiemetics. However, antiemetics should be avoided if possible during this time because of possible harmful effects on embryo development.

Urinary Frequency

Urinary frequency is a common discomfort of pregnancy. It occurs early in pregnancy and again during the third trimester because of pressure of the enlarging uterus on the bladder. While urinary frequency is considered normal during the first and third trimesters, the woman should report signs of bladder infection such as pain, burning with voiding, or blood in the urine to her health care provider. The woman should also be encouraged to maintain an adequate fluid intake—at least 2000 mL per day.

Fatigue

Marked fatigue is so common in early pregnancy that it is considered a presumptive sign of pregnancy. It is aggravated if the woman has to arise each night because of urinary frequency. Typically it resolves after the end of the first trimester.

Breast Tenderness

Sensitivity of the breasts occurs early and continues throughout the pregnancy. Increased levels of estrogen and progesterone contribute to soreness and tingling of the breasts and increased sensitivity of the nipples.

COMMUNITY IN FOCUS The Pregnancy Wellness Program

Pregnancy education programs offered at the workplace have been effective in improving pregnancy outcomes, reducing health care costs, and decreasing the amount of employee absenteeism. The Oster/Sunbeam Appliance Company is a classic example of such a success story. In 1986 the company began a mandatory prenatal education program for all pregnant employees. After 3 years of implementation, the company reported no preterm births and a decrease in the average cost of maternity from $27,000 to $3,000 per pregnancy (Guastini and Marshall 1989).

Pitt County Memorial Hospital in Greenville, North Carolina, a large tertiary medical center, employs over 2,800 women. Over 40 percent of these women are within their childbearing years, and analysis of costs revealed that a significant portion of the hospital's health insurance dollars was spent to cover complications related to pregnancy. To address this issue, in 1991 the hospital began to offer a Pregnancy Wellness Program to pregnant employees and pregnant spouses of employees. The program has several goals (Walden et al 1996):

- to increase each pregnant woman's knowledge about pregnancy
- to encourage women to begin and maintain prenatal care
- to reduce complications related to pregnancy and birth
- to promote lifestyle behaviors that are healthy and conducive to a favorable pregnancy outcome
- to encourage a positive pregnancy environment by providing management's support for employees

The program, offered three times a year, consists of three parts:

1. *Pregnancy Wellness classes.* These classes, coordinated and taught by a clinical nurse specialist, are offered at noon one day per week for 12 weeks. Scheduled as brown bag sessions, the classes last an hour and focus on topics such as nutrition, positive lifestyle behaviors, discomforts of pregnancy, preparation for labor and birth, and newborn care.
2. *Baby Quest.* In this program surveys are sent to each participant once each semester and during the postpartum period. Based on the input, each woman receives an individualized packet of educational materials.
3. *Follow-up contact with a Women's Services Division clinical nurse specialist.*

To encourage employee/spouse participation, incentives are provided. Those who register for the program before the end of the first trimester of pregnancy, and who then complete the entire Baby Quest Program and at least 75 percent of the Pregnancy Wellness classes, may choose to receive a $100 reduction in their annual medical insurance cost or $100 in baby-related gifts (Walden et al 1996).

The program is quite successful. Participants have demonstrated increased knowledge of pregnancy and have had shorter mean length of stay than nonparticipants. Moreover, insurance claim costs for participants were 37 percent lower than for nonparticipants (Walden et al 1996). Hopefully, success stories such as this one will encourage employers to actively support health-focused, effective programs. They make sense and make a difference, too!

Increased Vaginal Discharge

Increased whitish vaginal discharge, called **leukorrhea,** is common in pregnancy. It occurs as a result of hyperplasia of the vaginal mucosa and increased mucus production by the endocervical glands. The increased acidity of the secretions encourages the growth of *Candida albicans,* so the woman is more susceptible to monilial vaginitis.

Nasal Stuffiness and Epistaxis

Once pregnancy is well established, elevated estrogen levels may produce edema of the nasal mucosa. This results in nasal stuffiness, nasal discharge, and obstruction. Epistaxis (nosebleeds) may also result. Cool-air vaporizers may help, but the problem is often unresponsive to treatment. Women experiencing these problems find it difficult to sleep and may resort to nasal sprays and decongestants. Such interventions can increase nasal stuffiness and create other discomforts. Pregnant women should avoid using any medications if possible.

Ptyalism

Ptyalism is a rare discomfort of pregnancy in which excessive, often bitter saliva is produced. The cause is unknown, and effective treatments are limited.

Second and Third Trimesters

It is more difficult to classify discomforts as specifically occurring in the second or third trimesters, since many problems represent individual variations in women. The discomforts discussed in this section usually do not appear until the third trimester in primigravidas, but occur earlier with each succeeding pregnancy.

Heartburn (Pyrosis)

Heartburn is the regurgitation of acidic gastric contents into the esophagus. It creates a burning sensation in the esophagus and sometimes leaves a bad taste in the mouth. Heartburn appears to be primarily a result of the displacement of the stomach by the enlarging uterus. The increased production of progesterone in pregnancy, decreases in gastrointestinal motility, and relaxation of the cardiac (esophageal) sphincter also contribute to heartburn.

The caregiver may recommend a low-sodium antacid, such as aluminum hydroxide (Amphojel) or a combination of aluminum hydroxide and magnesium hydroxide (Maalox). Because aluminum alone tends to cause constipation and magnesium alone is associated with diarrhea, the combined approach is more desirable.

Sodium bicarbonate (baking soda) and Alka-Seltzer should be avoided because they may lead to electrolyte imbalance.

If maternal heartburn is severe, not relieved by antacids, and accompanied by gastrointestinal reflux, an antisecretory agent (H_2 blocker) may be indicated. In such cases ranitidine (Zantac) or famotidine (Pepcid) are preferred because some research suggests that cimetidine (Tagamet) may have a feminizing effect on a male fetus (Larson and Rayburn 1996).

Ankle Edema

Most women experience ankle edema in the last part of pregnancy because of the increasing difficulty of venous return from the lower extremities. Prolonged standing or sitting and warm weather increase the edema. It is also associated with varicose veins. Ankle edema becomes a concern only when accompanied by hypertension or proteinuria or when the edema is not postural in origin.

Varicose Veins

Varicose veins are a result of weakening of the walls of veins or faulty functioning of the valves. Poor circulation in the lower extremities predisposes to varicose veins in the legs and thighs, as does prolonged standing or sitting. Pressure of the gravid uterus on the pelvic veins prevents good venous return and may therefore aggravate existing problems or contribute to obvious changes in the veins of the legs (Figure 9–1).

Treatment of varicose veins by the injection method or by surgery is not recommended during pregnancy. The woman should be aware that treatment may be needed after pregnancy because the problem will be aggravated by a succeeding pregnancy.

Although they are less common, varicosities in the vulva and perineum may also develop. They produce aching and a sense of heaviness. Support for vulvar varicosities is sometimes achieved by wearing two sanitary pads inside the underpants. The woman may relieve uterine pressure on the pelvic veins by resting on her side.

Hemorrhoids

Hemorrhoids are varicosities of the veins in the lower rectum and the anus. During pregnancy, the gravid uterus presses on the veins and interferes with venous circulation. In addition, the straining that accompanies constipation is frequently a contributing cause of hemorrhoids.

Some women may not be bothered by hemorrhoids until the second stage of labor, when the hemorrhoids appear as they push. These usually become asymptomatic a few days after the birth.

Symptoms of hemorrhoids include itching, swelling, pain, and bleeding. Women who have had hemorrhoids before pregnancy will probably experience difficulties with them during pregnancy.

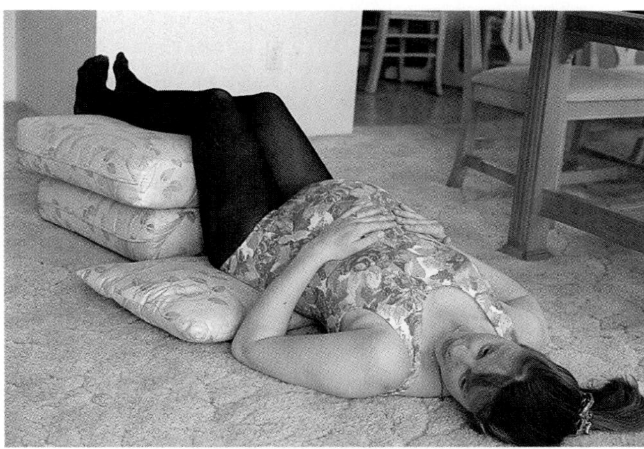

FIGURE 9–1 Swelling and discomfort from varicosities can be decreased by lying down with the legs and one hip elevated (to avoid compression of the vena cava).

It is possible to find relief by gently reinserting the hemorrhoid. The woman lies on her side, places some lubricant on her finger, and presses against the hemorrhoids, pushing them inside. She holds them in place for 1–2 minutes and then gently withdraws her finger. The anal sphincter should then hold them inside the rectum. The woman will find it especially helpful if she can maintain a side-lying (Sims') position for a time, so this method is best done before bed or a daily rest period.

Constipation

Conditions that predispose the pregnant woman to constipation include general bowel sluggishness caused by increased progesterone and steroid metabolism; displacement of the intestines, which increases with the growth of the fetus; and the oral iron supplements most pregnant women need.

In severe or preexisting cases of constipation, the physician may prescribe stool softeners, mild laxatives, or suppositories.

Backache

Many pregnant women experience backache, due primarily to exaggeration of the lumbosacral curve that occurs as the uterus enlarges and becomes heavier. The use of good posture and proper body mechanics throughout pregnancy is important in preventing backache. The woman should avoid bending over to pick up objects and should bend from the knees instead (Figure 9–2). She should place her feet 12–18 inches apart to maintain body balance. If the woman uses work surfaces that require her to bend, the nurse should advise the woman to adjust the height of the surfaces.

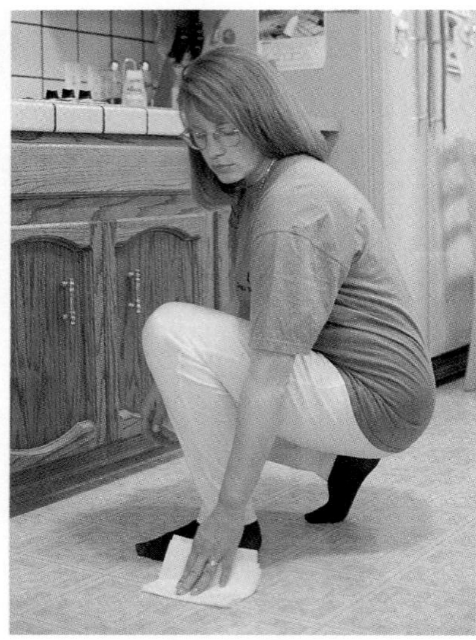

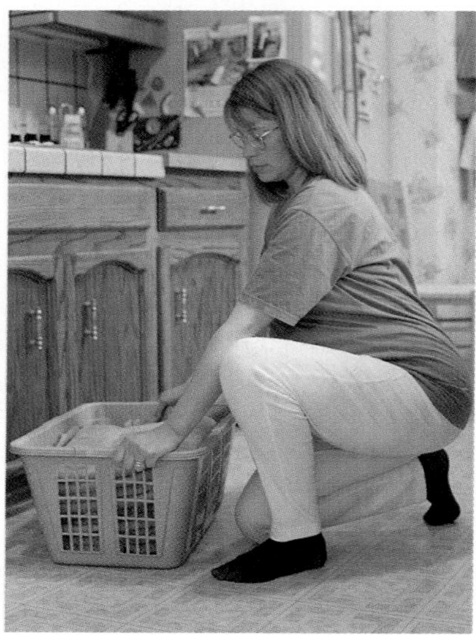

FIGURE 9–2 When picking up objects from floor level or lifting objects, the pregnant woman must use proper body mechanics.

Leg Cramps

Leg cramps are painful muscle spasms in the gastrocnemius muscles. They occur most frequently after the woman has gone to bed at night but may occur at other times. Extension of the foot can often cause leg cramps; the nurse should warn the pregnant woman not to extend the foot during childbirth preparation exercises or during rest periods. The exact cause of leg cramps is not known, but they may be caused by changes in calcium and phosphorous metabolism or by pressure of the enlarged uterus on pelvic nerves or blood vessels leading to the legs.

Leg cramps are more common in the third trimester because of increased weight of the uterus on the nerves supplying the lower extremities. Fatigue and poor circulation in the lower extremities contribute to this problem.

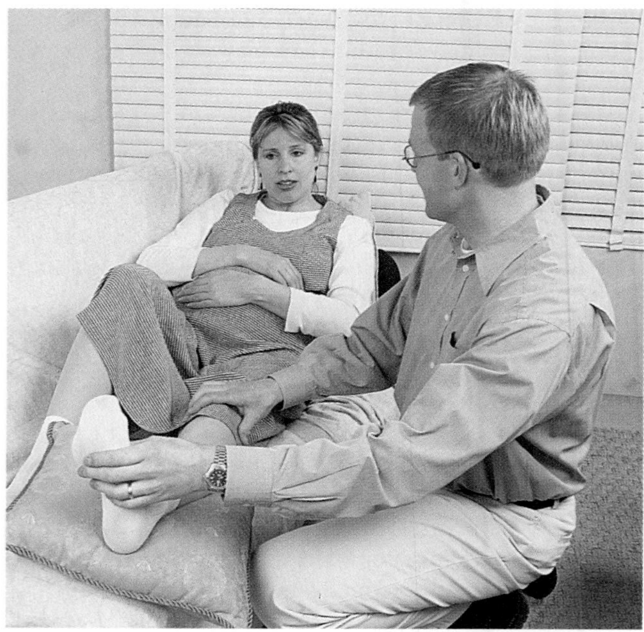

FIGURE 9–3 The expectant father can help relieve the woman's painful leg cramps by massaging her calf.

Immediate relief of the muscle spasm is achieved by stretching the muscle. With the woman lying on her back, another person presses the woman's knee down to straighten her leg while pushing her foot toward her leg. The woman may also stand and put her foot flat on the floor. Massage and warm packs can alleviate the discomfort of leg cramps (Figure 9–3).

The physician may recommend that the woman drink no more than a pint of milk daily and take calcium carbonate or that she drink a quart of milk daily and take aluminum hydroxide gel. This stops the action of phosphorus on calcium by absorbing the phosphorus and eliminating it directly through the intestinal tract. The treatment recommended depends on the frequency of the leg cramps.

Faintness

Many pregnant women occasionally feel faint, especially in warm, crowded areas. Faintness is caused by changes in the blood volume and postural hypotension due to pooling of blood in the dependent veins. Sudden change of position or standing for prolonged periods can also cause this sensation, and fainting can occur.

If a woman begins to feel faint from prolonged standing or from being in a stuffy room, she should sit down and lower her head between her legs. If this procedure does not help, the woman needs to be assisted to an area where she can lie down and get fresh air. When arising from a resting position, it is important that she move slowly. Women whose jobs require standing in one place for long periods should march in place regularly to increase venous return from the legs.

Shortness of Breath (Dyspnea)

Shortness of breath occurs as the uterus rises into the abdomen and causes pressure on the diaphragm. This problem worsens in the last trimester as the enlarged uterus presses directly on the diaphragm, decreasing vital capacity. In the last few weeks of pregnancy in the primigravida, the fetus and uterus move down in the pelvis, and the woman experiences considerable relief. This feeling is called **lightening.** Because the multigravida does not usually experience lightening until labor, she will tend to feel short of breath throughout the latter part of her pregnancy.

Flatulence

Flatulence is caused by decreased gastrointestinal motility, leading to delayed emptying of the bowel, and by pressure of the growing uterus on the large intestine. Air swallowing may also contribute to the problem.

Round Ligament Pain

As the uterus enlarges during pregnancy, the round ligaments stretch, hypertrophy, and lengthen as the uterus rises up in the abdomen. The woman may feel concern when she first experiences round ligament pain, because it is often intense and causes a "grabbing" sensation in the lower abdomen and inguinal area. The nurse should warn the pregnant woman of this possible discomfort. Once the caregiver has determined the cause of the pain is not a medical complication such as appendicitis, the woman may find that a heating pad to the abdomen brings relief.

Carpal Tunnel Syndrome

Carpal tunnel syndrome causes numbness, tingling, or burning in the fleshy part of the hand near the thumb and is due to compression of the median nerve in the carpal tunnel of the wrist. The syndrome is aggravated by repetitive hand movements such as typing, and may disappear following birth. Surgery is indicated in severe cases if more conservative approaches are not effective.

Promotion of Self-Care During Pregnancy

Fetal Activity Monitoring

Many caregivers encourage pregnant women to monitor their unborn child's well-being by regularly assessing fetal activity. Vigorous fetal activity generally provides reassurance of fetal well-being, while a marked decrease in activity or cessation of movement may indicate possible fetal compromise that requires immediate evaluation. Fetal activity is affected by sound, drugs, cigarette smoking, fetal sleep, blood glucose level, and time of day. There are times when minimal or no fetal activity occurs with a healthy fetus. A variety of methods for tracking fetal activity have been developed. They focus on having the woman keep **fetal movement records (FMR)** or a **fetal activity diary (FAD).** The Cardiff Count-to-Ten method is a widely used, noninvasive technique that permits the pregnant woman to monitor fetal well-being easily and without expense. She then records her findings. See Teaching Guide: What to Tell the Pregnant Woman About Assessing Fetal Activity on p 208.

Breast Care

Whether the pregnant woman plans to bottle- or breastfeed her infant, proper support of the breasts is important to promote comfort, retain breast shape, and prevent back strain, particularly if the breasts become large and pendulous. The sensitivity of the breasts in pregnancy is also relieved by good support.

A well-fitting, supportive brassiere has the following qualities:

- The straps are wide and do not stretch (elastic straps soon lose their tautness with the weight of the breasts and frequent washing).
- The cup holds all breast tissue comfortably.
- The brassiere has tucks or other devices that allow it to expand, thus accommodating the enlarging chest circumference.
- The brassiere supports the nipple line approximately midway between the elbow and shoulder but is not pulled up in the back by the weight of the breasts.

Cleanliness of the breasts is important, especially as the woman begins producing colostrum. Colostrum that crusts on the nipples should be removed with warm water. The woman planning to breastfeed should not use soap on her nipples because of its drying effect.

Nipple preparation, generally begun during the third trimester, helps prevent soreness during the first few days of breastfeeding. Nipple preparation helps distribute the natural lubricants produced by Montgomery's tubercles, stimulates blood flow to the breast, and helps develop the protective layer of skin over the nipple. Women who are planning to nurse can begin by occasionally going braless and by exposing their nipples to sunlight and air. Rubbing the nipples removes protective oils and should be avoided; but rolling the nipple—grasping it between thumb and forefinger and gently rolling it for a short time each day—helps prepare for breastfeeding. A woman with a history of preterm labor is advised *not* to do this because nipple stimulation triggers the release of oxytocin. (See Chapter 14 for further discussion of the effects of nipple stimulation on contractions.)

Text continues on page 210

TEACHING GUIDE What To Tell the Pregnant Woman About Assessing Fetal Activity

ASSESSMENT

The nurse focuses on the woman's prior knowledge and former use of fetal movement assessment methods, the week of gestation, and her communication and ability to understand and process information.

NURSING DIAGNOSIS

The key nursing diagnosis will probably be: Knowledge deficit related to lack of information about fetal movement assessment methods.

NURSING PLAN AND IMPLEMENTATION

The goal of the teaching sessions is to provide general information regarding fetal movement and assessment methods.

CLIENT GOALS

At the completion of the teaching session the woman will:

- Discuss the types of fetal assessment methods, reasons for assessment, how to accomplish the assessment, and methods of record keeping.
- Demonstrate the use of a fetal movement record.
- Identify resources to call if questions arise.
- Agree to bring the fetal movement record to each prenatal visit.

Teaching Plan

CONTENT

The expectant woman needs to know that fetal movements are first felt around 18 weeks' gestation. From that time the fetal movements get stronger and easier to detect. A slowing or stopping of fetal movement may be an indication that the fetus needs some attention and evaluation. The normal amount of movement varies considerably; however, most healthy fetuses move at least ten times in 3 hours.

TEACHING METHOD

Describe procedures and demonstrate how to assess fetal movement. Sit beside woman and show her how to place her hand on the fundus to feel fetal movement.

Provide a written teaching sheet for the woman's use at home.

Cardiff Count-to-Ten (Figure 9–4)

The woman begins these assessments in the 27th week of gestation. The woman chooses what time she will start each day but keeps the time relatively consistent. She can either place a mark for each fetal movement until ten have been recorded or place an X at the beginning of the counting period and then again at the time ten movements have been felt.

It will be advantageous for the woman to schedule the counting periods about 1 hour past eating and to combine the counting period with rest. A side-lying position provides optimal circulation to the uterus-placenta-fetus unit. In addition the fetus's movements are felt more readily while lying on the side. Later in the pregnancy some women may be bothered by indigestion after eating. In this case they can prop up the upper body but still maintain a side-lying position.

Demonstrate how to record fetal movements on Cardiff Count-to-Ten scoring card.

Watch woman fill out record as examples are provided. Encourage her to complete the record each day and bring it with her to each prenatal visit. Assure her that the record will be discussed at each prenatal visit, and questions may be addressed at that time if desired.

When to Contact the Care Provider

When there are questions or concerns.

If there are fewer than ten movements in 3 hours.

If overall the fetus's movements are slowing, and it takes much longer each day to note ten movements.

Provide the woman with a name and phone number in case she has further questions.

What Happens Next

The care provider will probably suggest a nonstress test (NST) to further evaluate the fetus. Additional testing may include a contraction stress test (CST), tests for pulmonary maturity, and ultrasound. (These tests are discussed in Chapter 14.)

TEACHING GUIDE continued

EVALUATION

The nurse may evaluate learning by having the woman explain the method to the nurse and by asking the woman to fill the card in using a fictitious situation. At each prenatal visit the expectant woman's record is reviewed, and this provides another opportunity for evaluation of learning. Asking about the record at each visit will demonstrate that it is an important part of the woman's care. Review of the record provides opportunities for questions and clarification.

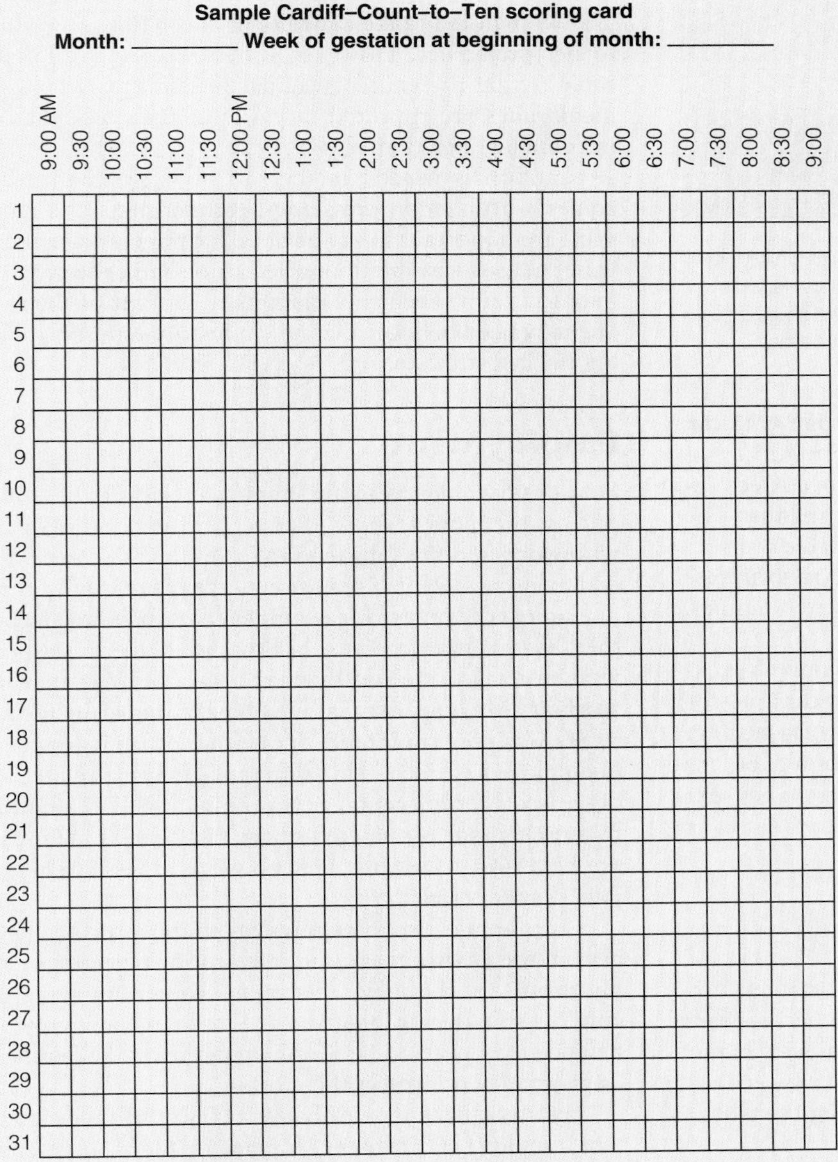

Sample Cardiff–Count–to–Ten scoring card

Month: ________ Week of gestation at beginning of month: ________

	9:00 AM	9:30	10:00	10:30	11:00	11:30	12:00 PM	12:30	1:00	1:30	2:00	2:30	3:00	3:30	4:00	4:30	5:00	5:30	6:00	6:30	7:00	7:30	8:00	8:30	9:00
1																									
2																									
3																									
4																									
5																									
6																									
7																									
8																									
9																									
10																									
11																									
12																									
13																									
14																									
15																									
16																									
17																									
18																									
19																									
20																									
21																									
22																									
23																									
24																									
25																									
26																									
27																									
28																									
29																									
30																									
31																									

FIGURE 9–4 Fetal movement assessment method: the Cardiff Count-to-Ten scoring card (adaptation).

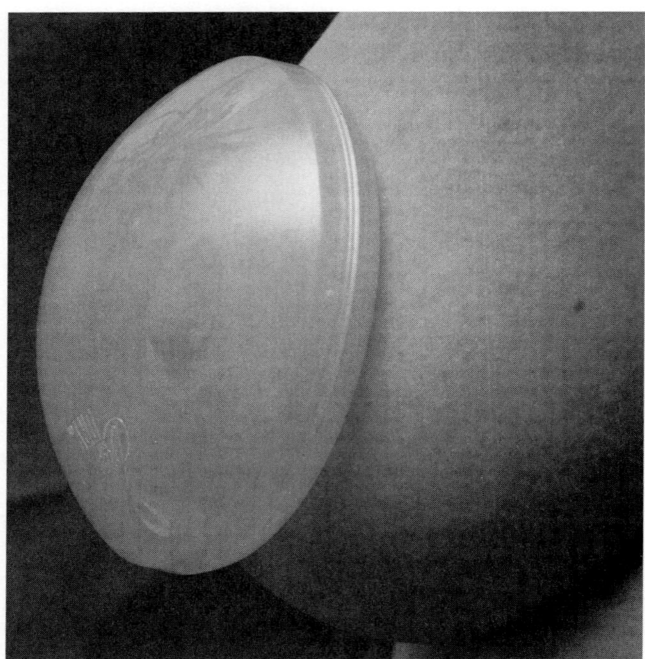

FIGURE 9–5 This breast shield is designed to increase the protractility of inverted nipples. Worn the last 3 to 4 months of pregnancy, it exerts gentle pulling pressure at the edge of the areola, gradually forcing the nipple through the center of the shield. They may be used after birth if still necessary.

Nipple-rolling is more difficult for women with flat or inverted nipples, but it is still a useful preparation for breast-feeding. Breast shields designed to correct inverted nipples can be worn during pregnancy. The shields appear to be the only currently available measure that offers some help to women with inverted nipples (Figure 9–5). For further discussion of inverted nipples, see Chapter 24.

Oral stimulation of the nipple by the woman's partner during sex play is also an excellent technique for toughening the nipple in preparation for breast-feeding. The couple who enjoy this stimulation should be encouraged to continue it throughout the pregnancy, except when the woman has a history of preterm labor, as discussed earlier.

Clothing

Clothing in pregnancy is generally an important factor in the woman's feelings about herself and her appearance. Maternity clothes can be expensive, however, and are worn for a relatively short time. Women may economize by sharing clothes with friends, sewing their own garments, or buying used maternity clothes.

Clothes should be loose and nonconstricting. Maternity girdles are seldom worn today and are not necessary for most women. Some women athletes who maintain a light workout schedule during pregnancy use a girdle to provide support. Women who have large, pendulous abdomens may also benefit from a well-fitting, supportive girdle. Tight leg bands on girdles must be avoided.

High-heeled shoes aggravate back discomfort by increasing the curvature of the lower back. They should not be worn if the woman experiences backache or has problems with balance. Shoes should fit properly and feel comfortable.

Bathing

Daily bathing is important because perspiration and mucoid vaginal discharge increase during pregnancy. The woman may take showers or tub baths, according to her preference. However, tub baths are contraindicated in the presence of vaginal bleeding or when the membranes are ruptured, because of the possibility of introducing infection.

Caution is needed in the tub because balance becomes a problem in pregnancy. Rubber mats and hand grips are important safety devices. Extremely warm bath water causes vasodilation; after a hot bath, the woman may feel faint when she attempts to get out of the tub. She may need help getting out of the tub, especially during the last trimester.

Employment

Studies of women who are employed outside the home during pregnancy show distinct differences. Women who work in office jobs tend to have slightly lower odds of having a small-for-gestational-age (SGA) baby than unemployed women, for example. This may be because they have better access to health care or because these women tend to be healthier as a group. Women who work at strenuous manual jobs have a higher incidence of SGA or preterm infants than either office workers or unemployed women. This difference may be related to decreased uteroplacental perfusion as blood is shunted to muscle tissue or may reflect the fact that women who are better off financially tend to work at less strenuous jobs (Launer et al 1990).

Overfatigue, excessive physical strain, fetotoxic hazards in the environment, and medical or obstetric complications are the major deterrents to certain types of employment during pregnancy. Employment involving balance may need to be terminated during the last half of pregnancy to protect the mother.

Fetotoxic hazards are always a concern to the expectant couple. The pregnant woman (or the woman contemplating pregnancy) who works in industry should contact her company physician or nurse about possible hazards in her work environment and should do her own reading and research on environmental hazards as well.

Travel

If medical or pregnancy complications are not present, there are no restrictions on travel. Pregnant women should avoid travel if there is a history of bleeding or pregnancy-induced hypertension or if multiple births are anticipated.

Travel by automobile can be especially fatiguing, aggravating many of the discomforts of pregnancy. The pregnant woman needs frequent opportunities to get out of the car and walk. (A good pattern is to stop every 2 hours and walk around for approximately 10 minutes.) She should wear both lap and shoulder belts; the lap belt should fit snugly and be positioned under the abdomen and across the upper thighs. Seat belts play an important role in preventing maternal mortality with subsequent fetal loss (Cunningham 1997). To decrease the risk of bladder trauma in the event of an accident, the woman should be encouraged to void regularly while traveling.

As pregnancy progresses, long-distance trips are best taken by plane or train. The availability of medical care at the destination is an important factor for the near-term woman who travels.

Activity and Rest

Normal participation in exercise can continue throughout an uncomplicated pregnancy. The woman should check with her certified nurse-midwife/physician about taking part in strenuous sports, such as skiing, diving, and horseback riding. In general, however, the skilled sportswoman is no longer discouraged from participating in these activities if her pregnancy is uncomplicated. However, pregnancy is not the appropriate time to learn a new or strenuous sport.

Exercise helps prevent constipation, increase energy, improve sleep, control weight gain, condition the body, and maintain a healthy mental state. It is especially important during pregnancy not to overdo it.

Certain conditions do contraindicate exercise. These include preterm rupture of the membranes, pregnancy-induced hypertension, incompetent cervix (cerclage), persistent second or third trimester bleeding, a history of preterm labor in a prior or the current pregnancy, or intrauterine growth retardation. Women with other obstetric conditions or preexisting medical conditions such as chronic hypertension or cardiac or pulmonary disease should be evaluated carefully to determine whether any form of exercise is appropriate (ACOG 1994).

The American College of Obstetricians and Gynecologists (ACOG) has developed guidelines about exercise during pregnancy (ACOG 1994), including

- Even mild to moderate exercise is beneficial during pregnancy. Regular exercise, which occurs at least three times a week, is preferred.
- After the first trimester women should avoid exercising in the supine position. In most pregnant women, the supine position is associated with decreased cardiac output. Since uterine blood flow is reduced during exercise as blood is shunted from the visceral organs to the muscles, the remaining cardiac output is further decreased. Similarly, women should also avoid standing motionless for prolonged periods.
- Because decreased oxygen is available for aerobic exercise during pregnancy, women should modify the intensity of their exercise based on their symptoms, should stop when they become fatigued, and should avoid exercising to the point of exhaustion. Non-weight-bearing exercises such as swimming or cycling are recommended because they decrease the risk of injury and provide fitness with comfort.
- As pregnancy progresses and the center of gravity changes, especially in the third trimester, women should avoid exercises in which the loss of balance could pose a risk to mother or fetus. Similarly, women should avoid any type of exercise that might result in even mild abdominal trauma for the woman.
- A normal pregnancy requires an additional 300 kcal per day. Women who exercise regularly during pregnancy should be careful to ensure that they consume an adequate diet.
- To augment heat dissipation, especially during the first trimester, pregnant women who exercise should wear appropriate clothing, ensure adequate hydration, and avoid the prolonged overheating associated with vigorous exercise in hot, humid weather. By the same token, they should avoid hot tubs and saunas. Research suggests that maternal exposure to heat (hot tubs, sauna, or fever) in the first trimester is associated with an increased risk of neural tube defects, mental deficiencies, seizures, facial abnormalities, and external ear anomolies in the fetus/newborn (Rogers and Davis 1995).

CRITICAL THINKING IN ACTION

Constance Petrowski, a 24-year-old, G1P0, world-class marathon runner, is 11 weeks pregnant when she sees the nurse-midwife for her first prenatal exam. Because of her low body fat, her menses had always been irregular, and it had not occurred to Constance that she might be pregnant. Constance tells the certified nurse-midwife that she has just begun serious training for a marathon, which is to take place when Constance is about 22 weeks pregnant. Constance says that she has been told that it is fine to continue any physical activity at which one is proficient and says that she would like to compete in the marathon because she believes she has a chance to come in as one of the top three women runners. What should the nurse tell Constance about competing in the marathon?

Answers can be found in Appendix H.

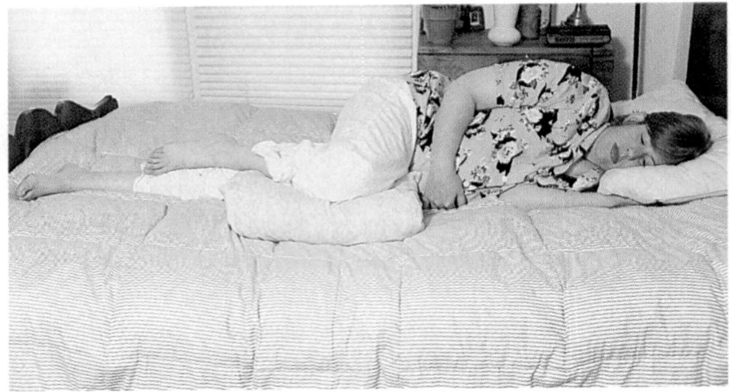

FIGURE 9–6 Position for relaxation and rest as pregnancy progresses.

In addition to the ACOG (1994) recommendations, the nurse may suggest that the woman wear a supportive bra and appropriate shoes when exercising. She should be advised to warm up and stretch to help prepare the joints for activity and cool down with a period of mild activity to help restore circulation and avoid pooling of blood. A moderate, rhythmic exercise routine involving large muscle groups such as swimming, cycling, walking, or cross-country skiing is best. Jogging or running is acceptable for women already conditioned to this activity.

Warning signs include back pain, absent fetal movement, difficulty walking, dizziness or faintness, pain, palpitations, pubic pain, shortness of breath, tachycardia, uterine contractions, vaginal bleeding, or fluid loss (Artal and Buckenmeyer 1995). The woman should stop exercising if these occur and modify her exercise program. If the symptoms persist, the woman should contact her caregiver.

Adequate rest in pregnancy is important for both physical and emotional health. Women need more sleep throughout pregnancy, particularly in the first and last trimesters, when they tire easily. Without adequate rest, pregnant women have less resilience.

Finding time to rest during the day may be difficult for women who work outside the home or who have small children. The nurse can help the expectant mother examine her daily schedule to develop a realistic plan for short periods of rest and relaxation.

Sleeping becomes more difficult during the last trimester because of the enlarged abdomen, increased frequency of urination, and greater activity of the fetus. Finding a comfortable position becomes difficult for the pregnant woman. Figure 9–6 shows a position most pregnant women find comfortable. Progressive relaxation techniques similar to those taught in prepared childbirth classes can help prepare the woman for sleep.

Exercises to Prepare for Childbirth

Certain exercises help strengthen muscle tone in preparation for birth and promote more rapid restoration of muscle tone after birth. Some physical changes of pregnancy can be minimized by faithfully practicing prescribed body-conditioning exercises. Many body-conditioning exercises for pregnancy are taught; a few of the more common ones are discussed here.

The **pelvic tilt,** or pelvic rocking, helps prevent, or at least reduce, back strain as it strengthens abdominal muscles. To do the pelvic tilt, the pregnant woman lies on her back and puts her feet flat on the floor. This flexes the knees and helps prevent strain or discomfort. She decreases the curvature in her back by pressing her spine toward the floor. With her back pressed to the floor, the woman tightens her abdominal muscles as she tightens and tucks in her buttocks. The woman can also perform the pelvic tilt on her hands and knees (Figure 9–7), while sitting in a chair, or while standing with her back against a wall. The body alignment that results when the pelvic tilt is correctly done should be maintained as much as possible throughout the day.

Abdominal Exercises

A basic exercise to increase abdominal muscle tone is tightening abdominal muscles with each breath. It can be done in any position, but it is best learned while the woman lies supine. With knees flexed and feet flat on the floor, the woman expands her abdomen and slowly takes a deep breath. Exhaling slowly, she gradually pulls in her abdominal muscles until they are fully contracted. She relaxes for a few seconds, and then repeats the exercise.

Partial sit-ups strengthen abdominal muscle tone and are done according to individual comfort levels. A partial sit-up must be done with the knees flexed and the feet flat on the floor to avoid strain on the lower back. The woman stretches her arms toward her knees as she slowly pulls her head and shoulders off the floor to a comfortable level (if she has poor abdominal muscle tone, she may not be able to pull up very far). She then slowly returns to the starting position, takes a deep breath, and repeats the exercise. To strengthen the oblique abdominal muscles, she repeats the process, but stretches the left arm to the side of her right knee, returns to the floor, takes a deep breath, and then reaches with the right arm to the left knee.

These exercises can be done approximately five times in a sequence, and the sequence can be repeated at other times during the day as desired. It is important to do the exercises slowly to prevent muscle strain and overtiring.

Perineal Exercises

Perineal muscle tightening, also called **Kegel's exercises,** strengthens the pubococcygeus muscle and increases its elasticity (Figure 9–8). The woman can feel the specific muscle group to be exercised by stopping urination midstream. Doing Kegel's exercises while urinating is discouraged, however, because this practice has been associated with urinary stasis and urinary tract infection.

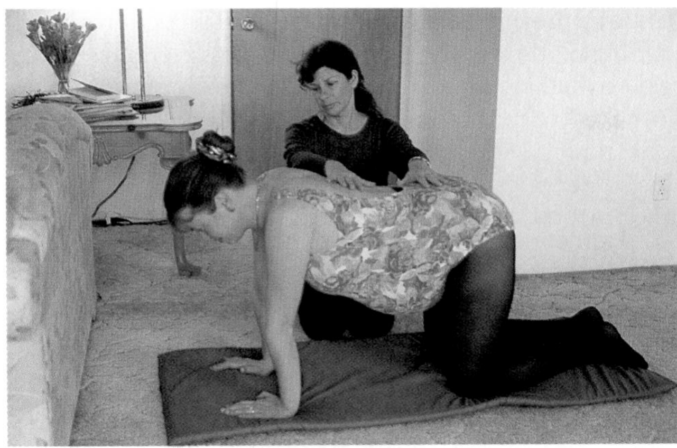

A

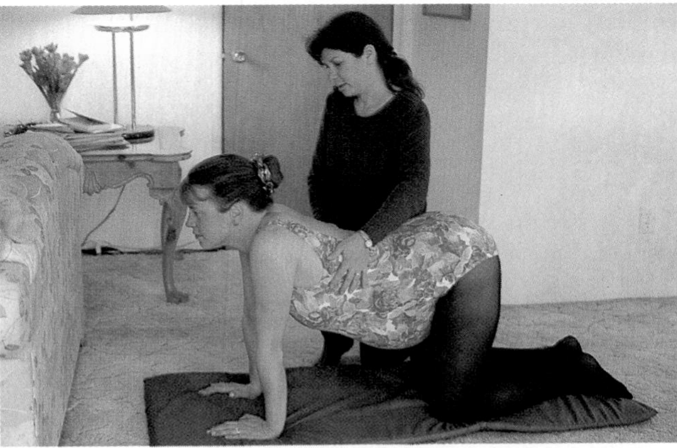

B

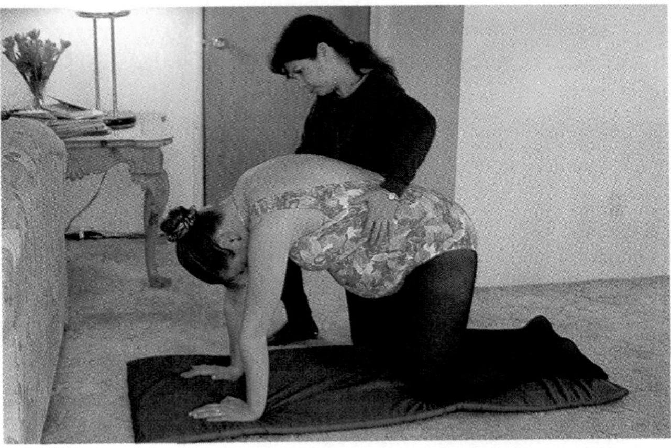

C

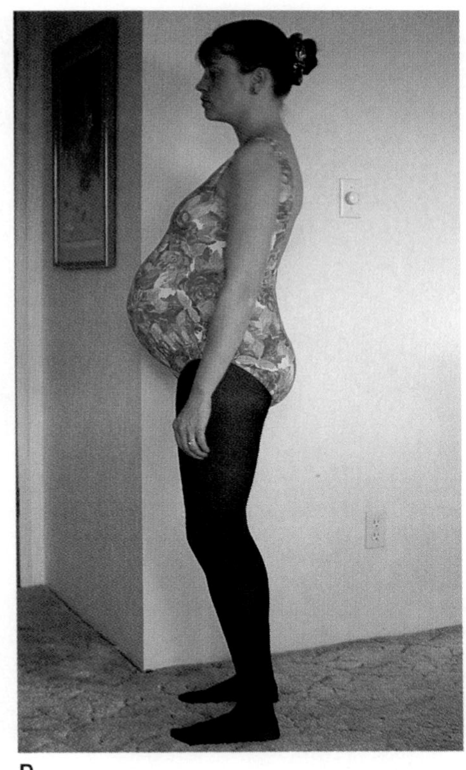

D

FIGURE 9–7 ***A*** Starting position when the pelvic tilt is done on hands and knees. The back is flat and parallel to the floor, the hands are below the head, and the knees are directly below the buttocks. ***B*** A prenatal yoga instructor offers pointers for proper positioning for the first part of the tilt: head up, neck long and separated from the shoulders, buttocks up, and pelvis thrust back, allowing the back to drop and release on an inhaled breath. ***C*** The instructor helps the woman assume the correct position for the next part of the tilt. It is done on a long exhalation, allowing the pregnant woman to arch her back, drop her head loosely, push away from her hands, and draw in the muscles of her abdomen to strengthen them. Note that in this position the pelvis and buttocks are tucked under, and the buttock muscles are tightened. ***D*** Proper posture. The knees are slightly bent but not locked, and the pelvis and buttocks are tucked under, thereby lengthening the spine and helping support the weighty abdomen. With her chin tucked in, this woman's neck, shoulders, hips, knees, and feet are all in a straight line perpendicular to the floor. Her feet are parallel. This is also the starting position for doing the pelvic tilt while standing.

Childbirth educators sometimes use the following technique to teach Kegel's exercises. They tell the woman to think of her perineal muscles as an elevator. When she relaxes, the elevator is on the first floor. To do the exercises, she contracts, bringing the elevator to the second, third, and fourth floors. She keeps the elevator on the fourth floor for a few seconds, and then gradually relaxes the area. If the exercise is properly done, the woman does not contract the muscles of the buttocks and thighs.

Kegel's exercises can be done at almost any time. Some women use ordinary events—for instance, stopping at a red light—as a cue to remember to do the exercise. Others do Kegel's exercises while waiting in a checkout line, talking on the telephone, or watching television.

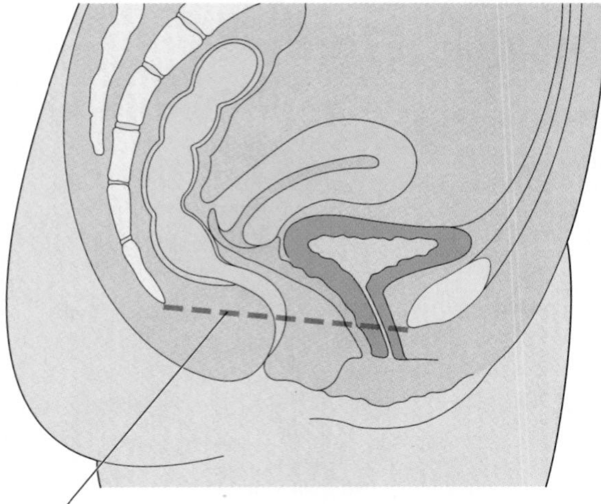

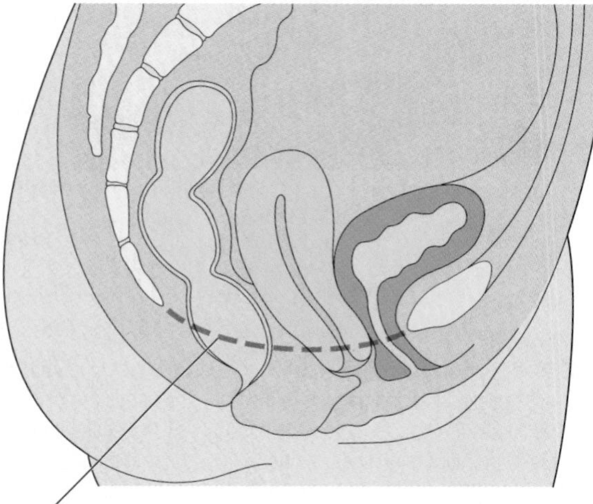

FIGURE 9–8 Kegel's exercises. The woman learns to tighten the pubococcygeus muscle, which improves support to the pelvic organs.

Inner Thigh Exercises

The pregnant woman should assume a cross-legged sitting position whenever possible. This "tailor sit" stretches the muscles of the inner thighs in preparation for labor and birth.

Sexual Activity

As a result of the physiologic, anatomic, and emotional changes of pregnancy, couples usually have many questions and concerns about sexual activity during pregnancy. Often, these questions are about possible injury to the baby or the woman during intercourse and about changes in the desire each partner feels for the other.

In the past, couples were frequently warned to avoid sexual intercourse during the last 6 to 8 weeks of pregnancy to prevent complications such as infection or premature rupture of the membranes. However, these fears seem to be unfounded. In a healthy pregnancy, there is no valid reason to limit sexual activity. Intercourse is contraindicated only when bleeding is present or membranes are ruptured. Women with a history of preterm labor or premature rupture of the membranes and those who experience strong uterine contractions following orgasm should be advised of the possible risks of coitus after 32 weeks' gestation (Kochenour 1994).

The expectant mother may experience changes in sexual desire and response. Often, these are related to the various discomforts that occur throughout pregnancy. For instance, during the first trimester fatigue or nausea and vomiting may decrease desire, while breast tenderness may make the woman less responsive to fondling of her breasts. During the second trimester, many of the discomforts have lessened, and, with the vascular congestion of the pelvis, the woman may experience greater sexual satisfaction than she experienced before pregnancy.

During the third trimester, interest in coitus may again decrease as the woman becomes more uncomfortable and fatigued. In addition, shortness of breath, painful pelvic ligaments, urinary frequency, leg cramps, and decreased mobility may lessen sexual desire and activity. If they are not already doing so, the couple should consider coital positions other than male superior, such as side-by-side, female superior, and vaginal rear entry.

Sexual activity does not have to include intercourse. Many of the nurturing and sexual needs of the pregnant woman can be satisfied by cuddling, kissing, and being held. The warm, sensual feelings that accompany these activities can be an end in themselves. Her partner, however, may choose to masturbate more frequently than before.

The sexual desires of men are also affected by many factors in pregnancy. These include the previous relationship with the partner, acceptance of the pregnancy, attitudes toward the partner's change of appearance, and concern about hurting the expectant mother or baby. Some men find it difficult to view their partners as sexually appealing while they are adjusting to the concept of them as mothers. Other men find their partner's pregnancy arousing and experience feelings of increased happiness, intimacy, and closeness.

The expectant couple should be aware of their changing sexual desires, the normality of these changes, and the importance of communicating these changes to each other so that they can make nurturing adaptations. The nurse has an important role in helping the expectant couple adapt. The couple must feel free to express concerns about sexual activity, and the nurse must be able to respond and give anticipatory guidance in a comfortable manner. See Teaching Guide: Sexual Activity During Pregnancy on p 216.

Dental Care

Proper dental hygiene is important in pregnancy. In spite of such discomforts as nausea and vomiting, gum hypertrophy and tenderness, possible ptyalism, and heartburn, regular oral hygiene must not be neglected.

The pregnant woman is encouraged to have a dental checkup early in her pregnancy. General dental repair and extractions can be done during pregnancy, preferably under local anesthetic. The woman should inform her dentist of her pregnancy so that she is not exposed to teratogenic substances. Dental x-ray examinations or extensive dental work should be delayed until after the birth when possible.

Immunizations

All women of childbearing age should be aware of the risks of receiving certain immunizations if pregnancy is possible. Immunizations with attenuated live viruses, such as rubella vaccine, should not be given in pregnancy because of the teratogenic effect of the live viruses on the developing embryo. Vaccinations using killed viruses may be used, however.

Teratogenic Substances

Substances that adversely affect the normal growth and development of the fetus are called **teratogens.** Many of these effects are readily apparent at birth, but others may not be identified for years. A well-known example is the development of cervical cancer in adolescent females whose mothers took diethylstilbestrol (DES) during pregnancy.

Many substances are known or suspected to be teratogens, including certain medications, cigarettes, psychotropic drugs, and alcohol. The harmful effects of others, such as some pesticides or exposure to x-rays in the first trimester of pregnancy, have been documented. During pregnancy, women need to have a realistic attitude about environmental hazards. Factors that are suspected to be hazardous to the general population should obviously be avoided if possible.

Medications

The use of medications during pregnancy, including both prescription and over-the-counter drugs, is of great concern. Many pregnant women need medication for therapeutic purposes, such as the treatment of infections, allergies, or other pathologic processes. In these situations, the problem can be extremely complex. Known teratogenic agents are not prescribed and usually can be replaced by medications considered safe. Even when a woman is highly motivated to avoid taking any medications, she may have taken potentially teratogenic medications before her pregnancy was confirmed, especially if she has an irregular menstrual cycle.

The greatest potential for gross abnormalities in the fetus occurs during the first trimester of pregnancy, when fetal organs are first developing. The classic period of teratogenesis in a woman with a 28-day cycle extends from day 31 after the LMP (17 days after fertilization) to day 71 (54 days after fertilization) (Niebyl 1994). Many factors influence teratogenic effects, including timing and duration of exposure to the medication as correlated with specific organ development; route of administration; individual metabolic and circulatory factors in the mother, placenta, and fetus; concurrent exposure to other agents; and species susceptibility to the effects (Kochenour 1992). For example, the commonly prescribed acne medication isotretinoin (Accutane) is associated with a high incidence of spontaneous abortion and congenital malformations if taken early in pregnancy. Valproic acid, an anticonvulsant, is associated with an increased risk of spina bifida. Table 9–3 on page 218 identifies the possible effects of selected drugs on the fetus and newborn. To provide information for caregivers and clients, the Food and Drug Administration has developed the following classification system for medications administered during pregnancy:

Category A: Controlled studies in women have demonstrated no associated fetal risk. Few drugs fall into this category.

Category B: Animal studies show no risk, but there are no controlled studies in women; or animal studies indicate a risk, but controlled human studies fail to demonstrate a risk. Heparin and the penicillins fall into this category.

Category C: No adequate animal or human studies are available; or animal studies show teratogenic effects, but no controlled studies in women are available. Many drugs fall into this category, which, because of the lack of information, is a problematic one for caregivers. Epinephrine, beta-blockers, and acyclovir fall into this category.

Category D: Evidence of human fetal risk does exist, but the benefits of the drug in certain situations are thought to outweigh the risks. Examples of drugs in this category include tetracycline, vincristine, lithium, and hydrochlorothiazide.

Category X: The demonstrated fetal risks clearly outweigh any possible benefit. Examples of drugs in this category include isotretinoin (Accutane), estrogens, and clomiphene.

If a woman has taken a drug in category D or X, she should be informed of the risks associated with that drug and of her alternatives. Similarly, a woman who has taken a drug in the safer categories can be reassured.

Although the first trimester is the critical period for teratogenesis, some medications are known to have a teratogenic effect when taken in the second and third trimesters. For example, tetracycline taken in late pregnancy is commonly associated with staining of teeth in

Text continues on page 218

TEACHING GUIDE Sexual Activity During Pregnancy

ASSESSMENT

Occasionally a woman indicates her beliefs about sexual activity during pregnancy by asking a direct question. This is most likely to occur if the woman and the nurse have a good rapport. Often, however, the nurse must ask some general questions to determine the woman's level of understanding. A general statement may trigger a discussion and help the nurse make a determination. In many cases teaching about this topic is coupled with ongoing assessment of the woman's understanding of sexual activity during pregnancy.

NURSING DIAGNOSIS

The key nursing diagnosis will probably be: knowledge deficit related to lack of information about changes in sexuality and sexual activity during pregnancy.

NURSING PLAN AND IMPLEMENTATION

The teaching plan will generally focus on discussion or use of a "question and answer" format. The presence of both partners may be beneficial in fostering communication between them and is acceptable unless personal or cultural factors indicate otherwise.

CLIENT GOALS

At the completion of the teaching the woman will:

- Relate the changes in sexuality and sexual response that may occur during pregnancy to changes in technique, frequency, and response that may be indicated.
- Explore personal attitudes, beliefs, and expectations about sexual activity during pregnancy.
- Cite maternal factors that would contraindicate sexual intercourse.

Teaching Plan

CONTENT	TEACHING METHOD
Begin by explaining that the pregnant woman may experience changes in desire during the course of pregnancy. During the first trimester, discomforts such as nausea, fatigue, and breast tenderness may make intercourse less desirable for many women. Other women may have fewer discomforts and may find that their sexual desire is unchanged. In the second trimester, as symptoms decrease, desire may increase. In the third trimester, discomfort and fatigue may lead to decreased desire in the woman.	Universal statements that give permission, such as "Many couples experience changes in sexual desire during pregnancy. What kind of changes have you experienced?" are often effective in starting discussion. Depending on the woman's (or couple's) level of knowledge and sophistication, part or all of this discussion may be necessary.
Men may notice changes in their level of desire, too. Among other things, this may be related to feelings about their partner's changing appearance, their belief about the acceptability of sexual activity with a pregnant woman, or concern about hurting the woman or fetus. Some men find the changes of pregnancy erotic; others must adjust to the notion of their partners as mothers.	If the partner is present, approach him in the same nonjudgmental way used above. If not, ask the woman if she has noticed any changes in her partner or if he has expressed any concerns.
Explain that the woman may notice that orgasms are much more intense during the last weeks of pregnancy and may be followed by cramping. Because of the pressure of the enlarging uterus on the vena cava, the woman should not lie flat on her back for intercourse after about the fourth month. If the couple prefer that position, a pillow should be placed under her right hip to displace the uterus. Alternate positions such as side-by-side, female superior, or vaginal rear entry may become necessary as her uterus enlarges.	Deal with any specific questions about the physical and psychologic changes that the couple may have.

TEACHING GUIDE Sexual Activity During Pregnancy continued

Teaching Plan *continued*

Stress that sexual activities that both partners enjoy are generally acceptable. It is not advisable for couples who favor anal sex to go from anal penetration to vaginal penetration because of the risk of introducing *E coli* into the vagina.

Discussion about various sexual activities requires that nurses be comfortable with their sexuality and be tactful. Often the nurse may find it advisable to volunteer such information to show that discussion of sexual variations is acceptable.

Alternative methods of expressing intimacy and affection such as cuddling, holding and stroking each other, and kissing may help maintain the couple's feelings of warmth and closeness.

The couple may be content with these approaches to meeting their sexual needs, or they may require assurance that such approaches are indeed "normal."

If the man feels desire for further sexual release, his partner may help him masturbate to ejaculation, or he may prefer to masturbate in private.

The woman who is interested in masturbation as a form of gratification should be advised that the orgasmic contractions may be especially intense in later pregnancy.

Stress that sexual intercourse is contraindicated once the membranes are ruptured or if bleeding is present. Women with a history of preterm labor may be advised to avoid intercourse because the oxytocin that is released with orgasm stimulates uterine contractions and may trigger preterm labor. Because oxytocin is also released with nipple stimulation, fondling the breasts may also be contraindicated in those cases.

An explanation of the contraindications accompanied by their rationale provides specific guidelines that most couples find helpful.

A discussion of sexuality and sexual activity should stress the importance of open communication so that the couple feel comfortable expressing their feelings, preferences, and concerns.

Some couples are skilled at expressing their feelings about sexual activity. Others find it difficult and can benefit from specific suggestions. The nurse should provide opportunities for discussion throughout the talk.

Specific handouts on sexual activity are also helpful for couples and may address topics that were not discussed.

EVALUATION

The nurse determines the effectiveness of teaching by evaluating the woman's (or couple's) response to information throughout the discussion. The nurse may also ask the woman to express information such as the contraindications to intercourse in her own words. Follow-up sessions and questions from the woman also provide information about teaching effectiveness.

TABLE 9–3 Possible Effects of Selected Drugs on the Fetus and Neonate

Maternal Drug	Effects on Fetus and Neonate
Risk outweighs benefits if the following drugs are given in the first trimester:	
Thalidomide	Limb, auricle, eye, and visceral malformations
Tolbutamide (Orinase)	Increase of anomalies
Streptomycin	Eighth nerve damage; multiple skeletal anomalies
Tetracycline	Inhibition of bone growth; syndactyly; discoloration of teeth
Iodide	Congenital goiter; hypothyroidism; mental retardation
Methotrexate	Multiple anomalies
Diethylstilbestrol	Clear-cell adenocarcinoma of the vagina and cervix; genital tract anomalies
Warfarin (Coumadin)	Skeletal and facial anomalies; mental retardation
Risk vs. benefits uncertain in the first trimester:	
Gentamicin	Eighth cranial nerve damage
Kanamycin	Eighth cranial nerve damage
Lithium	Goiter; eye anomalies; cleft palate
Barbiturates	Increase of anomalies
Quinine	Increase of anomalies
Septra or Bactrim	Cleft palate
Cytotoxic drugs	Increase of anomalies
Benefit outweighs risk in the first trimester:	
Clomiphene (Clomid)	Increase of anomalies; neural tube defects; Down syndrome
Glucocorticoids	Cleft palate; cardiac defects
General anesthesia	Increase of anomalies
Tricyclic antidepressants	CNS and limb malformations
Sulfonamides	Cleft palate; facial and skeletal defects
Antacids	Increase of anomalies
Salicylates	Central nervous system, visceral, and skeletal malformations
Acetaminophen	None
Heparin	None
Terbutaline	None
Phenothiazines	None
Insulin	Skeletal malformations
Penicillins	None
Chloramphenicol	None
Isoniazid (INH)	Increase of anomalies

Source: Adapted from Howard FM, Hill JM: *Obstet Gynecol Survey* 1979; 34:643.

children and has been shown to depress skeletal growth, especially in premature infants. Sulfonamides taken in the last few weeks of pregnancy are known to compete with bilirubin attachment of protein-binding sites, increasing the risk of jaundice in the newborn (Niebyl 1994). Warfarin (Coumadin), a commonly prescribed anticoagulant, is associated with CNS defects following fetal exposure during the second and third trimesters (Kochenour 1992).

Pregnant women should avoid all medication if possible. If no alternative exists, it is wisest to select a well-known medication rather than a newer drug whose potential teratogenic effects may not be known. When possible, the oral form of a drug should be used, and it should be prescribed in the lowest possible therapeutic dose for the shortest time possible. Finally, the caregiver should carefully consider the multiple components of the medication. Caution is the watchword for nurses caring for pregnant women who have been taking medications. It is essential that the pregnant woman check with her certified nurse-midwife/physician about medications she was taking when pregnancy occurred and about any nonprescription drugs she is thinking of using. The advantage of using a particular medication must outweigh the risks. Any medication with possible teratogenic effects must be avoided.

Tobacco

Infants of mothers who smoke cigarettes tend to have a lower birth weight and a higher incidence of preterm birth than infants of mothers who do not smoke (Cunningham et al 1997). These findings increase significantly as maternal age increases. In addition, mothers who smoke have an increased risk of spontaneous abortion, preterm birth, placenta previa, abruptio placentae, and premature rupture of the membranes. The risk is related to the number of cigarettes smoked (ACOG 1993). Research also links maternal smoking, both during pregnancy and afterward, with an increased risk of sudden infant death syndrome (SIDS), as well as with pneumonia and other respiratory infections (Petersen et al 1992).

The specific mechanism of smoking's effect on the fetus is not known. Smoking appears to decrease placental blood flow and plasma volume. In addition, changes found in the placentas of smokers suggest toxicity related to elements in tobacco smoke and ischemia due to the vasoconstrictive effects of nicotine on uterine vessels. Smoking may also interfere with maternal absorption or metabolism of calcium, vitamin C, vitamin B_{12}, and perhaps vitamins A, B_6, and B_1 (Aaronson and MacNee 1989).

Fewer women smoke today than did 20 years ago, although approximately 25 percent of women still continue to smoke during pregnancy (Floyd et al 1991). Women who do smoke tend to stop smoking or at least reduce their intake once pregnancy is confirmed. Unfortunately, a majority of women who quit smoking during pregnancy do resume following birth, although this percentage is lower for women who quit early in pregnancy. This finding suggests that although women are aware of the potential impact of smoking on the fetus they may be less knowledgeable about the effects of passive smoke on the baby (Fingerhut 1990).

Studies demonstrate that any decrease in smoking during pregnancy improves the fetal outcome, and researchers continue to explore approaches designed to help women quit smoking (O'Connor et al 1992; Petersen et al 1992). Pregnancy may be a difficult time for a woman to stop smoking, but the nurse should encourage her to reduce the number of cigarettes she smokes daily. The need to protect her unborn child may increase her motivation.

Alcohol

Alcohol is now considered one of the primary teratogens in the Western world. Fetuses of women who are heavy drinkers are at increased risk of developing **fetal alcohol syndrome (FAS)** (Chapter 25). Furthermore, malnutrition (common in heavy drinkers) and alcohol-induced maternal hypoglycemia may also contribute to fetal problems (Niebyl 1994).

The effects of moderate intake of alcohol during pregnancy are unclear. Research indicates an increased incidence of lowered birth weight and some neurologic effects, such as attention deficit disorder. Evidence suggests that the risk of teratogenic effects increases proportionately with increased average daily intake of alcohol. Although studies indicate that light drinkers (fewer than seven drinks per week) have a degree of risk for adverse pregnancy effects similar to that of nondrinkers, no safe level of drinking during pregnancy has been identified, and caregivers recommend that pregnant women abstain from all alcohol during pregnancy (Bruce et al 1993).

In most cases, once a woman becomes aware of her pregnancy, she decreases her consumption of alcohol. However, the alcohol consumed after conception and before pregnancy is diagnosed remains a cause for concern.

Assessment of alcohol intake should be a chief part of every woman's medical history, with questions asked in a direct and nonjudgmental manner. All women should be counseled about the role of alcohol in pregnancy. If heavy consumption is involved, the nurse refers the pregnant woman immediately to an alcoholic treatment program. Counselors in these programs need to be made aware of a woman's pregnancy before drug therapy is suggested, since certain drugs may be harmful to the developing fetus. For example, the drug disulfiram (Antabuse), often used in conjunction with alcohol treatment, is suspected to be a teratogenic agent.

Caffeine

Current research reveals no evidence that caffeine has teratogenic effects in humans (Cunningham et al 1997). However, maternal coffee consumption does decrease iron absorption and may increase the risk of anemia (Niebyl 1994). Until more definitive data are available, nurses should advise women about common sources of caffeine, including coffee, tea, colas, and chocolate, and suggest that they moderate caffeine intake.

Marijuana

Teratogenic effects of marijuana use during pregnancy have not been documented (Cunningham et al 1997). However, the prevalence of marijuana use in our society raises many concerns about its effect on the fetus. Doing research on marijuana use in pregnancy is difficult because it is an illegal drug. Unreliability of reporting, lack of a representative population, inability to determine strength or composition of the marijuana used (including the presence of herbicides), and use of other drugs at the same time are major factors complicating the research being done.

Cocaine

A woman who uses cocaine during pregnancy is at increased risk for acute myocardial infarction, cardiac arrhythmias, ruptured ascending aorta, seizures, cerebrovascular accidents, hyperthermia, bowel ischemia, and sudden death (AAP and ACOG 1992). Cocaine use during pregnancy has been related to abruptio placentae, preterm birth, fetal distress, low birth weight, neonatal withdrawal, and SIDS (Blume et al 1993). Several congenital anomalies in the neonate have also been linked to maternal cocaine use, including genitourinary anomalies, congenital heart defects, limb reduction defects, CNS anomalies, prune belly syndrome, and segmental intestinal atresia (Cunningham et al 1997). (See also Chapter 12.)

As cocaine becomes more widely used by women of childbearing age, health care providers must be alert to early signs of cocaine use. It is often difficult for a nurse or physician to face the fact that a client is using cocaine, but ongoing alertness and an open, nonjudgmental approach are important in early detection. Urine screening for cocaine is valuable, but because cocaine is metabolized rapidly, the drug screen is negative within 24–48 hours after cocaine use. Thus it is probable that many abusers are missed. It is possible to use radioimmunoassays (RIA) of meconium to detect cocaine. This tool is valuable in detecting potential addiction in newborns of cocaine-abusing women (Dombrowski and Sokol 1990).

Evaluation

Throughout the antepartal period, evaluation is an ongoing and essential part of effective nursing care. As nurses ask questions of the pregnant woman and her family or make observations of physical changes, they are evaluating the results of previous interventions. In evaluating the effectiveness of the interactions, the nurse should not be afraid to try creative solutions if they are logical and carefully thought out. This is especially important in dealing with families from other cultures. If a practice is important to a woman and not harmful, the culturally sensitive nurse will not discourage it.

In completing an evaluation, the nurse must also recognize situations that require referral for further evaluation. For example, a woman who has gained 4 pounds in a single week does not require counseling about nutrition; she needs further assessment for PIH. The nurse who has a sound knowledge of theory will recognize this and act immediately.

The ongoing and cyclic nature of the nursing process is especially evident in the prenatal setting. However, throughout the course of pregnancy certain criteria can be used to determine the quality of care provided. In essence, nursing care has been effective if

- The common discomforts of pregnancy are quickly identified and are relieved or lessened effectively.
- The woman is able to discuss the physiologic and psychologic changes of pregnancy.
- The woman implements appropriate self-care measures if they are indicated during pregnancy.
- The woman avoids substances and situations that pose a risk to her well-being or that of her child.
- The woman seeks regular prenatal care.

CHAPTER HIGHLIGHTS

- The nurse provides anticipatory guidance for the expectant father and siblings, as well as for the expectant mother.
- Culturally based practices and proscribed activities may have a major impact on the childbearing family.
- The common discomforts of pregnancy occur as a result of physiologic and anatomic changes. The nurse provides the pregnant woman with information about self-care activities aimed at reducing or relieving discomfort.
- Maternal assessment of fetal activity keeps the woman in touch with her fetus and provides ongoing assessment of fetal status.
- To make appropriate self-care choices and ensure healthful habits, a pregnant woman requires accurate information about a range of subjects from exercise to sexual activity, bathing, and immunizations.
- Teratogenic substances are substances that adversely affect the normal growth and development of the fetus.
- A pregnant woman should avoid taking medications or using over-the-counter preparations during pregnancy.
- Evidence exists that smoking, consuming alcohol, or using social drugs during pregnancy may be harmful to the fetus.

REFERENCES

Aaronson LS, MacNee CL: Tobacco, alcohol, and caffeine use during pregnancy. *JOGNN* 1989; 18(4):279.

American Academy of Pediatrics (AAP) and the American College of Obstetricians and Gynecologists (ACOG): *Guidelines for Perinatal Care,* 3rd ed. Elk Grove Village, IL: AAP, 1992.

American College of Obstetricians and Gynecologists (ACOG): Exercise during pregnancy and the postpartum period. *ACOG Technical Bulletin 189*. Washington, DC: ACOG, February 1994.

American College of Obstetricians and Gynecologists (ACOG): Smoking and reproductive health. *ACOG Technical Bulletin 180*. Washington, DC: ACOG, May 1993.

Artal R, Buckenmeyer PJ: Exercise during pregnancy and postpartum. *Contemp OB/GYN* May 1995; 40(5):62.

Blackburn ST, Loper DL: *Maternal, Fetal, and Neonatal Physiology: A Clinical Perspective.* Philadelphia: Saunders, 1992.

Blume SB et al: When you first suspect substance abuse. *Contemp OB/GYN* March 1993; 38(3):74.

Brown MS: A cross-cultural look at pregnancy, labor, and delivery. *JOGNN* September/October 1976; 5:35.

Bruce FC et al: Alcohol use before and during pregnancy. *Am J Prev Med* 1993; 9(5):267.

Carrington BW: The Afro American. In: *Culture, Childbearing, Health Professionals.* Clark AL (editor). Philadelphia: Davis, 1978.

Cunningham FG et al: *Williams Obstetrics,* 20th ed. Stamford, CT: Appleton & Lange, 1997.

Dombrowski MP, Sokol RJ: Cocaine and abruption. *Contemp OB/GYN* April 1990; 35:13.

Fingerhut LA et al: Smoking before, during, and after pregnancy. *Am J Public Health* May 1990; 80(5):541.

Floyd RL et al: Smoking during pregnancy: Prevalence, effects, and intervention strategies. *Birth* March 1991; 18(1):48.

Guastini D, Marshall K. Million dollar babies. *Personnel J* November 1989; 1965:1.

Kochenour NK: Medication in pregnancy: Minimize the risks. *Contemp OB/GYN* February 1992; 37(2):59.

Kochenour NK: Normal pregnancy and prenatal care. In: *Danforth's Obstetrics and Gynecology,* 7th ed. Scott JR et al (editors). Philadelphia: Lippincott, 1994.

Larson JD, Rayburn WF: Gestational heartburn: What role for medications? *Contemp OB/GYN* August 1996; 41(8):95.

Launer LJ et al: The effect of maternal work on fetal growth and duration of pregnancy: A prospective study. *Br J Obstet Gynaecol* January 1990; 97:62.

Niebyl JR: Teratology and drug use during pregnancy and lactation. In: *Danforth's Obstetrics and Gynecology,* 7th ed. Scott JR et al (editors). Philadelphia: Lippincott, 1994.

O'Connor AM et al: Effectiveness of a pregnancy smoking cessation program. *JOGNN* September/October 1992; 21(5):385.

Petersen L et al: Smoking reduction during pregnancy by a program of self-help and clinical support. *Obstet Gynecol* June 1992; 79(6):924.

Rogers J, Davis BA: How risky are hot tubs and saunas for pregnant women? *MCN* May/June 1995; 20(3):137.

Spector RE: *Cultural Diversity in Health and Illness,* 3rd ed. Norwalk, CT: Appleton & Lange, 1991.

Stringer M et al: Maternal-fetal physical assessment in the home setting: Role of the advanced practice nurse. *JOGNN* October 1994; 23(8):720.

Walden CM et al: Perinatal effects of a pregnancy wellness program in the workplace. *MCN* November/December 1996; 21:288.

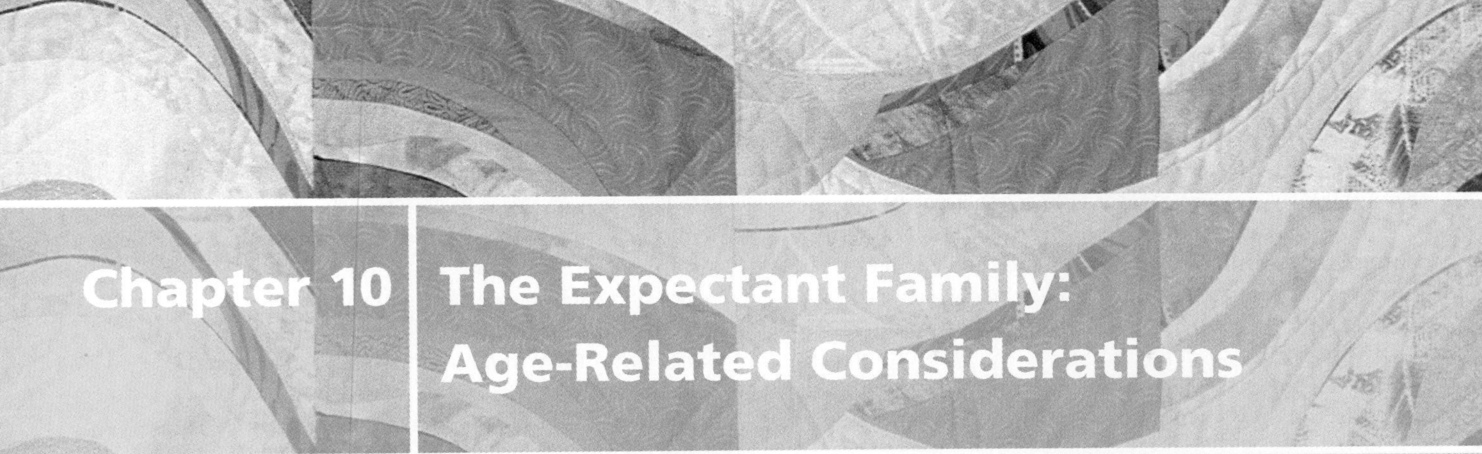

Chapter 10 The Expectant Family: Age-Related Considerations

OBJECTIVES

- Summarize the physical, psychologic, and sociologic risks faced by an adolescent who is pregnant.
- Compare the effects of pregnancy on the adolescent mother and the adolescent father.
- Identify common parental reactions to adolescent pregnancy.
- Relate the use of the nursing process to the provision of effective care for the pregnant adolescent.
- Describe factors that have contributed to the increased incidence of pregnancy in women over age 35.
- Discuss some of the special concerns felt by older expectant couples.
- Relate the use of the nursing process to the provision of effective care for the older expectant couple.

KEY TERMS

Blended family
Early adolescence
Emancipated minors
Late adolescence
Middle adolescence

Pregnancy is a challenging time for all women as they adjust to the changes they experience and prepare to assume a new role as the mother of one child or of two or more children. Even if a woman chooses to terminate her pregnancy, the very fact of being pregnant has a lasting effect on her. Age at the time of pregnancy may be a factor in a woman's adjustment, both physically and psychologically. This chapter explores the special needs and concerns of pregnant adolescents and of women who become pregnant after age 35.

Care of the Pregnant Adolescent

In the United States each year over one million teenage girls become pregnant, and most of these pregnancies are unintended (Adolescent unintended pregnancy 1994). Although the overall teenage birth rate has remained stable, nonmarital adolescent births have increased from 33 to 81 percent. This change reflects a trend toward later marriages. Because fewer young people are marrying, the majority of teens are single when they have their first intercourse (Contraception and adolescents 1995).

First intercourse occurs during the middle to late teenage years for many adolescents. Almost three-quarters of men (73%) and more than half of women (56%) have had intercourse by the age of 18 (Alan Guttmacher Institute 1994). Unfortunately only about 50 percent of adolescents use contraception at first intercourse, and, while condom use among adolescents has increased, it is still inconsistent (Keller et al 1996).

The incidence of teenage sexual activity in the United States is similar to that among industrialized European nations and Canada. However, the incidence of teen pregnancy, therapeutic abortion, and births among adolescents is significantly higher in the United States (Blume 1996). Researchers suggest that these countries may have lower adolescent pregnancy rates because of family influences, the greater availability of contraceptives, and the strong emphasis on sex education (Crooks and Baur 1993).

The decision to terminate a pregnancy is not uncommon among the teenage population. Statistics indicate that for every ten teenage pregnancies there were approximately five live births, four abortions, and one miscarriage (Blume 1996). When abortion rates for whites and other races were compared, the percentages were essentially the same during the teenage years (US Bureau of the Census 1993).

Many factors contribute to this high teen pregnancy rate. These factors include earlier onset of menarche, earlier age of first sexual intercourse, lack of knowledge about conception and contraception, lack of easy access to contraception, and lessened stigma associated with adolescent pregnancy in some populations.

The pregnant adolescent faces a tremendous challenge at a time when her physical growth may still be incomplete, she has not yet completed the developmental tasks of adolescence, her available support systems may be limited, and her education is unfinished. The health care community must address the consequences of adolescent pregnancy for the young woman, her partner, and their families, as well as the implications for society, if the incidence of teen pregnancy is to be reduced.

Overview of the Adolescent Period

Physical Changes

Puberty, the period of time during which an individual becomes capable of reproduction, lasts from 1.5 to 6 years. Menarche, the first menstrual period, usually occurs in the latter half of this process with an average age of 12–13 years. Initial menstrual cycles may be anovulatory, although they are not always so. Because of this, contraception is important during this time for all adolescents who are sexually active.

Psychosocial Development

Developmental tasks of adolescence have been described by many writers and are based on a variety of classic theories. Steinberg (1993) includes among these tasks

- Developing an identity
- Gaining autonomy and independence
- Developing intimacy in a relationship
- Developing comfort with one's own sexuality
- Developing a sense of achievement

Although theorists have identified average ages for the completion of tasks, these ages are somewhat arbitrary and are affected by many factors such as culture, religion, and socioeconomic status. In **early adolescence** (age 14 and under) teens still see authority in parents. During **middle adolescence** (15–17 years) teens rely on the peer group for authority and decision making. Middle adolescence is a critical time for challenging: Experimenting with drugs, alcohol, and sex are avenues for rebellion. In **late adolescence** (18–19 years) teens are more at ease with their individuality and decision making.

Cognitive development is another crucial change of adolescence. Young people move from the concrete and egocentric thinking of childhood to abstract conceptualization. The ability of the young adolescent to see herself in the future or to foresee the consequences of her behavior is minimal. She perceives her focus of control as external; that is, she believes that her destiny is controlled by others, especially parents and other authority figures. As she matures and learns to solve problems, conceptualize, and make decisions, she gradually comes

TABLE 10–1 Initial Reaction to Awareness of Pregnancy

Age	Adolescent Behavior	Nursing Implications
Early adolescent (14 and under)	Fears rejection by family and peers. Enters health care system with an adult, most likely mother (parents still seen as locus of control). Value system still closely reflects that of parents, so still turns to parents for decision or approval of decision. Pregnancy probably not result of intimate relationship. Self-conscious about normal adolescent changes in body. Self-consciousness and low self-esteem likely to increase with rapid breast enlargement and abdominal enlargement of pregnancy.	Nonjudgmental in approach to care. Focus on needs and concerns of adolescent teenager, but if parent accompanies daughter, include parent in plan of care. Encourage both to express concerns and feelings about pregnancy and options: abortion, maintaining pregnancy, adoption. Be realistic and concrete in discussing implications of each option. During physical exam of adolescent respect increased sense of modesty. Explain in simple and concrete terms physical changes that are produced by pregnancy versus puberty. Explain each step of physical exam in simple and concrete terms.
Middle adolescent (15–17 years)	Fears rejection by peers and parents. Unsure in whom to confide. May seek confirmation of pregnancy on own with increased awareness of options and services, such as over-the-counter pregnancy kits and Planned Parenthood. If in an ongoing, caring relationship with partner (peer), may choose him as confidant. Economic dependence on parents may determine if and when parents are told. Future educational plans, perception of parental support or lack of support are significant factors in decision regarding termination or maintenance of the pregnancy. Possible conflict in parental and own developing value system.	Nonjudgmental in approach to care. Reassure regarding confidentiality. Help adolescent identify significant individuals in whom she can confide to help make a decision about the pregnancy. Need to be aware of state laws regarding requirement of parental notification if abortion intended. Also need to be aware of state laws regarding requirements for marriage: usually minimum age 18 for both parties; 16- and 17-year-olds only with consent of parents. Encourage adolescent to be realistic about parental response to pregnancy.
Late adolescent (18–19 years)	Most likely to confirm pregnancy on own and at an earlier date due to increased acceptance and awareness of consequences of behavior. Likely to use pregnancy kit for confirmation. Relationship with father of baby, future educational plans, own value system are among significant determinants about pregnancy.	Nonjudgmental in approach to care. Reassure regarding confidentiality. Encourage adolescent to identify significant individuals in whom she can confide. Refer to counseling as appropriate. Encourage adolescent to be realistic about parental response to pregnancy.

to see herself as having control and can see the consequences of her behavior. Table 10–1 suggests typical behaviors of the early, middle, and late adolescent when she becomes aware of her pregnancy. Other factors may influence the age at which these behaviors are seen.

The Adolescent Mother

There are many possible explanations for adolescent pregnancy. The conflicts of adolescence may provide motivation: The adolescent girl may be using pregnancy to maintain dependence on her own mother. Deficits in ego functioning have also been suggested as a cause for acting out sexually. The adolescent may have little sense of self-worth and some hopelessness regarding the future. Other psychologic rationales include unstable family relationships, needing someone to love, competition with mother, punishment of parents, desire for emancipation from an undesirable home situation, and attention seeking. Pregnancy may be a young woman's form of acting out.

Cultural values may cause a young woman to desire pregnancy. Many cultures equate evidence of fertility with adult status. Duany and Pittman (1990) suggest that the formation of families and onset of employment occur at an earlier age for Latinos than for either white or black youths and are marks of adult success. Similarly, many Native American teenagers believe that early pregnancy validates the female role and is therefore valued by their culture. In contrast, many white adolescent mothers believe that early motherhood is not accepted by their culture and see it as an indication of failure.

Another school of thought suggests that pregnancy is a result of unmotivated accidents. The adolescent has sex infrequently, often without planning it, and therefore does not consider contraception. She may have guilt feelings surrounding sex and may not be able to admit she is sexually active. She is incapable of understanding how pregnancy will affect her future. Her rationale may include "I don't have sex often enough (to get pregnant)," or "It was the safe time of the month." Many adolescent girls have no idea when they ovulate or what would cause them to conceive.

Teenage pregnancy can also result from an incestuous relationship. The psychologic turmoil experienced by the incest victim may obliterate thought of the risk of pregnancy, especially for the young adolescent. Older adolescents may fear the possibility of pregnancy but for a variety of psychologic reasons deny the reality. In the very young adolescent, incest or sexual abuse should be suspected as a possible cause of pregnancy. Repeat pregnancies in adolescent mothers are influenced by such factors as marital status, educational achievement, parental relationships, and contraceptive practices.

Physiologic Risks

Adolescents over age 15 who receive early, thorough prenatal care are at no greater risk during pregnancy than women over 20 years. Unfortunately, many adolescents fail to seek early prenatal care and fail to cooperate with recommendations they receive. Thus risks for pregnant adolescents include preterm births, low-birth-

TABLE 10–2 The Early Adolescent's Response to the Developmental Tasks of Pregnancy

Stage	Developmental Tasks of Pregnancy	Early Adolescent's Response to Pregnancy	Nursing Implications
First trimester	Pregnancy confirmation. Seeking early prenatal care as a confirmation tool. Begins to evaluate her diet and general health habits. Initial ambivalence common. Usually seeks supportive partner.	May delay confirmation of pregnancy until late part of first trimester—unaware of pregnancy, fear of confiding in anyone, or denial. Rapid enlargement and sensitivity of breasts embarrassing and frightening to early adolescent—may be perceived as changes of puberty. If confiding in mother, may be experiencing family turmoil in response to pregnancy.	Explain physiologic changes of pregnancy versus those associated with puberty. Explain that ambivalence is normal with any pregnancy, but recognize it as a much greater concern with adolescent pregnancy. Emphasize need for good nutrition as important for her well-being as much as infant's (prevention of PIH and anemia). Use simple explanations and lots of audiovisuals. Have adolescent listen to FHR with Doppler.
Second trimester	Experiences beginning of changes in physical appearance and fetal movement, causing pregnancy to be experienced as a reality. Begins wearing maternity clothes to accommodate the physical changes. As a result of quickening she perceives her fetus as a real baby and begins preparing for the maternal role and new relationships with her partner and members of her family.	Some teenagers may delay validation of pregnancy until now, with family turmoil occurring at this time. Abdominal enlargement and quickening may be perceived as loss of control over body image. May try to maintain prepregnant weight and wear restrictive clothing to control and conceal changing body. Becomes dependent on her own mother for support. Egocentric; unable to develop a maternal role at this time.	Continue to discuss importance of good nutrition and adequate weight gain as noted above. Discuss ways of using common teenage clothing (large sweatshirts, blouses) to promote comfort but preserve adolescent image to some degree. Discuss plans being made for baby, continued educational plans, and role of teen's parents.
Third trimester	At end of second trimester begins to view fetus as separate from self. Buys baby clothes and supplies. Prepares a place for the baby. Realistic about what baby is like. Prepares to give birth to infant. Anxiety increases as labor and birth approach, and she has concerns about well-being of fetus.	May focus on "wanting it to be over." May have trouble individuating fetus. May have fantasies, dreams, or nightmares about childbirth. Natural fears of labor and birth greater than with older primigravida. Probably has not been in a hospital, and may associate this with negative experiences.	Assess whether mother is preparing for baby by buying supplies and preparing a place in the home. Provide childbirth education and hospital tour. Assess for discomforts of pregnancy, such as heartburn and constipation. Adolescent may be uncomfortable mentioning these and other problems.

weight (LBW) infants, cephalopelvic disproportion (CPD), pregnancy-induced hypertension (PIH) and its sequelae, and iron deficiency anemia. In the adolescent age group, prenatal care is the critical factor that most influences pregnancy outcome.

Teens between ages 15 and 19 have a high incidence of sexually transmitted infections, including herpesvirus, syphilis, and gonorrhea. The incidence of chlamydial infection is also increased in this age group. The presence of such infections during pregnancy greatly increases risks to the fetus. Other problems seen in adolescents are cigarette smoking and alcohol and drug abuse. By the time pregnancy is confirmed in young women, the fetus may already be damaged by these substances.

Psychologic Risks

The major psychologic risk to the pregnant adolescent is the interruption in her developmental tasks. Add to this the tasks of pregnancy, and the young woman has an overwhelming amount of psychologic work to do, the completion of which will affect her own and her newborn's future.

Table 10–2 identifies the early adolescent's responses to the developmental tasks of pregnancy. Middle and older adolescents would respond differently, reflecting their progression through the developmental tasks. In addition to her maturational level, the amount of nurturing the pregnant adolescent receives is a critical factor in the way she handles pregnancy and motherhood.

Sociologic Risks

Being forced into adult roles before completing adolescent developmental tasks causes a series of events that affect the adolescent's entire life. These events may result in a prolonged dependency on parents, lack of stable relationships with the opposite sex, and lack of economic and social stability. Furthermore, the closer the pregnancy occurs to the changes of puberty and menarche, the more difficulty the teen will have in becoming comfortable with her body image, given the continuing physical changes that do not fit her image of a "normal" teenager.

Many adolescents who become pregnant drop out of school and never complete their education, reducing the jobs available to them. Programs for pregnant adolescents and adolescent mothers may help this problem.

Failure to limit family size is often a problem for pregnant adolescents. The younger the adolescent at her first pregnancy, the more likely she is to become pregnant again while still an adolescent. In fact, 25 percent of adolescents who give birth become pregnant again within one year (Blume 1996). These young women frequently fail to establish stable families. Their family structure tends to be single-parent and matriarchal, often the same family structure in which they were raised. Certainly situations of poverty aggravate this problem. Failure to be self-supporting logically follows lack of education and lost career goals. Many adolescents with children end up on welfare.

Some pregnant adolescents choose to marry the father of the baby, who is often also a teenager. Unfortunately the majority of adolescent marriages end in divorce (Steinburg 1993). This fact should not be surprising because pregnancy and marriage interrupt adolescents' "childhood" and basic education. Lack of maturity in dealing with an intimate relationship also contributes to marital breakdown in this age group.

Finally, adolescents are at risk for having unhealthy babies. The younger the teen when she gives birth, the greater the probability that she and her infant will experience health-related complications due in large part to poor nutrition, late onset of prenatal care, and other lifestyle factors (Planned Parenthood 1993).

The Adolescent Father

The adolescent father must complete the developmental tasks of his age group, and he faces similar sociologic and psychologic risks as the adolescent mother if he attempts to assume his responsibilities as a father.

Adolescent fathers are usually within three to four years of the age of the adolescent mother. The mother and father are generally from similar socioeconomic backgrounds and have similar education. Many are involved in meaningful relationships. Frequently, the fathers are involved in the decision making about abortion or adoption. Many fathers are very involved in the pregnancy and childrearing.

Adolescent males do become sexually active at an earlier age than adolescent females but many know less about contraception and reproduction, feeling this is a woman's domain (Marsiglio 1993).

Psychologic and sociologic risks to the adolescent father are similar to those of adolescent mothers. Adolescent fathers tend to achieve less formal education than older fathers, and they enter the labor force earlier with less education. They tend to pursue less prestigious careers and have less job satisfaction. Adolescent fathers often marry at a younger age and have larger families than older fathers. In addition, the divorce rate of adolescent fathers is greater than that of fathers who have postponed childbearing and marriage (Fielding and Williams 1991).

Psychologically, the adolescent father's developmental tasks will be interrupted. Because he is not yet mature, his level of cognitive development and decision-making skills will influence whether he remains supportive or flees the situation. Certainly he will be more vulnerable to emotional stressors than an adult man. The stresses of pregnancy on the adolescent male come from many sources. He faces negative reactions from people in his own family and in the family of the young woman. Feelings of anger, shame, and disappointment will be aimed at him. He will feel isolated and alone, and if the young woman's parents refuse to allow him to see her, his sole emotional support may be gone.

Another source of stress arises from changes in his life. His educational and career goals may be threatened as he anticipates marriage or quitting school to support the young woman and his forthcoming child. His relationship with his peers may be altered as well.

A third stressor will be his concerns about the health of the young woman and the fetus. He may be protective but may not understand the physical and psychologic changes of pregnancy.

The implications for the health care team are important. Even if the couple has severed their relationship, the father should be sought to assess how he is coping and to offer him counseling. He may not understand why he needs to come to the clinic, and the nurse must let him know that the staff would like to help him too.

If the couple is still together, the father should be told that his participation is important, that he is an excellent support person for the young woman, and that he is welcome to attend clinic and classes. Many clinics routinely interview the couple on the first prenatal visit.

Even if the couple has a good relationship, it is not unusual for the adolescent female to want her mother as her primary support person during labor and birth. This is especially true of young adolescents. It is important to support her wishes, while also seeing to the needs of the young father. The practice of permitting more than one support person helps address this issue.

The young man will need education about pregnancy, childbirth, child care, and parenting. Some clinics have couples attend classes together; others offer "father" classes. In becoming parents, men need to learn rates of growth and development so they understand their newborn's potential and do not become frustrated and dissatisfied with the child's behavior.

In the first few months after birth, many adolescent males have daily contact with the adolescent mother and their baby. Unfortunately, by five years after the birth, 60 percent remain in contact but only about 30 percent have regular interaction. While these young fathers seem to mean well, they may lack strong models of fatherhood and may become caught up in stereotypical models of male noninvolvement. If they are to learn to be effective parents, they need help in understanding and valuing their role as fathers.

As part of his counseling, the nurse should assess the young man's stressors, support systems, plans for involvement in the pregnancy and childrearing, future plans, and health care needs. He should be referred to social services for an opportunity to be counseled regarding his educational and vocational future. When the

COMMUNITY IN FOCUS **The School Community Sexual Risk Reduction Model**

The high incidence of adolescent pregnancy is of great concern nationwide, and communities have employed a variety of approaches to address the issue. The School/Community Sexual Risk Reduction Model is a comprehensive, multidisciplinary, community-wide model that has achieved significant success in reducing the incidence of unintended pregnancy among never-married teenagers and pre-teens. The model is designed to provide regular doses of multiple interventions directed at the adolescent population in general with higher levels of intervention for at-risk adolescents. The Model was originally developed and implemented in two South Carolina counties—Bamberg County and Hampton County. Evaluation of the success of the effort revealed a 54 percent decrease in the estimated pregnancy rate for teens aged 14–17 (Vincent et al 1987).

The Model is designed to address issues related to adolescent pregnancy through a variety of interventions including the following: training and workshops about sexuality for parents, community members, and other professionals; graduate-level course work about sexuality education for teachers; age-appropriate, comprehensive school-based sexuality education for students in grades K to 12; student access to contraceptives and health services; use of mass media approaches to increase community awareness and involvement; close cooperation with school officials to plan school-based interventions; peer support and education programs; and student activities focused on awareness of alternatives and skill development.

When teen pregnancy became a focus of concern in Kansas, the Kansas Health Foundation, an organization committed to improving the quality of health in Kansas, decided to support initiatives to reduce adolescent pregnancy rates. The Foundation reviewed the literature and sought out "success stories" of models that used community-based approaches, stressed primary prevention, and were sustainable long term. The Foundation was impressed with the results achieved by the South Carolina School/Community Model and decided to support a replication project in selected Kansas counties. To ensure fidelity to the major components of the model, the Model's co-director and originator was employed as a co-director for the Kansas project.

Following a Request for Proposal (RFP) process, three counties were selected for implementation: a rural county, an urban county, and a county with a major military facility and resultant transient population. To promote feelings of ownership, each county selected its own name for the project and minor modifications were made to address the specific issues unique to each site. The Kansas-based co-director of the project works closely with the three sites to provide technical assistance, guidance, and support.

The School/Community Model is an exciting, dynamic approach to addressing an important problem. Equally exciting, however, is the Kansas approach—one of respect for success, a willingness to learn from others, and a commitment to implementing faithfully the South Carolina model. This type of sharing forms the basis for the spread of successful models and is a credit to both states.

Sources: Personal communication with Dr. Adrienne Paine-Andrews, Program Co-Director and Courtesy Assistant Professor, Department of Human Development, University of Kansas, Lawrence, Kansas. Also adapted from information found in: Paine-Andrews A et al: Replicating a community initiative for preventing adolescent pregnancy: From South Carolina to Kansas. *Fam Community Health* April 1996; 19(1):14; and Vincent M et al: Reducing adolescent pregnancy through school and community-based education. *JAMA* 1987; 257:3382.

father is involved in the pregnancy, the young mother feels less deserted, more confident in her decision making, and better able to discuss her future.

Reactions of Family and Social Supports to Adolescent Pregnancy

Telling her parents that she is pregnant is often very difficult for the adolescent, and she may avoid it until her pregnancy is obvious. Her mother is usually the first to find out and often attempts to prevent the young woman's father from discovering his daughter's pregnancy. Unfortunately, little research is available on the reactions of the father of pregnant adolescents.

Parents' initial reactions to the news are usually shock, anger, shame, guilt, and sorrow. If the mother accompanies her daughter to the clinic, the nurse should assess any disharmony and explain the process of adaptation that follows.

The mother frequently feels guilty about her daughter's pregnancy and feels that she has been an inadequate parent. She may also be angry about having to help her daughter deal with a crisis just as her children are growing up and she is experiencing a new sense of freedom. The idea of being a grandmother may also be upsetting. Once these reactions are faced, normalcy returns to the mother-daughter relationship. The mother may become involved in decision making and in dealing with the father-to-be and his family.

As the pregnancy progresses, the adolescent's mother begins to take on the grandmother role. She may buy presents for the newborn and plan for the future. She may participate in prenatal care and classes and can be an excellent support for her daughter. She should be encouraged to participate if the mother-daughter relationship is positive. The mother should be updated on maternity care to clarify any misconceptions she might have. During labor and birth, the mother will be a key figure for her daughter. She can offer reassurance and instill confidence in the adolescent.

The last stages of a mother's acceptance occur after her daughter's child is born. As the mother attempts to integrate her role of grandmother, an initial blurring of roles occurs. The grandmother should now see her daughter as a mother, and the daughter should begin to identify herself as a mother. However, role confusion may develop and sometimes continues for years. The grandmother may do essentially all the mothering and caretaking activities for the newborn, while the daughter remains only a daughter and becomes a sibling of her newborn. Until the daughter is able to internalize her role as mother, the grandmother will be unable to completely identify as a grandmother.

This new role development is clouded by the adolescent's struggle to complete her tasks of adolescence. The wise mother will gently encourage a balance between helping her daughter to be a parent and allowing her to complete the tasks of adolescence. As her daughter becomes more confident in the role of parent, the grandmother can gradually encourage her to be more independent.

The pregnant adolescent must also deal with the reactions of siblings and other family members and friends who form her social network. Their concern and caring can be a significant factor in her ability to deal with the pregnancy and make needed decisions. Those teens who decide not to tell anyone about the pregnancy face a stressful period without normal support systems. This increases the crisis nature of the situation unless the young woman is able to develop a new support network during the pregnancy.

APPLYING THE NURSING PROCESS

Nursing Assessment

The nurse must establish a database to plan interventions for the adolescent mother-to-be. Areas of assessment include a history of personal and family physical health, developmental level and impact of pregnancy, availability of emotional and financial support systems, and the father's degree of involvement in the pregnancy.

Physical Health

It is important to have general physical health information in the prenatal period. Often this is the first time an adolescent has ever provided a health history. Consequently the nurse may find it helpful to ask very specific questions and give examples when necessary.

The following areas should be assessed:

- Family and personal health history
- Medical history
- Menstrual history
- Obstetric and gynecologic history

Developmental Level and the Impact of Pregnancy

The developmental tasks common to pregnancy and their impact on the adolescent are listed in Table 9–2. Personal maturity may vary widely within any age group, so it is important to consider maturational level individually. Significant factors that need to be assessed include the mother's self-concept (including body image), her relationship with the significant adults in her life, her attitude toward her pregnancy, her degree of understanding of the realities of teenage pregnancy and parenting, and her coping methods in the situation.

Support Systems

The socioeconomic status of the pregnant adolescent often places her baby at risk throughout life, beginning with conception. It is essential to assess emotional and financial support systems.

Adolescent lifestyles and support systems vary tremendously. It is imperative that the interdisciplinary health team have information about expectant adolescents' feelings and perceptions about themselves, their sexuality, and the coming baby; their knowledge of, attitude toward, and anticipated ability to care for and support the infant; and their maturational level and needs.

Nursing Diagnosis

Nursing diagnoses that may apply to the pregnant adolescent are similar to those that apply to any pregnant woman. Appropriate diagnoses are influenced by the adolescent's age, support systems, health, and personal maturity. Nursing diagnoses more specific to the pregnant adolescent include the following:

- Altered nutrition: Less than body requirements related to poor eating habits
- Self-esteem disturbance related to unanticipated pregnancy

Nursing Plan and Implementation

Early and thorough prenatal care is the strongest and most critical determinant for reducing risk to the adolescent mother and her newborn. The nurse must understand the special needs of the adolescent mother to meet this challenge successfully. See Key Facts to Remember: The Pregnant Adolescent on the next page.

Issue of Confidentiality

Most states in the United States have passed legislation that confirms the right of some minors to assume the rights of adults. These adolescents are known as **emancipated minors.** An adolescent may be considered emancipated if he or she is self-supporting and living away

KEY FACTS TO REMEMBER

The Pregnant Adolescent

- The rate of adolescent pregnancy in the United States is among the highest of all the developed countries of the world.
- Early, regular, and excellent prenatal care can prevent many of the risks associated with adolescent pregnancy, especially for the young adolescent.
- Prenatal education especially designed for adolescents also plays a significant role in increasing an adolescent's knowledge and in decreasing maternal and perinatal complications.

from home, married, pregnant or a parent, or in the military service (Cohn 1991). The pregnant adolescent, even if very young, is considered emancipated and has the right and responsibility to consent to health care for herself and, later, for her child. She is entitled to respect and confidentiality in dealing with health care providers. Only with her agreement can caregivers include other adults, including her parents, in communication.

Development of a Trusting Relationship with the Pregnant Adolescent

The first visit to the clinic or caregiver's office for diagnosis of the pregnancy or beginning of prenatal care may make the young woman feel anxious and vulnerable. Making the experience as positive as possible will encourage the adolescent to return for follow-up care and cooperate with her caregivers, and will help ensure her recognition of the importance of health care for herself and her baby.

An overview of what the young woman will experience over the prenatal course, including thorough explanations and rationale for each procedure as it occurs, will improve the client's understanding and give her a feeling of control. Actively involving the young woman in her care will give her a sense of participation and responsibility in her own health care (Figure 10–1).

Since this first office or clinic visit may include the young woman's first pelvic examination, a thorough explanation of the procedure is essential to lessen the inevitable anxiety provoked by this situation. Gentle and thoughtful examination technique will help put her at ease. A mirror is useful in allowing the client to see her cervix, educating her about her anatomy, and giving her an active role in the examination. Clinical pelvimetry is an important tool in predicting CPD, but it may be postponed until a later visit if the adolescent is extremely nervous and uncomfortable during the first pelvic exam.

Developing a trusting relationship with the pregnant adolescent is essential. Honesty and respect for the young woman and a caring attitude promote self-esteem. As a role model, the nurse's attitudes about self-care and responsibility affect the adolescent's maturation process.

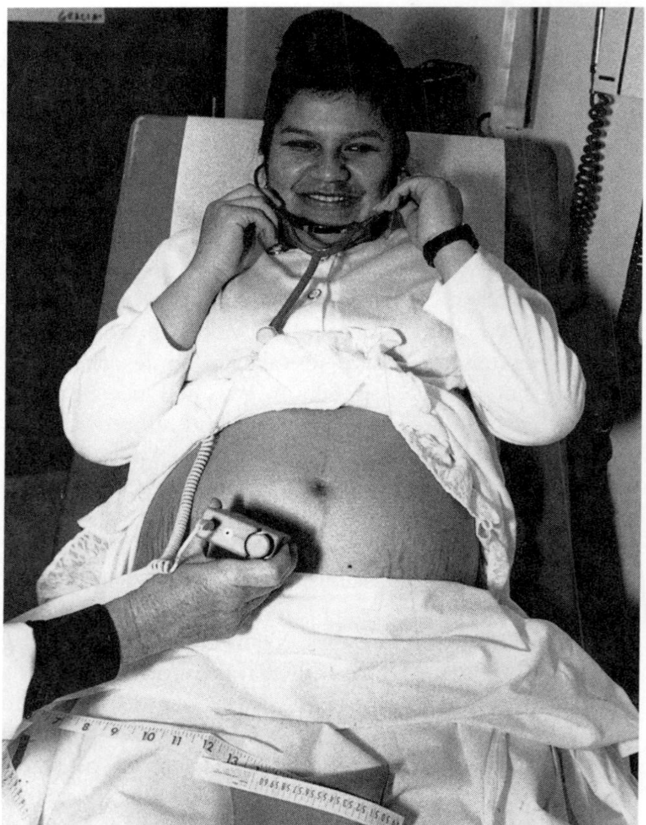

FIGURE 10–1 The nurse gives this young mother an opportunity to listen to her baby's heartbeat.

Promotion of Self-Esteem and Problem-Solving Skills

The adolescent must meet the developmental tasks of pregnancy in addition to the developmental tasks of adolescence. The nurse assists the adolescent in her decision-making and problem-solving skills so that she can proceed with her developmental tasks and begin to assume responsibility for her life.

If the adolescent is accompanied by a parent or boyfriend, the nurse should first visit with her alone to assess her concerns without the presence or influence of another person. Because incest is a possibility in the early adolescent, it is important to explore family relationships.

Many adolescents are not aware of all the legally available options in dealing with an unplanned pregnancy. The teen should be given information about her alternatives: terminating the pregnancy, maintaining the pregnancy, and choosing whether to parent or relinquish the child. The nurse can encourage the young woman to share her feelings about each alternative and the projected consequences as they relate to her situation in life. The nurse can also provide information about community resources available with help for each alternative. The nurse should provide information in an open, nonjudgmental way without imposing personal values on the teen. Once the adolescent has decided on a course, health care providers should respect her decision and support her efforts to achieve her goals.

If the adolescent chooses to maintain her pregnancy, the nurse should give her an overview of what she will experience over the course of her pregnancy and should provide a thorough explanation and rationale for each procedure as it occurs. If she elects to terminate the pregnancy, the nurse should give her information about abortions, including what to expect, costs, applicable state laws about parental notification, and so forth. This approach fosters the adolescent's understanding and gives her some measure of control.

Early adolescents tend to be egocentric and oriented to the present. They may not regard as important the fact that their health and habits affect the fetus. Consequently, it is often useful to emphasize the effects of these practices on the client herself. The young woman will also need help in problem solving and in visualizing the future so she can plan effectively.

The middle adolescent is developing the ability to think abstractly and can recognize that actions may have long-term consequences. She may not yet have acquired assertive communication skills, however, and may be reluctant to ask questions. Nurses should anticipate this unwillingness to ask questions and initiate discussion by asking the teen directly if she has any concerns (Drake 1996). The middle adolescent can absorb more detailed health teaching and apply it.

The late adolescent can think abstractly, plan for the future, and function in a manner comparable to older pregnant women. She can handle complex information and apply it.

Promotion of Physical Well-Being

Baseline weight and blood pressure measurements are valuable in assessing weight gain and predisposition to PIH. The nurse can encourage the adolescent to take part in her care by measuring and recording her own weight. The nurse may use this time as an opportunity to assist the young woman in problem solving: "Have I gained too much or too little weight?" "What influence does my diet have on my weight?" "How can I change my eating habits?"

Another way to introduce the subject of nutrition is during measurement of baseline and subsequent hemoglobin and hematocrit values. Because the adolescent is at risk for anemia, she will need education about the importance of iron in her diet. A nutritional consultation is indicated for all adolescents. Group classes are helpful because peer pressure is strong among this age group.

> **CRITICAL THINKING IN ACTION**
>
> Cindy Lenz, a 15-year-old Gr1P0, is 16 weeks pregnant when she arrives for her second prenatal visit. She is drinking diet soda and eating potato chips as she waits for her appointment. Her 18-year-old boyfriend is with her. In reviewing her history the nurse remembers that Cindy had tried to get pregnant for several months. Her boyfriend, a high school dropout, has a part-time job. As a result Cindy is still living at home, although she does not get along with her mother or sister. Cindy plans to stay in school until her baby is born because she has two other friends at school who are also pregnant. As the nurse weighs Cindy she asks a few questions about her nutritional habits and finds that Cindy eats lots of junk food and very few vegetables or fruits. How should the nurse discuss Cindy's nutritional needs with her?
>
> *Answers can be found in Appendix H.*

Adolescents may fear laboratory tests, which can evoke early childhood memories of being "stuck" with needles or hurt. Explanations help relieve anxiety and coordination of services will avoid multiple venous punctures.

Pregnancy-induced hypertension represents the most prevalent medical complication of pregnant adolescents. The criteria of blood pressure readings of 140/90 mm Hg are not acceptable as the determinant of PIH in adolescents. Women aged 14 to 20 years without evidence of high blood pressure usually have diastolic readings between 50 and 66 mm Hg. Gradual increases from the prepregnant diastolic readings, along with excessive weight gain, must be evaluated as precursors to PIH. This is one reason why early prenatal care is vital to management of the adolescent.

Adolescents have an increased incidence of sexually transmitted infections. The initial prenatal examination should include gonococcal and chlamydial cultures; wet prep for *Candida, Trichomonas,* and *Gardnerella;* and tests for syphilis. Education about sexually transmitted infections is important, as is careful observation of herpetic lesions or other symptoms throughout the young woman's pregnancy. Research indicates that while today's teens are knowledgeable about AIDS, they know much less about other STIs, especially with regard to symptoms and risk reduction (Witwer 1990). If the adolescent's history indicates that she is at increased risk for HIV, she should be given information about it and offered HIV screening.

The nurse should also discuss substance abuse with adolescents. It is important to review the risks associated with the use of tobacco, caffeine, drugs, cocaine, marijuana, and alcohol. The adolescent should be aware of the effects of these substances on her development as well as on the development of the fetus.

Ongoing care should include the same assessments that the older pregnant woman receives. The nurse should pay special attention to evaluating fetal growth by determining when quickening occurs and by measuring fundal height, fetal heart tones, and fetal movement. Corresponding dates of auscultating fetal heart tones with the date of last menstrual period and quickening can be helpful in determining correct estimations of time of birth. If there is a question of size–date discrepancy by 2 cm either way, an ultrasound is warranted to establish fetal age so that instances of intrauterine growth retardation (IUGR) can be diagnosed and treated early.

For adolescents, the incidence of a subsequent pregnancy is very high. Thus, despite the pregnant teen's strong assertion that she will not be sexually active again, contraception is an important consideration during the postpartal period. Because of the risks of thrombophlebitis associated with immediate postpartum use of oral contraceptives, many caregivers recommend that the adolescent use barrier methods of contraception (foam and condoms). Postpartal visits are then scheduled at 2 weeks to assess for problems and at 4 weeks to discuss and initiate contraception if it is acceptable to her, often using oral contraceptives (Reedy 1991).

Promotion of Family Adaptation

The nurse assesses the family situation during the first prenatal visit and determines what level of involvement the adolescent desires from each of her family members and from the father of the child, as well as her perception of their present support. A sensitive approach to the daughter-mother relationship helps motivate their communication. If the mother and daughter agree, the mother should be included in the client's care. Encouraging the mother to become part of the maternity team, join grandmother crisis support groups, and obtain counseling helps the mother adapt to her role and support her daughter.

The nurse should also help the mother assess and meet her daughter's needs. Some adolescents become more dependent during pregnancy, and some become more independent. The mother can ease and encourage her daughter's self-growth by understanding how to respond to and support her.

The adolescent's relationship with her father will also be affected by her pregnancy. The nurse can provide information to the father and encourage his involvement to whatever degree is acceptable to both daughter and father.

The father of the adolescent's infant should not be forgotten in promoting the family's adaptation to the pregnancy. He should be included to the extent that he wishes and the teenage mother finds acceptable.

Community-Based Nursing Care

Educational programs for adolescents address two areas: pregnancy prevention and, if pregnancy occurs, prenatal education. Ideally these programs are community based and include the clinic or the caregiver's office, community agencies, and the school system. Many adolescents cite school as the preferred agency for education.

Effective pregnancy prevention programs generally include a focus on abstinence or on delaying sexual initiation, information about human sexuality and contraceptive options, and training in negotiation and decision-making skills. Research suggests that the programs are most effective when they target early adolescents (Frost and Forrest 1995).

The most effective method for education during pregnancy and early parenting appears to be mainstreaming the pregnant adolescent in academic classes with her peers and adding classes appropriate to her needs. Classes about growth and development beginning with the newborn and early infancy can help teenage parents have more realistic expectations of their infants and may help decrease child abuse. Mainstreaming pregnant adolescents in school is also an ideal way to help them complete their education while learning the skills they need to cope with childbearing and parenting. Vocational guidance in this setting is also most beneficial to their future.

Regardless of the sponsorship or setting of prenatal classes for pregnant teenagers and adolescent fathers, the adolescent's developmental tasks must be considered. For example, methods for teaching this age group should be somewhat different from regular prenatal classes (Figure 10–2). The younger adolescent tends to be a more concrete thinker than the older, more mature pregnant adult. Increased use of audiovisuals appropriate to their social situation and age is helpful. More demonstrations may be required, and they need to be simple and direct.

Areas that might be included in prenatal classes are anatomy and physiology, sex education, exercises for pregnancy and after birth, maternal and infant nutrition, growth and development of the fetus, labor and birth, family planning, and infant development. Adolescents may want to participate in the teaching of these classes and should be encouraged to do so. Peer support and friendships can blossom among these young women, helping them all to mature.

The clinic can offer rap sessions, pamphlets, or films in the waiting room. Giving the clients something to do while they wait for their appointments may encourage them to return and also help them learn. Decorating the clinic with attractive educational posters and creating an informal atmosphere establishes an environment where adolescents feel free to interact with professionals.

Ideally, prenatal classes for the adolescent are oriented to more than just pregnancy, childbirth, and immediate newborn care (Figure 10–2). The goals of many of these classes are expanding to deal with more complex social issues that result from adolescent pregnancies. A multidisciplinary team approach is important in planning and implementing these classes. Goals for many of them now include promoting self-esteem; helping participants identify and prepare for the problems and conflicts of teenage parenting; educating participants about sexuality, relationships, and contraception to deter unwanted pregnancies; teaching participants parenting skills, including information about community resources and other resources available to teenage parents; and helping participants develop more adaptive coping skills.

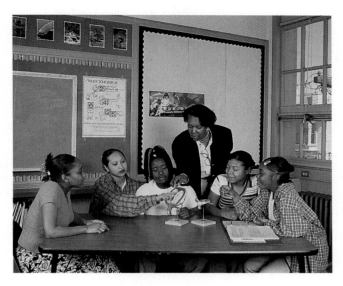

FIGURE 10–2 Young adolescents may benefit from prenatal classes designed for them.

Evaluation

Anticipated outcomes of nursing care include

- A trusting relationship is established with the pregnant adolescent.
- The adolescent is able to use her problem-solving abilities to make appropriate choices.
- The adolescent follows the recommendations of the health care team and receives effective health care throughout her pregnancy, the birth, and the postpartum period.
- The adolescent, her partner (if he is involved), and their families are able to cope successfully with the effects of the pregnancy.
- The adolescent is able to discuss pregnancy, prenatal care, and childbirth.
- The adolescent demonstrates developmental and pregnancy progression within established normal parameters.
- The adolescent develops skill in child care and parenting.

Care of the Expectant Couple over Age 35

Today an increasing number of women over age 35 are choosing to give birth for the first time. In fact, the rate of first births to women between ages 35 and 39 more than doubled between 1970 and 1992 in the United States. For women between the ages of 40 and 44, the birth rate increased by 40 percent during the same period (US Bureau of the Census 1993). Many factors contributed to this trend, including the following:

- The availability of effective birth control methods
- The women's liberation movement and its emphasis on expanded roles for women
- The increased number of women obtaining advanced education, pursuing careers, and delaying parenthood until they are established professionally
- The increased incidence of later marriage and second marriage
- The high cost of living, which causes some young couples to delay childbearing until they are more secure financially
- The increase in the population of women in this age group
- The increased availability of specialized fertilization procedures, which offers opportunities for women previously considered infertile

There are advantages to having a first baby after the age of 35. Single women or couples who delay childbearing until they are older tend to be well educated and financially secure. Usually their decision to have a baby was deliberately and thoughtfully made. Given their greater life experiences, they are much more aware of the realities of having a child and what it means to have a baby at their age (Figure 10–3). Many of the women have experienced fulfillment in their careers and feel secure enough to take on the added responsibility of a child. Some women are ready to make a change in their lives, desiring to stay home with a new baby. Those who plan to continue working are able to afford good child care.

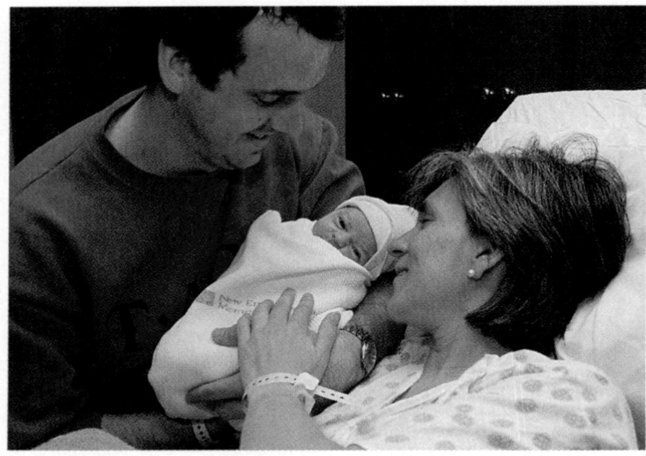

FIGURE 10–3 For older couples, the decision to have a child may be very rewarding.

Medical Risks

In the United States and Canada over the past 30 years, the risk of fetal death has declined dramatically for women of all ages. However, the risk remains highest among women over age 35. Recent research indicates that women age 35 and older, with a fetal loss of 6 deaths per 1000 births, are approximately twice as likely to have a stillbirth as women under age 35 (3 deaths per 1000 births) (Fretts et al 1995). This may be due in part to the decreased ability of the uterine blood vessels of the older woman to accommodate the needs of pregnancy. It may also be related to the fact that older women may experience multiple gestation (a risk factor for fetal death) after fertility-enhancing therapy (Fetal loss 1996).

Preexisting medical conditions such as hypertension or diabetes probably play a more significant role than age in maternal well-being and outcome of pregnancy. Research is mixed, however. A study of white first-born infants suggests a modest increase of low-birth-weight babies and preterm births with increased maternal age when high risk factors were not present (Aldous and Edmonson 1993).

Medical conditions associated with the reproductive organs, such as uterine fibroids, occur with greater frequency in women in their late thirties, and fertility decreases in women as they grow older. The incidence of spontaneous abortion also increases with maternal age, as does the incidence of cesarean birth, gestational diabetes, PIH, abruptio placenta, and placenta previa (Maroulis 1993). The increased cesarean birth rate may actually be due to the reluctance of physicians to take chances with the outcome of a long-awaited pregnancy in this age group (Berkowitz et al 1990).

The risk of conceiving a child with Down syndrome does increase with age, especially over age 35. The use of amniocentesis or chorionic villus sampling (CVS) is routinely offered to all women over age 35 to permit the early detection of several chromosomal abnormalities including Down syndrome.

Research has also focused on the use of multiple marker screening to detect Down syndrome and trisomy 18. This involves a blood test to detect levels of specific serum markers, namely, alpha-fetoprotein (AFP), human chorionic gonadotropin (hCG), and unconjugated estriol. When these tests in combination show certain patterns of increase or decrease, they are considered positive and the woman is advised to consider amniocentesis. While these tests are not as definite as amniocentesis or chorionic villus sampling in detecting abnormalities, they are safer and less expensive (Rose and Mennuti 1995).

Special Concerns of the Older Expectant Couple

No matter what their age, most expectant couples have concerns regarding the well-being of the fetus and their ability to parent. The older couple has additional concerns related to their age. Some couples are concerned about whether they will have enough energy to care for a new baby. Of greater concern is their ability to deal with the needs of the older child when they, too, are older.

The financial concerns of the older couple are usually different from those of the younger couple. The older couple is generally more financially secure than the younger couple. However, when their "baby" is ready for college, the older couple may be close to retirement and may not have the means to provide for their child.

While considering their financial future and future retirement, the older couple may be forced to face their own mortality. Certainly this is not uncommon in midlife, but instead of confronting this issue at 40 to 45 years of age or later, the older expectant couple may confront the issue several years earlier as they consider what will happen as their child grows.

The older expectant couple facing pregnancy following a late or second marriage or after therapy for infertility may find themselves somewhat isolated socially. They may feel "different" because they are often the only couple in their peer group expecting their first baby. In fact, many of their peers are parents of adolescents or young adults and may even be grandparents.

The response of older couples who already have children to learning that the woman is pregnant may vary greatly depending on whether the pregnancy was planned or unexpected. Other factors influencing their response include the attitude of their children, family, and friends to the pregnancy; the impact on their lifestyle; and the financial implications of having another child. Sometimes couples who had previously been married to other mates will choose to have a child together. The concept of **blended family** applies to situations in which "her" children, "his" children, and "their" children come together as a new family group.

Health care professionals may treat the older expectant couple differently than they would a younger couple, especially if the woman is having her first child. Older women may be asked to submit to more medical procedures, such as amniocentesis and ultrasound, than younger women. An older woman may be prevented from using a birthing room or birthing center even if she is healthy, because her age is considered to put her at risk.

The woman who has delayed pregnancy may be concerned about the limited amount of time that she has to bear children. When pregnancy does not occur as quickly as she hoped, the older woman may become increasingly anxious as time slips away on her "biological clock." When an older woman becomes pregnant but experiences a spontaneous abortion, her grief for the loss of her unborn child is exacerbated by her anxiety about her ability to conceive again in her remaining time of fertility.

APPLYING THE NURSING PROCESS

Nursing Assessment

In working with a woman in her thirties or forties who is pregnant, the nurse makes the assessments that are appropriate in caring for any woman who is pregnant. These include assessment of physical status, the woman's understanding of pregnancy and the changes that accompany it, any health teaching needs, the degree of support the woman has available to her, and her knowledge of infant care. In addition, the nurse explores the woman's and her partner's attitudes about the pregnancy and their expectations of the impact a baby will have on their lives.

Nursing Diagnosis

The nursing diagnoses that are applicable to any pregnant woman apply to the pregnant woman who is over age 35. Other nursing diagnoses that may apply include the following:

- Decisional conflict related to unexpected pregnancy
- Impaired social interaction related to unplanned pregnancy

Nursing Plan and Implementation

Once an older couple has made the decision to have a child, it is the nurse's responsibility to respect and support the couple in this decision. As with any client, risks need to be discussed, concerns need to be identified, and strengths need to be promoted. The woman's age should not be made an issue. To promote a sense of well-being, the nurse should treat the pregnancy as "normal" unless specific health risks are identified.

As the pregnancy continues, the nurse should identify and discuss concerns the woman may have related to her age or to specific health problems. The older woman who has made a conscious decision to become pregnant often has carefully thought through potential problems and may actually have fewer concerns than a younger woman or one with an unplanned pregnancy.

Childbirth education classes are important in promoting adaptation to the event of childbirth for expectant couples of any age. However, older expectant couples, who are still in the minority, often feel uncomfortable in classes where the majority of participants are much younger. Because of the differences in age and life experiences, many of the needs of the older couple may not be met in the class. The nurse teaching a childbirth education class should try to anticipate the informational needs of the older couple. As the number of expectant older couples increases, the nurse may find it useful to offer an "over 35" childbirth education class to accommodate the specific needs of older couples.

Women who are over 35 years of age and having their first baby are often better educated than other health care consumers. These clients frequently know the kind of care and services they want and are assertive in their interactions with the health care system. The nurse should not be intimidated by these individuals or assume that anticipatory guidance and support are unnecessary. Instead the nurse should support the couple's strengths and be sensitive to their individual needs.

Provision of Support if Amniocentesis Is Advised

In working with older expectant couples or an older single woman, the nurse must be sensitive to special needs. A particularly difficult issue these individuals face is the possibility of bearing an unhealthy child. Because of the risk of Down syndrome, amniocentesis is often suggested. Chorionic villus sampling (CVS) may also be suggested if available in the area. The decision to have amniocentesis can be difficult merely because of its possible risk to the fetus. But that becomes almost a minor concern when the couple thinks of the implications of a finding of Down syndrome or other chromosomal abnormalities. The finding of abnormalities means that the couple may be faced with the even more difficult decision whether to continue the pregnancy.

A couple's decision to have amniocentesis is usually related to their beliefs and attitudes about abortion. Amniocentesis is usually not even considered by couples who are strongly opposed to abortion for any reason. Health professionals must respect their decision and take a nonjudgmental approach to their continued care.

KEY FACTS TO REMEMBER

Pregnancy in Women over Age 35

- Couples who choose pregnancy at a later age are usually financially secure and have made a thoughtful, planned choice.
- If the woman has no existing health problems, her risk during pregnancy is not appreciably higher than that of the general population.
- The decreased fertility of women over age 35 may make conception more difficult.
- The incidence of Down syndrome does increase somewhat in women over age 35 and significantly over age 40.
- The couple may choose to have amniocentesis or CVS to gain information about the health of their fetus.

For the couple who agree to amniocentesis, the first few months can be a difficult time. Amniocentesis cannot be done until 14 weeks of pregnancy and then the studies take about 2 weeks to complete. Research suggests that older women who undergo amniocentesis may suppress any feelings of attachment to the fetus until they are sure that the results of the amniocentesis are normal (Harker and Thorpe 1992).

The nurse can support couples who decide to have amniocentesis in several ways:

- The nurse should make sure that the couple is aware of the risks of amniocentesis and why it is being performed.
- The nurse who is present during the amniocentesis procedure can offer comfort and emotional support to the expectant woman. The nurse can also provide information about the procedure as it is being performed.
- The nurse can facilitate a support group for women during the difficult waiting period between the procedure and the results.
- If the results indicate that the fetus has Down syndrome or another genetic abnormality, the nurse can ensure that the couple has complete information about the condition, its range of possible manifestations, and its developmental implications.
- The nurse can support the couple in their decision to continue or terminate the pregnancy. It is essential that the nurse and other health professionals involved not impose on the couple their philosophical or political beliefs about abortion. The decision is the couple's, and it should be based on their belief system and a nonbiased presentation of risks and choices from caregivers.

Key Facts to Remember: Pregnancy in Women over Age 35 summarizes key points about pregnancy in this age group.

Evaluation

Anticipated outcomes of nursing care include

- The woman and her partner are knowledgeable about the pregnancy and make appropriate health care choices.
- The expectant couple (and their other children) are able to cope successfully with the pregnancy and its implications for the future.
- The woman receives effective health care throughout her pregnancy and during and after birth.
- The woman and her partner develop skills in child care and parenting as necessary.

CHAPTER HIGHLIGHTS

- The pregnant adolescent must deal with the developmental tasks of adolescence as well as the developmental tasks of pregnancy. Pregnant adolescents face the risks of prolonged dependence on parents, lack of stable relationships with the opposite sex, and lack of economic and social stability.
- Factors affecting an adolescent's response to pregnancy include her degree of achievement of the developmental tasks of adolescence (which can be closely associated with age) and cultural, religious, and socioeconomic factors.
- The adolescent father who wants to be involved is often overlooked by health care providers. If he assumes accountability, however, he is also at increased risk for social and economic problems.
- Often the adolescent has little understanding of pregnancy, childbirth, or parenting. Consequently, education is a primary responsibility of the nurse.
- Childbirth among women over 35 is becoming increasingly common. It poses fewer health risks than previously believed and offers definite advantages for the woman or couple who make the choice.
- A major risk for the older expectant couple relates to the increased incidence of Down syndrome in children born to women over age 35 or 40. Amniocentesis can provide information about whether the fetus has Down syndrome or other genetic abnormalities. The couple can then decide whether they wish to continue the pregnancy.

REFERENCES

Adolescent unintended pregnancy: The scope of the problem. *Contraception Report* May 1994; 5(2):4.

Alan Guttmacher Institute: *Sex and America's Teenagers.* New York: Author, 1994.

Aldous MB, Edmonson MB: Maternal age at first childbirth and risk of low birth weight and preterm delivery in Washington state. *JAMA* December 1993; 270:2574.

Berkowitz GS et al: Delayed childbearing and the outcome of pregnancy. *N Engl J Med* March 1990; 322:659.

Blume GT: *Teenage Pregnancy Facts—Reference Collected for NAE4-HA Task Force on Youth with Special Needs.* Van Horn J (editor). Penn State: Document No. 28507918, January 3, 1996. Available from gopher://psupena.psu.edu/0%24d%2028507918.

Cohn SD: The evolving law of adolescent health care. *Clin Issues Perinatal Women Health Nurs* 1991; 2(2):201.

Contraception and adolescents: Highlights from the NASPAG conference. *Contraception Report* July 1995; 6(3):4.

Crooks R, Baur K: *Our Sexuality,* 5th ed. Redwood City, CA: Benjamin/Cummings, 1993.

Drake P: Addressing developmental needs of pregnant adolescents. *JOGNN* July/August 1996; 25(6):518.

Duany L, Pittman K: Latino youths at a crossroads. *Children's Defense Fund: An Adolescent Pregnancy Prevention Clearinghouse Report.* (ISSN 0899-5591) January/February 1990.

Fetal loss is a relatively uncommon experience, but risk doubles among women aged 35 and older. *Family Plan Perspect* March/April 1996; 28(2):86.

Fielding JE, Williams CA: Adolescent pregnancy in the United States: A review and recommendations for clinicians and research needs. *Am J Preventive Med* 1991; 7:47.

Fretts RC et al: Increased maternal age and the risk of fetal death. *New Engl J Med* 1995; 333:953.

Frost JJ, Forrest JD: Understanding the impact of effective teenage pregnancy prevention programs. *Fam Plan Perspect* September/October 1995; 27(5):188.

Harker L, Thorpe K: "The last egg in the basket?" Elderly primiparity—A review of the findings. *Birth* March 1992; 19(1):23.

Keller ML et al: Adolescents' views of sexual decision making. *Image* Summer 1996; 28(2):125.

Maroulis GB: Fertility, pregnancy, and the older woman. *Contemp OB/GYN* May 1993; 38(5):101.

Marsiglio W: Adolescent males' orientation toward paternity and contraception. *Fam Plan Perspect* January/February 1993; 25:22.

Planned Parenthood: *Pregnancy and Childbearing Among US Teens.* Planned Parenthood Fact Sheet; Planned Parenthood Federation of America, 1993. Available from http://www.ppfa.org/ppfa/teenpreg.html.

Reedy NJ: The very young pregnant adolescent. *Clin Issues Perinatal Women Health Nurs* 1991; 2(2):209.

Rose NC, Mennuti MT: Multiple marker screening for women 35 and older. *Contemp OB/GYN* September 1995; 40(9):55.

Steinburg L: *Adolescence,* 3rd ed. New York: McGraw-Hill, 1993.

US Bureau of the Census: *Statistical Abstract of the United States 1993,* 13th ed. Washington, DC, 1993.

Witwer M: Survey finds teenagers know more about AIDS than about other STDs. *Fam Plan Perspect* May/June 1990; 22:138.

Chapter 11 Maternal Nutrition

OBJECTIVES

- Identify the role of specific nutrients in the diet of the pregnant woman.
- Compare nutritional needs during pregnancy, the postpartum period, and lactation with nonpregnant requirements.
- Plan adequate prenatal vegetarian diets based on the nutritional requirements of pregnancy.
- Describe ways in which various physical, psychosocial, and cultural factors can affect nutritional intake and status.
- Compare recommendations for weight gain and nutrient intakes in the pregnant adolescent with those for the mature pregnant adult.
- Discuss basic factors a nurse should consider when offering nutritional counseling to a pregnant adolescent.
- Compare nutritional counseling issues for nursing and nonnursing mothers.
- Identify women at nutritional risk during pregnancy.
- Formulate a nutritional care plan for pregnant women based on a diagnosis of nutritional problems.

KEY TERMS

Calorie
Folic acid
Lactase deficiency
Lacto-ovovegetarian
Lactose intolerance
Lactovegetarian
Pica
Recommended dietary allowances (RDA)
Vegan

A woman's nutritional status before and during pregnancy can significantly influence her health and that of her fetus. In most prenatal clinics and offices, nurses offer nutritional counseling directly or work closely with the nutritionist in providing necessary nutritional assessment and teaching.

This chapter focuses on the nutritional needs of a normal pregnant woman. Special sections consider the nutritional needs of the pregnant adolescent and the woman after birth.

Good prenatal nutrition is the result of proper eating for a lifetime, not just during pregnancy. Many factors influence a woman's ability to achieve good prenatal nutrition:

- *General nutritional status prior to pregnancy.* Nutritional deficits present at the time of conception and continuing into the early prenatal period may influence the outcome of the pregnancy.
- *Maternal age.* An expectant adolescent must meet her own growth needs in addition to the nutritional needs of pregnancy. This may be especially difficult because teenagers often have nutritional deficiencies.
- *Maternal parity.* The mother's nutritional needs and the outcome of the pregnancy are influenced by the number of pregnancies she has had and the interval between them.

Fetal growth occurs in three overlapping stages: (1) growth by increase in cell number, (2) growth by increases in cell number and cell size, and (3) growth by increase in cell size alone. Nutritional problems that interfere with cell division may have permanent consequences. If the nutritional insult occurs when cells are mainly enlarging, the changes are usually reversible when normal nutrition resumes.

Growth of fetal and maternal tissues requires increased quantities of essential dietary components. Table 11–1 presents the **recommended dietary allowances (RDA)** for nonpregnant, pregnant, and lactating adolescent and adult women. Most of the recommended nutrients can be obtained by eating a well-balanced diet each day. A daily food plan for pregnancy and lactation is presented in Table 11–2.

Maternal Weight Gain

Researchers suggest that an increased maternal weight gain reduces the risk of intrauterine growth retardation (IUGR) in the fetus and newborn. The optimal weight

TABLE 11–1 Recommended Dietary Allowances (RDAs) for Nonpregnant, Pregnant, and Lactating Females, revised 1989*

						Fat-Soluble Vitamins				*Water-Soluble Vitamins*							*Minerals*						
Age (years) and Group	Weight† kg	Weight† lb	Height† cm	Height† in	Protein	Vitamin A	Vitamin D	Vitamin E	Vitamin K	Vitamin C	Thiamine	Riboflavin	Niacin	Vitamin B_6	Folate	Vitamin B_{12}	Calcium	Phosphorous	Magnesium	Iron	Zinc	Iodine	Selenium
					g	μgR‡	μg§	mg α-TE‖	μg	← mg	mg	mg →	mg NE¶	mg	← μg	μg →	← mg	mg	mg	mg	mg →	← μg	μg →
Females																							
11–14	46	101	157	62	46	800	10	8	45	50	1.1	1.3	15	1.4	150	2.0	1200	1200	280	15	12	150	45
15–18	55	120	163	64	44	800	10	8	55	60	1.1	1.3	15	1.5	180	2.0	1200	1200	300	15	12	150	50
19–24	58	128	164	65	46	800	10	8	60	60	1.1	1.3	15	1.6	180	2.0	1200	1200	280	15	12	150	55
25–50	63	138	163	64	50	800	5	8	65	60	1.1	1.3	15	1.6	180	2.0	800	800	280	15	12	150	55
51+	65	143	160	63	50	800	5	8	65	60	1.0	1.2	13	1.6	180	2.0	800	800	280	10	12	150	55
Pregnant					60	800	10	10	65	70	1.5	1.6	17	2.2	400	2.2	1200	1200	320	30	15	175	65
Lactating																							
1st 6 months					65	1300	10	12	65	95	1.6	1.8	20	2.1	280	2.6	1200	1200	355	15	19	200	75
2nd 6 months					62	1200	10	11	65	90	1.6	1.7	20	2.1	260	2.6	1200	1200	340	15	16	200	75

*The allowances, expressed as average daily intakes over time, are intended to provide for individual variations among most normal persons as they live in the United States under usual environmental stresses. Diets should be based on a variety of common foods to provide other nutrients for which human requirements have been less well defined.

†Weights and heights of reference adults are actual medians for the US population of the designated age, as reported by NHANES II. The median weights and heights of those under 19 years of age were taken from Hamill PVV et al: Physical growth. National Center for Health Statistics Percentiles. *Am J Clin Nutr* 1979; 32:607. The use of these figures does not imply that the height-to-weight ratios are ideal.

‡Retinol equivalents. 1 retinol equivalent = 1 μg retinol or 6 μg β-carotene.

§As cholecalciferol. 10 μg cholecalciferol = 400 IU of vitamin D.

‖α-Tocopherol equivalents. 1 mg d-α tocopherol = 1 α-TE.

¶1 NE (niacin equivalent) is equal to 1 mg of niacin or 60 mg of dietary tryptophan.

Source: *Recommended Dietary Allowances,* 10th ed. 1989 National Academy of Sciences, National Research Council, Washington, DC.

TABLE 11–2 Daily Food Plan for Pregnancy and Lactation

Food Group	Nutrients Provided	Food Source	Recommended Daily Amount During Pregnancy	Recommended Daily Amount During Lactation
Dairy products	Protein; riboflavin; vitamins A, D, and others; calcium; phosphorous; zinc; magnesium	Milk—whole, 2%, skim, dry, buttermilk Cheeses—hard, semisoft, cottage Yogurt—plain, low-fat Soybean milk—canned, dry	Four (8 oz) cups (5 for teenagers) used plain or with flavoring, in shakes, soups, puddings, custards, cocoa Calcium in 1 cup milk equivalent to 1 1/2 cups cottage cheese, 1 1/2 oz hard or semisoft cheese, 1 cup yogurt, 1 1/2 cups ice cream (high in fat and sugar)	Four (8 oz) cups (5 for teenagers); equivalent amount of cheese, yogurt and so forth
Meat and meat alternatives	Protein; iron; thiamine, niacin, and other vitamins; minerals	Beef, pork, veal, lamb, poultry, animal organ meats, fish, eggs; legumes; nuts, seeds, peanut butter, grains in proper vegetarian combination (vitamin B_{12} supplement needed)	Three servings (one serving = 2 oz), combination in amounts necessary for same nutrient equivalent (varies greatly)	Two servings
Grain products, whole grain or enriched	B vitamins; iron; whole grain also has zinc, magnesium, and other trace elements; provides fiber	Breads and bread products such as cornbread, muffins, waffles, hotcakes, biscuits, dumplings, cereals, pastas, rice	Six to 11 servings daily: one serving = one slice bread, 3/4 cup or 1 oz dry cereal, 1/2 cup rice or pasta	Same as for pregnancy
Fruits and fruit juices	Vitamins A and C; minerals; raw fruits for roughage	Citrus fruits and juices, melons, berries, all other fruits and juices	Two to four servings (one serving for vitamin C): one serving = one medium fruit, 1/2–1 cup fruit, 4 oz orange or grapefruit juice	Same as for pregnancy
Vegetables and vegetable juices	Vitamins A and C; minerals; provides roughage	Leafy green vegetables; deep yellow or orange vegetables such as carrots, sweet potatoes, squash, tomatoes; green vegetables such as peas, green beans, broccoli; other vegetables such as beets, cabbage, potatoes, corn, lima beans	Three to five servings (one serving of dark green or deep yellow vegetable for vitamin A): one serving = 1/2–1 cup vegetable, two tomatoes, one medium potato	Same as for pregnancy
Fats	Vitamins A and D; linoleic acid	Butter, cream cheese, fortified table spreads; cream, whipped cream, whipped toppings; avocado, mayonnaise, oil, nuts	As desired in moderation (high in calories): one serving = 1 tbsp butter or enriched margarine	Same as for pregnancy
Sugar and sweets		Sugar, brown sugar, honey, molasses	Occasionally, if desired	Same as for pregnancy
Desserts		Nutritious desserts such as puddings, custards, fruit whips, and crisps; other rich, sweet desserts and pastries	Occasionally, if desired	Same as for pregnancy
Beverages		Coffee, decaffeinated beverages, tea, bouillon, carbonated drinks	As desired, in moderation	Same as for pregnancy
Miscellaneous		Iodized salt, herbs, spices, condiments	As desired	Same as for pregnancy

Note: The pregnant woman should eat regularly, three meals a day, with nutritious snacks of fruit, cheese, milk, or other foods between meals if desired. (More frequent but smaller meals are also recommended.) Four to 6 (8 oz) glasses of water and a total of 8–10 (8 oz) cups total fluid intake should be consumed daily. Water is an essential nutrient.

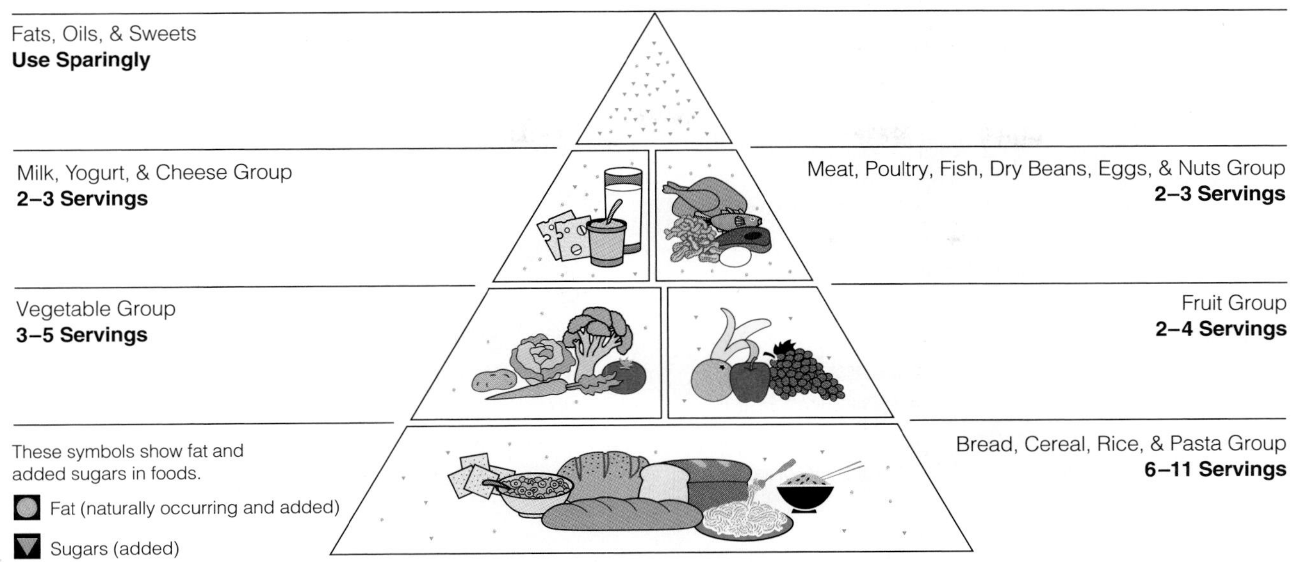

FIGURE 11–1 The Food Guide Pyramid provides a quick reference for people interested in healthy eating. The largest portion of the pyramid is devoted to grains, rice, bread, and pasta, while the smallest portion of the pyramid is devoted to fats, oils, and sweets, which should be used sparingly.

Source: US Dept of Agriculture; US Dept of Health and Human Services.

gain depends on the woman's weight for height (body mass index [BMI]) and her prepregnant nutritional state. An adequate weight gain indicates an adequate caloric intake. It does not, however, ensure that the woman has a sufficient nutrient intake. The pregnant woman must maintain the nutritional quality of her diet as her weight gain progresses.

The Institute of Medicine (1992) recommends weight gains in terms of optimum ranges. Their recommendations are as follows:

- Underweight woman: 28–40 lb (12.5–18 kg)
- Normal weight woman: 25–35 lb (11.5–16 kg)
- Overweight woman: 15–25 lb (7–11.5 kg)
- Obese woman: 15 lb (7.0 kg) or more

The average maternal weight gain is distributed as follows:

5 kg (11 lb)	Fetus, placenta, amniotic fluid
0.9 kg (2 lb)	Uterus
1.8 kg (4 lb)	Increased blood volume
1.4 kg (3 lb)	Breast tissue
2.3–4.5 kg (5–10 lb)	Maternal stores

The ideal pattern of weight gain during pregnancy consists of a gain of 2–5 lb (1–2.3 kg) during the first trimester, followed by a gain of about 1 lb (0.4–0.5 kg) per week during the second and third trimesters.

The pattern of weight gain is important. A woman should generally gain 10–13 lb (4.5–6 kg) by 20 weeks' gestation. If she has not, the nurse should offer further nutritional evaluation and counseling. Sudden, sharp increases (weight gains of 3–5 lb [1.4–2.3 kg] in one week) may indicate excessive fluid retention related to pregnancy-induced hypertension (PIH) and should be evaluated. Inadequate gains (less than 2.2 lb [1 kg] per month during the second and third trimesters) or excessive gains (more than 6.6 lb [3 kg] per month) should be assessed and the need for nutritional counseling considered.

Sometimes a woman will gain excessively during the first two-thirds of her pregnancy because of overeating. Dieting is not advised at this time, however, because the third trimester is the time of maximum fetal growth. Consequently nutritional counseling is directed toward helping the woman plan her diet to gain up to a pound per week. Calorie intake should focus on the RDA guidelines.

There are special concerns for weight gain in the obese woman (one who weighs 20 percent or more above her recommended prepregnant weight). Obese women (even if not diabetic) have an increased risk of having a large baby. Women who weigh 50 percent above their recommended weight also have an increased risk of chronic hypertension, increased blood lipids, and gestational diabetes. Obese women may have diets that are high in energy (from carbohydrates and fats) but low in protein, vitamins, and minerals. Pregnancy is not a time for dieting, and severe weight restrictions during pregnancy can result in maternal ketosis, a threat to fetal well-being. Counseling for the pregnant woman who is obese usually focuses on encouraging her to eat according to the Food Group Pyramid (Figure 11–1). Thus the emphasis is on adequate nutrition rather than on the amount of weight gained.

Women who are 10 percent or more below their recommended weight before conception have an increased

TEACHING GUIDE Helping the Pregnant Woman Add 300 kcal to Her Diet

ASSESSMENT

The nurse recognizes that the notion of "eating for two" may cause a woman to overestimate the amount of food she should consume during pregnancy. The nurse assesses the pregnant woman's knowledge of basic nutrition, including the use of the Food Guide Pyramid (Figure 11–1), and assesses her awareness of the best way to increase the nutrients in her diet.

NURSING DIAGNOSIS

The key nursing diagnosis will probably be: Knowledge deficit related to lack of information about nutritional needs during pregnancy.

NURSING PLAN AND IMPLEMENTATION

The teaching plan focuses on providing information about the Food Guide Pyramid and about the most effective way to use the additional 300 kcal that a woman needs daily during pregnancy.

CLIENT GOALS

At the completion of the teaching the woman will:

1. Identify the Food Guide Pyramid categories and the foods included in each
2. Cite the increase in kcal indicated during pregnancy
3. Discuss the most nutritionally sound way to use the additional calories
4. Use the information she has gained to plan a nutritionally sound sample menu

Teaching Plan

CONTENT

The food groups include the following:

Grains: 6 to 11 servings (one serving = one slice bread, 1/2 hamburger roll, 1 oz dry cereal, 1 tortilla, 1/2 cup pasta, rice, grits)

Fruits: Two to four servings; one should be a good source of vitamin C (one serving = 1 medium-sized piece of fruit, 1/2 cup juice)

Vegetables: Three to five servings (one serving = 1 cup raw vegetable, 1 cup green leafy vegetable, 1/2 cup cooked vegetable)

Dairy: Two to three servings (one serving = 1 cup milk or yogurt, 1.5 oz hard cheese, 2 cups cottage cheese, 1 cup pudding made with milk)

TEACHING METHOD

Ask woman if she has received nutritional information using this approach before. Discuss her understanding of it. Use that information to plan the amount of detail you will use.

Use a chart or colorful handout to explain the basic food groups and to give examples of equivalent foods.

risk of giving birth to a low-birth-weight infant and have an increased risk of developing PIH (Institute of Medicine 1990). Simply advocating the traditional weight gain is not adequate counseling for the underweight woman who is pregnant. The nurse first assesses why the woman is underweight. Once the cause is determined, the nurse can usually plan intervention with the woman. The underweight woman is generally advised to increase her caloric intake by 500 kilocalories (kcal) above the nonpregnant RDA, as opposed to the 300 kcal increase. She should also consume 20 g additional protein. This is often difficult for the underweight woman, especially if she has a small appetite, and she will require support and encouragement from family and health care providers.

Nutritional Requirements

The RDA for almost all nutrients increases during pregnancy, although the amount of increase varies with each nutrient. These increases reflect the additional requirements of both the mother and the developing fetus (Table 11–1).

Folic acid and iron are the only nutritional supplements generally recommended during pregnancy. The increased need for other vitamins and minerals can usually be met with an adequate diet. To avoid possible deficiencies, however, many health care professionals still recommend a daily vitamin supplement.

Calories

The term **calorie** (cal) designates the amount of heat required to raise the temperature of 1 gram of water 1 degree Celsius. The *kilocalorie* (kcal) is equivalent to 1000 cal and is the unit used to express the energy value of food.

The RDA for energy requirements during pregnancy recommends no increase during the first trimester, but an increase of 300 kcal/day during the second and third trimesters. Prepregnant weight, height, maternal age, health status, and activity level all influence caloric

TEACHING GUIDE continued

Meats and alternatives: Two to three servings (one serving = 2 oz cooked lean meat, poultry, or fish; 2 eggs; 1/2 cup cottage cheese; 1 cup cooked legumes [kidney, lima, garbanzo, or soy beans, split peas]; 6 oz tofu; 2 oz nuts or seeds; 4 tbsp peanut butter)

Not all foods that are nutritionally equivalent have the same number of calories; it is important to consider that when making food choices.	Use a calorie-counting guide to compare the calories in a variety of foods that are equivalent, such as 2 oz beef and 2 oz fish or 1 cup low-fat milk and 1 cup whole milk.
The Food Guide Pyramid is designed to represent the food groups needed to make a balanced diet. The grain, fruit, and vegetable groups are at the base of the pyramid and should account for the majority of the food selections. Fewer servings of dairy and meat or meat alternative are required in the diet, and these groups fall in the middle portion of the pyramid. The very top of the pyramid represents fats, oils, and sweets. These items do not have a high nutritional value and should be used sparingly.	Use a similar approach to evaluate the calories in fats, oils, and sweets, but also evaluate their nutrient content, especially levels of nutrients such as vitamin C, iron, and calcium.
Emphasize that a woman only has to add 300 kcal/day during pregnancy. This can be achieved by adding two milk servings and one serving of meat or alternative. Because of the varying caloric value a woman needs to consider the advisability of using low-fat milk, lean cuts of meat, or fish broiled or baked instead of fried.	In planning the woman's diet to get optimum nutrition without too many additional calories, it is often helpful to ask her to plan and evaluate a sample menu.
Foods can be combined. For example, 1 cup spaghetti with a 2 oz meatball would count as 1 serving meat, 3/4 cup spaghetti = 1 grain, and 1/4 cup tomato sauce = 1/2 serving vegetable.	Provide handouts on which the woman can list the foods she has eaten and check off the corresponding nutrient categories. Have her bring her completed handouts to a subsequent visit.

EVALUATION

Teaching has been effective if all the identified goals are achieved and if the woman seems comfortable planning her diet to provide for the best nutrition possible.

needs, and weight should be monitored regularly during the pregnancy. The Teaching Guide: Helping the Pregnant Woman Add 300 kcal to Her Diet offers suggestions for providing basic nutritional information to pregnant women.

Carbohydrates

Carbohydrates provide protective functions, fiber, and energy. Carbohydrates contribute to the total caloric intake required. If the total caloric intake is not adequate, the body uses protein for energy. Protein then becomes unavailable for growth needs. In addition, protein breakdown leads to ketosis. Ketosis can be a problem, especially in diabetic women, due to glycosuria, reduced alkaline reserves, and lipidemia.

The carbohydrate and caloric needs of the pregnant woman increase, especially during the last two trimesters. Carbohydrate intake promotes weight gain and growth of the fetus, placenta, and other maternal tissues. Dairy products, fruits, vegetables, and whole-grain cereals and breads all contain carbohydrates and other important nutrients.

Protein

Protein supplies the amino acids (nitrogen) required for the growth and maintenance of tissue and other physiologic functions. Protein also contributes to the body's overall energy metabolism.

The body uses the increased protein that is retained, beginning in early pregnancy, for hyperplasia and hypertrophy of maternal tissues such as the uterus and breasts, and to meet fetal needs. The fetus makes its greatest demands during the last half of pregnancy, when fetal growth is greatest.

The protein requirement for the pregnant woman is 60 g/day, a 14 g increase. Animal products such as meat, fish, poultry, and eggs are sources of high-quality protein. Dairy products are also important protein sources.

A quart of milk supplies 32 g of protein, more than half the average daily protein requirement. Milk can be incorporated into the diet in a variety of dishes, including soups, puddings, custards, sauces, and yogurt. Beverages such as hot chocolate and milk-and-fruit drinks can also be included, but they are high in calories. Various kinds of hard and soft cheeses and cottage cheese are excellent protein sources, although cream cheese is categorized as a fat source only.

Women who have allergies to milk, are **lactose intolerant,** or practice vegetarianism may find dried or canned soy milk acceptable. It can be used in cooked dishes or as a beverage. Tofu, or soybean curd, can replace cottage cheese.

If little or no protein comes from animal sources, it is necessary to combine foods of plant origin to obtain the amino acids necessary for a complete protein. Examples of combined proteins are beans and rice, peanut butter on whole grain bread, and whole grain cereal and milk. Except in unusual medical situations, the pregnant woman should obtain dietary protein through natural foods and avoid using protein and amino acid supplements.

Fat

Fats are valuable sources of energy for the body. Fats are more completely absorbed during pregnancy, resulting in a marked increase in serum lipids, lipoproteins, and cholesterol and decreased elimination of fat through the bowel. Fat deposits in the fetus increase from about 2 percent at midpregnancy to almost 12 percent at term. The RDA for fat is less than 30 percent of daily caloric intake, of which less than 10 percent should be saturated fat.

Minerals

Increased minerals needed for the growth of new tissue during pregnancy are obtained by improved mineral absorption and an increase in mineral allowances.

Calcium and Phosphorus

Calcium and phosphorus are involved in mineralization of fetal bones and teeth, energy and cell production, and acid-base buffering. Calcium is absorbed and used more efficiently during pregnancy. Some calcium and phosphorus are required early in pregnancy, but most fetal bone calcification occurs during the last 2–3 months. Teeth begin to form at about the eighth week of gestation and are formed by birth. The 6-year molars begin to calcify just before birth.

The RDA for calcium for the pregnant or lactating woman, regardless of age, is 1200 mg/day. If calcium intake is low, fetal needs will be met at the mother's expense by demineralization of maternal bone.

A diet that includes 4 cups of milk or an equivalent dairy alternative will provide sufficient calcium. Smaller amounts of calcium are supplied by legumes, nuts, dried fruits, and dark green leafy vegetables (such as kale, cabbage, collards, and turnip greens). It is important to remember that some of the calcium in beet greens, spinach, and chard is bound with oxalic acid, which makes it unavailable to the body.

The RDA for phosphorus is the same as the RDA for calcium: 1200 mg/day for the pregnant or lactating woman. As phosphorus is so widely available in foods, the dietary intake of phosphorus frequently exceeds calcium intake.

An excess of phosphorus can result in a disturbance of the calcium-phosphorus ratio in the body, decreased calcium absorption, and increased excretion of calcium. Excess phosphorus can be reduced by avoiding the snack foods, processed meats, and cola drinks in which it abounds. However, if vitamin D and magnesium are adequate, most adults can tolerate relatively wide variations in dietary calcium-phosphorus ratios.

Iodine

Inorganic iodine is excreted in the urine during pregnancy. Enlargement of the thyroid gland may occur if iodine is not replaced by adequate dietary intake or an additional supplement. Moreover, cretinism may occur in the infant if the mother has a severe iodine deficiency. The iodine allowance of 175 g/day can be met by using iodized salt. When sodium is restricted, the physician may prescribe an iodine supplement.

Sodium

The sodium ion is essential for proper metabolism. Sodium intake in the form of salt is never entirely curtailed during pregnancy, even when hypertension or PIH is present. The pregnant woman may season food to taste during cooking but should avoid using extra salt at the table. She can avoid excessive intake by eliminating salty foods such as potato chips, ham, sausages, and sodium-based seasonings.

Zinc

Zinc is involved in protein metabolism and the synthesis of DNA and RNA. The RDA for pregnancy is 15 mg. Sources include milk, liver, shellfish, and wheat bran. Zinc deficiency during pregnancy may affect embryonic growth and result in malformation (Rosso 1990).

Magnesium

Magnesium is essential for cellular metabolism and structural growth. The RDA for pregnancy is 320 mg.

Sources include milk, whole grains, beet greens, nuts, legumes, and tea.

Iron

Anemia in pregnancy is mainly caused by low iron stores, although it may also be caused by inadequate intake of other nutrients, such as vitamins B_6 and B_{12}, folic acid, ascorbic acid, copper, and zinc. Iron deficiency anemia is generally defined as a decrease in the oxygen-carrying capacity of the blood. Anemia leads to a significant reduction in hemoglobin in the volume of packed red cells per deciliter of blood (hematocrit), or in the number of erythrocytes.

The normal hematocrit in the nonpregnant woman is 38 to 47 percent. In the pregnant woman, the level may drop as low as 34 percent, even when nutrition is adequate. This condition is called the *physiologic anemia of pregnancy* (Chapter 7).

Fetal demands for iron further contribute to symptoms of anemia in the pregnant woman. The fetal liver stores iron, especially during the third trimester. The infant needs this stored iron during the first 4 months of life to compensate for the normally inadequate levels of iron in breast milk and non-iron-fortified formulas.

To prevent anemia, the woman must balance iron requirements and intake. This is a problem for nonpregnant women and a greater one for pregnant women. By carefully selecting foods high in iron, the woman can increase her daily iron intake considerably. Lean meats, dark green leafy vegetables, eggs, and whole-grain and enriched breads and cereals are the usual food sources of iron. Other iron sources include dried fruits, legumes, shellfish, and molasses.

Iron absorption is generally higher for animal products than for vegetable products. However, absorption of iron from nonmeat sources may be enhanced by combining them with meat or a food rich in vitamin C. The RDA for iron during pregnancy is 30 mg/day, but this intake is almost impossible to achieve through diet alone. Thus the pregnant woman should take a supplement of simple iron salt, such as ferrous gluconate, ferrous fumarate, or ferrous sulfate during the second and third trimesters when fetal demand is the greatest. Supplements are not usually given during the first trimester because the increased demand is still minimal, and iron may increase the woman's nausea.

Vitamins

Vitamins are organic substances necessary for life and growth. They are found in small amounts in specific foods and generally cannot be synthesized by the body.

Vitamins are grouped according to solubility. Those vitamins that dissolve in fat are A, D, E, and K; those soluble in water include vitamin C and the B complex. An adequate intake of all vitamins is essential during pregnancy; however, several are required in larger amounts to fulfill specific needs.

Fat-Soluble Vitamins

The fat-soluble vitamins A, D, E, and K are stored in the liver and thus are available should the dietary intake become inadequate. The major complication related to these vitamins is not deficiency but toxicity due to overdose. Unlike water-soluble vitamins, excess amounts of A, D, E, and K are not excreted in the urine. Symptoms of vitamin toxicity include nausea, gastrointestinal upset, dryness and cracking of the skin, and loss of hair.

Vitamin A is involved in the growth of epithelial cells, which line the entire gastrointestinal tract and compose the skin. Vitamin A plays a role in the metabolism of carbohydrates and fats. In the absence of A, the body cannot synthesize glycogen, and the body's ability to handle cholesterol is also affected. The protective layer of tissue surrounding nerve fibers does not form properly if vitamin A is lacking.

Probably the best-known function of vitamin A is its effect on vision in dim light. A person's ability to see in the dark depends on the eye's supply of retinol, a form of vitamin A. In this manner, vitamin A prevents night blindness. Vitamin A is associated with the formation and development of healthy eyes in the fetus.

If maternal stores of vitamin A are adequate, the overall effects of pregnancy on the woman's vitamin A requirements are not remarkable. The blood serum level of vitamin A decreases slightly in early pregnancy, rises in late pregnancy, and falls before the onset of labor. The RDA for vitamin A does not increase during pregnancy.

Excessive intake of preformed vitamin A is toxic to both children and adults. There are indications that excessive intake of vitamin A in the fetus can cause eye, ear, and bone malformation, cleft palate, possible renal anomalies, and central nervous system damage (Luke and Keith 1992). Rich plant sources of vitamin A include deep green and yellow vegetables; animal sources include liver, liver oil, kidney, egg yolk, cream, butter, and fortified margarine.

Vitamin D is best known for its role in the absorption and use of calcium and phosphorus in skeletal development. To supply the needs of the developing fetus, the pregnant woman should have a vitamin D intake of 10 μg/day.

Various degrees of vitamin D deficiency can affect the development of the fetus. Symptoms can range from a reduction of fetal bone calcification to hypoplasia of dental enamel or, in cases of severe deficiency, intrauterine rickets (Rosso 1990).

Main food sources of vitamin D include fortified milk, margarine, butter, liver, and egg yolks. Drinking a quart of milk daily provides the vitamin D needed during pregnancy.

Excessive intake of vitamin D is not usually a result of eating but of taking high-potency vitamin preparations. Overdoses during pregnancy can cause hypercalcemia or high blood calcium levels due to withdrawal of calcium from the skeletal tissue. In the fetus, cardiac defects, especially aortic stenosis, may occur (Luke and Keith 1992). Continued overdose can also cause hypercalcemia and eventually death, especially in young children. Symptoms of toxicity are excessive thirst, loss of appetite, vomiting, weight loss, irritability, and high blood calcium levels.

The major function of *vitamin E,* or tocopherol, is antioxidation. Vitamin E takes on oxygen, thus preventing another substance from undergoing chemical change. For example, vitamin E helps spare vitamin A by preventing its oxidation in the intestinal tract and in the tissues. It decreases the oxidation of polyunsaturated fats, thus helping to retain the flexibility and health of the cell membrane. In protecting the cell membrane, vitamin E affects the health of all cells in the body.

Vitamin E is also involved in certain enzymatic and metabolic reactions. It is an essential nutrient for the synthesis of nucleic acids required in the formation of red blood cells in the bone marrow. Vitamin E is beneficial in treating certain types of muscular pain and intermittent claudication, in surface healing of wounds and burns, and in protecting lung tissue from the damaging effects of smog. These functions may help explain the abundant claims and cures attributed to vitamin E, many of which have not been scientifically proved.

The newborn's need for vitamin E is widely recognized. Human milk provides adequate vitamin E, whereas cow's milk is lower in vitamin E content. Deficiency symptoms of vitamin E are related to long-term inability to absorb fats. In humans, malabsorption problems exist in cases of cystic fibrosis, liver cirrhosis, postgastrectomy, obstructive jaundice, pancreatic problems, and sprue.

The recommended intake of vitamin E increases from 8 international units (IU) for nonpregnant females to 10 IU for pregnant women. The vitamin E requirement varies with the polyunsaturated fat content of the diet. Vitamin E is widely distributed in foodstuffs, especially vegetable fats and oils, whole grains, greens, and eggs.

Some pregnant women use vitamin E oil on the abdominal skin to make it supple and possibly prevent permanent stretch marks. It is questionable whether taking high doses internally will accomplish this goal or satisfy any other claims related to vitamin E's role in reproduction or virility. Excessive intake of vitamin E has been associated with abnormal coagulation in the newborn.

Vitamin K, or menadione as used synthetically in medicine, is an essential factor for the synthesis of prothrombin; its function is thus related to normal blood clotting. Synthesis occurs in the intestinal tract by the *Escherichia coli* bacteria normally inhabiting the large intestine. However, the body's need for vitamin K is not totally met by synthesis. Green leafy vegetables and liver are excellent sources. The RDA for vitamin K does not increase during pregnancy. Newborn infants, having a sterile intestinal tract and receiving sterile feeding, lack vitamin K. Thus newborns often receive a dose of menadione as a protective measure to prevent hemorrhage.

Intake of vitamin K is usually adequate in a well-balanced prenatal diet. Secondary problems may arise if an illness is present that results in malabsorption of fats or if antibiotics are used for an extended period, which would inhibit vitamin K synthesis by destroying intestinal *E coli.*

Water-Soluble Vitamins

Water-soluble vitamins are excreted in the urine. Since only small amounts are stored, there is little protection from dietary inadequacies. Thus adequate amounts must be ingested daily. During pregnancy, the concentration of water-soluble vitamins in the maternal serum falls, whereas high concentrations are found in the fetus.

The RDA for *vitamin C* (ascorbic acid) increases in pregnancy from 60 to 70 mg. The major function of vitamin C is to aid the formation and development of connective tissue and the vascular system. Ascorbic acid is essential to the formation of collagen, which binds cells together. If the collagen begins to disintegrate because of a lack of ascorbic acid, cell functioning is disturbed and cell structure breaks down, resulting in muscular weakness, capillary hemorrhage, and eventual death. These are symptoms of scurvy, the disease caused by vitamin C deficiency. Infants fed mainly cow's milk become deficient in vitamin C, and they are the main population that develops these symptoms. Surprisingly, newborns of women who have taken megadoses of vitamin C may experience a rebound form of scurvy.

Maternal plasma levels of vitamin C progressively decline during pregnancy, with values at term being about half those at midpregnancy. It appears that ascorbic acid concentrates in the placenta; levels in the fetus are 50 percent or more above maternal levels.

A nutritious diet should meet the pregnant woman's needs for vitamin C without additional supplementation. Common food sources of vitamin C include citrus fruit, tomatoes, cantaloupe, strawberries, potatoes, broccoli, and other leafy greens. Ascorbic acid is readily destroyed by water and oxidation. Therefore, foods containing vitamin C must be stored and cooked properly.

The *B vitamins* include thiamine (B_1), riboflavin (B_2), niacin, folic acid, pantothenic acid, vitamin B_6, and vitamin B_{12}. These vitamins serve as vital coenzyme factors in many reactions such as cell respiration, glucose oxidation, and energy metabolism. The quantities needed, therefore, invariably increase as caloric intake increases to meet the metabolic and growth needs of the pregnant woman.

The *thiamine* requirement increases from the pre-pregnant level of 1.1 mg/day to 1.5 mg/day. Sources include pork, liver, milk, potatoes, enriched breads, and cereals.

Riboflavin deficiency is manifested by cheilosis (fissures and cracks of the lips and corners of the mouth) and other skin lesions. During pregnancy, women may excrete less riboflavin and still require more, because of increased energy and protein needs. An additional 0.3 mg/day is recommended. Sources include milk, liver, eggs, enriched breads, and cereals.

Niacin intake should increase 2 mg/day during pregnancy and 5 mg/day during lactation. Sources of niacin include meat, fish, poultry, liver, whole grains, enriched breads, cereals, and peanuts.

Folic acid is directly related to the outcome of pregnancy and to maternal and fetal health. It promotes adequate fetal growth and prevents the macrocytic, megalobastic anemia of pregnancy. Inadequate intake of folic acid has been associated with neural tube defects (NTD) (spina bifida, meningomyelocele). Because adequate folic acid can prevent most NTDs, all women of child-bearing age should consume 0.4 mg of folic acid daily. Unfortunately the average US intake of folic acid is only half that amount. Consequently, a 0.4 mg folic acid daily supplement is recommended. Women who have given birth previously to an infant with a NTD should receive a daily supplement of 4 mg (Niebyl 1995). Supplementation should begin, if possible, one to three months before conception and should continue for at least the first 3 months of pregnancy (Rayburn et al 1996).

Megaloblastic anemia due to folate deficiency is rarely found in the United States, but those caring for pregnant women must be aware that it does occur. Folate deficiency can also be present in the absence of overt anemia.

The best food sources of folates are fresh green leafy vegetables, kidney, liver, food yeasts, and peanuts. Cow's milk contains a small amount of folic acid, but goat's milk contains none. Therefore, infants and children who are given goat's milk must receive a folate supplement to prevent a deficiency.

The folic acid content of foods can be altered by preparation methods. Because folic acid is a water-soluble nutrient, care must be taken in cooking. Loss of the vitamin can be considerable when vegetables and meats are cooked in large amounts of water.

No allowance has been set for *pantothenic acid* in pregnancy, but 5 mg/day is considered a safe, adequate intake. Sources include liver, egg yolk, yeast, and whole-grain cereals and breads.

Vitamin B_6 (pyridoxine) has long been associated biochemically with pregnancy. The RDA for vitamin B_6 during pregnancy is 2.2 mg, an increase of 0.6 mg over the allowance for nonpregnant women. Because pyridoxine is associated with amino acid metabolism, a higher-than-average protein intake requires increased pyridoxine intake. Generally, the slightly increased need can be supplied by dietary sources, which include wheat germ, yeast, fish, liver, pork, potatoes, and lentils.

Vitamin B_{12}, or cobalamin, is the cobalt-containing vitamin found only in animal sources. Women of reproductive age rarely have a B_{12} deficiency. Vegans can develop a deficiency, however, so it is essential that their dietary intake be supplemented with this vitamin. Occasionally vitamin B_{12} levels decrease during pregnancy but increase again after childbirth. The RDA during pregnancy is 2.2 μg/day. A deficiency may be due to inability to absorb vitamin B_{12}. Pernicious anemia results; infertility is a complication of this type of anemia.

Fluid

Water is essential for life, and it is found in all body tissues. It is necessary for many biochemical reactions. It also serves as a lubricant, as a medium of transport for carrying substances in and out of the body, and as an aid in temperature control. A pregnant woman should consume at least 8–10 (8 oz) glasses of fluid each day, of which 4–6 glasses are water.

Because of their sodium content, diet sodas should be consumed in moderation. Caffeinated beverages have a diuretic effect, which may be counterproductive to increasing fluid intake.

Vegetarianism

Vegetarianism is the dietary choice of many people for religious, health, and ethical reasons. There are several types of vegetarians. **Lacto-ovovegetarians** include milk, dairy products, and eggs in their diet. **Lactovegetarians** include dairy products but no eggs in their diets. **Vegans** are "pure" vegetarians who will not eat any food from animal sources.

The expectant woman who is vegetarian must eat the proper combination of foods to obtain adequate nutrients. If her diet allows, a woman can obtain ample and complete proteins from dairy products and eggs. An adequate, pure vegetarian diet contains protein from unrefined grains (brown rice and whole wheat), legumes (beans, split peas, lentils), nuts in large quantities, and a variety of cooked and fresh vegetables and fruits. Seeds may be used in the vegetarian diet if the quantity is large enough. If the vegetarian woman's diet contains sufficient calories, it will also contain sufficient protein if she follows the recommendations for complementing proteins.

Because vegans use no animal products, a daily supplement of 4 μg of vitamin B_{12} is necessary. If the

TABLE 11–3 Vegetarian Food Groups

Food Group	Mixed Diet	Lacto-ovovegetarian	Lacto-vegetarian	Vegan
Grain	Bread, cereal, rice, pasta	Bread, cereal, rice, pasta	Bread, cereal, rice, pasta	Bread, cereal, rice, pasta
Fruit	Fruit, fruit juices	Fruit, fruit juices	Fruit, fruit juices	Fruit, fruit juices
Vegetable	Vegetables, vegetable juices	Vegetables, vegetable juices	Vegetables, vegetable juices	Vegetables, vegetable juices
Dairy	Milk, yogurt, cheese	Milk, yogurt, cheese	Milk, yogurt, cheese	Fortified soy milk
Meat and meat alternatives	Meat, fish, poultry, eggs, legumes, tofu, nuts, nut butters	Eggs, legumes, tofu, nuts, nut butters	Legumes, tofu, nuts, nut butters	Legumes, tofu, nuts, nut butters

woman uses soy milk, only partial supplementation may be needed. If she uses no soy milk, she needs daily supplements of 1200 mg of calcium and 10 μg of vitamin D.

Because the best sources of iron and zinc are animal products, vegan diets may also be low in these minerals. In addition, a high fiber intake may reduce mineral (calcium, iron, and zinc) bioavailability. Emphasis should be placed on use of foods containing these nutrients. A vegetarian food group guide appears in Table 11–3.

Factors Influencing Nutrition

Besides having knowledge of nutritional needs and food sources, the nurse must be aware of other factors that affect a client's nutrition. What is the age, lifestyle, and culture of the pregnant woman? What food beliefs and habits does she have? What a person eats is determined by availability, economics, and symbolism. These factors and others influence the expectant mother's acceptance of the nurse's intervention.

Lactase Deficiency (Lactose Intolerance)

Some individuals have difficulty digesting milk and milk products. This condition, known as **lactase deficiency (lactose intolerance)**, results from an inadequate amount of the enzyme lactase, which breaks down the milk sugar lactose into smaller digestible substances.

Lactose intolerance is found in many people of African, Mexican, Native American, Ashkenazic Jewish, and Asian descent. People who are not affected are mainly of northern European heritage. Symptoms include abdominal distention, discomfort, nausea, vomiting, loose stools, and cramps.

In counseling pregnant women who might be intolerant of milk and milk products, the nurse should be aware that even one glass of milk can produce symptoms. Milk in cooked form, such as custards, is sometimes tolerated, as are cultured or fermented dairy products such as buttermilk, cheese, or yogurt. In some instances, the enzyme lactase may be taken to alleviate this problem. It is available as a chewable tablet to be taken before ingesting milk products, or as a liquid to add to milk itself. Lactase-treated milk is also available commercially in some grocery stores, although it may be more expensive than regular milk.

Pica

Pica is the persistent eating of substances such as dirt, clay, starch, freezer frost, burnt matches, or ashes that are not ordinarily considered edible or nutritionally valuable. Most women who practice pica in pregnancy eat such substances only during that time.

Iron-deficiency anemia is the most common concern in pica. The ingestion of laundry starch or certain types of clay may contribute to iron deficiency because it interferes with iron absorption. The ingestion of large quantities of clay could fill the intestine and cause fecal impaction, while the ingestion of starch may be associated with excessive weight gain.

Nurses should be aware of pica and its implications for the woman and fetus. Assessment for the practice of pica is an important part of a nutritional history. Nurses may detect this practice as they help determine appropriate and effective relief measures for discomforts the woman is experiencing. A nonjudgmental approach and reeducation of the expectant woman are important in helping her to decrease or eliminate this practice.

Common Discomforts of Pregnancy

Gastrointestinal functioning can be altered at various times throughout pregnancy. Although these changes can be uncomfortable for the woman, they are seldom a major problem. Minor dietary modifications may provide relief (see also Chapter 9).

Many women experience nausea and vomiting during the first few months of their pregnancy. Dietary modifications for nausea and vomiting encourage the use of easy-to-digest foods and the avoidance of spicy and fatty food.

Heartburn is an uncomfortable, burning sensation that results when stomach contents back up into the esophagus. It is usually caused by the expanding uterus pushing against the digestive tract. Dietary modifications that control the amount and type of food in the stomach may help control the symptoms. The woman should also avoid lying down after eating.

Constipation may occur in pregnancy as a result of hormonal influence on the muscles of the digestive tract and pressure exerted on the intestines by the expanding uterus. Iron supplements may also contribute to constipation. Adequate fluid and fiber intake are recommended dietary modifications. Pregnant women should avoid using laxatives unless they are recommended by a health care provider.

Cultural, Ethnic, and Religious Influences

Cultural, ethnic, and occasionally religious backgrounds determine one's experiences with food and influence food preferences and habits (Figure 11–2). People of different nationalities are accustomed to eating different foods because of the kinds of foodstuffs available in their countries of origin. The way food is prepared varies, depending on the customs and traditions of the ethnic and cultural group. In addition, the laws of certain religions sanction particular foods, prohibit others, and direct the preparation and serving of meals.

In each culture, certain foods have symbolic significance. Generally these symbolic foods are related to major life experiences such as birth, death, or developmental milestones. Although generalizations have been made about the food practices of ethnic and religious groups, there are many variations. The extent to which traditional ethnic foods and customs are continued is affected by the extent of exposure to other cultures; the availability, quality, and cost of traditional foods; and the recency of immigration.

The relationship of food to pregnancy is reflected in beliefs or sayings. For example, nurses frequently hear that the pregnant woman must eat for two. Less frequently, nurses may hear that the woman believes that craving one food excessively can cause the baby to be "marked," and that the shape of the birthmark echoes the shape of the food the mother craved during pregnancy.

Many groups, especially those of Asian and Hispanic cultures, accept the concept of hot and cold. Certain conditions are considered hot or cold, and believed to be best treated with foods of the opposite temperature in order to maintain balance or harmony. For many of the Hmongs of Cambodia, for example, birth is viewed as a cold experience. To counteract it, pregnant women eat warm foods such as chicken and soup with rice and avoid cold drinks (Rairdan and Higgs 1992).

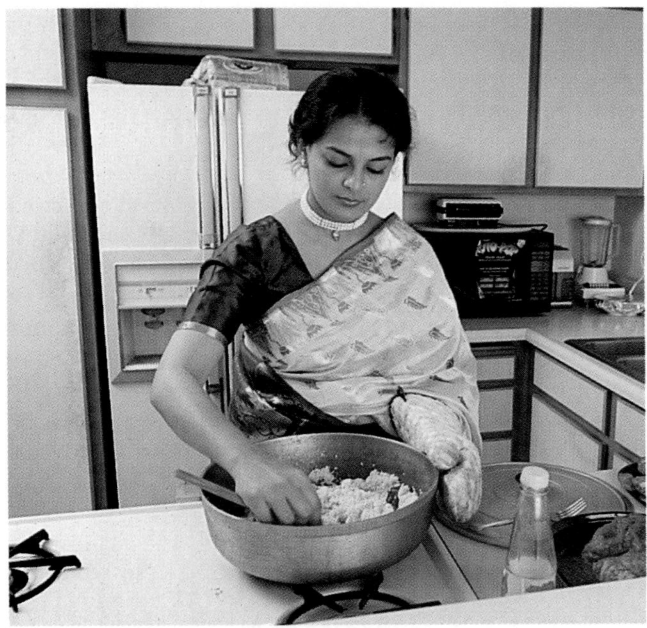

FIGURE 11–2 Food preferences and habits are affected by cultural factors.

Many traditional Chinese believe that a balance of two elements, yin (female, darkness, cold) and yang (male, light, hot) is essential for good health. Yin conditions such as menstruation, pregnancy, and the postpartal period are treated with yang foods to restore balance and rebuild lost strength. Examples of yang foods include broiled meat, chicken soup, garlic, onions, and sesame oil. Noodles, soft rice, and sweets are neutral and may also be eaten (Boyle and Andrews 1989).

It is common for health care providers to give dietary advice from their own cultural context. When working with pregnant women from any ethnic background, it is important to understand the impact of her cultural beliefs on her eating habits and to identify any beliefs she may have about food and pregnancy. The nurse can use generalizations about ethnic food preferences as an introduction to food customs and can determine the level of adherence to the traditional food customs by talking with the client. Dietary advice can then be given in a manner that is meaningful to the woman and her family.

Psychosocial Factors

The nurse should be aware of the various psychosocial factors that influence a woman's food choices. Some foods and food practices are associated with status. Some foods are prepared "just for company"; others are served only on special occasions or holidays.

Socioeconomic level may be a determinant of nutritional status. Poverty-level families cannot afford the same foods that higher-income families can. Thus pregnant women with low incomes are frequently at risk for poor nutrition.

Knowledge about the basic components of a balanced diet is essential. Often educational level is related to economic status, but even people on very limited incomes can prepare well-balanced meals if their knowledge of nutrition is adequate.

The expectant woman's attitudes and feelings about her pregnancy influence her nutritional status. The woman who is depressed or does not wish to be pregnant may manifest these feelings in loss of appetite or improper food practices such as overindulgence in sweets or alcohol.

Nutritional Care of the Pregnant Adolescent

Nutritional status is an important, controllable factor that influences the outcome of all pregnancies, but especially adolescent pregnancies. Good maternal weight gain during adolescent pregnancy significantly improves fetal growth and reduces mortality without increasing the overall risk of cesarean birth or complications.

Many adolescents are nutritionally at risk because of a variety of complex and interrelated emotional, social, and economic factors. Important nutrition-related factors to assess in pregnant adolescents include low prepregnant weight, low weight gain during pregnancy, younger age with regard to menarche, smoking, excessive prepregnant weight, anemia, unhealthy lifestyle (drugs, alcohol use), chronic disease, and history of an eating disorder (ADA 1989).

Estimates of the nutritional needs of adolescents are generally determined by using the RDA for nonpregnant teenagers and adding nutrient amounts recommended for all women (see Table 11–1). If mature (more than 4 years since menarche), the pregnant adolescent's nutritional needs approach those reported for pregnant adults. However, adolescents who become pregnant less than 4 years after menarche are at high biologic risk due to their physiologic and anatomic immaturity. They are more likely to be growing, which can impact the fetus's development. Growing adolescents have infants who weigh less than those of nongrowing adolescents and women 19 to 29 years of age (Scholl and Hediger 1993). Thus young adolescents (age 14 and under) need to gain more weight than older adolescents (18 years and older) to produce babies of equal size.

In determining the optimal weight gain for the pregnant adolescent, the nurse adds the recommended weight gain for an adult pregnancy to that expected during the postmenarcheal year in which the pregnancy occurs. If the teenager is underweight, additional weight gain is recommended to bring her to a normal weight for her height.

Specific Nutrient Concerns

Caloric needs of pregnant adolescents will vary widely. Major factors in determining calorie needs include whether growth has been completed and the physical activity level of the individual. Figures as high as 50 kcal/kg have been suggested for young, growing teens who are very active physically. A satisfactory weight gain will confirm adequacy of caloric intake in most cases.

Inadequate iron intake is a major concern with the adolescent diet. Iron needs are high for the pregnant teen due to the requirement for iron by the enlarging muscle mass and blood volume. Iron supplements—providing between 30 and 60 mg of elemental iron—are definitely indicated.

Calcium is another nutrient that demands special attention from pregnant adolescents. Inadequate intake of calcium is frequently a problem in this age group. To provide for these needs, an intake of 1200 mg/day of calcium is recommended to promote bone mineralization in the adolescent and support fetal skeletal growth. This is 400 mg/day more than the recommended amount for pregnant adults. An extra serving of dairy products is usually suggested for teenagers. Calcium supplementation is indicated for teens with an aversion to milk, unless other dairy products or significant calcium sources are consumed in sufficient quantities.

Because folic acid plays a role in cell reproduction, it is also an important nutrient for pregnant teens. As previously indicated, a supplement is usually suggested for all pregnant females, whether adult or teenager.

Other nutrients and vitamins must be considered when evaluating the overall nutritional quality of the teenager's diet. Nutrients that have frequently been found to be deficient in this age group include zinc and vitamins A, D, and B_6. Inclusion of a wide variety of foods—especially fresh and lightly processed foods—is helpful in obtaining adequate amounts of trace minerals, fiber, and other vitamins.

Dietary Patterns

Healthy adolescents often have irregular eating patterns. Many skip breakfast, and most tend to be frequent snackers. Teens rarely follow the traditional three-meals-a-day pattern. Their day-to-day intake often varies drastically, and they eat food combinations that may seem bizarre to adults. Despite this, adolescents usually achieve a better nutritional balance than most adults would expect.

In assessing the diet of the pregnant adolescent, the nurse should consider the eating pattern over time, not simply a single day's intake. Once the pattern is identified, counseling can be directed toward correcting deficiencies.

Eating Disorders

Two serious eating disorders, anorexia nervosa and bulimia nervosa, develop most commonly in adolescent girls and young women. For anorexia nervosa, the median age of onset is 16 to 17 years; for bulimia nervosa it is 18 years (Halmi et al 1994). Both conditions are psychologic disorders that can have a major impact on physiologic well-being.

Anorexia nervosa is an eating disorder characterized by an extreme fear of weight gain and fat. People with this problem have distorted body images and perceive themselves as fat even when they are extremely underweight. Their dietary intake is very restrictive in both variety and quantity. They may also engage in excessive exercise to prevent weight gain.

Individuals with anorexia nervosa do not often become pregnant because of the physiologic changes that affect their reproductive systems. If they do, they may suffer from hypokalemia, ketosis, and weight loss. In most cases the newborn's birth weight is severely depressed (Rosso 1990).

Bulimia is characterized by binging (secretly consuming large amounts of food in a short time) and purging. Self-induced vomiting is the most common method of purging; laxatives and/or diuretics may also be used. Individuals with bulimia nervosa often maintain normal or near normal weight for their height, so it is difficult to know whether binging and purging occur.

Women with bulimia do become pregnant. Their self-induced vomiting may produce many of the same complications as hyperemesis gravidarum.

In both anorexia nervosa and bulimia, a multidisciplinary approach to treatment is indicated involving medical, nursing, psychiatric, and dietetic practitioners. The pregnant adolescent or young woman with an eating disorder needs to be closely monitored and supported throughout her pregnancy.

Community-Based Nursing Care

Counseling about nutrition and healthy eating practices is an important element of care for pregnant teenagers that nurses can effectively provide in a community setting. This counseling may be individualized, involve other teens, or provide a combination of both approaches. Clinics and schools often offer classes and focused activities designed to address this topic.

The pregnant teenager will soon become a parent, and her understanding of nutrition will influence not only her well-being but also that of her child. However, teens tend to live in the present, and counseling that stresses long-term changes may be less effective than more concrete approaches. In many cases group classes are effective, especially those with other teens. In a group atmosphere, adolescents often work together to plan adequate meals including foods that are special favorites.

If the adolescent's mother does most of the meal preparation, it may be useful to include her in a discussion if the teen agrees. Involving the expectant father in counseling may also be beneficial. If the teen is remaining in school, cooperation can also be sought from the school cafeteria personnel.

Postpartum Nutrition

Nutritional needs will change following childbirth. Nutrient requirements will vary depending on whether the mother decides to breastfeed. An assessment of postpartal nutritional status is necessary before nutritional guidance is given.

Postpartal Nutritional Status

Determination of postpartal nutritional status is based primarily on the new mother's weight, hemoglobin and hematocrit levels, clinical signs, and dietary history. As mentioned previously, an ideal weight gain during pregnancy is 25–35 lb (11.5–16 kg). After birth there is a weight loss of approximately 10–12 lb. Additional weight loss is most rapid during the next few weeks as the body adjusts to the completion of pregnancy. The mother's weight will then begin to stabilize. This may take 6 months or longer.

The increased weight gain now recommended during pregnancy may have important implications for women postpartally unless they receive adequate counseling. Research indicates that women who gain between 25 and 35 lb while pregnant have a net gain of 3.5 lb (1.6 kg) 6 months after childbirth. Furthermore, multiparous women tend to lose less weight postpartally than primiparas; women who return to work outside the home tend to lose more weight than those who do not (Schauberger et al 1992). The mother's weight should be considered in terms of ideal weight, prepregnancy weight, and weight gain during pregnancy. Women who desire information about weight reduction can be referred to a dietitian.

Hemoglobin and erythrocyte levels should return to normal within 2 to 6 weeks. Hematocrit levels gradually rise due to hemoconcentration as extracellular fluid is excreted. Iron supplements are generally continued for 2 to 3 months following birth to replenish depleted stores.

The nurse assesses clinical symptoms the new mother may be experiencing. Constipation, in particular, is a common problem following birth. The nurse can encourage the woman to maintain a high fluid intake to keep the stool soft. Dietary sources of fiber, such as whole grains, fruits, and vegetables, are also helpful in preventing constipation.

The nurse obtains specific information on dietary intake and eating habits directly from the woman. Visiting the mother during mealtimes provides an opportunity for unobtrusive nutritional assessment. Which foods has the woman selected? Is her diet nutritionally sound? A comment focusing on a positive aspect of her meal selection may initiate a discussion of nutrition.

The nurse should inform the dietitian of any woman whose cultural or religious beliefs require specific foods so appropriate meals can be prepared for her. The nurse may also refer women with unusual eating habits or numerous questions about good nutrition to the dietitian. In all cases, the nurse should provide literature on nutrition so that the woman will have a source of appropriate information at home.

Nutritional Care of Nonnursing Mothers

After birth, the nonnursing mother's dietary requirements return to prepregnancy levels (see Table 11–1). If the mother has a good understanding of nutritional principles, it is sufficient to advise her to reduce her daily caloric intake by about 300 kcal and to return to prepregnancy levels for other nutrients.

If the mother has a poor understanding of nutrition, now is the time to teach her the basic principles and the importance of a well-balanced diet. Her eating habits and dietary practices will eventually be reflected in the diet of her child.

If the mother has gained excessive weight during pregnancy (or perhaps was overweight before pregnancy), a referral to the dietitian is appropriate. The dietitian can design weight-reduction diets to meet nutritional needs and food preferences. Weight loss goals of 1–2 lb per week are usually suggested.

In addition to meeting her own nutritional needs, the new mother will be interested in learning how to provide for her infant's nutritional needs. A discussion of infant feeding that includes topics such as selecting infant formulas, formula preparation, and vitamin and mineral supplementation is appropriate and generally well received.

Nutritional Care of Nursing Mothers

Nutrient needs are increased during breastfeeding. Table 11–1 lists the RDA during breastfeeding for specific nutrients. Table 11–2 provides a sample daily food guide for lactating women. It is especially important for the nursing mother to consume sufficient calories, because inadequate caloric intake can reduce milk volume. However, milk quality generally remains unaffected. The nursing mother should increase her calories by about 200 kcal over her pregnancy requirement, or 500 kcal over her prepregnancy requirement.

Because protein is an important ingredient in breast milk, an adequate intake while breastfeeding is essential. An intake of 65 g/day during the first 6 months of breastfeeding and 62 g/day during the second 6 months is recommended. As in pregnancy, it is important to consume adequate nonprotein calories to prevent the use of protein as an energy source.

Calcium is an important ingredient in milk production, and requirements remain the same as during pregnancy—an increase of 1200 mg/day. If the intake of calcium from food sources is not adequate, calcium supplements are recommended.

Because iron is not a principal mineral component of milk, the needs of lactating women are not substantially different from those of nonpregnant women. As previously mentioned, however, supplementation for 2 to 3 months after childbirth is advisable to replenish maternal stores depleted by pregnancy.

Liquids are especially important during lactation, since inadequate fluid intake may decrease milk volume. Fluid recommendations while breastfeeding are 8–10 (8 oz) glasses daily, including water, juice, milk, and soups.

In addition to counseling nursing mothers on how to meet their increased nutrient needs during breastfeeding, it is important to discuss a few issues related to infant feeding. For example, many mothers are concerned about how specific foods they eat will affect their babies during breastfeeding. Generally there are no foods the nursing mother must avoid except those to which she might be allergic. Occasionally, however, some nursing mothers find that their babies are affected by certain foods. Onions, turnips, cabbage, chocolate, spices, and seasonings are commonly listed as offenders. The best advice to give the nursing mother is to avoid those foods she suspects cause distress in her infant. For the most part, however, she should be able to eat any nourishing food she wants without fear that her baby will be affected. For further discussion of successful infant feeding see Chapter 24.

APPLYING THE NURSING PROCESS

Nursing Assessment

Assessment of nutritional status is necessary to plan an optimal diet with each woman. From the woman's chart and by interviewing her, the nurse gathers information about (a) the woman's height and weight, as well as her weight gain during pregnancy; (b) pertinent laboratory values, especially hemoglobin and hematocrit; (c) clinical signs that have possible nutritional implications, such as constipation, anorexia, or heartburn; and (d) dietary history to evaluate the woman's views on nutrition as well as her specific nutrient intake.

During the data-gathering process, the nurse has an opportunity to discuss important aspects of nutrition within the context of the family's needs and lifestyle. The nurse also seeks information about psychologic, cultural, and socioeconomic factors that may influence food intake.

The nurse can use a nutritional questionnaire to gather and record important facts. This information provides a database the nurse can use to develop an intervention plan to fit the woman's individual needs. The sample questionnaire shown in Figure 11–3 has been filled in to demonstrate this process.

Nursing Diagnosis

Once the data are obtained, the nurse begins to analyze the information, formulate appropriate nursing diagnoses, and develop client goals. For a woman during the first trimester, for example, the diagnosis may be "Altered nutrition: less than body requirements related to nausea and vomiting." The diagnosis may be related to excessive weight gain. In such cases the diagnosis might be "Altered nutrition: more than body requirements related to excessive intake of calories." Although these diagnoses are broad, the nurse must be specific in addressing issues such as inadequate intake of nutrients like iron, calcium, or folic acid; problems with nutrition because of a limited food budget; problems related to physiologic alterations like anorexia, heartburn, or nausea; and behavioral problems related to excessive dieting, binge eating, and so on. In some instances, the category "knowledge deficit" may seem most appropriate.

Nursing Plan and Implementation

After the nursing diagnosis is made, the nurse can plan an approach to correct any nutritional deficiencies or improve the overall quality of the diet. To be truly effective, this plan must be made in cooperation with the woman. The following example demonstrates ways in which the nurse can plan with the woman based on the nursing diagnosis.

CRITICAL THINKING IN ACTION

Jane is 14 weeks pregnant. The rate and total amount of her weight gain during the first trimester have been consistent with recommendations. She has gained an average of 0.5 kg (1 lb) per week during both of the past 2 weeks. Her appetite is good, and she consumes three meals per day and snacks between meals on occasion.

Jane has altered her diet because she is concerned about her weight gain becoming excessive. She told the nurse that she has decreased her intake from the bread and dairy groups in order to limit her calorie intake. Since she has omitted most dairy products, she has increased her consumption of salads and broccoli to provide sources of calcium.

A diet history revealed the following:

Grain	3–4 servings, mainly cereal and rice
Fruit	2–4 servings, fresh fruit
Vegetables	3–5 servings, salads, peas, corn, broccoli
Meat	4–5 servings, beef, pork, chicken
Dairy	occasionally cheese, ice cream, pudding
Fats, oils, sweets	occasionally salad dressings, margarine, desserts
Beverages	8–10 servings, soda, juices, water

After assessing her diet history, what is your evaluation of Jane's diet? How could you counsel her?

Answers can be found in Appendix H.

Diagnosis: Altered nutrition: less than body requirements related to low intake of calcium.

Goal: The woman will increase her daily intake of calcium to the minimum RDA levels.

Implementation:

1. Plan with the woman additional milk or dairy products that can reasonably be added to the diet (specify amounts).
2. Encourage the use of other calcium sources such as leafy greens and legumes.
3. Plan for the addition of powdered milk in cooking and baking.
4. If none of the above are realistic or acceptable, consider the use of calcium supplements.

Most families can benefit from guidance about food purchasing and preparation. Women should be advised to plan food purchases thoughtfully by preparing general menus and a list before shopping. It is also helpful to advise clients to monitor sales, compare brands, and be cautious when purchasing "convenience" foods, which tend to be expensive. Other techniques for keeping food costs down without jeopardizing quality include buying food in season, using bulk foods when appropriate, using whole-grain or enriched products,

FIGURE 11–3 Sample nutritional questionnaire used in nursing management of a pregnant woman.

NUTRITIONAL QUESTIONNAIRE

Name Susan Longmont   Date 1-4-98

Age 20

Ethnic group Caucasian

Religion Protestant

Gravida $\dot{\bar{\text{I}}}$ Para $\dot{\bar{0}}$ EDB 8-10-98

Age of youngest child? NA

Birth weights of previous children? NA

Usual nonpregnant weight 115   Present weight 125

Weight gain during last pregnancy? NA

Vitamin supplements? none

Current medications? aspirin for headache

Do you smoke? yes   How much per day? 1-1½ packs

Eating patterns:

1. How many meals per day? 2 when 12:30 pm 6:30 pm
2. How many snacks per day? 3 when 10:30 am 4:00 pm 10:00 pm
3. What other foods are important to your usual diet? chocolate and candy bars
4. Amount per day 4 bars/week
5. Do you have any different food preferences now? no
6. Do you eat nonfoods such as:

		Amount
laundry starch	no	NA
ice	yes	10 cubes/day
other (name)	no	NA

7. What foods do you dislike or do not eat? spinach and dried beans
8. For added information complete a typical daily intake (24 hour recall is suggested).

Do you have special problems in food preparation such as:

1. Physical disability yes ___ no ✓ Explain ___
2. Cooking appliances yes ___ no ✓ Explain ___
3. Refrigeration of food yes ___ no ✓ Explain ___

Who does the meal planning? I do.   shopping? We both do.

cooking? I do most of the time but my husband likes to help.

Are there transportation problems? We have only one car but we go in the evening.

Financial situation: My husband is working and going to school. I am not working.   Foodstamps yes   w/c no

Do you have any previous nutritional problems? No. I have never paid much attention to food before, but now I have lots of questions.

Are there any problems with this pregnancy? Nausea Yes, in the morning.

Constipation No   Other NA

Assessment by the nurse following the completion of the questionnaire.

Basic estimated nutrient and caloric value of typical daily intake.

Please circle one of the following:

Protein intake was	low	(adequate)	high
Caloric intake was	low	adequate	(high)
Calcium intake was	(low)	adequate	high
Iron intake was	(low)	adequate	high
Vitamin C intake was	low	(adequate)	high

buying lower-grade eggs (grading has no relation to the egg's nutritional value but indicates color of the shell, delicacy of flavor, etc), and avoiding fancy grades of food and foods in elaborate packaging.

Community-Based Nursing Care

Food is a significant portion of a family's budget, and meeting nutritional needs may be a challenge for families on limited incomes. Community-based services offered through clinics, local agencies, schools, and volunteer organizations are effective in addressing these needs. Increasingly nurses play an important role in managing such community-based services, especially those services focusing on client education. In addition, most communities offer special assistance to qualifying families to meet their nutritional needs. The Food Stamp Program provides stamps or coupons for participating households whose net monthly income is below a specified level. These stamps can be used to purchase food for the household each month.

The Special Supplemental Food Program for Women, Infants, and Children (WIC) is designed to provide nutritious food for pregnant or breastfeeding women with low incomes and for their children under age 5. The program provides food assistance, nutrition education, and referrals to health care providers. The food distributed, including eggs, cheese, milk, fortified cereals, juice, and infant formula, is designed to provide good sources of iron, protein, and certain vitamins for individuals with an inadequate diet. The WIC program is credited with helping reduce the incidence of low birth weight in infants and in decreasing the incidence of anemia in the infants and young children of low-income families (General Accounting Office 1992).

Evaluation

Once a plan has been developed and implemented, the nurse and client may wish to identify ways of evaluating its effectiveness. Evaluation may involve keeping a food journal, writing out weekly menus, returning for weekly weigh-ins, and the like. If anemia is a special problem, periodic hematocrit assessments are also indicated. Key Facts to Remember: Prenatal Nutrition summarizes key points that the pregnant woman should thoroughly understand.

Women with serious nutritional deficiencies are referred to a dietitian. The nurse can then work closely with the dietitian and the client to improve the pregnant woman's health by modification of her diet.

KEY FACTS TO REMEMBER

Prenatal Nutrition

- The pregnant woman should eat regularly, three meals a day, and snack on fruits, cheese, milk, or other nutritious foods between meals if desired.
- More frequent but smaller meals are also recommended.
- The woman should diet *only* under the guidance of her primary health care provider.
- Water is an essential nutrient. The woman should drink 4–6 (8 oz) glasses of water and a total of 8–10 glasses of fluid daily.
- If the diet is adequate, iron is the only supplement necessary during pregnancy.
- A multivitamin supplement is indicated for women with a poor diet and for those at high nutritional risk.
- To avoid possible deficiencies, many caregivers also recommend a daily vitamin supplement.
- Taking megadoses of vitamins during pregnancy is unnecessary and potentially dangerous.

CHAPTER HIGHLIGHTS

- Maternal weight gains averaging 25–35 lb (11.5–16 kg) for a normal-weight woman are associated with the best reproductive outcomes.
- If the diet is adequate, folic acid and iron are the only supplements generally recommended during pregnancy.
- Women should not undertake caloric restriction to reduce weight during pregnancy.
- Pregnant women should be encouraged to eat regularly and to eat a wide variety of foods, especially fresh and lightly processed foods.
- Taking megadoses of vitamins during pregnancy is unnecessary and potentially dangerous.
- In vegetarian diets, special emphasis should be placed on obtaining ample proteins, calories, calcium, iron, vitamin D, vitamin B_{12}, and zinc through food sources, or supplementation if necessary.
- Evaluation of physical, psychosocial, and cultural factors that affect food intake is essential before the nurse can determine nutritional status and plan nutritional counseling.
- Adolescents who become pregnant less than 4 years after menarche have higher nutritional needs and are considered to be at high biologic risk.

- Weight gains during adolescent pregnancy must accommodate recommended gains for a normal pregnancy plus necessary gains due to growth.
- After giving birth, the nonnursing mother's dietary requirements return to prepregnancy levels.
- Nursing mothers require an adequate calorie and fluid intake to maintain ample milk volume.

REFERENCES

American Dietetic Association: Position of the American Dietetic Association: Nutrition management of adolescent pregnancy. *J Am Diet Assoc* January 1989; 89:104.

Boyle JS, Andrews MM: *Transcultural Concepts in Nursing Care.* Glenview IL: Scott, Foresman/Little, Brown, 1989.

General Accounting Office: *Early Intervention: Federal Investments Like WIC Can Produce Savings.* Document HRD 92-18. Washington DC, May 1992.

Halmi KA et al: Recognizing and treating eating disorders. *Contemp OB/GYN* June 15, 1994;39S:28.

Institute of Medicine, Subcommittee for a Clinical Application Guide. *Nutrition During Pregnancy and Lactation: An Implementation Guide.* Washington DC, National Academy Press, 1992.

Institute of Medicine, National Academy of Sciences, Food and Nutrition Board: *Nutrition during Pregnancy.* Part 1: Weight gain. Washington, DC: National Academy Press, 1990.

Luke B, Keith L: *Principles and Practice of Maternal Nutrition.* Park Ridge NJ: Parthenon, 1992.

National Research Council: *Recommended Dietary Allowances,* 10th ed. Washington, DC: National Academy Press, 1989.

Niebyl JR: Folic acid supplementation to prevent birth defects. *Contemp OB/GYN* June 1995; 40(6):43.

Rairdan B, Higgs ZR: When your patient is a Hmong refugee. *AJN* March 1992; 92(3):52.

Rayburn WF et al: Periconceptional folate intake and neural tube defects. *J Am Coll Nutr* 1996; 15(2):121.

Rosso P: *Nutrition and Metabolism in Pregnancy.* New York: Oxford University Press, 1990.

Schauberger CW et al: Factors that influence weight loss in the puerperium. *Obstet Gynecol* March 1992; 79(3):424.

Scholl TO, Hediger ML: A review of the epidemiology of nutrition and adolescent pregnancy: Maternal growth during pregnancy and its effect on the fetus. *J Am Coll Nutr* 1993; 12:101.

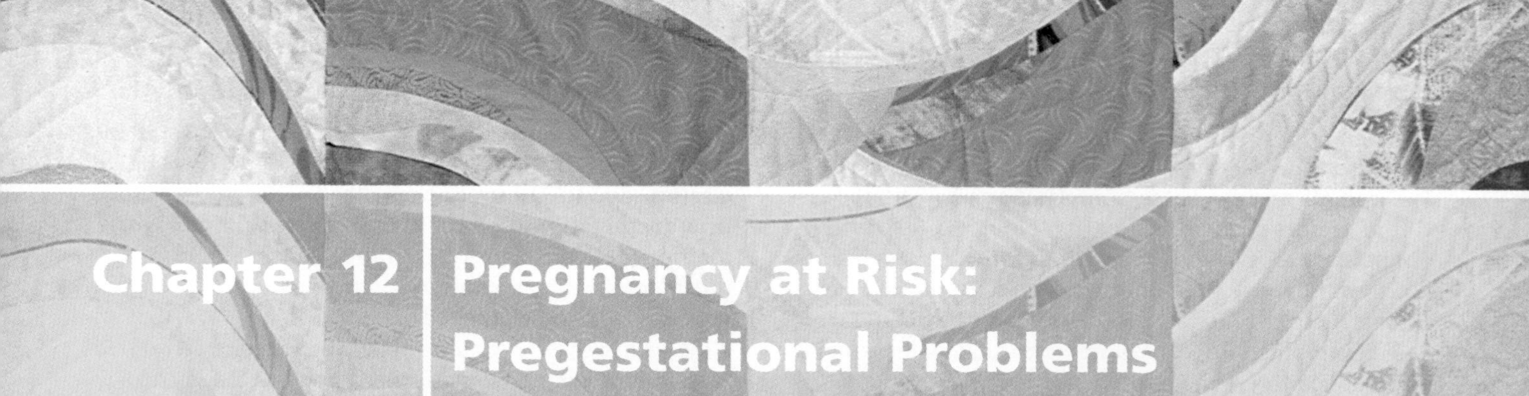

Chapter 12 Pregnancy at Risk: Pregestational Problems

OBJECTIVES

- Describe the effects of various heart disorders on pregnancy, including their implications for nursing care.
- Relate the pathology and medical treatment of diabetes mellitus in pregnancy to the implications for nursing care.
- Discriminate among the types of anemia associated with pregnancy regarding signs, treatment, and implications for pregnancy.
- Discuss acquired immunodeficiency syndrome (AIDS), including care of the pregnant woman who is HIV positive, fetal implications, and ramifications for the childbearing family.
- Summarize the effects of alcohol and illicit drugs on the childbearing woman and her fetus/newborn.
- Delineate the effects of selected pregestational medical conditions on pregnancy.

KEY TERMS

Acquired immunodeficiency syndrome (AIDS)
Crack
Gestational diabetes mellitus
Macrosomia

For some women, pregnancy may become a life-threatening event because of potential or existing complications. These complications can be the result of factors such as age, parity, blood type, socioeconomic status, psychologic health, or preexisting chronic illnesses. Effective prenatal care is directed toward identifying factors that increase a pregnant woman's risk and developing supportive therapies that will promote optimal health for the mother and her fetus.

This chapter focuses on women with pregestational medical disorders and the possible effects of these disorders on the pregnancy.

Care of the Woman with Heart Disease

Pregnancy results in increased cardiac output, heart rate, and blood volume. The normal heart is able to adapt to these changes without undue difficulty. The woman with heart disease, however, has decreased cardiac reserve, making it more difficult for her heart to accommodate the higher work load of pregnancy.

Approximately 1 percent of pregnant women are at risk because of preexisting heart disease (Landon 1996). The pathology found in a pregnant woman with heart disease varies with the type of disorder. The more common conditions are discussed briefly here.

Congenital heart defects now constitute at least half of all cases of heart disease encountered during pregnancy (Cunningham et al 1997). Congenital heart defects most commonly seen in pregnant women include atrial septal defect, ventricular septal defect, patent ductus arteriosus, coarctation of the aorta, and tetralogy of Fallot.

For women with congenital heart disease, the implications of pregnancy depend on the specific defect. If the heart defect has been surgically repaired and no evidence of organic heart disease remains, pregnancy may be undertaken with confidence. In such cases, antibiotic prophylaxis is recommended to prevent subacute bacterial endocarditis at the time of birth. Women with congenital heart disease who experience cyanosis should be counseled to avoid pregnancy because the risk to mother and fetus is high.

Rheumatic fever, which may develop in untreated streptococcal infections, is an inflammatory connective tissue disease that can involve the heart, joints, central nervous system, skin, and subcutaneous tissue. Once it occurs, rheumatic fever can recur; it is serious primarily because of the permanent damage it can do to the heart—rheumatic heart disease.

Rheumatic heart disease results when recurrent inflammation from bouts of rheumatic fever causes scar-tissue formation on the valves. The scarring results in stenosis (failure of the valve to open completely), regurgitation due to failure of the valve to close completely, or a combination of both, thereby increasing the workload of the heart. Although mitral valve stenosis is the most commonly seen lesion, the aortic or tricuspid valves may also be affected.

The increased blood volume of pregnancy, coupled with the pregnant woman's need for increased cardiac output, stresses the heart of a woman with mitral stenosis and increases her risk of developing congestive heart failure. Even the woman who has no symptoms at the onset of her pregnancy is at risk.

Rheumatic heart disease has declined rapidly in the last four decades, primarily because of prompt identification of pharyngeal infections caused by group A beta-hemolytic streptococcus and the availability of antibiotics for treatment.

Mitral valve prolapse (MVP) is usually an asymptomatic condition that is found in about 12 percent of women of childbearing age (Landon 1996). The condition is more common in women than in men and seems to run in families. In MVP, the mitral valve leaflets tend to prolapse into the left atrium during ventricular systole because the chordae tendineae that support them are long, stretched, and thin. As a result, some mitral regurgitation may occur.

Women with MVP usually tolerate pregnancy well. Most women require assurance that they can continue with normal activities. A few women experience symptoms—primarily palpitations, chest pain, and dyspnea—which are often due to arrhythmias. They are usually treated with propranolol hydrochloride (Inderal). Limiting caffeine intake also helps decrease palpitations. Antibiotics are given prophylactically at the time of birth to prevent bacterial endocarditis.

Peripartum cardiomyopathy is a dysfunction of the left ventricle that occurs in the last month of pregnancy or the first 5 months postpartum in a woman with no previous history of heart disease. The symptoms are similar to those in congestive heart failure: dyspnea, orthopnea, chest pain, palpitations, weakness, and edema. The cause is unknown. Treatment includes digitalis, diuretics, anticoagulants, and bed rest. The condition may resolve with bed rest as the heart gradually returns to normal size. Subsequent pregnancy is strongly discouraged because the disease tends to recur during pregnancy.

Medical Therapy

The primary goal of medical therapy is early diagnosis and ongoing management of the woman with cardiac disease. Echocardiogram, chest x-ray, auscultation of heart sounds, and sometimes cardiac catheterization are essential for establishing the type and severity of the heart disease. The severity of the disease can also be determined by the individual's ability to perform ordinary physical activity. The following classification of functional capacity has been standardized by the Criteria Committee of the New York Heart Association (1979):

- *Class I.* Asymptomatic. No limitation of physical activity.
- *Class II.* Slight limitation of physical activity. Asymptomatic at rest; symptoms occur with heavy physical activity.
- *Class III.* Moderate to marked limitation of physical activity. Symptomatic during less-than-ordinary physical activity.
- *Class IV.* Inability to carry on any physical activity without discomfort. Even at rest the person experiences symptoms of cardiac insufficiency or anginal pain.

Women in classes I and II usually experience a normal pregnancy and have few complications, whereas those in classes III and IV are at risk for more severe complications. Because anemia increases the work of the heart, it should be diagnosed early and treated if present. Infections, even if minor, also increase cardiac workload and should be treated.

Drug Therapy

The pregnant woman with heart disease may need drug therapy in addition to the iron and vitamin supplements ordinarily prescribed to maintain health during pregnancy. Antibiotics, usually penicillin if not contraindicated by allergy, are used during pregnancy to prevent recurrent bouts of rheumatic fever and subsequent heart valve damage. Antibiotics are also recommended during labor and the early postpartum period to prevent bacterial endocarditis in women with either acquired or congenital disease. If the woman develops coagulation problems, the anticoagulant heparin may be used. Heparin offers the greatest safety to the fetus because it does not cross the placenta. The thiazide diuretics and furosemide (Lasix) may be used to treat congestive heart failure if it develops. Digitalis glycosides and common antiarrhythmic drugs may be used to treat cardiac failure and arrhythmias. These agents do cross the placenta but have no reported teratogenic effect.

Medical Interventions During Labor

Spontaneous natural labor with adequate pain relief is usually recommended for women in classes I and II. Those in classes III and IV may have labor induced and may need to be hospitalized before the onset of labor for cardiac stabilization. They also require invasive cardiac monitoring during labor via a pulmonary artery (Swan-Ganz) catheter or central venous pressure catheter.

Medical Interventions During Birth

Use of low forceps provides the safest method of birth, with lumbar epidural anesthesia to reduce the stress of pushing. Cesarean birth is used only if fetal or maternal indications exist, not on the basis of heart disease alone.

APPLYING THE NURSING PROCESS

Nursing Assessment

The stress of pregnancy on the functional capacity of the heart is assessed during every antepartal visit. The nurse notes the category of functional capacity assigned to the woman, takes the woman's pulse, respirations, and blood pressure, and compares them to the normal values expected during pregnancy. The nurse then determines the woman's activity level, including rest, and any changes in the pulse and respirations that have occurred since previous visits. Because it is also an early sign of decompensation, the nurse should ask the woman about any increased fatigue with activity. The nurse also identifies and evaluates other factors that would increase strain on the heart. These might include anemia, infection, anxiety, lack of a support system, and household and career demands.

The following symptoms, if they are progressive, are indicative of congestive heart failure:

- Cough (frequent, with or without blood-stained sputum [hemoptysis])
- Dyspnea (progressive, upon exertion)
- Edema (progressive, generalized, including extremities, face, eyelids)
- Heart murmurs (heard on auscultation)
- Palpitations
- Rales (auscultated in lung bases)
- Weight gain (related to fluid retention)

This cycle is progressive because some of these same behaviors are seen to a minor degree in a pregnancy without cardiac problems.

Nursing Diagnosis

Nursing diagnoses that might apply to the pregnant woman with heart disease include the following:

- Decreased cardiac output: easy fatigability
- Impaired gas exchange related to pulmonary edema secondary to cardiac decompensation
- Fear related to the effects of the maternal cardiac condition on fetal well-being

Nursing Plan and Implementation

Nursing care is directed toward maintaining a balance between cardiac reserve and cardiac workload.

Antepartal Nursing Care

Nursing actions are designed to meet the physiologic and psychosocial needs of the pregnant woman with heart disease. The priority of nursing action varies based on the severity of the disease process and the individual needs of the woman determined by the nursing assessment.

The woman and her family should thoroughly understand her condition and its management and should recognize signs of potential complications. This will increase their understanding and decrease anxiety. When the nurse provides thorough explanations, uses printed material, and provides frequent opportunities to ask questions and discuss concerns, the woman is better able to meet her own health care needs and seek assistance appropriately.

As part of health teaching, the nurse explains the purposes of the dietary and activity changes that are required. A diet is instituted that is high in iron, protein, and essential nutrients but low in sodium, with adequate calories to ensure normal weight gain. Such a diet best meets the nutrition needs of the client with cardiac disease. To help preserve her cardiac reserves, the woman may need to restrict her activities. In addition, 8–10 hours of sleep, with frequent daily rest periods, is essential. Because upper respiratory infections may tax the heart and lead to decompensation, the woman must avoid contact with sources of infection.

During the first half of pregnancy, the woman is seen approximately every 2 weeks to assess cardiac status. During the second half of pregnancy, the woman is seen weekly. These assessments are especially important between weeks 28 and 30 when the blood volume reaches its maximum. If symptoms of cardiac decompensation occur, prompt medical intervention is indicated to correct the cardiac problem.

Intrapartal Nursing Care

Labor and birth exert tremendous stress on the woman and her fetus. This stress could be fatal to the fetus of a woman with cardiac disease, because the fetus may be receiving a decreased oxygen and blood supply. Thus the intrapartal care of a woman with cardiac disease is aimed at reducing physical exertion and accompanying fatigue.

The nurse evaluates maternal vital signs frequently to determine the woman's response to labor. A pulse rate greater than 100 beats/min or respirations greater than 25/min may indicate the onset of cardiac decompensation and require further evaluation. The nurse also auscultates the woman's lungs frequently for evidence of rales and carefully observes for other signs of developing decompensation.

To ensure cardiac emptying and adequate oxygenation, the nurse encourages the laboring woman to assume either a semi-Fowler's or side-lying position with her head and shoulders elevated. Oxygen by mask, diuretics to reduce fluid retention, sedatives and analgesics, prophylactic antibiotics, and digitalis may also be used as indicated by the woman's status.

The nurse remains with the woman to support her. It is essential that the nurse keep the woman and her family informed of labor progress and management plans, collaborating with them to fulfill their wishes for the birth experience as much as possible. The nurse needs to maintain an atmosphere of calm to lessen the anxiety of the woman and her family.

Continuous electronic fetal monitoring is used to provide ongoing assessment of the fetal response to labor. To prevent overexertion and the accompanying fatigue, the nurse encourages the woman to sleep and relax between contractions and provides her with emotional support and encouragement. Epidural anesthesia is often used to decrease exertion. During pushing, the nurse encourages the woman to use shorter, more moderate open-glottis pushing, with complete relaxation between pushes. Forceps or vacuum extraction may be used if pushing is too difficult. Vital signs are monitored closely during the second stage.

Postpartal Nursing Care

The postpartal period is a most significant time for the woman with cardiac disease. As extravascular fluid returns to the bloodstream for excretion, cardiac output and blood volume increase. This physiologic adaptation places great strain on the heart and may lead to decompensation, especially in the first 48 hours after birth.

So that the health team can detect any possible problems, the woman remains in the hospital for approximately a week to rest and recover. Her vital signs are monitored frequently and she is assessed for signs of decompensation. She stays in the semi-Fowler's or side-lying position, with her head and shoulders elevated, and begins a gradual, progressive activity program. Appropriate diet and stool softeners facilitate bowel movement without undue strain.

The postpartum nurse gives the woman opportunities to discuss her birth experience and helps her deal with any feelings or concerns that distress her. The nurse also encourages maternal-infant attachment by providing frequent opportunities for the mother to interact with her child.

No evidence exists that breastfeeding compromises cardiac output. Thus the only concern about breastfeeding for women with cardiovascular disease is related to medications the mother may be taking (Lawrence 1989). These should be evaluated for the likelihood of

COMMUNITY IN FOCUS Gestational Diabetes Program

The Memorial HealthCare System (MHCS) is a ten-hospital, community-based, not-for-profit, integrated health care system located in Houston, Texas. A large system, each year MHCS has about 12,000 births; it also serves approximately 400 women with gestational diabetes mellitus. To address the special health care needs of women with gestational diabetes, the system established the Gestational Diabetes Program, which is managed totally by diabetes nurse educators.

Pregnant women with gestational diabetes are referred directly to the program by their caregiver. Each woman is seen individually by a diabetes nurse educator for assessment and one-on-one education. The educational services provided include blood sugar testing, use of the glucometer, documentation of blood sugars, pathophysiology of diabetes in pregnancy, pharmacology of insulin, administration of insulin, signs and symptoms of hypo- and hyperglycemia, danger signs of pregnancy, fetal assessment, and explanation of the medical and nursing care of women with gestational diabetes. The diabetes nurse educators coordinate services with the dietitians, who perform nutritional assessments and dietary planning and counseling. Educational protocols are standardized throughout the system. In addition, group classes are offered on selected topics.

Diabetes educators also provide 24-hour on-call services so that a knowledgeable educator is always available to answer questions or address concerns. During the postpartum period, a diabetes nurse educator visits each woman with gestational diabetes in the hospital and continues to work with her until her blood glucose levels are normalized and she no longer requires insulin therapy.

The multidisciplinary team members involved in the care of women with gestational diabetes mellitus include diabetes nurse educators, dietitians, physicians and their staff, home health nurses, social workers, pharmacists, perinatologists, neonatologists, ultrasonographers, and chaplains. The Gestational Diabetes Program was recently credentialed by the American Diabetic Association. Evaluation data to date reveal overwhelmingly positive maternal and fetal outcomes for women who participate in the program.

Source: Personal communication with Vicki Lucas, PhD, RNC, Director of Women's and Children's Services, Memorial HealthCare System, Houston, Texas.

passing into the milk or affecting lactation. The nurse can assist the breastfeeding mother to a comfortable side-lying position with her head moderately elevated or to a semi-Fowler's position. To conserve the mother's energy, the nurse should position the newborn at the breast and be available to burp the baby and reposition him or her at the other breast.

In addition to providing the normal postpartum discharge teaching, the nurse should ensure that the woman and her family understand the signs of possible problems from her heart disease or other postpartal complications. The nurse also plans an activity schedule with the woman and her family. Visiting nurse referrals may be necessary, depending on the woman's health status.

Evaluation

Anticipated outcomes of nursing care include

- The woman is able to discuss her condition and its possible impact on pregnancy, labor and birth, and the postpartal period.
- The woman participates in developing an appropriate health care regimen and follows it throughout her pregnancy.
- The woman gives birth to a healthy infant.
- The woman avoids congestive heart failure, thromboembolism, and infection.
- The woman is able to identify signs and symptoms of possible postpartum complications.
- The woman is able to care effectively for her newborn infant.

Care of the Woman with Diabetes Mellitus

Diabetes mellitus, an endocrine disorder of carbohydrate metabolism resulting from inadequate production or use of insulin, occurs in about 4 percent of all pregnancies (Gabbe 1996). Insulin, produced by the β cells of the islets of Langerhans in the pancreas, lowers blood glucose levels by enabling glucose to move from the blood into muscle and adipose tissue cells.

Carbohydrate Metabolism in Normal Pregnancy

In early pregnancy the rise in serum levels of estrogen, progesterone, and other hormones stimulates increased insulin production by the maternal pancreas, and increased tissue response to insulin. Thus an anabolic (building up) state exists during the first half of pregnancy, with storage of glycogen in the liver and other tissues.

In the second half of pregnancy, placental secretion of human placental lactogen (hPL) and prolactin (from the decidua), as well as elevated cortisol and glycogen, cause increased resistance to insulin and decreased glucose tolerance. This decreased effectiveness of insulin results in a catabolic (destructive) state during fasting periods, such as during the night or after meal absorption. Fat is metabolized more readily at these times, and ketones may be present in the urine.

The delicate system of checks and balances that exists between glucose production and glucose use is stressed by the growing fetus, who derives energy from

TABLE 12–1 Classification of Diabetes Mellitus (DM) and Other Categories of Glucose Intolerance

Diabetes mellitus
- Type I, insulin-dependent (IDDM)
- Type II, noninsulin-dependent (NIDDM)
  - Nonobese NIDDM
  - Obese NIDDM
- Secondary diabetes

Impaired glucose tolerance (IGT)

Gestational diabetes mellitus (GDM)

Source: National Diabetes Data Group of National Institutes of Health, *Diabetes* 1979; 28:1039. Adapted with permission from the American Diabetes Association Inc.

glucose taken solely from maternal stores. This stress is known as the diabetogenic effect of pregnancy. Thus any preexisting disruption in carbohydrate metabolism is augmented by pregnancy, and any diabetic potential may precipitate gestational diabetes mellitus.

Pathophysiology of Diabetes Mellitus

In diabetes mellitus, the pancreas does not produce enough insulin to allow necessary carbohydrate metabolism. Without adequate insulin, glucose does not enter the cells and they become energy depleted. Blood glucose levels remain high (hyperglycemia), and the cells break down their stores of fats and protein for energy. Protein breakdown results in a negative nitrogen balance; fat metabolism causes ketosis.

These pathologic developments cause the four cardinal signs and symptoms of diabetes mellitus: polyuria, polydipsia, polyphagia, and weight loss. Polyuria (frequent urination) results because water is not reabsorbed by the renal tubules due to the osmotic activity of glucose. Polydipsia (excessive thirst) is caused by dehydration from polyuria. Polyphagia (excessive hunger) is caused by tissue loss and a state of starvation, which results from the inability of the cells to use the blood glucose. Weight loss (seen in insulin-dependent diabetes mellitus [IDDM], also called type I diabetes) is due to the use of fat and muscle tissue for energy.

Classification

States of altered carbohydrate metabolism have been classified in several ways. Table 12–1 shows the currently accepted classification, a result of the 1979 report of a special committee of the National Institutes of Health (National Diabetes Data Group 1979). This classification contains three main categories: diabetes mellitus (DM), impaired glucose tolerance (IGT), and gestational diabetes mellitus (GDM).

TABLE 12–2 White's Classification of Diabetes in Pregnancy

Class	Criterion
A	Chemical diabetes
B	Maturity onset (age over 20 years), duration under 10 years, no vascular lesions
C_1	Age 10 to 19 years at onset
C_2	10 to 19 years' duration
D_1	Under 10 years at onset
D_2	Over 20 years' duration
D_3	Benign retinopathy
D_4	Calcified vessels of legs
D_5	Hypertension
E	No longer sought
F	Nephropathy
G	Many failures
H	Cardiopathy
R	Proliferating retinopathy
T	Renal transplant (added by Tagatz and colleagues of the University of Minnesota)

Source: White P: Classification of obstetric diabetes. *Am J Obstet Gynecol* 1978; 130:228. Used with permission.

Gestational diabetes mellitus is diabetes mellitus that has its onset or is first diagnosed during pregnancy. Except for showing an impaired tolerance to glucose, the woman may remain asymptomatic or may have a mild form of the disease. Diagnosis of GDM is very important, however, because even mild diabetes causes increased risk for perinatal morbidity and mortality.

Table 12–2 shows White's classification of diabetes in pregnancy. This classification is useful for describing the extent of the disease.

Influence of Pregnancy on Diabetes

Pregnancy can affect diabetes significantly because the physiologic changes of pregnancy can drastically alter insulin requirements. In addition, pregnancy may alter the progress of vascular disease secondary to diabetes. Pregnancy can affect diabetes in the following ways:

1. Diabetic control
   a. Change in insulin requirements
      (1) Frequently, the need for insulin decreases during the first trimester. Levels of hPL, an insulin antagonist, are low, and the woman and developing fetus use more glycogen and glucose.
      (2) Nausea and vomiting may cause dietary fluctuations and increase the risk of hypoglycemia or insulin shock.

(3) Insulin requirements begin to rise in the second trimester and may double or quadruple by the end of pregnancy as a result of placental maturation and hPL production.

(4) Increased energy needs during labor may require increased insulin to balance intravenous glucose.

(5) Usually an abrupt decrease in insulin requirement occurs after the passage of the placenta and the resulting loss of hPL in maternal circulation.

b. Decreased renal threshold for glucose

c. Increased risk of ketoacidosis, insulin shock, and coma

2. Possible accelerations of vascular disease

   a. Hypertension: increase in blood pressure of greater than 30 mm Hg systolic and 15 mm Hg diastolic

   b. Nephropathy: renal impairment

   c. Retinopathy

ESSENTIAL PRECAUTIONS FOR PRACTICE

A Pregnant Woman with Diabetes Mellitus

In caring for a pregnant woman with diabetes mellitus, all the precautions apply that are established for any hospitalized pregnant, laboring, or postpartal woman. In addition, remember the following specifics:

- Gloves should be worn when doing finger-sticks for glucose levels, when starting IVs, when testing urine for ketones, or when drawing blood for other laboratory tests.
- When teaching a woman to do her own blood glucose testing, gloves should be available and put on if it becomes necessary for the nurse to help the woman obtain a blood sample. The woman does not need to wear gloves during the procedure.
- Needles, syringes, lancets, and other sharp objects should be disposed of in appropriately labeled containers.

REMEMBER to wash your hands prior to putting the disposable gloves on and AGAIN immediately after you remove the gloves.

For further information consult OSHA and CDC guidelines.

Influence of Diabetes on Pregnancy Outcome

The pregnancy of a woman who has diabetes carries a higher risk of complications, especially perinatal mortality. This risk has been reduced by the recent recognition of the importance of tight metabolic control (glucose between 70 mg/dL and 120 mg/dL). New techniques for monitoring blood glucose, delivering insulin, and monitoring the fetus have also reduced perinatal mortality.

Maternal Risks

The prognosis for the pregnant woman with gestational, type I, or type II diabetes (see Table 12–1) without significant vascular damage is positive. However, diabetic pregnancy still carries a higher risk of complications than normal pregnancy.

Hydramnios, or an increase in the volume of amniotic fluid, occurs in 10 to 20 percent of pregnant diabetic women. The exact mechanism causing the increase is unknown, although it is thought to be a result of excessive fetal urination because of fetal hyperglycemia (Mandeville 1992). Premature rupture of membranes and onset of labor may occasionally be a problem with hydramnios.

Pregnancy-induced hypertension (PIH) occurs more often in diabetic pregnancies, especially when diabetes-related vascular changes already exist.

Hyperglycemia can lead to ketoacidosis as a result of the increase in ketone bodies (which are acidic) released in the blood from the metabolism of fatty acids. Decreased gastric motility and the contrainsulin effects of hPL also predispose the woman to ketoacidosis. Ketoacidosis usually develops slowly but, if untreated, it can lead to coma and death for mother and fetus.

Fetal-Neonatal Risks

It is now clear that many of the problems of the neonate result directly from high maternal plasma glucose levels. In the presence of untreated maternal ketoacidosis, the risk of fetal death increases to 50 percent (Spellacy 1994). Fetal enzyme systems cease functioning in an acidic environment.

The incidence of congenital anomalies in diabetic pregnancies is 6 to 10 percent and is the major cause of death for infants of diabetic mothers. Research suggests that this increased incidence of congenital anomalies is related to high glucose levels in early pregnancy (before week 7 of gestation) (Reece et al 1995). Most anomalies involve the heart, central nervous system, and skeletal system. One anomaly, sacral agenesis, appears almost exclusively in infants of diabetic mothers. In sacral agenesis, the sacrum and lumbar spine fail to develop and the lower extremities develop incompletely. To reduce the incidence of congenital anomalies, preconception counseling and strict diabetes control before conception are indicated.

Characteristically, infants of type I diabetic mothers (or classes A, B, and C, see Table 12–2) are large for gestational age (LGA) as a result of the high maternal levels of blood glucose, from which the fetus derives its glucose. These elevated levels continually stimulate the fetal islets of Langerhans to produce insulin. This hyperinsulin state causes the fetus to use the available glucose.

This leads to excessive growth (known as **macrosomia**) and fat deposits. If born vaginally, the macrosomic infant is at increased risk for shoulder dystocia, traumatic birth injuries, and asphyxia (Landon 1996).

After birth the umbilical cord is severed and the generous maternal blood glucose supply eliminated. However, continued islet cell hyperactivity leads to excessive insulin levels and depleted blood glucose (hypoglycemia) in 2 to 4 hours. Macrosomia can be significantly reduced by tight maternal blood glucose control.

Infants of mothers with advanced diabetes (vascular involvement) may demonstrate intrauterine growth retardation (IUGR). This occurs because vascular changes in the diabetic woman decrease the efficiency of placental perfusion and the fetus is not as well sustained in utero.

Respiratory distress syndrome appears to result from inhibition, by high levels of fetal insulin, of some fetal enzymes necessary for surfactant production. Polycythemia (excessive number of red blood cells) in the newborn is due primarily to the diminished ability of glycosylated hemoglobin in the mother's blood to release oxygen. Hyperbilirubinemia is a direct result of the inability of immature liver enzymes to metabolize the increased bilirubin resulting from the polycythemia.

Medical Therapy

Screening for the detection of diabetes is a standard part of prenatal care. If caregivers suspect the possibility of diabetes, further testing is undertaken for diagnosis.

Detection and Diagnosis of Gestational Diabetes

Two screening tests are commonly administered to pregnant women:

1. Urine testing. Tes-Tape and Diastix are generally used to test the pregnant woman's urine at the first prenatal visit and again on subsequent visits. Because the renal threshold is lower during pregnancy, glucose may spill into the urine when blood glucose levels are 130 mg/dL. Thus glycosuria is not considered diagnostic of diabetes, but it does indicate the need for further testing.
2. 50 g oral glucose tolerance test. It has become common practice to screen all pregnant women for gestational diabetes between 24 and 28 weeks' gestation (Reece et al 1995). Women with risk factors (age over 30; family history of diabetes; a prior macrosomic, malformed, or stillborn infant; obesity; hypertension; or glycosuria) should be screened when first seen for prenatal care (Spellacy 1994). To do this test, the woman ingests a 50 g oral glucose solution. One hour later a blood sample is obtained. If the plasma glucose level exceeds 140 mg/dL, a 3-hour oral glucose tolerance test (GTT) is necessary. The 50 g screen test is convenient because the woman does not need to be fasting, and the test does not need to be done after a meal.

During pregnancy, gestational diabetes mellitus is diagnosed by using a 3-hour, 100 g oral glucose tolerance test. To do this test the woman eats a high-carbohydrate (greater than 200 g carbohydrate daily) diet for 3 days before her scheduled test. The woman ingests a 100 g oral glucose solution in the morning after an overnight fast of at least 8 hours but not more than 14 hours. Plasma glucose levels are determined fasting and at 1, 2, and 3 hours. Gestational diabetes is diagnosed if two or more of the following values are equaled or exceeded:

Fasting	105 mg/dL
1 hr	190 mg/dL
2 hr	165 mg/dL
3 hr	145 mg/dL

Laboratory Assessment of Long-Term Glucose Control

Measurement of glycosylated hemoglobin levels provides information about the long-term (previous 4–8 weeks) control of hyperglycemia. It measures the percentage of glycohemoglobin in the blood. Glycohemoglobin or HbA_{1c} is the hemoglobin to which a glucose molecule is attached. Because glycosylation is a rather slow and essentially irreversible process, the level of HbA_{1c} gives an indication of previous average serum glucose concentrations. For a woman who is a known diabetic, this test should be done at preconception counseling, again at the first prenatal visit, and once each succeeding trimester.

Management of Diabetes During Pregnancy

The major goals of medical care for a pregnant woman with diabetes are: (a) to maintain a physiologic equilibrium of insulin availability and glucose utilization during pregnancy, and (b) to ensure an optimally healthy mother and newborn. To achieve these goals, good prenatal care using a team approach must be a top priority. The woman with gestational diabetes may find the diagnosis shocking and upsetting. She needs clear explanations and teaching to enlist her cooperation in ensuring a good outcome. The nurse educator plays a major role in this counseling. The woman with pregestational diabetes needs to understand what changes she can expect during pregnancy; she should receive such teaching in preconception counseling.

Antepartal Period During the antepartal period, medical therapy focuses on the following:

1. Dietary regulation. The pregnant woman with diabetes needs to increase her caloric intake by about 300 kcal/day. During the first trimester she generally requires about 30 kcal/kg of ideal body weight

(IBW). During the second and third trimesters she needs about 35 kcal/kg IBW. Approximately 50 to 60 percent of the calories should come from complex carbohydrates, 12 to 20 percent from protein, and 25 to 30 percent from fats (Landon 1996). The food is divided among three meals and three snacks. The bedtime snack is the most important and should include both protein and complex carbohydrates to prevent nighttime hypoglycemia. A nutritionist should work out meal plans with the woman based on the woman's lifestyle, culture, and food preferences. The woman should also be familiar with the use of food exchanges so she can plan her own meals.

2. Glucose monitoring. Glucose monitoring is essential to determine the need for insulin and assess glucose control. Many physicians have the woman come in for weekly assessment of her fasting glucose levels and one or two postprandial levels. In addition, frequent self-monitoring of glucose levels is paramount in maintaining good glucose control. Self-monitoring is discussed in the sections on "Promotion of Effective Insulin Use" and "Community-Based Nursing Care."
3. Insulin administration. Many women with gestational diabetes require insulin to maintain normal glucose levels. Individuals with pregestational diabetes usually have type I diabetes, which requires insulin administration. In either case, human insulin should be used because it is less likely to cause an allergic reaction. Insulin is given either in multiple injections or by continuous subcutaneous infusion. Multiple injections are used more commonly, and with excellent results. Often a mixture of intermediate-acting (NPH) and short-acting (regular) insulin is taken twice a day. Usually two-thirds of the total insulin dose is taken just before breakfast in a 2:1 ratio of NPH to regular insulin. The remaining third is taken in the evening before dinner. Some centers now use a three-dose approach in which two-thirds of the insulin dose is taken before breakfast in a 2:1 NPH to regular insulin ratio; the remaining regular insulin dose is then taken before dinner, and the remaining NPH dose is taken at bedtime. This approach is used to avoid episodes of nocturnal hypoglycemia (Landon 1996).
4. Evaluation of fetal status. Information about the well-being, size, and maturation of the fetus is important for planning the course of pregnancy and the timing of birth. Maternal serum α-fetoprotein (AFP) screening is done at 16 to 18 weeks' gestation to detect neural tube defects such as spina bifida, because pregnancies complicated by diabetes are at increased risk of neural tube defects in the fetus. Ultrasound is done at 18 weeks to establish gestational age and detect anomalies. It is then repeated about every 4 to 6 weeks to evaluate fetal growth for IUGR or macrosomia (Landon 1996). Some agencies do fetal biophysical profiles (BPP) (ultrasound evaluation of fetal well-being in which fetal breathing movements; fetal activity, reactivity, and muscle tone; and amniotic fluid volume are assessed) as part of an ongoing evaluation of fetal status.

   Daily maternal evaluation of fetal activity is begun at about 28 weeks, as is weekly nonstress testing (NST) using a fetal monitor. NSTs are increased to twice a week at 32 weeks' gestation (Gabbe 1996). If the NST is nonreactive, a fetal biophysical profile or contraction stress test is performed (Gabbe 1996). For an explanation of these tests, see Chapter 14.

Intrapartal Period During the intrapartal period, medical therapy focuses on the following:

1. Timing of birth. Most pregnant women with diabetes are allowed to go to term, with spontaneous labor, if their diabetes is in good metabolic control. In pregnancies in which there is evidence of fetal macrosomia, fetal compromise, poor maternal metabolic control, worsening maternal hypertension, or hydramnios, elective induction of labor may be done after confirming fetal lung maturity (Reece et al 1995). To determine fetal lung maturity, amniotic fluid (obtained by amniocentesis) is evaluated for lecithin/sphingomyelin (L/S) ratio and concentration of saturated phosphatidylcholine (SPC). See Chapter 14.

   Preterm induced birth, often by cesarean, must be considered if prenatal testing indicates the fetal condition is deteriorating.
2. Labor management. Maternal insulin requirements are not always predictable during labor. To maintain normal glucose levels (euglycemia), an intravenous infusion of 1000 mL of 5 percent dextrose solution is begun. Insulin is added to the solution and infused at a rate that maintains glucose levels at approximately 100 mg/dL (about 100–125 mL/hr) (Landon 1996). Maternal glucose levels are measured hourly to determine insulin need. Because insulin clings to plastic IV bags and tubing, the tubing should be flushed with insulin before the prescribed amount is added to the intravenous bag of dextrose and water. During the second stage of labor and the immediate postpartal period, the woman may not need additional insulin. The intravenous insulin is discontinued with the completion of the third stage of labor.

Postpartal Period Maternal insulin requirements fall significantly during the postpartal period because, with placental separation, hormone levels fall and the anti-insulin effect ceases. For the first 24 hours the diabetic

CRITICAL THINKING IN ACTION

Patti Chang is a 35-year-old, gravida 3, para 2, well-educated, active Chinese American woman with no history of glucose intolerance. Her two children were born healthy at 36 weeks' gestation. She receives the usual 50 g glucose tolerance test at 26 weeks gestation, and her plasma level is 160 mg/dL. She seems irritated and frustrated when her obstetrician tells her that it would be best to perform a 3-hour fasting glucose tolerance test. After the physician leaves the room, Patti asks the nurse the following questions: Will the glucose hurt my baby? What will the treatment be? How will the nurse answer the questions? Why does Patti seem so upset?

Answers can be found in Appendix H.

mother may require no insulin or only 25 to 50 percent of her normal dose. Then insulin needs are reestablished based on blood glucose testing.

The establishment of parent-child relationships is a high priority. If the newborn requires a special-care nursery, the parents need ongoing information, support, and encouragement to visit and be involved in the newborn's care.

Breastfeeding is encouraged as beneficial to both mother and baby. Calorie needs increase during lactation to 500–800 kcal above prepregnant requirements, and insulin must be adjusted accordingly. Home blood glucose monitoring should continue for the insulin-dependent diabetic.

The couple should also receive information on family planning. Barrier methods of contraception (diaphragm, cervical cap, condom) used with a spermicide are safe, effective, and economical and are the method of choice for insulin-dependent diabetic women. The use of oral contraceptives (OC) by diabetic women is controversial. Some evidence suggests that women with diabetes may be at greater risk for OC complications such as myocardial infarction and thrombophlebitis (Landon 1996). Many physicians who prescribe low-dose OCs to women with diabetes restrict them to women who have no vascular disease and do not smoke. The progesterone-only pill has a higher failure rate but is otherwise safer. Many couples who have completed their families choose sterilization.

APPLYING THE NURSING PROCESS

Nursing Assessment

Whether diabetes (usually type I) has been diagnosed before pregnancy occurs or the diagnosis is made during pregnancy (GDM), careful assessment of the disease process and the woman's understanding of diabetes is important. Thorough physical examination—including assessment for vascular complications of the disease, any signs of infectious conditions, and urine and blood testing for glucose—is essential on the first prenatal visit. Follow-up visits are usually scheduled twice a month during the first two trimesters and once a week during the last trimester.

Assessment also yields vital information about the woman's ability to cope with the combined stress of pregnancy and diabetes and to follow a recommended regimen of care. It is necessary to determine the woman's knowledge about diabetes and self-care before formulating a teaching plan.

Nursing Diagnosis

Nursing diagnoses that may apply to the pregnant woman with diabetes include the following:

- Risk for altered nutrition: More than body requirements related to imbalance between intake and available insulin
- Risk for injury related to possible complications secondary to hypoglycemia or hyperglycemia
- Altered family processes related to client's DM and the need for hospitalization

Nursing Plan and Implementation

Provision of Prepregnancy Counseling

A nurse and a physician may provide counseling using a team approach. Ideally they see the couple before pregnancy so that the diabetes can be evaluated. The outlook for pregnancy is good if the diabetes is of recent onset without vascular complications and if glucose levels can be controlled.

Promotion of Effective Insulin Use

Based on the assessment of the couple's level of knowledge, the nurse ensures that the couple understands the purpose of insulin, the types of insulin to be used, and the correct procedure for administering it. The woman's partner is also instructed about insulin administration in case it should be necessary for the partner to give it. For some highly motivated women whose glucose levels are not well controlled with multiple injections, the continuous infusion pump may improve glucose control.

The nurse teaches the woman how and when to monitor her blood glucose, the desired range of blood glucose levels, and the importance of good control (Figure 12–1 on page 266). The woman may use either a visual method of glucose testing or a glucose meter. With either method she is taught to follow the manufacturer's directions exactly; to wash her hands thoroughly before puncture; to touch the blood droplet, not her finger, to the test pad on the strip; and to store the test strips as directed and discard them after the expiration date.

CRITICAL PATHWAY FOR A WOMAN WITH DIABETES MELLITUS

Category	Antepartal Management	Intrapartal Management*	Postpartal Management*
Referral	• Perinatologist • Endocrinologist • Neonatologist • Social worker • Psych clinical nurse practitioner • Diabetes nurse educator • Dietary/nutritionist • Physical therapy, occupational therapy	• Obtain prenatal record	• Home nursing referral if indicated • Diabetes nurse educator
Assessment	• Electronic fetal monitoring as indicated • Nonstress test as indicated • Ultrasound as indicated • Amniocentesis for lung maturity at 34–36 weeks • Alpha-fetoprotein (done usually at 16 weeks)	• Assess for signs and symptoms (s/sx) of hypoglycemia (sweating, periodic tingling, disorientation, shakiness, pallor, clammy skin, irritability, hunger, headache and blurred vision) during labor • Continuous electronic fetal monitoring • Assess glucose levels with glucometer as ordered or if s/sx of hypoglycemia occur	• Assess glucose levels with glucometer—generally insulin requirements fall significantly in the postpartum phase • Continue normal postpartum assessment q8h • Feeding technique with newborn: should be progressing • Vital signs assessment: q8h; all WNL; report temperature >38C (100.4F) • Continue assessment of comfort level
Comfort	• Assess for discomfort • Provide comfort measures as needed	• Assess for discomfort • Provide comfort measures as needed	• Continue with pain management techniques
Teaching/ psychosocial	• Room orientation • Notify RN of s/sx of hyper/hypoglycemia, uterine contractions, decreased fetal movement, vaginal leaking and/or bleeding, dysuria • Assess family status and/or additional psychosocial needs • Eval of client teaching • Importance of following diet • Tour of ICN • Prebirth teaching for vag and/or CS • Evaluation of teaching effectiveness	• Evaluation of teaching effectiveness	• Complete normal postpartum teaching (see Chapter 28)
Therapeutic nursing interventions and reports	• CBC • UA/dipstick for protein and ketones • Biochemistry profile • Glycosylated hemoglobin level ($HbgA_1C$) daily • 24 hour urine for protein and creatinine clearance • Fingerstick BS, every am, before meals, and 2 hours after meals • Vital signs q4h • Fundal height weekly • Daily weight	• Glucose levels monitored hourly	• Continue sitz bath prn • May shower if ambulating without difficulty • DC buffalo cap if present
Activity	• Bed rest with bathroom privileges • Diversional activity	• Bed rest	• Up ad lib
Nutrition	• ADA per order • Encourage fluids	• Ice chips	• Encourage breastfeeding • Increase calorie needs 500–800 kcal • Continue diet and fluids

*Interventions for a woman with a normal labor and birth and during the early postpartum period may be found in those appropriate critical pathways.

CRITICAL PATHWAY FOR A WOMAN WITH DIABETES MELLITUS continued

Category	Antepartal Management	Intrapartal Management*	Postpartal Management*
Elimination	• Review measures to prevent UTI		
Medications	• IV ____ @ ____ mL/h/buffalo cap • Insulin as ordered → ____________ • Prenatal vitamins and iron	• Two IV lines are usually used, one with 5% dextrose solution and one with a saline solution (saline line is used for insulin if needed) • The IV insulin is usually discontinued with completion of 3rd stage of labor	• May take own prenatal vitamins • RhoGAM and rubella vaccine administered if indicated
Discharge planning/ home care	• Explain purpose of scheduled tests and procedures • Include family in diabetic teaching • Assess family support	• Assess family support	• Review discharge instruction sheet and check list • Describe postpartum warning signs and when to call CNM/physician • Provide prescriptions. Gift pack given to woman. • Arrangements made for baby pictures if desired • Postpartum visit scheduled • Newborn check scheduled
Family Involvement	• Identify available support persons • Assess family perceptions of situation	• Involve support persons in care	• Evidence of parental bonding behaviors apparent • Involve support persons in care: teaching • Plans being made for providing support to mother following discharge
Date			

*Interventions for a woman with a normal labor and birth and during the early postpartum period may be found in those appropriate critical pathways.

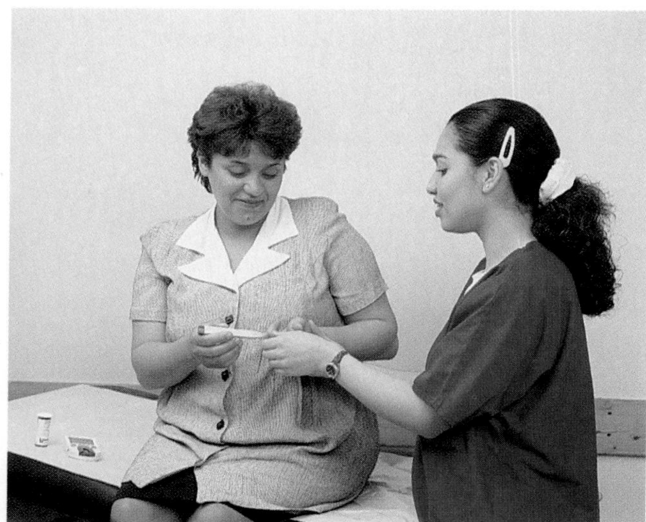

FIGURE 12–1 The nurse teaches the pregnant woman with gestational diabetes mellitus how to do home glucose monitoring.

The nurse can provide the following tips regarding finger puncture: (a) various spring-loaded devices are available that make puncturing easier; (b) letting the arm hang down for 30 seconds increases blood flow to the fingers; and (c) the sides of fingers should be punctured instead of the ends because the ends contain more pain-sensitive nerves.

Diabetic clients need to keep a record of each blood sugar reading as a guide for management. Specific record sheets are available for this purpose. The woman is instructed to bring the record sheet with her for each visit.

Promotion of a Planned Exercise Program

Exercise is encouraged for the woman's overall well-being. If she is accustomed to a regular exercise program, she is encouraged to continue. She is advised to exercise after meals when blood sugar levels are high, to wear diabetic identification, to carry a simple sugar such as hard candy (because of the possibility of exercise-induced hypoglycemia), to monitor her blood glucose levels regularly, and to avoid injecting insulin into an extremity that will soon be used during exercise.

If she has not been following a regular exercise plan, the nurse can encourage her to begin gradually. Due to alterations in metabolism with exercise, the woman's blood glucose should be well controlled before she begins an exercise program.

Community-Based Nursing Care

In many cases, women with gestational diabetes are stabilized in the hospital and necessary teaching for self-care is begun. Women with preexisting diabetes may also require hospitalization for stabilization of their diabetes. In either case, the majority of ongoing teaching and supervision of pregnant women with diabetes is then carried out by nurses in clinics, community agencies, and the women's homes.

- *Glucose monitoring.* Home monitoring of blood glucose levels is the most accurate and convenient method for determining insulin dose and assessing control. Women are taught self-monitoring techniques that they perform 4–6 times a day according to a specified schedule. They then regulate their insulin dosage based on blood glucose values and anticipated activity level. Women are encouraged to maintain blood glucose levels in the following ranges if possible: fasting blood glucose, 60–90 mg/dL; before other meals, 60–105 mg/dL; two hours after a meal, 120 mg/dL (Landon 1996).
- *Symptoms of hypoglycemia and ketoacidosis.* The pregnant diabetic woman must recognize symptoms of changing glucose levels and take appropriate action by immediately checking her capillary blood glucose level. If it is less than 60 mg/dL, she is advised to take 20 g of carbohydrate, wait 20 minutes, and then retest her glucose level. The necessary carbohydrate can be obtained by drinking 14.5 oz whole milk, 12 oz orange or apple juice, or 13.3 oz cola (Mandeville 1992). Many people overtreat their symptoms by continuing to eat. This can cause a rebound hyperglycemia. The woman should carry a snack at all times and should have other fast sources of glucose (simple carbohydrates) at hand to treat an insulin reaction when milk is not available. Family members are also taught how to inject glucagon in the event that food does not work or is not feasible, for instance, in the presence of severe morning sickness.
- *Smoking.* Smoking has harmful effects on both the maternal vascular system and the developing fetus and is contraindicated for both pregnancy and diabetes.
- *Travel.* Insulin can be kept at room temperature while traveling. Insulin supplies should be kept with the traveler and not packed in the baggage. Special meals can be arranged by notifying most airlines a few days before departure. The woman should wear a diabetic identification bracelet or necklace and should check with her physician for any instructions or advice before traveling.
- *Hospitalization.* Hospitalization may become necessary during the pregnancy to evaluate blood glucose levels and adjust insulin dosages.
- *Support groups.* Many communities have diabetes support groups or education classes that can be most helpful to women with newly diagnosed diabetes.
- *Cesarean birth.* Chances for a cesarean birth increase if the pregnant woman is diabetic. The possibility should be anticipated; caregivers may suggest enrollment in cesarean birth preparation classes. Many hospitals offer classes, and information is available through organizations such as Cesarean/Support Education and Concern (C/Sec, Inc); Cesarean Birth Council; or the Cesarean Association for Research, Education, Support and Satisfaction in Birthing (CARESS). The couple may prefer simply to discuss cesarean birth with the nurse and their obstetrician and read some books on the topic.

Evaluation

Anticipated outcomes of nursing care include

- The woman is able to discuss her condition and its possible impact on her pregnancy, labor and birth, and postpartal period.
- The woman participates in developing a health care regimen to meet her needs and follows it throughout her pregnancy.
- The woman gives birth to a healthy newborn.
- The woman avoids developing hypoglycemia or hyperglycemia.
- The woman is able to care for her newborn.

Care of the Woman with Anemia

Anemia indicates inadequate levels of hemoglobin (Hb) in the blood. The CDC defines anemia as hemoglobin less than 11 g/dL in the first and third trimesters and less than 10.5 g/dL in the second trimester. The common anemias of pregnancy are due either to insufficient hemoglobin production related to nutritional deficiency in

TABLE 12–3 Anemia and Pregnancy

Condition	Brief Description	Maternal Implications	Fetal/Neonatal Implications
Iron deficiency anemia	Condition caused by inadequate iron intake resulting in hemoglobin levels below 11g/dL. To prevent this, most women are advised to take supplemental iron during pregnancy.	Pregnant woman with this anemia tires easily, is more susceptible to infection, has increased chance of PIH and postpartal hemorrhage, and cannot tolerate even minimal blood loss during birth.	Risk of low birth weight, prematurity, stillbirth, and neonatal death increases in women with severe iron deficiency anemia (maternal Hb less than 6 g/dL). Fetus may be hypoxic during labor due to impaired uteroplacental oxygenation.
Sickle cell anemia	Recessive autosomal disease present in about 1 in 600 of African-Americans in the US (the sickle cell trait is carried by 8%). The disease is characterized by sickling of the RBCs in the presence of decreased oxygenation. Condition may be marked by crisis with profound anemia, jaundice, high temperature, infarction, and acute pain. Crisis is treated by partial exchange transfusion, rehydration with IV fluids, antibiotics, and analgesics. The fetus is monitored throughout.	Pregnancy may aggravate anemia and bring on more crises. Risk of developing preeclampsia increases. Risk of urinary tract infection, pneumonia, congestive heart failure, and pulmonary infarction also increases. The goal of treatment is to reduce the anemia and maintain good health. Oxygen supplementation should be used continuously during labor. Additional blood should be available if transfusion is necessary following birth.	Abortion, fetal death, and prematurity may occur. IUGR is also a characteristic finding in newborns of women with sickle cell anemia.
Folic acid deficiency anemia	Folic acid deficiency is the most common cause of megaloblastic anemia. In the absence of folic acid, immature RBCs fail to divide, become enlarged (megaloblastic), and are fewer in number. Increased folic acid metabolism during pregnancy and lactation can result in deficiency. Because the condition is difficult to diagnose, the best approach is prevention by supplementing with 0.4 mg folate daily (generally found in prenatal vitamin supplements). The condition is treated with 1 mg folate daily.	Folate deficiency is the second most common cause of anemia in pregnancy. Severe deficiency increases the risk that the mother may need a blood transfusion following birth due to anemia. She also has an increased risk of hemorrhage due to thrombocytopenia, and is more susceptible to infection. Folic acid is readily available in foods such as fresh leafy green vegetables, red meat, fish, poultry, and legumes, but it is easily destroyed by overcooking or cooking with large quantities of water.	Early studies suggested a link between folate deficiency and complications such as spontaneous abortion or abruptio placentae with resultant fetal death, but newer studies have not replicated these findings. Generally the fetus is not anemic at birth even in the presence of severe maternal anemia.

iron or folic acid during pregnancy, or to hemoglobin destruction in an inherited disorder such as sickle cell anemia. Table 12–3 describes these common anemias.

Care of the Woman with HIV Infection

Human immunodeficiency virus (HIV) infection is one of today's major health concerns. HIV is a progressive disease that ultimately results in the development of **acquired immunodeficiency syndrome (AIDS)**. AIDS has become the fourth leading cause of death among women ages 25–44 and is now the seventh leading cause of death for children ages 1–4. In 1994 women accounted for 18 percent of newly reported cases of HIV infection, up from 10.4 percent in 1990. These rates are even higher among black and Hispanic women (HRSA Program Advisory 1995). Although intravenous drug use remains a significant source of HIV transmission, currently over 50 percent of women who become HIV-positive acquire the infection through heterosexual contact. Because HIV/AIDS is increasing more rapidly among women than among men, experts believe that HIV/AIDS in the United States is beginning to reflect the more gender-equal patterns of infection seen in third world countries (Eyler 1996).

Pathophysiology of HIV/AIDS

HIV, which causes AIDS, typically enters the body through blood, blood products, or other bodily fluids such as semen, vaginal fluid, breast milk, and urine. HIV affects specific T-cells, thereby decreasing the body's immune responses. This makes the affected person susceptible to opportunistic infections such as *Pneumocystis carinii,* which causes a severe pneumonia, candidiasis, cytomegalovirus, tuberculosis, and toxoplasmosis (Duff 1996). Opportunistic infections are most often the cause of death in individuals with AIDS.

HIV disease is progressive. Initially, the individual infected with HIV is already infectious but has not yet developed detectable antibody levels. Antibodies usually develop within 6 to 12 weeks after exposure, although in some people this latent period is longer. Once antibodies develop, an individual is classified as HIV-positive, and screening tests such as the ELISA (enzyme-linked immunosorbent assay) and the Western blot test become positive. However, the individual often remains unaware that he or she is infected. The duration of this latent, asymptomatic phase is approximately 5 to 10 years (Duff 1996). The majority of pregnant women fall in this category.

In women, recurrent gynecologic disorders such as candidiasis or nonhealing vaginal ulcers may be the initial sign of altered immunity (Cohn 1993). As symptoms develop, the HIV-infected person may experience fatigue, lymphadenopathy, weight loss, fever, night sweats, and so forth. AIDS-defining diseases that are more common in women than men include wasting syndrome, esophogeal candidiasis, and herpes simplex virus disease. Kaposi's sarcoma is rare in women.

Many women who are HIV positive choose to avoid pregnancy because of the risk of infecting the fetus and the likelihood of dying before the child is raised. Women who do become pregnant should be advised that pregnancy is not believed to accelerate the progression of HIV/AIDS, that the use of zidovudine (ZDV) during pregnancy significantly reduces the risk of transmitting the HIV to the fetus, and that most medications used to treat HIV can be taken during the pregnancy (Eyler 1995).

Fetal-Neonatal Risks

AIDS may develop in infants whose mothers are seropositive, usually due to perinatal transmission. Perinatal transmission occurs transplacentally, at birth when the infant is exposed to maternal blood and vaginal secretions, and via breast milk (Lindberg 1995). The risk to infants born to mothers who are HIV-positive is estimated to be about 25 percent. However, findings of the NIH AIDS Clinical Trials Group (ACTG) Protocol 076 of zidovudine showed a significant reduction in fetal transmission; 8.3 percent in women who received zidovudine compared to 25.5 percent among women in the placebo group (HRSA Program Advisory 1995). Although the long-term effects of zidovudine are not yet known, no other treatment currently available is as effective in reducing the perinatal spread of HIV infection (Eyler 1996).

Often infants will have a positive antibody titer for up to 15 months due to the passive transfer of maternal antibodies. For further discussion of the infant who is HIV-positive, see Chapter 25.

Medical Therapy

The goal for antenatal care is identification of the pregnant woman at risk for HIV infection. All women who are pregnant or planning a pregnancy should be offered voluntary HIV antibody testing using ELISA. If the results are positive, the Western blot test is used to confirm the diagnosis. Women who test positive should be counseled about the implications of the diagnosis for themselves and their fetus to ensure an informed reproductive choice. A woman who chooses to continue her pregnancy needs excellent prenatal care.

The HIV-infected woman should be evaluated and treated for other sexually transmitted infections. She should also have a tuberculin skin test done and, if the results are positive, a chest x-ray to identify any pulmonary disease. If there is no history of hepatitis B, she should receive the hepatitis vaccine, as well as vaccines for hemophilus B influenza, pneumococcal infection, and viral influenza (Duff 1996).

At each prenatal visit, asymptomatic, HIV-infected women should be monitored for early signs of complications, such as weight loss in the second or third trimesters or fever. The mouth should be inspected for signs of infections such as thrush (candidiasis) or hairy leukoplakia; the lungs should be auscultated for signs of pneumonia; the lymph nodes, the liver, and the spleen should be palpated for signs of enlargement. Each trimester the woman should have a visual examination and a fundoscopic examination to detect such complications as toxoplasmosis retinitis.

In addition to routine prenatal testing, the woman who is HIV-positive should be assessed regularly for serologic changes indicating that HIV/AIDS is progressing. This includes the absolute CD4 lymphocyte count, which provides the number of helper T4 cells. When the CD4 count reaches a level of 200/mm^3 or lower, opportunistic infections are more likely to develop. The ratio of CD4 to CD8 (helper to suppressor) T-cell lymphocytes is also obtained. This ratio tends to be reversed in women who are showing symptoms of AIDS.

Asymptomatic HIV-positive women should be given information about the potential benefits and unknown long-term side effects of the ACTG Protocol 076, which demonstrated the success of prophylactic zidovudine in decreasing perinatal HIV transmission. This protocol involves the oral administration of zidovudine (100 mg 5 times/day) beginning after the first trimester; continuous intravenous administration of zidovudine during labor and birth; and the oral administration of zidovudine to the newborn every 6 hours for the first 6 weeks of life (HRSA Program Advisory 1995). Zidovudine suppresses bone marrow function and can have major side effects such as thrombocytopenia and anemia. Thus women who choose to take zidovudine should have monthly CBC and liver function tests, and the CD4 count should be determined each trimester (Eyler 1996).

Women with CD4 counts below 200/mm^3 should also be offered treatment with oral zidovudine. Because opportunistic infections such as *Pneumocystis carinii* pneumonia are more likely to develop in these women, prophylactic treatment should be started using oral trimethoprim-sulfamethoxazole (Duff 1996).

Text continues on page 272

CRITICAL PATHWAY FOR A WOMAN WITH HIV/AIDS

Category	Antepartal Management	Intrapartal Management*	Postpartal Management*
Referral	• Perinatologist • Internist • Social worker • Psych clinical nurse practitioner • Dietary/nutritionist • Infectious disease consult	• Obtain prenatal record	• Home nursing referral if indicated

Assessment	• Obtain course of present pregnancy
	• Assess estimated gestational age
	• Assess any sensitivity to medications
	• Obtain history of any infections
	• Obtain complete physical examination to include
	  • Fetal size, fetal status (FHR), and fetal maturity
	  • Signs of fatigue, weakness, recurrent diarrhea, pallor, night sweats
	  • Lymphadenopathy
	  • Present weight and amount of weight gain or weight loss
	  • Presence of nonproductive cough, fever, sore throat, chills, shortness of breath (*Pneumocystis carinii* pneumonia)
	  • Dark purplish marks or lesions, especially on the lower extremities (Kaposi's sarcoma)
	  • Oral, gingival lesions
	• Obtain diagnostic studies:
	  • Ultrasound
	  • Fetal maturity studies (L/S ratio, PG creatinine)
	  • Hemoglobin and hematocrit
	  • WBC
	  • HIV-I
	  • CD4+ T lymphocyte count
	  • ESR
	  • Differential
	  • Platelet count
		• Assess for signs of infection	• Monitor daily Hct
			• Continue normal postpartum assessment q8h
			• Feeding technique with newborn: should be progressing
			• TPR assessment: q8h; all WNL; report temperature >38C (100.4F)
			• Continue assessment of comfort level

Comfort	• Assess for discomfort • Provide comfort measures as needed	• Assess for discomfort • Provide comfort measures as needed	• Continue with pain management techniques
Teaching/ psychosocial	• Room orientation • Explain signs and symptoms (s/sx) of worsening disease & importance of notifying RN • Explain s/sx of labor • Increase pt awareness of fetal monitoring • Evaluation of client teaching	• Tour of ICN • Discuss with woman: a. Mode of childbirth b. Postpartum expectation	• Implement normal postpartum teaching and psychosocial support (see Chapter 28)
Therapeutic nursing interventions and reports	• Assess emotional response so that support and teaching can be planned accordingly • Weigh woman • Obtain food history • Establish rapport • Provide opportunities to talk without interruption • Monitor for signs of infection • Maintain appropriate isolation precautions	• Ongoing monitoring of blood pressure • Electronic fetal monitoring in place • Try to have same nurses caring for woman during her hospitalization • Maintain appropriate isolations precautions • Monitor for signs of infection	• Continue sitz baths prn • May shower if ambulating without difficulty • DC buffalo cap (heparin lock) if present • Maintain appropriate isolation precautions • Monitor for signs of infection

CRITICAL PATHWAY continued

Category	Antepartal Management	Intrapartal Management*	Postpartal Management*
Activity	• Decreased stimulation in room • Limit visitors		• Up ad lib
Nutrition	• Plan high-protein, high-calorie diet	• Ice chips; popsicles	• Continue diet and fluids
Elimination			
Medications		• Continuous IV infusion	• May take own prenatal vitamins • RhoGAM administered if indicated • Rubella vaccine administered if indicated

Discharge planning/ home care	• Assess home care needs
	• If the client is asymptomatic, the primary nursing activity is client teaching regarding
	  • Disease process
	  • Screening and health care for sex partners as appropriate
	  • Impact of disease on pregnancy
	  • Methods of HIV transmission
	  • Precautions to take in preventing the spread of infection
	  • Options in regard to pregnancy
	  • Available community resources
	  • Signs and symptoms to report to health care provider including common discomforts of pregnancy such as nausea and fatigue and complications such as premature rupture of membranes, vaginal bleeding, and preterm labor
	  • Importance of regular prenatal visits
	• Provide teaching regarding nutritional needs
	• Refer to community resources
	• Discuss disease process, impact on pregnancy, and pregnancy options
	• Provide support and counseling
			• Review discharge instruction sheet and check list
			• Describe postpartum warning signs and when to call CNM/physician
			• Provide prescriptions. Gift pack given to woman.
			• Arrangements made for baby pictures if desired
			• Postpartum visit scheduled
			• Newborn check scheduled
			• Discuss the implications of breastfeeding (current information suggests that the virus may be spread in breast milk)
			• Provide information on transmission of HIV and measures to prevent infection. Discuss household safety issues (eg, it is acceptable to use same dishes, safe to sleep in same bed, safe to use same bathroom, can hold and hug children, should avoid using razors and tooth-brushes and should wear gloves and use 10% bleach solution to clean spills of body fluids or disinfect bathroom). Inform the woman that sexual abstinence is safest; otherwise latex condoms should be used.

Family Involvement	• Assess woman's major concerns ie: losing fetus, relationship with other children, relationship with partner • Assess support systems	• Encourage family member to stay with the woman as long as possible throughout labor and childbirth	• Family members urged to visit • Continue to involve support persons in teaching • Evidence of parental bonding behaviors present • Plans made for providing support to mother following discharge. Support persons verbalize understanding of need for woman to rest, eat nutritionally, recover.
Date			

*Interventions for a woman with a normal labor and birth and during the early postpartum period may be found in those appropriate critical pathways.

A pregnancy complicated by HIV infection, even if asymptomatic, is considered high-risk, and the fetus is monitored closely. Weekly nonstress testing is begun at 32 weeks' gestation, and serial ultrasounds are done to detect intrauterine growth retardation (IUGR). Biophysical profiles are also indicated (see Chapter 14). Invasive procedures such as amniocentesis are avoided when possible to prevent the contamination of a noninfected infant.

Intrapartal care is similar to that for all pregnant women, although strict adherence to universal precautions is crucial to avoid nosocomial infection. To prevent exposure of an uninfected infant to HIV during labor and birth, the fetal membranes should be left unruptured until birth if possible and invasive procedures such as fetal scalp electrode monitoring and fetal scalp pH sampling should be avoided (Duff 1996). Studies to date do not indicate that cesarean birth decreases the risk of fetal infection; as a result cesarean is used only for obstetric reasons (ACOG 1992).

Women who are HIV-positive are at increased risk for complications such as intrapartal or postpartal hemorrhage, postpartal infection, poor wound healing, and infections of the genitourinary tract. Thus they need careful monitoring and appropriate therapy as indicated. Research suggests that breastfeeding increases the risk of HIV transmission to the newborn. Consequently, the HIV-positive woman should be cautioned against breastfeeding her infant (Duff 1996).

Because of the profound implications of HIV infection for the woman, her family, the child, and her health care providers, screening is recommended for women who are at increased risk, including the following: prostitutes; women whose current or previous sexual partners have been bisexual, have abused IV drugs, had hemophilia, or tested positive for HIV; and women from countries where heterosexual transmission is common. In addition, clinical facilities that are located in areas with a large population of people who test HIV-positive may require routine HIV screening of all prenatal clients.

APPLYING THE NURSING PROCESS

Nursing Assessment

A woman who tests positive for HIV may be asymptomatic or may present with any of the following signs or symptoms: fatigue, anemia, malaise, progressive weight loss, lymphadenopathy, diarrhea, fever, neurologic dysfunction, cell-mediated immunodeficiency, or evidence of Kaposi's sarcoma (purplish, reddish-brown lesions either externally or internally).

If a woman tests HIV-positive or is involved in a relationship that places her at high risk, the nurse should assess the woman's knowledge level about the disease, its implications for her and her fetus, and self-care measures the woman can take.

Nursing Diagnosis

Examples of nursing diagnoses that might apply for a pregnant woman who tests HIV-positive include the following:

- Knowledge deficit related to lack of information about AIDS and its long-term implications for the woman and her unborn child
- Risk for infection related to altered immunity secondary to HIV infection
- Ineffective family coping related to the implications of a positive HIV test in one of the family members

Nursing Plan and Implementation

Providing Anticipatory Guidance

Nurses need to help women understand that HIV/AIDS is a fatal disease. HIV infection can be avoided if women avoid sharing IV drug needles and practice safe sex, including insisting that their partners wear a latex condom for each act of intercourse.

Women at high risk for AIDS should have premarital and prenatal screening for HIV before considering a pregnancy. In many instances, the nurse will be responsible for counseling the woman about the test and its implications for her, her partner, and a child should she become pregnant.

Monitoring the Asymptomatic Pregnant Woman

In monitoring the asymptomatic pregnant woman who is HIV-positive, the nurse should be alert for nonspecific symptoms such as fever, weight loss, fatigue, persistent candidiasis, diarrhea, cough, skin lesions, and behavior changes. These may be signs of developing symptomatic HIV infection. Laboratory findings such as decreased hemoglobin, hematocrit, and CD4 lymphocytes; elevated erythrocyte sedimentation rate (ESR); and abnormal complete blood count, differential, and platelets may indicate complications such as infection or progression of the disease.

Education about optimal nutrition and maintenance of wellness are important and should be reviewed frequently with the woman.

Reducing the Risk of Transmission

The nurse is faced with the important task of taking the precautions necessary to protect staff, other clients, and families, while meeting the needs of the childbearing woman who is HIV-positive.

In 1987 the Centers for Disease Control (CDC) stated that the increasing prevalence of HIV/AIDS and the risk of exposure faced by health care workers is significant enough that precautions should be taken with all clients (not only those with known HIV infection), especially in dealing with blood and body fluids (MMWR Supplement 1987). These precautions are now called *universal precautions*.

Nurses who deal with childbearing families are exposed frequently to blood and body fluids, and should pay careful attention to the CDC guidelines, including the following:

1. Caregivers should wear disposable latex gloves when having contact with a client's mucous membranes, nonintact skin, body fluids, or blood. Contact includes, for example, changing chux pads, peripads, diapers, or dressings; starting or discontinuing intravenous fluids; and drawing blood.
2. After giving care to a client, gloves should be removed and hands should be washed before caring for another client.
3. In addition to gloves, protective coverings such as a plastic apron, gown, mask, and eye or face shield should be worn during any procedures that frequently result in contamination from splashing of body fluids. These include amniotomy, vaginal examination, vaginal or cesarean birth, suctioning, and care of the newborn until after the initial bath has been done. (Note: Full-size glasses are considered sufficient eye protection. While agencies are required to provide eye shields, nurses may choose to purchase their own goggles and clean them with soap and water.)
4. At birth, the newborn should be suctioned with a disposable bulb syringe or mucus extractor attached to wall suction at a low setting. DeLee mucus traps with mouth suction are not used because of the risk of inadvertently ingesting secretions.
5. Similar care should be taken during any resuscitation procedures. To avoid the need for mouth-to-mouth resuscitation, sufficient mouthpieces and ventilation equipment should be available. Disposable resuscitation masks are recommended.
6. Syringes and needles are disposed of in a special puncture-resistant container. Needles are never recapped using two hands; a one-handed scoop technique is acceptable. Needles should never be twisted or broken by hand.
7. In the event that a glove is torn it should be removed, the hands should be washed, and new gloves should be applied.
8. Gloves and protective coverings should also be worn during any cleaning procedures.

See Key Facts to Remember: The Pregnant Woman with HIV Infection.

KEY FACTS TO REMEMBER

The Pregnant Woman with HIV Infection

- Following initial infection, antibodies usually become detectable within about 6–12 weeks, but it may take 6 months or longer. *Despite this, the woman is infected, and infectious.*
- HIV infection is spread primarily through sexual contact, exposure to contaminated blood, and (perinatally) from infected mother to child.
- Many women who are HIV-positive are asymptomatic and may be unaware they have the infection. *Universal precautions are indicated in caring for all pregnant women.*
- A pregnant woman found to be HIV-positive should receive prenatal counseling about the possible implications of HIV for the fetus so that she can make an informed choice about continuing her pregnancy. Her choice should be supported.
- During pregnancy, caregivers should be alert to nonspecific symptoms such as weight loss and fatigue, which may indicate progression of HIV disease.
- Invasive procedures during the intrapartal period increase the risk of exposure to HIV for the fetus (who may be uninfected) and should be undertaken only after carefully weighing the advantages and risks.
- **The cardinal rule in caring for pregnant women is: If it's wet and it's not yours, use protection when handling it!**

Providing Emotional Support

The psychologic implications of HIV/AIDS for the childbearing family are staggering. The woman is faced with the knowledge that she and her newborn, if infected, have a decreased life expectancy. If her infant is not infected, she must face the probability that others will raise her child. The couple must deal with the impact of the illness on the partner, who may or may not be infected, and on other children. The woman and her family may have feelings of fear, helplessness, anger, and isolation.

The nonjudgmental, supportive nurse plays an essential role in preserving confidentiality and the client's right to privacy. In addition, the nurse can help ensure that the woman receives complete, accurate information about her condition and ways she might cope. This usually involves a referral to social services for follow-up care.

Evaluation

Anticipated outcomes of nursing care include

- The woman discusses the implications of her HIV infection, its implications for her unborn child and for herself, the method of transmission, and the treatment options.

TABLE 12–4 Possible Effects of Selected Drugs of Abuse/Addiction on Fetus and Neonate

Maternal Drug	Effect on Fetus and Neonate
Depressants	
Alcohol	Cardiac anomalies, IUGR, potential teratogenic effects, FAS, FAE
Narcotics	
Heroin	Withdrawal symptoms, convulsions, death, IUGR, respiratory alkalosis, hyperbilirubinemia
Methadone	Fetal distress, meconium aspiration; with abrupt termination of the drug, severe withdrawal symptoms, neonatal death
Barbiturates	Neonatal depression, increased anomalies; teratogenic effect; withdrawal symptoms, convulsions, hyperactivity, hyperreflexia, vasomotor instability
Phenobarbital	Bleeding (with excessive doses)
"T's and Blues" (combination of the following)	
Talwin (narcotic)	Safe for use in pregnancy; depresses respiration if taken close to time of birth
Amytal (barbiturate)	See barbiturates
Tranquilizers	
Phenothiazine derivatives	Withdrawal, extrapyramidal dysfunction, delayed respiratory onset, hyperbilirubinemia, hypotonia or hyperactivity, decreased platelet count
Diazepam (Valium)	Hypotonia, hypothermia, low Apgar score, respiratory depression, poor sucking reflex, possible cleft lip
Antianxiety drugs	
Lithium	Congenital anomalies; lethargy and cyanosis in the newborn
Stimulants	
Amphetamines	
Amphetamine sulfate (Benzedrine)	Generalized arthritis, learning disabilities, poor motor coordination, transposition of the great vessels, cleft palate
Dextroamphetamine sulfate (dexedrine sulfate)	Congenital heart defects, hyperbilirubinemia
Cocaine	Learning disabilities, poor state organization, decreased interactive behavior, CNS anomalies, cardiac anomalies, genitourinary anomalies, SIDS
Caffeine (more than 600 mg/day)	Spontaneous abortion, IUGR, increased incidence of cleft palate; other anomalies
Nicotine (half to one pack cigarettes/day)	Increased rate of spontaneous abortion, increased incidence of placental abruption, SGA, small head circumference, decreased length, SIDS
Psychotropics	
PCP ("angel dust")	Flaccid appearance, poor head control, impaired neurologic development
LSD	Chromosomal breakage
Marijuana	IUGR, potential impaired immunologic mechanisms

- The woman uses information about social services (or other agency referral) for follow-up assistance and counseling.
- The woman begins to verbalize her feelings about her condition and its implications for her and her family.

Care of the Woman Practicing Substance Abuse

As discussed in Chapter 9, drugs that adversely affect fetal growth and development are called teratogens. Table 12–4 identifies common addictive drugs and their effects on the fetus or newborn.

Drugs that are commonly misused include alcohol, amphetamines, barbiturates, hallucinogens, marijuana, cocaine, crack, and heroin and other narcotics. Abuse of these drugs constitutes a major threat to the successful completion of pregnancy.

Indiscriminate drug use during pregnancy, particularly in the first trimester, may adversely affect the health of the woman and the growth and development of the fetus. Originally it was thought that the placenta acted as a protective barrier to keep the drugs ingested by the woman from reaching the fetal system. This is not true. The degree to which a drug is passed to the fetus depends on the drug's chemical properties, including molecular weight, and on whether it is administered alone or in combination with other drugs.

Drug use during pregnancy may be the most frequently missed diagnosis in all of maternity care. The reported incidence of drug use in pregnancy is related to the thoroughness of the prenatal assessments done by health care professionals. Unfortunately, substance-abusing women often wait until late in pregnancy to seek health care. Moreover, the substance-abusing woman who seeks early prenatal care may not voluntarily reveal her addiction, so caregivers should be alert for a history or physical signs that suggest substance abuse.

Substances Commonly Abused During Pregnancy

Alcohol

The use of alcohol during pregnancy has been described as the major preventable cause of birth defects (Horton 1992). The incidence of alcohol abuse is highest among women 20 to 40 years old; alcoholism is also seen in teenagers. Chronic abuse of alcohol can undermine maternal health by causing malnutrition (especially folic acid and thiamine deficiencies), bone marrow suppression, increased incidence of infections, and liver disease. As a result of alcohol dependence, the woman may have withdrawal seizures in the intrapartal period as early as 12–48 hours after she stops drinking. Delirium tremens may occur in the postpartal period, and the newborn may suffer a withdrawal syndrome.

The effects of alcohol on the fetus may result in a group of signs known as fetal alcohol syndrome (FAS). The syndrome has characteristic physical and mental abnormalities that vary in severity and combination. (The abnormalities and care of these infants are discussed in Chapter 25.) There is no definitive answer to how much alcohol a woman can safely consume during pregnancy. The expectant woman should play it safe by avoiding alcohol completely during the early weeks of pregnancy when organogenesis is occurring. During the remainder of pregnancy, she may have an occasional drink, although none at all is safest.

The nursing staff in the maternal-newborn unit must be aware of the manifestations of alcohol abuse so they can prepare for the client's special needs. The care regimen includes sedation to decrease irritability and tremors, seizure precautions, intravenous fluid therapy for hydration, and preparation for an addicted newborn. Although high doses of sedatives and analgesics may be necessary for the woman, caution is advised because these can cause fetal depression.

Breastfeeding generally is not contraindicated, although alcohol is excreted in breast milk. Excessive alcohol consumption may intoxicate the infant and inhibit maternal let-down reflex. Discharge planning for the alcohol-addicted mother and newborn should be correlated with the social service department of the hospital.

Cocaine/Crack

Cocaine use is one of the most serious epidemics affecting the childbearing family. Approximately 1 in 10 pregnant women is believed to use cocaine, with even higher rates reported in urban areas (Weathers et al 1993). Cocaine acts at the nerve terminals to prevent the re-uptake of dopamine and norepinephrine, which in turn results in vasoconstriction, tachycardia, and hypertension. Placental vasoconstriction decreases blood flow to the fetus.

Cocaine is usually taken in three ways: snorting, smoking, and intravenous injection. **Crack** is a form of freebase cocaine that is made up of baking soda, water, and cocaine mixed into a paste and cooked to form a rock. The rock can then be smoked in a pipe. Many women, especially those in low-income areas, favor this form of the drug over other forms because it is readily available and cheaper than other forms of cocaine. In addition, smoking crack leads to a quicker, more intense high because the drug is absorbed through the large surface area of the lungs.

The onset of cocaine effects occurs rapidly, but the euphoria lasts only about 30 minutes. Euphoria and excitement are usually followed by irritability, depression, pessimism, fatigue, and a strong desire for more cocaine. This pattern often leads the user to take repeated doses to sustain the effect. Cocaine metabolites may be present in the urine of a pregnant woman for as long as 4 to 7 days after use.

The cocaine user is difficult to identify prenatally. Because cocaine is an illegal substance, many women are reluctant to volunteer information about their drug use. The nurse who is familiar with the woman may recognize subtle signs of cocaine use (including mood swings and appetite changes) and withdrawal symptoms such as depression, irritability, nausea, lack of motivation, and psychomotor changes.

Major adverse maternal effects of cocaine use include seizures and hallucinations, pulmonary edema, cerebral hemorrhage, respiratory failure, and heart problems. Women who use cocaine have an increased incidence of spontaneous abortion, abruptio placentae, preterm birth, and stillbirth (Niebyl 1996).

Exposure of the fetus to cocaine in utero increases the risk of IUGR, small head circumference, shorter body length, altered brain development, malformations of the genitourinary tract, and lower Apgar scores. Newborns who were exposed to cocaine in utero may have neurobehavioral disturbances, marked irritability, an exaggerated startle reflex, labile emotions, and an increased risk of sudden infant death syndrome (SIDS). These newborns have poor interactive behaviors, have difficulty responding appropriately to voices, and fail to respond well to consoling behaviors. These complications may interfere with maternal-infant attachment and increase the infant's risk of abuse and neglect (Zaichkin et al 1993).

Cocaine crosses into breast milk and may cause symptoms in the breastfeeding infant, including extreme irritability, vomiting, diarrhea, dilated pupils, and apnea. Women who continue to use cocaine after childbirth should avoid nursing.

Marijuana

Approximately 15 percent of pregnant women use marijuana, often in conjunction with alcohol and tobacco. To date, there is no evidence that marijuana has any teratogenic effects on the fetus. One study did report an increase in precipitous labors (less than 3 hours) in heavy marijuana users, but these results have not been confirmed (Niebyl 1996). The impact of heavy marijuana use on pregnancy is difficult to evaluate because of the variety of social factors that may influence the results.

Infants exposed to marijuana in utero have been reported to have increased fine tremors, prolonged startles, irritability, and poor habituation to visual stimuli, but these symptoms were not present in follow-up at 12 and 24 months of age (Cunningham et al 1997).

TABLE 12–5 Less Common Medical Conditions and Pregnancy

Condition	Brief Description	Maternal Implications	Fetal/Neonatal Implications
Rheumatoid arthritis	Chronic inflammatory disease believed to be caused by a genetically influenced antigen-antibody reaction. Symptoms include fatigue, low-grade fever, pain and swelling of joints, morning stiffness, pain on movement. Treated with salicylates, physical therapy, and rest. Corticosteroids used cautiously if not responsive to above.	Usually there is remission of rheumatoid arthritis symptoms during pregnancy, often with a relapse postpartum. Anemia may be present due to blood loss from salicylate therapy. Mother needs extra rest, particularly to relieve weight-bearing joints, but needs to continue range-of-motion exercises. If in remission, may stop medication during pregnancy.	Possibility of prolonged gestation and longer labor with heavy salicylate use. Possible teratogenic effects of salicylates.
Epilepsy	Chronic disorder characterized by seizures; may be idiopathic or secondary to other conditions, such as head injury, metabolic and nutritional disorders such as PKU or vitamin B_6 deficiency, encephalitis, neoplasms, or circulatory interferences. Treated with anticonvulsants.	Vast majority of pregnancies in women with seizure disorders are uneventful and have an excellent outcome. Women with more frequent seizures before pregnancy may have exacerbations during pregnancy but this may be related to lack of cooperation with drug regimen or sleep deprivation. During pregnancy the woman should continue to be treated with the medication that best controls her seizures. Folic acid therapy should be started prior to conception if possible. Folic acid and vitamin D are indicated throughout pregnancy (Samuels 1996b).	There is an increased incidence of stillbirth in women with epilepsy. Also, anticonvulsant medications are associated with increased incidence of congenital anomalies, especially cleft lip and heart defects, although the incidence has decreased in recent years. This may be due to the fact that the current ability to determine blood levels of medications has led to more accurate dosages and the resultant use of a single medication; consequently multiple medications are used less often (Samuels 1996b).
Hepatitis B	Hepatitis B, caused by the hepatitis B virus (HBV), is a major, growing health problem. Groups at risk include those from areas with a high incidence (primarily developing countries), illegal IV drug users, prostitutes, homosexuals, those with multiple sex partners, or occupational exposure to blood, although many infected people have no identifiable source of infection. HBV transmission is blood borne, primarily sexually and perinatally transmitted. Because of the dramatic increase and the difficulty of vaccinating high-risk individuals before they become infected, the CDC now recommends (1) testing all pregnant women for the presence of hepatitis B surface antigen (HBsAG), (2) providing immunoprophylaxis to the newborns of HBsAg-positive women, (3) providing routine vaccinations to all neonates born to HBsAg-negative women (CDC 1993).	Hepatitis B does not usually affect the course of pregnancy. However, chronic HBV carriers have a great potential for infecting others when exposure to blood and bodily fluids occurs. In addition chronic carriers may develop long-term sequelae, such as chronic liver disease and liver cancer. Approximately 4000 to 5000 deaths are caused annually by liver disease associated with chronic HBV infection. It is now recommended that all pregnant women be tested for the presence of hepatitis B surface antigen (HBsAg). A woman who is negative may be given the hepatitis vaccine.	Perinatal transmission most often occurs at or near the time of childbirth. More important, the risk of becoming a chronic carrier of the HBV is inversely related to the age of the individual at the time of initial infection (Crawford and Pruss 1993). Therefore infants infected perinatally have the highest risk of becoming chronically infected if not treated. Recommendations now include routine vaccination of all neonates born to HBsAg-negative women and immunoprophylaxis to all newborns of HBsAg-positive women.
Hyperthyroidism (thyrotoxicosis)	Enlarged, overactive thyroid gland; increased T_4:TBG ratio and increased BMR. Symptoms include muscle wasting, tachycardia, excessive sweating, and exophthalmos. Treatment by antithyroid drug propylthiouracil (PTU) while monitoring free T_4 levels. Surgery used only if drug intolerance exists.	Mild hyperthyroidism is not dangerous. Increased incidence of PIH and postpartum hemorrhage if not well controlled. Serious risk related to thyroid storm characterized by high fever, tachycardia, sweating, and congestive heart failure. Now occurs rarely. When diagnosed during pregnancy, may be transient or permanent.	Neonatal thyrotoxicosis is rare. Even low doses of antithyroid drug in mother may produce a mild fetal/neonatal hypothyroidism; higher dose may produce a goiter or mental deficiencies. Fetal loss not increased in euthyroid women. If untreated, rates of abortion, intrauterine death, and stillbirth increase. Breastfeeding contraindicated for women on antithyroid medication because it is excreted in the milk (may be tried by woman on low dose if neonatal T_4 levels are monitored).
Hypothyroidism	Characterized by inadequate thyroid secretions (decreased T_4:TBG ratio), elevated TSH, lowered BMR, and enlarged thyroid gland (goiter). Symptoms include lack of energy, excessive weight gain, cold intolerance, dry skin, and constipation. Treated by thyroxine replacement therapy.	Long-term replacement therapy usually continues at same dosage during pregnancy as before. Weekly NST after 35 weeks' gestation.	If mother untreated, fetal loss 50%; high risk of congenital goiter or true cretinism. Therefore newborns are screened for T_4 level. Mild TSH elevations present little risk because TSH does not cross the placenta.

TABLE 12–5 Less Common Medical Conditions and Pregnancy continued

Condition	Brief Description	Maternal Implications	Fetal/Neonatal Implications
Maternal phenylketonuria (PKU) (hyperphenylalaninemia)	Inherited recessive single gene anomaly causing a deficiency of the liver enzyme needed to convert the amino acid phenylalanine to tyrosine, resulting in high serum levels of phenylalanine. Brain damage and mental retardation occur if not treated early.	Low phenylalanine diet is mandatory before conception and during pregnancy. The woman should be counseled that her children will either inherit the disease or be carriers, depending on the zygosity of the father for the disease. Treatment at a PKU center is recommended.	Risk to fetus if maternal treatment not begun preconception. In untreated women increased incidence of fetal mental retardation, microcephaly, congenital heart defects, and growth retardation. Fetal phenylalanine levels are approximately 50% higher than maternal levels.
Multiple sclerosis	Neurologic disorder characterized by destruction of the myelin sheath of nerve fibers. The condition occurs primarily in young adults, more commonly in females, and is marked by periods of remission; progresses to marked physical disability in 10 to 20 years.	Associated with remission during pregnancy, but with slighly increased relapse rate postpartum (Rice and Ebers 1995). Rest is important; help with child care should be planned. Uterine contraction strength is not diminished, but because sensation is frequently lessened, labor may be almost painless.	Increased evidence of a genetic predisposition. Therefore reproductive counseling is recommended (Rice and Ebers 1995).
Systemic lupus erythematosus (SLE)	Chronic autoimmune collagen disease, characterized by exacerbations and remissions; symptoms range from characteristic rash to inflammation and pain in joints, fever, nephritis, depression, cranial nerve disorders, and peripheral neuropathies.	Women are generally advised that SLE should be in remission for at least 5–7 months before conceiving. Pregnancy does not appear to alter the long-term prognosis of women with SLE, but maternal morbidity and mortality increase. They also face an increased risk of permanent renal deterioration after pregnancy. Most maternal deaths occur in the postpartal period and are caused by pulmonary hemorrhage or lupus pneumonitis (Samuels 1996a).	Increased incidence of spontaneous abortion, stillbirth, prematurity, and IUGR. Infants born to women with SLE may have characteristic skin rash, which usually disappears by 12 months. Infants are at increased risk for complete congenital heart block, a condition that can be diagnosed prenatally. Fetal echocardiography is then performed to rule out other cardiac defects (Samuels 1996a).
Tuberculosis (TB)	Infection caused by *Mycobacterium tuberculosis;* inflammatory process causes destruction of lung tissue, increased sputum, and coughing. Associated primarily with poverty and malnutrition and may be found among refugees from countries where TB is prevalent. Treated with isoniazid and either ethambutol or rifampin or both.	The incidence of tuberculosis has begun to increase significantly since the late 1980s, and it is increasingly associated with HIV infection (Simpkins et al 1996). If TB inactive due to prior treatment, relapse rate no greater than for nonpregnant women. When isoniazid is used during pregnancy, the woman should take supplemental pyridoxine (vitamin B_6). Extra rest and limited contact with others is required until disease becomes inactive.	If maternal TB is inactive, mother may breastfeed and care for her infant. If TB is active, neonate should not have direct contact with mother until she is noninfectious. Isoniazid crosses the placenta, but most studies show no teratogenic effects. Rifampin crosses the placenta. Possibility of harmful effects still being studied.

Heroin

Heroin is an illicit CNS depressant narcotic that alters perception and produces euphoria. It is an addictive drug that is generally administered intravenously, although a snortable form of heroin called Karachi is available. Pregnancy in women who use heroin is considered high risk because of the increased incidence in these women of poor nutrition, iron deficiency anemia, and PIH. There is also an increased rate of breech position, abnormal placental implantation, abruptio placentae, preterm labor, premature rupture of the membranes (PROM), and meconium staining. These women also have a higher incidence of sexually transmitted infection because many rely on prostitution to support their drug habits.

The fetus of a heroin-addicted woman is at increased risk for IUGR, meconium aspiration, and hypoxia. The newborn frequently shows signs of heroin addiction such as restlessness; shrill, high-pitched cry; irritability; fist sucking; vomiting; and seizures. Signs of withdrawal usually appear within 72 hours and may last for several days. The newborn may exhibit poor consolability for 3 months or more. These behaviors may interfere with successful maternal-infant attachment and increase the potential for parenting problems in an already high-risk mother.

Methadone

Methadone is the most commonly used drug in the treatment of women who are dependent on opioids such as heroin. Methadone blocks withdrawal symptoms and the craving for street drugs. Dosage should be individualized at the lowest possible therapeutic level. Methadone does cross the placenta and has been associated with problems such as PIH, hepatitis, placental problems, and abnormal fetal presentation.

Prenatal exposure to methadone may result in reduced head circumference, poor motor coordination, increased body tension, and delayed achievement of motor skills. Approximately 60 to 90 percent of newborns experience withdrawal symptoms, which are often more severe than those associated with heroin (Briggs et al 1990).

Medical Therapy

A misconception exists that alcohol and drug use is found primarily in lower income or minority groups. Research indicates that in the United States there is no difference in the prevalence of drug use among whites, African Americans, and Hispanics or among private and public clinic clients (Svikis and Huggins 1996). Thus, it is wisest to screen all pregnant women for substance use during the initial prenatal visit.

Antepartal care of the pregnant addict involves medical, socioeconomic, and legal considerations. The use of a team approach allows for the comprehensive management necessary to provide safe labor and childbirth for the woman and her child.

The management of drug addiction may include hospitalization as necessary to initiate detoxification. "Cold turkey" withdrawal is not advisable during pregnancy because of potential risk to the fetus. Maintenance and support therapy are given during weekly prenatal visits. Urine screening is also done regularly throughout pregnancy if the woman is a known or suspected substance abuser. This testing helps caregivers identify the type and amount of drug being abused.

APPLYING THE NURSING PROCESS

Nursing Assessment

The nurse should be alert for clues in the history or appearance of the woman that suggest substance abuse. If abuse is suspected, the nurse needs to ask direct questions, beginning with less threatening questions about use of tobacco, caffeine, and over-the-counter medications. The nurse can then progress to questions about alcohol consumption, and finally to questions focusing on past and current use of illicit drugs. The nurse who is matter-of-fact and nonjudgmental in approach is more likely to elicit honest responses.

Nursing assessment of the woman who is a known substance abuser focuses on the woman's general health status, with specific attention to nutritional status, susceptibility to infections, and evaluation of all body systems. The nurse also assesses the woman's understanding of the impact of substance abuse on herself and her pregnancy. Some women are reluctant to discuss their substance abuse, while others are quite open about it. After establishing a relationship of trust, the nurse can gain information that can be used to plan the woman's ongoing care.

Nursing Diagnosis

Examples of nursing diagnoses that may apply include the following:

- Altered nutrition: less than body requirements related to inadequate food intake secondary to substance abuse
- Risk for infection related to use of inadequately cleaned syringes and needles secondary to IV drug use
- Knowledge deficit related to a lack of information about the impact of substance abuse on the fetus

Nursing Plan and Implementation

Prevention of substance abuse during pregnancy is the ideal nursing goal and is best accomplished through client education. Unfortunately, many women who are substance abusers do not receive regular health care and may not seek care until they are far along in pregnancy.

The nurse's role in providing prenatal care for the woman who is a substance abuser focuses on ongoing assessment and client teaching. The nurse can provide information about the relationship between substance abuse and existing health problems and the implications for the woman's unborn child. By establishing a relationship of trust and support, the nurse may be effective in ensuring the woman's cooperation.

Preparation for labor and birth should be part of prenatal planning. Relief of fear, tension, or discomfort may be achieved through nonnarcotic psychologic support and careful explanation of the labor process. If pain medication is necessary, it should not be withheld; the notion that it will contribute to further addiction is mistaken (Lynch and McKeon 1990). Preferred methods of pain relief include the use of psychoprophylaxis and regional or local anesthetics such as pudendal block and local infiltration. These techniques are preferred to decrease risk of additional fetal respiratory depression. Immediate intensive care should be available for the newborn, who will probably be depressed, small-for-gestational-age (SGA), and premature. For care of the addicted newborn, see Chapter 25.

Evaluation

Anticipated outcomes of nursing care include

- The woman is able to describe the impact of her substance abuse on herself and her unborn child.
- The woman successfully participates in a drug therapy program.
- The woman gives birth to a healthy infant.
- The woman agrees to cooperate with a referral to social services (or another appropriate community agency) for follow-up care after discharge.

Other Medical Conditions and Pregnancy

A woman with a preexisting medical condition should be aware of the possible impact of pregnancy on her condition, as well as the impact of her condition on the successful outcome of her pregnancy. Table 12–5, on pages 276–277, discusses some of the less common medical conditions vis-à-vis pregnancy.

CHAPTER HIGHLIGHTS

- Almost any health problem that a person can have when not pregnant can coexist with pregnancy. Some problems, such as anemias, may be exacerbated by pregnancy. Others, such as collagen disease, may go into temporary remission with pregnancy. Regardless of the health problem, careful health care is needed throughout pregnancy to improve the outcome for mother and fetus.
- The diagnosis of high-risk pregnancy can shock an expectant couple. Providing emotional support, teaching about the condition and prognosis, and educating for self-care are important nursing measures that help clients cope.
- Cardiac disease during pregnancy requires careful assessment, limitation of activity, and knowing and reporting signs of impending cardiac decompensation by both client and nurse.
- The key point in the care of the pregnant diabetic is scrupulous maternal plasma glucose control. This is best achieved by home blood glucose monitoring, multiple daily insulin injections, and a careful diet. To reduce incidence of congenital anomalies and other problems in the newborn, the woman should maintain a normal blood glucose before conception and throughout the pregnancy. Diabetics more than most other clients need to be educated about their condition and involved with their own care.
- HIV infection, which is transmitted via blood and body fluids, may also be transmitted transplacentally to the fetus. Currently there is no definitive treatment for HIV/AIDS. Nurses should employ blood and body fluid precautions (universal precautions) in caring for all women to avoid potential spread of infection.
- Substance abuse (either drugs or alcohol) not only is detrimental to the mother's health but also may have profound lasting effects on the fetus. Nurses need to be alert to signs of substance abuse and nonjudgmental in their care of women who practice substance abuse.

REFERENCES

ACOG: *Human Immunodeficiency Virus Infections.* ACOG Technical Bulletin June 1992; No. 169.

Briggs GG et al: *Drugs in Pregnancy and Lactation,* 3rd ed. Baltimore: Williams & Wilkins, 1990.

Centers for Disease Control and Prevention: 1993 sexually transmitted disease treatment guidelines. *MMWR* 1993; 42(RR-14):4.

Cohn JA: Human immunodeficiency virus and AIDS 1993 update. *J Nurse Midwifery* March/April 1993; 38(2):65.

Crawford N, Pruss A: Preventing neonatal hepatitis B infection during the perinatal period. *JOGNN* 1993: 22(6):491.

Criteria Committee of the New York Heart Association, Inc: *Nomenclature and Criteria for Diagnosis of Diseases of the Heart and Great Vessels,* 8th ed. New York: New York Heart Association, 1979.

Cruikshank DP: Cardiovascular, pulmonary, renal, and hematologic diseases in pregnancy. In: *Danforth's Obstetrics and Gynecology,* 7th ed. Scott JR et al (editors). Philadelphia: Lippincott, 1994.

Cunningham FG et al: *Williams Obstetrics,* 20th ed. Stamford, CT: Appleton & Lange, 1997.

Duff P: Maternal and perinatal infection. In: *Obstetrics: Normal and Problem Pregnancies,* 3rd ed. Gabbe SG et al (editors). New York: Churchill Livingstone, 1996.

Eyler AE: Current issues in the primary care of women with HIV. *Female Patient* April 1996; 21:14.

Eyler AE: Current issues in the primary care of women with HIV. *Female Patient* July 1995; 20:15.

Gabbe SG: High risk pregnancy: Diabetes mellitus. *Contemp OB/GYN* July 1996; 41(7):13.

Horton JA (editor): *The Women's Health Data Book.* Washington, DC: Elsevier, 1992.

HRSA Program Advisory: *Use of zidovudine (ZDV) to Reduce Perinatal HIV Transmission in HRSA-Funded Programs.* Washington DC: US Dept. of Health and Human Services Health Resources and Services Administration, December 1995.

Landon MB: Diabetes mellitus and other endocrine diseases. In: *Obstetrics: Normal and Problem Pregnancies,* 3rd ed. Gabbe SG et al (editors). New York: Churchill Livingstone, 1996.

Landon MB, Samuels P: Cardiac and pulmonary disease. In: *Obstetrics: Normal and Problem Pregnancies,* 3rd ed. Gabbe SG et al (editors). New York: Churchill Livingstone, 1996.

Lawrence RA: Breastfeeding and medical disease. *Med Clin North Am* May 1989; 73:583.

Lindberg CE: Perinatal transmission of HIV: How to counsel women. *MCN* July/August 1995; 20:207.

Lynch M, McKeon VA: Cocaine use during pregnancy. *JOGNN* July/August 1990; 19:285.

Mandeville LK: Diabetes mellitus in pregnancy. In: *High-Risk Intrapartum Nursing.* Mandeville LK, Troiano NH (editors). Philadelphia: Lippincott, 1992.

Morbidity and Mortality Weekly Report: Supplement. Recommendations for prevention of HIV transmission in health care settings. *MMWR* August 21, 1987; 36(25):2.

National Diabetes Data Group: *Classification of Diabetes Mellitus and Other Categories of Glucose Intolerance.* Washington, DC: NIH, 1979.

Niebyl JR: Drugs in pregnancy and lactation. In: *Obstetrics: Normal and Problem Pregnancies,* 3rd ed. Gabbe SG et al (editors). New York: Churchill Livingstone, 1996.

Reece EA et al: When the pregnancy is complicated by diabetes. *Contemp OB/GYN* June 1995; 40(7):43.

Samuels P: Collagen vascular diseases. In: *Obstetrics: Normal and Problem Pregnancies,* 3rd ed. Gabbe SG et al (editors). New York: Churchill Livingstone, 1996a.

Samuels P: Neurologic disorders. In: *Obstetrics: Normal and Problem Pregnancies,* 3rd ed. Gabbe SG et al (editors). New York: Churchill Livingstone, 1996b.

Simpkins SM et al: Management of the obstetric patient with tuberculosis. *JOGNN* May 1996; 25(4):305.

Spellacy WN: Diabetes mellitus and pregnancy. In: *Danforth's Obstetrics and Gynecology,* 7th ed. Scott JR et al (editors). Philadelphia: Lippincott, 1994.

Svikis D; Huggins G: Substance abuse in pregnancy: Screening and intervention. *Contemp OB/GYN* April 1996; 41(4):32.

Weathers WT et al: Cocaine use in women from a defined population: Prevalence at delivery and effects on growth in infants. *Pediatrics* 1993; 91(2):350.

Zaichkin J et al: The drug-exposed mother and infant: A regional center experience. *Neonatal Network* 1993; 12(3):41.

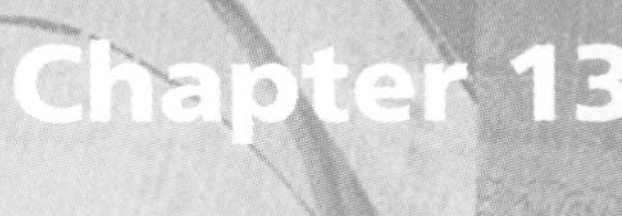

Chapter 13 Pregnancy at Risk: Gestational Onset

OBJECTIVES

- Discuss the medical therapy and nursing care of a woman with hyperemesis gravidarum.
- Contrast the etiology, medical therapy, and nursing interventions for the various bleeding problems associated with pregnancy.
- Identify the medical therapy and nursing interventions indicated in caring for a woman with an incompetent cervix.
- Delineate the nursing care needs of a woman experiencing premature rupture of the membranes or preterm labor.
- Describe the development and course of hypertensive disorders associated with pregnancy.
- Explain the cause and prevention of hemolytic disease of the newborn secondary to Rh incompatibility.
- Compare Rh incompatibility to ABO incompatibility with regard to occurrence, treatment, and implication for the fetus/newborn.
- Summarize the effects of surgical procedures on pregnancy and explain ways in which pregnancy may complicate diagnosis.
- Discuss the implications of trauma due to accidents or battering for the pregnant woman and her fetus.
- Describe the effects of infections on the pregnant woman and her unborn child.

KEY TERMS

Abortion
Eclampsia
Ectopic pregnancy
Erythroblastosis fetalis
Gestational trophoblastic disease (GTD)
HELLP syndrome
Hydatidiform mole
Hydrops fetalis
Hyperemesis gravidarum
Incompetent cervix
Miscarriage
Preeclampsia
Pregnancy-induced hypertension (PIH)
Premature rupture of membranes (PROM)
Preterm labor
Rh immune globulin (RhoGAM)
Tocolysis

Pregnancy is usually an uncomplicated experience. In some cases, however, problems arise during the pregnancy that place the woman and her unborn child at risk. Regular prenatal care serves to detect these potential complications quickly so that effective care can be provided. This chapter focuses on problems that primarily occur during pregnancy, those with a *gestational onset.*

Care of the Woman with Hyperemesis Gravidarum

Hyperemesis gravidarum is excessive vomiting during pregnancy. It may be mild at first, but true hyperemesis may progress to a point at which the woman not only vomits everything she swallows, but retches between meals.

Although the exact cause of hyperemesis is unclear, it may be related to increased levels of human chorionic gonadotropin (hCG) and estradiol (Long and Russell 1993). Other variables under investigation include a possible dysfunction of the pituitary-adrenal axis or a transient increase in thyroid function (Varner 1994). It may sometimes be stimulated or exaggerated by psychologic factors.

In severe cases, the pathology begins with dehydration, which leads to fluid-electrolyte imbalance and alkalosis from loss of hydrochloric acid. Hypovolemia, hypotension, tachycardia, increased hematocrit and blood urea nitrogen (BUN), and decreased urine output can also occur. If untreated, metabolic acidosis may develop. Severe potassium loss may disrupt cardiac functioning. Starvation causes muscle wasting and severe protein and vitamin deficiencies. Fetal or embryonic death may result, and the woman may suffer irreversible metabolic changes or death.

Medical Therapy

The goals of treatment include control of vomiting, correction of dehydration, restoration of electrolyte balance, and maintenance of adequate nutrition. Initially the woman is given nothing by mouth (NPO). Intravenous fluids containing glucose, vitamins (B-complex, C, A, and D), and electrolytes are administered. Agents commonly used to control the nausea and vomiting of hyperemesis gravidarum include the phenothiazines (prochlorperazine, chlorpromazine, and pyridoxine) and antihistamines such as meclizine and trimethobenzamide (Varner 1994). Typically the woman remains NPO for 48 hours. IV therapy continues until all vomiting stops. If her condition does not improve, total parenteral nutrition may be needed. She then begins controlled oral feedings.

APPLYING THE NURSING PROCESS

Nursing Assessment

When a woman is hospitalized for control of vomiting, the nurse regularly assesses the amount and character of any emesis, intake and output, fetal heart rate, evidence of jaundice or bleeding, and the woman's emotional state.

Nursing Diagnosis

Nursing diagnoses that may apply to a woman with hyperemesis gravidarum include the following:

- Altered nutrition: less than body requirements related to persistent vomiting secondary to hyperemesis
- Fear related to the effects of hyperemesis on fetal well-being

Nursing Plan and Implementation

Nursing care should be supportive and directed at maintaining a relaxed, quiet environment away from food odors or offensive smells. Once oral feedings resume, food should be attractively served. Oral hygiene is important because the mouth is dry and may be irritated from vomitus. Because emotional factors have been found to play a major role in this condition, psychotherapy may be recommended. With proper treatment, prognosis is favorable.

Evaluation

Anticipated outcomes of nursing care include

- The woman is able to explain hyperemesis gravidarum, its therapy, and its possible effects on her pregnancy.
- The woman's condition is corrected and possible complications are avoided.

Care of the Woman with a Bleeding Disorder

During the first and second trimesters of pregnancy, the major cause of bleeding is **abortion.** This is the expulsion of the fetus prior to viability, which is considered to be 20 weeks' gestation. Abortions are either *spontaneous* (occurring naturally) or *induced* (occurring as a result of artificial or mechanical interruption). **Miscarriage** is a lay term applied to spontaneous abortion.

Other complications that can cause bleeding in the first half of pregnancy are ectopic pregnancy and gestational trophoblastic disease. In the second half of pregnancy, particularly in the third trimester, the two major causes of bleeding are placenta previa and abruptio placentae. They are discussed in detail in Chapter 19.

General Principles of Nursing Intervention

Spotting is relatively common during pregnancy and usually occurs following sexual intercourse or exercise because of trauma to the highly vascular cervix. However, the woman is advised to report for evaluation any spotting or bleeding that occurs during pregnancy.

It is often the nurse's responsibility to make the initial assessment of bleeding. In general, the following nursing measures should be implemented for pregnant women being treated for bleeding disorders:

- Monitor blood pressure and pulse frequently.
- Observe woman for behaviors indicative of shock, such as pallor, clammy skin, perspiration, dyspnea, or restlessness.
- Count pads to assess amount of bleeding over a given time period; save any tissue or clots expelled.
- If pregnancy is of 12 weeks' gestation or beyond, assess fetal heart tones with a Doppler.
- Prepare for intravenous therapy. There may be standing orders to begin IV therapy on bleeding clients.
- Prepare equipment for examination.
- Have oxygen therapy available.
- Collect and organize all data, including antepartal history, onset of bleeding episode, and laboratory studies (hemoglobin, hematocrit, and hormonal assays).
- Assess coping mechanisms of woman in crisis. Give emotional support to enhance her coping abilities by continuous, sustained presence; by clear explanation of procedures; and by communicating her status to her family. Most importantly, prepare the woman for possible fetal loss. Assess her expressions of anger, denial, silence, guilt, depression, or self-blame.

Spontaneous Abortion

Many pregnancies end in the first trimester because of spontaneous abortion. Often the woman assumes she is having a heavy menstrual period when she is really having an early abortion. Thus statistics are inaccurate, but the incidence is about 10 to 12 percent for clinically recognized pregnancies and about 16 percent overall (Simpson 1996).

At least 50 percent of early spontaneous abortions are related to chromosomal abnormalities (Simpson 1996). Other causes include teratogenic drugs, faulty implantation due to abnormalities of the female reproductive tract, a weakened cervix, placental abnormalities, chronic maternal diseases, endocrine imbalances, and maternal infections from the TORCH group. Research does not support the belief that accidents or psychic trauma are primary causes of spontaneous abortion.

Spontaneous abortion can be extremely distressing to the couple desiring a child. Chances for carrying the next pregnancy to term after one spontaneous abortion are as good as they are for the general population. Thereafter, however, chances of successful pregnancy decrease with each succeeding spontaneous abortion.

Classification

Spontaneous abortions are subdivided into the following categories to differentiate them clinically:

1. *Threatened abortion.* The fetus is jeopardized by unexplained bleeding, cramping, and backache. The cervix is closed. Bleeding may persist for days. It may be followed by partial or complete expulsion of the products of pregnancy (Figure 13–1).
2. *Imminent abortion.* Bleeding and cramping increase. The internal cervical os dilates. Membranes may rupture. The term *inevitable abortion* also applies.
3. *Complete abortion.* All the products of conception are expelled.
4. *Incomplete abortion.* Some of the products of conception are retained, most often the placenta. The internal cervical os is dilated slightly.
5. *Missed abortion.* The fetus dies in utero but is not expelled. Uterine growth ceases, breast changes regress, and the woman may report a brownish vaginal discharge. The cervix is closed. Diagnosis is based on history, pelvic examination, and a negative pregnancy test and may be confirmed by ultrasound if necessary. If the fetus is retained beyond 6 weeks, the breakdown of fetal tissues results in the release of thromboplastin, and disseminated intravascular coagulation (DIC) may develop.
6. *Habitual abortion.* Abortion occurs consecutively in three or more pregnancies.

Medical Therapy

One of the more reliable indicators of potential spontaneous abortion is the presence of pelvic cramping and backache. These symptoms are usually absent in

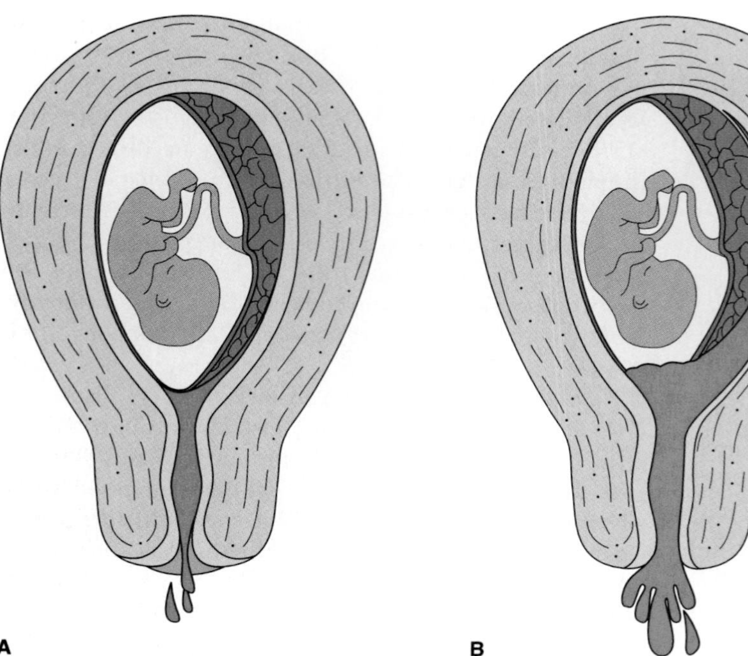

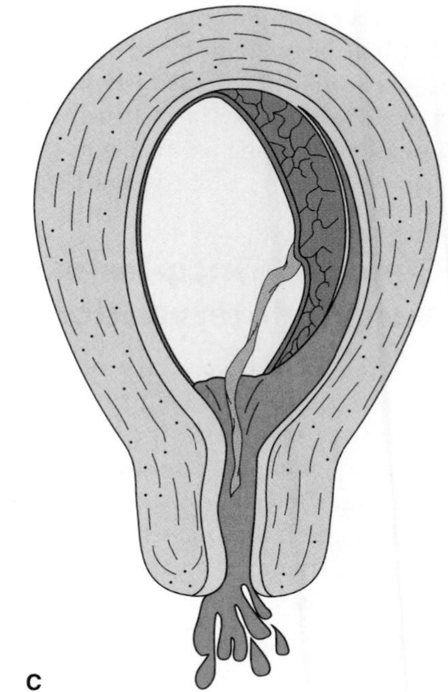

FIGURE 13–1 Types of spontaneous abortion. ***A*** Threatened. The cervix is not dilated, and the placenta is still attached to the uterine wall, but some bleeding occurs. ***B*** Imminent. The placenta has separated from the uterine wall, the cervix has dilated, and the amount of bleeding has increased. ***C*** Incomplete. The embryo/fetus has passed out of the uterus; however, the placenta remains.

bleeding caused by polyps, ruptured cervical blood vessels, or cervical erosion. Ultrasound scanning may be used to detect the presence of a gestational sac if the cause of bleeding is unclear. Results of human chorionic gonadotropin (hCG) levels are not particularly helpful, because hCG levels fall slowly after fetal death and therefore cannot confirm a live embryo/fetus. Hemoglobin and hematocrit are obtained to assess blood loss. Blood is typed and crossmatched for possible replacement needs.

The therapy prescribed for the pregnant woman with bleeding is abstinence from coitus and perhaps sedation. If bleeding persists and abortion is imminent or incomplete, the woman may be hospitalized, intravenous therapy or blood transfusions may be started to replace fluid, and dilatation and curettage or suction evacuation is performed to remove the remainder of the products of conception. If the woman is Rh-negative and not sensitized, anti-D Rh immune globulin is given within 72 hours (see discussion on Rh sensitization later in this chapter).

In missed abortions, the products of conception eventually are expelled spontaneously. If this does not occur within 4–6 weeks after fetal death, hospitalization is necessary. Dilatation and curettage or suction evacuation is done if the pregnancy is in the first trimester. Beyond 12 weeks' gestation, induction of labor by intravenous oxytocin and prostaglandins may be used to expel the dead fetus.

APPLYING THE NURSING PROCESS

Nursing Assessment

The nurse assesses the woman's vital signs, amount of bleeding, level of comfort, and physical health. The nurse also assesses the responses of the woman and her family to this crisis and evaluates their coping mechanisms and ability to comfort each other.

Nursing Diagnosis

Examples of nursing diagnoses that may apply include the following:

- Fear related to possible pregnancy loss
- Pain related to abdominal cramping secondary to threatened abortion
- Anticipatory grieving related to expected loss of unborn child

Nursing Plan and Implementation

The physical pain of the cramps and the amount of bleeding may be more severe than a couple anticipates, even when they are prepared for the possibility of an abortion. Nurses can provide support by explaining why the discomfort is occurring and by providing analgesics for pain relief.

Providing emotional support is an important task for nurses caring for women who have spontaneously aborted, because the attachment process already begun is disrupted. Feelings of shock or disbelief are normal at first. Couples who approached the pregnancy with feelings of joy and a sense of expectancy now feel grief, sadness, and possibly anger.

Because many women, even with planned pregnancies, feel some ambivalence initially, guilt is a common emotion. These feelings may be even stronger for women who were negative about their pregnancies. The woman may harbor negative feelings about herself or even believe that the abortion may be a punishment for some wrongdoing.

The nurse can offer invaluable psychologic support to the woman and her family by encouraging them to talk about their feelings, allowing them the privacy to grieve, and listening sympathetically to their concerns about this pregnancy and future ones. The nurse may help decrease feelings of guilt or blame by informing the woman and her family about the causes of spontaneous abortion. The nurse can also refer them to other health care professionals for additional help as necessary.

The grieving period following a spontaneous abortion usually lasts 6 to 24 months. Many couples can be helped during this period by an organization or support group established for parents who have lost a fetus or newborn.

Evaluation

Anticipated outcomes of nursing care include

- The woman is able to explain spontaneous abortion, the treatment measures employed in her care, and long-term implications for future pregnancies.
- The woman suffers no complications.
- The woman and her partner are able to begin verbalizing their grief and acknowledge that the grieving process usually lasts several months.

Ectopic Pregnancy

Ectopic pregnancy is the implantation of the blastocyst in a site other than the endometrial lining of the uterus. It has many causes, including tubal damage caused by pelvic inflammatory disease (PID); previous pelvic or tubal surgery; endometriosis; previous ectopic pregnancy; presence of an IUD; high levels of estrogen and progesterone, which can alter the motility of the egg in the fallopian tube; congenital anomalies of the tube; and blighted ovum (Hammond and Bachus 1994).

The incidence of ectopic pregnancy has increased dramatically in the past several years. Currently there is 1 ectopic pregnancy for every 44 live births in the United States (Hammond and Bachus 1994). This increased incidence may be related in part to improved diagnostic technology. Approximately 10 percent of maternal mortality is due to ectopic pregnancy (Simpson 1996).

Ectopic pregnancy occurs when the fertilized ovum is prevented or slowed in its passage through the tube. The fertilized ovum then implants elsewhere. The most common location for implantation is the ampulla of the fallopian tube. Figure 13–2 identifies other implantation sites.

Initially the normal symptoms of pregnancy may be present, specifically amenorrhea, breast tenderness, and nausea. The hormone hCG is present in the blood and urine. As the pregnancy progresses, the chorionic villi grow into the wall of the tube or site of implantation and a blood supply is established. When the embryo outgrows this space, the tube ruptures and there is bleeding into the abdominal cavity. This bleeding irritates the peritoneum, causing the characteristic symptoms of sharp, one-sided pain, syncope, and referred shoulder pain. The woman may also experience lower abdominal pain. Vaginal bleeding, a common finding, occurs when the embryo dies and the decidua begins to slough.

Physical examination usually reveals adnexal tenderness. (The adnexae are the areas of the lower abdomen located over each ovary and fallopian tube.) An adnexal mass is palpable about half the time. Bleeding tends to be slow and chronic, and the abdomen gradually becomes rigid and very tender. With extensive bleeding into the abdominal cavity, pelvic examination causes extreme pain, and a mass of blood may be palpated in the cul-de-sac of Douglas.

Laboratory tests may reveal low hemoglobin and hematocrit levels and rising leukocyte levels. The hCG titers are lower than in intrauterine pregnancy.

Medical Therapy

Diagnosis of ectopic pregnancy begins with an assessment of menstrual history, including the last menstrual period (LMP), followed by a careful pelvic exam to identify any abnormal pelvic masses and tenderness. Ultrasound may be useful in confirming an intrauterine pregnancy or in identifying a gestational sac in an unruptured tubal pregnancy. Laparoscopy may reveal an extrauterine pregnancy and is especially helpful in diagnosing an unruptured tubal pregnancy.

Two laboratory tests aid in diagnosis:

- *Serial testing of serum hCG levels.* In normal pregnancy, hCG levels double every 48–72 hours, while in ectopic pregnancy they increase more slowly and then begin to diminish.
- *Serum progesterone levels.* Progesterone concentrations tend to be lower in ectopic pregnancy (< 5 ng/mL) than in normal intrauterine pregnancies, which typically are ≥ 25 ng/mL (Simpson 1996).

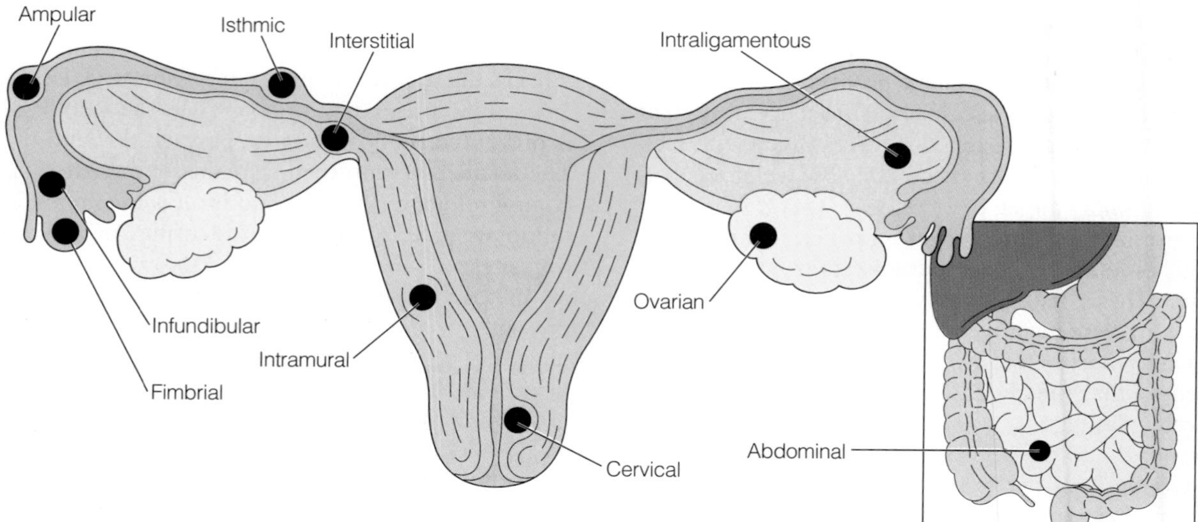

FIGURE 13–2 Various implantation sites in ectopic pregnancy. The most common site is within the fallopian tube, hence the name "tubal pregnancy." Implantation may also occur within the abdominal cavity.

Formerly culdocentesis was used as the primary tool for diagnosing ectopic pregnancy. In culdocentesis, a needle is inserted through the posterior vaginal vault into the cul-de-sac of Douglas. If nonclotting blood (blood that was clotted and then fibrinolysed) is aspirated, it is indicative of ectopic pregnancy. Currently, culdocentesis is used if ultrasound is not available.

Once the diagnosis of ectopic pregnancy is made, surgery is usually necessary. Conservative treatment involves salpingostomy via a laparoscope. This method involves using a laser to make a linear incision in the tube, and then gently removing the products of conception through the laparoscope. The surgical incision is left open and allowed to close by secondary intention (Simpson 1996). If the ectopic pregnancy is too advanced, laparotomy is indicated. If the tube is badly damaged, total salpingectomy is performed, leaving the ovary in place unless it is damaged. If rupture and massive infection are found, it is sometimes necessary to remove the uterus, tubes, and ovaries.

Intravenous therapy and blood transfusion are used to replace fluid loss. During surgery the most important risk to be considered is potential hemorrhage. Bleeding must be controlled and replacement therapy should be on hand. The Rh-negative nonsensitized woman is given Rh immune globulin to prevent sensitization.

Recently, drug therapy to induce dissolution of the ectopic pregnancy has been attempted with some success. The drug used is usually methotrexate, a folic acid antagonist, which acts by inhibiting cell division. The drug, which is given intramuscularly, has the advantage of being less expensive than surgery when done on an outpatient basis. Tubal healing is improved, and there is a greater chance of maintaining fertility (Maiolatesi and Peddicord 1996).

APPLYING THE NURSING PROCESS

Nursing Assessment

When the woman with a suspected ectopic pregnancy is admitted to the hospital, the nurse assesses the appearance and amount of vaginal bleeding, and monitors vital signs for evidence of developing shock.

The nurse assesses the woman's emotional state and coping abilities, and determines the couple's informational needs. The woman may experience marked abdominal discomfort, so the nurse also determines the woman's level of pain. If surgery is necessary, the nurse performs the ongoing assessments appropriate postoperatively.

Nursing Diagnosis

Nursing diagnoses that may apply for a woman with an ectopic pregnancy include the following:

- Anticipatory grieving related to the loss of the pregnancy
- Pain related to abdominal bleeding secondary to tubal rupture
- Knowledge deficit related to lack of information about treatment of ectopic pregnancy and its long-term implications

Nursing Plan and Implementation

Once a diagnosis of ectopic pregnancy is made and surgery is scheduled, the nurse starts an IV as ordered and begins preoperative teaching. The nurse should immediately report signs of developing shock. If the woman is experiencing severe abdominal pain, the nurse can administer appropriate analgesics and evaluate their effectiveness.

Teaching is an important part of the nursing care. The woman may want her condition and various procedures explained. She may need instruction about measures to prevent infection, symptoms to report (pain, bleeding, fever), and her follow-up visit.

The woman and her family will need emotional support during this difficult time. Their feelings and responses to this crisis will probably be similar to those that occur in cases of spontaneous abortion. As a result, similar nursing actions are required for these women.

Evaluation

Anticipated outcomes of nursing care include

- The woman is able to explain ectopic pregnancy, treatment alternatives, and implications for future childbearing.
- The woman and her caregivers detect possible complications of therapy early and manage them successfully.
- The woman and her partner are able to begin verbalizing their loss and acknowledge that the grieving process usually lasts several months.

Gestational Trophoblastic Disease

Gestational trophoblastic disease (GTD) includes hydatidiform mole, invasive mole (chorioadenoma destruens), and choriocarcinoma.

Hydatidiform mole (molar pregnancy) is a disease in which (a) the chorionic villi of the placenta become swollen, fluid-filled (hydropic), grapelike clusters, while a central fluid-filled space forms in the placenta (central cistern formation); and (b) the trophoblastic tissue proliferates. The disease results in the loss of the pregnancy and the possibility, though remote, of developing choriocarcinoma from the trophoblastic tissue.

Molar pregnancies are classified into two types, complete and partial, both of which meet the above criteria. In the United States, complete moles are more common than partial moles, occurring in about 1 in 2000 pregnancies (Urbanski et al 1996). A complete mole develops from an ovum containing no maternal genetic material that is fertilized by a normal sperm. The embryo dies very early, no circulation is established, the hydropic vesicles are avascular, and no embryonic tissue or membranes are found. Choriocarcinoma seems to be associated exclusively with the complete mole.

The partial mole usually has a triploid karyotype (69 chromosomes), generally because of failure of either the ovum or sperm to undergo the first meiotic division. There may be a fetal sac or even a fetus with a heartbeat. The fetus has multiple anomalies because of the triploidy and little chance for survival. The villi are often vascularized and may be hydropic in only portions of the placenta. Often partial moles are recognized only after spontaneous abortion, and they may go unnoticed even then.

Invasive mole (chorioadenoma destruens) is similar to a complete mole, but it involves the uterine myometrium. Treatment is the same as for complete mole.

Medical Therapy

Initially the clinical picture is similar to that of pregnancy. However, classic signs soon appear. Vaginal bleeding occurs almost universally. It is often brownish (like prune juice) due to liquefaction of the uterine clot, but it may be bright red. Because of the rapid proliferation of the trophoblastic cells that occurs with complete moles, uterine enlargement may be greater than expected for gestational age. Hydropic vesicles may be passed, and, if so, are diagnostic. With a partial mole the vesicles are often smaller and may not be noticed. In addition, because serum hCG levels are higher than with normal pregnancy, the woman may experience hyperemesis gravidarum. Symptoms of pregnancy-induced hypertension (PIH) prior to 24 weeks' gestation strongly suggest a molar pregnancy. No fetal heart tones are heard and no fetal movement is palpated. Ultrasound is the primary diagnostic tool and may reveal a characteristic molar pattern.

Therapy begins with evacuation of the mole and curettage of the uterus to remove all fragments of the placenta. Early evacuation decreases the possibility of other complications. If the woman is older and has completed her childbearing, or if there is excessive bleeding, hysterectomy may be the treatment of choice to reduce the risk of choriocarcinoma.

The woman treated for hydatidiform mole should receive follow-up therapy for a year. Follow-up care includes baseline chest x-ray exam to detect metastasis, physical exam including pelvic exam, and regular measurements of serum hCG levels. The woman avoids pregnancy during that time because the elevated hCG levels associated with pregnancy would cause confusion about whether choriocarcinoma had developed.

Continued high or rising hCG titers are abnormal. If they occur, dilatation and curettage is performed, and the tissue is examined. If malignant cells are found, treatment at a center specializing in GTD is advised. Chemotherapy for choriocarcinoma is started using methotrexate alone or in combination with other chemotherapy agents. If therapy is ineffective, the choriocarcinoma has a tendency to metastasize rapidly.

If, after a year of monitoring, the hCG serum titers are within normal limits, a couple may be assured that subsequent normal pregnancy can be anticipated with a low probability of recurring hydatidiform mole.

COMMUNITY IN FOCUS Healthy Beginnings

More and more communities are acting proactively to improve the parenting skills of their residents and decrease the incidence of child abuse and neglect. One especially successful program is the Healthy Beginnings Program in Hastings, Nebraska. Established in 1990, the program, which is the first mainland replication of the successful Hawaii Healthy Start Program, is a home visitation program designed to help parents be "the best they can be." The program is voluntary and free to participants.

Families enter the program prenatally or up to three months following the birth of a child. Approximately 75 percent of families are referred to the program by a health care professional; the remainder are self-referred or referred by another agency. Once a contact is made, each family is seen by a nurse and paraprofessional for an interview and initial assessment. The Family Stress Checklist, developed in 1978 by Smith and Carroll of the University of Colorado Health Sciences Center, is used to screen families as low, moderate, or high risk for parenting problems. All moderate and high-risk families are invited to join the program.

The program offers long-term and intensive services. Prenatally, parents participate in a series of nursing home visits to discuss a wide variety of topics related to pregnancy and parenting. Additional nursing visits are scheduled in the home following childbirth and again within the first month. The emphasis of these early visits is on adjustment to the newborn and on learning to read and respond appropriately to the baby's cues. Moreover, six times during the first two years, nurses complete developmental assessments of each child and make appropriate referrals if they identify any concerns or developmental delays. Nurses also regularly assess and educate parents about issues such as age-appropriate developmental expectations and activities, and parent-child interactions and communication.

In addition, the family is visited weekly by a specially trained paraprofessional who helps the family develop skill in parenting. To ensure consistency and promote a sense of trust, the family works with the same paraprofessional and nurse throughout the duration of services. These weekly visits last up to a year or more and then progress to bi-weekly and quarterly visits as the family gains skills and confidence. Visits continue until the child is five years old. Throughout the process, families receive case management services including community and professional referrals and networking, health, nutritional and safety assessments, and encouragement to use the health care system appropriately (clinic, ER, phone support). Results to date are impressive. Of the families served by Healthy Beginnings:

- 98 percent have no child abuse or neglect requiring court involvement.
- 97 percent of the children are up-to-date on their well child care and immunizations.
- At least 98 percent of the families have no unintended repeat pregnancies.
- Over 80 percent of the families are either employed, furthering their education, or both.

Source: Personal communication with Paula Witt, RN, PNP, Director of the Healthy Beginnings Program, and printed program materials.

APPLYING THE NURSING PROCESS

Nursing Assessment

It is important for nurses involved in antepartal care to be aware of symptoms of hydatidiform mole and observe for them at each antepartal visit. The classic symptoms used to diagnose molar pregnancy are found more frequently with the complete than with the partial mole. Before evacuation, the partial mole may be difficult to distinguish from a missed abortion. If a molar pregnancy is diagnosed, the nurse should assess the woman's (or the couple's) understanding of the condition and its implications.

Nursing Diagnosis

Nursing diagnoses that may apply to a woman with a hydatidiform mole include the following:

- Fear related to the possible development of choriocarcinoma
- Anticipatory grieving related to the loss of the pregnancy

Nursing Plan and Implementation

When a molar pregnancy is suspected, the woman needs support. The nurse can relieve some of the woman's anxiety by answering questions about the condition and explaining what ultrasound and other diagnostic procedures will entail. If a molar pregnancy is diagnosed, the nurse supports the childbearing family as they deal with their grief about the lost pregnancy. Health care counselors, the hospital chaplain, or their own clergy may be able to help them deal with this loss.

When the woman is hospitalized for evacuation of the mole, the nurse must monitor vital signs and vaginal bleeding for evidence of hemorrhage. In addition, the nurse determines whether abdominal pain is present and evaluates the woman's emotional state and coping ability. Typed and crossmatched blood must be available for surgery because of previous blood loss and the potential for hemorrhage. Oxytocin is administered to keep the uterus contracted and prevent hemorrhage. If the woman is Rh-negative and not sensitized, she is given Rh immune globulin to prevent antibody formation.

The woman needs to understand the importance of the follow-up visits. She is advised to delay becoming pregnant again until after the follow-up program is completed.

Evaluation

Anticipated outcomes of nursing care include

- The woman has a smooth recovery following successful evacuation of the mole.
- The woman is able to explain GTD, its treatment, follow-up, and long-term implications for pregnancy.
- The woman and her partner are able to begin verbalizing their grief at the loss of their anticipated child.
- The woman can discuss the importance of follow-up assessment and indicates her willingness to cooperate with the regimen.

Care of the Woman with an Incompetent Cervix

Incompetent cervix refers to the premature dilatation of the cervix, usually in the fourth or fifth month of pregnancy. It is associated with repeated second-trimester abortions. Possible causes include cervical trauma associated with previous surgery or birth, congenital cervical structural defects, or uterine anomalies.

Diagnosis is established by eliciting a positive history of repeated, relatively painless and bloodless second trimester abortions. Serial pelvic exams early in the second trimester reveal progressive effacement and dilatation of the cervix and bulging of the membranes through the cervical os. If incompetent cervix is suspected, serial ultrasound provides information on dilatation of the internal cervical os before a dilated external os is detected.

Incompetent cervix is managed surgically with a Shirodkar-Barter operation (cerclage)—or a modification of it by McDonald—which reinforces the weakened cervix by encircling it at the level of the internal os with suture material. A purse-string suture is placed in the cervix between 14 and 18 weeks of gestation. Once the suture is in place, a cesarean birth may be planned (to prevent repeating the procedure in subsequent pregnancies), or the suture may be released at term and vaginal birth permitted. The woman must understand the importance of contacting her physician immediately if her membranes rupture or labor begins. The physician can remove the suture to prevent possible complications. The success rate for carrying the pregnancy to term is 80 to 90 percent (Scott 1994a).

Care of the Woman with Premature Rupture of Membranes

Premature rupture of membranes (PROM) is spontaneous rupture of the membranes and leakage of amniotic fluid prior to the onset of labor. Preterm PROM (PPROM) is defined as rupture of membranes that occurs before 37 weeks' gestation. PROM is associated with infection, previous history of PROM, hydramnios, multiple pregnancy, UTI, amniocentesis, placenta previa, abruptio placentae, trauma, incompetent cervix, bleeding during pregnancy, and maternal genital tract anomalies.

Maternal risk is related to infection, specifically chorioamnionitis (intra-amniotic infection resulting from bacterial invasion before birth) and endometritis (postpartal infection of the endometrium).

Fetal-newborn implications include risk of

- Respiratory distress syndrome (with PPROM)
- Fetal sepsis due to ascending pathogens
- Malpresentation
- Prolapse of the umbilical cord
- Increased perinatal morbidity and mortality

Medical Therapy

After confirming with nitrazine paper and a microscopic examination (ferning test) that the membranes have ruptured, the gestational age of the fetus is calculated. Single or combination methods of calculation may be used, including Nägele's rule, fundal height, ultrasound to measure the fetal biparietal diameter (BPD) and femur length, and amniocentesis to identify lung maturity (Chapter 14). The gestational age of the fetus and the presence or absence of infection determine the direction of treatment for PROM. If maternal signs and symptoms of infection are evident, antibiotic therapy (usually by intravenous infusion) is initiated immediately, and the fetus is born vaginally or by cesarean regardless of the gestational age. Upon admission to the nursery, the newborn is assessed for sepsis and placed on antibiotics. Chapter 26 provides further information about the newborn with sepsis.

Management of PROM in the absence of infection and gestation of less than 37 weeks is usually conservative. The woman is hospitalized on bed rest. On admission, complete blood cell count (CBC), C-reactive protein, and urinalysis are obtained. Continuous electronic fetal monitoring may be ordered at the beginning of treatment, but usually is discontinued after a few hours, unless the fetus is estimated to be very low birth weight (VLBW). Daily prolonged nonstress test (NST)

DRUG GUIDE Betamethasone (Celestone Solupan)

Overview of Maternal-Fetal Action

Studies have provided ample evidence that glucocorticoids such as betamethasone are capable of inducing pulmonary maturation and decreasing the incidence of respiratory distress syndrome in preterm infants. The mechanism by which corticosteroids accelerate fetal lung maturity is unclear, but it is related to the stimulation of enzyme activity by the drug. The enzyme is required for biosynthesis of surfactant by the type II pneumocytes. Surfactant is of major importance to the proper functioning of the lung in that it decreases the surface tension of the alveoli. Glucocorticoids also increase the rate of glycogen depletion, which leads to thinning of the interalveolar septa and increases the size of the alveoli. The thinning of the epithelium brings the capillaries into closer proximity with the air spaces and improves oxygen exchange (Blackburn and Loper 1992). Black female newborns have shown the largest decrease in respiratory distress syndrome after this therapy; white males have been much less responsive (Williams 1991). Only firstborn twin appears to benefit from antenatal steroid therapy (Briggs et al 1994).

Route, Dosage, Frequency

Prenatal maternal intramuscular injections of 12 mg of betamethasone are given once a day for 2 days. Dexamethasone may also be given in doses of 6 mg every 12 hours for four doses (NIH Development Conference 1994). To obtain maximum results, birth should be delayed for at least 24 hours after completing the first round of treatment. The effect of corticosteroids may be transient. Currently, it is suggested that the treatment regimen be repeated every week up to 34 weeks' gestation for the undelivered fetus with an immature lung profile.

Contraindications

Inability to delay birth for 24 to 48 hours
Adequate L/S ratio
Presence of a condition that necessitates immediate birth (eg, maternal bleeding)
Presence of maternal infection, diabetes mellitus, hypertension
Gestational age greater than 34 completed weeks

Maternal Side Effects

Bishop (1981) reports that suspected maternal risks include (1) initiation of lactation; (2) increased risk of infection; (3) augmentation of placental insufficiency in hypertensive women; (4) gastrointestinal bleeding; (5) inability to use estriol levels to assess fetal status; (6) possible pulmonary edema when used concurrently with tocolytics (such as ritodrine)
May cause Na^+ retention, K^+ loss, weight gain, edema, indigestion
Increased risk of infection if PROM present (Briggs et al 1994)
May mask signs and symptoms of infection

Effects on Fetus/Neonate

Lowered cortisol levels at birth, but rebound occurs by 2 hours of age (Briggs et al 1994)
Hypoglycemia
Increased risk of neonatal sepsis (Briggs et al 1994)
Animal studies have shown serious fetal side effects such as reduced head circumference, reduced weight of the fetal adrenal and thymus glands, and decreased placental weight (Briggs et al 1994). Human studies have not shown these effects, however.

Nursing Considerations

Assess for presence of contraindications.
Provide education regarding possible side effects.
Administer betamethasone deep into gluteal muscle, avoiding injection into deltoid (high incidence of local atrophy). (Dexamethasone may be administered I/M or I/V.)
Periodically evaluate BP, pulse, weight, and edema.
Assess lab data for electrolytes and blood glucose.
Although concomitant use of betamethasone and tocolytic agents has been implicated in increased risk of pulmonary edema, the betamethasone has little mineral corticoid activity; therefore it probably doesn't add significantly to the salt and water retention effects of beta-adrenergic agonists. Other causes of noncardiogenic pulmonary edema should also be investigated if pulmonary edema develops during administration of betamethasone to a woman in preterm labor.

and regular biophysical profiles are used to monitor fetal well-being until labor begins or cesarean birth becomes necessary (Kappy et al 1993). (These tests are discussed in Chapter 14). Maternal blood pressure (BP), pulse, and temperature, and FHR are assessed every 4 hours. A white blood cell count (WBC) and CRP are ordered daily. Vaginal exams are avoided to decrease the chance of infection. As the gestation approaches 34 weeks, an amniocentesis may be done weekly to evaluate lecithin/sphingomyelin (L/S) ratio and phosphatidylglycerol (PG) (see Chapter 14).

Opinions about the value of administering glucocorticoids (betamethasone or dexamethasone) prophylactically are sharply divided. However, when gestation is between 34 and 36 weeks, medical practice has been to delay birth for 24 hours to allow natural elevation of maternal-fetal blood glucocorticoids, thereby contributing to fetal lung maturity. If gestation is less than 32 weeks—or between 32 and 34 weeks (if lung immaturity has been determined)—and labor can be delayed 24–48 hours, betamethasone is frequently given. Glucocorticoids are not administered in the presence of uterine infection. (See Drug Guide: Betamethasone.)

Weekly nonstress tests should be continued until delivery.

APPLYING THE NURSING PROCESS

Nursing Assessment

Determining the duration of the rupture of the membranes is a significant component of the intrapartal assessment. The nurse asks the woman when her membranes ruptured and when labor began, because the risk of infection may be directly related to the time involved. Gestational age is determined to prepare for the possibility of a preterm birth. The nurse observes the mother for signs and symptoms of infection, especially by reviewing her WBC, temperature, pulse rate, and the character of her amniotic fluid. If the mother has a fever, hydration status should be checked. When a preterm or cesarean birth is anticipated, the nurse evaluates the childbirth preparation and coping abilities of the woman and her partner.

Nursing Diagnosis

Nursing diagnoses that may apply to a woman with PROM include the following:

- Risk for infection related to premature rupture of membranes
- Impaired gas exchange in the fetus related to compression of the umbilical cord secondary to prolapse of the cord
- Risk for ineffective individual coping related to unknown outcome of the pregnancy

Nursing Plan and Implementation

Nursing actions should focus on the woman, her partner, and the fetus. The nurse records the time her membranes ruptured and the time of labor onset. In addition, the nurse observes the woman for signs and symptoms of infection by frequently monitoring her vital signs (especially temperature and pulse), describing the character of the amniotic fluid, and reporting elevated WBC to the certified nurse-midwife/physician. Uterine activity and fetal response to the labor are evaluated, but vaginal exams are not done unless absolutely necessary. The woman is encouraged to rest on her left side to promote optimal uteroplacental perfusion. Comfort measures may help promote rest and relaxation. The nurse must also ensure that hydration is maintained, particularly if the woman's temperature is elevated.

Education is another important aspect of nursing care. The women and her partner, if he is involved, need to understand the implications of PROM and all treatment methods. It is important to address side effects and alternative treatments. The couple needs to know that although the membranes are ruptured, amniotic fluid continues to be produced.

Providing psychologic support for the couple is critical. The nurse may reduce anxiety by listening empathetically, relaying accurate information, and providing explanations of procedures. Preparing the couple for a cesarean birth, a preterm newborn, and the possibility of fetal or newborn demise may be necessary.

Community-Based Nursing Care

After initial treatment and observation, if leaking of fluid ceases, some women may be discharged and followed at home by home health care nurses. The nurse encourages the woman to continue bed rest as ordered (with bathroom privileges). The nurse also teaches the woman to monitor and record her temperature four times daily and to avoid intercourse, douches, and tampons. In addition, the nurse advises the woman to contact her physician and return to the hospital if she has fever, uterine tenderness and/or contractions, increased leakage of fluid, decreased fetal movement, or a foul vaginal discharge.

Evaluation

Anticipated outcomes of nursing care include

- The woman's risk of infection and cord prolapse decrease.
- The couple is able to discuss the implications of PROM and all treatments and alternative treatments.
- The pregnancy is maintained without trauma to the mother or her baby.

Care of the Woman at Risk Due to Preterm Labor

Labor that occurs between 20 and 37 completed weeks of pregnancy is called **preterm labor.** Prematurity continues to be the number one perinatal and neonatal problem in the United States today—it is estimated that 7 to 10 percent of all live births in the United States occur prematurely (Parsons and Spellacy 1994). The causes may be maternal, fetal, or placental factors. Maternal factors include cardiovascular or renal disease, diabetes, pregnancy-induced hypertension (PIH), abdominal surgery during pregnancy, a blow to the abdomen, uterine anomalies, cervical incompetence, DES exposure, history of cone biopsy, and maternal infection. Fetal factors include multiple pregnancy, hydramnios, and fetal infection. Placental factors include placenta previa and abruptio placentae.

A correlation exists between preterm birth and low socioeconomic status, a history of preterm births, poor antenatal care, and maternal smoking (especially more than one pack per day) (Lipshitz et al 1993).

Maternal implications of preterm labor include

- Psychologic stress related to the baby's condition
- Stress of unplanned hospitalization
- Administration of additional medications such as tocolytics (medications used to stop labor)

Fetal-neonatal implications include

- Increased morbidity and mortality, especially due to respiratory distress syndrome (RDS)
- Increased risk of trauma during birth
- Maturational deficiencies (fat storage, heat regulation, immaturity of organ systems)

Medical Therapy

Women who are at risk for preterm labor are taught to recognize the symptoms associated with preterm labor and, if any symptoms are present, to notify their certified nurse-midwife/physician immediately. Prompt diagnosis is necessary to stop preterm labor before it progresses to the point at which intervention will be ineffective.

In 1995 a fetal fibronectin (fFN) assay was approved by the FDA for use in screening for preterm labor. Fetal fibronectin is a protein normally found in fetal tissue, membranes, amniotic fluid, and the decidua. It is found in cervicovaginal fluid during the first half of pregnancy, as the gestational sac implants and develops, and again in the two to three weeks before childbirth. It is absent through midpregnancy and most of the third trimester. Women who demonstrate symptoms of preterm labor and who have a positive fFN assay are likely to give birth within one week. Thus this test helps identify women who are likely to benefit from aggressive treatment, close observation, and corticosteroid administration to promote fetal lung maturity. Conversely, the test may also be useful in screening asymptomatic, high-risk women. Preliminary research indicates that negative results when cervical sampling for fFN is done every two weeks is quite accurate in ruling out impending premature birth (Garite and Lockwood 1996).

Diagnosis of preterm labor is confirmed by documented uterine contractions (4 in 20 min or 6–8 in 1 hr), cervical dilatation of 2 cm (or documented cervical change), and cervical effacement of 80 percent. Uterine contractions and ruptured membranes also are diagnostic of preterm labor (Creasy and Resnik 1989).

Labor is not interrupted if one or more of the following conditions are present: severe PIH, eclampsia (convulsions), maternal hemodynamic instability, fetal anomalies incompatible with life, chorioamnionitis, hemorrhage, fetal maturity, fetal death, severe abruptio placentae, severe fetal growth retardation, or acute fetal distress.

The use of medications to attempt to stop labor is called **tocolysis,** and the medications that are given are termed *tocolytics.* Drugs currently used for tocolysis include the β-adrenergic agonists also called β-mimetics), magnesium sulfate ($MgSO_4$), prostaglandin synthetase inhibitors, and calcium channel blockers. The β-mimetics (ritodrine [Yutopar] and terbutaline sulfate [Brethine]) and magnesium sulfate ($MgSO_4$) are the most widely used tocolytics. Although not FDA-approved for tocolysis, terbutaline sulfate is the most widely used of the β-mimetics. It is effective and has the added advantage of being available for administration subcutaneously as well as intravenously and orally.

Although tocolytic drugs suppress uterine contractions and allow pregnancy to continue, the β-mimetics, $MgSO_4$, and prostaglandin synthetase inhibitors do cause maternal side effects; the most serious is pulmonary edema. Efforts to maintain the effectiveness of the β-adrenergic agonists while decreasing the incidence of side effects have focused on using as little of the drug as necessary and reducing drug levels as soon as possible after labor stops. Once uterine activity stops, the woman is placed on oral forms of the medication (terbutaline or magnesium gluconate) for long-term maintenance.

Because it is effective and has fewer side effects than β-adrenergic agonists, magnesium sulfate, which has long been used in the treatment of PIH, has been gaining favor in the treatment of preterm labor. The usual recommended loading dose is 4–6 g IV using an infusion pump over 20 minutes, followed by a constant dose of 2–4 g/hr until contractions cease, when the dose is further decreased to 1–2 g/hr (Iams 1996). The therapy is continued for 12 to 24 hours at the lowest rate that maintains cessation of contractions.

Side effects with the loading dose may include flushing, a feeling of warmth, headache, nystagmus, nausea, and dizziness. Other side effects include lethargy, sluggishness, and pulmonary edema (see Drug Guide: Magnesium Sulfate). Fetal side effects may include hypotonia and lethargy that persists for 1 or 2 days following birth (Lipshitz et al 1993).

Compared to IV ritodrine, magnesium sulfate has less effect on systolic or diastolic blood pressure (mean blood pressure and uteroplacental perfusion are maintained), no alteration of maternal heart rate (though it may cause a slight decrease in the fetal heart rate), no effect on cardiac output, and only a slight increase in placental blood flow.

Long-term oral therapy may be accomplished with magnesium gluconate. The therapeutic dose is usually 1 g every 2–4 hours.

One calcium channel blocker, nifedipine, is becoming increasingly popular as a tocolytic because it is easily administered orally or sublingually and has few serious maternal side effects. It decreases smooth muscle contractions by blocking the slow calcium channels at the cell surface. It should not be used with magnesium because both drugs block calcium and simultaneous administration has been implicated in serious maternal side effects related to low calcium levels.

Prostaglandin synthesis inhibitors (PSI) such as indomethacin (Indocin) are being investigated and used for tocolysis in selected instances. However, potential fetal side effects, such as premature closure of the ductus

DRUG GUIDE Magnesium Sulfate ($MgSO_4$)

Pregnancy Risk Category: B

Overview of Obstetric Action

$MgSO_4$ acts as a CNS depressant by decreasing the quantity of acetylcholine released by motor nerve impulses and thereby blocking neuromuscular transmission. This action reduces the possibility of convulsion, which is why $MgSO_4$ is used in the treatment of preeclampsia. Because magnesium sulfate secondarily relaxes smooth muscle, it may decrease the blood pressure, although it is not considered an antihypertensive. $MgSO_4$ may also decrease the frequency and intensity of uterine contractions; as a result it is also used as a tocolytic in the treatment of preterm labor.

Route, Dosage, Frequency

$MgSO_4$ is generally given intravenously to control dosage more accurately and prevent overdosage. An occasional physician still prescribes intramuscular administration. However, it is painful and irritating to the tissues and does not permit the close control that IV administration does. The intravenous route allows for immediate onset of action. It must be given by infusion pump for accurate dosage.

For Treatment of Preterm Labor

Loading dose: 6 g $MgSO_4$ in 250 mL solution administered over a 30-minute period (Parsons and Spellacy 1994).
Maintenance dose: 2–4 g/hour via infusion pump (Parsons and Spellacy 1994).

For Treatment of Preeclampsia

Loading dose: 4–6 g $MgSO_4$ as a 20% solution is administered over a 15–20 minute period (Arias 1993).
Maintenance dose: 1–2 g/hour via infusion pump (Mandeville and Troiano 1992).
Note: $MgSO_4$ is excreted via the kidneys. Because women in preterm labor typically have normal renal function, they generally require higher levels of magnesium to achieve a therapeutic range than women who have preeclampsia and may have compromised renal function (Parsons and Spellacy 1994).

Maternal Contraindications

Diagnosed maternal myasthenia gravis is the only absolute contraindication to the administration of $MgSO_4$ (Mandeville and Troiano 1992). A history of myocardial damage or heart block is a relative contraindication to use of the drug because of the effects on nerve transmission and muscle contractility. Extreme care is necessary in administration to women with impaired renal function because the drug is eliminated by the kidneys, and toxic magnesium levels may develop quickly.

Maternal Side Effects

Most maternal side effects are dose related. Lethargy and weakness related to neuromuscular blockade are common. Sweating, a feeling of warmth, flushing, and nasal congestion may be related to peripheral vasodilation. Other common side effects include nausea and vomiting, constipation, visual blurring, headache, and slurred speech. Signs of developing toxicity include depression or absence of reflexes, oliguria, confusion, respiratory depression, circulatory collapse, and respiratory paralysis. Rapid administration of large doses may cause cardiac arrest.

Effects on Fetus/Neonate

The drug readily crosses the placenta. Some authorities suggest that transient decrease in FHR variability may occur; others report that no change occurred. In general $MgSO_4$ therapy does not pose a risk to the fetus. Occasionally, the newborn may demonstrate neurologic depression or respiratory depression, loss of reflexes, and muscle weakness (Briggs et al 1994). Ill effects in the newborn may actually be related to fetal growth retardation, prematurity, or perinatal asphyxia (Knuppel and Drukker 1993).

Nursing Considerations

1. Monitor the blood pressure closely during administration.
2. Monitor maternal serum magnesium levels as ordered (usually every 6–8 hours). Therapeutic levels are in the range of 4–8 mg/dL. Reflexes often disappear at serum magnesium levels of 8–10 mg/dL; respiratory depression occurs at levels of 10–15 mg/dL; cardiac conduction problems occur at levels above 15 mg/dL (Scott 1994b).
3. Monitor respirations closely. If the rate is less than 12/minute, magnesium toxicity may be developing, and further assessments are indicated. Many protocols require stopping the medication if the respiratory rate falls below 12/minute.
4. Assess knee jerk (patellar tendon reflex) for evidence of diminished or absent reflexes. Loss of reflexes is often the first sign of developing toxicity (Sibai 1990). Also note marked lethargy or decreased level of consciousness and hypotension.
5. Determine urinary output. Output less than 30 mL/hour may result in the accumulation of toxic levels of magnesium.
6. If the respirations or urinary output fall below specified levels or if the reflexes are diminished or absent, no further magnesium should be administered until these factors return to normal.
7. The antagonist of magnesium sulfate is calcium. Consequently, an ampule of calcium gluconate should be available at the bedside. The usual dose is 1 g given IV over a period of about 3 minutes.
8. Monitor fetal heart tones continuously with IV administration.
9. Continue $MgSO_4$ infusion for approximately 24 hours after birth as prophylaxis against postpartum seizures if given for PIH.
10. If the mother has received $MgSO_4$ close to birth, the newborn should be closely observed for signs of magnesium toxicity for 24–48 hours.

Note: Protocols for magnesium sulfate administration may vary somewhat according to agency policy. Consequently, individuals are referred to their own agency protocols for specific guidelines.

arteriosus, have been reported. Consequently, indomethacin is used for only a brief course of therapy in women with preterm labor occurring before 32 weeks' gestation (Iams 1996).

HOME CARE OF WOMEN WITH PRETERM LABOR

Once uterine activity stops, the woman is placed on oral tocolysis or subcutaneous terbutaline via infusion pump for long-term maintenance. She may then be discharged and followed by home care nurses or as part of a specialized prematurity prevention program.

Home care frequently involves programs that combine home monitoring of uterine activity with daily contact between a woman and nurse. In these programs women at high risk record uterine activity on a home monitor once or twice daily. This recording is transmitted via the telephone to a nurse specially prepared to identify the signs and symptoms of preterm labor. If uterine activity is excessive or if symptoms are reported, the woman is referred to her certified nurse-midwife/physician for prompt evaluation. Although this combination of the electronic monitor and nursing care seems to be effective, it is not yet clear whether the value lies in the monitor itself or in the close contact and follow-up by the nurse (Devoe 1996). Because of this lack of clarity, the American College of Obstetricians and Gynecologists does not currently recommend the routine clinical use of the electronic uterine activity monitor at home (Lantz and Porter 1995).

APPLYING THE NURSING PROCESS

Nursing Assessment

During the antepartal period, the nurse identifies the woman at risk for preterm labor by noting the presence of predisposing factors. During the intrapartal period, the nurse assesses the progress of labor and the physiologic impact of labor on the mother and fetus.

Nursing Diagnosis

Nursing diagnoses that may apply to the woman with preterm labor include the following:

- Knowledge deficit related to lack of information about causes, identification, and treatment of preterm labor
- Fear related to risk of early labor and birth
- Ineffective individual coping related to need for constant attention to pregnancy

Nursing Plan and Implementation

Community-Based Nursing Care

Once the woman at risk for preterm labor has been identified, she needs to be taught about the importance of preventing the onset of labor (see Teaching Guide: Preterm Labor, p 296). This teaching is often provided by clinic nurses or home care nurses. Increasing the woman's awareness of the subtle symptoms of preterm labor is one of the most important teaching objectives of the nurse. The signs and symptoms of preterm labor include

- Uterine contractions that occur every 10 minutes or less with or without pain
- Mild menstrual-like cramps felt low in the abdomen
- Constant or intermittent feelings of pelvic pressure that may feel like the baby pressing down
- Constant or intermittent low backache
- A change in the vaginal discharge (an increase in amount, a change to more clear and watery, or a pinkish tinge)
- Abdominal cramping with or without diarrhea

The woman is also taught to evaluate contraction activity once or twice a day. She does so by lying down tilted to one side with a pillow behind her back for support. The woman places her fingertips on the fundus of the uterus, which is above the umbilicus (navel). She checks for contractions (hardening or tightening in the uterus) for about 1 hour. It is important for the pregnant woman to know that uterine contractions occur occasionally throughout the pregnancy. If they occur every 10 minutes for 1 hour, however, the cervix could begin to dilate, and labor could ensue.

The nurse ensures that the woman knows when to report signs and symptoms. If contractions occur every 10 minutes (or less) for 1 hour, if any of the other signs and symptoms are present for 1 hour, or if clear fluid begins leaking from the vagina, the woman should telephone her physician/certified nurse-midwife, clinic, or hospital birthing unit and make arrangements to be checked for ongoing labor.

Caregivers need to be aware that the woman is knowledgeable and attuned to changes in her body, and her call must be taken seriously. When a woman is at risk for preterm labor, she may have many episodes of contractions and other signs or symptoms. If she is treated positively, she will feel freer to report problems as they arise.

Preventive self-care measures are also very important. The nurse has a vital role in communicating the self-care measures described in Table 13–1.

During home visits the nurse completes physical assessments similar to those done in the hospital. If a terbutaline pump is being used, the pump regime is adjusted based on the daily uterine activity records.

The home care nurse needs to be alert to any signs that the woman is failing to achieve the emotional and developmental tasks of pregnancy, such as lack of maternal attachment. The nurse can also provide the woman with information about support groups and other community resources for women at risk for preterm birth.

Promotion of Maternal-Fetal Physical Well-Being During Labor

Provision of supportive nursing care to the woman in preterm labor is important during hospitalization. This care consists of promoting bed rest, monitoring vital signs (especially blood pressure and respirations), measuring intake and output, and continuous monitoring of FHR and uterine contractions. Placing the woman on her left side facilitates maternal-fetal circulation. Vaginal examinations are kept to a minimum. If tocolytic agents are being administered, the mother and fetus are monitored closely for any adverse effects.

Whether preterm labor is arrested or proceeds, the woman and her partner experience intense psychologic stress. Decreasing the anxiety associated with the risk of a preterm newborn by providing emotional support is a primary aim of the nurse. With empathetic communication, the nurse can facilitate the couple's expression of their feelings, which commonly include guilt and anxiety, thereby helping the couple identify and implement coping mechanisms. The nurse also keeps the couple informed about the labor progress, the treatment regimen, and the status of the fetus, so that their full cooperation will be elicited. In the event of imminent vaginal or cesarean birth, the couple should be offered brief but ongoing explanations to prepare them for the actual birth process and the events following the birth.

Evaluation

Anticipated outcomes of nursing care include

- The woman is able to discuss the cause, identification, and treatment of preterm labor.
- The woman states that she feels comfortable in her ability to cope with her situation and has resources to call on.
- The woman can describe appropriate self-care measures and can identify characteristics that need to be reported to her caregiver.
- The woman and her baby have a safe labor and birth.

TABLE 13–1 Self-Care Measures to Prevent Preterm Labor

Rest two or three times a day lying on your left side.

Drink 2 to 3 quarts of water or fruit juice each day. Avoid caffeine drinks. Filling a quart container and drinking from it will eliminate the need to keep track of numerous glasses of fluid.

Empty your bladder at least every 2 hours during waking hours.

Avoid lifting heavy objects. If small children are in the home, work out alternatives for picking them up, such as sitting on a chair and having them climb on your lap.

Avoid prenatal breast preparation such as nipple rolling or rubbing nipples with a towel. This is not meant to discourage breastfeeding but to avoid the potential increase in uterine irritability.

Pace necessary activities to avoid overexertion.

Sexual activity may need to be curtailed or eliminated.

Find pleasurable ways to help compensate for limitations of activities and boost the spirits.

Try to focus on 1 day or 1 week at a time rather than on longer periods of time.

If on bed rest, get dressed each day and rest on a couch rather than becoming isolated in the bedroom.

Source: Prepared in consultation with Susan Bennett, RN, ACCE, Coordinator of the Prematurity Prevention Program.

Care of the Woman with a Hypertensive Disorder

A number of hypertensive disorders can occur during pregnancy. Various attempts have been made to classify these disorders. The following classification is recommended by the American College of Obstetricians and Gynecologists (Sibai 1996):

1. Preeclampsia and eclampsia
2. Chronic hypertension (of any etiology preceding pregnancy)
3. Chronic hypertension with superimposed preeclampsia
4. Transient hypertension

Preeclampsia and Eclampsia

Preeclampsia is the most common hypertensive disorder in pregnancy. It is characterized by the development of hypertension, proteinuria, and edema. Because only hypertension may be present early in the disease process, that finding is therefore the basis for diagnosis.

The definition of preeclampsia is an increase in systolic blood pressure of 30 mm Hg and/or diastolic of 15 mm Hg over baseline. These blood pressure changes must be noted on at least two occasions 6 hours or more apart for the diagnosis to be made. In the absence of baseline values, a blood pressure of 140/90 has been accepted as hypertension (Sibai 1996).

TEACHING GUIDE Preterm Labor

ASSESSMENT

During the antepartal period the woman generally is screened for factors that place her at risk for preterm labor. The nurse then spends time with the woman and assesses her understanding of the danger of preterm labor, signs of preterm labor, and actions she can take to prevent it. If she is on a home monitoring program, the nurse assesses the woman's understanding of the purpose and rationale for the program.

NURSING DIAGNOSIS

The key nursing diagnosis will probably be: Knowledge deficit related to lack of information about the risks of preterm labor and self-care measures to prevent it.

NURSING PLAN AND IMPLEMENTATION

Teaching will focus on the risks of preterm labor, the functions of and procedures for home monitoring, and self-care activities to decrease the risk of preterm labor.

CLIENT GOALS

At the completion of the teaching the woman will be able to

1. Discuss the risks of preterm labor
2. Describe the purpose of home monitoring
3. Demonstrate the correct procedures for doing home monitoring
4. Explain self-care measures that help decrease the risk of preterm labor

Teaching Plan

CONTENT	TEACHING METHOD
Describe the dangers of preterm labor, especially the risk of prematurity in the infant, and all the potential problems.	Discuss the risks specifically. Many people understand in a general way that prematurity can be dangerous, but they fail to understand how the baby is affected.
Stress the value of home monitoring in evaluating uterine activity on a regular basis. Emphasize that many of the early symptoms of labor such as backache and increased bloody show may be subtle initially. Home monitoring can often detect increased uterine activity in the early stages before cervical changes progress to the point where it is impossible to stop labor.	Use handouts during the discussion. Help the woman clearly understand the value of the program because, to be successful, it requires a real commitment on her part.
Recent studies have demonstrated that home uterine monitoring programs offer little or no significant difference in preterm birth compared with women followed by daily patient-nurse contact and no home uterine monitoring (Grimes and Shultz 1992; Lipshitz et al 1993).	Teach the woman how to palpate for uterine contractions.
If the woman is to be part of a home monitoring program, the monitoring nurse will usually do the initial teaching. Be prepared to reinforce the information provided and answer questions that may arise.	Do a demonstration, and ask for a return demonstration.
Summarize self-care measures such as excellent fluid intake (2 to 3 quarts daily), voiding every 2 hours, avoiding lifting and overexertion, avoiding nipple stimulation or orgasm, limiting sexual activity, and cooperating with activity restrictions and bed rest requirements.	Use a handout during the discussion. Provide opportunities for discussion. If the woman has concerns about certain recommendations, try to modify the approach to best meet her needs.

EVALUATION

At the end of the teaching session the woman will be able to discuss the risks of preterm labor, demonstrate home monitoring techniques and explain their rationale, and implement self-care activities to decrease the risks of preterm labor.

Preeclampsia, typically categorized as mild or severe, is a progressive disorder. In its most severe form, eclampsia, generalized seizures or coma develop. If a woman has a seizure, she is considered eclamptic. Preeclampsia and eclampsia are sometimes collectively labeled **pregnancy-induced hypertension (PIH).** Most often preeclampsia is seen in the last 10 weeks of gestation, during labor, or in the first 48 hours after childbirth. Although birth of the fetus is the only known cure for PIH, it can be controlled with early diagnosis and careful management. Preeclampsia occurs in about 5 percent of all pregnancies in the United States. However the incidence is significantly higher among primigravidas (Scott 1994b). Preeclampsia is seen more often in teenagers and in women over 35, especially if they are primigravidas. Women with a history of preeclampsia are at increased risk, as are women with a large placental mass associated with multiple gestation, GTD, Rh incompatibility, and diabetes mellitus.

Pathophysiology of Preeclampsia

The cause of preeclampsia-eclampsia remains unknown despite decades of research. The condition was previously called "toxemia" because of a theory that a toxin produced in a pregnant woman's body caused the disease. This term is no longer used because the theory has not been substantiated.

Preeclampsia affects all the major systems of the body. The following pathophysiologic changes are associated with the disease:

- In normal pregnancy, the lowered peripheral vascular resistance and the increased maternal resistance to the pressor effects of angiotensin II result in lowered blood pressure. In preeclampsia, blood pressure begins to rise after 20 weeks' gestation, probably due to a gradual loss of resistance to angiotensin II. This response has been linked to the ratio between the prostaglandins prostacyclin and thromboxane. Prostacyclin is a potent vasodilator. It is decreased in preeclampsia, allowing the potent vasodilator and platelet-aggregating effects of thromboxane to dominate.
- The loss of normal vasodilation of uterine arterioles results in decreased placental perfusion. The effect on the fetus may be growth retardation, decrease in fetal movement, and chronic hypoxia or fetal distress.
- In preeclampsia, normal renal perfusion is decreased. With a reduction of glomerular filtration rate (GFR), serum levels of creatinine, BUN, and uric acid begin to rise from normal pregnant levels, while urine output decreases. Sodium is retained in increased amounts, which results in increased extracellular volume, increased sensitivity to angiotensin II, and edema. Stretching of the capillary walls of the glomerular endothelial cells allows the large protein molecules, primarily albumin, to escape in the urine, decreasing serum albumin. The decreased serum albumin causes decreased plasma colloid osmotic pressure. This results in a further movement of fluid to the extracellular spaces, which also contributes to the development of edema.
- The decreased intravascular volume causes increased viscosity of the blood and a corresponding rise in hematocrit.

HELLP Syndrome (*h*emolysis, *e*levated *l*iver enzymes, and *l*ow *p*latelet count) is sometimes associated with severe preeclampsia. Women who experience this multiple organ failure syndrome have high morbidity and mortality rates, as do their offspring.

The hemolysis that occurs is termed *microangiopathic hemolytic anemia.* It is thought that red blood cells are distorted or fragmented during passage through small, damaged blood vessels. Elevated liver enzymes occur from blood flow that is obstructed due to fibrin deposits. Hyperbilirubinemia and jaundice may also be seen. Liver distension causes epigastric pain. Thrombocytopenia (low platelet count) is a frequent finding in preeclampsia. Vascular damage is associated with vasospasm, and platelets aggregate at sites of damage, resulting in low platelet count (less than 100,000). Symptoms may include nausea, vomiting, flu-like symptoms or epigastric pain (Knuppel and Drukker 1993).

Women with HELLP syndrome are best cared for in a tertiary care center. Initially the mother's condition should be assessed and stabilized, especially if her platelets are very low. Platelet transfusions are indicated for platelet counts below 20,000/mm^3. The fetus is also assessed, using a nonstress test and biophysical profile. Once HELLP is diagnosed and the woman's condition is stable, expeditous birth of the child is indicated.

Maternal Risks

Central nervous system changes associated with PIH are hyperreflexia, headache, and seizures. Hyperreflexia may be due to increased intracellular sodium and decreased intracellular potassium levels. Cerebral vasospasm causes headaches, and cerebral edema and vasoconstriction are responsible for seizures.

Women with severe preeclampsia-eclampsia are at increased risk for renal failure, abruptio placentae, disseminated intravascular coagulation (DIC), ruptured liver, and pulmonary embolism.

Fetal-Neonatal Risks

Infants of women with hypertension during pregnancy tend to be small for gestational age (SGA). The cause is related specifically to maternal vasospasm and hypovolemia, which result in fetal hypoxia and malnutrition. In addition, the neonate may be premature because of the necessity for early birth. Perinatal mortality associated with preeclampsia is approximately 10 percent, and that associated with eclampsia is 20 percent.

At birth, the newborn may be oversedated because of medications administered to the woman. The newborn may also have hypermagnesemia due to treatment of the woman with large doses of magnesium sulfate.

Medical Therapy

The goals of medical management are prompt diagnosis of the disease; prevention of cerebral hemorrhage, seizures, hematologic complications, and renal and hepatic diseases; and birth of an uncompromised newborn as close to term as possible. Reduction of elevated blood pressure is essential in accomplishing these goals.

Clinical Manifestations and Diagnosis

Mild Preeclampsia Women with mild preeclampsia may exhibit few if any symptoms. The blood pressure is elevated to 140/90 or more, or increases 30 mm Hg systolic and 15 mm Hg diastolic above baseline on two occasions at least 6 hours apart. Thus a young woman who normally has a blood pressure of 90/60 would be hypertensive at 120/76. Therefore, a baseline blood pressure obtained early in the pregnancy is essential.

Generalized edema, seen as puffy face, hands, and dependent areas such as the ankles, may be present. Edema is identified by a weight gain of more than 3.3 lb/month (1.5 kg) in the second trimester or more than 1.1 lb/week (0.5 kg) in the third trimester. Edema is assessed on a 1+ to 4+ scale. Urine testing may show a 1+ to 2+ albumin, although proteinuria is often the last of the three cardinal signs to appear.

Severe Preeclampsia Severe preeclampsia may develop suddenly. Edema becomes generalized and readily apparent in hands, face, sacral area, lower extremities, and the abdominal wall. Edema is also characterized by an excessive weight gain of more than 2 lb (0.9 kg) over a couple of days to a week. Blood pressure is 160/110 or higher, a dipstick albumin measurement is 3+ to 4+, and the 24-hour urine protein is greater than 5 g. Hematocrit, serum creatinine, and uric acid levels are elevated. Other characteristic symptoms are frontal headaches, blurred vision, scotomata (spots before the eyes), nausea, vomiting, irritability, hyperreflexia, cerebral disturbances, oliguria (less than 400 mL of urine in 24 hours), pulmonary edema with moist breath sounds and dyspnea, cyanosis, retinal edema (retinas appear wet and glistening), narrowed segments on the retinal arterioles when examined with an ophthalmoscope, and, finally, epigastric pain. Epigastric pain is often the sign of impending convulsion and is thought to be caused by increased vascular engorgement of the liver.

Eclampsia **Eclampsia,** characterized by a grand mal seizure or coma, may occur before the onset of labor, during labor, or early in the postpartal period. The seizure usually has a tonic phase, then a clonic phase. The tonic phase is marked by pronounced muscular contraction, so that the women's arms and legs stiffen, her back arches, and her jaw snaps shut. Her respirations cease due to thoracic muscle contraction, and she may become cyanotic. The clonic phase is marked by alternate contraction and relaxation of the muscles, which causes the woman to thrash about wildly. As the convulsive movements gradually cease, the woman often slips into a coma that may last for an hour or more. In other cases, the coma may be quite brief and, if the woman is not treated, seizures may recur in a few minutes. Some women experience only one seizure. Others have several. Unless they occur quite frequently, the woman often regains consciousness between seizures.

Antepartal Management The medical therapy for PIH depends on the severity of the disease.

Home Care of Mild Preeclampsia In general, women with preeclampsia should be admitted to the hospital. However, changes in health care have given more attention to decreasing inpatient hospital days and for women whose symptoms allow, home care is now an option. A woman can be considered for management at home if she meets the following criteria: blood pressure ≤ 150/100, proteinuria less than 1 g/24 hr or less than 3+ dipstick, platelet count greater than 120,000/mm^3, and normal fetal growth if not at term or showing signs of complicating factors such as vaginal bleeding. She must have a basic understanding of her condition, be able to recognize the signs and symptoms of worsening preeclampsia, be able to accurately count fetal movements, and know when to call the physician. She is not restricted to bed rest (Frangieh and Sibai 1996). The woman monitors her blood pressure, weight, and urine protein daily. Home uterine monitoring may be used and remote transmission of NSTs may be performed on a daily to biweekly basis. Home care nurses are in regular contact with the woman and her family. Any woman with worsening symptoms or severe preeclampsia should be hospitalized.

Hospital Care of Mild Preeclampsia The woman is placed on bed rest, primarily in the left lateral recumbent position, to decrease pressure on the vena cava, thereby increasing venous return, circulatory volume, and placental and renal perfusion. Improved renal blood flow helps decrease angiotensin II levels, promotes diuresis, and lowers blood pressure.

Diet should be well balanced and moderate to high in protein (80–100 g/day, or 1.5 g/kg/day) to replace protein lost in the urine. Sodium intake should be moderate, not to exceed 6 g/day. Excessively salty foods should be avoided, but sodium restriction and diuretics are no longer used in treating PIH.

Tests to evaluate fetal status are done more frequently as PIH progresses. Monitoring fetal well-being is essential to achieving a safe outcome for the fetus. The following tests are used:

- Fetal movement record
- Nonstress test (NST)
- Ultrasonography every 3 or 4 weeks for serial determination of growth
- Biophysical profile
- Serum creatinine determinations
- Amniocentesis to determine fetal lung maturity
- Doppler velocimetry beginning at 30 to 32 weeks to screen for fetal compromise

These tests are described in detail in Chapter 14.

Severe Preeclampsia The woman should be hospitalized. If the uterine environment is considered detrimental to fetal well-being, birth may be the treatment of choice for both mother and fetus, even if the fetus is immature. Other medical therapies for severe preeclampsia include the following:

- *Bed rest.* Bed rest must be complete. Stimuli that may bring on a seizure should be reduced.
- *Diet.* A high-protein, moderate-sodium diet is given as long as the woman is alert and has no nausea or indication of impending seizure.
- *Anticonvulsants.* Magnesium sulfate (MgSO) is the treatment of choice for convulsions. Its CNS-depressant action reduces the possibility of seizure (see Drug Guide: Magnesium Sulfate).
- *Fluid and electrolyte replacement.* The goal of fluid intake is to achieve a balance between correcting hypovolemia and preventing circulatory overload. Fluid intake may be oral or supplemented with intravenous therapy. Intravenous fluids may be started "to keep lines open" in case they are needed for drug therapy even when oral intake is adequate. Electrolytes are replaced as indicated by daily serum electrolyte levels.
- *Medication.* A sedative such as diazepam (Valium) or phenobarbital is sometimes given to encourage quiet bed rest.
- *Antihypertensives.* Hydralazine (Apresoline), labetelol, and nifedipine (Procardia) are the antihypertensives most commonly used. In general, antihypertensive therapy is given for diastolic blood pressures of 110 or above (Sibai 1996).

Eclampsia An eclamptic seizure requires immediate effective treatment. A bolus of magnesium sulfate is given intravenously to control convulsions. Sedatives such as diazepam or amobarbitol are used only if the seizures are not controlled by magnesium sulfate. The lungs are auscultated for pulmonary edema. The woman is observed for circulatory and renal failure and signs of cerebral hemorrhage. Furosemide (Lasix) may be given for pulmonary edema, digitalis for circulatory failure. Urinary output is monitored.

The woman is observed for signs of labor. She is also checked every 15 minutes for evidence of vaginal bleeding and abdominal rigidity, which might indicate abruptio placentae. While she is comatose, she is positioned on her side with the side rails up.

Because of the severity of her condition, the woman is often cared for in an intensive care unit. Invasive hemodynamic monitoring of either central venous pressure (CVP) or pulmonary artery wedge pressure (PAWP) may be started using a Swan-Ganz catheter. Both these procedures carry risk for the woman, and the decision to use them should be made carefully. When the condition of the woman and the fetus are stabilized, induction of labor is considered, because birth is the only known cure for PIH. The woman and her partner should be given a careful explanation about her status and that of her unborn child and the treatment they are receiving. Plans for further treatment and for birth must be discussed with them.

ESSENTIAL PRECAUTIONS FOR PRACTICE

A Woman with PIH

In caring for a woman with PIH, all the precautions established for any hospitalized pregnant, laboring, or postpartal woman apply. In addition remember the following specifics.

- Gloves should be worn when testing urine for proteinuria, starting IV for $MgSO_4$ therapy, doing finger-sticks to test hematocrit, or drawing blood for other laboratory tests.
- If eclampsia occurs and the woman convulses, gloves should be worn when removing the airway.
- If incontinence occurs during the convulsion, a splash apron and gloves should be worn when cleansing the woman and changing the bedding.
- Needles, syringes, lancets, and other sharp objects should be disposed of in appropriately labeled containers.

REMEMBER to wash your hands before putting disposable gloves on and AGAIN immediately after you remove the gloves.

For further information, consult OSHA and CDC guidelines.

Intrapartal Management If preeclampsia is diagnosed, labor may be induced by intravenous oxytocin when there is evidence of fetal maturity and cervical readiness. In very severe cases, cesarean birth may be necessary even if the fetus is immature.

The woman may receive intravenous oxytocin and magnesium sulfate simultaneously. Infusion pumps should be used and bags and tubing should be carefully labeled.

Meperidine (Demerol) or fentanyl may be given intravenously for labor. A pudendal block is often used for vaginal birth. An epidural block may be used if it is administered by a skilled anesthesiologist who is knowledgeable about preeclampsia.

Birth in the Sims' or semi-sitting position should be considered. If the lithotomy position is used, a wedge should be placed under the right buttock to displace the uterus. The wedge should also be used if birth is by cesarean. Oxygen is administered to the woman during labor if the need is indicated by fetal response to the contractions.

A pediatrician or neonatal nurse practitioner must be available to care for the newborn at birth. This caregiver must be informed of all amounts and times of medication the woman has received during labor.

Postpartum Management The woman with PIH usually improves rapidly after giving birth, although seizures can still occur during the first 48 hours postpartum. When the hypertension is severe, the woman may continue to receive hydralazine or magnesium sulfate postpartally.

APPLYING THE NURSING PROCESS

Nursing Assessment

Blood pressure is taken and recorded during each antepartal visit. If the blood pressure rises, or if the normal slight decrease in blood pressure expected between 8 and 28 weeks of pregnancy does not occur, the woman should be followed closely. The woman's urine is checked for proteinuria at each visit.

If hospitalization becomes necessary, the nurse then assesses the following:

- *Blood pressure.* Blood pressure should be determined every 2 to 4 hours—more frequently if indicated by medication or other changes in the woman's status.
- *Temperature.* Temperature should be determined every 4 hours; every 2 hours if elevated.
- *Pulse and respirations.* Pulse rate and respiration should be determined along with blood pressure.
- *Fetal heart rate.* The fetal heart rate should be determined with the blood pressure or monitored continuously with the electronic fetal monitor if the situation indicates.
- *Urinary output.* Every voiding should be measured. The woman frequently has an indwelling catheter. In this case, urine output can be assessed hourly. Output should be 700 mL or greater in 24 hours, or at least 30 mL per hour.
- *Urine protein.* Urinary protein is determined hourly if an indwelling catheter is in place or with each voiding. Readings of 3+ or 4+ indicate loss of 5 g or more of protein in 24 hours.
- *Urine specific gravity.* Specific gravity of the urine should be determined hourly or with each voiding. Readings over 1.040 correlate with oliguria and proteinuria.
- *Edema.* The face (especially eyelids and cheekbone area), fingers, hands, arms (ulnar surface and wrist), legs (tibial surface), ankles, feet, and sacral area are inspected and palpated for edema. The degree of pitting is determined by pressing over bony areas.
- *Weight.* The woman is weighed daily at the same time, wearing the same robe or gown and slippers. Weighing may be omitted if the woman is to maintain strict bed rest.
- *Pulmonary edema.* The woman is observed for coughing. The lungs are auscultated for moist respirations.
- *Deep tendon reflexes.* The woman is assessed for evidence of hyperreflexia in the brachial, wrist, patellar, or Achilles tendons (Table 13–3). The patellar reflex is the easiest to assess (Procedure 13–1). Clonus should also be assessed by vigorously dorsiflexing the foot while the knee is held in a fixed position. Normally no clonus is present. If it is present, it is measured as beats and recorded as such.
- *Placental separation.* The woman should be assessed hourly for vaginal bleeding and/or uterine rigidity.
- *Headache.* The woman should be questioned about the existence and location of any headache.
- *Visual disturbance.* The woman should be questioned about any visual blurring or changes, or scotomata. The results of the daily fundoscopic exam should be recorded on the chart.
- *Epigastric pain.* The woman should be asked about any epigastric pain. It is important to differentiate it from simple heartburn, which tends to be familiar and less intense.
- *Laboratory blood tests.* Daily tests of hematocrit to measure hemoconcentration; blood urea nitrogen, creatinine, and uric acid levels to assess kidney function; clotting studies for any indication of thrombocytopenia or DIC; liver enzymes; and electrolyte levels for deficiencies are all indicated.
- *Level of consciousness.* The woman is observed for alertness, mood changes, and any signs of impending convulsion or coma.
- *Emotional response and level of understanding.* The woman's emotional response should be carefully assessed, so that support and teaching can be planned accordingly.

In addition, the nurse continues to assess the effects of any medications administered. Since the administration of prescribed medications is an important aspect of

TABLE 13–2 Deep Tendon Reflex Rating Scale

Rating	*Assessment*
4+	Hyperactive; very brisk, jerky, or clonic response; abnormal
3+	Brisker than average; may not be abnormal
2+	Average response; normal
1+	Diminished response; low normal
0	No response; abnormal

PROCEDURE 13–1 Assessing Deep Tendon Reflexes and Clonus

Nursing Action	Rationale
Objective: Assemble and prepare the equipment.	
• Obtain a percussion hammer. If one is not available, you may use the side of your hand.	A percussion hammer permits accurate delivery of a brisk tap.
Objective: Prepare the woman.	
• Explain the procedure, indications for the procedure, and the information that will be obtained.	Explanation decreases anxiety and increases cooperation.
Objective: Elicit the reflexes.	
See below for the correct technique.	
Objective: Grade the reflexes.	
• Reflexes are graded on a scale of 1+ to 4+. See the reflex rating scale in Table 13–2.	
Objective: Assess for clonus.	
See page 302 for the correct technique.	
Objective: Report and record your findings.	
Sample recordings: DTRs 2+, no clonus DTRs 4+, 2 beats clonus	Provides a permanent record.

Assessing Deep Tendon Reflexes (DRTs)

DTRs are assessed to gain information about CNS status and to assess the effects of $MgSO_4$ if the woman is receiving it. At the minimum, the patellar reflex should be checked. Most nurses check a second reflex such as the biceps, triceps, or brachioradialis.

Eliciting the Biceps Reflex

Correct positioning and technique is essential to elicit this reflex. The correct position causes the muscle to stretch; when the tendon is stretched with the tap, the muscle should contract.

- Place your thumb on the woman's biceps tendon and flex her arm at the elbow.
- Strike your thumb in a slightly downward motion and assess the response. Normal response is flexion of the arm.

Eliciting the Patellar Reflex

- Position the woman with her legs hanging over the edge of the bed or the examining table. Her feet should not be touching the floor. See Figure 13–3. She may also lie supine with her knees slightly flexed and supported.
- Briskly strike the patellar tendon, which is located just below the patella. Normal response is extension or thrusting forward of the foot.

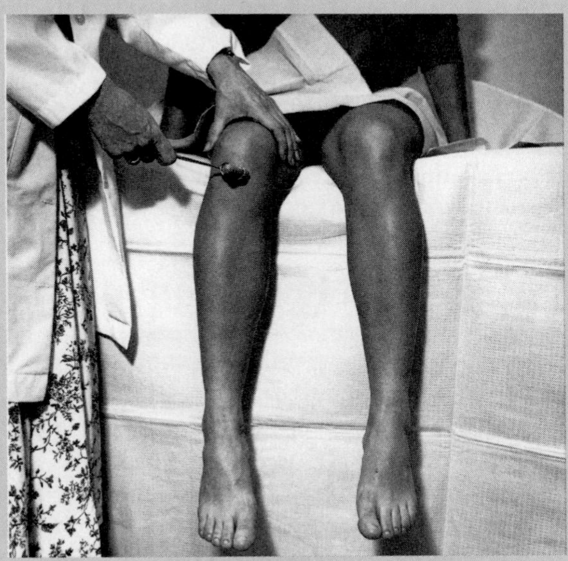

FIGURE 13–3 Correct sitting position for eliciting patellar reflex.

PROCEDURE 13–1 Assessing Deep Tendon Reflexes and Clonus continued

Assessing for Clonus

Clonus manifests as more pronounced hyperreflexia and is indicative of CNS irritability.

- Flex and support the woman's leg.
- Vigorously dorsiflex the foot. Maintain the dorsiflexion momentarily and then release. See Figure 13–4.

  Normal response: The foot returns to its normal position of plantar flexion.

  Clonus: The foot "jerks" or taps against the examiner's hand.
- Record the number of taps or beats of clonus, if present.

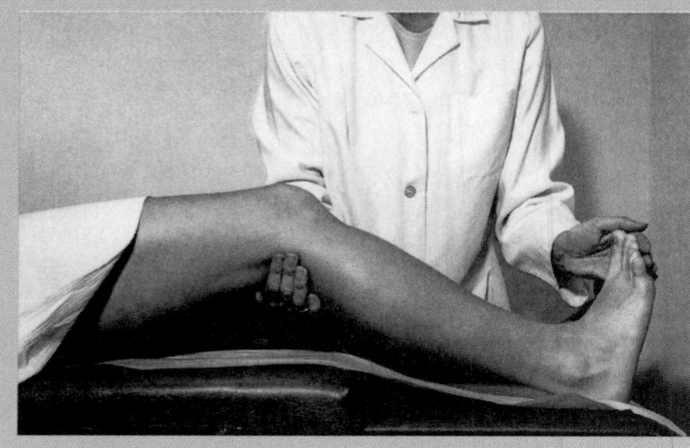

FIGURE 13–4 To elicit clonus, sharply dorsiflex the foot.

care, the nurse is, of course, familiar with the more commonly used medications, their purpose, implications, and associated untoward or toxic effects.

Nursing Diagnosis

Examples of nursing diagnoses that might apply to the woman with preeclampsia include the following:

- Fluid volume deficit related to fluid shift from intravascular to extravascular space secondary to vasospasm
- Risk for injury related to the possibility of seizure secondary to cerebral vasospasm or edema
- Knowledge deficit related to lack of information about preeclampsia, its treatment, and its implications for the woman and her fetus

Nursing Plan and Implementation

Community-Based Nursing Care

When a woman with mild preeclampsia is cared for as an outpatient, regular nursing contact is essential. A variety of approaches have been used, including home care programs, day-care programs, and perinatal outpatient monitoring services using a device designed to monitor a variety of information (Frangieh and Sibai 1996). Nursing contact varies from daily to weekly depending on physician request. The nurse must ensure that the woman clearly understands her condition and its implications. In addition, during visits the nurse assesses blood pressure and fetal heart rate, tests the urine for proteinuria, and reviews fetal movement records. At each visit, the nurse assesses the woman for signs that her preeclampsia is worsening. In addition, the woman should know which symptoms are significant and should be reported at once. Usually the woman with mild preeclampsia is seen once or twice a week, but she may need to come in earlier if symptoms indicate that her condition is worsening.

Provision of Support and Teaching

A woman with preeclampsia has several major concerns. She may fear losing her fetus; she may worry about her personal relationship with her other children and her personal and sexual relationship with her partner; she may be concerned about finances; she may also feel bored and a little resentful if she faces prolonged bed rest. If she has small children, she may have trouble providing for their care. The nurse should help the couple identify and discuss their concerns. The nurse can offer information and explanations if certain aspects of therapy cause difficulty. The nurse can also refer the woman and her family to community resources such as support groups or homemaker services as appropriate.

The development of severe preeclampsia is a cause for increased concern for the woman and her family. The most immediate concerns usually are about the prognosis for the woman and her fetus. The nurse can explain medical therapy and its purpose and offer honest, hopeful information. The nurse should keep the couple informed of fetal status and should also take the time to discuss other concerns the couple may express. The nurse provides as much information as possible and seeks other sources of information or aid for the family as needed. The nurse can offer to contact a member of the clergy or hospital chaplain for additional support if the couple so chooses.

Prevention of Seizure

The nurse maintains a quiet, low-stimulus environment for the woman. The woman should be placed in a private room in a quiet location where she can be watched closely. Visitors are limited to close family or main support persons. The woman should maintain the left lateral recumbent position most of the time, with side rails up for her protection. Unlimited phone calls are avoided because the phone ringing unexpectedly may be too jarring. To avoid a sense of isolation, however, some women find it preferable to limit calls to a certain time of day. Bright lights and sudden loud noises may precipitate seizures in the woman with severe preeclampsia.

Provision of Effective Care and Support if Eclampsia Develops

The occurrence of a convulsion is frightening to any family members who may be present, although the woman will not be able to recall it when she becomes conscious. Therefore, it is essential to offer explanations to the family member and the woman herself later.

When the tonic phase of the contraction begins, the woman should be turned to her side (if she is not already in that position) to aid circulation to the placenta. Her head should be turned face down to allow saliva to drain from her mouth. Attempting to insert a padded tongue blade is no longer advocated in many facilities. In others it is used if it can be done without force because it may prevent injury to the woman's mouth. The side rails should be padded, or a pillow put between the woman and each side rail.

After 15 to 20 seconds the clonic phase starts. When the thrashing subsides, intensive monitoring and therapy begin. An oral airway is inserted, the woman's nasopharynx is suctioned, and oxygen administration is begun by nasal catheter. Fetal heart tones are monitored continuously. Maternal vital signs are monitored every 5 minutes until they are stable, then every 15 minutes.

Promotion of Maternal and Fetal Well-Being During Labor and Birth

The laboring woman with preeclampsia must receive all the care and precautions necessary for normal labor, as well as those required for managing preeclampsia. The woman is kept positioned on her left side as much as possible. Both the woman and the fetus are monitored carefully throughout labor. The nurse notes the progress of labor and is alert to signs of worsening PIH or its complications.

During the second stage of labor, the woman is encouraged to push in the side-lying position if possible. If she is unable to do so comfortably or effectively, she can be helped to a semisitting position for pushing, and can then resume the lateral position between contractions. Birth is in the side-lying position or in the lithotomy position with a wedge placed under the woman's right hip.

A family member or other support person is encouraged to stay with the woman as much as possible. The woman in labor and the support person should be kept informed of the progress and plan of care. Their wishes concerning the birth experience should be respected whenever possible. If at all possible, the woman should be cared for by the same nurses throughout her hospital stay.

Promotion of Maternal Well-Being During the Postpartal Period

Because the woman with preeclampsia is hypovolemic, even normal blood loss can be serious. The amount of vaginal bleeding must be assessed and the woman observed for signs of shock. Blood pressure and pulse are monitored every 4 hours for 48 hours. Hematocrit is checked daily. The woman is assessed for any further signs of preeclampsia. Intake and output are measured. Normal postpartum diuresis helps eliminate edema and is a favorable sign.

Postpartal depression can develop after such a difficult pregnancy. To help prevent it, opportunities are provided for frequent maternal-infant contact and family members are encouraged to visit. The couple may have many questions and the nurse should be available for discussion. The couple should be given family-planning information. Oral contraceptives may be used if the woman's blood pressure has returned to normal by the time they are prescribed (usually 4 to 6 weeks after birth).

For a brief summary of PIH, see Key Facts to Remember: Preeclampsia-Eclampsia on page 306.

Evaluation

Anticipated outcomes of nursing care include

- The woman is able to explain PIH, its implications for her pregnancy, the treatment regimen, and possible complications.
- The woman suffers no eclamptic seizures.
- The woman and her caregivers detect early evidence of increasing severity of the PIH or possible complications, so that appropriate treatment measures can be instituted.
- The woman gives birth to a healthy newborn.

Chronic Hypertensive Disease

Chronic hypertension exists when the blood pressure is 140/90 or higher before pregnancy or before the 20th week of gestation, or hypertension persists for more than 42 days following childbirth (Sibai 1996). If the diastolic blood pressure is greater than 80 mm Hg during

Text continues on page 306

CRITICAL PATHWAY FOR A WOMAN WITH PREGNANCY-INDUCED HYPERTENSION

Category	Antepartal Management	Intrapartal Management*	Postpartal Management
Referral	• Perinatologist • Internist • Social worker • Psych clinical nurse practitioner • Dietary/nutritionist	• Obtain prenatal record	• Home nursing referral if indicated
Assessment	• Electronic fetal monitoring (EFM) ___ q4h ___ q8h ___ Continuous • NST: ___ qd • Ultrasound as indicated • Assess for headache, visual disturbances, epigastric pain, edema, DTRs, clonus, and protein in urine	• Assess prenatal BP readings and compare to baseline reading • Assess for headache, visual disturbances, epigastric pain, edema, DTRs, clonus, and protein in urine	• BP q4h for first 48h then q8h until discharge • Monitor daily Hct • Continue normal postpartum assessment q8h • Feeding technique with newborn: should be progressing • TPR assessment: q8h; all WNL: report temperature >38C (100.4F) • Continue assessment of comfort level • Assess for headache, visual disturbances, epigastric pain, edema, DTRs, clonus, and protein in urine
Comfort	• Assess for discomfort • Provide comfort measures as needed	• Assess for discomfort • Provide comfort measures as needed	• Continue with pain management techniques
Teaching/ psychosocial	• Room orientation • Explain of signs and symptoms (s/sx) of worsening disease and importance of notifying RN • Explain s/sx of labor • Increase pt awareness of fetal monitoring, importance of bed rest and lying on left side • Evaluation of client teaching	• Tour of ICN • Discuss with woman: a. Mode of childbirth b. Progression of disease and possible use of $MgSO_4$ prior to birth c. Postpartum expectation	• Implement normal postpartum teaching and psychosocial support (see Chapter 28)

Therapeutic nursing interventions and reports	• CBC daily
	• Biochemical profile
	• U/A/Dipstick for protein and ketones with each void as well as specific gravity
	• 24 hour urine for total protein and creatinine clearance
	• VS q4h or more frequently if indicated
	• I&O q8h; fluid restriction ___ mL as ordered
	• DTR and clonus q4h; report 3+ or 4+ results
	• Daily weight
	• Seizure precautions
	  • Headache, visual distress, epigastric pain → report abnormal findings
	  • Edema (ongoing)
	  • Auscultate lungs for moist respirations and report
	• Assess hourly for vaginal bleeding and/or uterine irritability or contractions
	• Observe for alertness, mood changes, and signs of impending convulsion or coma
	• Assess emotional response so that support and teaching can be planned accordingly
		• Ongoing monitoring of blood pressure
		• Ongoing monitoring of edema
		• Assess urine for proteinuria every shift
		• Electronic fetal monitoring in place
		• Assess woman for worsening signs of PIH (placental separation, pulmonary edema, renal failure, and fetal distress)
		• Try to have same nurses caring for woman during her hospitalization
			• Continue sitz bath prn
			• May shower if ambulating without difficulty
			• DC buffalo cap (heparin lock) if present
			• Continue to monitor VS, breath sounds, edema, epigastric pain, DTRs, clonus, and protein in urine until return to normal limits

CRITICAL PATHWAY FOR A WOMAN WITH PREGNANCY-INDUCED HYPERTENSION continued

Category	Antepartal Management	Intrapartal Management*	Postpartal Management
Activity	• BR with BRP • Decreased stimulation in room • Limit visitors • Encourage left lateral recumbent position	• Positioned on side • Encouraged to push while lying on side • Birth is in a side-lying position if possible	• Up ad lib when VS have stabilized
Nutrition	• Reg diet	• Ice chips	• Continue diet and fluids
Elimination	• Report urine output <30 mL/hr or urine specific gravity >1.040	• Monitor urine output	• Monitor urine output • I/O recorded for 48h after birth

Medications	• Buffalo cap or IV
	• If gestational age indicates:
	  • Celestone Soluspan
	  • TRH
	• $MgSO_4$ per infusion pump if indicated
		• Continuous IV infusion
		• $MgSO_4$ infusion pump if indicated
			• Continue $MgSO_4$ as indicated
			• May take own prenatal vitamins
			• RhoGAM and rubella vaccine administered if indicated

Discharge planning/ home care	• Assess home care needs		• Review discharge instruction and checklist • Describe postpartum warning signs and when to call CNM/physician • Provide prescriptions. Gift pack given to woman. • Arrangements made for baby pictures if desired • Postpartum visit scheduled • Newborn check scheduled
Family Involvement	• Assess woman's major concerns: ie, fear for fetus, relationship with other children, relationship with partner	• Encourage family member to stay with the woman as long as possible throughout labor and childbirth	• Family members urged to visit • Continue to involve support persons in teaching • Evidence of parental bonding behaviors apparent • Plans being made for providing support to mother following discharge. Support persons verbalize understanding of need for woman to rest, eat nutritionally, recover.
Date			

*Interventions for a woman with a normal labor and birth and during the early postpartum period may be found in those appropriate critical pathways.

KEY FACTS TO REMEMBER

Preeclampsia-Eclampsia

- Preeclampsia, which occurs after the 20th week of pregnancy, involves elevated BP, edema, and proteinuria. It may be mild or severe.
- A woman with preeclampsia who has a seizure is said to have eclampsia.
- The exact cause of preeclampsia is unknown.
- Vasospasm is responsible for most of the clinical manifestations, including the CNS signs of headache, hyperreflexia, and convulsion. Vasospasm also causes poor placental perfusion, which leads to IUGR.
- The only known cure for preeclampsia is birth of the infant, but symptoms may develop up to 48 hours postpartum.
- Management is supportive and includes anticonvulsant therapy, generally with $MgSO_4$; prevention of renal, hepatic, and hematologic complications; and careful assessment of fetal well-being.
- Nursing care focuses on implementing appropriate interventions based on the data gathered from regular assessment of vital signs, reflexes, degree of edema and proteinuria, response to therapy, fetal status, detection of developing complications, knowledge level and psychologic state of the woman and her family.

the second trimester, chronic hypertension should be suspected. The cause of chronic hypertension has not been determined. In most chronic hypertensive women the disease is mild.

The goals of care are to prevent the development of preeclampsia and to ensure normal growth of the fetus. The woman is seen regularly for prenatal care (at least every 2 weeks). Ultrasound is done at 10 to 14 weeks to date the pregnancy and then at 20 to 26 weeks and at 32 weeks to detect IUGR. Creatinine clearance is determined early in pregnancy and repeated every 2 months if renal disease is suspected.

The woman is taught the importance of daily rest periods in the left lateral recumbent position and also learns to monitor her blood pressure at home. A diet that provides a protein intake of 1.5 g/kg body weight/day is recommended if proteinuria is significant. Moderate salt intake is acceptable. Antihypertensive medication is continued throughout pregnancy in women with severe chronic hypertension (blood pressure $>$ 100 Hg diastolic). The drug of choice is methyldopa (Aldomet) (Scott 1994b).

Nursing care is directed at providing sufficient information that the woman can meet her health care needs. She is given information about her diet, the importance of regular rest, her medications, the need for blood pressure control, and any procedures used to monitor the well-being of her fetus.

Chronic Hypertension with Superimposed Preeclampsia

Preeclampsia may develop in a woman previously found to have chronic hypertension. Close monitoring and careful management are indicated if the following signs develop:

- Elevations of systolic blood pressure 30 mm Hg above the baseline or diastolic blood pressure 15–20 mm Hg above the baseline, on two occasions at least 6 hours apart
- Proteinuria
- Edema occurring in the upper half of the body

A woman with chronic hypertension who develops superimposed preeclampsia often progresses quickly to eclampsia, sometimes before 30 weeks of pregnancy.

Late or Transient Hypertension

Late hypertension exists when transient elevation of blood pressure occurs during labor or in the early postpartal period, returning to normal within 10 days after birth.

Care of the Woman at Risk for Rh Sensitization

The Rh blood group is present on the surface of erythrocytes of a majority of the population. When it is present, a person is designated as Rh-positive. Those without the factor are designated as Rh-negative. If an Rh-negative individual is exposed to Rh-positive blood, an antigen-antibody response occurs, and the person forms anti-Rh agglutinin and is said to be sensitized. Subsequent exposure to Rh-positive blood can then cause a serious reaction that results in agglutination and hemolysis of red blood cells. Sensitization most commonly occurs when an Rh-negative woman carries an Rh-positive fetus, either to term or to termination by spontaneous or induced abortion. It can also occur if an Rh-negative nonpregnant woman receives an Rh-positive blood transfusion.

The red blood cells from the fetus invade the maternal circulation, thereby stimulating the production of Rh antibodies. Because this usually occurs at birth, the first offspring is not affected. In a subsequent pregnancy, however, Rh antibodies cross the placenta and enter the fetal circulation, causing severe hemolysis. The destruction of fetal red blood cells causing anemia in the fetus is proportional to the extent of maternal sensitization (Figure 13–5).

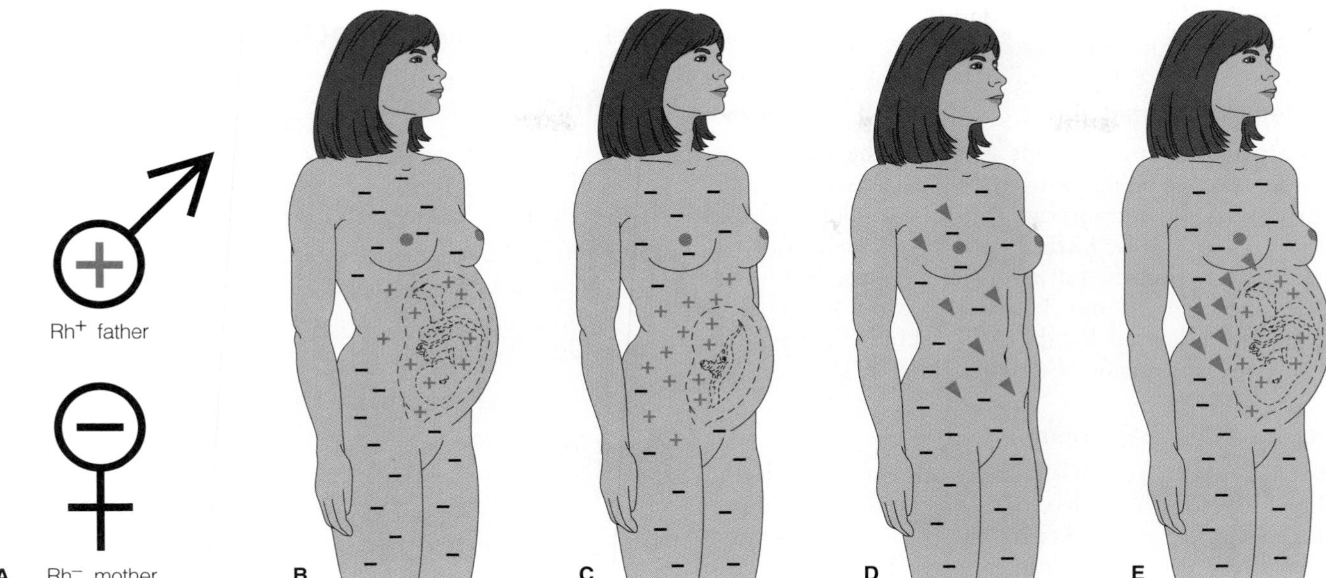

FIGURE 13–5 Rh isoimmunization sequence. ***A*** Rh-positive father and Rh-negative mother. ***B*** Pregnancy with Rh-positive fetus. Some Rh-positive blood enters the mother's blood. ***C*** As the placenta separates, the mother is further exposed to the Rh-positive blood. ***D*** The mother is sensitized to the Rh-positive blood; anti-Rh-positive antibodies (triangles) are formed. ***E*** In subsequent pregnancies with an Rh-positive fetus, Rh-positive red blood cells are attacked by the anti-Rh-positive maternal antibodies, causing hemolysis of red blood cells in the fetus.

Fetal-Neonatal Risks

Although maternal sensitization can now be prevented by appropriate administration of Rh immune globulin, infants still die of Rh hemolytic disease. If treatment is not initiated, the anemia resulting from this disorder can cause marked fetal edema, called **hydrops fetalis.** Congestive heart failure may result, as well as marked jaundice (called *icterus gravis*), which can lead to neurologic damage (kernicterus). This severe hemolytic syndrome is known as **erythroblastosis fetalis.**

Screening for Rh Incompatibility and Sensitization

At the first prenatal visit, caregivers (a) take a history of previous sensitization, abortions, blood transfusions, or children who developed jaundice or anemia during the newborn period; (b) determine maternal blood type (ABO) and Rh factor and do a routine Rh antibody screen; and (c) identify other medical complications such as diabetes, infections, or hypertension.

When assessment identifies an Rh-negative woman who may be pregnant with an Rh-positive fetus, an antibody screen (indirect Coombs' test) is done to determine if the woman is sensitized (has developed isoimmunity) to the Rh antigen. The indirect Coombs' test measures the number of antibodies in the maternal blood.

Negative antibody titers and a negative indirect Coombs' test can consistently identify the fetus not at risk. However, the titers cannot reliably point out the fetus in danger, since titer level does not correlate with the severity of the disease. Antibody titers are determined periodically throughout the pregnancy. If the maternal antibody titer is 1:16 or greater, an optical density (ΔOD) analysis of the amniotic fluid is performed. This optical density analysis measures the amount of pigment from the breakdown of red blood cells and can determine the severity of the hemolytic process.

Ultrasound should be done at 14 to 16 weeks to determine gestational age. Then serial ultrasounds and amniotic fluid analysis should be done to follow fetal progress. The presence of ascites and subcutaneous edema are signs of severe fetal involvement (Scott and Branch 1994). Other indicators of the fetal condition include an increase in fetal heart size and hydramnios. Placental size and texture are also useful in evaluating fetal condition.

Medical Therapy

The goal of medical management is the birth of a mature fetus who has not developed severe hemolysis in utero. This requires early identification and treatment of maternal conditions that predispose to hemolytic disease, identification and evaluation of the Rh-sensitized woman, coordinated obstetric-pediatric treatment for the seriously affected newborn, and prevention of Rh sensitization if none is present.

Antepartal Management

Two primary interventions can help the fetus whose blood cells are being destroyed by maternal antibodies: early birth and intrauterine transfusion, both of which carry risks. Ideally, birth should be delayed until fetal maturity is confirmed at about 36–37 weeks. Only fetuses between 23 and 32 weeks with a prognosis of death as indicated by the ΔOD should be given intrauterine transfusion (Cunningham et al 1997).

Postpartal Management

The Rh-negative mother who has no antibody titer (indirect Coombs' negative, nonsensitized) and has given birth to an Rh-positive fetus (direct Coombs' negative) is given an intramuscular injection of **Rh immune globulin (RhoGAM).** The Rh immune globulin provides passive antibody protection against Rh antigens. This "tricks" the body, which does not then produce antibodies of its own (active immunity). The woman must receive RhoGAM (HypRho-D) within 72 hours of childbirth so she does not have time to produce antibodies to fetal cells that entered her bloodstream when the placenta separated. Administration of Rh immune globulin in a dose of 300 μg generally provides temporary passive immunity to the mother, which prevents the development of permanent active immunity (antibody formation).

When the woman is Rh-negative and not sensitized and the father is Rh-positive or unknown, Rh immune globulin is also given after each abortion, ectopic pregnancy, or amniocentesis. If abortion or ectopic pregnancy occurs in the first trimester, a smaller (50 μg) dose of Rh immune globulin (MICRhoGAM or Mini-Gamulin Rh) is used. A full dose is used following second trimester amniocentesis.

Since transplacental hemorrhage is possible during pregnancy, an antibody screen is performed on an Rh-negative woman at 28 weeks. If it is negative, Rh immune globulin is administered prophylactically. Rh immune globulin is not given to the newborn or the father. It is not effective for, and should not be given to, a previously sensitized woman. However, sometimes after birth or an abortion the results of the blood test do not clearly show whether the mother is already sensitized to the Rh antigen. In such cases, the Rh immune globulin should be given; it will cause no harm. For the major considerations in caring for an Rh-negative woman, see Key Facts to Remember: Rh Sensitization. The treatment of the newborn with isoimmune hemolytic disease is discussed in Chapter 25.

KEY FACTS TO REMEMBER

Rh Sensitization

When trying to work through Rh problems, the nurse should remember the following:

- A potential problem exists when an Rh− mother and an Rh+ father conceive a child who is Rh+.
- In this situation, the mother may become sensitized or produce antibodies to her fetus's Rh+ blood.

The following tests are used to detect sensitization:

- Indirect Coombs' test—done on the mother's blood to measure the number of Rh+ antibodies.
- Direct Coombs' test—done on the infant's blood to detect antibody-coated Rh+ RBCs.

Based on the results of these tests, the following may be done:

- If the mother's indirect Coombs' test is negative and the infant's direct Coombs' test is negative, the mother is given Rh immune globulin within 72 hours of birth.
- If the mother's indirect Coombs' test is positive and her Rh+ infant has a positive direct Coombs' test, Rh immune globulin is *not* given; in this case the infant is carefully monitored for hemolytic disease.
- It is recommended that Rh immune globulin be given at 28 weeks antenatally to decrease possible transplacental bleeding concerns.
- Rh immune globulin is also administered after each abortion (spontaneous or therapeutic), ectopic pregnancy, or amniocentesis.

APPLYING THE NURSING PROCESS

Nursing Assessment

As part of the initial prenatal history, the nurse asks the mother if she knows her blood type and Rh factor. Many women are aware that they are Rh-negative and that this status has implications for pregnancy. If the woman knows she is Rh-negative, the nurse can assess the woman's knowledge of what that means. The nurse can also ask the woman if she has ever received Rh immune globulin, if she has had any previous pregnancies and what their outcome was, and if she knows her partner's Rh factor. Should the partner be Rh-negative, there is no risk to the fetus, who will also be Rh-negative.

If the woman does not know what Rh type she is, intervention cannot begin until the initial laboratory data are obtained. Once that is done, the nurse plans interventions based on the findings.

If the woman becomes sensitized during her pregnancy, nursing assessment focuses on the knowledge level and coping skills of the woman and her family. The nurse also provides ongoing assessment during procedures to evaluate fetal well-being, such as ultrasound and amniocentesis.

After birth, the nurse reviews data about the Rh type of the fetus. If the newborn is Rh-positive, the mother is Rh-negative, and no sensitization has occurred, nursing assessment reveals the need to administer Rh immune globulin.

Nursing Diagnosis

Nursing diagnoses that might apply to the pregnant woman at risk for Rh sensitization include the following:

- Knowledge deficit related to a lack of understanding of the need to receive Rh immune globulin and when it should be administered
- Ineffective individual coping related to depression secondary to the development of indications of the need for fetal exchange transfusion

Nursing Plan and Implementation

During the antepartal period the nurse explains the mechanisms involved in isoimmunization and answers any questions the woman and her partner have. It is imperative that the woman understand the importance of receiving Rh immune globulin after every spontaneous or therapeutic abortion or ectopic pregnancy. The nurse also explains the purpose of the Rh immune globulin administered at 28 weeks' gestation if the woman is not sensitized.

If the woman is sensitized to the Rh factor, it poses a threat to any Rh-positive fetus she carries. The nurse provides emotional support to the family to help them deal with their grief and any feelings of guilt about the infant's condition. Should an intrauterine transfusion become necessary, the nurse continues to provide emotional support while also assuming responsibility as part of the health care team.

During labor, the nurse caring for an Rh-negative woman who has not been sensitized ensures that the woman's blood is assessed for any antibodies and also has been crossmatched for Rh immune globulin. On the postpartum unit the nurse generally is responsible for administering the Rh immune globulin intramuscularly if the newborn is Rh-positive (see Procedure 13–2).

Evaluation

Anticipated outcomes of nursing care include

- The woman is able to explain the process of Rh sensitization and its implications for her unborn child and for subsequent pregnancies.
- If the woman has not been sensitized, she is able to discuss the importance of receiving Rh immune globulin when necessary and cooperates with the recommended dosage schedule.
- The woman gives birth to a healthy newborn.
- If complications develop for the fetus (or newborn) they are detected quickly and therapy is instituted.

Care of the Woman at Risk Due to ABO Incompatibility

ABO incompatibility is rather common (occurring in 12 percent of pregnancies), but it rarely causes significant hemolysis. In most cases ABO incompatibility is limited to type O mothers with a type A or B fetus. Group O infants, because they have no antigenic sites on the red blood cells, are never affected regardless of the mother's blood type. The incompatibility occurs as a result of the interaction of antibodies present in maternal serum and the antigen sites on the fetal red blood cells.

Anti-A and anti-B antibodies are naturally occurring; that is, women are naturally exposed to the A and B antigens through the foods they eat and through exposure to infection by gram-negative bacteria. As a result, some women have high serum anti-A and anti-B titers before they become pregnant. Once the woman becomes pregnant, the maternal serum anti-A and anti-B antibodies cross the placenta and produce hemolysis of the fetal red blood cells. With ABO incompatibility, the first infant is frequently involved, and no relationship exists between the appearance of the disease and repeated sensitization from one pregnancy to the next.

Unlike Rh incompatibility, antepartal treatment is never warranted. As part of the initial assessment, however, the nurse should note whether the potential for an ABO incompatibility exists. This alerts caregivers so that, following birth, the newborn can be assessed carefully for the development of hyperbilirubinemia (see Chapter 26).

Care of the Woman Requiring Surgery During Pregnancy

Elective surgery should be delayed until the postpartal period; however, essential surgery can generally be undertaken during pregnancy. Surgery does pose some risks. The incidence of spontaneous abortion is increased for women who have surgery in the first trimester. There is also an increased incidence of fetal mortality and of low-birth-weight (less than 2500 g)

PROCEDURE 13–2 Administering Rh Immune Globulin (RhIgG, RhoGAM, HypRho-D)

Rh Immune Globulin

Immunization with Rh immune globulin is indicated anytime there is a potential for maternal exposure to Rh positive blood. It is given prophylactically at 28 weeks' gestation, within 72 hours after the birth of an Rh positive Coombs' negative child, and following any spontaneous or therapeutic abortion, ectopic pregnancy, or amniocentesis.

Medication is administered intramuscularly. It causes passive immunity to occur and "tricks" the body into believing that it is not necessary to develop antibodies. The normal dose of 300 μg provides passive immunity following exposure of up to 15 mL of transfused RBCs or 30 mL or fetal blood. If a larger bleed is expected to occur (as in cases of severe abruptio placentae), additional doses may be administered at one time using multiple sites or at regular intervals as long as all doses are given within 72 hours of childbirth.

Nursing Action	Rationale
Objective: Confirm that Rh immune globulin is needed.	
• Confirm that the mother is Rh-negative by checking her prenatal or intrapartal record, and confirm that sensitization has not occurred (maternal indirect Coombs' test is negative).	When an Rh-negative woman is exposed to Rh-positive blood, sensitization—development of antibodies to the Rh-positive blood—occurs. The antibodies can attack the fetal red blood cells, causing profound anemia.
• Confirm that the infant is Rh-positive (a sample of the infant's cord blood is usually sent to the lab immediately after birth for typing and crossmatching), and confirm that sensitization has not occurred (direct Coombs' is negative).	If the direct and the indirect Coombs' tests are negative, sensitization has not occurred and Rh immune globulin is indicated.
Objective: Confirm that the woman does not have a history of allergy to immune globulins or blood products.	
• Review any entries on medication allergies in the client's chart, and ask the woman if she has ever had any allergic reactions to medications, globulins, or blood products.	Rh immune globulin is made from the plasma portion of blood; thus allergic reactions are possible.
Objective: Prepare the woman.	
• Explain the procedure, its purpose, and its potential side effects (erythema and tenderness at the injection site and allergic responses).	Explanation of the procedure decreases anxiety.
• Ascertain that the woman clearly understands the purpose of the procedure, its rationale, and the risks associated with it.	Many women, especially primigravidas, are not aware of the risks for an Rh-positive fetus of a sensitized Rh-negative mother. They must understand the importance of receiving medication for each pregnancy to ensure continued protection.
• Ask the woman to sign a consent form if your agency requires one.	Many agencies require informed consent before administering Rh immune globulin.
Objective: Obtain the correct medication.	
• Obtain the medication from the blood bank or pharmacy according to agency policy.	
• Check to make sure that the lot numbers for the drug and the crossmatch are the same.	Blood products are involved in the preparation, so careful verification is essential.
Objective: Confirm client identity and administer the medication in the deltoid muscle.	
Objective: Complete education for self-care.	
• Encourage the woman to ask questions and express concerns.	
Objective: Complete the client record.	
• Chart according to agency procedure. Most agencies chart lot number, route, dose, site, and provision of client education.	Provides a permanent record.

infants. Finally, when pelvic surgery is necessary, the incidence of preterm labor increases.

Although general preoperative and postoperative care is similar for gravid and nongravid women, special considerations must be kept in mind whenever the surgical client is pregnant. The early second trimester is the best time to operate because there is less risk of causing spontaneous abortion or early labor, and the uterus is not so large as to impinge on the abdominal field.

To prevent uterine compression of major blood vessels while the woman is supine, the caregiver must place a wedge under her right hip to tilt the uterus during both surgery and recovery. The decreased intestinal motility and delayed gastric emptying that occur in pregnancy increase the risk of vomiting when anesthetics are given and during the postoperative period. Thus inserting a nasogastric tube is recommended before a pregnant woman has major surgery. An indwelling urinary catheter prevents bladder distention, decreases risk of injury to the bladder, and permits convenient monitoring of output.

Pregnancy causes increased secretions of the respiratory tract and engorgement of the nasal mucous membrane, often making breathing through the nose difficult. Because of this, pregnant women often need an endotracheal tube for respiratory support during surgery.

Caregivers must guard against maternal hypoxia. During surgery, uterine circulation decreases, and fetal oxygenation may be reduced quickly. Fetal heart rate must be monitored electronically before, during, and after surgery. Blood loss is also closely monitored throughout the procedure and following it.

Postoperatively, the nurse encourages the woman to turn, breathe deeply, and cough regularly and to use any ventilation therapy such as incentive spirometry to avoid developing pneumonia. The pregnant woman is at increased risk for thrombophlebitis, so the nurse applies antiembolism stockings, encourages leg exercises while the woman is confined to bed, and introduces ambulation as soon as possible.

Discharge teaching is especially important. The woman and her family should clearly understand what to expect regarding activity level, discomfort, diet, medications, and any special considerations. In addition, they should know the warning signs they need to report to the physician immediately.

Care of the Woman Suffering Trauma from an Accident

Trauma complicates approximately 6 to 7 percent of all pregnancies. Motor vehicle accidents are by far the most common cause of trauma, accounting for two-thirds of injuries, with falls and assaults accounting for most of the remaining cases (Pearlman 1996). Domestic violence, which may be the etiology of trauma, is discussed in the next section.

Fortunately, most accidents produce minor injuries, and the outcome of the pregnancy is seldom affected. Late in pregnancy, when balance and coordination are adversely affected, the woman may fall. Her protruding abdomen is vulnerable to a variety of minor injuries. The fetus is usually well protected by the amniotic fluid, which distributes the force of a blow equally in all directions, and by the muscle layers of the uterus and abdominal wall. In early pregnancy, while the uterus is still in the pelvis, it is shielded from blows by the surrounding pelvic organs, muscles, and bony structures.

Trauma that causes concern includes blunt trauma, from an automobile accident, for example; penetrating abdominal injuries, such as knife and gunshot wounds; and the complications of maternal shock, premature labor, and spontaneous abortion. Maternal mortality most often occurs from head trauma or hemorrhage. Uterine rupture may result from strong deceleration forces in an automobile accident with or without seat belts. Traumatic separation of the placenta can occur; it causes a high rate of fetal mortality. Premature labor is another serious hazard to the fetus, often following rupture of membranes during an accident. Premature labor can ensue even if the woman is not injured.

Treatment of major injuries during pregnancy focuses initially on life-saving measures for the woman. Such measures include establishing an airway, controlling external bleeding, and administering intravenous fluid to alleviate shock. The woman must be kept on her left side to avoid further hypotension. Fetal heart rate is monitored. Exploratory surgery may be necessary following abdominal trauma to determine the extent of injuries. If the fetus is near term and the uterus has been damaged, cesarean birth is indicated. If the fetus is still immature, the uterus can often be repaired, and the pregnancy continues until term.

In cases of trauma in which the mother's life is not directly threatened, fetal monitoring for four hours should be sufficient if there are no contractions, vaginal bleeding, uterine tenderness, or leaking amniotic fluid.

Abruptio placentae may occur following a blow to the abdomen. Increased uterine irritability in the first few hours after trauma helps identify women who may be at risk for this potentially catastrophic complication.

Care of the Battered Pregnant Woman

Female partner abuse, the intentional injury of a woman by her partner, also called battering, often begins or increases during pregnancy. Battering often includes injuries to the breasts, blows to the abdomen, trauma to the genitals, and sexual assault (Parker and McFarlane 1991). It may cause loss of pregnancy, preterm labor, low-birth-weight infants, injury to the fetus, and fetal death (Bohn 1990). The first step toward helping the battered woman is to identify her. She needs support, confidence in her decision making, and the recognition that she can help herself.

Chronic psychosomatic symptoms can be an indicator of abuse. The woman may have nonspecific or vague complaints. It is important to assess old scars around the head, chest, arms, abdomen, and genitalia. Any bruising or evidence of pain is also evaluated. The nurse should be especially alert for signs of bruising or injury to the woman's breasts, abdomen, or genitalia because these areas are common targets of violence during pregnancy. Other indicators include a decrease in eye contact; silence when the partner is in the room; and a history of nervousness, insomnia, drug overdose, or alcohol problems. Frequent visits to the emergency room and a history of accidents without understandable causes are possible indicators of abuse.

The goals of treatment are to identify the woman at risk, increase her decision-making abilities to decrease the potential for further abuse, and provide a safe environment for the pregnant woman and her unborn child. It is important to provide an environment that is private, accepting, and nonjudgmental so the woman can express her concerns. She needs to be aware of community resources available to her, such as emergency shelters; police, legal, and social services; and counseling. Nurses need to recognize that, ultimately, it is the woman's decision to either seek assistance or return to old patterns.

Because abuse often begins during pregnancy, it may be a new and unexpected experience for the woman. She may believe it is an isolated incidence. She needs to know that battering may well occur following childbirth and may extend to the child as well. This is an important time for the nurse to provide information and establish a trusted link for the woman with a health professional. For further discussion see Chapter 5.

Care of the Woman with a TORCH Infection

The TORCH group of infectious diseases are those identified as causing serious harm to the embryo-fetus. These are: toxoplasmosis *(TO),* rubella *(R),* cytomegalovirus *(C),* and herpesvirus type 2 *(H).* (Some sources identify the O as "other infections.") The TORCH identification has been useful in assessing major areas of risk, but, because so many major infections such as HIV, hepatitis, syphilis, and the parvovirus, are not included, the acronym may lead to an underappreciation of the variety of organisms that can cause congenital infections (McMillan 1992).

The importance of understanding what these infections are, and identifying risk factors, cannot be overemphasized. Exposure of the woman during the first 12 weeks of gestation may cause developmental anomalies in the fetus.

Toxoplasmosis

Toxoplasmosis is caused by the protozoan *Toxoplasma gondii.* It is innocuous in adults, but when contracted in pregnancy, it can profoundly affect the fetus. The pregnant woman may contract the organism by eating raw or poorly cooked meat or by contact with the feces of infected cats, either through the cat litter box or by gardening in areas frequented by cats.

Fetal-Neonatal Risks

Maternal infection with toxoplasmosis during the first trimester is associated with the lowest incidence of fetal infection but the highest risk of fetal brain damage. In general it increases the incidence of abortion, prematurity, stillbirths, newborn deaths, and severe congenital anomalies. About two-thirds of infants born with congenital toxoplasmosis are asymptomatic at birth but develop symptoms of the disease weeks or months later (Freij and Sever 1996). The infection may vary from mild to severe. In very mild cases, retinochoroiditis (inflammation of the retina and choroid of the eye) may be the only recognizable damage, and it and other manifestations may not appear until adolescence or young adulthood. Severe neonatal disorders associated with congenital infection include convulsions, coma, encephalitis, microcephaly, and hydrocephalus. The infant with a severe infection may die soon after birth. Survivors are often blind, deaf, and severely retarded.

Medical Therapy

The goal of medical treatment is to identify the woman at risk for toxoplasmosis and to treat the disease promptly if diagnosed. Diagnosis can be made by detecting Toxoplasma-specific IgM antibodies using the indirect fluorescent antibody (IFA) test or the IgM ELISA coupled with high IgG titers as measured by the IFA or Sabin-Feldman dye test. IgM titers become positive within 1 to 2 weeks after infection and may persist for months or years (Freij and Sever 1996).

Prenatal diagnosis of toxoplasmosis is possible using amniocentesis and ultrasound-guided cordocentesis to obtain a sample of fetal blood, which is then tested for Toxoplasma-specific IgM. If diagnosis is established, the woman may be treated with sulfadiazine, pyrimethamine, and spiramycin. Treatment of the mother can reduce the incidence of fetal infection significantly.

If toxoplasmosis is diagnosed before 20 weeks' gestation, therapeutic abortion may be considered if it is acceptable to the parents, because damage to the fetus is generally more severe than it is when the disease is acquired later in the pregnancy.

Infants infected with toxoplasmosis are treated with a combination of pyrimethamine, sulfadiazine, and leucovorin calcium.

APPLYING THE NURSING PROCESS

Nursing Assessment

The incubation period for the disease is 10 days. The woman with acute toxoplasmosis may be asymptomatic, or she may develop myalgia, malaise, rash, splenomegaly, and enlarged posterior cervical lymph nodes. Symptoms usually disappear in a few days or weeks.

Nursing Diagnosis

Nursing diagnoses that might apply to the pregnant woman with toxoplasmosis include the following:

- Risk for altered health maintenance related to lack of knowledge about ways in which a pregnant woman can contract toxoplasmosis
- Anticipatory grieving related to potential effects on infant of maternal toxoplasmosis

Nursing Plan and Implementation

The nurse caring for women during the antepartal period has the primary opportunity to discuss methods of preventing toxoplasmosis. The woman must understand the importance of avoiding poorly cooked or raw meat, especially pork, beef, lamb, and, in the arctic region, caribou. Fruits and vegetables should be washed. She should avoid contact with the cat litter box and have someone else clean it frequently, since it takes approximately 48 hours for a cat's feces to become infectious. The nurse should also discuss the importance of wearing gloves when gardening and of avoiding garden areas frequented by cats.

Evaluation

Anticipated outcomes of nursing care include

- The woman is able to discuss toxoplasmosis, its methods of transmission, the implications for her fetus, and measures she can take to avoid contracting it.
- The woman implements health measures to avoid contracting toxoplasmosis.
- The woman gives birth to a healthy newborn.

Rubella

The effects of rubella (German measles) are no more severe, and there are no greater complications in pregnant women than in nonpregnant women of comparable age. However, the effects of this infection on the fetus and newborn are great because rubella causes a chronic infection that begins in the first trimester of pregnancy and may persist for months after birth.

Fetal-Neonatal Risks

The period of greatest risk for the teratogenic effects of rubella on the fetus is the first trimester. Clinical signs of congenital infection are congenital heart disease, IUGR, and cataracts. Cardiac complications most often seen are patent ductus arteriosus and narrowing of peripheral pulmonary arteries. Cataracts may be unilateral or bilateral and may be present at birth or develop in the newborn period. A petechial rash is seen in some infants, and hepatosplenomegaly and hyperbilirubinemia are frequently seen. Other abnormalities, such as mental retardation or cerebral palsy, may become evident in infancy. Diagnosis in the newborn can be conclusively made in the presence of these conditions and with an elevated rubella IgM antibody titer at birth.

Infants born with congenital rubella syndrome are infectious and should be isolated. These infants may continue to shed the virus for months.

The expanded rubella syndrome relates to effects that may develop for years after the infection. These include an increased incidence of insulin-dependent diabetes mellitus; sudden hearing loss; glaucoma; and a slow, progressive form of encephalitis.

Medical Therapy

The best therapy for rubella is prevention. Live attenuated vaccine is available and should be given to all children. Women of childbearing age should be tested for immunity and vaccinated if susceptible once it is established that they are not pregnant.

As part of the prenatal laboratory screen, the woman is evaluated for rubella using hemagglutination inhibition (HAI), a serology test. The presence of a 1:16 titer or greater is evidence of immunity. A titer less than 1:8 indicates susceptibility to rubella.

Because the vaccine is made with attenuated virus, pregnant women are not vaccinated. However, it is considered safe for newly vaccinated children to have contact with pregnant women.

If a woman becomes infected during the first trimester, therapeutic abortion is an alternative.

APPLYING THE NURSING PROCESS

Nursing Assessment

A woman who develops rubella during pregnancy may be asymptomatic or may show signs of a mild infection including a maculopapular rash, lymphadenopathy, muscular achiness, and joint pain. The presence of IgM antirubella antibody is diagnostic of a recent infection. These titers remain elevated for approximately 1 month after infection.

Nursing Diagnosis

Nursing diagnoses that may apply to the woman who develops rubella early in her pregnancy include the following:

- Ineffective family coping due to an inability to accept the possibility of fetal anomalies secondary to maternal rubella exposure
- Risk for altered health maintenance related to lack of knowledge about the importance of rubella immunization before becoming pregnant

Nursing Plan and Implementation

Nursing support and understanding are vital for the couple contemplating abortion due to a diagnosis of rubella. Such a decision may initiate a crisis for the couple who have planned their pregnancy. They need objective data to understand the possible effects on their unborn fetus and the prognosis for the offspring.

Evaluation

Anticipated outcomes of nursing care include

- The woman is able to describe the implications of rubella exposure during the first trimester of pregnancy.
- If exposure occurs in a woman who is not immune, she is able to identify her options and make a decision about continuing her pregnancy that is acceptable to her and her partner.
- The nonimmune woman receives the rubella vaccine during the early postpartal period.
- The woman gives birth to a healthy infant.

Cytomegalovirus

Cytomegalovirus (CMV) belongs to the herpesvirus group and causes both congenital and acquired infections referred to as *cytomegalic inclusion disease (CID)*. The significance of this virus in pregnancy is related to its ability to be transmitted by asymptomatic women across the placenta to the fetus or by the cervical route during birth.

CID is probably the most prevalent infection in the TORCH group. Nearly half of adults have antibodies for the virus. The virus can be found in urine, saliva, cervical mucus, semen, and breast milk. It can be passed between humans by any close contact such as kissing, breastfeeding, and sexual intercourse. Asymptomatic CMV infection is particularly common in children and gravid women. It is a chronic, persistent infection in that the individual may shed the virus continually over many years. The cervix can harbor the virus, and an ascending infection can develop after birth. Although the virus is usually innocuous in adults and children, it may be fatal to the fetus.

Accurate diagnosis in the pregnant woman depends on the presence of CMV in the urine, a rise in IgM levels, and identification of the CMV antibodies within the serum IgM fraction. At present, no treatment exists for maternal CMV or for the congenital disease in the neonate.

The cytomegalovirus is the most frequent agent of viral infection in the human fetus. It infects 0.5 to 2.5 percent of newborns, and of these about 5–10 percent develop serious manifestations (Faro and Pastorek 1993). Subclinical infections in the newborn may produce mental retardation and auditory deficits, sometimes not recognized for several months, or learning disabilities not seen until childhood. CMV may be the most common cause of mental retardation.

For the fetus, this infection can result in extensive intrauterine tissue damage that leads to fetal death; in survival with microcephaly, hydrocephaly, cerebral palsy, or mental retardation; or in survival with no damage at all. The infected newborn is often small for gestational age (SGA). The principal tissues and organs affected are the blood, brain, and liver. However, virtually all organs are potentially at risk. Hemolysis leads to anemia and hyperbilirubinemia. Thrombocytopenia and hepatosplenomegaly may also develop.

Herpes Simplex Virus

Herpes simplex virus (HSV-I or HSV-2) infection can cause painful lesions in the genital area. Lesions may also develop on the cervix. This condition and its implications for nonpregnant women are discussed in Chapter 5. However, because the presence of herpes lesions in the genital tract may profoundly affect the fetus, herpes infection as it relates to a pregnant woman is discussed here as part of the TORCH complex of infections.

Fetal-Neonatal Risks

The risk of transmission to the newborn is highest among women who contract their first herpes infection near the time of birth. It is lower among women with recurrent herpes (CDC 1993). Transmission of HSV-2 to the fetus almost always occurs after the membranes rupture, as the virus ascends from active lesions. It also occurs during vaginal birth, when the fetus comes in contact with genital lesions. Transplacental infection is rare.

Primary genital HSV infection during pregnancy has been associated with spontaneous abortion, preterm birth, and intrauterine growth retardation. Approximately 40 percent of all infants who are born vaginally when the mother is experiencing a primary HSV infection and shedding HSV in her vagina or cervix develop some form of herpes infection. Of these infants, approximately half will die if untreated, and 35–40 percent will have severe neurologic problems (Duff 1996).

Infants born to women with a primary HSV infection should have cultures taken of the nasopharynx, conjunctivae, urine, stool, and cerebrospinal fluid. The infected infant is often asymptomatic at birth but develops symptoms of fever (or hypothermia), jaundice, seizures, and poor feeding after an incubation period of 2 to 12 days. Approximately half of infected infants develop the characteristic vesicular skin lesions. To date no definitive treatment exists. However, a positive culture or abnormal CSF finding in a newborn older than 48 hours should be treated with intravenous acyclovir (Brown 1995).

Medical Therapy

The vesicular lesions of herpes have a characteristic appearance and they rupture easily. Definitive diagnosis is made by culturing active lesions. Because cultures are expensive and not always available, many caregivers obtain a discharge from the lesion and prepare a slide as for a Pap test. The presence of multinucleated giant cells indicates herpes.

Treatment is directed first toward relieving the woman's vulvar pain. If the attack is severe, walking, sitting, and even wearing clothing may be painful. The woman may be most comfortable in bed during the peak of the infection. Sitz baths 3–4 times daily, followed by air drying of the vulva, may promote healing and help prevent secondary infection. Cotton underwear helps keep the genital area dry.

Although acyclovir (Zovirax) does not cure the infection or prevent recurrence, it does reduce healing time of the initial attack and shortens the time that the live virus is in the lesions, thereby reducing the infectious period. Currently it is not recommended for use during pregnancy, however.

HSV has not been found in breast milk. Present experience shows that breastfeeding is acceptable if the mother washes her hands well to prevent any direct transfer of the virus.

Because most infants become infected when they pass through the birth canal, it was formerly the practice to do serial cervical cultures. Recently the Infectious Disease Society for Obstetrics and Gynecology issued new guidelines for the management of HSV-2 in pregnancy. The society recommends that caregivers should obtain and record a history of HSV infection in the woman or her partner at the first prenatal visit. Weekly cultures are not recommended for women with a history of HSV but with no visible lesions. When she is admitted for childbirth the woman should be asked about the presence of any prodromal symptoms and examined carefully for vulvar, vaginal, or cervical lesions. For women with no symptoms and no visible lesions, vaginal birth should be attempted. For women with symptoms or visible lesions, cesarean birth is indicated to reduce the risk of newborn infection. Cesarean birth is best attempted within 4 to 6 hours of rupture of membranes to decrease the risk of ascending infection. However, cesarean birth is still recommended, regardless of the time elapsed in women with visible lesions.

APPLYING THE NURSING PROCESS

Nursing Assessment

During the initial prenatal visit it is important to learn whether the woman or her partner have had previous herpes infections. If so, ongoing assessment by means of cervical cultures is indicated as pregnancy progresses.

Nursing Diagnosis

Nursing diagnoses that may apply to the pregnant woman with HSV infection include the following:

- Sexual dysfunction related to unwillingness to engage in sexual intercourse secondary to the presence of active herpes lesions
- Ineffective individual coping related to depression secondary to the risk to the fetus if herpes lesions are present at birth

Nursing Plan and Implementation

Nurses need to be particularly concerned with client education about this fast-spreading disease. Women should be informed of the association of HSV infection with spontaneous abortion, newborn mortality and morbidity, and the possibility of cesarean birth. A woman needs to inform her future health care providers of her infection. She should also know of the possible

TABLE 13–3 Infections that Put Pregnancy at Risk

Condition and Causative Organism	Signs and Symptoms	Treatment	Implications for Pregnancy
Urinary Tract Infections			
Asymptomatic bacteriuria (ASB): *E coli, Klebsiella, Proteus* most common	Bacteria present in urine on culture with no accompanying symptoms.	Oral sulfonamides early in pregnancy, ampicillin and nitrofurantoin (Furadantin) in late pregnancy.	Women with ASB in early pregnancy may go on to develop cystitis or acute pyelonephritis by third trimester if not treated. Oral sulfonamides taken in the last few weeks of pregnancy may lead to neonatal hyperbilirubinemia and kernicterus.
Cystitis (lower UTI): Causative organisms same as ASB	Dysuria, urgency, frequency; low-grade fever and hematuria may occur. Urine culture (clean catch) show ↑ leukocytes. Presence of 10^5 (100,000) or more colonies bacteria per mL urine.	Same.	If not treated, infection may ascend and lead to acute pyelonephritis.
Acute pyelonephritis: Causative organisms same as ASB	Sudden onset. Chills, high fever, flank pain. Nausea, vomiting, malaise. May have decreased urine output, severe colicky pain, dehydration. Increased diastolic BP, positive FA test, low creatinine clearance. Marked bacteremia in urine culture, pyuria, WBC casts.	Hospitalization; IV antibiotic therapy. Other antibiotics safe during pregnancy include carbenicillin, methenamine, cephalosporins. Catheterization if output is ↓. Supportive therapy for comfort. Follow-up urine cultures are necessary.	Increased risk of premature birth and IUGR. These antibiotics interfere with urinary estriol levels and can cause false interpretations of estriol levels during pregnancy.
Vaginal Infections			
Vulvovaginal candidiasis (yeast infection): *Candida albicans*	Often thick, white, curdy discharge, severe itching, dysuria, dyspareunia. Diagnosis based on presence of hyphae and spores in a wet mount preparation of vaginal secretions.	Intravaginal insertion of miconazole or clotrimazole suppositories at bedtime for 1 week. Cream may be prescribed for topical application to the vulva if necessary.	If the infection is present at birth and the fetus is born vaginally, the fetus may contract thrush.
Bacterial vaginosis: *Gardnerella vaginalis*	Thin, watery, yellow-gray discharge with foul odor often described as "fishy." Wet mount preparation reveals "clue cells." Application of KOH (potassium hydroxide) to a specimen of vaginal secretions produces a pronounced fishy odor.	Nonpregnant women treated with metronidazole (Flagyl). In first trimester, pregnant women treated with clindamycin. In second and third trimesters, metronidazole vaginal gel or clindamycin cream preferred (CDC 1993).	Metronidazole has potential teratogenic effects. Possible ↑ risk of PROM and preterm birth. Confirmatory studies needed (CDC 1993).
Trichomoniasis: *Trichomonas vaginalis*	Occasionally asymptomatic. May have frothy greenish-gray vaginal discharge, pruritus, urinary symptoms. Strawberry patches may be visible on vaginal walls or cervix. Wet mount preparation of vaginal secretions shows motile flagellated trichomonads.	During early pregnancy symptoms may be controlled with clotrimazole vaginal suppositories. Both partners are treated, but no adequate treatment exists. After first trimester, a single 2 g dose of metronidazole may be used (CDC 1993).	Metronidazole has potential teratogenic effects. Associated with ↑ risk of PROM and preterm birth (CDC 1993).

association of genital herpes with cervical cancer and the importance of a yearly Pap smear.

The woman who acquired HSV infection as an adolescent may be devastated as a mature young adult who wants to have a family. Clients may be helped by counseling that allows them to express the anger, shame, and depression often experienced by herpes victims. Literature may be helpful and is available from Planned Parenthood and many public health agencies. The American Social Health Association has established the HELP program to provide information and the latest research results on genital herpes. The association has a quarterly journal, *The Helper*, for nurses and clients with HSV infection.

Evaluation

Anticipated outcomes of nursing care include

- The woman is able to describe her infection with regard to its method of spread, therapy and comfort measures, implications for her pregnancy, and long-term implications.
- The woman has appropriate cultures done as recommended throughout her pregnancy.
- The woman successfully gives birth to a healthy infant.

TABLE 13–3 Infections that Put Pregnancy at Risk continued

Condition and Causative Organism	Signs and Symptoms	Treatment	Implications for Pregnancy
Sexually Transmitted Infections			
Chlamydial infection: *Chlamydia trachomatis*	Women are often asymptomatic. Symptoms may include thin or purulent discharge, urinary burning and frequency, or lower abdominal pain. Lab test available to detect monoclonal antibodies specific for *Chlamydia*.	Although nonpregnant women are treated with tetracycline, it may permanently discolor fetal teeth. Thus pregnant women are treated with erythromycin ethyl succinate.	Infant of woman with untreated chlamydial infection may develop newborn conjunctivitis, which can be treated with erythromycin eye ointment (but not silver nitrate). Infant may also develop chlamydial pneumonia. May be responsible for premature labor and fetal death.
Syphilis: *Treponema pallidum,* a spirochete	Primary stage: chancre, slight fever, malaise. Chancre lasts about 4 weeks, then disappears. Secondary stage: occurs 6 weeks to 6 months after infection. Skin eruptions (condyloma lata); also symptoms of acute arthritis, liver enlargement, iritis, chronic sore throat with hoarseness. Diagnosed by blood tests such as VDRL, RPR, FTA-ABS. Dark-field examination for spirochetes may also be done.	For syphilis less than 1 year in duration: 2.4 million U benzathine penicillin G IM. For syphilis of more than 1 year's duration: 2.4 million U benzathine penicillin G once a week for 3 weeks. Sexual partners should also be screened and treated.	Syphilis can be passed transplacentally to the fetus. If untreated, one of the following can occur: second trimester abortion, stillborn infant at term, congenitally infected infant, uninfected live infant.
Gonorrhea: *Neisseria gonorrhoeae*	Majority of women asymptomatic; disease often diagnosed during routine prenatal cervical culture. If symptoms are present they may include purulent vaginal discharge, dysuria, urinary frequency, inflammation and swelling of the vulva. Cervix may appear eroded.	Nonpregnant women are treated with ceftriaxone plus doxycycline. Pregnant women are treated with ceftriaxone plus erythromycin (CDC 1993). If the woman is allergic to ceftriaxone, spectinomycin is used. All sexual partners are also treated.	Infection at time of birth may cause ophthalmia neonatorum in the newborn.
Condyloma acuminata: caused by a papovavirus	Soft, grayish-pink lesions on the vulva, vagina, cervix, or anus.	Podophyllin not used during pregnancy. Trichloroacetic acid, liquid nitrogen, or cryotherapy CO_2 laser therapy done under colposcopy is also successful (CDC 1993).	Possible teratogenic effect of podophyllin. Large doses have been associated with fetal death.

Other Infections in Pregnancy

In addition to the TORCH infections, other infections contribute to risk during pregnancy. Spontaneous abortion is frequently the result of a severe maternal infection. Some evidence links infection and prematurity. In addition, if the pregnancy is carried to term in the presence of infection, the risk of maternal and fetal morbidity and mortality increases. Thus it is essential to maternal and fetal health that infection be diagnosed and treated promptly.

Urinary tract, vaginal, and sexually transmitted infections are discussed in detail in Chapter 5. Table 13–3 provides a summary of these infections and their implications for pregnancy.

CHAPTER HIGHLIGHTS

- Hyperemesis gravidarum, excessive vomiting during pregnancy, may cause fluid and electrolyte imbalance, dehydration, and signs of starvation in the mother, and, if severe enough, death of the fetus. Treatment is aimed at controlling the vomiting, correcting fluid and electrolyte imbalance, correcting dehydration, and improving nutritional status.

- Several health problems associated with bleeding arise from the pregnancy itself, such as spontaneous abortion, ectopic pregnancy, and gestational trophoblastic disease. The nurse needs to be alert to early signs of these situations, to guard the woman against heavy bleeding and shock, to facilitate the medical treatment, and to provide educational and emotional support.
- Incompetent cervix, the premature dilatation of the cervix, is the most common cause of second trimester abortion. It is treated surgically with a Shirodkar-Barter operation (cerclage), which involves placing a purse-string suture in the cervix to keep it closed.
- Both premature rupture of the membranes and preterm labor place the fetus at risk. Women with PROM and no signs of infection are managed conservatively with bed rest and careful monitoring of fetal well-being. Women with a history of preterm labor are often placed on home fetal monitoring programs. If preterm labor develops, tocolytics are often effective in stopping labor, but they do have associated side effects.
- Hypertension may exist before pregnancy or, more often, may develop during pregnancy. Preeclampsia can lead to growth retardation for the fetus, and if untreated may lead to convulsions (eclampsia) and even death for the mother and fetus. A woman's understanding of the disease process helps motivate her to maintain the required rest periods in the left lateral position. Antihypertensive or anticonvulsive drugs may be part of the therapy.
- Rh incompatibility can exist when an Rh− woman and an Rh+ partner conceive a child who is Rh+. The use of Rh immune globulin has greatly decreased the incidence of severe sequelae due to Rh because the drug "tricks" the body into thinking antibodies have been produced in response to the Rh antigen.
- The impact of surgery, trauma, or battering on the pregnant woman and her fetus is related to timing in the pregnancy, seriousness of the situation, and other factors influencing the situation.
- Physical violence often begins or continues during pregnancy. The nurse needs to be alert for signs of abuse, including bruising or injury to the breasts, abdomen, or genitalia. The woman should be given information about female partner abuse and about community resources available to assist her.
- Urinary tract infections are a common problem in pregnancy. If untreated, the infection may ascend, causing more serious illness for the mother. Urinary tract infections are also associated with an increased risk of premature labor.
- TORCH is an acronym standing for toxoplasmosis, rubella, cytomegalovirus, and herpes, all of which pose a grave threat to the fetus.
- Sexually transmitted infections pose less of a threat to the fetus if detected and treated quickly.

REFERENCES

Arias F: *Practical Guide to High-Risk Pregnancy and Delivery,* 2nd ed. St. Louis: Mosby Year Book, 1993.

Bishop EH: Acceleration of fetal pulmonary maturity. *Obstet Gynecol* 1981; 58(suppl):48.

Blackburn ST, Loper DL: *Maternal, Fetal and Neonatal Physiology: A Clinical Perspective.* Philadelphia: Saunders, 1992.

Bohn DK: Domestic violence and pregnancy: Implications for practice. *J Nurse-Midwifery* March/April 1990; 35:86.

Briggs GC et al: *Drugs in Pregnancy and Lactation,* 4th ed. Baltimore: Williams & Wilkins, 1994.

Brown ZA: Preventing vertical transmission of herpes simplex. *Contemp OB/GYN* July 1995; 40(7):27.

Centers for Disease Control and Prevention: 1993 Sexually transmitted disease treatment guidelines. *MMWR* 1993; 42(RR-14):4.

Creasy RK, Resnik R: *Maternal-Fetal Medicine: Principles and Practices.* Philadelphia: Saunders, 1989.

Cunningham FG et al: *Williams Obstetrics,* 20th ed. Stamford, CT: Appleton & Lange, 1997.

Devoe LD: Home uterine activity monitoring. *Contemp OB/GYN* April 15, 1996; 41:72.

Duff P: Maternal and perinatal infection. In: *Obstetrics: Normal and Problem Pregnancies,* 3rd ed. Gabbe SG et al (editors). New York: Churchill Livingstone, 1996.

Faro, F, Pastorek JG: Perinatal infections. In: *High-Risk Pregnancy: A Team Approach,* 2nd ed. Knuppel RA, Drukker JE (editors). Philadelphia: Saunders, 1993.

Frangieh AY, Sibai BM: Outpatient management of mild gestational hypertension and preeclampsia. *Contemp OB/GYN* August 1996; 41(8):67.

Freij BJ, Sever JL: What do we know about toxoplasmosis? *Contemp OB/GYN* February 1996; 41(2):41.

Garite TJ, Lockwood CJ: A new test for diagnosis and prediction of preterm delivery. *Contemp OB/GYN* January 1996; 41(1):77.

Grimes DA, Shultz KF: Randomized controlled trials of home uterine activity monitoring: A review and critique. *Obstet Gynecol* 1992; 79(1):137.

Hammond CB, Bachus KE: Ectopic pregnancy. In: *Danforth's Obstetrics and Gynecology,* 7th ed. Scott JR et al (editors). Philadelphia: Lippincott, 1994.

Harvey CJ, Burke ME: Hypertensive disorders in pregnancy. In: *High Risk Intrapartum Nursing.* Mandeville LK, Troiano NH (editors). Philadelphia: Lippincott, 1992.

Iams JD: Preterm birth. In: *Obstetrics: Normal and Problem Pregnancies,* 3rd ed. Gabbe SG et al (editors). New York: Churchill Livingstone, 1996.

Kappy KA et al: Premature rupture of the membranes. In: *High-Risk Pregnancy: A Team Approach,* 2nd ed. Knuppel RA, Drukker JE (editors). Philadelphia: Saunders, 1993.

Knuppel RA, Drukker JE: Hypertension in pregnancy. In: *High-Risk Pregnancy: A Team Approach,* 2nd ed. Knuppel RA, Drukker JE (editors). Philadelphia: Saunders, 1993.

Lantz ME, Porter KB: Home uterine activity monitoring. *Female Patient* September 1995; 20(9):80.

Lipshitz J et al: Preterm labor. In: *High-Risk Pregnancy: A Team Approach,* 2nd ed. Knuppel RA, Drukker JE (editors). Philadelphia: Saunders, 1993.

Long P, Russell L: Hyperemesis gravidarum. *Perinatal Neonatal Nurs* 1993; 6(4):21.

Maiolatesi CR, Peddicord K: Methotrexate for nonsurgical treatment of ectopic pregnancy: Nursing implications. *JOGNN* March/April 1996; 25(3):205.

Mandeville LK, Troiano NH: *High Risk Intrapartum Nursing.* Philadelphia: Lippincott, 1992.

McMillan JA: Why TORCH no longer sheds light. *Contemp OB/GYN* November 1992; 37(11):83.

Morbidity and Mortality Weekly Report: Supplement. Recommendations for prevention of HIV transmission in health care settings. *MMWR* August 21, 1987; 36(25):2.

NAACOG: Preterm labor and tocolytics. *OGN Nurs Pract Res* September 1984; 10.

Neal AD, Bockman VC: Preterm labor and preterm rupture of membranes. In: *High Risk Intrapartum Nursing.* Mandeville LK, Troiano NH (editors). Philadelphia: Lippincott, 1992.

Niebyl JR: Detecting incompetent cervix. *Contemp OB/GYN* October 1990; 35:37.

NIH: Effect of corticosteroids for fetal maturation on perinatal outcomes. *National Institutes of Health Consensus Development Conference Statement.* February 28–March 2, 1994.

Nursing 93: *Nursing 93 Drug Handbook.* Springhouse, PA: Springhouse Corp, 1993.

Parker B, McFarlane J: Identifying and helping battered pregnant women. *MCN* May/June 1991; 16(3):161.

Parsons MT, Spellacy WN: Causes and management of preterm labor. In: *Danforth's Obstetrics and Gynecology,* 7th ed. Scott JR et al (editors). Philadelphia: Lippincott, 1994.

Pauerstein CJ: *Clinical Obstetrics.* New York: Wiley, 1987.

Paulson JD: The use of carbon-dioxide laser laparoscopy in the treatment of tubal ectopic pregnancy. *Am J Obstet Gynecol* 1992; 167:382.

Pearlman MD: Management of trauma during pregnancy. *Female Patient* August 1996; 21:79.

Scott JR: Early pregnancy loss. In: *Danforth's Obstetrics and Gynecology,* 7th ed. Scott JR et al (editors). Philadelphia: Lippincott, 1994a.

Scott JR: Hypertensive disorders of pregnancy. In: *Danforth's Obstetrics and Gynecology,* 7th ed. Scott JR et al (editors). Philadelphia: Lippincott, 1994b.

Scott JR: Immunologic disorders in pregnancy. In: *Danforth's Obstetrics and Gynecology,* 7th ed. Scott JR et al (editors). Philadelphia: Lippincott, 1994c.

Scott JR, Branch DW: Immunologic disorders in pregnancy. In: *Danforth's Obstetrics and Gynecology,* 7th ed. Scott JR et al (editors). Philadelphia: Lippincott, 1994.

Shortliffe LMD: UTI during pregnancy: It's not the same. *Contemp OB/GYN* October 1992; 37(10):69.

Sibai BM: Preeclampsia-eclampsia: Valid treatment approaches. *Contemp OB/GYN* August 1990; 35:84.

Sibai BM: Hypertension in pregnancy. In: *Obstetrics: Normal and Problem Pregnancies,* 3rd ed. Gabbe SG et al (editors). New York: Churchill Livingstone, 1996.

Simpson JL: Fetal wastage. In: *Obstetrics: Normal and Problem Pregnancies,* 3rd ed. Gabbe SG et al (editors). New York: Churchill Livingstone, 1996.

Soper JT, Hammond CB: Nonmetastatic gestational trophoblastic disease. *Obstet Gynecol Clin North Am* September 1990; 15:505.

Urbanski TK et al: Caring for a woman with a hydatidiform mole and coexisting pregnancy. *MCN* March/April 1996; 21:85.

Varner MW: General medical and surgical diseases in pregnancy. In: *Danforth's Obstetrics and Gynecology,* 7th ed. Scott JR et al (editors). Philadelphia: Lippincott, 1994.

Williams MC: Premature rupture of membranes. In: *Manual of Obstetrics: Diagnosis and Therapy.* Niswander KR, Evans AT (editors). Boston: Little, Brown, 1991.

Chapter 14 Assessment of Fetal Well-Being

OBJECTIVES

- List indications for ultrasonic examination and the information that can be obtained from this procedure.
- Discuss current prenatal tests such as biophysical profile (BPP), nonstress test (NST), fetal acoustic stimulation (FAST), and Doppler blood flow studies.
- Outline pertinent information to be discussed with the woman regarding her assessment of fetal activity and methods of recording fetal activity.
- Discuss the use of amniocentesis as a diagnostic tool.
- Describe the tests that can be done on amniotic fluid.

KEY TERMS

Amniocentesis
Biophysical profile (BPP)
Contraction stress test (CST)
Lecithin/sphingomyelin (L/S) ratio
Nonstress test (NST)
Phosphatidylglycerol (PG)
Surfactant
Ultrasound

Over the past 15 to 20 years the problems of the high-risk pregnant woman and her baby have received increasing attention. It has been demonstrated that perinatal morbidity (sickness) and mortality (death) can be significantly reduced when there is early diagnosis of pregnancy and of high-risk factors, and ongoing prenatal care of the pregnant woman.

Several tests can be used to assess fetal well-being during the pregnancy. These tests include diagnostic ultrasound, fetal stress tests, and amniocentesis for lung maturity studies. In addition, after the seventh month of pregnancy the expectant woman can assess fetal movement each day. The tests and assessment methods provide information about fetal well-being, normal growth of the fetus, the presence of congenital anomalies, the location of the placenta, and fetal lung maturity (Table 14–1). At times just one test will be done, and in other circumstances a combination of the tests is beneficial.

Some of these tests pose risks to the fetus and possibly to the pregnant woman, and these risks should be considered before a particular test is done. The health care provider must be certain that the advantages outweigh the potential risks and added expense. In addition, the diagnostic accuracy and applicability of these tests may vary. Certainly not all high-risk pregnancies require the same tests. Conditions that indicate a high-risk pregnancy include

- Maternal age less than 16 or more than 35 years
- Chronic maternal hypertension, preeclampsia, diabetes mellitus, or heart disease
- Presence of Rh isoimmunization
- A maternal history of unexplained stillbirth
- Suspected intrauterine growth retardation (IUGR)
- Pregnancy prolonged past 42 weeks' gestation
- Multiple gestation

See Chapter 7 for further discussion of prenatal high-risk factors and Chapters 12 and 13 for descriptions of various conditions that may threaten the successful completion of pregnancy.

Using the Nursing Process During Diagnostic Testing

Because many of the diagnostic tests are completed on an outpatient basis, the nurse may have only brief contact with the woman and her support person. Nevertheless, the nurse uses the nursing process to guide nursing care during these interactions.

TABLE 14–1 Summary of Screening and Diagnostic Tests

Goal	*Test*	*Timing*
To validate the pregnancy	Ultrasound: gestational sac volume	5 and 6 weeks after LMP by endovaginal ultrasound
To determine how advanced the pregnancy is	Ultrasound: crown-rump length Ultrasound: biparietal diameter, femur length, abdomen circumference	6 to 10 weeks' gestation 13 to 40 weeks' gestation
To identify normal growth of the fetus	Ultrasound: biparietal diameter Ultrasound: head:abdomen ratio Ultrasound: estimated fetal weight	Most useful from 20 to 30 weeks' gestation 13 to 40 weeks' gestation About 24 to 40 weeks' gestation
To detect congenital anomalies and problems	Ultrasound Chorionic villus sampling Amniocentesis Fetoscopy Percutaneous blood sampling Triple test	18 to 40 weeks' gestation 8 to 12 weeks' gestation 16 to 18 weeks' gestation 18 weeks' gestation Second and third trimesters About 10 weeks' gestation
To localize the placenta	Ultrasound	Usually in third trimester or before amniocentesis
To assess fetal status	Biophysical profile Maternal assessment of fetal activity Nonstress test Contraction stress test	Approximately 28 weeks to birth About 28 weeks to birth Approximately 28 weeks to birth After 28 weeks
To diagnose cardiac problems	Fetal echocardiography	Second and third trimesters
To assess fetal lung maturity	Amniocentesis L/S ratio Phosphatidylglycerol Phosphatidylcholine	33 to 40 weeks 33 weeks to birth 33 weeks to birth 33 weeks to birth
To obtain more information about breech presentation	Ultrasound	Just before labor is anticipated or during labor

APPLYING THE NURSING PROCESS

Nursing Assessment

The nursing assessment begins with a history of the prenatal course and identification of possible indications for the particular test. The nurse assesses the woman's and her partner's knowledge about the test and the presence of any factors that may influence the teaching process. During the test, the nurse completes assessments needed to monitor the status of the mother and her unborn child.

Nursing Diagnosis

The primary nursing diagnoses are directed toward the woman's knowledge about the diagnostic test and any risks to herself and her unborn child. The woman may also be fearful of the outcome of the tests, and the nurse can play an important role in providing support and counseling. Examples of nursing diagnoses that may apply include the following:

- Knowledge deficit related to lack of information about the fetal assessment test, purpose, benefits, risks, and alternatives
- Fear related to concern about negative test results

Nursing Plan and Implementation

The nursing plan of care is directed toward each specific nursing diagnosis. The nurse generally plays a vital role in providing information about the diagnostic test. The nurse assesses the woman's knowledge of the test and then provides information as needed. Some of the tests require written informed consent; in these cases the certified nurse-midwife/physician is responsible for informing the woman about all aspects of the test. The nurse can reinforce information and clarify information that the woman does not fully understand (Table 14–2).

Contact with the expectant woman may be very brief. The nurse uses basic knowledge of communication, developmental psychology, cultural factors, and so forth to establish a trusting relationship with the woman and her support person. The nurse also functions as an advocate for the expectant woman by helping her clarify question areas and obtain needed information. The nurse frequently knows the areas about which most women have questions and can anticipate many of their fears. When the woman is not able to verbalize questions, the nurse can assist by bringing up questions other women have had.

During the testing sessions, the nurse addresses the woman's fear by providing support and comfort measures. The presence of the nurse reassures the woman and helps her cope with the tests.

TABLE 14–2 Sample Nursing Approaches to Pretest Teaching

Assess whether the woman knows the reason the screening or diagnostic test is being recommended.
Examples:
"Has your doctor/nurse-midwife told you why this test is necessary?"
"Sometimes tests are done for many different reasons. Can you tell me why you are having this test?"
"What is your understanding about what the test will show?"

Provide an opportunity for questions.
Examples:
"Do you have any questions about the test?"
"Is there anything that is not clear to you?"

Explain the test procedure, paying particular attention to any preparation the woman needs to do prior to the test.
Example:
"The test that has been ordered for you is designed to . . . " (Add specific information about the particular test. Give the explanation in simple language.)

Validate the woman's understanding of the preparation.
Example:
"Tell me what you will have to do to get ready for this test."

Give permission for the woman to continue to ask questions if needed.
Example:
"I'll be with you during the test. If you have any questions at any time, please don't hesitate to ask."

Evaluation

The expected outcomes for the woman who is having diagnostic testing are that she understands the reasons for the test and the test results and has had support during the test. In addition, the tests have been done without complication and the safety of the mother and her unborn child has been maintained.

Maternal Assessment of Fetal Activity

Assessment of fetal movement patterns has been used as a screening procedure in the evaluation of fetal status since 1971, when the clinical significance of various types of fetal activity was first described (Sadovsky 1985b). Clinicians now generally agree that vigorous fetal activity provides reassurance of fetal well-being and that marked decrease in activity or cessation of movement may indicate possible fetal compromise requiring immediate follow-up evaluation. Although there is considerable variation among individuals, the average number of daily movements during the third trimester is approximately 720 (or 30 gross fetal body movements/hour) (Druzin and Gabbe 1996). In women with a multiple gestation, daily fetal movements are significantly higher. During the last few weeks of gestation the fetus spends 60–70 percent of its time in an active sleep state.

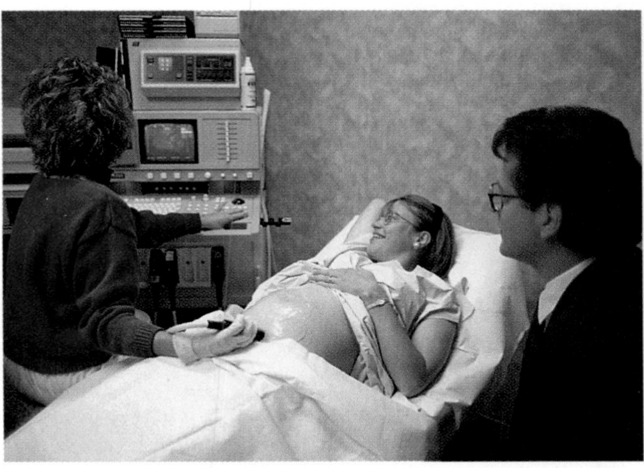

FIGURE 14–1 Ultrasound scanning permits visualization of the fetus in utero.

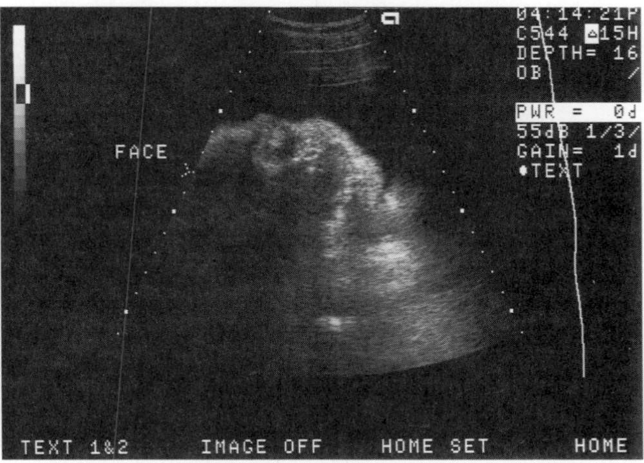

FIGURE 14–2 Ultrasound of fetal face.

The fetus has abrupt movements of its limbs, trunk and head. (Druzin and Gabbe 1996).

Fetal activity is affected by many factors, including sound, drugs, cigarette smoking, sleep states of the fetus, blood glucose levels, and time of day. The expectant mother's perception of fetal movements and her commitment to completing the movement record may vary. When the woman understands the purpose of the assessment, how to complete the form, whom to call with questions, and what to report—and has the opportunity for follow-up during each visit—she will also see this as an important activity. (See Teaching Guide—What to Tell the Pregnant Woman About Assessing Fetal Activity, in Chapter 9.) The nurse can also help the woman devise a daily record on which she can record fetal movements. The nurse is available to answer questions and clarify areas of concern.

Ultrasound

Valuable information about the fetus may be obtained from pulsed echo **ultrasound** testing. Intermittent ultrasonic waves (high-frequency sound waves) are transmitted by an alternating current to a transducer, which is applied to the woman's abdomen. The ultrasonic waves deflect off tissues within the woman's abdomen, showing structures of varying densities (Figures 14–1 and 14–2).

The most common type of perinatal ultrasound is *real-time scanning,* in which a transducer produces a rapid sequence of fixed images on a small screen similar to a television screen. A real-time scan shows movement as it happens, so that a beating fetal heart can be visualized. The ultrasound operator may freeze an image on the screen and photograph it for a permanent record. Real-time ultrasound is particularly helpful for assessing functions that can be detected through movement, such as fetal breathing, cardiac activity, and bladder function. Real-time ultrasound equipment is small and easily moved and need not be used in the x-ray department. Thus it is frequently kept in birthing areas, so a pregnant woman can have the procedure done without the inconvenience of a trip to a different department.

In recent years considerable effort and research have centered on validating the usefulness of ultrasound in pregnancy. Common arguments in favor of routine scanning include early detection of unsuspected fetal anomalies and multiple gestation; accurate determination of gestational age, leading to improved diagnosis and management of postdatism and fetal growth retardation; and decreased perinatal mortality rate (Chervenak and Gabbe 1996). Routine ultrasonography early in pregnancy is used to date the gestation and therefore can reduce the incidence of labor induction for suspected postterm gestation and the frequency of undiagnosed major fetal anomalies and twins.

Diagnostic ultrasound has several advantages. It is noninvasive, painless, and nonradiating to both the woman and the fetus, and it has no known harmful effects to either (Chervenak and Gabbe 1996). Serial studies (several ultrasound tests done over a span of time) may be done for assessment and comparison. Soft tissue masses can be differentiated. The practitioner obtains results immediately. Finally, ultrasound does not pose the same risk as other diagnostic or medical procedures (such as amniocentesis or intrauterine surgery) yet allows the clinician to visualize the fetus.

Procedures

The two most common methods of real-time ultrasound scanning are transabdominal and endovaginal.

Transabdominal Ultrasound

In the transabdominal approach, a transducer is moved across the woman's abdomen. The woman is usually scanned with a full bladder, except when ultrasound is used to localize the placenta before amniocentesis. When the bladder is full, the examiner can assess other structures, especially the vagina and cervix, in relation to the bladder. This is particularly important when vaginal bleeding is noted and placenta previa is the suspected cause. The woman is advised to drink 1–1.5 quarts of water approximately 2 hours before the examination, and she is asked to refrain from emptying her bladder. If the bladder is not sufficiently filled, she is asked to drink 3–4 (8 oz) glasses of water and is rescanned 30–45 minutes later. Mineral oil or a transmission gel is generously spread over the woman's abdomen, and the sonographer slowly moves a transducer over the abdomen to obtain a picture of the contents of the uterus. Ultrasound testing takes 20–30 minutes. The woman may feel discomfort due to pressure applied over a full bladder. In addition, if the woman lies on her back during the test, shortness of breath can develop. This may be relieved by elevating her upper body during the test.

Endovaginal Ultrasound

The endovaginal approach uses a probe inserted into the vagina. Once inserted, the endovaginal probe is close to the structures being imaged and so produces a better, clearer image. The improved images obtained by endovaginal ultrasound have enabled sonographers to identify structures and fetal characteristics earlier in pregnancy than was possible with the transabdominal approach (Chervenak and Gabbe 1996).

After the procedure is fully explained to the woman, she is prepared in the same manner as for a pelvic examination: in lithotomy position, with appropriate drapes to provide privacy and a female attendant in the room. It is important that her buttocks are at the end of the table so that, once inserted, the probe can be moved in various directions. The small, lightweight vaginal transducer is covered with a specially fitted sterile sheath, a condom, or one finger of a glove. Ultrasound coupling gel is then applied to the covering, making insertion into the vagina easier and providing a medium for enhancing the ultrasound image (Goldstein 1992). In addition to providing a clearer image than the transabdominal method, the endovaginal procedure can be accomplished with an empty bladder. Most women do not feel discomfort during the ultrasound exam. The probe is smaller than a speculum, so insertion is usually completed with ease. The woman may feel some movement of the probe during the exam as various structures are imaged. Some women may want to insert the probe themselves to enhance their comfort, while others would feel embarrassed even to be asked. The certified nurse-midwife, physician, or ultrasonographer offers the choice based on their comfort level and the rapport they have with the woman.

A less common scanning method, translabial ultrasound, may be used in combination with transabdominal ultrasound. The transducer is placed on the woman's labia but is not inserted into the vaginal vault.

Clinical Applications

Ultrasound testing can be of benefit in the following ways:

- *Early identification of pregnancy.* (Pregnancy may be detected as early as the fifth or sixth week following the last menstrual period [LMP].)
- *Identification of more than one embryo/fetus.*
- *Measurement of the biparietal diameter of the fetal head or the fetal femur length.* These measurements help determine the gestational age of the fetus and identify IUGR.
- *Detection of fetal anomalies.* Two major abnormalities that may be detected are anencephaly and hydrocephalus.
- *Detection of hydramnios (or polyhydramnios) or oligohydramnios.* The presence of more or less than normal amounts of amniotic fluid is frequently associated with fetal anomalies.
- *Identification of amniotic fluid index (AFI).* The maternal abdomen is divided into quadrants. The umbilicus is used to divide the upper and lower sections and the linea nigra divides the right and left sections. The vertical diameter of the largest amniotic fluid pocket in each quadrant is measured. All measurements are totaled to obtain AFI in centimeters. The mean AFI at 36–42 weeks is 12.9 ± 4.6 cm. Women with AFI of more than 20 cm are considered to have hydramnios and women with less than 5 cm at term are considered to have oligohydramnios. Both hydramnios and oligohydramnios are associated with increased risk to the fetus (Phelan et al 1987).
- *Location of the placenta.* This is done before amniocentesis to avoid puncturing the placenta. Ultrasound is also used to determine the presence of placenta previa.
- *Observation of fetal heartbeat and fetal breathing movements.* Fetal breathing movements (FBM) have been observed as early as the 11th week of gestation.
- *Placental grading.* As the fetus matures, the placenta calcifies. These changes can be visualized by ultrasound and graded according to the degree of calcification and amount of chorionic convolutions (Treacy et al 1990).

- *Detection of fetal death.* Inability to visualize the fetal heart beating and the separation of the bones in the fetal head are signs of fetal death.
- *Determination of fetal position and presentation.* Ultrasound images give information about position and presentation.
- Accompanying procedures such as amniocentesis, periumbilical blood sampling, intrauterine procedures, and other procedures to be discussed shortly.

Risks of Ultrasound

Ultrasound has been used clinically for over 25 years, and to date no clinical studies verify harmful effects to the mother, fetus, or newborn. Early studies with animals suggested that ultrasound may retard fetal growth and cause cell damage, but the ultrasound levels used in these studies were much higher than the levels used in medical diagnosis of pregnancy and pregnancy-related conditions (Chervenak and Gabbe 1996).

Role of the Nurse

It is important for the nurse to ascertain whether the woman understands why the ultrasound is being suggested. The nurse provides an opportunity for the woman to ask questions and acts as an advocate if there are questions or concerns that need to be addressed before the ultrasound examination.

The nurse explains the preparation needed and ensures that adequate preparation is done. After the test is completed, the nurse can assist with clarifying or interpreting test results to the woman.

Doppler Blood Flow Studies (Umbilical Velocimetry)

Recent advantages in ultrasound technology have made it possible noninvasively to study blood flow changes that occur in maternal and fetal circulations to assess placental function. An ultrasound beam, like that provided by the pocket Doppler (a hand-held ultrasound device) is directed at the umbilical artery (in some cases a maternal vessel such as the arcuate can also be used). The signal is reflected off the red blood cells moving within the vessels, and creates a "picture" (waveform) that looks like a series of waves (Figures 14–3 and 14–4). The highest velocity peak of the waves is the systolic measurement and the lowest point is the diastolic velocity. To interpret the waveforms, the systolic (S) peak is divided by the end diastolic (D) component. This calculation is called the S/D ratio. The normal S/D ratio is below 2.6 by 26 weeks' gestation and below 3 at term. When uteroplacental perfusion decreases (because of

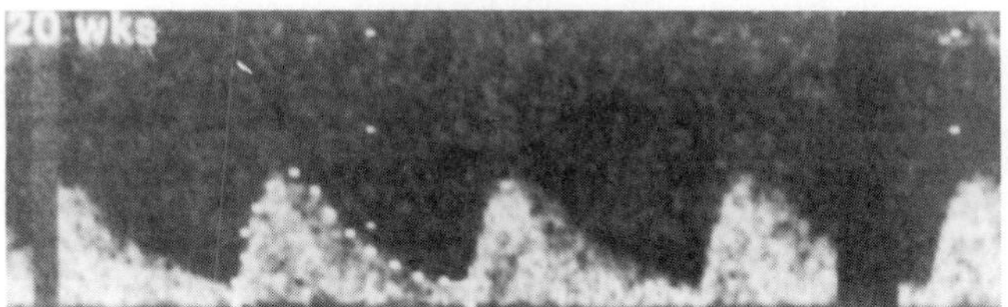

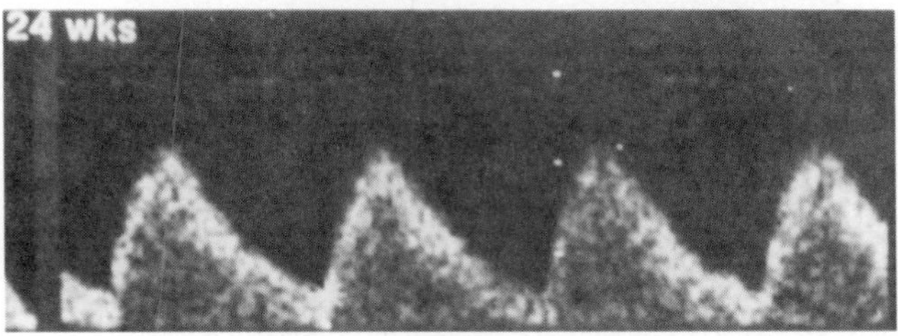

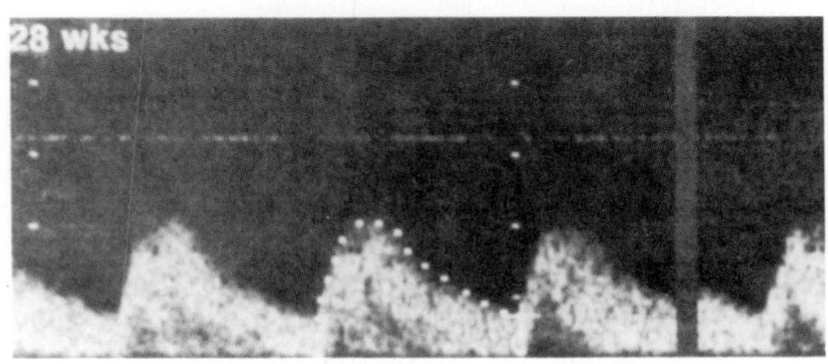

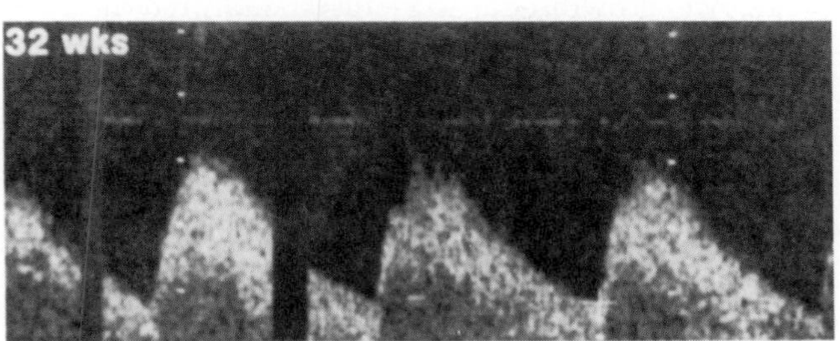

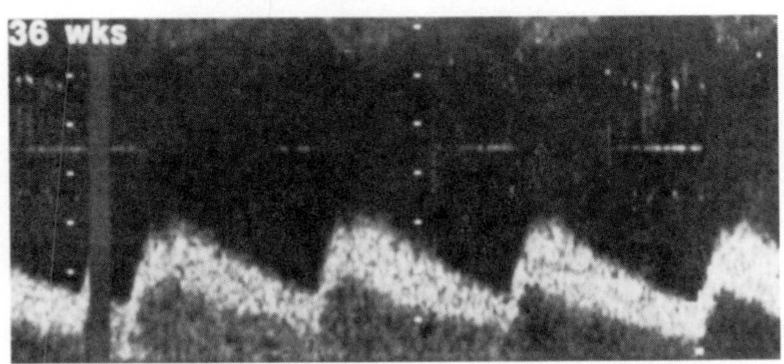

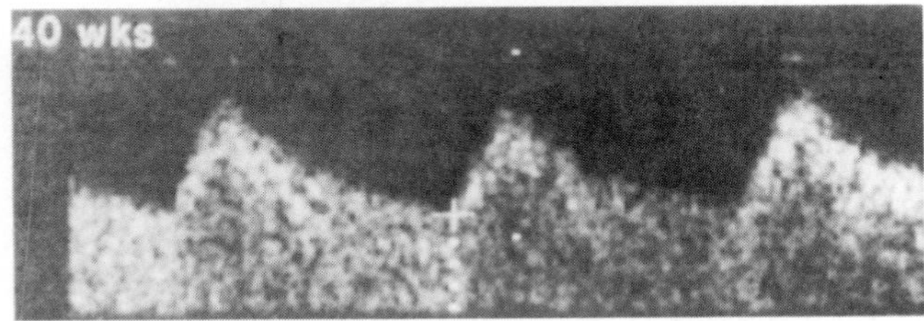

FIGURE 14–3 Serial studies of the umbilical artery velocity waveforms in a normal pregnancy from one client.

Source: Cundiff JL, Haybrich KL, Hinzman HG: Umbilical artery Doppler flow studies during pregnancy. *JOGNN* November/December 1990; 19(6):475, fig 3.

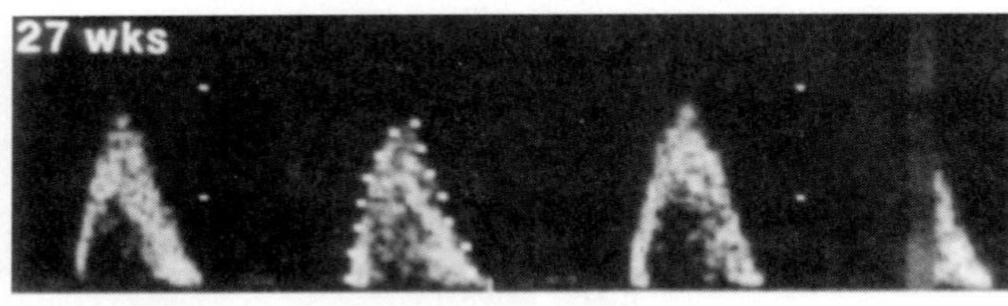

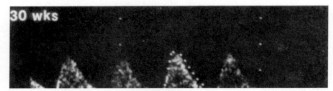

FIGURE 14–4 Two examples of abnormal umbilical artery velocity waveforms taken from a client with intrauterine growth retardation.

Source: Cundiff JL, Haybrich KL, Hinzman HG: Umbilical artery Doppler flow studies during pregnancy. *JOGNN* November/December 1990; 19(6):475, fig 4.

narrowing of the vessels), it causes an increase in placental bed resistance and a decrease in diastolic flow, resulting in an elevated S/D ratio (Druzin and Gabbe 1996). Abnormal elevations are considered to be 3.0 and above.

Doppler blood flow studies are helpful in assessing and managing multiple gestation, diabetes, prolonged pregnancy, growth-retarded fetuses, and preterm labor (Maulik 1995).

Doppler blood flow studies are relatively easy to obtain. The woman lies supine with a wedge under the left hip (to promote uteroplacental perfusion). Warmed transducer gel is applied to the abdomen and a pulsed-wave Doppler device is used to ascertain the blood flow. The Doppler flow study takes about 15 to 20 minutes. Doppler flow studies can be initiated at 16 to 18 weeks' gestation and done at regular intervals for women at risk.

Nonstress Test

The **nonstress test (NST)** has become a widely used method of evaluating fetal status. The nonstress test is based on the knowledge that when the fetus has adequate oxygenation and an intact central nervous system, there will be accelerations of the fetal heart rate (FHR) with fetal movement. An NST requires an electronic fetal monitor to observe these accelerations (see discussion of acceleration in Chapter 16.) The advantages of the NST are as follows:

- It is quick to perform.
- It permits easy interpretation.
- It is inexpensive.
- It can be done in an office or clinic setting.
- There are no known side effects.

The disadvantages of the NST include the following:

- It is sometimes difficult to obtain a suitable tracing.
- The woman has to lie relatively still for at least 20 minutes.

Procedure for NST

The test can be done with the woman in a reclining chair or in bed in a semi-Fowler's or side-lying position. An electronic fetal monitor is used to obtain a tracing of FHR and fetal movement (FM). The examiner puts two belts on the woman's abdomen. One belt holds a device that detects uterine or fetal movement. The other belt holds a device that detects the FHR. As the NST is done, each fetal movement is documented, so that associated or simultaneous FHR changes can be evaluated. Women with a high-risk factor will probably begin having NSTs at 30 to 32 weeks of pregnancy. They probably will be continued once or twice a week until birth of the baby (Paul and Miller 1995).

Interpretation of NST Results

The results of the NST are interpreted as follows:

- *Reactive test.* A reactive NST shows at least two accelerations of FHR with fetal movements, of 15 beats per minute, lasting 15 seconds or more, over 20 minutes (Figure 14–5). This is the desired result.
- *Nonreactive test.* In a nonreactive test, the reactive criteria are not met. For example, the accelerations are not as much as 15 beats per minute or do not last 15 seconds and so on (Figure 14–6).
- *Unsatisfactory test.* An unsatisfactory NST has data that cannot be interpreted or inadequate fetal activity.

Criteria for the reactive NST appear to vary somewhat from one report to another. Most require two accelerations of FHR in 20 minutes; others require two in 15 minutes. See Key Facts to Remember: Nonstress Test.

KEY FACTS TO REMEMBER

Nonstress Test

Diagnostic value: Demonstrates fetus's ability to respond to its environment by acceleration of FHR with movement.

Results:

- Reactive test: Accelerations of 15 beats per min above the baseline, lasting 15 sec in a 20-min window, are present, indicating fetal well-being.
- Nonreactive test: Accelerations are not present, indicating that the fetus is sick or asleep.

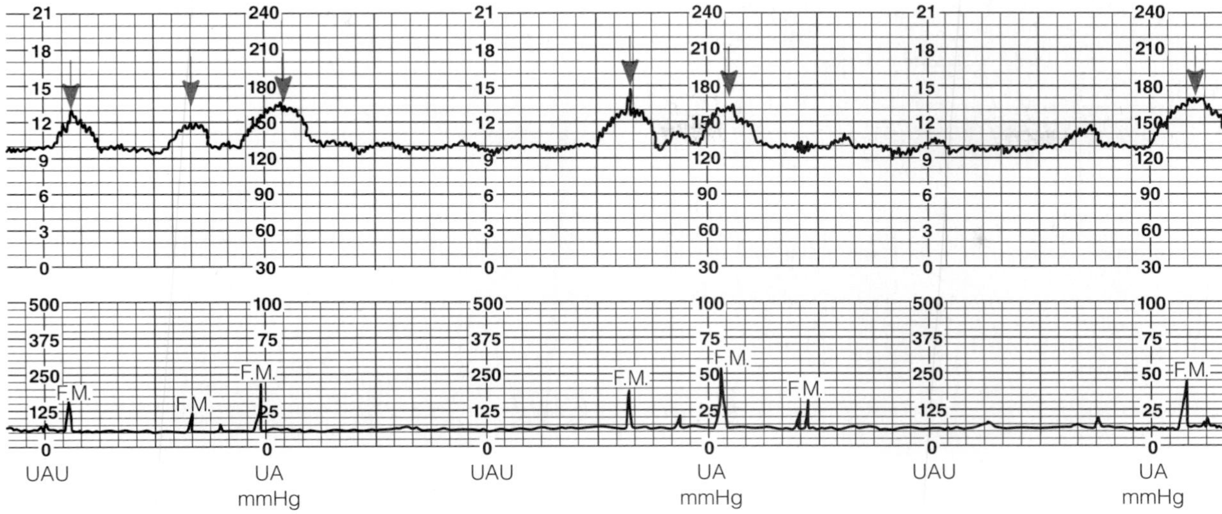

FIGURE 14–5 Example of a reactive nonstress test (NST). Accelerations of 15 bpm lasting 15 seconds with each fetal movement (FM). Top of strip shows FHR; bottom of strip shows uterine activity tracing. Note that FHR increases (above the baseline) at least 15 beats and remains at that rate for at least 15 seconds before returning to the former baseline.

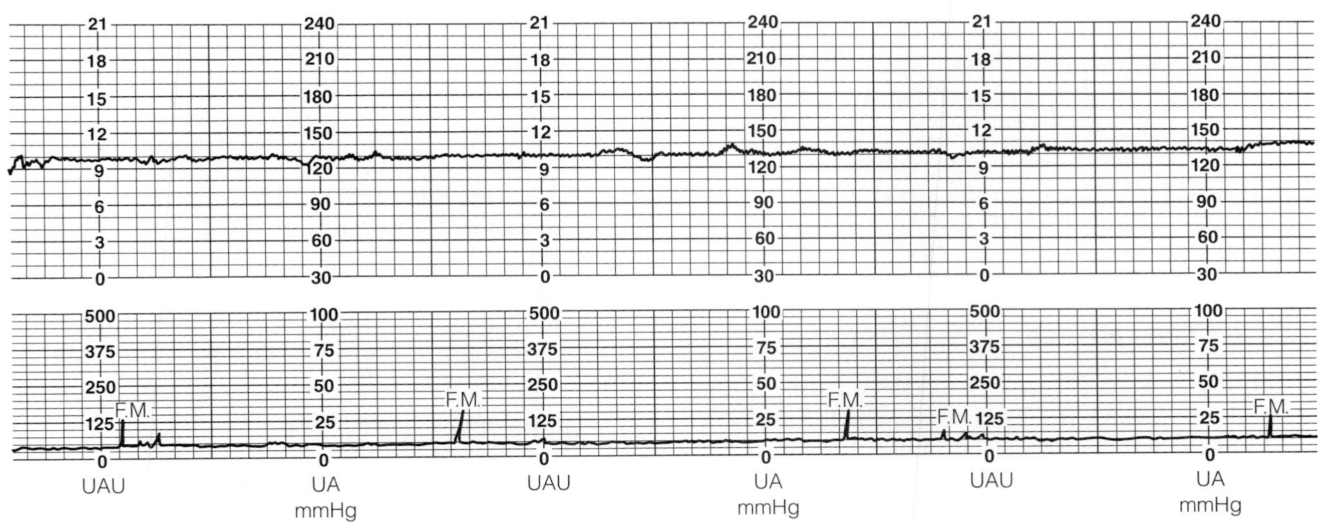

FIGURE 14–6 Example of a nonreactive NST. There are no accelerations of FHR with FM. Baseline FHR is 130 bpm. The tracing of uterine activity is on the bottom of the strip.

It is particularly important that anyone who performs the NST also understand the significance of any decelerations of the FHR during testing. If decelerations are noted, the certified nurse-midwife/physician should be notified for further evaluation of fetal status. (See Chapter 16 for further discussion of FHR decelerations.)

Management

The clinical management of potential fetal distress may vary somewhat among clinicians. Devoe (1989) recommends the following: If the NST is reactive in less than 30 minutes, the test is concluded and rescheduled as indicated by the high-risk condition that is present; if it is nonreactive, the test time is extended for 30 minutes at a time until the results are reactive, and then the test is rescheduled as indicated, or, if the FHR is still nonreactive, additional testing (such as diagnostic ultrasound and BPP or CST) or immediate birth is considered; if the NST is nonreactive and spontaneous decelerations of the FHR are present, diagnostic ultrasound and BPP are recommended (Figure 14–7). Paul and Miller (1995) note that many testing guidelines vary between once or

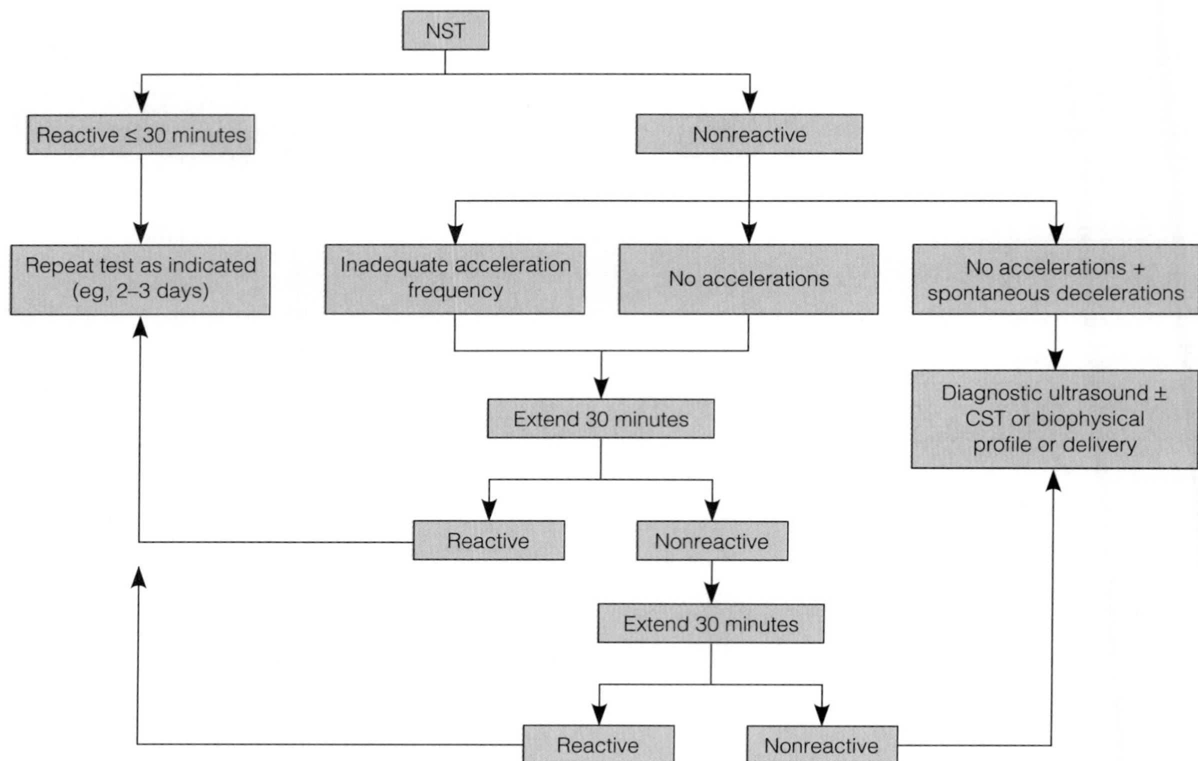

FIGURE 14–7 NST management scheme.

Source: Devoe LD: Nonstress and contraction stress testing. In: *Gynecology and Obstetrics, Vol 3.* Depp R, Eschenbach DA, Sciarri JJ (editors). Philadelphia: Lippincott, 1989 (Ch 78, Figure 5, p 9).

twice a week depending upon the at-risk condition that is present. In some situations, such as preterm premature rupture of membranes, daily testing may be done.

Role of the Nurse

The nurse ascertains the woman's understanding of the NST and the possible results. The reasons for the NST and the procedure are reviewed before beginning the test. The nurse administers the NST, interprets the results, and reports the findings to the certified nurse-midwife/physician and the expectant woman.

Fetal Acoustic Stimulation Test (FAST) and Vibroacoustic Stimulation Test (VST)

Use of acoustic (sound) and vibroacoustic (vibration and sound) stimulation of the fetus is used as an adjunct to the NST. A hand-held, battery-operated device is applied to the woman's abdomen over the area of the fetal head. This device generates a low-frequency vibration and a buzzing sound that are intended to induce movement and associated accelerations of FHR in those fetuses who have a nonreactive NST—and in the fetus with decreased variability of FHR during labor. (See discussion of variability in Chapter 16.) The sound stimulus persists for 2–5 seconds and is then repeated at 1-minute intervals up to 3 times if no accelerations occur (Smith 1995). Two FHR accelerations of 15 beats per minute, lasting 15 seconds, in a 10-minute period, is designated a reactive test (Garite 1992). Advantages of FAST and VST are:

- They are noninvasive techniques.
- Results are rapidly available.
- Time for the NST is shortened.
- The test is easy to perform.

Whether the fetus responds more to the vibration or to the sound is not known.

Biophysical Profile

The **biophysical profile (BPP),** also called fetal biophysical profile (FBPP), is an assessment of five biophysical variables: fetal breathing movement, fetal movements of body or limbs, fetal tone (extension and flexion of extremities), amniotic fluid volume (visualized as pockets of fluid around the fetus), and reactive FHR with activ-

TABLE 14–3 Biophysical Profile Scoring: Technique and Interpretation

Biophysical Variable	Normal (Score = 2)	Abnormal (Score = 0)
Fetal breathing movements	≥1 episode of ≥30 seconds in 30 minutes	Absent or no episode of ≥30 seconds in 30 minutes
Gross body movements	≥3 discrete body/limb movements in 30 minutes (Episodes of active continuous movement considered as single movement.)	≤2 episodes of body/limb movements in 30 minutes
Fetal tone	≥1 episode of active extension with return to flexion of fetal limb(s) or trunk (Opening and closing of hand considered normal tone.)	Either slow extension with return to partial flexion or movement of limb in full extension or absent fetal movement
Reactive fetal heart rate	≥2 episodes of acceleration of ≥15 bpm and of ≥15 seconds associated with fetal movement in 20 minutes	<2 episodes of acceleration of fetal heart rate or acceleration of <15 bpm in 20 minutes
Qualitative amniotic fluid volume	≥1 pocket of fluid measuring ≥1 cm in two perpendicular planes	Either no pockets or a pocket <1 cm in two perpendicular planes

Management Based on Biophysical Profile Score

Attained Score	Intervention
10 of 10 or 8 of 10, with normal amniotic fluid volume	No intervention is needed, normal finding.
8 of 10 with abnormal amniotic fluid volume	If fetal renal function is normal and membranes are intact, delivery is indicated.
6 of 10 with normal amniotic fluid volume	Deliver fetus if it is mature. If immature, repeat test within 24 hours. If score is 6 of 10 or below, deliver fetus.
4 of 10, 2 of 10, or 0 of 10	Deliver fetus.

Sources: Manning FA et al: Fetal assessment based on fetal biophysical profile scoring: Experience in 12,620 referred high-risk pregnancies. *Am J Obstet Gynecol* 1985; 151(3):344; Manning FA: The biophysical profile: Contemporary use. *Tenth International Symposium on Perinatal Medicine and Obstetrical Ultrasound, April 9–12, 1990, Las Vegas, NV.*

ity (reactive NST). The first four variables are assessed by ultrasound scanning; FHR reactivity is assessed with the NST. By combining these five assessments, the BPP helps to identify the compromised fetus and confirm the healthy fetus (Druzin and Gabbe 1996). Specific criteria for normal and abnormal assessments are presented in Table 14–3. A score of 2 is assigned to each normal finding, and 0 to each abnormal one, for a maximum score of 10. The absence of a specific activity is difficult to interpret, since it may be indicative of CNS depression, or simply the resting state of a healthy fetus. Scores of 8 (with normal amniotic fluid) and 10 are considered normal (Druzin and Gabbe 1996). Such scores seem to have the least chance of being associated with a compromised fetus unless a decrease in the amount of amniotic fluid is noted, in which case the infant's birth is indicated (Manning 1995). A management protocol regarding BPP is outlined in Figure 14–7. Currently there is some variation in management recommendations; however there is a consensus that the BPP is more accurate than any other test in identifying the compromised fetus (Garite 1992).

Contraction Stress Test

The **contraction stress test** (CST) is a means of evaluating the respiratory function (oxygen and carbon dioxide exchange) of the placenta. It enables the health care team to identify the fetus at risk for intrauterine asphyxia by observing the response of the FHR to the stress of uterine contractions (spontaneous or induced). During contractions, intrauterine pressure increases. Blood flow to the intervillous space of the placenta is reduced momentarily, thereby decreasing oxygen transport to the fetus. A healthy fetus usually tolerates this reduction well. If the placental reserve is insufficient, fetal hypoxia, depression of the myocardium, and a decrease in FHR occur. (See Figure 16–14*B*.)

The CST is indicated when there is risk of placental insufficiency or fetal compromise because of the following:

- IUGR
- Diabetes mellitus
- Heart disease
- Chronic hypertension
- Preeclampsia-eclampsia (pregnancy-induced hypertension, or PIH)
- Sickle cell anemia

- Suspected postmaturity (more than 42 weeks' gestation)
- History of previous stillbirths
- Rh sensitization
- Abnormal estriol excretion
- Hyperthyroidism
- Renal disease
- Nonreactive NST

The CST is contraindicated if there is third trimester bleeding from placenta previa or marginal abruptio placentae, previous cesarean with classical uterine incision, risk of precipitating premature labor outweighing the advantage of the CST, premature rupture of the membranes, incompetent cervix, or multiple gestation.

The advantages of the CST are as follows:

- The test provides information about how the fetus will react to the stress of uterine contractions.
- It can show that the fetal environment is deteriorating.

The disadvantages include the following:

- The test needs to be administered in a birthing setting.
- It is an invasive procedure if an intravenous line is used.
- It may initiate uterine contractions that precipitate labor.

Procedure

A necessary component of the CST is the presence of uterine contractions. They may occur spontaneously (which is unusual), or they may be induced (stimulated) with oxytocin. The most common method of stimulating uterine contractions for a CST is through intravenous administration of oxytocin (Pitocin). Consequently, the CST used to be called the *oxytocin challenge test (OCT)*. Another method of obtaining oxytocin is through the use of breast stimulation during a breast self-stimulation test (also called nipple stimulation). This method is based on the knowledge that the posterior pituitary produces oxytocin in response to stimulation of the breasts or nipples.

The procedure for CST, reasons for administering the test, equipment used, and normal variations in monitoring that occur during the test should be clearly explained to the woman before the test. A consent form is signed. The woman should empty her bladder before the CST is begun, because she may be unable to move about for 1.5–2 hours. The woman is positioned in a sitting or side-lying position to maintain optimum uteroplacental circulation and to enhance the quality of the uterine contractions as they occur.

An electronic fetal monitor is used to provide continuous data regarding the fetal heart rate and uterine contractions. Maternal blood pressure and pulse are assessed as the recording is begun. After a 15-minute baseline recording of uterine activity and FHR, the tracing is evaluated for evidence of spontaneous contractions. If three spontaneous contractions of good quality and lasting 40–60 seconds occur in a 10-minute period, the results are evaluated, and the test is concluded. If no contractions occur or they are insufficient for interpretation, oxytocin is administered intravenously or breast stimulation is done to produce contractions of good quality. If a hyperstimulation pattern occurs (contractions occur more frequently than every 2 minutes, or last more than 90 seconds), the CST should be discontinued, the side-lying position maintained, the FHR carefully observed, and the certified nurse-midwife/physician notified. Oxygen may be administered. The woman's blood pressure and pulse should be assessed. In the presence of a hyperstimulation pattern, the nurse should also be prepared to administer tocolytics or prepare for emergency birth in the event of unresolved fetal distress.

CST with Intravenous Oxytocin

An electrolyte solution such as lactated Ringer's solution is started as a primary infusion. The nurse attaches a piggyback infusion of oxytocin in a similar solution. An infusion pump is used so that the amount of oxytocin being infused can be measured accurately. The administration procedure is the same for inducing labor through oxytocin administration (see Chapter 20). Oxytocin is administered until three uterine contractions lasting 40–60 seconds occur in a 10-minute period. If late decelerations are repetitive or occur more than three times, the oxytocin infusion should be discontinued. The woman and fetus are monitored until contractions cease and no late decelerations are noted.

CST with Breast Self-Stimulation Test (BSST)

In BSST, the breasts are stimulated by applying warm washcloths or manually rolling one nipple. When the contractions are sufficient to allow interpretation, the test is concluded. Continued assessment is maintained until contractions subside. The results are reviewed, recorded, and explained to the woman.

If a decrease in the fetal heart rate occurs with a uterine contraction, nipple stimulation is discontinued. The woman and fetus are monitored until contractions cease and no late decelerations are noted.

Interpretation of CST Results

The CST is classified as follows:

- *Negative.* A negative CST shows three contractions of good quality lasting 40 or more seconds in 10 minutes without evidence of late decelerations. This is the desired result. It implies that the fetus can handle the hypoxic stress of uterine contractions.

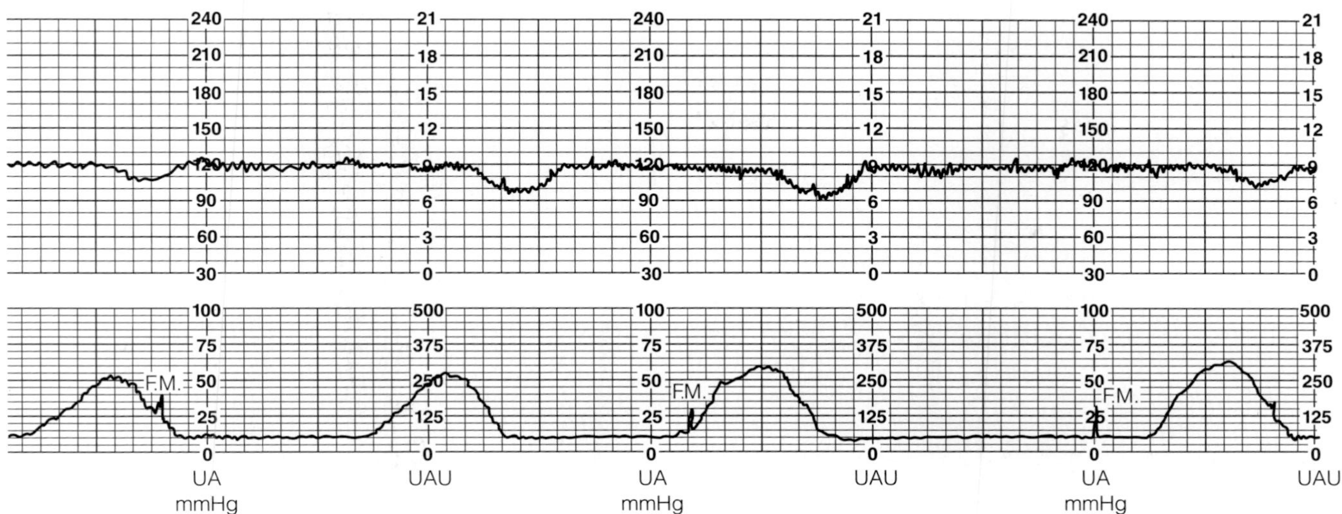

FIGURE 14–8 Example of a positive contraction stress test (CST). Repetitive late decelerations occur with each contraction. Note that there are no accelerations of FHR with three fetal movements (FM). The baseline FHR is 120 bpm. Uterine contractions (bottom half of strip) occurred four times in 12 minutes.

- *Positive.* A positive CST shows repetitive persistent late decelerations with more than 50 percent of the contractions (Figure 14–8). This is *not* a desired result. The hypoxic stress of the uterine contraction causes a slowing of the FHR. The pattern will not improve and will most likely get worse with additional contractions.
- *Equivocal/suspicious.* An equivocal/suspicious test has nonpersistent late decelerations or decelerations that are associated with hyperstimulation (contraction frequency of <2 minutes or duration of ≥90 seconds. When this test result occurs, more information is needed.

Clinical Application

CSTs are most commonly done as a follow-up for questionable or nonreactive NSTs. However, some physicians may choose to do a CST as a primary fetal assessment test. In this case, the CSTs are usually begun at approximately 32 to 34 weeks' gestation and are repeated at weekly intervals until intervention is necessary or the baby is born. A woman with diabetes or other medical condition that might change rapidly may be tested more frequently (Lagrew 1995).

A negative CST implies that the placenta is functioning normally and fetal oxygenation is adequate. As long as additional complications do not develop, data suggest that the incidence of perinatal death within 7 days following a negative CST is less than 1/1000 (Druzin and Gabbe 1996). A negative CST also suggests that the fetus is able to withstand the stress of labor, should it occur within the ensuing week.

A positive CST may indicate a fetus who has compromised placental circulation and decreased fetal oxygenation. Although a negative CST is reliable in predicting fetal status, a positive result may or may not indicate a problem. As many as 50 percent of fetuses with positive CSTs may tolerate labor without any further signs of fetal stress (a false-positive result). If labor is allowed to proceed, the fetus is carefully assessed for signs of stress, and all interventions to maximize placental–fetal blood flow are used (maternal side-lying position, maintenance of adequate fluid volume with IV fluid, oxygen by mask as needed) (Huddleston 1990).

If the CST is positive, FHR variability is minimal, FHR accelerations do not occur with fetal movement, and the fetal lungs are mature (as demonstrated by lecithin/sphingomyelin [L/S] ratio or phosphatidylglycerol [PG, discussed later in this chapter]), the fetus must be delivered immediately. Whether the woman with a positive CST should have a cesarean birth instead of a vaginal birth depends on the speed with which the fetus must be delivered to avoid severe fetal distress, the adequacy of cervical dilatation and effacement at the time the decision is being made, and the woman's condition. See Key Facts to Remember: Contraction Stress Test.

Role of the Nurse

The nurse ascertains the woman's understanding of the CST and the possible results and reviews the reasons for the CST and the procedure before the test begins. Written consent is required in some settings. In this case, the certified nurse-midwife/physician is responsible for fully informing the woman about the test. The nurse administers the CST, interprets the results, and reports the

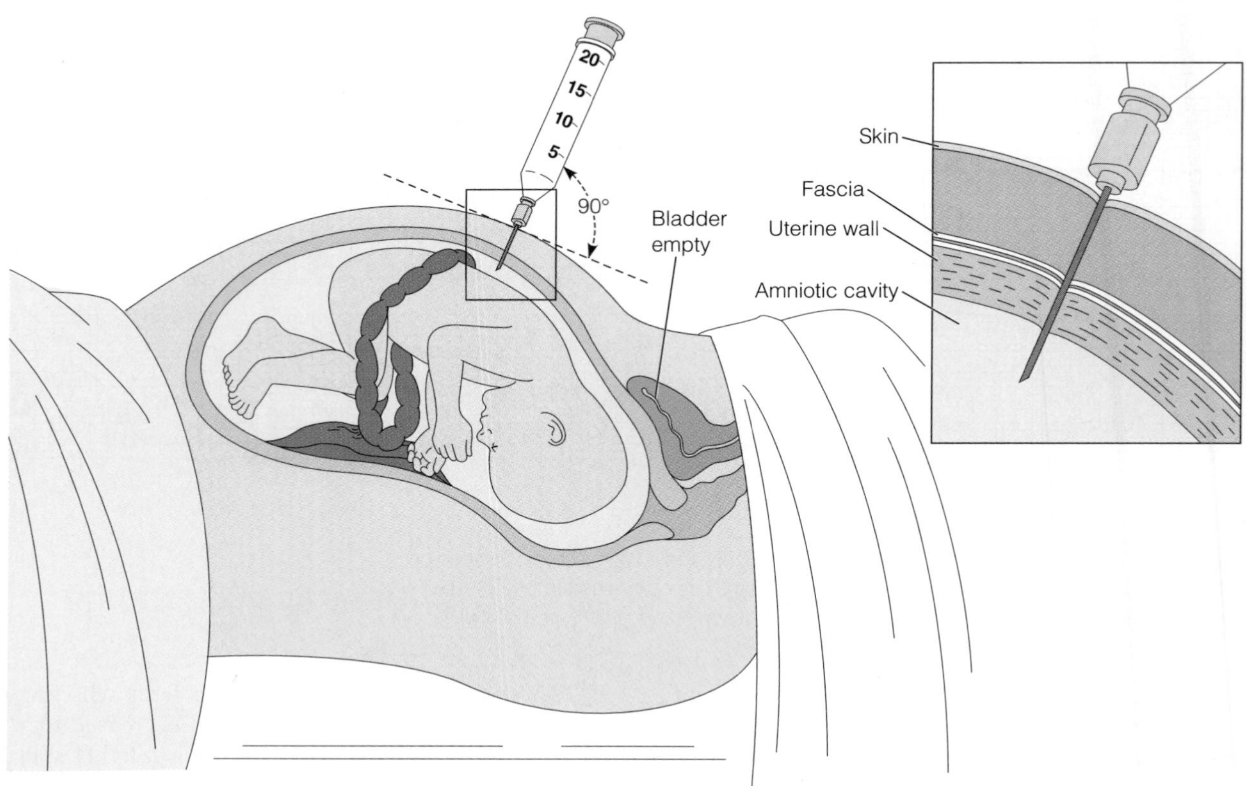

FIGURE 14–9 Amniocentesis. The woman is scanned by ultrasound to determine the placental site and to locate a pocket of amniotic fluid. Then the needle is inserted into the uterine cavity to withdraw amniotic fluid.

findings to the certified nurse-midwife/physician and the expectant woman. Throughout the whole procedure, the nurse provides continual reassurance to the woman and her support person. The nurse is also available to clarify any further treatment ordered by the certified nurse-midwife/physician.

KEY FACTS TO REMEMBER

Contraction Stress Test

Diagnostic value: Demonstrates reaction of FHR to stress of uterine contraction.

Results:

- Negative test: Stress of uterine contraction does not cause a late deceleration of the FHR.
- Positive test: Stress of uterine contraction is associated with a late deceleration of the FHR.

Amniotic Fluid Analysis

Procedure

Amniocentesis is a procedure used to obtain amniotic fluid. The analysis of amniotic fluid provides valuable information about fetal status. The amniotic fluid is withdrawn by a needle inserted through the abdominal wall into the uterus (Figure 14–9). Amniocentesis is a fairly simple procedure, although complications do occur rarely (less than 1 percent of cases). Procedure 14–1 describes the nursing interventions during amniocentesis.

Role of the Nurse

The nurse assists the physician during the amniocentesis and supports the woman undergoing the procedure. Although the physician has explained the amniocentesis procedure in advance so that the woman can give informed consent, the woman is likely to be apprehensive —both about the amniocentesis and about the information it will reveal. She may become anxious during the procedure and need additional emotional support. The nurse can provide this by further clarifying the physician's instructions or explanations, by relieving the

PROCEDURE 14–1 Assisting During Amniocentesis

Nursing Action	Rationale
Objective: Prepare the woman.	
• Explain the procedure and reassure the woman.	Explanation of the procedure decreases anxiety.
• Ask the woman to sign a consent form.	It is the physician's responsibility to obtain informed consent. The woman's signature indicates her awareness of risks and gives her consent to the procedure.
Objective: Assemble the equipment.	
• Prepare and arrange the following items so that they are easily accessible:	
• 22-gauge spinal needle with stylet	
• 10 mL and 20 mL syringes	
• 1% xylocaine	
• Betadine	
• Three 10 mL test tubes with tops (amber colored or covered with tape)	Amniotic fluid must be shielded from light to prevent breakdown of bilirubin.
Objective: Monitor the woman's vital signs.	
• Obtain baseline data on maternal BP, temperature, pulse, respirations, and FHR; then monitor every 15 minutes.	
Objective: Locate the fetus and the placenta.	
• Assist with real-time ultrasound to assess needle insertion during the procedure.	Amniocentesis is usually performed laterally in the area of fetal small parts, where pockets of amniotic fluid are often seen. Real-time ultrasound will identify fetal parts and locate pockets of amniotic fluid.
Objective: Cleanse the woman's abdomen.	Cleansing the woman's abdomen will decrease the incidence of infection.
Objective: Collect the amniotic fluid specimen.	
See Essential Precautions for Practice: During Amniocentesis.	
• Obtain the test tubes from the physician.	
• Label the tubes with the correct identification and send to the lab with the appropriate lab slips.	
Objective: Monitor the woman and reassess her vital signs.	It is important to determine if the fetus was inadvertently punctured.
• Determine the woman's BP, pulse, respirations, and FHR.	
• Palpate the woman's fundus to assess for uterine contractions.	
• Monitor the woman with an external fetal monitor for 20–30 minutes after the amniocentesis.	
• Determine a treatment course to counteract any supine hypotension and to increase venous return and cardiac output.	
• Assess the woman's blood type and determine any need for RhoGAM.	
• Have woman lie on her left side.	

PROCEDURE 14–1 Assisting During Amniocentesis continued

Nursing Action	Rationale
Objective: Reassure the woman and provide self-care education.	
• Instruct the woman to report any of the following side effects to her primary caretaker: • Unusual fetal hyperactivity or lack of movement • Vaginal discharge—clear drainage or bleeding • Uterine contractions or abdominal pain • Fever or chills	The woman will know how to recognize side effects or conditions that warrant further treatment.
• Encourage the woman to engage in only light activity for 24 hours.	A decrease in maternal activity will decrease uterine irritability and increase uteroplacental circulation.
• Encourage the woman to increase her fluid intake.	Increased hydration will replace the amniotic fluid through the uteroplacental circulation.
Objective: Complete the client record.	Provides a permanent record.
• Record the type of procedure, the date and time, and the name of the physician who performed the procedure.	
• Record the maternal-fetus response, disposition of the specimen, and discharge teaching.	

woman's physical discomfort when possible, and by responding verbally and physically to the woman's need for reassurance.

During the amniocentesis, the nurse follows CDC guidelines to avoid exposure to the amniotic fluid. (See Essential Precautions: During Amniocentesis.)

Following the amniocentesis, the nurse reiterates explanations given by the physician and provides opportunities for questions. The nurse reviews the experience with the woman and presents self-care measures.

ESSENTIAL PRECAUTIONS FOR PRACTICE

During Amniocentesis

The nurse should wear goggles or eye covering with side panels, a splash apron, and disposable gloves while assisting with an amniocentesis and handling amniotic fluid specimens. The amniotic fluid specimen should be clearly labeled so that laboratory personnel can take appropriate precautions while handling the specimen.

REMEMBER to wash your hands before putting on the disposable gloves and AGAIN immediately after you remove the gloves.

For further information consult OSHA and CDC guidelines.

Evaluation of Fetal Maturity

A number of studies can be performed on amniotic fluid. These tests can provide genetic information about the fetus (see Chapter 4) as well as information about the health and maturity of the fetus. The remainder of the section describes the amniotic fluid studies.

When managing a high-risk pregnancy, the caregiver is faced with the possibility of naturally occurring preterm labor or the need to terminate the pregnancy by induction of labor or cesarean birth. Indications for early termination of pregnancy include premature rupture of membranes and developing amnionitis, severe preeclampsia or eclampsia, bleeding problems, worsening Rh sensitization, and placental insufficiency. When an infant is born before the lungs are mature, the risk of such complications as respiratory distress syndrome is high.

Concentrations of certain substances in amniotic fluid reflect the health status of the fetus. For example, the triple test assesses alpha-fetoprotein (AFP), human chorionic gonadotrophin (hCG), and unconjugated estriol (UE3) in relation to maternal age. This test is used to screen for Down syndrome (trisomy 21), trisomy 18, and neural tube defect (NTD).

Because gestational age, birth weight, and the rate of development of organ systems do not necessarily correspond, amniotic fluid may also be analyzed to determine the maturity of the fetal lungs.

Lecithin/Sphingomyelin (L/S) Ratio

The alveoli of the lungs are lined with a substance called **surfactant,** which is composed of phospholipids. Surfactant lowers the surface tension of the alveoli when the newborn exhales. When a newborn with mature pulmonary function takes its first breath, a tremendously high pressure is needed to open the lungs. By lowering the alveolar surface tension, surfactant stabilizes the alveoli, and a certain amount of air always remains in the alveoli during expiration. Thus, when the infant exhales, the lungs do not collapse. An infant born before synthesis of surfactant is complete is unable to maintain lung stability. Each breath requires the same effort as the first. This results in underinflation of the lungs and development of respiratory distress syndrome.

Fetal lung maturity can be ascertained by determining the ratio of two components of surfactant—lecithin and sphingomyelin. Early in pregnancy, the sphingomyelin concentration in amniotic fluid is greater than the concentration of lecithin, and so the **lecithin/sphingomyelin (L/S) ratio** is low (lecithin levels are low and sphingomyelin levels are high). At about 32 weeks' gestation, sphingomyelin levels begin to fall and the amount of lecithin begins to increase. By 35 weeks' gestation, an L/S ratio of 2:1 (also reported as 2.0) is usually achieved in the normal fetus. A 2:1 L/S ratio indicates that the risk of RDS is very low (Druzin and Gabbe 1996). Under certain conditions of stress (a physiologic problem in the mother, placenta, and/or fetus), the fetal lungs mature more rapidly. Some conditions that may accelerate lung maturation are chronic maternal hypertension, severe pregnancy-induced hypertension, placental infarction, prolonged rupture of amniotic membranes, and intrauterine growth retardation (Jobe 1992).

KEY FACTS TO REMEMBER

L/S Ratio and PG

Diagnostic value: Provides information to help determine fetal lung maturity.

Results: L/S ratio of 2:1 and presence of PG correlate with 35 weeks' gestation.

An L/S ratio lower than 2:1 and/or an absence of PG may indicate underinflation of lungs and an increased risk for development of RDS.

There are also pregnancy-related conditions that act to delay maturation of the fetal lung. These conditions include diabetes mellitus and Rh isoimmunization with hydrops fetalis (Jobe 1992). In the presence of these conditions, an L/S ratio of 3:1 may be necessary to ensure adequate fetal lung maturity.

Phosphatidylglycerol

Phosphatidylglycerol (PG) is another phospholipid in surfactant. PG is not present in the fetal lung fluid early in gestation. It appears when fetal lung maturity has been attained, at about 35 weeks' gestation. Since the presence of PG is associated with fetal lung maturity, when it is present the risk of RDS is very low (Jobe 1992). PG determination is also useful in blood-contaminated specimens. Since PG is not present in blood or vaginal fluids, its presence is reliable in predicting lung maturity (Druzin and Gabbe 1996). See Key Facts to Remember: L/S Ratio and PG.

TABLE 14–4 Additional Diagnostic Techniques

Diagnostic Technique	*Purpose of Test*	*When Test May Be Done*
Chorionic Villus Sampling (CVS) A sample of chorionic villi from the placenta is obtained by introducing an aspiration catheter through the cervix. The whole procedure is guided and monitored by ultrasound.	To obtain tissue for genetic studies, sex determination. When a genetic problem is anticipated.	Between 8 and 12 weeks.
Fetoscopy Ultrasound is used to locate an area through which to insert a cannula and trochar into the uterus. Following insertion, an endoscope is introduced to find the desired part of the fetus for viewing and sampling.	To observe the fetus and obtain skin and/or blood samples (PUBS).	During the second and third trimesters.
Percutaneous Umbilical Blood Sampling An ultrasound scan is used to locate the fetal umbilical cord. A needle is introduced through the maternal abdomen into the umbilical cord and blood is aspirated.	To obtain a fetal blood sample for use in diagnosis of hemophilias, hemoglobinopathies, congenital rubella, and toxoplasmosis—and in fetal karyotyping.	In the second and third trimesters.
Fetal Echocardiography Ultrasound is used to examine fetal cardiac structures so that, if abnormalities are found, treatment can be initiated. Used primarily for high-risk women who are suspected of carrying a fetus with anomalies or a heart problem.	To identify cardiac anomalies.	During second or third trimesters.

Creatinine Level

Amniotic creatinine progressively increases as pregnancy advances, apparently because of increasing fetal muscle mass and maturing fetal renal function. Creatinine levels of 2 mg/dL of amniotic fluid seem to correlate closely with a pregnancy of 37 weeks or more (Creasy and Resnik 1990).

Other Fetal Diagnostic Techniques

In high-risk centers additional diagnostic techniques may be used to assess fetal status. *Chorionic villus sampling* (CVS) is used early in pregnancy to obtain tissue for genetic studies. It can be done much earlier than a genetic amniocentesis (between 8 and 12 menstrual weeks, rather than 16 to 18 weeks) and can provide needed information more quickly (Druzin and Gabbe 1996). There is a 1 in 3000 risk of fetal digital deficiency (a portion of a finger or toe missing) with the majority of defects occurring when CVS was performed before 7 weeks' gestation (Druzin and Gabbe 1996).

Fetoscopy allows the examiner to observe the fetus and to obtain skin or blood samples for further study. While a fetoscopy is done, the physician may obtain a blood specimen from the umbilical cord, a procedure called *percutaneous umbilical blood sampling (PUBS)*. *Computed tomography (CT) scanning* and *magnetic resonance imaging (MRI)* may also be used in some circumstances. See also Table 14–4 on page 335.

CHAPTER HIGHLIGHTS

- Maternal assessment of fetal activity can be used as a screening procedure in evaluation of fetal status.
- Ultrasound offers a valuable means of assessing intrauterine fetal growth because the growth can be followed over a period of time. It is noninvasive and painless, allows the certified nurse-midwife/physician to study the gestation serially, is nonradiating to both the woman and her fetus, and has no known harmful effects.
- A nonstress test (NST) is based on the knowledge that the FHR normally increases in response to fetal activity. The desired result is a reactive test.
- A fetal biophysical profile includes five variables (fetal breathing movement, fetal body movement, fetal tone, amniotic fluid volume, and FHR reactivity) to assess the fetus at risk for intrauterine compromise.
- A contraction stress test (CST) provides a method for observing the response of the FHR to the stress of uterine contractions. The desired result is a negative test.
- Amniocentesis can be used to obtain amniotic fluid to test for L/S ratio, PG, and creatinine.
- The L/S ratio can be used to assess fetal lung maturity. The presence of PG also provides information about fetal lung maturity.

REFERENCES

Chervenak FA, Gabbe SG. Obstetric ultrasound: Assessment of fetal growth and anatomy. In: *Obstetrics: Normal and Problem Pregnancies.* 3rd ed. Gabbe SG, Niebyl JR, Simpson JL (editors). New York: Churchill Livingstone, 1996.

Creasy RK, Resnik R: *Maternal Fetal Medicine.* Philadelphia: Saunders, 1989.

Cundiff JL et al: Umbilical artery Doppler flow studies during pregnancy. *JOGNN* November/December 1990; 19(6):475.

Dahmus M, Amon E: The biophysical profile. In: *Gynecology and Obstetrics, Vol. 3.* Depp R, Eschenbach DA, Sciarra JJ (editors). Philadelphia: Harper & Row, 1992.

Druzin ML, Gabbe SG. Antepartum fetal evaluation. In: *Obstetrics: Normal and Problem Pregnancies.* 3rd ed. Gabbe SG, Neibyl JR, Simpson JL (editors). New York: Churchill Livingstone, 1996.

Goldstein ST: Practical aspects of vaginal sonography. *Eleventh International Symposium on Perinatal Medicine and Obstetrical Ultrasound,* March 30–April 2, 1992, Las Vegas, Nevada.

Huddleston JF: Antepartum assessment of fetal well-being. In: *Manual of Clinical Problems in Obstetrics and Gynecology.* Revlin ME, Morrison JC, Bates GW (editors). Boston: Little, Brown, 1990.

Jobe AH: The respiratory system. In: *Neonatal-Perinatal Medicine,* 5th ed. Fanaroff AA, Martin RJ (editors). St Louis: Mosby, 1992.

Lagrew DC: The contraction stress test. *Clin Obstet Gynecol* March 1995; 38:11.

Manning FA: Dynamic ultrasound-based fetal assessment: The fetal biophysical profile score. *Clin Obstet Gynecol* March 1995; 38:26.

Manning FA: The biophysical profile: Contemporary use. *Tenth International Symposium on Perinatal Medicine and Obstetrical Ultrasound,* April 9–12, 1990, Las Vegas, Nevada.

Maulik D: Doppler ultrasound velocimetry for fetal surveillance. *Clin Obstet Gynecol* March 1995; 38:91.

Paul RH, Miller DA: Nonstress test. *Clin Obstet Gynecol* March 1995; 38:3.

Saari-Kemppainen A et al: Ultrasound screening and perinatal mortality: Controlled trial of systematic one-stage screening in pregnancy. The Helsinki Ultrasound Trial. *Lancet* August 18, 1990; 336(8712):387.

Smith CV: Vibroacoustic stimulation. *Clin Obstet Gynecol* March 1995; 38:68.

Treacy B et al: Ultrasound in labor and delivery. *Obstet Gynecol Survey* 1990; 45(4):213.

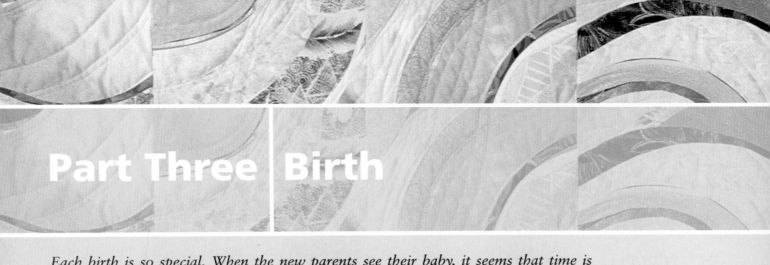

Part Three Birth

Each birth is so special. When the new parents see their baby, it seems that time is suspended. I watch as they gaze at their baby and reach out with their fingers to touch the baby's hands and fingers. I have been so fortunate to be a birthing room nurse and to share this experience with so many new families, but each time is like no other.

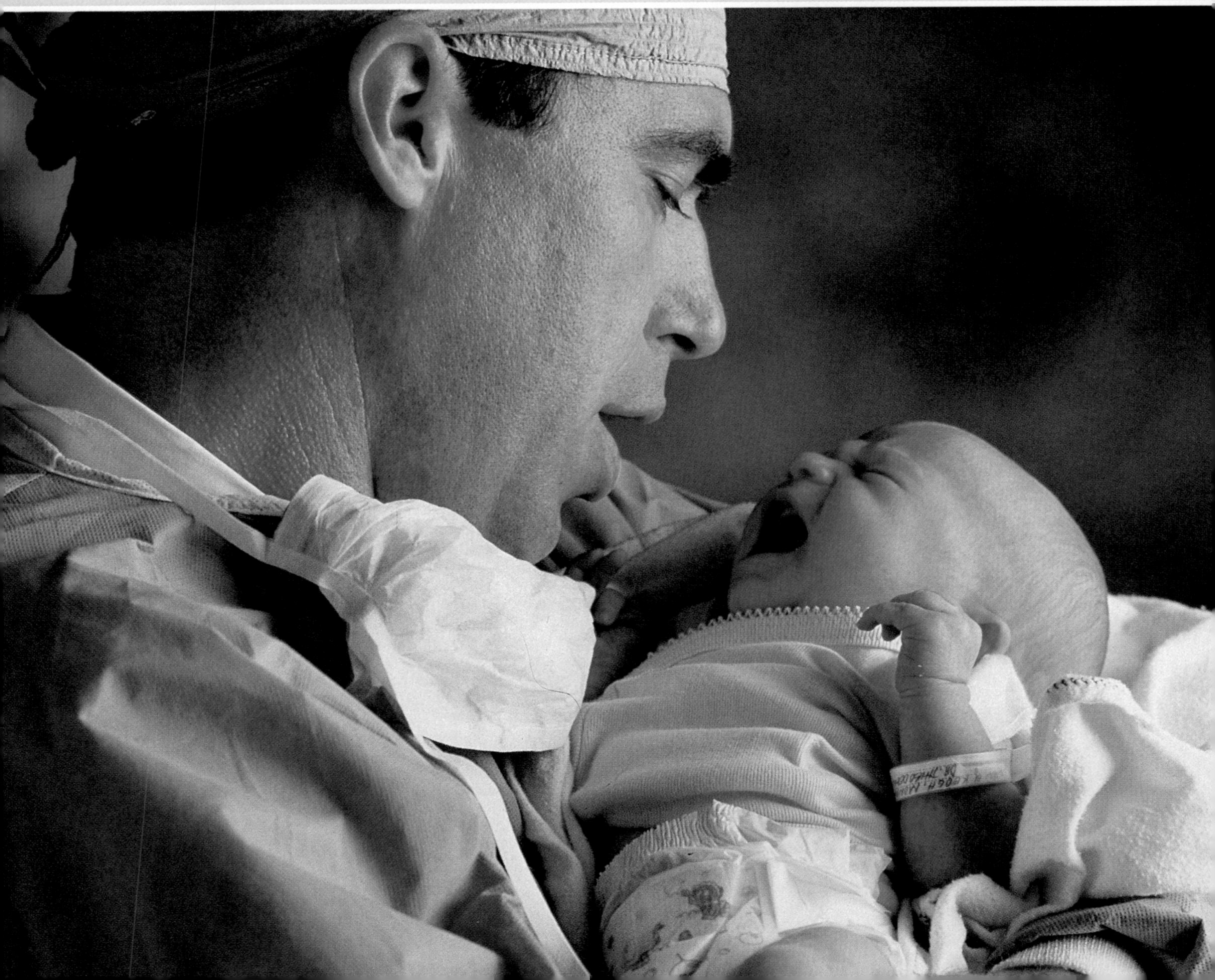

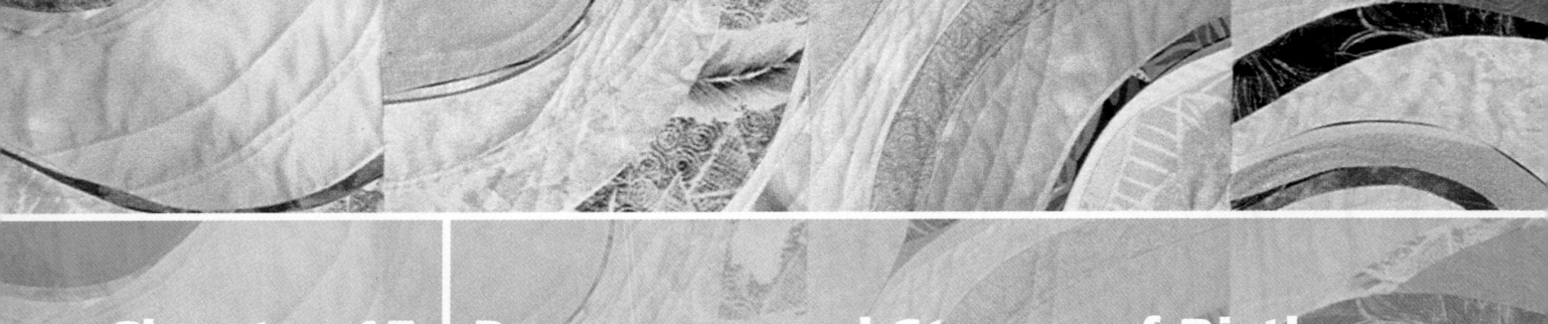

Chapter 15 Processes and Stages of Birth

OBJECTIVES

- Examine the four critical factors that influence labor.
- Describe the physiology of labor.
- Discuss premonitory signs of labor.
- Differentiate between false and true labor.
- Describe the physiologic and psychologic changes occurring in each of the stages of labor.
- Summarize maternal systemic responses to labor.
- Discuss fetal responses to labor.

KEY TERMS

Bloody show
Cardinal movements
Cervical dilatation
Crowning
Duration
Effacement
Engagement
Fetal attitude
Fetal lie
Fetal position
Fetal presentation
Fontanelles
Frequency
Intensity
Lightening
Malpositions
Malpresentations
Molding
Presenting part
Rupture of membranes (ROM)
Station
Sutures

At the end of the 40-week prenatal period, the zygote has grown into a baby ready for the independence of extrauterine life. The expectant woman has undergone numerous physiologic and psychologic changes that gradually prepared her for childbirth and for the role of mother. The moment has arrived for the birth of this new baby. As labor begins, so begins the process of moving this new individual into the world.

Critical Factors in Labor

Four factors are important in the process of labor and birth: the birth passage, the fetus, the forces of labor, and psychosocial considerations. These four factors are defined as follows:

1. The birth passage
   - Size of the pelvis (diameters of the pelvic inlet, midpelvis or pelvic cavity, and outlet)
   - Type of pelvis (gynecoid, android, anthropoid, platypelloid, or a combination)
   - Ability of the cervix to dilate and efface, and ability of the vaginal canal and the external opening of the vagina (the *introitus*) to distend
2. The fetus
   - Fetal head (size and presence of molding)
   - Fetal attitude (flexion or extension of the fetal body and extremities)
   - Fetal lie
   - Fetal presentation (the part of the fetal body entering the pelvis first in a single or multiple pregnancy)
   - Fetal position (relationship of the presenting part to one of the four quadrants of the maternal pelvis)
   - Placenta (implantation site)
3. Primary forces of labor
   - The frequency, duration, and intensity of uterine contractions as the fetus moves through the birth passage
   - The effectiveness of maternal pushing effort
   - The duration of labor
4. Psychosocial considerations
   - Physical preparation for childbirth
   - Sociocultural values and beliefs
   - Previous childbirth experience
   - Support from significant others
   - Emotional integrity

The progress of labor is critically dependent on the complementary relationship of these four factors. Abnormalities of the birth passage, the fetus, the forces of labor, or the psychosocial status of the woman can alter the outcome of labor and jeopardize both the expectant woman and her baby. Complications are discussed in Chapter 19.

The Birth Passage

The true pelvis, which forms the bony canal through which the fetus must pass, is divided into three sections: the inlet, the pelvic cavity (midpelvis), and the outlet. (*Note:* See Chapter 2 for discussion of each part of the pelvis and Chapter 8 for assessment techniques.)

The four classic types of pelvis are gynecoid, android, anthropoid, and platypelloid (Caldwell and Moloy 1933). The *gynecoid,* or female, pelvis is most common. All diameters of the gynecoid are adequate for childbirth. The *android,* or male, pelvis is usually not adequate for vaginal birth. The *anthropoid* pelvis is narrow from side to side, but is usually adequate for vaginal birth. The *platypelloid* pelvis, which is narrow from front to back, is usually not adequate.

The Fetus

Fetal Head

The fetal head is composed of bony parts that can either hinder childbirth or make it easier. Once the head (the least compressible and largest part of the fetus) has been born, the birth of the rest of the body is rarely delayed. The fetal skull has three major parts: the face, the base of the skull (cranium), and the vault of the cranium (roof). The bones of the face and cranial base are well fused and essentially fixed. The base of the cranium is composed of the two temporal bones, each with a sphenoid and ethmoid bone. The bones composing the vault are the two frontal bones, the two parietal bones, and the occipital bone (Figure 15–1). These bones are not fused, allowing this portion of the head to adjust in shape as the presenting part passes through the narrow portions of the pelvis. The cranial bones overlap under pressure of the powers of labor and the demands of the unyielding pelvis. This overlapping is called **molding.**

The **sutures** of the fetal skull are membranous spaces between the cranial bones. The intersections of the cranial sutures are called **fontanelles.** These sutures allow for molding of the fetal head and help the clinician to

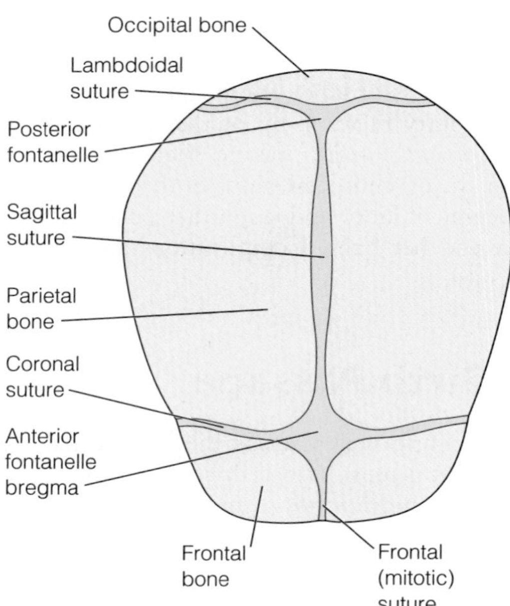

FIGURE 15–1 Superior view of the fetal skull.

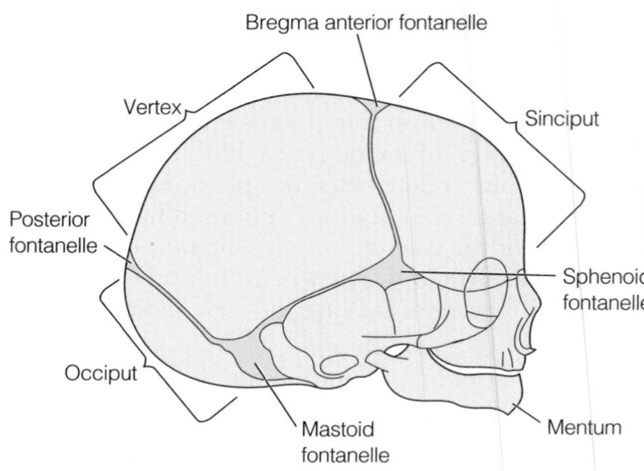

FIGURE 15–2 Lateral view of the fetal skull identifying the landmarks that have significance during birth.

identify the position of the fetal head during vaginal examination. The important sutures of the cranial vault are as follows (see Figure 15–1):

- *Mitotic suture:* Located between the two frontal bones; becomes the anterior continuation of the sagittal suture.
- *Sagittal suture:* Located between the parietal bones; divides the skull into left and right halves; runs anteroposteriorly, connecting the two fontanelles.
- *Coronal sutures:* Located between the frontal and parietal bones; extend transversely left and right from the anterior fontanelle.
- *Lambdoidal suture:* Located between the two parietal bones and the occipital bone; extends transversely left and right from the posterior fontanelle.

The anterior and posterior fontanelles are clinically useful in identifying the position of the fetal head in the pelvis and in assessing the status of the newborn after birth. The anterior fontanelle is diamond-shaped and measures about 2 by 3 cm. It permits growth of the brain by remaining unossified for as long as 18 months. The posterior fontanelle is much smaller and closes within 8–12 weeks after birth. It is shaped like a small triangle and marks the meeting point of the sagittal suture and the lambdoidal suture (Cunningham et al 1997).

Following are several important landmarks of the fetal skull (Figure 15–2):

- *Mentum:* The fetal chin.
- *Sinciput:* The anterior area known as the brow.
- *Bregma:* The large diamond-shaped anterior fontanelle.
- *Vertex:* The area between the anterior and posterior fontanelles.
- *Posterior fontanelle:* The intersection between posterior cranial sutures.
- *Occiput:* The area of the fetal skull occupied by the occipital bone, beneath the posterior fontanelle.

The diameters of the fetal skull vary considerably within normal limits. Some diameters shorten and others lengthen as the head is molded during labor. Fetal head diameters are measured between the various landmarks on the skull (Figure 15–3). For example, the suboccipitobregmatic diameter is the distance from the undersurface of the occiput to the center of the bregma, or anterior fontanelle. Fetal skull measurements are given in Figure 15–3.

Fetal Attitude

Fetal attitude refers to the relation of the fetal parts to one another. The normal attitude of the fetus is one of moderate flexion of the head, flexion of the arms onto the chest, and flexion of the legs onto the abdomen.

Changes in fetal attitude, particularly in the position of the head, cause the fetus to present larger diameters of the fetal head to the maternal pelvis. These deviations from a normal fetal attitude often contribute to difficult labor (see Figure 15–4).

Fetal Lie

Fetal lie refers to the relationship of the cephalocaudal axis of the fetus to the cephalocaudal axis of the woman. The fetus may assume either a longitudinal or a

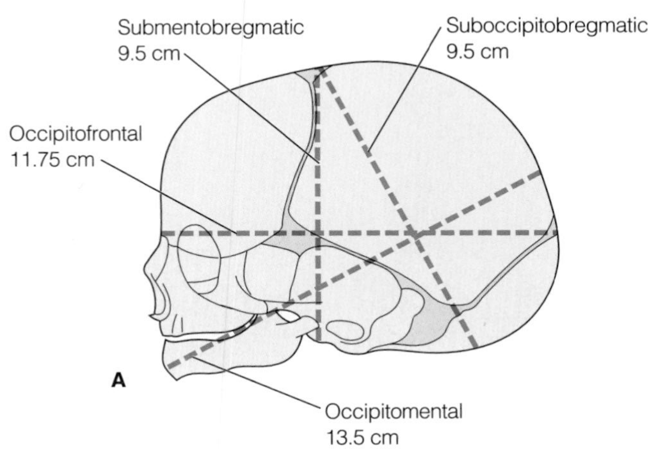

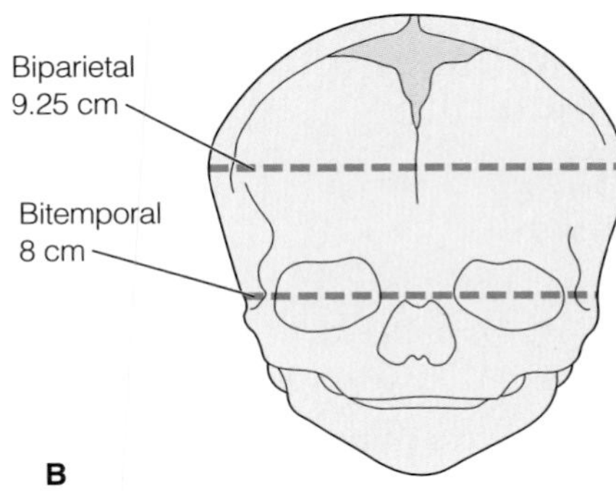

FIGURE 15–3 ***A*** Anteroposterior diameters of the fetal skull. When the vertex of the fetus presents and the fetal head is flexed with the chin on the chest, the smallest anteroposterior diameter (suboccipitobregmatic) enters the birth canal. ***B*** Transverse diameters of the fetal skull.

transverse lie. A *longitudinal lie* occurs when the cephalocaudal axis of the fetus is parallel to the woman's spine. A *transverse lie* occurs when the cephalocaudal axis of the fetus is at right angles to the woman's spine.

Fetal Presentation

Fetal presentation is determined by fetal lie and by the body part of the fetus that enters the pelvic passage first. This portion of the fetus is referred to as the **presenting part.** Fetal presentation may be cephalic, breech, or shoulder. The most common presentation is cephalic. When this presentation occurs, labor and birth are likely to proceed normally. Breech and shoulder presentations are associated with difficulties during labor and do not proceed as normal; therefore, they are called **malpresentations** (see Chapter 19 for discussion).

Cephalic Presentation

The fetal head presents itself to the passage in approximately 97 percent of term births. The cephalic presentation can be further classified according to the degree of flexion or extension of the fetal head (attitude).

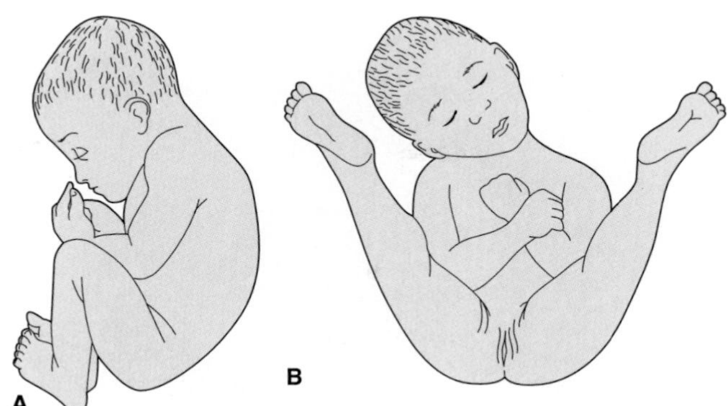

FIGURE 15–4 Fetal attitude. ***A*** The attitude (or relationship of body parts) of this fetus is normal. The head is flexed forward with the chin almost resting on the chest. The arms and legs are flexed. ***B*** In this view, the head is tilted to the right. Although the arms are flexed, the legs are extended.

Vertex Presentation

- Vertex is the most common type of presentation.
- The fetal head is completely flexed onto the chest.
- The smallest diameter of the fetal head (suboccipitobregmatic) presents to the maternal pelvis (Figure 15–5*A*).
- The occiput is the presenting part.

Military Presentation

- The fetal head is neither flexed nor extended.
- The occipitofrontal diameter presents to the maternal pelvis (Figure 15–5*B*).
- The top of the head is the presenting part.

Brow Presentation

- The fetal head is partially extended.
- The occipitomental diameter, the largest anteroposterior diameter, is presented to the maternal pelvis (Figure 15–5*C*).
- The sinciput (see Figure 15–2, p 340) is the presenting part.

Face Presentation

- The fetal head is hyperextended (complete extension).
- The submentobregmatic diameter presents to the maternal pelvis (Figure 15–5D).
- The face is the presenting part.

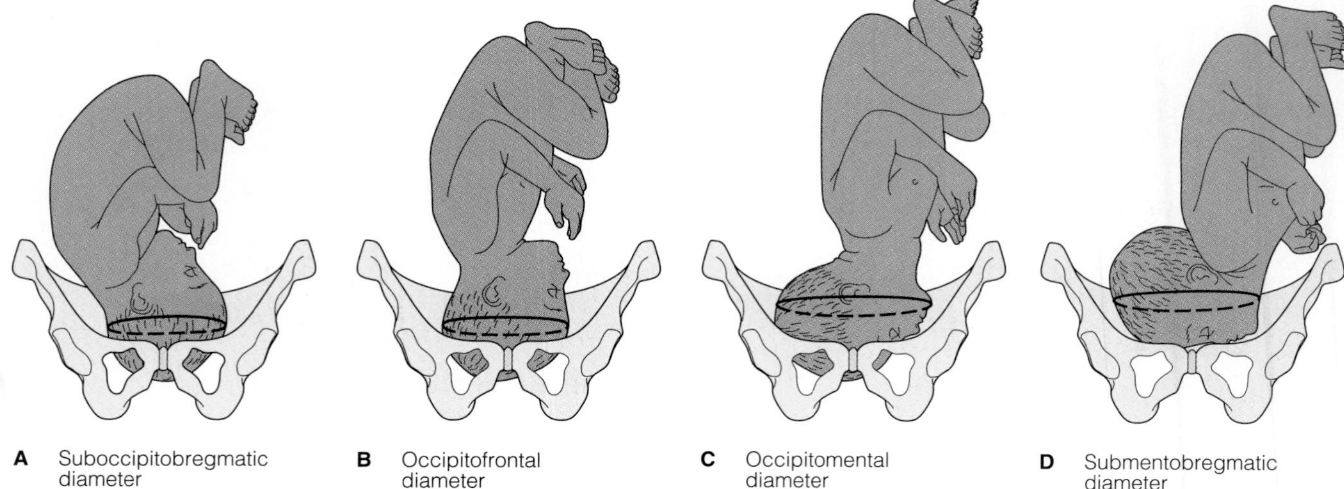

FIGURE 15–5 Cephalic presentation. ***A*** Vertex presentation. Complete flexion of the head allows the suboccipitrobregmatic diameter to present to the pelvis. ***B*** Military (median vertex) presentation with no flexion or extension. The occipitofrontal diameter presents to the pelvis. ***C*** Brow presentation. The fetal head is in partial (halfway) extension. The occipitomental diameter, which is the largest diameter of the fetal head, presents to the pelvis. ***D*** Face presentation. The fetal head is in complete extension, and the submentobregmatic diameter presents to the pelvis.

Breech Presentation

Breech presentations occur in 3 percent of term births. These presentations are classified according to the attitude of the fetus's hips and knees. In all variations of the breech presentation, the sacrum is the landmark to be noted.

Complete Breech

- The fetal knees and hips are both flexed; the thighs are on the abdomen, and the calves are on the posterior aspect of the thighs.
- The buttocks and feet of the fetus present to the maternal pelvis. (Refer to Chapter 19, Figure 19–7.)

Frank Breech

- The fetal hips are flexed, and the knees are extended.
- The buttocks of the fetus present to the maternal pelvis.

Footling Breech

- The fetal hips and legs are extended.
- The feet of the fetus present to the maternal pelvis.
- In a single footling, one foot presents; in a double footling, both feet present.

Shoulder Presentation

A shoulder presentation is also called a transverse lie. Most frequently, the shoulder is the presenting part and the acromion process of the scapula is the landmark to be noted. However, the fetal arm, back, abdomen, or side may present in a transverse lie. (Refer to Chapter 19, Figure 19–8.)

Functional Relationships of Presenting Part and Passage

Engagement

Engagement of the presenting part occurs when the largest diameter of the presenting part reaches or passes through the pelvic inlet (Figure 15–6). Engagement can be determined by vaginal examination. In primigravidas, engagement usually occurs 2 weeks before term. Multiparas, however, may experience engagement several weeks before the onset of labor or during the process of labor. Engagement confirms the adequacy of the pelvic inlet. Engagement does not, however, indicate whether the midpelvis and outlet are also adequate.

Station

Station refers to the relationship of the presenting part to an imaginary line drawn between the ischial spines of the maternal pelvis. In a normal pelvis, the ischial spines mark the narrowest diameter through which the fetus must pass. These spines are not sharp protrusions that harm the fetus, but blunted prominences at the midpelvis. The ischial spines as a landmark have been desig-

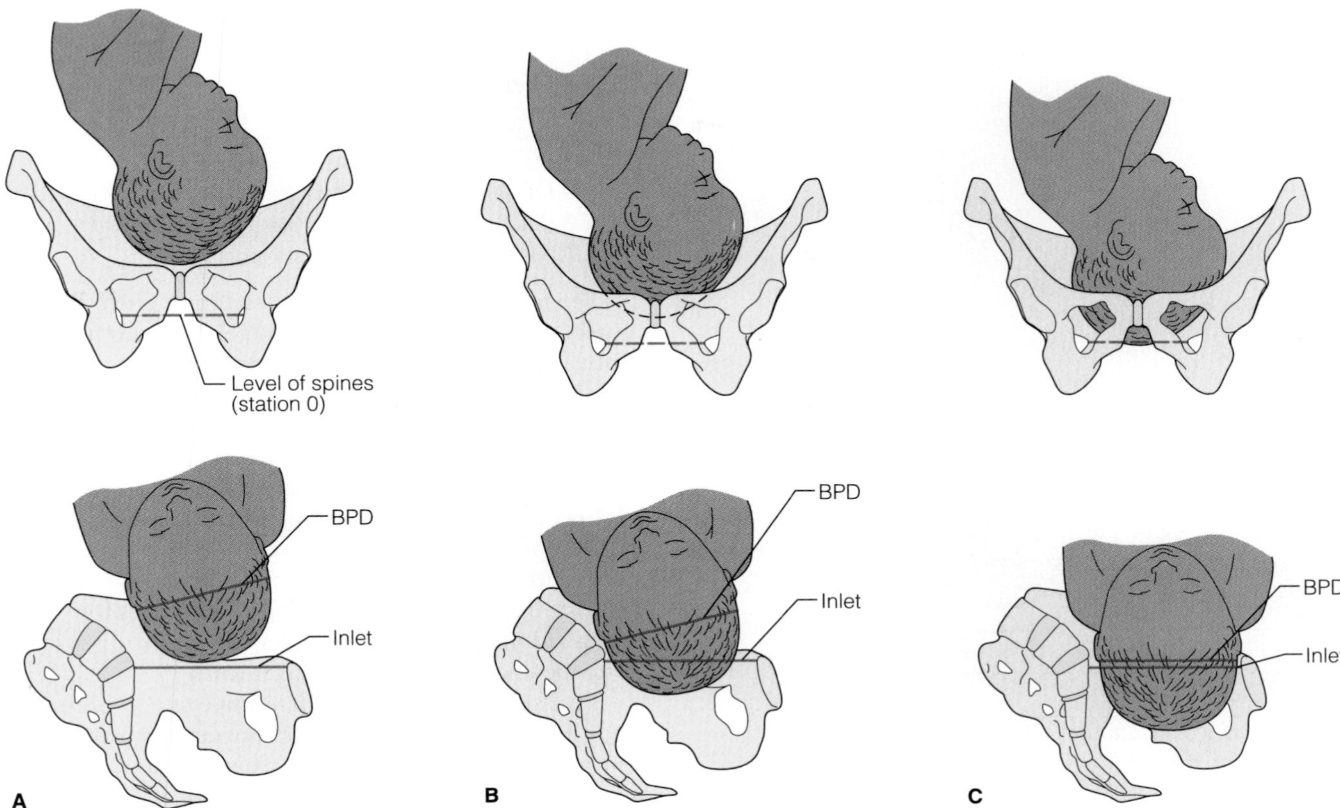

FIGURE 15–6 Process of engagement in cephalic presentation. ***A*** Floating. The fetal head is directed down toward the pelvis but can still easily move away from the inlet. ***B*** Dipping. The fetal head dips into the inlet but can be moved away by exerting pressure on the fetus. ***C*** Engaged. The biparietal diameter (BPD) of the fetal head is in the inlet of the pelvis. In most instances the presenting part (occiput) is at the level of the ischial spines (zero station).

nated as zero station (Figure 15–7). If the presenting part is higher than the ischial spines, a negative number is assigned, noting centimeters above zero station. Station −5 is at the inlet, and station +4 is at the outlet. If the presenting part can be seen at the woman's perineum, birth is imminent. During labor, the presenting part should move progressively from the negative stations to the midpelvis at zero station and into the positive stations. Failure of the presenting part to descend in the presence of strong contractions may be due to disproportion between the maternal pelvis and fetal presenting part or to a short or entangled umbilical cord.

Fetal Position

Fetal position refers to the relationship of the landmark on the presenting fetal part to the front, sides, or back of the maternal pelvis. The landmark on the fetal presenting part is related to four imaginary quadrants of the pelvis: left anterior, right anterior, left posterior, and right posterior. These quadrants designate whether the presenting part is directed toward the front, back, left, or right of the passage. The landmark chosen for vertex presentations is the occiput, and the landmark for face presentations is the mentum. In breech presentations, the sacrum is the designated landmark, and the acromion process on the scapula is the landmark in shoulder presentations. If the landmark is directed toward the center of the side of the pelvis, fetal position is designated as *transverse,* rather than anterior or posterior. Three notations are used to describe the fetal position:

1. Right (R) or left (L) side of the maternal pelvis.
2. The landmark of the fetal presenting part: occiput (O), mentum (M), sacrum (S), or acromion process (A).
3. Anterior (A), posterior (P), or transverse (T), depending on whether the landmark is in the front, back, or side of the pelvis.

The abbreviations of these notations help the health care team communicate the fetal position. Thus, when the fetal occiput is directed toward the back and to the left of the birth passage, the abbreviation used is LOP

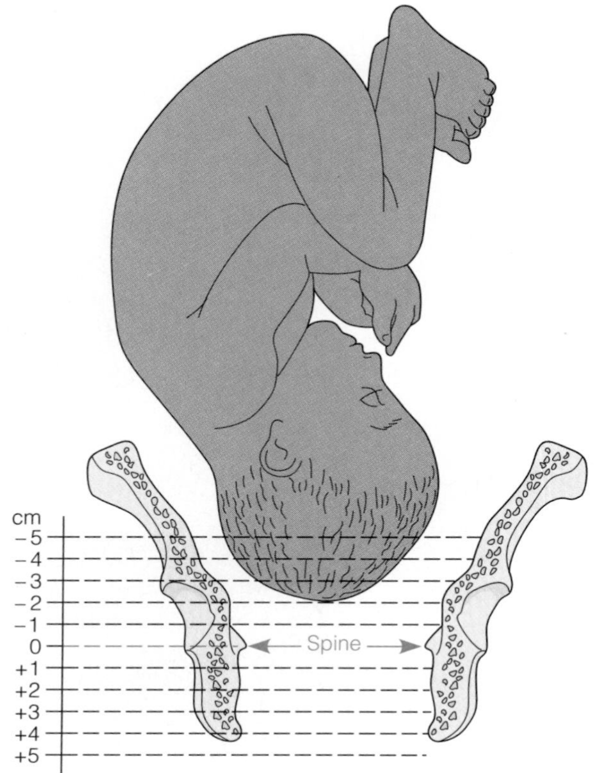

FIGURE 15–7 Measuring the station of the fetal head while it is descending. In this view the station is −2/ −3.

(left-occiput-posterior). The term *dorsal* (D) is used when denoting the fetal position in a transverse lie; it refers to the fetal back. Thus RADA indicates that the acromion process of the scapula is directed toward the woman's right and the fetus's back is anterior. Following is a list of the positions for various fetal presentations, some of which are illustrated in Figure 15–8.

Positions in vertex presentation:
ROA Right-occiput-anterior
ROT Right-occiput-transverse
ROP Right-occiput-posterior
LOA Left-occiput-anterior
LOT Left-occiput-transverse
LOP Left-occiput-posterior

Positions in face presentation:
RMA Right-mentum-anterior
RMT Right-mentum-transverse
RMP Right-mentum-posterior
LMA Left-mentum-anterior
LMT Left-mentum-transverse
LMP Left-mentum-posterior

Positions in breech presentation:
RSA Right-sacrum-anterior
RST Right-sacrum-transverse
RSP Right-sacrum-posterior
LSA Left-sacrum-anterior
LST Left-sacrum-transverse
LSP Left-sacrum-posterior

Positions in shoulder presentation:
RADA Right-acromion-dorsal-anterior
RADP Right-acromion-dorsal-posterior
LADA Left-acromion-dorsal-anterior
LADP Left-acromion-dorsal-posterior

The fetal position influences labor and birth. For example, the fetal head presents a larger diameter in a posterior position than in an anterior position. A posterior position increases the pressure on the maternal sacral nerves, causing the laboring woman to experience backache and pelvic pressure, which may lead her to bear down or push earlier than normal. The most common fetal position is occiput anterior. When this position occurs, labor and birth are likely to proceed normally. Positions other than occiput anterior are more frequently associated with problems during labor; therefore they are called **malpositions.** (See Chapter 19 for discussion of malpositions and their management.)

Assessment techniques to determine fetal position include inspection and palpation of the maternal abdomen and vaginal examination. (See Chapter 16 for further discussion of assessing fetal position.)

The Forces of Labor

Primary and secondary forces work together to achieve birth of the fetus, the fetal membranes, and the placenta. The *primary force* is uterine muscular contractions, which cause the changes of the first stage of labor—complete effacement and dilatation of the cervix. The *secondary force* is the use of abdominal muscles to push during the second stage of labor. The pushing augments the primary force after full dilatation.

In labor, uterine contractions are rhythmic but intermittent. Between contractions there is a period of relaxation. This allows uterine muscles to rest and provides respite for the laboring woman. It also restores uteroplacental circulation, which is important to fetal oxygenation and adequate circulation in the uterine blood vessels.

Each contraction has three phases: (a) *increment,* the "building up" of the contraction (the longest phase); (b) *acme,* or the peak of the contraction; and (c) *decrement,* or the "letting up" of the contraction. When describing uterine contractions during labor, caregivers use the terms *frequency, duration,* and *intensity.* **Frequency** refers to the time between the beginning of one contraction and the beginning of the next contraction. **Duration** is measured from the beginning of increment to the completion of decrement (Figure 15–9). In beginning labor, the duration is about 30 seconds. As labor continues,

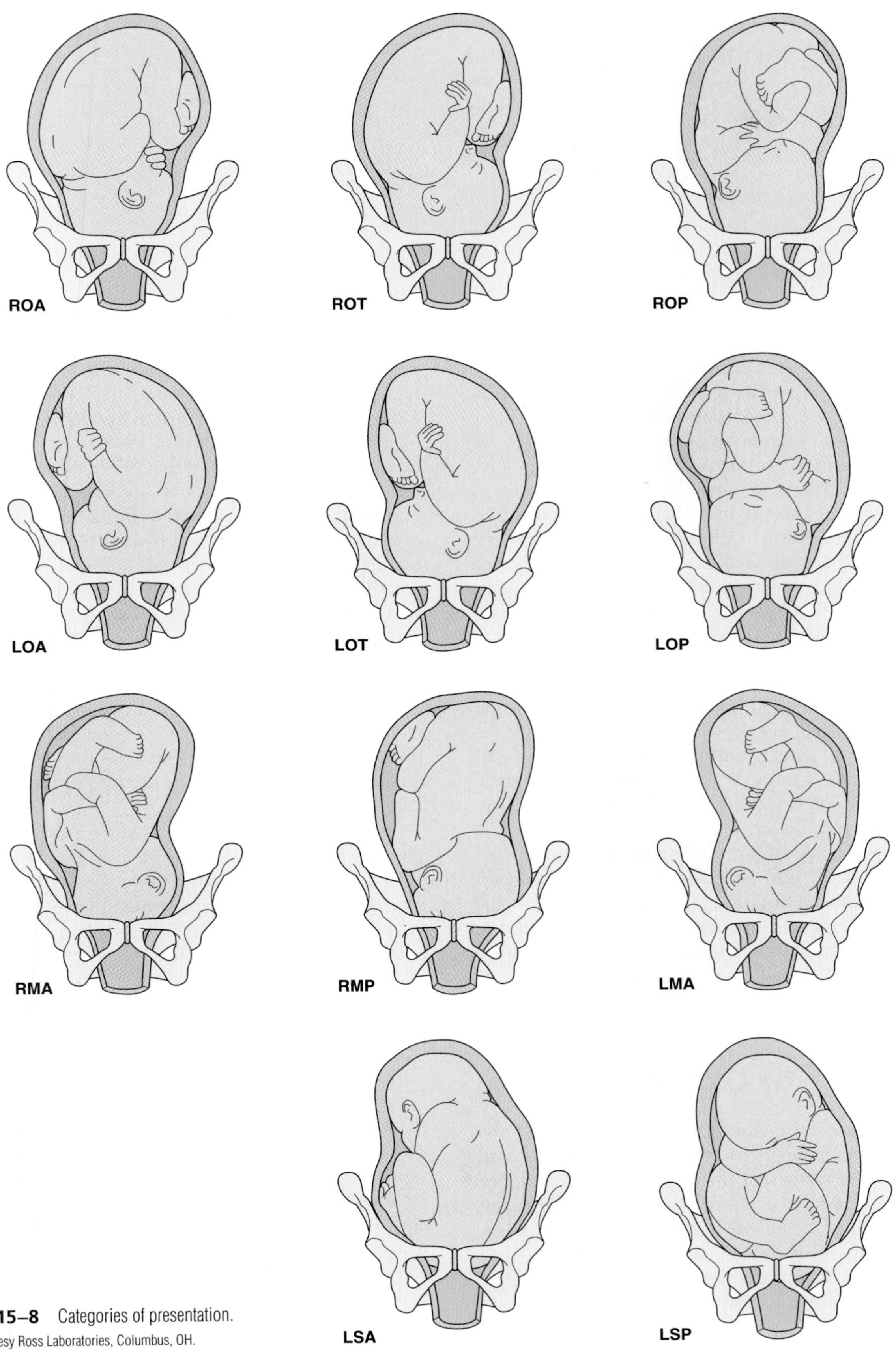

FIGURE 15–8 Categories of presentation.
Source: Courtesy Ross Laboratories, Columbus, OH.

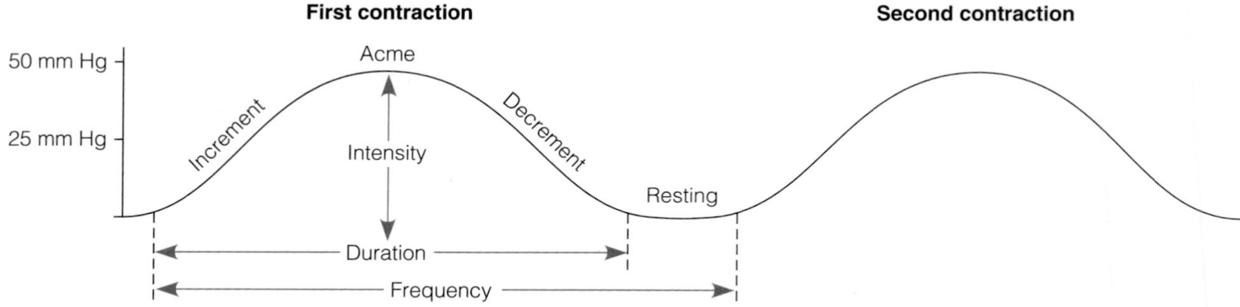

FIGURE 15–9 Characteristics of uterine contractions.

duration increases to an average of 60 seconds with a range of 45–90 seconds (Varney 1987).

Intensity refers to the strength of the contraction during acme. In most instances intensity is estimated by palpating the contraction, but it may be measured directly with an intrauterine catheter. When estimating intensity by palpation, the nurse determines whether it is mild, moderate, or strong by judging the amount of indentability of the uterine wall during the acme of a contraction. If the uterine wall can be indented easily, the contraction is considered mild. Strong intensity exists when the uterine wall cannot be indented. Moderate intensity falls between these two ranges. When intensity is measured with an intrauterine catheter, the normal resting pressure in the uterus (between contractions) averages 10–12 mm Hg. During acme the intensity ranges from 25–30 mm Hg in early labor, 25–70 mm Hg in active labor, 40–80 mm Hg during transition, and 80–110 mm Hg while the woman is pushing in the second stage (Murray 1989). (See Chapter 16 for further discussion of assessment techniques.)

At the beginning of labor, the contractions are usually mild, of short duration, and relatively infrequent. As labor progresses, duration of contractions lengthens, intensity increases, and frequency is every 2–3 minutes. Because the contractions are involuntary, the laboring woman cannot control their duration, frequency, or intensity.

Psychosocial Considerations

Similar psychosocial factors affect the mother and the father. Both are making a transition into a new role, and both have expectations of themselves during the labor and birth experience, as caregivers for their child and their new family. Although many prospective mothers and fathers attend childbirth preparation classes, they still tend to be concerned about what labor will be like, whether they will be able to perform the way they expect, whether the discomfort and pain will be more than the mother expects or can cope with, and whether the father can provide helpful support (McKay and Smith 1993; Nichols 1993; Tomlinson and Bryan 1996).

Every woman is uncertain about what her labor will be like: A woman anticipating her first labor faces a totally new experience, and even multiparas cannot be certain what each new labor will bring. The woman does not know whether she will live up to her expectations for herself in relation to her friends and relatives, whether she will be physically injured through laceration, episiotomy, or cesarean incision, or whether significant others will be as supportive as she hopes (Mercer 1995). The woman faces an irrevocable event—the birth of a new family member—and, consequently, disruption of lifestyle, relationships, and self-image. Finally, the woman must deal with concerns about her loss of control of bodily functions, emotional responses to an unfamiliar situation, and reactions to the pain associated with labor.

Various factors influence a woman's reaction to the physical and emotional crisis of labor (Table 15–1). Her accomplishment of the tasks of pregnancy, usual coping mechanisms in response to stressful life events, support system, preparation for childbirth, and cultural influences are all significant factors.

In her study of the psychosocial adaptations of pregnancy, Lederman (1996) found that expectant women prepared for labor through actions and imaginary rehearsal. The actions frequently consisted of "nesting behavior" (housecleaning, decorating the nursery) and a "psyching up" for the labor, which seemed to vary depending on the woman's self-confidence, self-esteem, and previous experiences with stress. Specific actions to prepare for labor are usually focused on becoming better informed and prepared. Nichols and Humenick (1988) suggest that mastery, or control, of the childbearing experience is the key factor in decreased pain and perceived satisfaction (Lowe 1996). Childbirth education helps increase positive reactions to the birth ex-

TABLE 15–1 Factors Associated with a Positive Birth Experience

Motivation for the pregnancy
Attendance at childbirth education classes
A sense of competence or mastery
Self-confidence and self-esteem
Positive relationship with mate
Maintaining control during labor
Support from mate or other person during labor
Not being left alone in labor
Trust in the medical/nursing staff
Having personal control of breathing patterns, comfort measures
Choosing a physician/certified nurse-midwife who has a similar philosophy of care
Receiving clear information regarding procedures

perience by giving the laboring woman and her support persons greater opportunities to control the experience of labor. DiMatteo, Kahn, and Berry (1993) suggest that women need to be prepared to face not only areas that are under their personal control, such as patterned breathing and certain comfort measures, but also experiences involving situational control, which include some procedures requested by the certified nurse-midwife/physician or birth-setting institutional protocols.

An important developmental step for expectant women is to anticipate the labor in fantasy. Just as a woman "tries on" the maternal role during pregnancy, fantasizing about labor seems to help her understand and become better prepared for it. Fantasies about the excitement of the baby's birth and the sharing of the experience involve the woman in constructive preparation. A woman who has a great deal of apprehension about becoming a mother or a high fear of pain during labor is unable to fantasize the labor in positive ways and may have many disturbing thoughts (Lederman 1996).

Many women fear the pain of contractions. They not only see the pain as threatening but also associate it with a loss of control over their bodies and emotions. When a woman is facing labor, especially for the first time, she may worry about her ability to withstand pain and maintain control over herself.

The laboring woman's support system may also influence the course of labor and birth. For some women, the presence of the father and other significant persons, including the nurse, tends to have a positive effect. Other women may prefer not to have a support person or family member with them. Interestingly, Berry (1988) reported that fathers often felt they had not been able to provide the type of support they had imagined and voiced feelings of failure in their expected role during the labor and birth. In a study by Khazoyan and Anderson (1994), Latina women identified the need for the partner's presence at the bedside for communication and showing love. Communication needs included talking and "affectionate and understanding words" from their partner. Showing love was described as holding their hand, hugging, or touching. The partner's presence at the bedside was interpreted as a "loving" gesture.

How the woman views the birth experience in hindsight may have implications for mothering behaviors. Mercer (1995) and Walker and Montgomery (1994) found a significant relationship between the birth experience and mothering behaviors. It appears that any activities by the expectant woman or by health care providers that enhance the birth experience will be beneficial. The father's experience of childbirth and his opportunities for bonding may also have important implications for fathering (Henderson and Brouse 1991).

The Physiology of Labor

Possible Causes of Labor Onset

The process of labor usually begins between the 38th and the 42nd week of gestation, when the fetus is mature and ready for birth. While the exact cause of onset is not clearly understood, researchers do know that labor is precipitated by complex interactions of progesterone, estrogen, oxytocin, prostaglandins, fetal cortisol, and uterine distention. The relationship of some of these factors is presented in Figure 15–10.

Progesterone

Progesterone exerts a relaxant effect on the uterine smooth muscle by interfering with the conduction of

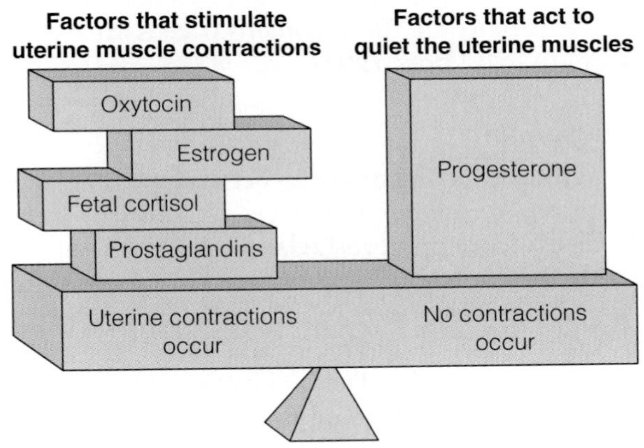

FIGURE 15–10 Factors affecting initiation of labor. The factors listed on the left have all been identified as providing stimulus to the beginning of labor. Progesterone exerts a relaxing effect, and a balance between all the factors keeps the uterus quiet, without contraction. When the relationship of factors changes, the balance is tipped and uterine labor begins.

impulses from one cell to the next. During pregnancy, progesterone exerts a quieting effect and the uterus generally is without contractions. The placenta produces progesterone, and, toward the end of gestation, biochemical changes decrease the availability of progesterone to myometrial cells (Blackburn and Loper 1992). With the decreased availability of progesterone, estrogen is better able to exert its effects.

Estrogen

Estrogen stimulates the smooth muscle of the uterus to contract. During pregnancy, the stimulating effects of estrogen are counterbalanced by the relaxing effects of progesterone. The balance between these two hormones keeps the uterine muscles from contracting in a regular pattern during pregnancy. At about 34–35 weeks' gestation, estrogen levels rise. Estrogen exerts an effect on the formation of gap junctions, which help propagate the contraction from one cell to the next; stimulates an increase in the sensitivity of the myometrium to oxytocin; and stimulates prostaglandin formation (Blackburn and Loper 1992). This leads first to increased irritability (a readiness to contract) of the uterine smooth muscle and then to promotion of actual contractions.

The stimulating effect is increased further because estrogen promotes the synthesis of prostaglandin in the decidua and the fetal membranes (amnion and chorion). Prostaglandins also stimulate the smooth muscle of the uterus (O'Brien and Cefalo 1996).

Oxytocin

Oxytocin is produced by the maternal posterior pituitary. One of the effects of oxytocin is to stimulate contractions of the smooth muscle of the uterus. The uterus becomes increasingly sensitive (responsive) to the effects of oxytocin as the pregnancy nears term (40 weeks). This increased responsiveness is due to a marked change in the sensitivity of the myometrial cells to oxytocin (Blackburn and Loper 1992).

Prostaglandin

Although the exact relationship between prostaglandins and the onset of labor is not yet established, there is growing evidence that prostaglandin involvement is significant. Prostaglandin is known to stimulate smooth muscle contractions. It may also stimulate the production and release of oxytocin and lower the uterine threshold to oxytocin. The production of prostaglandins increases just before labor begins (Challis 1994), most likely as a result of the interaction of such factors as increased estrogen and decreased progesterone, increased fetal cortisol (Nathanielsz 1994), and increased distention of the uterus, as noted earlier.

Fetal Cortisol

As the woman approaches term, the fetus produces more cortisol. Cortisol is thought to exert two effects. It (1) slows the production of progesterone by the placenta, and (2) stimulates the precursors to prostaglandins. These two effects decrease the relaxing effect of progesterone on the uterus and increase the stimulating effect of prostaglandins.

Uterine Distention

The uterus slowly increases in size during gestation, stretching its smooth muscle. Most smooth muscle contracts when stretched, but the uterine smooth muscle does not because of the effect of progesterone. As the woman approaches term, the decreased amount or effectiveness of progesterone increases uterine irritability and contractions. The irritability of the smooth muscle is enhanced by uterine distention, which stimulates the production of prostaglandins.

Myometrial Activity

In true labor, the uterus divides into two portions. This division is known as the *physiologic retraction ring*. The upper portion, which is the contractile segment, becomes progressively thicker as labor advances. The lower portion, which includes the lower uterine segment and cervix, is passive. As labor continues, the lower uterine segment expands and thins out.

With each contraction, the muscles of the upper uterine segment shorten and exert a longitudinal traction on the cervix, causing effacement. **Effacement** is the drawing up of the internal os and the cervical canal into the uterine side walls. The cervix changes progressively from a long, thick structure to a structure that is tissue-paper thin (Figure 15–11). In primigravidas, effacement usually precedes dilatation.

The uterus elongates with each contraction, decreasing the horizontal diameter. This elongation causes a straightening of the fetal body, pressing the upper portion against the fundus and thrusting the presenting part down toward the lower uterine segment and the cervix. The pressure exerted by the fetus is called the *fetal axis pressure*. As the uterus elongates, the longitudinal muscle fibers are pulled upward over the presenting part. This action and the hydrostatic pressure of the fetal membranes cause **cervical dilatation.** The cervical os and cervical canal widen from less than a centimeter to approximately 10 cm, allowing birth of the fetus. When the cervix is completely dilated and retracted up into the lower uterine segment, it can no longer be palpated.

The round ligament pulls the fundus forward, aligning the fetus with the bony pelvis.

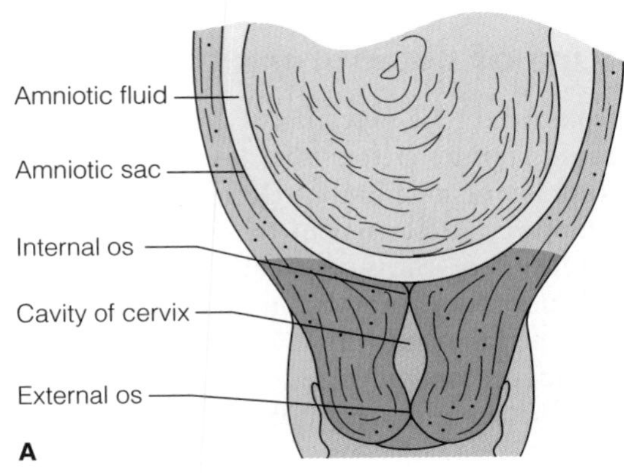

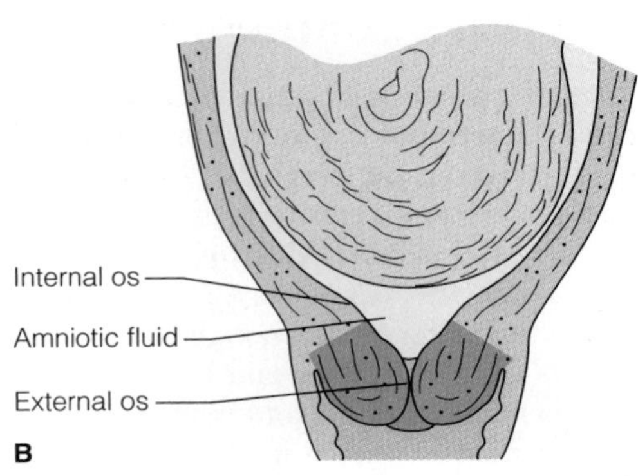

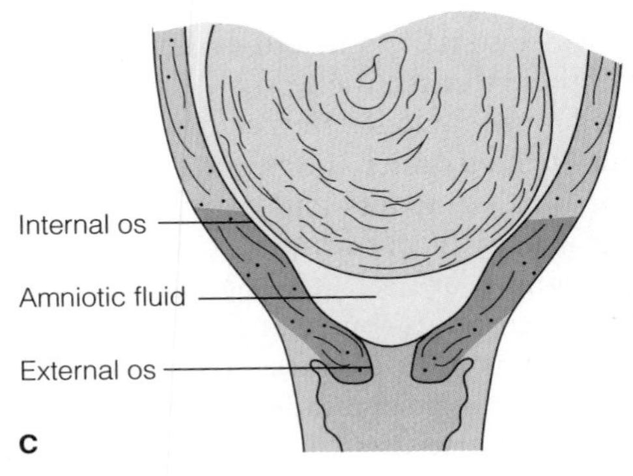

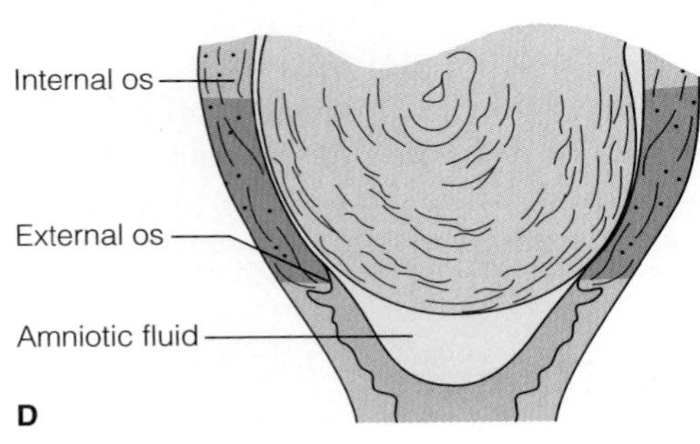

FIGURE 15–11 Effacement of the cervix in the primigravida. ***A*** Beginning of labor. There is no cervical effacement or dilatation. The fetal head is cushioned by amniotic fluid. ***B*** Beginning cervical effacement. As the cervix begins to efface, more amniotic fluid collects below the fetal head. ***C*** Cervix about one-half effaced and slightly dilated. The increasing amount of amniotic fluid exerts hydrostatic pressure. ***D*** Complete effacement and dilatation.

Intraabdominal Pressure

After the cervix is completely dilated, the maternal abdominal muscles contract as the woman pushes. This pushing aids in expulsion of the fetus and placenta. If the cervix is not completely dilated, however, bearing down can cause cervical edema (which retards dilatation), possible tearing and bruising of the cervix, and maternal exhaustion.

Musculature Changes in the Pelvic Floor

The levator ani muscle and fascia of the pelvic floor draw the rectum and vagina upward and forward with each contraction, along the curve of the pelvic floor. As the fetal head descends to the pelvic floor, the pressure of the presenting part causes the perineal structure, which was once 5 cm in thickness, to change to a structure of less than a centimeter. A normal physiologic anesthesia is produced as a result of the decreased blood supply to the area. The anus everts, exposing the interior rectal wall as the fetal head descends forward (Cunningham et al 1997).

Premonitory Signs of Labor

Most primigravidas and many multiparas experience the following signs and symptoms of impending labor.

Lightening

Lightening describes what happens when the fetus begins to settle into the pelvic inlet (engagement). With its descent, the uterus moves downward, and the fundus no longer presses on the diaphragm.

The woman can breathe more easily after lightening. With increased downward pressure of the presenting part, however, she may notice

- Leg cramps or pains due to pressure on the nerves that course through the obturator foramen in the pelvis
- Increased pelvic pressure
- Increased venous stasis leading to edema in the lower extremities
- Increased vaginal secretions resulting from congestion of the vaginal mucous membranes

Braxton Hicks Contractions

Before the onset of labor, Braxton Hicks contractions—the irregular, intermittent contractions that have been occurring throughout the pregnancy—may become uncomfortable. The pain seems to be in the abdomen and groin, but may feel like the "drawing" sensations experienced by some women with dysmenorrhea. When these contractions are strong enough for the woman to believe she is in labor, she is said to be in false labor. *False labor* is uncomfortable and may be exhausting as the woman wonders if "this is it." Since the contractions can be fairly regular, she has no way of knowing if they are the beginning of true labor. She may come to the hospital or birthing center for a vaginal examination to determine if cervical dilatation is occurring. Frequent episodes of false labor and trips back and forth to the certified nurse-midwife/physician's office or hospital may frustrate or embarrass the woman, who feels that she should know when she is really in labor. Reassurance by nursing staff can ease embarrassment.

Cervical Changes

Considerable change occurs in the cervix during the prenatal and intrapartal period. At the beginning of pregnancy the cervix is rigid and firm, and it must soften so that it can stretch and dilate to allow the fetus passage. This softening of the cervix is called *ripening.*

As term approaches, collagen fibers in the cervix are broken down by the action of enzymes such as collagenase and elastase. As the collagen fibers change, their ability to bind together decreases because of increasing amounts of hyaluronic acid, which loosely binds collagen fibrils, and decreasing amounts of dermatan sulfate, which tightly binds collagen fibrils. There is also an increase in the water content of the cervix. All these changes result in a weakening and softening of the cervix (Blackburn and Loper 1992, p 121).

Bloody Show

During pregnancy, cervical secretions accumulate in the cervical canal to form a mucous plug. With softening and effacement of the cervix, the mucous plug is often expelled, resulting in a small amount of blood loss from the exposed cervical capillaries. The resulting pink-tinged secretions are called **bloody show.** Bloody show is considered a sign of imminent labor, which usually begins within 24–48 hours. Vaginal examination that includes manipulation of the cervix may also result in a blood-tinged discharge, which is sometimes confused with bloody show.

Rupture of Membranes

In approximately 12 percent of women, the amniotic membranes rupture before the onset of labor. This is called **rupture of membranes (ROM).** After the membranes rupture, 80 percent of these women experience spontaneous labor within 24 hours. If membranes rupture and labor does not begin spontaneously within 12–24 hours, labor may be induced to avoid infection. Labor is induced only if the pregnancy is near term.

When the membranes rupture, the amniotic fluid may be expelled in large amounts. If engagement has not occurred, there is danger of the umbilical cord washing out with the fluid *(prolapsed cord).* In addition, the open pathway into the uterus causes danger of infection. Because of these threats, the woman is advised to notify her certified nurse-midwife/physician and proceed to the hospital or birthing center. In some instances, the fluid is expelled in small amounts and may be confused with episodes of urinary incontinence associated with urinary urgency, coughing, or sneezing. The discharge should be checked to ascertain its source and to determine further action. (See Chapter 16 for assessment techniques used to establish whether membranes are ruptured and for precautions the nurse uses to avoid exposure to amniotic fluid.)

Sudden Burst of Energy

Some women report a sudden burst of energy approximately 24–48 hours before labor. The cause of the energy spurt is unknown. In prenatal teaching the nurse should warn prospective mothers not to overexert themselves during this energy burst to avoid being excessively tired when labor begins.

Other Signs

Other premonitory signs include

- Weight loss of 1–3 lb resulting from fluid loss and electrolyte shifts produced by changes in estrogen and progesterone levels
- Increased backache and sacroiliac pressure from the influence of relaxin hormone on the pelvic joints
- Diarrhea, indigestion, or nausea and vomiting just before onset of labor

The causes of these signs are unknown.

Differences Between True and False Labor

The contractions of true labor produce progressive dilatation and effacement of the cervix. They occur regularly and increase in frequency, duration, and intensity.

The discomfort of true labor contractions usually starts in the back and radiates around to the abdomen. The pain is not relieved by ambulation (in fact, walking may intensify the pain).

The contractions of false labor do not produce progressive cervical effacement and dilatation. Classically, they are irregular and do not increase in frequency, duration, and intensity. The contractions may be perceived as a hardening or "balling up" without discomfort, or discomfort may occur mainly in the lower abdomen and groin. The discomfort may be relieved by ambulation. The woman will find it helpful to know the characteristics of true labor contractions as well as the premonitory signs of ensuing labor. However, many times the only way to differentiate accurately between true and false labor is to assess dilatation. The woman must feel free to come in for accurate assessment of labor and should never be allowed to feel foolish if the labor is false. The nurse must reassure the woman that false labor is common and that it often cannot be distinguished from true labor except by vaginal examination. (See Key Facts to Remember: Comparison of True and False Labor.)

KEY FACTS TO REMEMBER

Comparison of True and False Labor

True Labor	False Labor
Contractions are at regular intervals.	Contractions are irregular.
Intervals between contractions gradually shorten.	Usually no change.
Contractions increase in duration and intensity.	Usually no change.
Discomfort begins in back and radiates around to abdomen.	Discomfort is usually in abdomen.
Intensity usually increases with walking.	Walking has no or effect or lessens contractions.
Cervical dilatation and effacement are progressive.	No change.

Stages of Labor and Birth

There are three stages of labor. The *first stage* begins with the beginning of true labor and ends when the cervix is completely dilated at 10 cm. The *second stage* begins with complete dilatation and ends with the birth of the newborn. The *third stage* begins with the birth of the newborn and ends with the delivery of the placenta.

Some clinicians identify a *fourth stage.* During this stage, which lasts 1–4 hours after delivery of the placenta, the uterus effectively contracts to control bleeding at the placental site (Cunningham et al 1997). The care of the laboring woman is discussed in Chapter 17.

First Stage

The first stage of labor is divided into the latent, active, and transition phases. Each phase of labor is characterized by physical and psychologic changes.

Latent Phase

The *latent phase* begins with the onset of regular contractions. As the cervix begins to dilate, it also effaces, although little or no fetal descent is evident. For a woman in her first labor (nullipara), the latent phase averages 8.6 hours but should not exceed 20 hours. The latent phase in multiparas averages 5.3 hours but should not exceed 14 hours.

Uterine contractions become established during the latent phase and increase in frequency, duration, and intensity. They may start as mild contractions lasting 15–20 seconds with a frequency of 10–20 minutes and progress to moderate ones lasting 30–40 seconds with a frequency of 5–7 minutes. They average 40 mm Hg during acme from a baseline tonus of 10 mm Hg (Varney 1987).

In the early or latent phase of the first stage of labor, contractions are usually mild. The woman feels able to cope with the discomfort. She may be relieved that labor has finally started. Although she may be anxious, she is able to recognize and express those feelings of anxiety. The woman is often talkative and smiling and is eager to talk about herself and answer questions. Excitement is high, and her partner or other support person is often as elated as she is.

At the beginning of labor, the amniotic membranes bulge through the cervix in the shape of a cone. Spontaneous rupture of membranes (SROM) generally occurs at the height of an intense contraction with a gush of fluid out of the vagina. In many instances, the membranes are ruptured by the certified nurse-midwife/physician. This is called *amniotomy,* or *artificial rupture of membranes (AROM).*

Active Phase

During the *active phase,* the cervix dilates from about 3–4 cm to 8 cm. Fetal descent is progressive. The cervical dilatation should be at least 1.2 cm/hr in nulliparas, and 1.5 cm/hr in multiparas (Cunningham et al 1997).

Transition Phase

The *transition phase* is the last part of the first stage. Cervical dilatation slows as it progresses from 8 to 10 cm and the rate of fetal descent increases. The average rate of descent is at least 1 cm/hr in nulliparas and 2 cm/hr in multiparas. The transition phase should not be longer than 3 hours for nulliparas and 1 hour for multiparas (Cunningham et al 1997).

During the active and transition phases, contractions become more frequent and longer in duration, and increase in intensity. At the beginning of the active phase, contractions have a frequency of 2–3 minutes, a duration of 60 seconds, and strong intensity. During transition, contractions have a frequency of about every 2 minutes, a duration of 60–75 seconds, and strong intensity (Varney 1987).

When the woman enters the early active phase, her anxiety tends to increase as she senses the fairly constant intensification of contractions and pain. She begins to fear a loss of control and may use coping mechanisms to maintain control. Some women exhibit decreased ability to cope and a sense of helplessness. Women who have support persons and family available may experience greater satisfaction and less anxiety than those without support (Tomlinson and Bryan 1996).

When the woman enters the transition phase, she may demonstrate significant anxiety. She becomes acutely aware of the increasing force and intensity of the contractions. She may become restless, frequently changing position. She may fear being left alone, and it is crucial that the nurse be available as backup and relief for the support person. By the time the woman enters the transition phase, she is inner-directed and often tired. At the same time, the support person may be feeling the need for a break. The nurse should reassure the woman that she will not be left alone and should keep her informed about where her support people are and how to reach the nurse.

The woman may also fear that she will be "torn open" or "split apart" by the force of the contractions. Many clients experience a sensation of pressure so great with the peak of a contraction that it seems to them that their abdomens will burst open with the force. The nurse should inform the woman that this is a normal sensation and reassure her that such bursting will not happen. During transition the woman generally withdraws. She may increasingly doubt her ability to cope with labor and may become apprehensive and irritable. She may be terrified of being left alone, though she does not want anyone to talk to or touch her. However, with the next contraction she may ask for verbal and physical support. Other characteristics of this phase may include

- Hyperventilation, as the woman increases her breathing rate
- Restlessness
- Difficulty understanding directions
- A sense of bewilderment and anger at the contractions
- Statements that she "can't take it anymore"
- Requests for medication
- Hiccupping, belching, nausea, or vomiting
- Beads of perspiration on the upper lip
- Increasing rectal pressure

The woman in this phase is anxious to "get it over with." She may be amnesic and sleep between her now-frequent contractions. Her support persons may start to feel helpless and may turn to the nurse for increased participation as their efforts to alleviate her discomfort seem less effective.

As dilatation approaches 10 cm, there may be increased rectal pressure and uncontrollable desire to bear down, increased amount of bloody show, and rupture of membranes.

Second Stage

The second stage of labor is traditionally defined as beginning with complete cervical dilatation and ends with birth of the infant. Traditional thought suggests that the second stage should be completed within 2 hours after the cervix becomes fully dilated for primigravidas; multiparas average 15 minutes. Contractions continue with a frequency of about every 2 minutes, a duration of 60–75 seconds, and strong intensity (Varney 1987). Descent of the fetal presenting part continues until it reaches the perineal floor.

As the fetal head descends, the woman usually has the urge to push because of pressure of the fetal head on the sacral and obturator nerves. As she pushes, intraabdominal pressure is exerted from contraction of the maternal abdominal muscles. As the fetal head continues its descent, the perineum begins to bulge, flatten, and move anteriorly. The amount of bloody show may increase. The labia begin to part with each contraction. Between contractions the fetal head appears to recede. With succeeding contractions and maternal pushing effort, the fetal head descends farther. **Crowning** occurs when the fetal head is encircled by the external opening of the vagina (introitus), and it means birth is imminent.

A childbirth-prepared woman may feel some relief that the acute pain she felt during the transition phase is over (see Key Facts to Remember: Characteristics of Labor). She may also be relieved that the birth is near and she can push. Some women feel a sense of control now that they can be actively involved (Roberts and Woolley 1996). Others, particularly those without childbirth preparation, may become frightened. They may tend to fight each contraction and any attempt to encourage them to push with contractions. Such behavior may be frightening and disconcerting to the woman's support persons. The woman may feel she has lost control and become embarrassed and apologetic, or she may dem-

KEY FACTS TO REMEMBER

Characteristics of Labor

	First Stage			Second Stage
	Latent Phase	Active Phase	Transition Phase	
Nullipara	8.5 hours average (1–20 hours)	6 hours	2 hours	1–2 hours
Multipara	5 hours average	4.5 hours	1–1.5 hours	A few minutes to 1 hour
Cervical dilatation	0 to 3–4 cm	4–8 cm	8–10 cm	
Contractions				
Frequency	Every 10–20 minutes at the beginning, progressing to every 5–7 minutes	Every 2–3 minutes	Every 2 minutes	Every 2 minutes
Duration	15–20 second progressing to 30–40 seconds	40–60 seconds	60–75 seconds	60–75 seconds
Intensity	Begin as mild and progress to moderate	Begin as moderate and progress to strong	Strong	Strong

onstrate extreme irritability toward the staff or her supporters in an attempt to regain control over external forces against which she feels helpless. Some women feel acute, increasingly severe pain and a burning sensation as the perineum distends.

Spontaneous Birth (Vertex Presentation)

As the head distends the vulva with each contraction, the perineum becomes extremely thin and the anus stretches and protrudes. As extension occurs under the symphysis pubis, the head is born. When the anterior shoulder meets the underside of the symphysis pubis, a gentle push by the mother aids in birth of the shoulders. The body then follows.

Birth of a fetus in other than a vertex presentation is discussed in Chapter 9.

Cardinal Movements of the Fetus

For the fetus to pass through the birth canal, the fetal head and body must adjust to the passage by certain positional changes. These changes, called **cardinal movements** or *mechanisms of labor*, are described in the order in which they occur (Figure 15–12).

Descent Descent is thought to occur because of four forces: (a) pressure of the amniotic fluid, (b) direct pressure of the fundus on the breech, (c) contraction of the abdominal muscles, and (d) extension and straightening of the fetal body. The head enters the inlet in the occiput transverse or oblique position because the pelvic inlet is widest from side to side. The sagittal suture is an equal distance from the maternal symphysis pubis and sacral promontory.

Flexion Flexion occurs as the fetal head descends and meets resistance from the soft tissues of the pelvis, the muscles of the pelvic floor, and the cervix.

Internal Rotation The fetal head must rotate to fit the diameter of the pelvic cavity, which is widest in the anteroposterior diameter. As the occiput of the fetal head meets resistance from the levator ani muscles and their fascia, the occiput rotates—usually from left to right—and the sagittal suture aligns in the anteroposterior pelvic diameter.

Extension The resistance of the pelvic floor and the mechanical movement of the vulva opening anteriorly and forward assist with extension of the fetal head as it passes under the symphysis pubis. With this positional change, the occiput, then brow and face, emerge from the vagina.

Restitution The shoulders of the fetus enter the pelvis obliquely and remain oblique when the head rotates to the anteroposterior diameter through internal rotation. Because of this rotation, the neck becomes twisted. Once the head is born and is free of pelvic resistance, the neck untwists, turning the head to one side (restitution), and aligns with the position of the back in the birth canal.

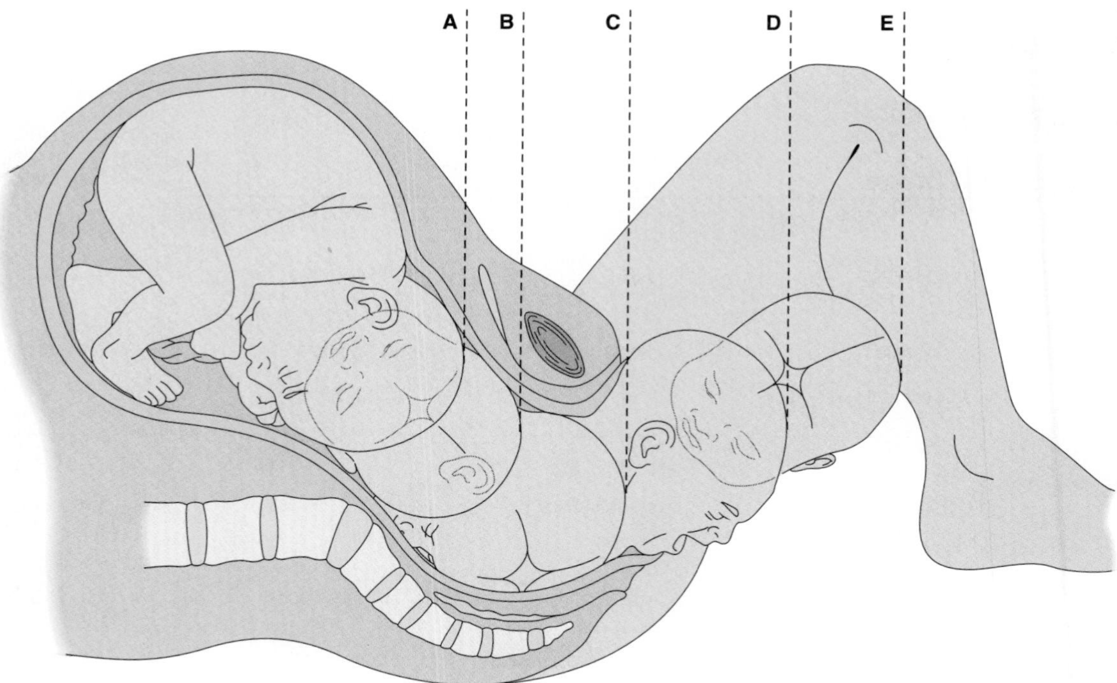

FIGURE 15–12 Mechanisms of labor. ***A, B*** Descent. ***C*** Internal rotation. ***D*** Extension. ***E*** External rotation.

External Rotation As the shoulders rotate to the anteroposterior position in the pelvis, the head turns farther to one side (external rotation).

Expulsion After the external rotation, and through the pushing efforts of the laboring woman, the anterior shoulder meets the undersurface of the symphysis pubis and slips under it. As lateral flexion of the shoulder and head occurs, the anterior shoulder is born before the posterior shoulder. The body follows quickly.

Third Stage

Placental Separation

After the infant is born, the uterus contracts firmly, diminishing its capacity and the surface area of placental attachment. The placenta begins to separate because of this decrease in surface area. As this separation occurs, bleeding results in the formation of a hematoma between the placental tissue and the remaining decidua. This hematoma accelerates the separation process. The membranes are the last to separate. They are peeled off the uterine wall as the placenta descends into the vagina. Signs of placental separation usually appear about 5 minutes after the birth of the newborn. These signs are (a) a globular-shaped uterus, (b) a rise of the fundus in the abdomen, (c) a sudden gush or trickle of blood, and (d) further protrusion of the umbilical cord out of the vagina.

Placental Delivery When the signs of placental separation appear, the woman may bear down to aid in placental expulsion. If this fails and the certified nurse-midwife/physician has ascertained that the fundus is firm, gentle traction may be applied to the cord while pressure is exerted on the fundus. The weight of the placenta as it is guided into the placental collection pan aids in the removal of the membranes from the uterine wall. A placenta is considered to be *retained* if 30 minutes have elapsed from completion of the second stage of labor.

If the placenta separates from the inside to the outer margins, it is delivered with the fetal (shiny) side presenting (Figure 15–13). This is known as the *Schultze mechanism* of placental delivery or, more commonly, *shiny Schultze.* If the placenta separates from the outer margins inward, it will roll up and present sideways with the maternal surface delivering first. This is known as the *Duncan mechanism* of placental delivery and is commonly called *dirty Duncan* because the placental surface is rough.

Nursing and medical interventions during the third stage of labor are discussed in detail in Chapter 17.

Fourth Stage

The fourth stage of labor is the time from 1 to 4 hours after birth, in which physiologic readjustment of the mother's body begins. With the birth, hemodynamic

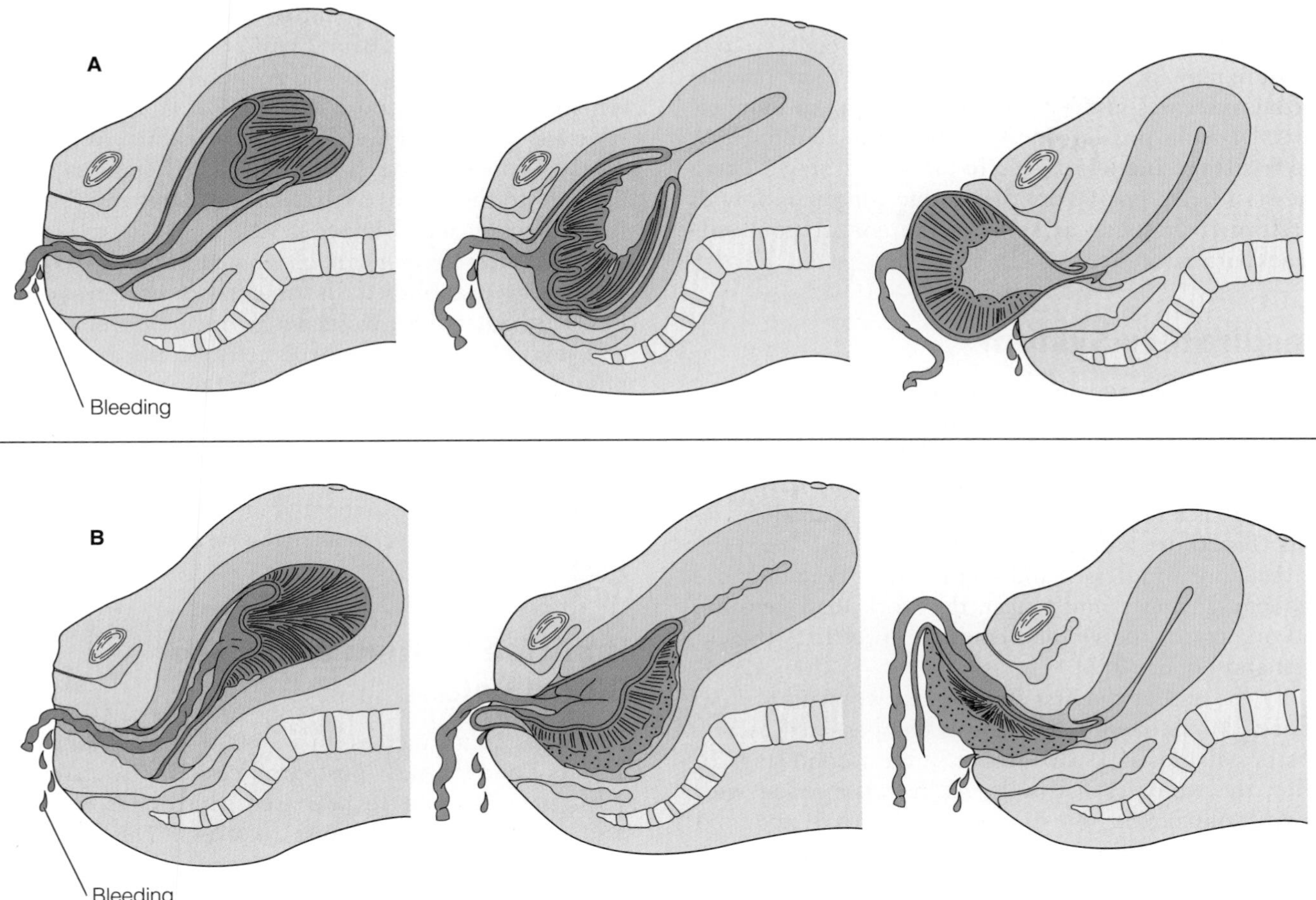

FIGURE 15–13 Placental separation and expulsion. ***A*** Schultze mechanism. ***B*** Duncan mechanism.

changes occur. Blood loss at birth ranges from 250 to 500 mL. With this blood loss and removal of the weight of the pregnant uterus from the surrounding vessels, blood is redistributed into venous beds. This results in a moderate drop in both systolic and diastolic blood pressure, increased pulse pressure, and moderate tachycardia (Albright et al 1986).

The uterus remains contracted in the midline of the abdomen. The fundus is usually midway between the symphysis pubis and umbilicus. Its contracted state constricts the vessels at the site of placental implantation. Immediately after birth of the placenta, the cervix is widely spread and thick.

Nausea and vomiting usually cease. The woman may be thirsty and hungry. She may experience a shaking chill, which is thought to be associated with the ending of the physical exertion of labor. The bladder is often hypotonic due to trauma during the second stage and/or the administration of anesthetics that may decrease sensations. Hypotonic bladder leads to urinary retention. Nursing care of this stage is discussed in Chapter 17.

Maternal Systemic Response to Labor

Cardiovascular System

The woman's cardiovascular system is stressed both by the uterine contractions and by the pain, anxiety, and apprehension she experiences. During labor there is a significant increase in cardiac output. With each contraction, 300–500 mL of blood volume is forced back into the maternal circulation, which results in an increase in cardiac output of as much as a 31 percent. Further increases in cardiac output occur as the laboring woman experiences pain with uterine contractions and her anxiety and apprehension increase.

Maternal position also affects cardiac output. In the supine position, cardiac output lowers, heart rate increases, and stroke volume decreases. When the woman turns to a lateral (side-lying) position, cardiac output increases by about 22 percent, the pulse rate decreases by about 6 beats per minute, and stroke volume increases by 27 percent (Blackburn and Loper 1992).

Blood pressure (both systolic and diastolic) increases during uterine contractions. In the first stage, systolic pressure may increase by 35 mm Hg, and there may be further increases in the second stage during pushing efforts. Diastolic pressure increases by about 25 mm Hg in the first stage and 65 mm Hg in the second stage. These increases begin just before the uterine contraction, with a return to baseline as soon as the contraction ends (Blackburn and Loper 1992).

Respiratory System

Oxygen demand and consumption increase at the onset of labor because of the presence of uterine contractions. As anxiety and pain from uterine contractions increase, hyperventilation frequently occurs. With hyperventilation there is a fall in $PaCO_2$ and respiratory alkalosis results (Blackburn and Loper 1992).

As labor progresses and contractions become more frequent, stronger, and longer, the work load, tension, and anxiety of the woman continue to change (Blackburn and Loper 1992).

By the end of the first stage, most women have developed a mild metabolic acidosis compensated by respiratory alkalosis. As she pushes in the second stage of labor, the woman's $PaCO_2$ levels may rise along with blood lactate levels (due to muscular activity), and mild respiratory acidosis occurs. By the time the baby is born (end of second stage), there is metabolic acidosis uncompensated by respiratory alkalosis (Blackburn and Loper 1992).

The changes in acid-base status that occur in labor are quickly reversed in the fourth stage because of changes in the woman's respiratory rate. Acid-base levels return to pregnancy levels by 24 hours after birth, and nonpregnant values are attained a few weeks after birth (Blackburn and Loper 1992, p 269).

Renal System

During labor there is an increase in maternal renin, plasma renin activity, and angiotensinogen. This elevation is thought to be important in the control of uteroplacental blood flow during birth and the early postpartal period (Blackburn and Loper 1992, p 345).

Structurally, the base of the bladder is pushed forward and upward when engagement occurs. The pressure from the presenting part may impair blood and lymph drainage from the base of the bladder, leading to edema (Cunningham et al 1997).

Gastrointestinal System

During labor, gastric motility and absorption of solid food are reduced. Gastric emptying time is prolonged and gastric volume (amount of contents that remain in the stomach) remains over 25 mL, regardless of the time the last meal was taken. The acidity of the gastric contents increases, and more than half of laboring women have a gastric pH of less than 2.5 (Blackburn and Loper 1992). Some narcotics also delay gastric emptying time and add to the risk of aspiration if general anesthesia is used (Blackburn and Loper 1992).

The fluid requirements of women in labor have not been clearly established. In some instances, intravenous fluids are ordered for women who are experiencing normal labor, either because the certified nurse-midwife/physician believes that intravenous fluids are needed, or so that an intravenous line will be available in case problems develop. When hypertonic glucose infusions are used, there is an increase in maternal blood glucose; this can lead to fetal hyperglycemia and hyperinsulinemia and to hypoglycemia in the newborn (Blackburn and Loper 1992).

Immune System and Other Blood Values

The WBC count increases to 25,000–30,000/mm during labor and the early postpartal period. The change in WBC is mostly due to increased neutrophils resulting from a physiologic response to stress. The increased WBC count makes it difficult to identify the presence of an infectious process.

Maternal blood glucose levels decrease because glucose is used as an energy source during uterine contractions. The decreased blood glucose levels lead to a decrease in insulin requirements (Blackburn and Loper 1992).

Pain

Theories of Pain

According to the *gate-control theory,* pain results from activity in several interacting specialized neural systems. The gate-control theory proposes that a mechanism in the dorsal horn of the spinal column serves as a valve or gate that increases or decreases the flow of nerve impulses from the periphery to the central nervous system (CNS). The gate mechanism is influenced by the size of the transmitting fibers and by the nerve impulses that descend from the brain. Psychologic processes such as past experiences, attention, and emotion may influence pain perception and response by activating the gate mechanism. The gates may be opened or closed by CNS activities, such as anxiety or excitement, or selective localized activity.

The gate-control theory has two important implications for care of the laboring woman. Pain may be controlled by tactile stimulation and can be modified by activities controlled by the central nervous system. These

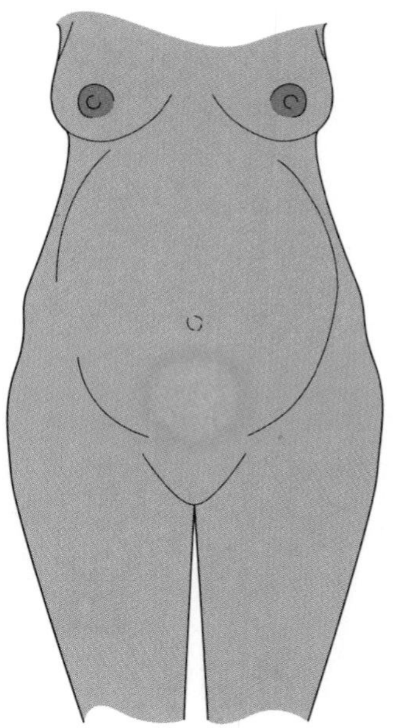
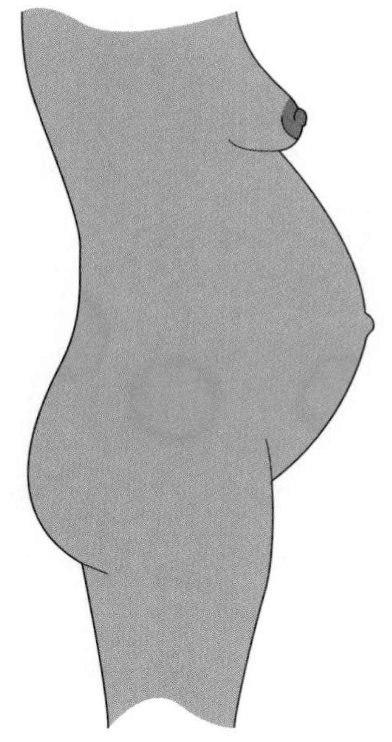
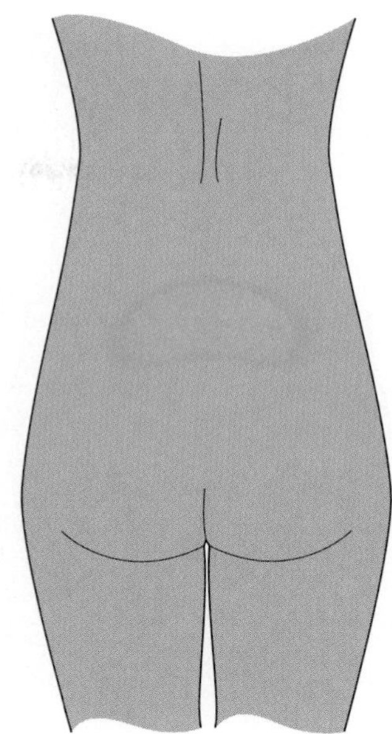

FIGURE 15–14 Area of reference of labor pain during the first stage. Pain is the most intense in the darker colored areas.
Source: Bonica JJ: *Principles and Practice of Obstetric Analgesia and Anesthesia.* Philadelphia: Davis, 1972, p 108.

include back rub, sacral pressure, effleurage, suggestion, distraction, and conditioning.

Causes of Pain During Labor

The pain associated with the first stage of labor is unique, in that it accompanies a normal physiologic process. Even though perception of the pain of childbirth varies among women, there is a physiologic basis for discomfort during labor. Pain during the first stage of labor arises from (a) dilatation of the cervix, which is the primary source of pain; (b) hypoxia of the uterine muscle cells during contraction; (c) stretching of the lower uterine segment; and (d) pressure on adjacent structures. The areas of pain include the lower abdominal wall and the areas over the lower lumbar region and the upper sacrum (Figure 15–14).

During the second stage of labor, discomfort is due to (a) hypoxia of the contracting uterine muscle cells, (b) distention of the vagina and perineum, and (c) pressure on adjacent structures. The area of pain increases as shown in Figures 15–15 and 15–16.

Pain during the third stage results from uterine contractions and cervical dilatation as the placenta is expelled. This stage of labor is short, and after it anesthesia is needed primarily for episiotomy repair.

Factors Affecting Response to Pain

Preparation for childbirth has been shown to reduce the need for analgesia during labor. Lowe (1996) reported that women who demonstrated greater knowledge of childbirth and indicated higher confidence after completing the classes reported a less painful childbirth.

Individuals tend to respond to painful stimuli in the way that is acceptable in their culture. In some cultures, it is natural to communicate pain, no matter how mild, while members of other cultures stoically accept pain out of fear or because it is expected (Weber 1996).

Another factor that may influence response to pain is *fatigue and sleep deprivation.* The fatigued woman has less energy and ability to use such strategies as distraction or imagination to deal with pain. As a result, she may lose her ability to cope with labor and choose analgesics or other medications to relieve the discomfort.

The woman's *previous experience* with pain also affects her ability to manage current and future pain. Those who have had experience with pain seem more sensitive to painful stimuli than those who have not.

Anxiety can affect a woman's response to pain. Unfamiliar surroundings and events can increase anxiety, as does separation from family and loved ones. Anticipation of discomfort and questions about whether she can cope with the contractions may also increase anxiety.

Both attention and distraction have an influence on the perception of pain. When pain sensation is the focus of attention, the perceived intensity is greater. A sensory stimulus such as a back rub can be a distraction that focuses the woman's attention on the stimulus rather than the pain.

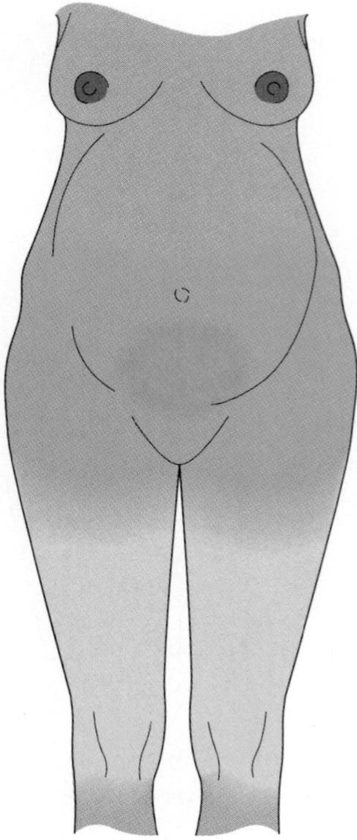

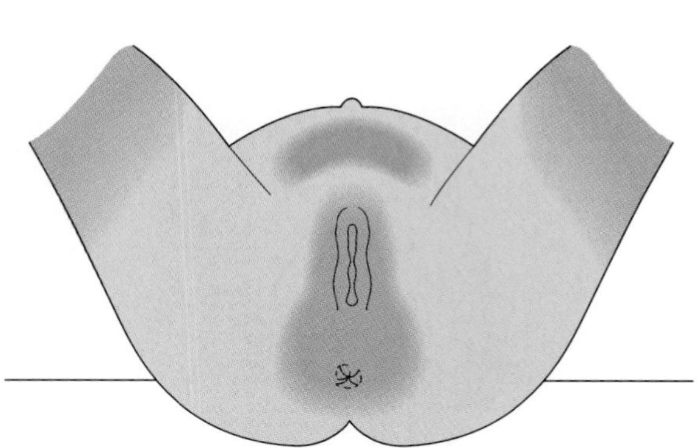

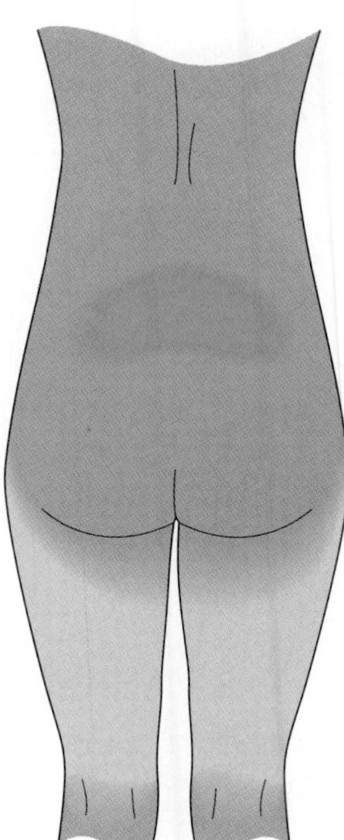

FIGURE 15–15 Distribution of labor pain during the later phase of the first stage and early phase of the second stage. The darkest colored areas indicate the location of the most intense pain; moderate color, moderate pain; and lighter color, mild pain. The uterine contractions, which at this stage are very strong, produce intense pain.

Source: Bonica JJ: *Principles and Practice of Obstetric Analgesia and Anesthesia.* Philadelphia: Davis, 1972, p 109.

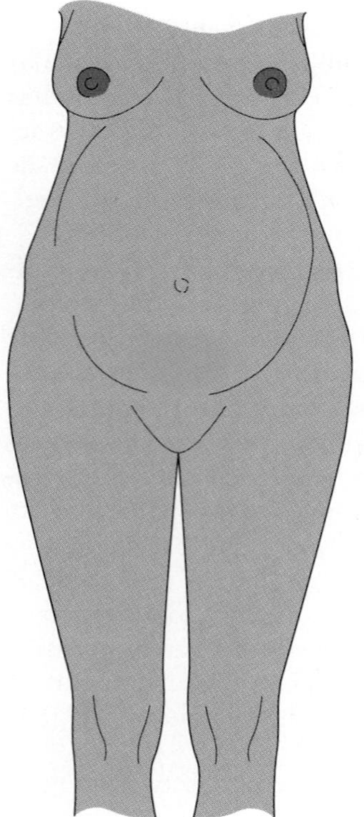

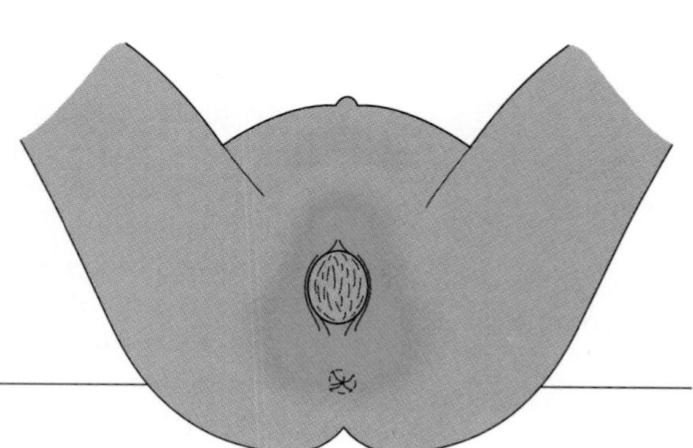

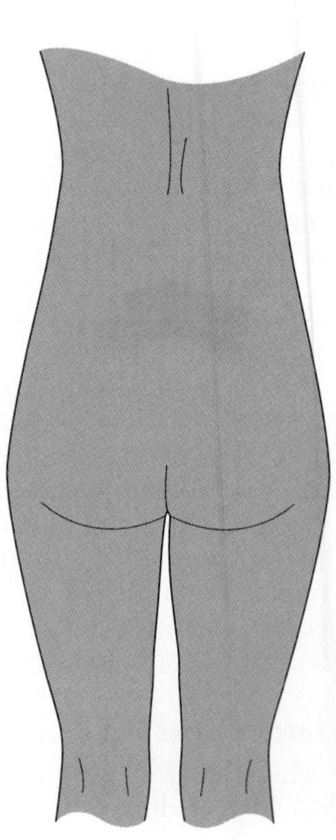

FIGURE 15–16 Distribution of labor pain during the later phase of the second stage and actual birth. The perineal component is the primary cause of discomfort. Uterine contractions contribute much less.

Source: Bonica JJ: *Principles and Practice of Obstetric Analgesia and Anesthesia.* Philadelphia: Davis, 1972, p 109.

Fetal Response to Labor

When the fetus is normal, the mechanical and hemodynamic changes of normal labor have no adverse effects.

Heart Rate Changes

Fetal heart rate decelerations can occur with intracranial pressures of 40–55 mm Hg. The currently accepted explanation of this early deceleration is hypoxic depression of the central nervous system, which is under vagal control. The absence of these head-compression decelerations (early decelerations) in some fetuses during labor is explained by the existence of a threshold that is reached more gradually in the presence of intact membranes and lack of maternal resistance.

Hemodynamic Changes

The adequate exchange of nutrients and gases in the fetal capillaries and intervillous spaces depends in part on the fetal blood pressure. Fetal blood pressure is a protective mechanism for the normal fetus during the anoxic periods caused by the contracting uterus during labor. The fetal and placental reserve is enough to see the fetus through these anoxic periods unharmed (Creasy and Resnik 1994).

CHAPTER HIGHLIGHTS

- Four factors that continuously interact during the process of labor and birth are the birth passage, the fetus, the uterine contractions and pushing efforts of the laboring woman (the forces of labor), and the emotional components the woman brings to the birth setting (psychosocial considerations).
- Important parts of the maternal pelvis include the pelvic inlet, pelvic cavity, and pelvic outlet.
- The fetal head contains bones that are not fused. This allows for some overlapping and molding to facilitate birth.
- Fetal *attitude* refers to the relation of the fetal parts to one another.
- Fetal *lie* refers to the relationship of the cephalocaudal axis of the fetus to the maternal spine. The fetal lie is either longitudinal or transverse.
- Fetal *presentation* is determined by the body part lying closest to the maternal pelvis. Fetal presentation can be cephalic, breech, or shoulder.
- Fetal *position* is the relationship of the landmark on the presenting fetal part to the front, sides, or back of the maternal pelvis.
- Engagement of the presenting part takes place when the largest diameter of the presenting part reaches or passes through the pelvic inlet.
- Station refers to the relationship of the presenting part to an imaginary line drawn between the ischial spines of the maternal pelvis.
- Each uterine contraction has an increment, acme, and decrement. Contraction frequency is the time from the beginning of one contraction to the beginning of the next contraction.
- Contraction duration is the time from the beginning to the end of one contraction.
- Contraction intensity is the strength of the contraction during acme. Intensity is termed mild, moderate, or strong.
- Factors that affect the woman's response to labor pain include education, cultural beliefs, fatigue and sleep deprivation, personal significance of pain, previous experience, anxiety, and the availability of coping techniques.
- Possible causes of labor include oxytocin stimulation, progesterone withdrawal, estrogen stimulation, fetal cortisol, uterine distention, and prostaglandin theory.
- Premonitory signs of labor include lightening, Braxton Hicks contractions, cervical softening and effacement, bloody show, sudden burst of energy, weight loss, and (sometimes) rupture of membranes.
- True labor contractions occur regularly with an increase in frequency, duration, and intensity. The contractions usually start in the back and radiate around the abdomen. The discomfort is not relieved by ambulation. False labor contractions do not produce progressive cervical effacement and dilatation. They are irregular and do not increase in intensity. The discomfort may be relieved by ambulation.
- There are four stages of labor and birth: first stage is from beginning of true labor to complete dilatation of the cervix; second stage is from complete dilatation of the cervix to birth; third stage is from birth to expulsion of the placenta; fourth stage is from expulsion of the placenta to a period of 1 to 4 hours after.
- Placental separation is indicated by lengthening of the umbilical cord, a small spurt of blood, change in uterine shape, and a rise of the fundus in the abdomen.
- The placenta is delivered by Schultze or Duncan mechanism. This is determined by the way it separates from the uterine wall.
- The fetus accommodates itself to the maternal pelvis in a series of movements called the cardinal movements of labor, which include descent, flexion,

internal rotation, extension, external rotation, expulsion, and restitution.

- Maternal systemic responses to labor involve the cardiovascular, respiratory, renal, gastrointestinal, and immune systems.
- The fetus is usually able to tolerate the labor process with no untoward changes.

REFERENCES

Albright GA et al: *Anesthesia in Obstetrics: Maternal, Fetal and Neonatal Aspects,* 2nd ed. Boston: Butterworth, 1986.

Berry LM: Realistic expectations of the labor coach. *JOGNN* 1988; 18:354.

Blackburn ST, Loper DL: *Maternal, Fetal and Neonatal Physiology.* Philadelphia: Saunders, 1992.

Caldwell WE, Moloy HC: Anatomical variations in the female pelvis and their effect on labor with a suggested classification. *Am J Obstet Gynecol* 1933; 26:479.

Challis JRG: Characteristics of parturition. In: *Maternal-Fetal Medicine,* 3rd ed. Creasy RK, Resnik RR (editors). Philadelphia: Saunders, 1994.

Creasy RK, Resnik R: *Maternal-Fetal Medicine,* 3rd ed. Philadelphia: Saunders, 1994.

Crowe K, Baeyer C: Predictors of a positive childbirth experience. *Birth* June 1989; 16:2.

Cunningham FG et al: *Williams Obstetrics,* 20th ed. Stamford, CT: Appleton & Lange, 1997.

DiMatteo, Kahn K, Berry SH: Narratives of birth and the postpartum: Analysis of the focus group responses of new mothers. *Birth* December 1993; 20(4):204.

Doering SG et al: Modeling the quality of women's birth experience. *J Health Social Behavior* March 1980; 21:12.

Henderson AD, Brouse AJ: The experience of new fathers during the first three weeks of life. *J Adv Nurs* 1991; 16:293.

Khazoyan CM, Anderson NLR: Latinas' expectations for their partners during childbirth. *MCN* July/Aug 1994; 19(4):226.

Lederman RP: *Psychosocial Adaptation in Pregnancy: Assessment of Seven Dimensions of Maternal Development,* 2nd ed. New York: Springer, 1996.

Lowe NK: The pain and discomfort of labor and birth. *JOGNN* January 1996; 25:82.

McKay S, Smith SY: "What are they talking about? Is something wrong?" Information sharing during the second stage of labor. *Birth* September 1993; 20(3):142.

Mercer RT: *Becoming a Mother.* New York: Springer, 1995.

Murray M: *Antepartal and Intrapartal Fetal Monitoring.* Washington, DC: NAACOG, 1989.

Nathanielsz PW: A time to be born: Implications of animal studies in maternal-fetal medicine. *Birth* September 1994; 21(3):163.

Nichols MR: Paternal perspectives of the childbirth experience. *MCN* 1993; 21(3):99.

O'Brien WF, Cefalo RC: Labor and delivery. In: *Obstetrics: Normal and Problem Pregnancies*, 3rd ed. Gabbe SG, Niebyl JR, Simpson JL (editors). New York: Churchill Livingstone, 1996.

Oxorn H: *Human Labor and Birth,* 5th ed. New York: Appleton-Century-Crofts, 1986.

Roberts J, Woolley D: A second look at the second stage of labor. *JOGNN* June 1996; 25:415.

Tomlinson PS, Bryan AA: Family centered intrapartum care: Revisiting an old concept. *JOGNN* May 1996; 25:331.

Varney H: *Nurse-Midwifery,* 2nd ed. Boston: Blackwell, 1987.

Walker LO, Montgomery E: Maternal identity and role attainment: Long-term relations to children's development. *Nurs Res* March/April 1994; 43(2):105.

Weber SE: Cultural aspects of pain in childbearing women. *JOGNN* January 1996; 25:67.

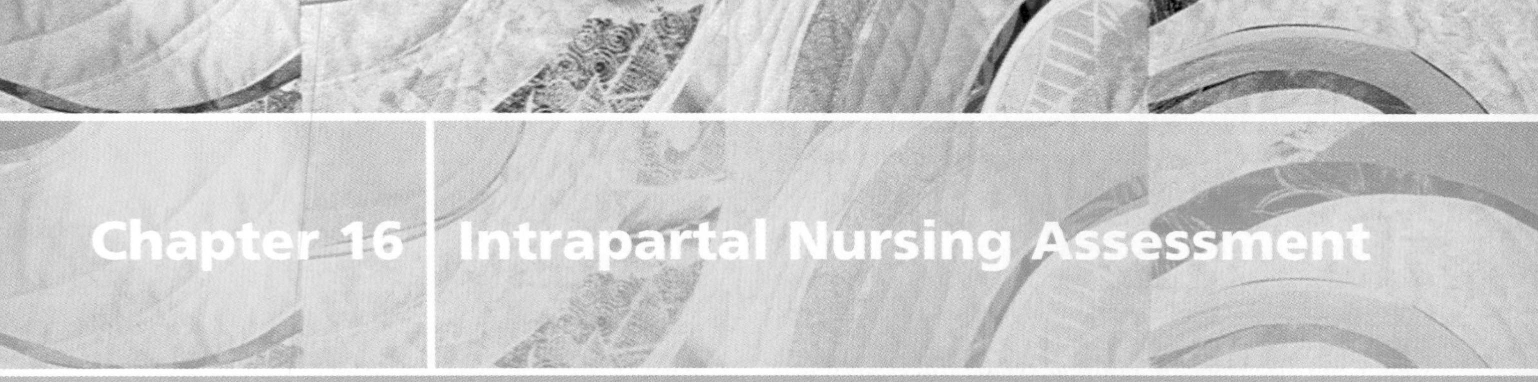

Chapter 16 Intrapartal Nursing Assessment

OBJECTIVES

- Discuss intrapartal assessment of maternal physical and psychosociocultural factors.
- Summarize methods used to evaluate the progress of labor.
- Describe the procedure for performing Leopold's maneuvers and the information that can be obtained.
- Differentiate between baseline and periodic changes in fetal monitoring, and describe the appearance and significance of each.
- Outline steps to be performed in the systematic evaluation of fetal heart rate tracings.
- Identify nonreassuring fetal heart rate patterns and nursing interventions that should be carried out in the management of fetal distress.
- Delineate the indications for fetal blood sampling, and state related pH values.
- Discuss psychologic reactions to electronic fetal monitoring.

KEY TERMS

Accelerations
Baseline rate
Baseline variability
Decelerations
Early deceleration
Fetal blood sampling
Fetal bradycardia
Fetal tachycardia
Late deceleration
Leopold's maneuvers
Sinusoidal pattern
Variable decelerations

The physiologic events that occur during labor call for many adaptations by the mother and fetus. Accurate and frequent assessment is crucial because the changes are rapid and involve two individuals, mother and child.

The number and effectiveness of intrapartal assessment techniques have increased over the years. In the past, observation, palpation, and auscultation were the only assessment techniques available. In current practice, these techniques are enhanced by the use of ultrasound and electronic monitoring. These tools can provide more detailed information for assessment.

Maternal Assessment

History

The nurse obtains a brief history when the woman is admitted to the birthing area. Each agency has its own admission forms, but they usually include the following information:

- Woman's name and age
- Attending physician/certified nurse-midwife (CNM)
- Personal data: blood type; Rh factor; results of serology testing; prepregnant and present weight; allergies to medications, foods, or substances; prescribed and over-the-counter medications taken during pregnancy; history of drug and alcohol use and smoking during the pregnancy
- History of previous illness, such as tuberculosis, heart disease, diabetes, convulsive disorders, thyroid disorders
- Problems in the prenatal period, such as elevated blood pressure, bleeding problems, recurrent urinary tract infections, other infections, or sexually transmitted infections
- Pregnancy data: gravida, para, abortions, neonatal deaths
- The method chosen for infant feeding
- Type of prenatal education classes
- Woman's requests regarding labor and birth, such as no enema, no analgesics or anesthetics, or the presence of the father or others in the birthing or delivery room
- Pediatrician or family practice physician
- Additional data: history of special tests such as NST, BPP, ultrasound; history of any preterm labor; onset of labor; amniotic fluid membrane status; and brief description of previous labor and birth

Assessment of psychosocial history is a critical component of intrapartal nursing assessment. The nurse begins the assessment when the woman is admitted to the birthing area by obtaining information such as

- What is her marital status? Who are her support people?
- Is she safe in her relationship with the baby's father? Was there any physical or emotional abuse before or during the pregnancy? If so, what interventions were made? In questioning the woman about safety and abuse issues it is important for the nurse to be aware that abuse affects one in six adult women and one in five teenagers during pregnancy (McFarland and Parker 1994). It is important to ensure that the woman is alone when the questions are asked so that she can answer freely. If she indicates there has been a problem, the questions from the Abuse Assessment Screen by McFarland and Parker (1994, p 322) could be used. The questions include
  1. Have you ever been emotionally or physically abused by your partner or someone important to you?
  2. Within the last year, have you been hit, slapped, kicked, or otherwise physically hurt by someone? If yes, by whom? Total number of times?
  3. Since you've been pregnant, have you been hit, slapped, kicked, or otherwise physically hurt by someone? If yes, by whom? Total number of times?
  4. Within the last year has anyone forced you to have sexual activities? If yes, who? Total number of times?
  5. Are you afraid of your partner or anyone you listed above?
- Has she had difficulty or problems with previous pregnancies, labors, or births that would increase her anxiety now?
- Have emotional problems been present during the past few months? What interventions have occurred?

Given the prevalence of sexual violence against women in our society (reported incidence is one in three women, regardless of age) the nurse needs to consider that the woman may have experienced sexual violence at some point in her life. In this case she may be anxious about the labor process, or anxiety may arise during labor. Because psychosocial factors may be complex, the woman's history may not be apparent until later in the labor and birth. The nurse needs to be aware of the following aspects of psychosocial history:

- Has the woman experienced rape or sexual abuse?
- Is there evidence of support between the woman and her partner?
- Is the partner controlling? Does the partner make decisions unilaterally?

One Family's Story

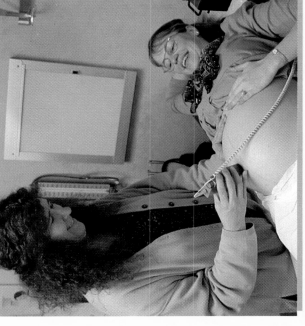

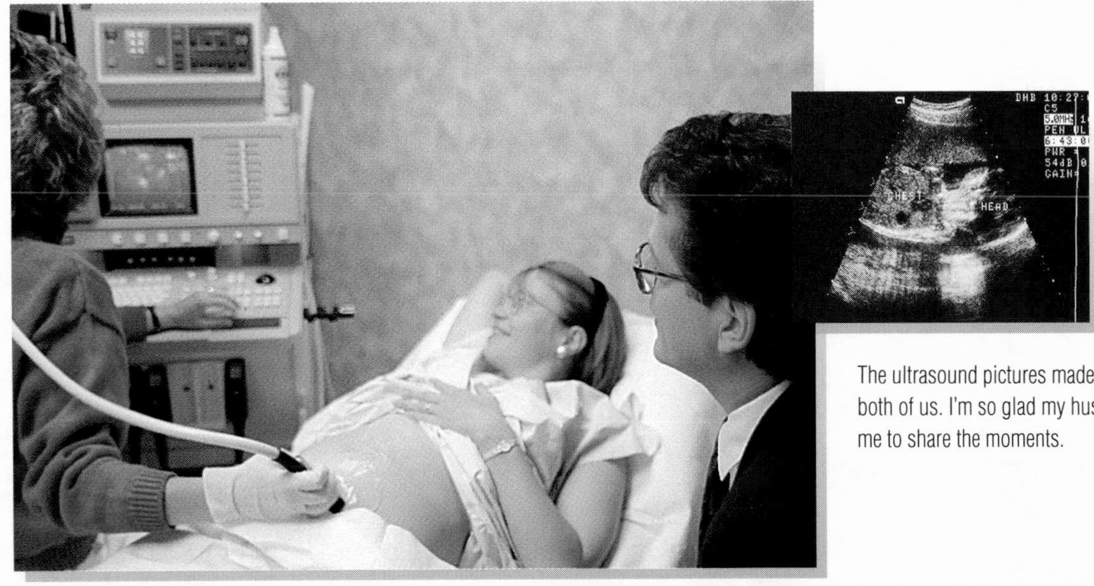

The ultrasound pictures made the baby seem real for both of us. I'm so glad my husband was able to be with me to share the moments.

We were so excited when we learned that I was pregnant. We had been waiting for this moment for some time, and we were ready to become parents. During the first trimester, I didn't look or feel pregnant, but when reading about the fetus' amazing development inside of me, I became very conscious of doing the best for our baby. I wonder if all parents feel the same?

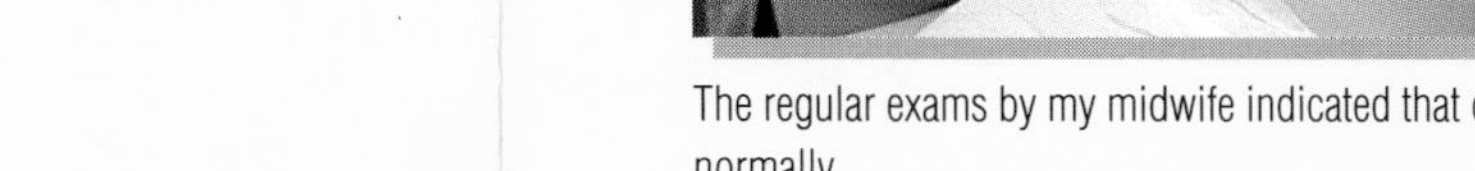

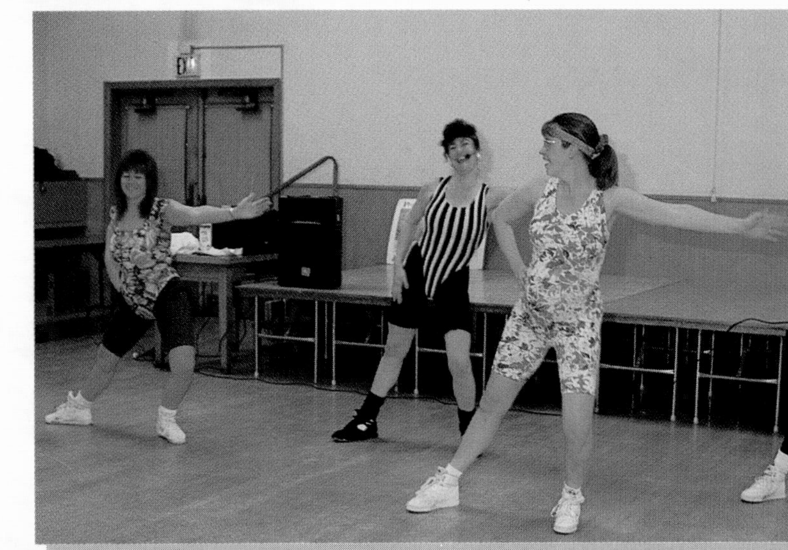

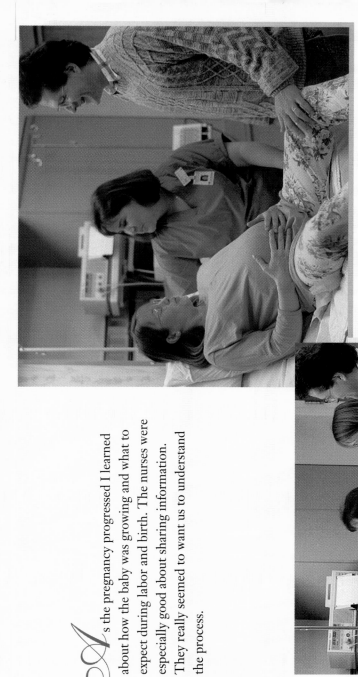

Exercise classes kept me fit and active. The instructor had me monitor my pulse to ensure that I didn't overdo.

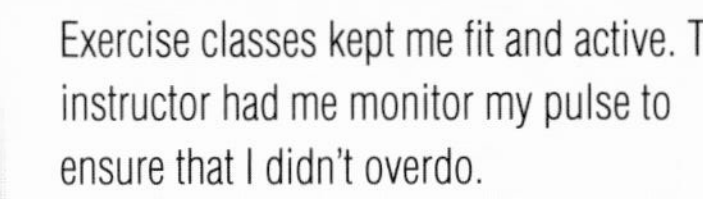

Childbirth preparation classes helped us learn to be a real team.

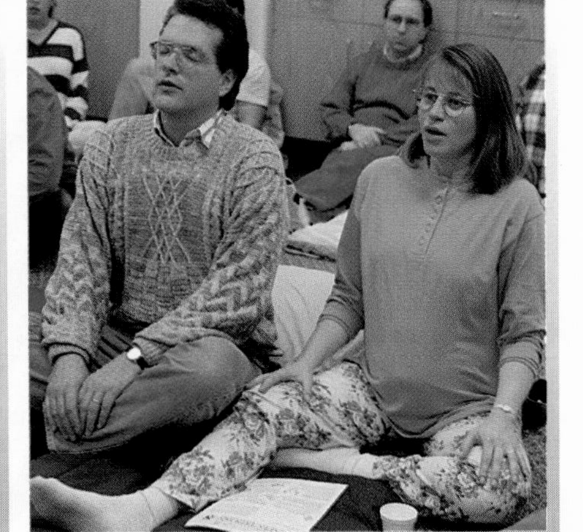

I was amazed at how fully involved my husband was. He did better at the breathing than I did!

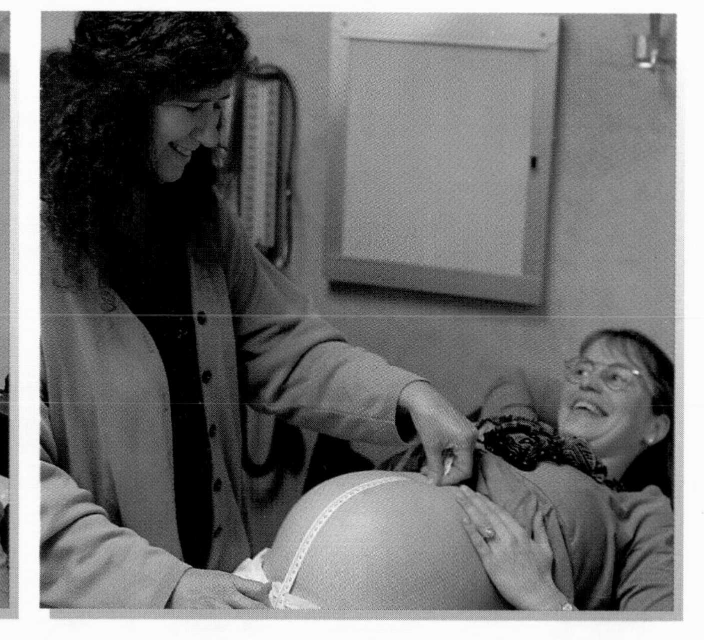

The regular exams by my midwife indicated that our baby was growing normally.

As the pregnancy progressed I learned about how the baby was growing and what to expect during labor and birth. The nurses were especially good about sharing information. They really seemed to want us to understand the process.

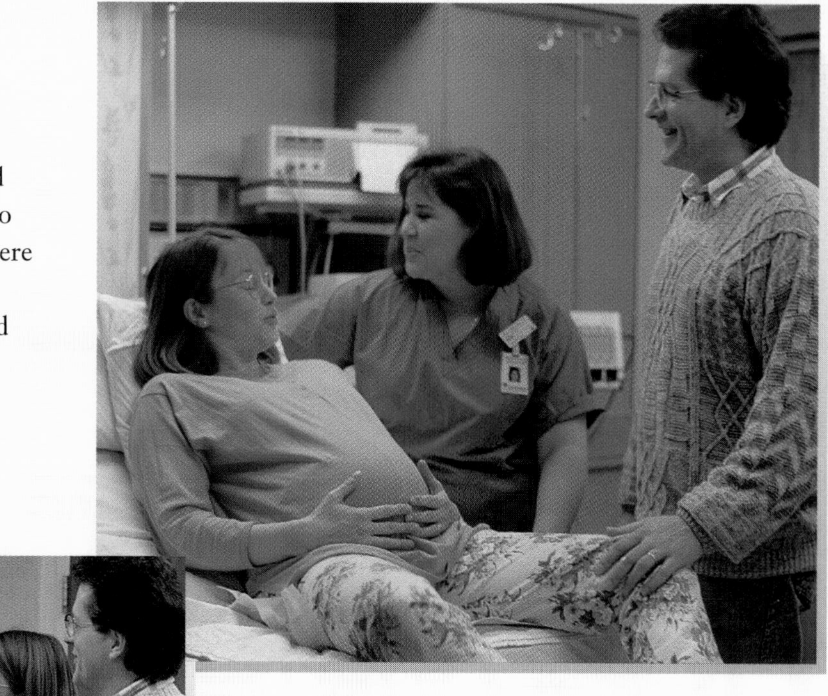

I loved listening to my baby's heartbeat.

Maternal-Fetal Development

Rows: Fetal Development · Maternal Changes · Client Teaching/Anticipatory Guidance

0 — Conception

Fetal Development

The sperm fertilizes the ovum, which then divides and burrows into the uterus.

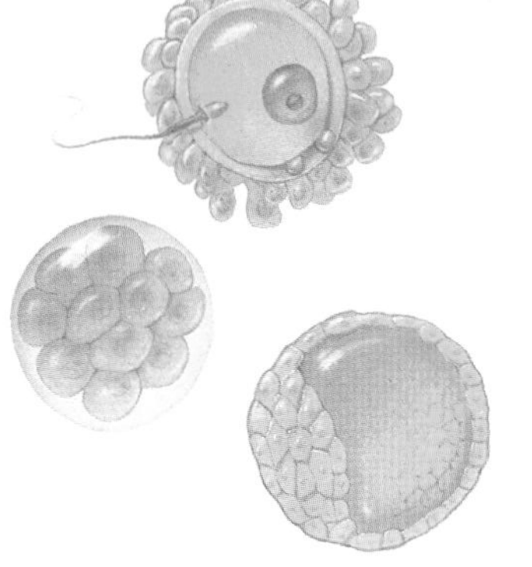

Maternal Changes

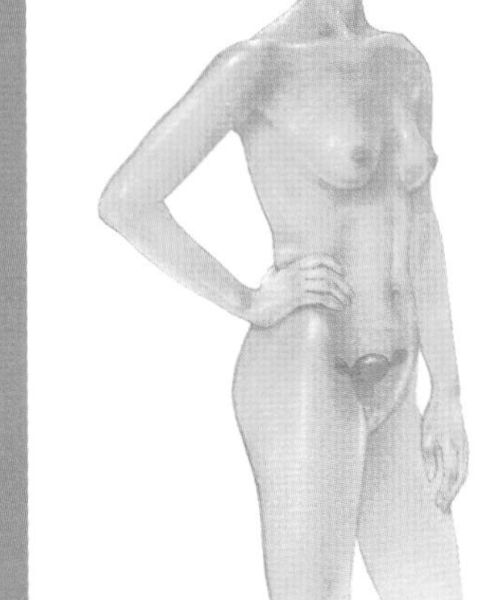

1 — 4 Weeks

Fetal Development

From the embryonic disk (ectoderm, entoderm, mesoderm), the first body segments appear that will eventually become the spine, brain, and spinal cord. Heart, blood circulation, and digestive tract take shape. Embryo is less than a quarter-inch long.

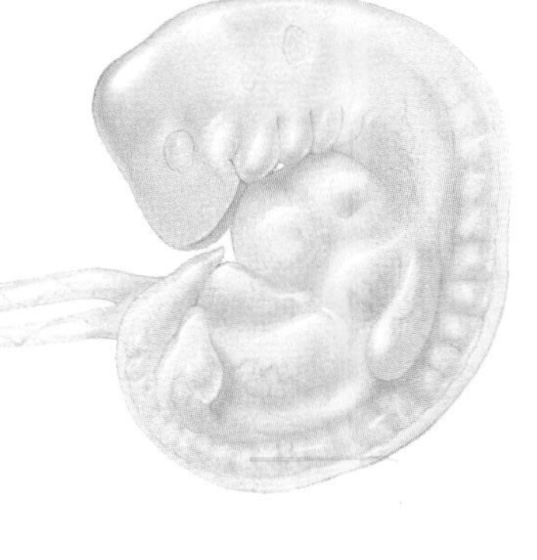

Maternal Changes

Mother misses first period; breasts become tender, may enlarge. Chronic fatigue and urinary frequency begin, may persist for three or more months. hCG in urine and serum 9 days after conception.

Client Teaching/Anticipatory Guidance

Supportive bra may ease discomfort. Increased rest and relaxation necessary now and throughout pregnancy. Increase fluids during the day; decrease fluid intake only at night to help prevent nocturia; sleep on side to decrease pressure on bladder. Avoid using any medications unless prescribed. Avoid use of social drugs; check with caregiver before using any OTC preparations.

2 — 8 Weeks

Fetal Development

Development is rapid; heart begins to pump blood; limb buds are well developed. Facial features and major divisions of the brain are discernible. Ears develop from skin folds; tiny bones and muscles are formed beneath the thin skin.

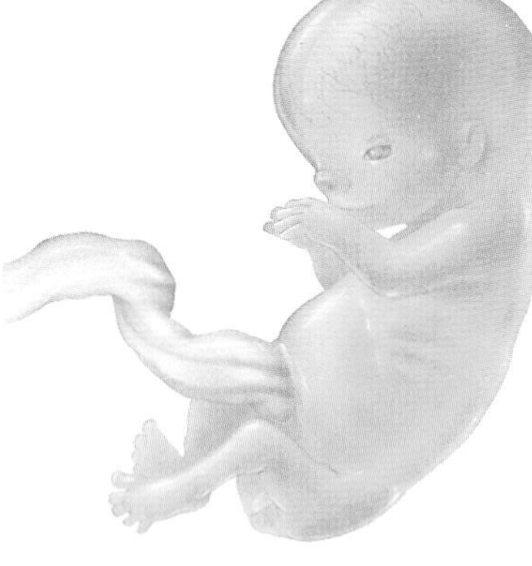

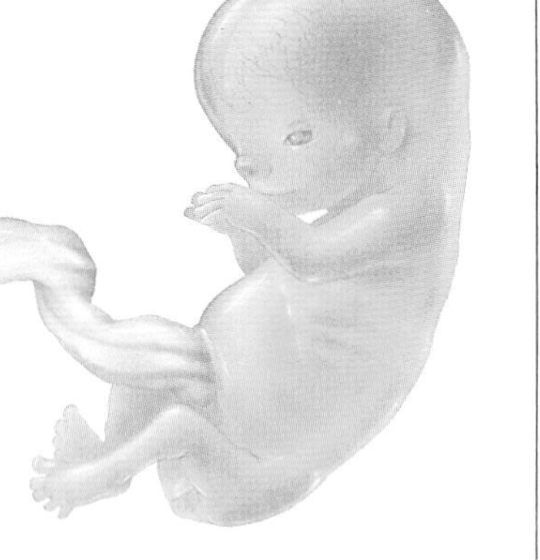

Maternal Changes

Morning sickness, may persist to 12 weeks. Uterus changes from pear to globular shape. Hegar's, Goodell's and Piskacek's signs appear. Cervix flexes; leukorrhea increases. Surprise and ambivalence about pregnancy may occur. No noticeable weight gain.

Client Teaching/Anticipatory Guidance

Eat dry crackers before arising; try frequent small, dry, low-fat meals with fluids taken between meals. Avoid use of hot tubs, saunas, and steam rooms throughout pregnancy.

Discuss attitudes toward pregnancy. Discuss value of early pregnancy classes that focus on what to expect during pregnancy. Provide information about childbirth preparation classes.

3 — 12 Weeks

Fetal Development

Embryo becomes a fetus, its beating heart discernible by ultrasound. Assumes a more human shape as lower body develops. At week 12, first movements begin. Sex is determinable. Kidneys produce urine.

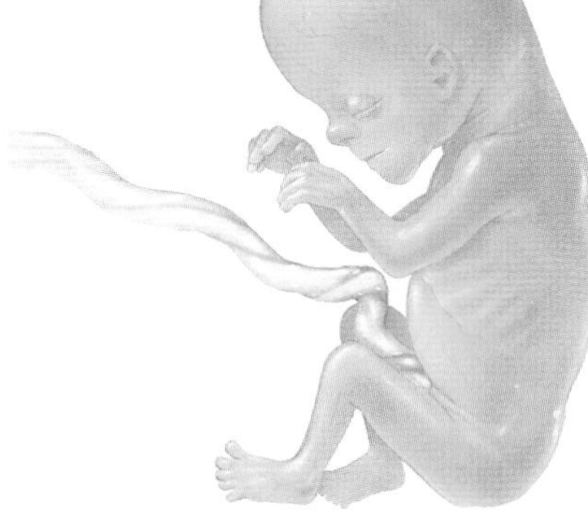

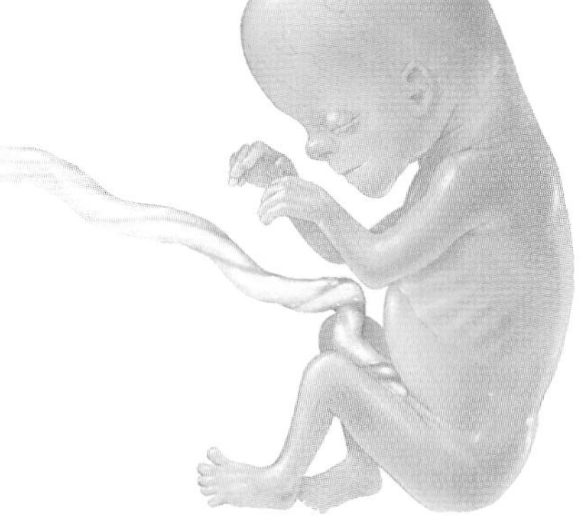

Maternal Changes

Chadwick's sign appears. Uterus rises above pelvic brim by 12 weeks. Braxton Hicks contractions may begin and continue throughout pregnancy. Potential for urinary tract infection (UTI) increases and exists throughout pregnancy. Weight gain of about 2½ to 4 lb during first trimester.

Placenta now fully functioning and producing hormones.

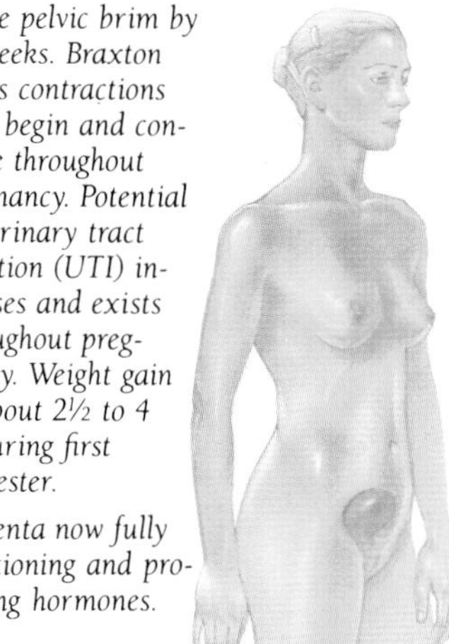

Client Teaching/Anticipatory Guidance

Adequate fluid intake and frequent voiding (every 2 hr while awake) help prevent UTI. Also helpful to void following intercourse. Wipe from front to rear.

Discuss nutrition and appropriate weight gain. Stress value of regular physical exercise, especially nonweightbearing activities or walking. Discuss possible effects of pregnancy on sexual relationship.

4 — 16 Weeks

Fetal Development

Musculoskeletal system has matured; nervous system begins to exert control. Blood vessels rapidly develop. Fetal hands can grasp; legs kick actively. All organs begin to mature and grow. Fetus weighs about 7 oz (½ lb). FHT discernible with Doppler. Pancreas produces insulin.

Maternal Changes

Fundus halfway between symphysis and umbilicus. Woman gains slightly less than 1 lb per wk for remainder of pregnancy. May feel more energetic. BPD measurement on ultrasound. Vaginal secretions increase. Itching, irritation, malodor suggest infection. Woman may begin wearing maternity clothes. Pressure on bladder lessens and urinary frequency decreases.

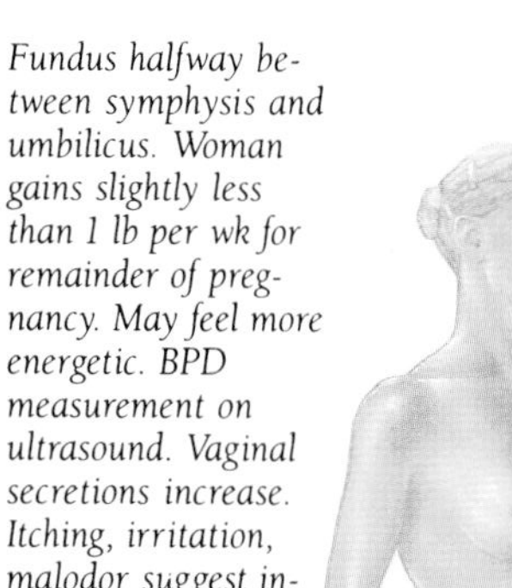

Client Teaching/Anticipatory Guidance

Daily shower or bath and thorough drying of vulva helpful; avoid douching during pregnancy. Consult caregiver if infection suspected; use only prescribed medications.

Review danger signs of pregnancy. Discuss infant feeding options; provide information on the value of breastfeeding. Provide information about clothing, shoes.

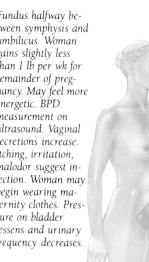

It is important for the nurse to obtain the history in a setting that promotes trust and the establishment of a relationship. Some of the questions are straightforward, but others require care and privacy (the nurse and the woman alone together) to ensure that the woman has a safe environment in which to address them.

Intrapartal High-Risk Screening

Screening for intrapartal high-risk factors is an integral part of assessing the normal laboring woman. As the history is obtained, the nurse notes the presence of any factors that may be associated with a high-risk condition. For example, the woman who reports a physical symptom such as intermittent bleeding needs further assessment to rule out abruptio placentae or placenta previa before the admission process continues. In addition to identifying the presence of a high-risk condition, the nurse must recognize the implications of the condition for the laboring woman and her fetus. For example, if an abnormal fetal presentation is present, the nurse understands that the labor may be prolonged, prolapse of the umbilical cord is more likely, and the possibility of a cesarean birth is increased.

Although physical conditions are frequently listed as the major factors that increase risk in the intrapartal period, sociocultural variables such as poverty, nutrition, the amount of prenatal care, cultural beliefs regarding pregnancy, and communication patterns may also precipitate a high-risk situation. The nurse can quickly review the prenatal record for number of prenatal visits; weight gain during pregnancy; progression of fundal height; assistance such as Medicaid and Women, Infants, and Children (WIC); and exposure to environmental agents.

The nurse can begin gathering data about sociocultural factors as the woman enters the birthing area. The nurse observes the communication pattern between the woman and her support person(s) and their responses to admission questions and initial teaching. If the woman and her support person(s) do not speak English and translators are not available within the birthing room staff, the course of labor and the nurse's ability to interact and provide support and education are affected. The couple needs information in their primary language to make informed decisions. Communication may also be affected by cultural practices such as beliefs about when to speak, who should ask questions, or whether it is acceptable to let others know if discomfort is occurring.

A partial list of intrapartal risk factors appears in Table 16–1. The factors precede the Intrapartal Assessment Guide because they must be kept in mind during the assessment.

ESSENTIAL PRECAUTIONS FOR PRACTICE

During Intrapartal Assessment

Examples of times when disposable gloves should be worn include:

- Assisting the woman as she removes any garments moist with bloody show and/or amniotic fluid
- Handling chux and bedding that are moist with bloody show and/or amniotic fluid
- Checking amniotic fluid–soaked materials with Nitrazine test tape
- Placing the elastic straps for the electronic monitor around a woman who has been lying in bedding moist with bloody show and/or amniotic fluid
- Assisting with fetal blood sampling and handling the lab tubes

Sterile gloves are worn when the nurse does a sterile vaginal exam and when fetal scalp electrodes are placed. The sterile gloves are used to maintain sterile asepsis. They protect the nurse from exposure to vaginal secretions, bloody show, and amniotic fluid.

REMEMBER to wash your hands before pulling the disposable gloves on and AGAIN immediately after you remove the gloves.

For further information consult OSHA and CDC guidelines.

Intrapartal Physical and Psychosociocultural Assessment

A physical examination is part of the admission procedure and part of the ongoing care of the client. Although the intrapartal physical assessment is not as complete and thorough as the initial prenatal physical examination (Chapter 8), it does involve assessment of some body systems and the actual labor process. The Intrapartal Assessment Guide on pages 365–370 provides a framework the maternity nurse can use when examining the laboring woman.

The physical assessment portion includes assessments performed immediately on admission as well as ongoing assessments. When labor is progressing very quickly, the nurse may not have time for a complete assessment. In this case, the critical physical assessments would include maternal vital signs, labor status, fetal status, and laboratory findings.

The cultural assessment portion provides a starting point for this increasingly important aspect of assessment. Individualized nursing care can best be planned and implemented when the values and beliefs of the laboring woman are known and honored. Frequently, however, the nurse feels uncertain about what to ask or consider, perhaps because there has been no personal

Text continues on page 371

TABLE 16–1 Intrapartal High-Risk Factors

Factor	Maternal Implication	Fetal-Neonatal Implication
Abnormal presentation	↑ Incidence of cesarean birth ↑ Incidence of prolonged labor	↑ Incidence of placenta previa Prematurity ↑ Risk of congenital abnormality Neonatal physical trauma ↑ Risk of intrauterine growth retardation
Multiple gestation	↑ Uterine distension → ↑ risk of postpartum hemorrhage ↑ Risk of cesarean birth ↑ Risk of preterm labor	Low birth weight Prematurity ↑ Risk of congenital anomalies Feto-fetal transfusion
Hydramnios	↑ Discomfort ↑ Dyspnea ↑ Risk of preterm labor Edema of lower extremities	↑ Risk of esophageal or other high alimentary tract atresias ↑ Risk of CNS anomalies (myelocele)
Oligohydramnios	Maternal fear of "dry birth"	↑ Incidence of congenital anomalies ↑ Incidence of renal lesions ↑ Risk of IUGR ↑ Risk of fetal acidosis ↑ Risk of cord compression Postmaturity
Meconium staining of amniotic fluid	↑ Psychologic stress due to fear for baby	↑ Risk of fetal asphyxia ↑ Risk of meconium aspiration ↑ Risk of pneumonia due to aspiration of meconium
Premature rupture of membranes	↑ Risk of infection (chorioamnionitis) ↑ Risk of preterm labor ↑ Anxiety Fear for the baby Prolonged hospitalization ↑ Incidence of tocolytic therapy	↑ Perinatal morbidity Prematurity ↓ Birth weight ↑ Risk of respiratory distress syndrome Prolonged hospitalization
Induction of labor	↑ Risk of hypercontractility of uterus ↑ Risk of uterine rupture ↑ Length of labor if cervix not ready ↑ Anxiety	Prematurity if gestational age not assessed correctly Hypoxia if hyperstimulation occurs
Abruptio placentae/placenta previa	Hemorrhage Uterine atony ↑ Incidence of cesarean birth	Fetal hypoxia/acidosis Fetal exsanguination ↑ Perinatal mortality
Failure to progress in labor	Maternal exhaustion ↑ Incidence of augmentation of labor ↑ Incidence of cesarean birth	Fetal hypoxia/acidosis Intracranial birth injury
Precipitous labor (< 3 hours)	Perineal, vaginal, cervical lacerations ↑ Risk of PP hemorrhage	Tentorial tears
Prolapse of umbilical cord	↑ Fear for baby Cesarean birth	Acute fetal hypoxia/acidosis
Fetal heart aberrations	↑ Fear for baby ↑ Risk of cesarean birth, forceps, vacuum Continuous electronic monitoring and intervention in labor	Tachycardia, chronic asphyxic insult, bradycardia, acute asphyxic insult Chronic hypoxia Congenital heart block
Uterine rupture	Hemorrhage Cesarean birth for hysterectomy ↑ Risk of death	Fetal anoxia Fetal hemorrhage ↑ Neonatal morbidity and mortality
Postdates (> 42 weeks)	↑ Anxiety ↑ Incidence of induction of labor ↑ Incidence of cesarean birth ↑ Use of technology to monitor fetus ↑ Risk of shoulder dystocia	Postmaturity syndrome ↑ Risk of fetal-neonatal mortality and morbidity ↑ Risk of antepartum fetal death ↑ Incidence/risk of large baby
Diabetes	↑ Risk of hydramnios ↑ Risk of hypoglycemia or hyperglycemia ↑ Risk of pregnancy-induced hypertension	↑ Risk of malpresentation ↑ Risk of macrosomia ↑ Risk of intrauterine growth retardation ↑ Risk of respiratory distress syndrome ↑ Risk of congenital anomalies
Pregnancy-induced hypertension	↑ Risk of seizures ↑ Risk of stroke ↑ Risk of HELLP	↑ Risk of small-for-gestational-age baby ↑ Risk of preterm birth ↑ Risk of mortality
AIDS/STD	↑ Risk of additional infections	↑ Risk of transplacental transmission

INTRAPARTAL ASSESSMENT GUIDE First Stage of Labor

Physical Assessment/ Normal Findings	Alterations and Possible Causes*	Nursing Responses to Data†
Vital Signs		
Blood pressure (BP): < 130 systolic and < 85 diastolic in adult 18 years of age or older or no more than 15–20 mm Hg rise in systolic pressure over baseline BP during early pregnancy (Johannsen 1993)	High blood pressure (essential hypertension, preeclampsia, renal disease, apprehension or anxiety) Low blood pressure (supine hypotension)	Evaluate history of preexisting disorders and check for presence of other signs of preeclampsia. Do not assess during contractions; implement measures to decrease anxiety and then reassess. Turn woman on her side and recheck blood pressure. Provide quiet environment. Have O_2 available.
Pulse: 60–90 bpm	Increased pulse rate (excitement or anxiety, cardiac disorders, early shock)	Evaluate cause, reassess to see if rate continues; report to physician.
Respirations: 14–22/minute (or pulse rate divided by 4)	Marked tachypnea (respiratory disease), hyperventilation in transition phase	Assess between contractions; if marked tachypnea continues, assess for signs of respiratory disease.
	Hyperventilation (anxiety)	Encourage slow breaths if woman is hyperventilating.
Temperature: 36.2–37.6 C (98–99.6 F)	Elevated temperature (infection, dehydration, prolonged rupture of membranes, epidural regional block)	Assess for other signs of infection or dehydration.
Weight 25–30 lb greater than prepregnant weight	Weight gain > 30 lb (fluid retention, obesity, large infant, diabetes mellitus, PIH), weight gain < 15 lb (SGA)	Assess for signs of edema. Evaluate pattern from prenatal record.
Lungs Normal breath sounds, clear and equal	Rales, rhonchi, friction rub (infection), pulmonary edema, asthma	Reassess; refer to physician.
Fundus At 40 weeks' gestation located just below xyphoid process	Uterine size not compatible with estimated date of birth (SGA, large for gestational age [LGA], hydramnios, multiple pregnancy)	Reevaluate history regarding pregnancy dating. Refer to physician for additional assessment.
Edema Slight amount of dependent edema	Pitting edema of face, hands, legs, abdomen, sacral area (preeclampsia)	Check deep tendon reflexes for hyperactivity; check for clonus; refer to physician.
Hydration Normal skin turgor, elastic	Poor skin turgor (dehydration)	Assess skin turgor; refer to physician for deviations.

*Possible causes of alterations are placed in parentheses.

†This column provides guidelines for further assessment and initial nursing interventions.

INTRAPARTAL ASSESSMENT GUIDE | First Stage of Labor continued

Physical Assessment/ Normal Findings	Alterations and Possible Causes*	Nursing Responses to Data†
Perineum		
Tissues smooth, pink color (see Prenatal Initial Physical Assessment Guide, Chapter 8)	Varicose veins of vulva, Herpes lesions	Exercise care while doing a perineal prep; note on client record need for follow-up in postpartal period; reassess after birth; refer to physician.
Clear mucus, may be blood tinged, earthy or human odor	Profuse, purulent, foul-smelling drainage	Suspected gonorrhea or chorioamnionitis; report to physician; initiate care to newborn's eyes; notify neonatal nursing staff and pediatrician.
Presence of small amount of bloody show that gradually increases with further cervical dilatation	Hemorrhage	Assess BP and pulse, pallor, diaphoresis; report any marked changes. (Note: Gaping of vagina or anus and bulging of perineum are suggestive signs of second stage of labor.) Universal precautions.
Labor Status		
Uterine contractions: regular pattern	Failure to establish a regular pattern, prolonged latent phase Hypertonicity Hypotonicity	Evaluate whether woman is in true labor; ambulate if in early labor. Evaluate client status and contractile pattern. Obtain a 20-minute EFM monitor strip. Notify physician/CNM.
Cervical dilatation: progressive cervical dilatation from size of fingertip to 10 cm (Procedure 16–1)	Rigidity of cervix (frequent cervical infections, scar tissue, failure of presenting part to descend)	Evaluate contractions, fetal engagement, position, and cervical dilatation. Inform client of progress.
Cervical effacement: progressive thinning of cervix (Procedure 16–1)	Failure to efface (rigidity of cervix, failure of presenting part to engage); cervical edema (pushing effort by woman before cervix is fully dilated and effaced, trapped cervix)	Evaluate contractions, fetal engagement, and position. Notify physician/certified nurse-midwife if cervix is becoming edematous; work with woman to prevent pushing until cervix is completely dilated. Keep vaginal exams to a minimum.
Fetal descent: progressive descent of fetal presenting part from station −5 to +4 (Figure 16–4 in Procedure 16–1)	Failure of descent (abnormal fetal position or presentation, macrosomic fetus, inadequate pelvic measurement)	Evaluate fetal position, presentation, and size. Evaluate maternal pelvic measurements.
Membranes: may rupture before or during labor	Rupture of membranes more than 12–24 hours before initiation of labor	Assess for ruptured membranes using Nitrazine test tape before doing vaginal exam. Follow BSI precautions. Instruct woman with ruptured membranes to remain on bed rest if presenting part is not engaged and firmly down against the cervix. Keep vaginal exams to a minimum to prevent infection. When membranes rupture in the birth setting, **the nurse immediately assesses FHR** to detect changes associated with prolapse of umbilical cord (FHR slows).

*Possible causes of alterations are placed in parentheses.

†This column provides guidelines for further assessment and initial nursing interventions.

INTRAPARTAL ASSESSMENT GUIDE continued

Physical Assessment/ Normal Findings	Alterations and Possible Causes*	Nursing Responses to Data†
Labor Status *continued*		
Findings on Nitrazine test tape: Membranes probably intact yellow pH 5.0 olive pH 5.5 olive green pH 6.0	False-positive results may be obtained if large amount of bloody show is present, previous vaginal examination has been done using lubricant, or tape is touched by nurse's fingers.	Assess fluid for consistency, amount, odor; assess FHR frequently. Assess fluid at regular intervals for presence of meconium staining. Follow BSI precautions while assessing amniotic fluid.
Membranes probably ruptured blue-green pH 6.5 blue-gray pH 7.0 deep blue pH 7.5		Teach woman that amniotic fluid is continually produced (to allay fear of "dry birth"). Teach woman that she may feel amniotic fluid trickle or gush with contractions. Change chux pads often.
Amniotic fluid clear, with earthy/human odor, no foul-smelling odor	Greenish amniotic fluid (fetal stress)	Assess FHR; do vaginal exam to evaluate for prolapsed cord; apply fetal monitor for continuous data; report to physician.
	Strong or foul odor (amnionitis)	Take woman's temperature and report to physician.
Fetal Status		
FHR: 120–160 bpm	<120 or >160 bpm (fetal stress); abnormal patterns on fetal monitor: decreased variability, late decelerations, variable decelerations, absence of accelerations with fetal movement	Initiate interventions based on particular FHR pattern.
Presentation: Cephalic, 97% Breech, 3%	Face, brow, breech, or shoulder presentation	Report to physician; after presentation is confirmed as face, brow, breech, or shoulder, woman may be prepared for cesarean birth.
Position: LOA most common	Persistent occipital-posterior (OP) position; transverse arrest	Carefully monitor maternal and fetal status.
Activity: fetal movement	Hyperactivity (may precede fetal hypoxia)	Carefully evaluate FHR; apply fetal monitor.
	Complete lack of movement (fetal distress or fetal demise)	Carefully evaluate FHR; apply fetal monitor. Report to physician/CNM.
Laboratory Evaluation		
Hematologic tests Hemoglobin: 12–16 g/dL	<12 g/dL (anemia, hemorrhage)	Evaluate woman for problems due to decreased oxygen-carrying capacity caused by lowered hemoglobin.
CBC Hematocrit: 38%–47% RBC: 4.2–5.4 million/μL WBC: 4500–11,000/μL, although leukocytosis to 20,000/μL is not unusual Platelets 150,000–400,000/mm^3	Presence of infection or blood dyscrasias, loss of blood (hemorrhage, DIC)	Evaluate for other signs of infection or for petechia, bruising, or unusual bleeding.

*Possible causes of alterations are placed in parentheses.

†This column provides guidelines for further assessment and initial nursing interventions.

INTRAPARTAL ASSESSMENT GUIDE First Stage of Labor continued

Physical Assessment/ Normal Findings	Alterations and Possible Causes*	Nursing Responses to Data†
Laboratory Evaluation *continued*		
Serologic testing STS or VDRL test: nonreactive	Positive reaction (Chapter 8, Initial Prenatal Physical Assessment Guide)	For reactive test notify newborn nursery and pediatrician.
Rh	Rh-positive fetus in Rh-negative woman	Assess prenatal record for titer levels during pregnancy. Obtain cord blood for direct Coombs' at birth.
Urinalysis Glucose: negative	Glycosuria (low renal threshold for glucose, diabetes mellitus)	Assess blood glucose; test urine for ketones; ketonuria and glycosuria require further assessment of blood sugars.‡
Ketones: negative	Ketonuria (starvation ketosis)	
Proteins: negative	Proteinuria (urine specimen contaminated with vaginal secretions, fever, kidney disease); proteinuria of 2+ or greater found in uncontaminated urine may be a sign of ensuing preeclampsia	Instruct woman in collection technique; incidence of contamination from vaginal discharge is common.
Red blood cells: negative	Blood in urine (calculi, cystitis, glomerulonephritis, neoplasm)	Assess collection technique (may be bloody show).
White blood cells: negative	Presence of white blood cells (infection in genitourinary tract)	Assess for signs of urinary tract infection.
Casts: none	Presence of casts (nephrotic syndrome)	

Cultural Assessment§	Variations to Consider	Nursing Responses to Data†
Cultural influences determine customs and practices regarding intrapartal care.	Individual preferences may vary.	
Ask the following questions: Who would you like to remain with you during your labor and birth?	She may prefer only her coach to remain or may also want family and/or friends.	Provide support for her wishes by encouraging desired people to stay. Provide information to others (with the woman's permission) who are not in the room.
What would you like to wear during labor?	She may be more comfortable in her own clothes.	Offer supportive materials such as chux if needed to protect her own clothing. Avoid subtle signals to the woman that she should not have chosen to remain in her own clothes. Have other clothing available if the woman desires. If her clothing becomes contaminated, it will be simple to place it in a plastic bag. The nurse can soak soiled clothing in cool water. The nurse needs to remember to wear disposable gloves and a plastic apron if splashing is anticipated.

§These are only a few suggestions. We do not mean to imply that this is a comprehensive cultural assessment; rather, it is a tool to encourage cultural sensitivity.

*Possible causes of alterations are placed in parentheses.

†This column provides guidelines for further assessment and initial nursing interventions.

‡Glycosuria should not be discounted. The presence of glycosuria necessitates follow-up.

INTRAPARTAL ASSESSMENT GUIDE continued

Cultural Assessment[§]	Variations to Consider	Nursing Responses to Data[†]
What activity would you like during labor?	She may want to ambulate most of the time, stand in the shower, sit in the jacuzzi, sit in a chair or on a stool, remain on the bed, and so forth.	Support the woman's wishes by providing encouragement and completing assessments in a manner so that the woman's activity and positional wishes are disturbed as little as possible.
What position would you like for the birth?	She may feel more comfortable in lithotomy with stirrups and her upper body elevated, or side-lying or sitting in birthing bed, or standing, or squatting, or on hands and knees.	Collect any supplies and equipment needed to support her in her chosen birthing position. Provide information to the coach regarding any changes that may be needed based on the chosen position.
Is there anything special you would like?	She may want the room darkened or to have curtains and windows open, music playing, a Leboyer birth, her coach to cut the umbilical cord, to save a portion of the umbilical cord, to save the placenta, to videotape the birth, and so forth.	Support requests, and communicate requests to any other nursing or medical personnel (so requests can continue to be supported and not questioned). If another nurse or physician does not honor the request, act as advocate for the woman by continuing to support her unless her desire is truly unsafe.
Ask the woman if she would like fluids, and ask what temperature she prefers.	She may prefer clear fluids other than water (tea, clear juice). She may prefer iced, room-temperature, or warmed fluids.	Provide fluids as desired.
Observe the woman's response when privacy is difficult to maintain and her body is exposed.	Some women do not seem to mind being exposed during an exam or procedure; others feel acute discomfort.	Maintain privacy and respect the woman's sense of privacy. If the woman is unable to provide specific information, the nurse may draw from general information regarding cultural variation: Southeast Asian women may not want any family member in the room during exam or procedures. Her partner may not be involved with coaching activities during labor or birth. Saudi women may need to remain covered during the labor and birth and avoid exposure of any body part. The husband may need to be in the room but remain behind a curtain or screen so he does not view his wife at this time.
If the woman is to breastfeed, ask if she would like to feed her baby immediately after birth.	She may want to feed her baby right away or may want to wait a little while.	

Psychosocial Assessment	Variations to Consider	Nursing Responses to Data[†]
Preparation for Childbirth Woman has some information regarding process of normal labor and birth	Some women do not have any information regarding childbirth.	Add to present information base.

[§]These are only a few suggestions. We do not mean to imply that this is a comprehensive cultural assessment; rather, it is a tool to encourage cultural sensitivity.

[†]This column provides guidelines for further assessment and initial nursing interventions.

INTRAPARTAL ASSESSMENT GUIDE | First Stage of Labor continued

Psychosocial Assessment	Variations to Consider	Nursing Responses to Data†
Preparation for Childbirth *continued* Woman has breathing and/or relaxation techniques to use during labor.	Some women do not have any method of relaxation or breathing to use, and some do not desire them.	Support breathing and relaxation techniques that client is using; provide information if needed.
Response to Labor Latent phase: relaxed, excited, anxious for labor to be well established	May feel unable to cope with contractions because of fear, anxiety, or lack of information	Provide support and encouragement; establish trusting relationship.
Active phase: becomes more intense, begins to tire Transitional phase: feels tired, may feel unable to cope, needs frequent coaching to maintain breathing patterns	May remain quiet and without any sign of discomfort or anxiety, may insist that she is unable to continue with the birthing process	Provide support and coaching if needed.
Coping mechanisms: Ability to cope with labor through utilization of support system, breathing, relaxation techniques	May feel marked anxiety and apprehension, may not have coping mechanisms that can be brought into this experience, or may be unable to use them at this time	Support coping mechanisms if they are working for the woman; provide information and support if woman is exhibiting anxiety or needs additional alternative to present coping methods.
	Survivors of sexual abuse may demonstrate fear of IV's or needles, may recoil when touched, may insist on a female caregiver, may be very sensitive to bodily fluids and cleanliness, and may be unable to labor lying down (Burrian 1995).	Encourage participation of coach/significant other if a supportive relationship seems apparent. Establish rapport and a trusting relationship. Provide information that is true and offer your presence.
Anxiety Some anxiety and apprehension is within normal limits	May show anxiety through rapid breathing, nervous tremors, frowning, grimacing, clenching of teeth, thrashing movements, crying, increased pulse and blood pressure	Provide support, encouragement, and information. Teach relaxation techniques; support controlled breathing efforts. May need to provide a paper bag to breathe into if woman says her lips are tingling. Note FHR.
Sounds During Labor	Some women are very quiet and others moan or make a variety of noises.	Provide a supportive environment. Encourage woman to do what is right for her.
Support System Physical intimacy of mother-father (or mother-support relationship): caretaking activities such as soothing conversation, touching	Some women would prefer no contact, others may show clinging behaviors.	Encourage caretaking activities that appear to comfort the woman; encourage support to the woman; if support is limited, the nurse may take a more active role.
Support person stays in close proximity	Limited interaction may come from a desire for quiet.	Encourage support person to stay close (if this seems appropriate).
Relationship of mother-father (or support person): involved interaction	The support person may seem to be detached and maintain little support, attention, or conversation.	Support interactions; if interaction is limited, the nurse may provide more information and support. Assure that coach/significant other has short breaks, especially prior to transition.

†This column provides guidelines for further assessment and initial nursing interventions.

opportunity to become aware of varying cultural values and beliefs.

The final section addresses psychosocial factors. The laboring woman's psychosocial status is an important part of the total assessment. The woman has previous ideas, knowledge, and fears about childbearing. By assessing her psychosocial status, the nurse can meet the woman's needs for information and support. The nurse can then support the woman and her partner; in the absence of a partner, the nurse may become the support person.

While performing the intrapartal assessment, it is imperative that the nurse follow CDC guidelines to prevent exposure to body substances. The nurse can provide information in a factual manner regarding the precautions. A statement such as the following is helpful: "I will be wearing gloves when I change the chux on which you are lying. This is to protect my hands from the discharge you are having and to protect you from any organisms that I may have on my hands." Sharing information with the laboring woman and her support person(s) will promote a supportive, caring environment. (See Essential Precautions for Practice: During Intrapartal Assessment on page 363 for further information.)

Methods of Evaluating Labor Progress

Contraction Assessment

Uterine contractions may be assessed by palpation or continuous electronic monitoring.

Palpation The nurse assesses contractions for frequency, duration, and intensity by placing one hand on the uterine fundus. The hand is kept relatively still because excessive movement may stimulate contractions or cause discomfort. The nurse determines the frequency of the contractions by noting the time from the beginning of one contraction to the beginning of the next. If contractions begin at 7:00, 7:04, and 7:08, for example, their frequency is every 4 minutes. To determine contraction duration, the nurse notes the time when tensing of the fundus is first felt (beginning of contraction) and again as relaxation occurs (end of contraction). During the acme of the contraction, intensity can be evaluated by estimating the indentability of the fundus. The nurse should assess at least three successive contractions to provide enough data to determine the contraction pattern. See Key Facts to Remember: Contraction Characteristics for review of characteristics in different phases of labor.

This is also a good time to assess the laboring woman's perception of pain. What is her affect? Is this contraction more uncomfortable than the last one? Is the nurse's palpation of intensity congruent with the woman's perception? (For instance, the nurse might evaluate a contraction as mild in intensity while the laboring woman evaluates it as very strong). A nurse's assessment is not complete without the laboring woman's affect and response to the contractions being charted.

KEY FACTS TO REMEMBER

Contraction Characteristics

Latent phase	Frequency: every 10–20 minutes Duration: 15–20 seconds Intensity: mild
progressing to	Frequency: every 5–7 minutes Duration: 30–40 seconds Intensity: moderate
Active phase	Frequency: every 2–3 minutes Duration: 40–60 seconds Intensity: moderate to strong
Transition phase	Frequency: every 2 minutes Duration: 60–75 seconds Intensity: strong

Source: Varney H: *Nurse Midwifery*, 2nd ed. Boston: Blackwell, 1987.

Electronic Monitoring of Contractions Electronic monitoring of uterine contractions provides continuous data. In many birth settings electronic monitoring is routine for all high-risk clients and women who are having oxytocin-induced labor; other facilities monitor all laboring women.

Electronic monitoring may be done externally, with a device that is placed against the maternal abdomen, or internally, with an intrauterine catheter. When monitoring by external means, the portion of the monitoring equipment called a *tocodynamometer,* or "toco," is placed against the fundus of the uterus and held in place with an elastic belt. The toco contains a flexible disk that responds to pressure. When the uterus contracts, the fundus tightens and the change in pressure against the toco is amplified and transmitted to the electronic fetal monitor (see Figure 16–1). The monitor displays the uterine contraction as a pattern on graph paper.

External monitoring provides a continuous recording of the frequency and duration of uterine contractions and is noninvasive. But it does not record the intensity of the uterine contraction; the woman may be bothered by the belt if it requires frequent readjustment when she changes position; and it is difficult to obtain an accurate fetal heart rate in some women, such as those who are very obese, those who have hydramnios (an abnormally large amount of amniotic fluid), or those whose fetus is very active.

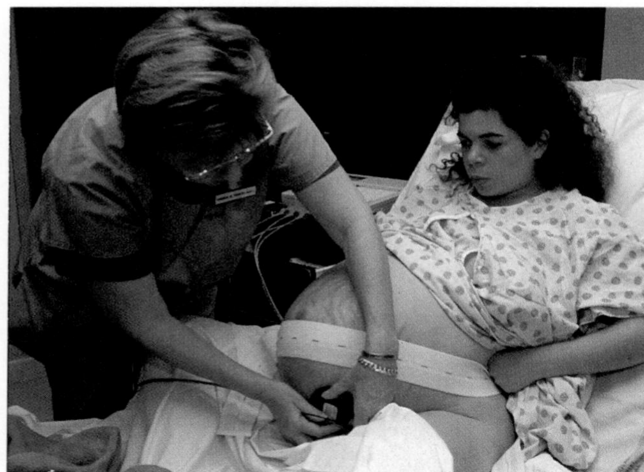

FIGURE 16–1 Woman in labor with external monitor applied

Internal intrauterine pressure electronic monitoring provides all this data and also provides accurate measurement of uterine contraction intensity (the strength of the contraction and the actual pressure within the uterus). After membranes have ruptured, the certified nurse-midwife/physician inserts the intrauterine pressure catheter into the uterine cavity and connects it by a cable to the electronic fetal monitor. The pressure within the uterus in the resting state and during each contraction is measured by a small micropressure device located in the tip of the catheter. Internal electronic monitoring is used when it is imperative to have accurate intrauterine pressure readings to evaluate the stress on the uterus.

Charting Contraction Assessments

Once labor contractions are assessed, the nurse notes them in the woman's record using an abbreviated method. For example, if assessed contractions have a frequency of 2–3 minutes and a duration of 60 seconds and are moderate in intensity, they are charted as: "every 2–3 × 60 moderate."

Cervical Assessment

Cervical dilatation and effacement are evaluated directly by vaginal examination (see Procedure 16–1: Intrapartal Vaginal Examination). The vaginal examination can also provide information about membrane status, fetal position, and station of the presenting part.

Fetal Assessment

Fetal Position

Fetal position is determined in several ways:

- Inspection and palpation of the woman's abdomen
- Auscultation of fetal heart rate
- A vaginal examination to determine the presenting part
- Ultrasound

Inspection

The nurse should observe the woman's abdomen for size and shape. The lie of the fetus should be assessed by noting whether the uterus projects up and down (longitudinal lie) or left to right (transverse lie).

Palpation: Leopold's Maneuvers

Leopold's maneuvers are a systematic way to evaluate the maternal abdomen (Figure 16–2). Frequent practice increases the examiner's skill in determining fetal position by palpation. Leopold's maneuvers may be difficult to perform on an obese woman or on a woman who has excessive amniotic fluid (hydramnios). Before performing Leopold's maneuvers: 1. Have the woman empty her bladder, and 2. Have the woman lie on her back with her feet on the bed and her knees bent.

First Maneuver Face the woman. Palpate the upper abdomen with both hands. Note the shape, consistency, and mobility of the palpated part. The fetal head is firm, hard, and round and moves independently of the trunk. The breech (buttocks) feels softer, and it moves with the trunk.

Second Maneuver Moving the hands down toward the pelvis, palpate the abdomen with gentle but deep pressure. The fetal back, on one side of the abdomen, feels smooth, and the fetal arms, legs, and feet, on the other side, feel knobby and bumpy.

Third Maneuver Place one hand just above the symphysis. Note whether the part palpated feels like the fetal head or the breech and whether the presenting part is engaged.

Fourth Maneuver Face the woman's feet. Place both hands on the lower abdomen, and move the fingers of both hands gently down the sides of the uterus toward the pubis. Note the cephalic prominence or brow.

Vaginal Examination and Ultrasound

Other assessment techniques to determine fetal position and presentation include vaginal examination and the use of ultrasound to visualize the fetus. During the vaginal examination, the examiner can palpate the presenting part if the cervix is dilated. Information about the position of the fetus and the degree of flexion of its head (in cephalic presentations) can also be obtained (see Procedure 16–1). Visualization by ultrasound is used when the fetal position cannot be determined by abdominal palpation (see Chapter 14).

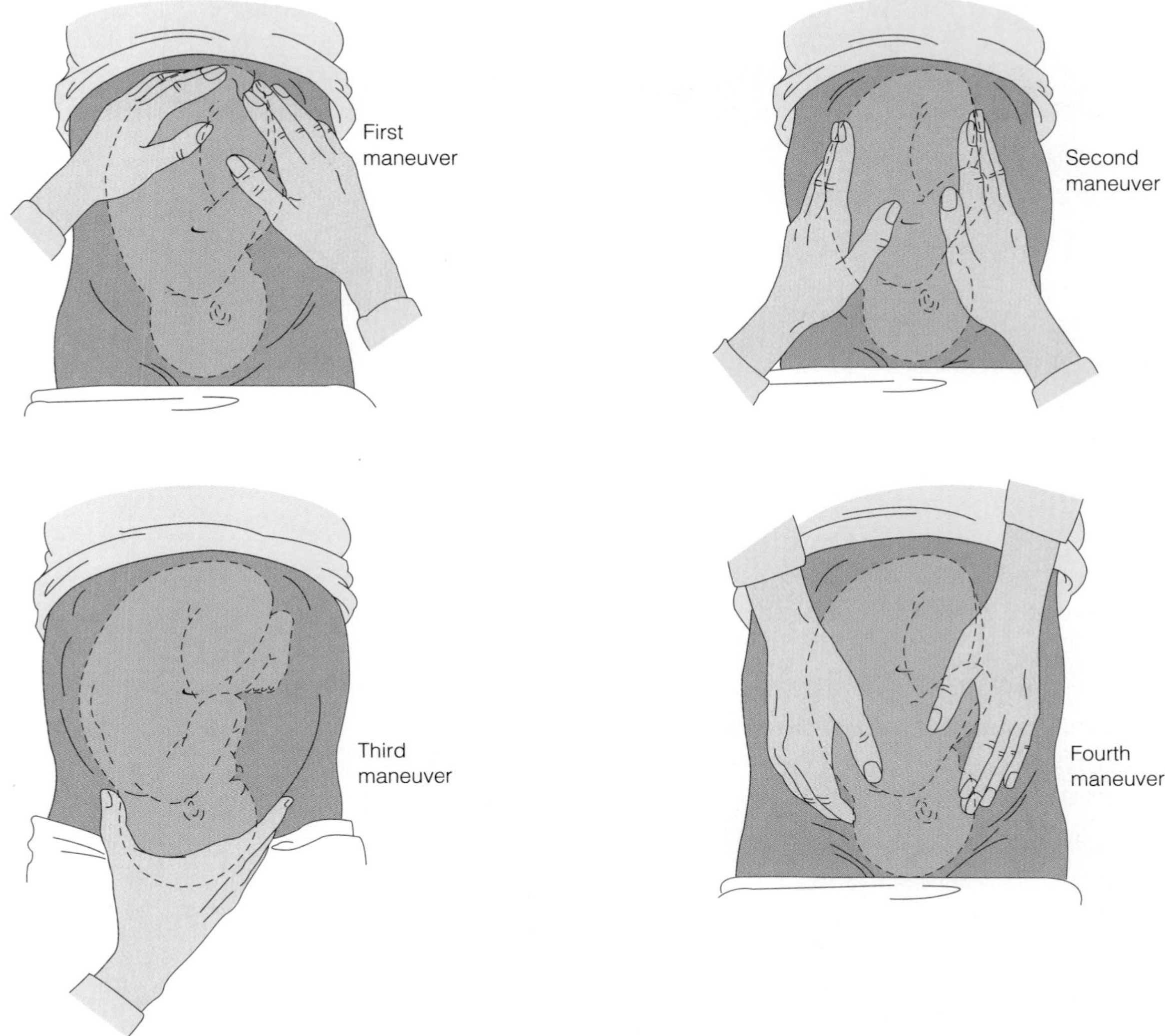

FIGURE 16–2 Leopold's maneuvers for determining fetal position and presentation.

Evaluation of Fetal Heart Rate

Auscultation of Fetal Heart Rate (FHR)

The fetoscope is used to auscultate the FHR between, during, and immediately after uterine contractions.

Instead of listening haphazardly over the client's abdomen for FHR, the nurse may choose to perform Leopold's maneuvers first. Leopold's maneuvers not only indicate the probable location of FHR but also help determine the presence of multiple fetuses, fetal lie, and fetal presentation. FHR is heard most clearly at the fetal back (see Figure 16–6 on page 377). Thus, in a cephalic presentation, FHR is best heard in the lower quadrant of the maternal abdomen. In a breech presentation, it is heard at or above the level of the maternal umbilicus. In a transverse lie, FHR may be heard best just above or just below the umbilicus. As the presenting part descends and rotates through the pelvic structure during labor, the location of the FHR tends to descend and move toward the midline.

After FHR is located, it is usually counted for 30 seconds and multiplied by 2 to obtain the number of beats per minute. The nurse should occasionally listen for a full minute, through and just after a contraction, to detect any abnormal heart rate, especially if the FHR is over 160 (tachycardia), under 120 (bradycardia), or irregular. If the FHR is irregular or has changed markedly from the last assessment, the nurse should listen for a full minute through and immediately after a contraction. See Procedure 16–2: Auscultating Fetal Heart Rate on pages 378–379, and Key Facts to Remember:

Text continues on page 376

PROCEDURE 16–1 Performing an Intrapartal Vaginal Examination

Nursing Action	Rationale
Objective: Assemble the equipment.	
Prepare and arrange the following items so that they are easily accessible:	Equipment organization facilitates the examination.
• Sterile or clean disposable gloves • Lubricant • Nitrazine test tape	If membranes are ruptured, sterile disposable gloves are used to decrease the chance of introducing bacteria during the examination. When membranes are intact, clean disposable gloves may be used.
Objective: Prepare the woman.	
• Explain the procedure, the indications for the exam, what the exam may feel like, and that it may cause discomfort.	Explanation of the procedure decreases anxiety and increases relaxation.
• Position the woman with her thighs flexed and abducted. Instruct her to put the heels of her feet together.	Position provides access to the vulvar area.
• Drape the woman with a sheet, leaving a flap so the perineum can be exposed.	Provides privacy.
• Encourage the woman to relax her muscles and legs during the procedure.	Decreases muscle tension and increases comfort.
• Inform the woman prior to touching her. Use gentleness.	This action communicates regard for the woman and her privacy.
Objective: Test for amniotic fluid leakage if indicated.	
• If fluid leakage has been reported or noted, use Nitrazine test tape before performing the exam.	As long as lubricant has not been used, Nitrazine tape registers a change in pH if amniotic fluid is present.
Objective: Use aseptic technique during the exam.	
• Pull glove onto dominant hand.	If sterile exam is needed, both hands will be gloved.
• Using your gloved hand, position the hand with the wrist straight and the elbow tilted downward.	This positioning allows the fingertips to point toward the umbilicus and find the cervix.
• Insert your well-lubricated second and index fingers of the gloved hand into the vagina until they touch the cervix. Avoid contaminating your hand by anal contact.	
• If the woman verbalizes discomfort, acknowledge it and apologize.	Acknowledgment decreases the passive role of the woman and validates that the woman is experiencing discomfort.
Objective: Determine the status of labor progress during and after contractions.	
• Perform the vaginal examination during and between contractions.	Cervical dilatation, effacement, and fetal station are affected by the presence of a contraction.
Objective: Identify the amount of cervical dilatation and effacement. (See Figure 16–3.)	
• Palpate for the opening, or what appears as a depression, in the cervix.	Allows determination of effacement and dilatation.
• Estimate the diameter of the depression to identify the amount of dilatation.	
Objective: Determine the status of the fetal membranes.	
• Palpate for a movable, bulging sac through the cervix.	If intact, the bag of waters will feel like a bulge.
• Observe for expression of amniotic fluid during the exam.	
Objective: Palpate the presenting part. (See Figure 16–4.)	Provides information regarding fetal descent and cardinal movements.
Objective: Assess the fetal descent. (See Figure 16–5.)	
• Assess the station and identify the position of the posterior fontanelle.	

PROCEDURE 16–1 Performing an Intrapartal Vaginal Examination continued

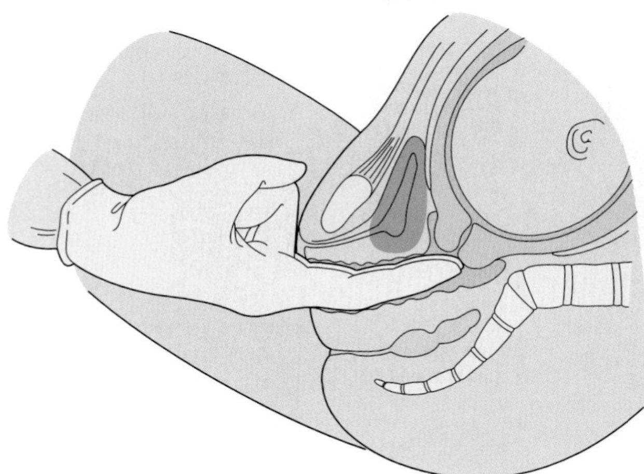

FIGURE 16–3 Determining cervical dilatation.

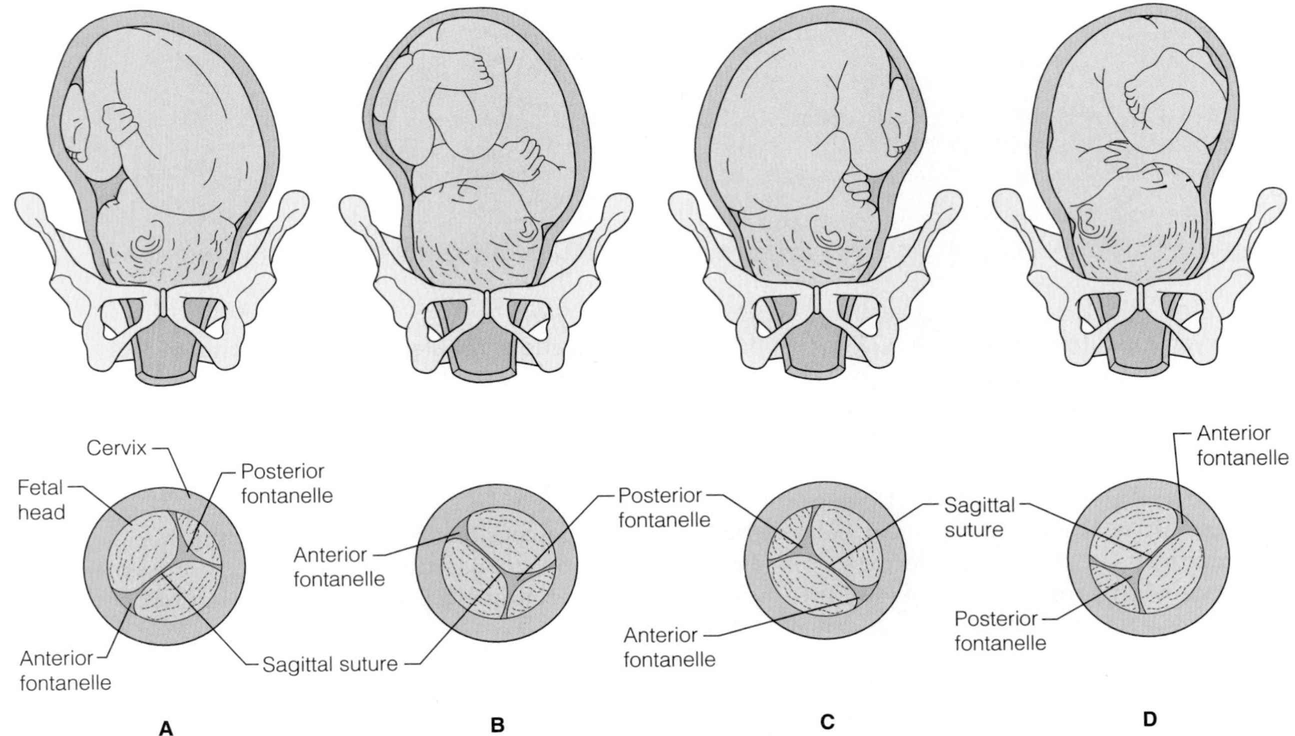

FIGURE 16–4 Palpating the presenting part (portion of the fetus that enters the pelvis first). ***A*** Left occiput anterior (LOA). The occiput (area over the occipital bone on the posterior part of the fetal head) is in the left anterior quadrant of the woman's pelvis. When the fetus is LOA, the posterior fontanelle (located just above the occipital bone and triangular in shape) is in the upper left quadrant of the maternal pelvis. ***B*** Left occiput posterior (LOP). The posterior fontanelle is in the lower left quadrant of the maternal pelvis. ***C*** Right occiput anterior (ROA). The posterior fontanelle is in the upper right quadrant of the maternal pelvis. ***D*** Right occiput posterior (ROP). The posterior fontanelle is in the lower right quadrant of the maternal pelvis. Note: The anterior fontanelle is diamond-shaped. Because of the roundness of the fetal head, only a portion of the anterior fontanelle can be seen in each of the views, so it appears to be triangular in shape.

PROCEDURE 16–1 Performing an Intrapartal Vaginal Examination continued

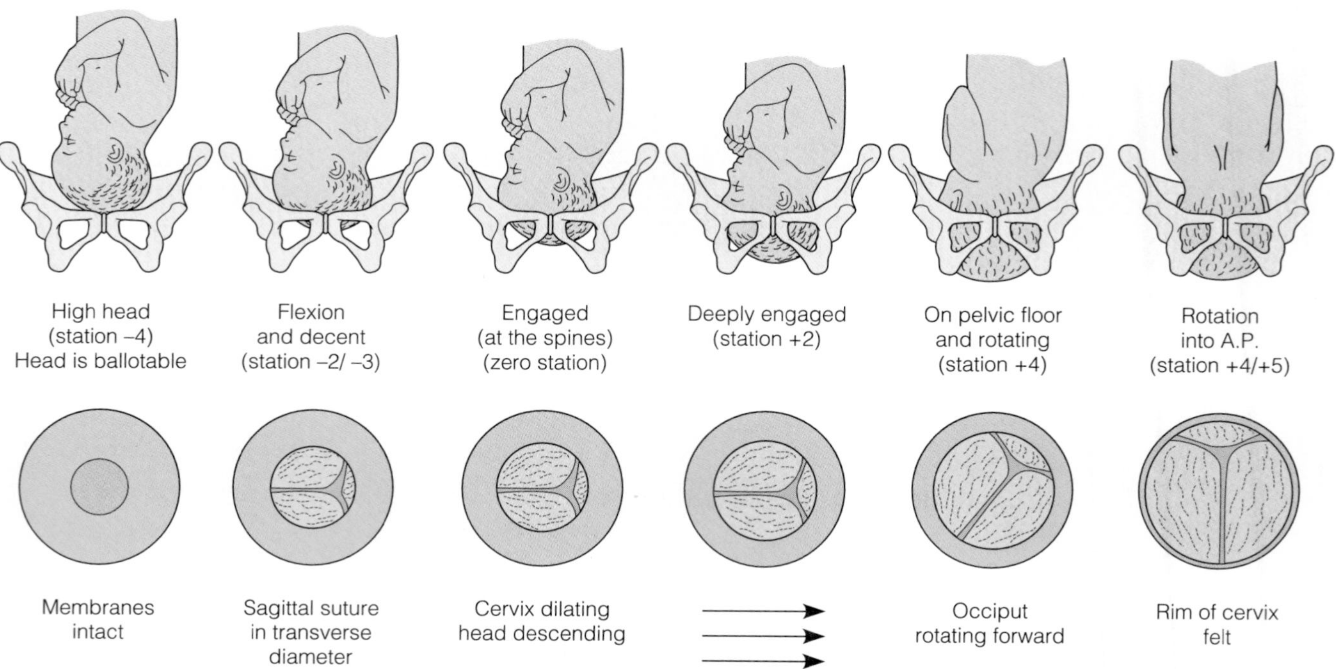

FIGURE 16–5 Top: The fetal head progressing through the pelvis. Bottom: The changes that the nurse will detect on palpation of the occiput through the cervix while doing a vaginal examination.
Source: Myles MF: *Textbook for Midwives.* Edinburgh, Scotland: Churchill Livingstone, 1975, p 246.

Frequency of Auscultation on page 377 for guidelines about how often to auscultate FHR.

The American Academy of Pediatrics and The American College of Obstetricians and Gynecologists (1992) have indicated that auscultation as outlined is equivalent to electronic fetal monitoring. Albers (1994, p 109) notes that "electronic fetal monitoring is not more effective than intermittent auscultation in reducing perinatal mortality or morbidity." Some nurses may feel that the one-on-one nursing required to follow the guidelines and the use of "old-fashioned," nonelectronic equipment is not desirable; however, auscultation by fetoscope is still a viable assessment that provides usable information and avoids additional exposure to ultrasound.

Electronic Monitoring of FHR

Electronic fetal monitoring (EFM) provides a visual assessment of fetal heart rate. It produces a continuous tracing of the FHR, allowing observation and evaluation of many characteristics of the FHR.

Indications for Electronic Monitoring of FHR If one or more of the following factors are present, the woman should be monitored by EFM:

1. Previous history of a stillborn (fetus dies in the uterus) at 38 or more weeks of gestation
2. Presence of a complication of pregnancy (eg, pregnancy-induced hypertension, placenta previa, abruptio placentae, multiple gestation)
3. Induction of labor (labor that is begun as a result of some type of intervention such as an intravenous infusion of pitocin)
4. Preterm labor (gestation less than 37 completed weeks)
5. Fetal stress or distress
6. Meconium staining of amniotic fluid (meconium has been released into the amniotic fluid by the fetus and may indicate a problem)

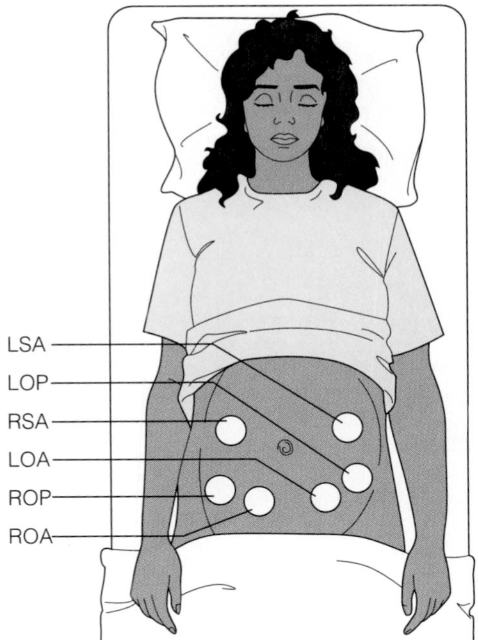

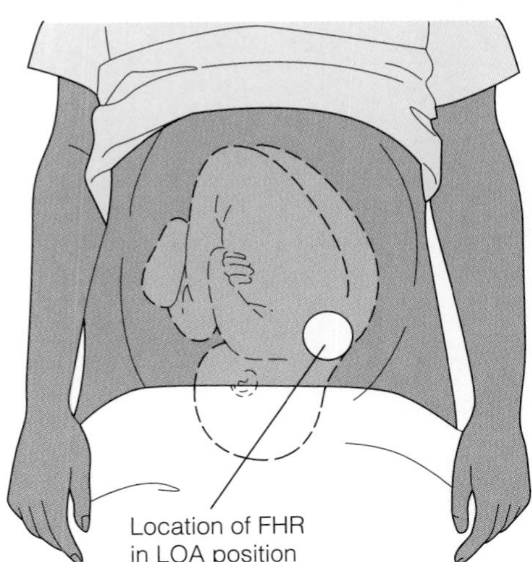

FIGURE 16–6 Location of FHR in relation to the more commonly seen fetal positions.

KEY FACTS TO REMEMBER

Frequency of Auscultation: Assessment and Documentation

Low-Risk Patients	High-Risk Patients
First Stage of Labor: q1h in latent phase q30min in active phase	First Stage of Labor q 30 min in latent phase q 15 min in active phase
Second Stage of Labor: q15min	Second Stage of Labor: q 5 min

Labor Events

Assess FHR prior to:
initiation of labor-enhancing procedures (eg, artificial rupture of membranes)
periods of ambulation
administration of medications
administration or initiation of analgesia/anesthesia

Assess FHR following:
rupture of membranes
recognition of abnormal uterine activity patterns, such as increased resting tone or contraction frequency < 2 min
evaluation of oxytocin (maintenance, increase, or decrease of dosage)
administration of medications (at time of peak action)
expulsion of enema
urinary catheterization
vaginal examination
periods of ambulation
evaluation of analgesia and/or anesthesia (maintenance, increase, or decrease of dosage)

Source: *NAACOG OGN Nursing Practice Resource, Fetal Heart Rate Auscultation,* March 1990. Washington, DC: NAACOG p 5; *AAP, AACOG Guidelines for Perinatal Care,* 1992.

Methods of Electronic Monitoring of FHR *External monitoring* of the fetus is usually accomplished by ultrasound. A transducer, which emits continuous sound waves, is placed on the maternal abdomen. When placed correctly, the sound waves bounce off the fetal heart and are picked up by the electronic monitor. The actual moment-by-moment FHR is displayed graphically on a screen (Figure 16–8 on page 380; see also Procedure 16–3 on page 381).

Recent advances in technology have led to the development of new ambulatory methods of external monitoring. Using a telemetry system, a small, battery-operated transducer transmits signals to a receiver connected to the monitor. This system, which is held in place with a shoulder strap, allows the woman to ambulate, helping her to feel more comfortable and less confined during labor. In contrast, the system depicted in Figure 16–8 requires the woman to remain confined, usually in bed.

Internal monitoring requires an internal spiral electrode. In order to place the spiral electrode on the fetal occiput, the amniotic membranes must be ruptured, the

Text continues on page 380

PROCEDURE 16–2 Auscultating Fetal Heart Rate

Nursing Action	Rationale
Objective: Assemble the equipment.	
• Obtain a fetoscope, which amplifies sound, or a Doppler, which uses ultrasound.	These devices amplify the fetal heart rate sounds.
Objective: Prepare the woman.	
• Explain the procedure, the indications for the procedure, and the information that will be obtained.	Explanation of the procedure decreases anxiety and increases relaxation.
• Uncover the woman's abdomen.	
Objective: Use the fetoscope or Doppler as indicated on the facing page and listen carefully for the FHR.	
Objective: Check the woman's pulse, then count the FHR.	
• Check the woman's pulse against the fetal sounds you hear. If the rates are the same, you have probably located maternal pulses and you need to readjust the fetoscope or ultrasound device.	
• If the rates are not similar, count the FHR for 1 full minute. Note that the fetal heart has a double rhythm and just one sound is counted.	
• If you do not find the FHR, move the fetoscope or ultrasound device laterally.	
• Explain to the parents what the FHR is and offer to help them listen if they would like to.	
Objective: Systematically evaluate the FHR.	
• Auscultate between, during, and for 30 seconds following a uterine contraction.	This evaluation provides the opportunity to assess the fetal status and response to the labor process.
NAACOG (1990) Frequency Recommendations Low-risk women: every 1 hour in the latent phase; every 30 minutes in the active phase, and every 15 minutes in the second stage. High-risk women: every 30 minutes in the latent phase, every 15 minutes in the active phase, and every 5 minutes in the second stage.	
Objective: Record the information on the woman's chart.	
• Document FHR data (rate and rhythm), characteristics of uterine activity, and any actions taken as a result of the FHR. Complete documentation is mandatory.	
Sample recordings are shown below.	

Sample Documentation

Sample entry documenting FHR, rhythm, and response to the labor process:

1-1-99 0730 FHR 140 by auscultation, regular rhythm. Maternal pulse 78. UC q3min × 60 sec strong. No increase or decrease in FHR noted during or following UC. J Smith RN

Sample entry documenting FHR, response to UC, nursing intervention, and fetal response:

1-1-99 0730 FHR 136 by auscultation with slowing to 130 bpm noted during the acme of UC and for 10 sec following the UC, STV present, LTV average. Client turned to left side. Maternal pulse 80, FHR 140, regular rhythm with no decrease during or following the next two UC. UC q3min × 60 sec strong. J Smith RN

PROCEDURE 16–2 continued

Using a Fetoscope or a Doppler Ultrasound Device

The Fetoscope

The fetoscope is an older assessment tool; however, some clinicians prefer it because it is "natural" and does not rely on ultrasound.

To use the fetoscope:

- Place the metal band of the fetoscope on your head; the diaphragm should extend out from your forehead.
- Place the diaphragm on the woman's abdomen halfway between the umbilicus and symphysis and in the midline. *You are most likely to hear the FHR in this area.*
- Without touching the fetoscope, listen carefully for the FHR (Figure 16–7*A*).

The Doppler

To use the Doppler:

- Place "ultrasonic gel" on the diaphragm of the Doppler. *Gel is used to maintain contact with the maternal abdomen and enhances conduction of ultrasound.*
- Place the diaphragm on the woman's abdomen halfway between the umbilicus and symphysis and in the midline. *You are most likely to hear the FHR in this area.*
- Listen carefully for the FHR (Figure 16–7*B*).

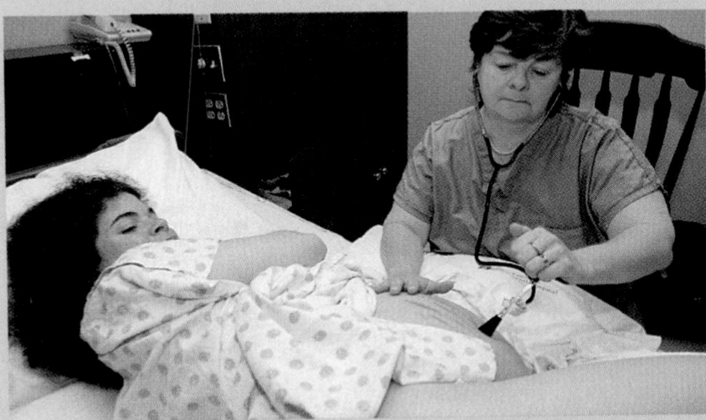

A

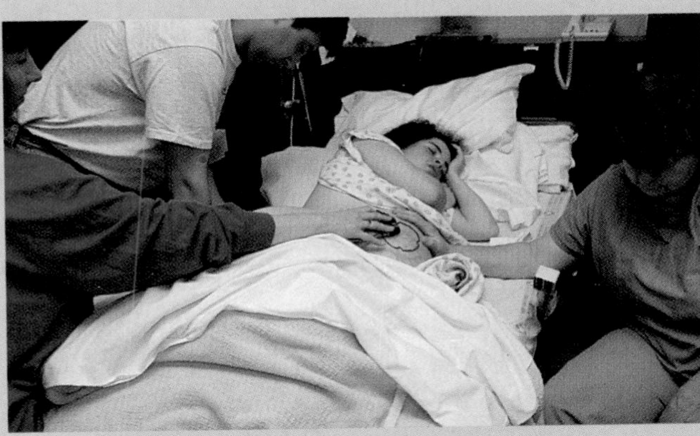

B

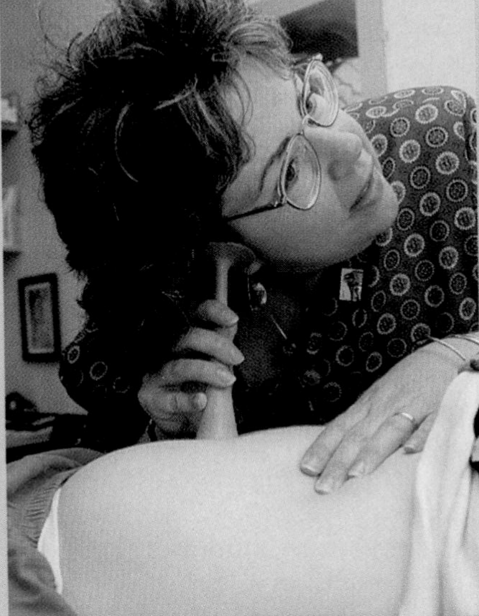

C

FIGURE 16–7 ***A*** The nurse holds the fetoscope as she places it against the maternal abdomen and then removes her fingers from the fetoscope while counting the fetal heartbeats. ***B*** When the fetal heart rate is picked up by the electronic monitor, the sound of the heartbeat can be heard by all persons in the room. ***C*** The Penar fetoscope can be easily used in outpatient or community settings.

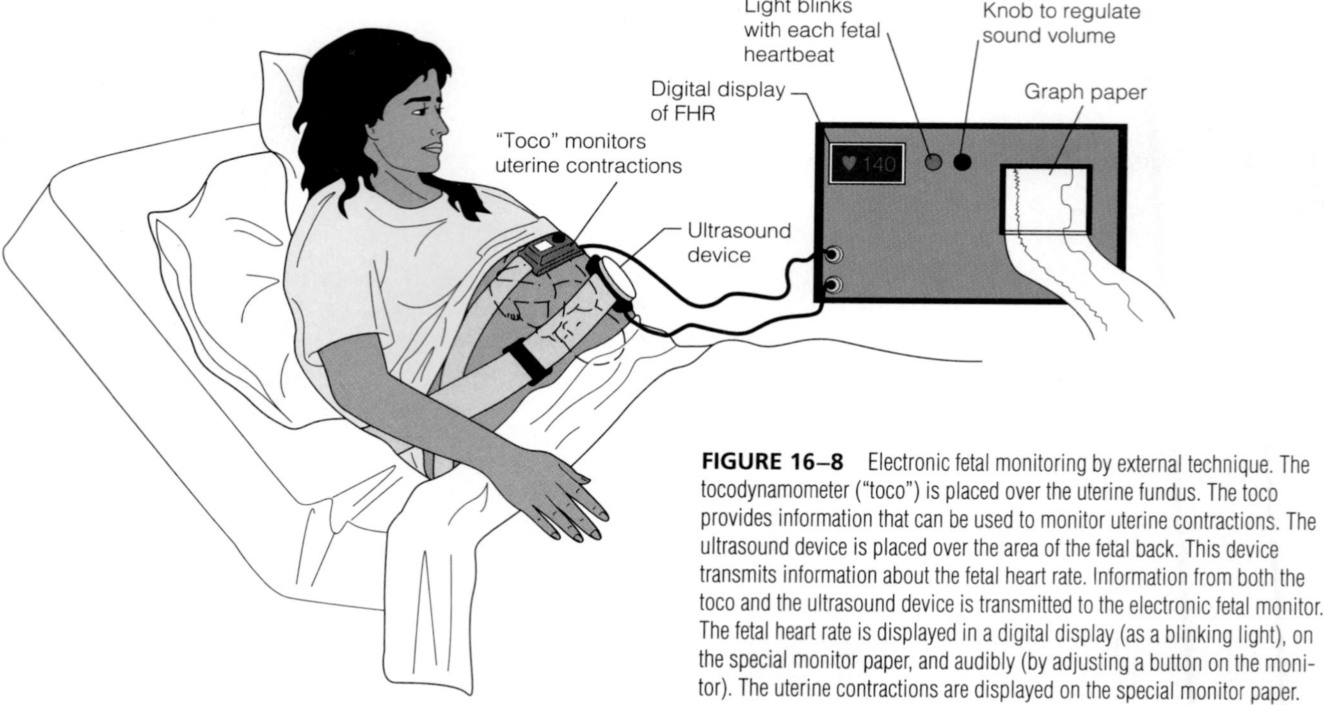

FIGURE 16–8 Electronic fetal monitoring by external technique. The tocodynamometer ("toco") is placed over the uterine fundus. The toco provides information that can be used to monitor uterine contractions. The ultrasound device is placed over the area of the fetal back. This device transmits information about the fetal heart rate. Information from both the toco and the ultrasound device is transmitted to the electronic fetal monitor. The fetal heart rate is displayed in a digital display (as a blinking light), on the special monitor paper, and audibly (by adjusting a button on the monitor). The uterine contractions are displayed on the special monitor paper.

cervix must be dilated at least 2 cm, the presenting part must be down against the cervix, and the presenting part must be known (ie, the nurse must be able to detect the actual part of the fetus that is down against the cervix). If all these factors are present, the labor and birth nurse, or the physician/certified nurse-midwife inserts a sterile internal spiral electrode into the vagina and places it against the fetal presenting part. The spiral electrode is rotated clockwise until it is attached to the presenting part. Wires that extend from the spiral electrode are attached to a leg plate (which is placed on the woman's thigh) and then attached to the electronic fetal monitor. This method of monitoring the FHR provides more accurate continuous data than external monitoring, because the signal is clearer and movement of the fetus or the woman does not interrupt it (Figure 16–9).

The FHR tracing at the top of Figure 16–10 was obtained by internal monitoring with a spiral electrode; the uterine contraction tracing at the bottom of the figure was obtained by external monitoring with a toco. Note the FHR is variable (the tracing moves up and down instead of in a straight line), and the tracing stays close to the line numbered 150. If the graph paper moves through the monitor at 3 cm/min, each vertical dark line represents 1 minute. The frequency of the uterine contractions (from the beginning of one contraction to the beginning of the next) is every 2½–3 minutes. The duration (length of each contraction) is 50–60 seconds.

FHR is evaluated by assessing an electronic monitor tracing for baseline rate, baseline variability, and periodic changes.

Baseline Fetal Heart Rates The **baseline rate** refers to the average FHR observed during a 10-minute period of monitoring. Normal FHR (baseline rate) ranges from 120 to 160 beats per minute. There are two abnormal variations of the baseline rate—those above 160 bpm (tachycardia) and those below 120 bpm (bradycardia). Another change affecting the baseline is called variability, which is a change in FHR over a few seconds to a few minutes.

Fetal tachycardia is a sustained rate of 160–179 beats/min, and marked tachycardia is 180 beats/min or more. Causes of tachycardia include the following (Tucker 1992, p 67):

- Early fetal hypoxia, which leads to stimulation of the sympathetic system as the fetus compensates for reduced blood flow.
- Maternal fever, which accelerates the metabolism of the fetus.
- Parasympatholytic drugs, such as atropine or Vistaril, which block the parasympathetic nervous system.
- Betasympathomimetic drugs such as ritodrine and isoxsuprine, which have a cardiac stimulant effect.
- Amnionitis. (Metabolism of fetal myocardium is accelerated due to increased maternal temperature.

PROCEDURE 16–3 Electronic Fetal Monitoring

Nursing Action	Rationale
Objective: Prepare the woman.	
• Explain the procedure, the indications for the procedure, and the information that will be obtained.	Explanation of the procedure decreases anxiety and increases relaxation.
Objective: Place the external fetal monitor.	
• Turn on the monitor.	
• Place two elastic belts around the woman's abdomen.	
• Place the "toco" over the uterine fundus in the midline and secure it with a belt so that it fits snugly.	The uterine fundus is the area of greatest contractility.
• Note the UC tracing. The resting tone tracing (without uterine contraction) should be recording on the 10 or 15 mm Hg pressure line.	If the tracing is on the zero line, there may be a constant grinding noise.
• Apply ultrasonic gel to the diaphragm of the ultrasound transducer.	Ultrasound gel is used to maintain contact with the maternal abdomen. The ultrasonic beam is directed toward the fetal heart.
• Place the diaphragm on the maternal abdomen in the midline between the umbilicus and the symphysis pubis.	
• Listen for the FHR, which will have a whip-like sound. When the FHR is located, attach the elastic belt snugly. Firm contact is necessary to maintain a continuous tracing.	
Objective: Identify the tracing. Place the following information on the beginning of the fetal monitor paper: date, time, client name, gravida, para, membrane status, physician/CNM name. Note: Each birthing area may have specific guidelines regarding additional information to include.	Ensures accurate identification.
Objective: Evaluate the EFM tracing. See the material below for evaluation guidelines.	
Objective: Report and record your findings.	Provides a permanent record.

Sample Documentation

Documenting reassuring FHR characteristics and response to UCs:

1-1-99 0700 FHR BL 135–140. STV and LTV present. Two accelerations of 20 bpm × 20 sec with fetal movement in 10 min. UC q3min × 50–60 sec of moderate intensity by palpation. No decelerations noted.

Documenting FHR rate, presence of variability, response of FHR to UC, the intervention used, and subsequent positive fetal response to the intervention.

0730 FHR BL 135–140. STV and LTV present. Late decelerations noted with decrease of FHR to 130 bpm for 20 sec. UC q3min × 50–60 sec of moderate intensity by palpation. Client turned to left side. No further deceleration with three subsequent UC. Two accelerations of 20 bpm × 20 sec noted with fetal movement. Client instructed to remain of left side.

Guidelines for Evaluating the EFM

Evaluation of the EFM tracing provides an opportunity to assess the fetal status and response to the labor process. The presence of reassuring characteristics is associated with good fetal outcome. Rapid identification of nonreassuring characteristics allows prompt interventions and the opportunity to determine the fetal response to the interventions.

For high-risk women, NAACOG (1988) recommends evaluating the EFM tracing every 15 minutes in the first stage, and every 5 minutes in the second stage. For low-risk women, specific time intervals have not been recommended by NAACOG (now known as AWHONN). However, evaluation every 15–30 minutes in the first stage and every 5–15 minutes in the second stage (as long as the FHR has reassuring characteristics) is frequently done. The time interval for evaluation needs to be shortened if any nonreassuring characteristics occur.

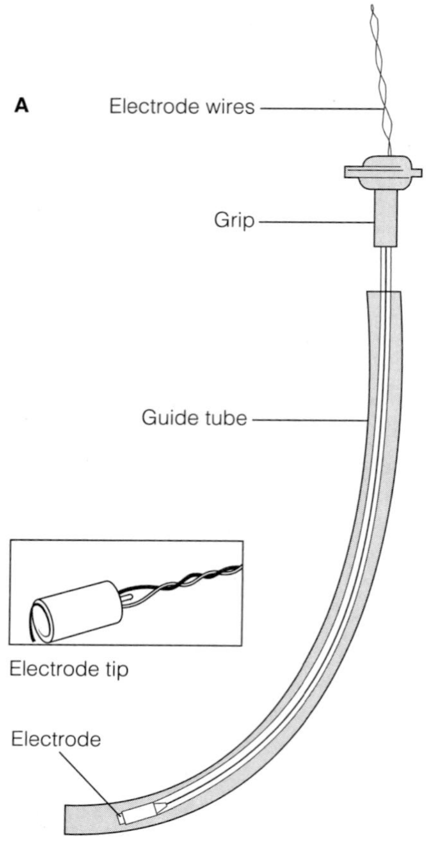

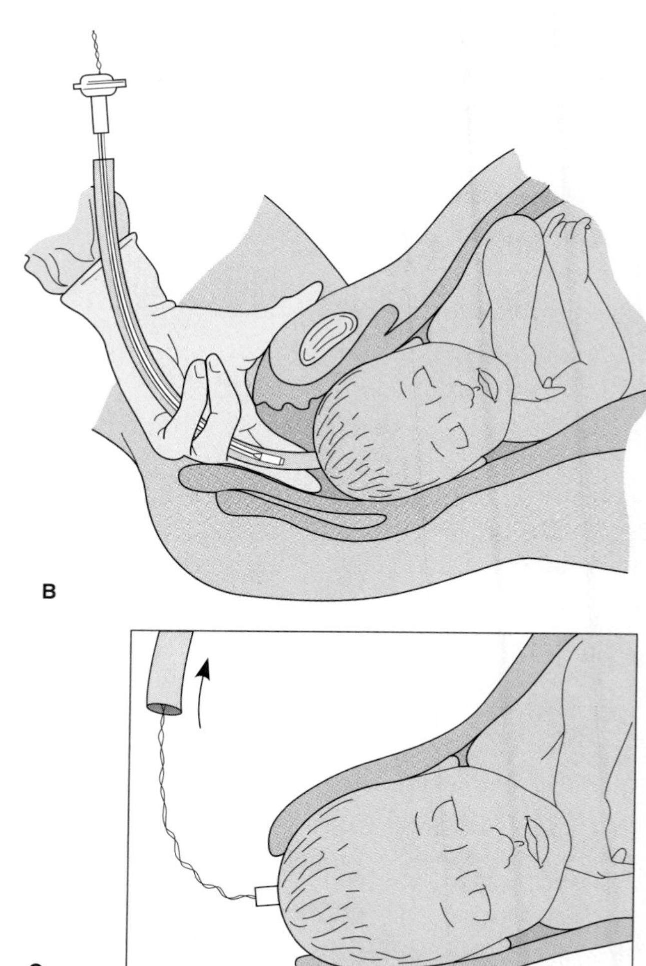

FIGURE 16–9 Technique for internal, direct fetal monitoring. ***A*** Spiral electrode. ***B*** Attaching the spiral electrode to the scalp. ***C*** Attached spiral electrode with the guide tube removed.

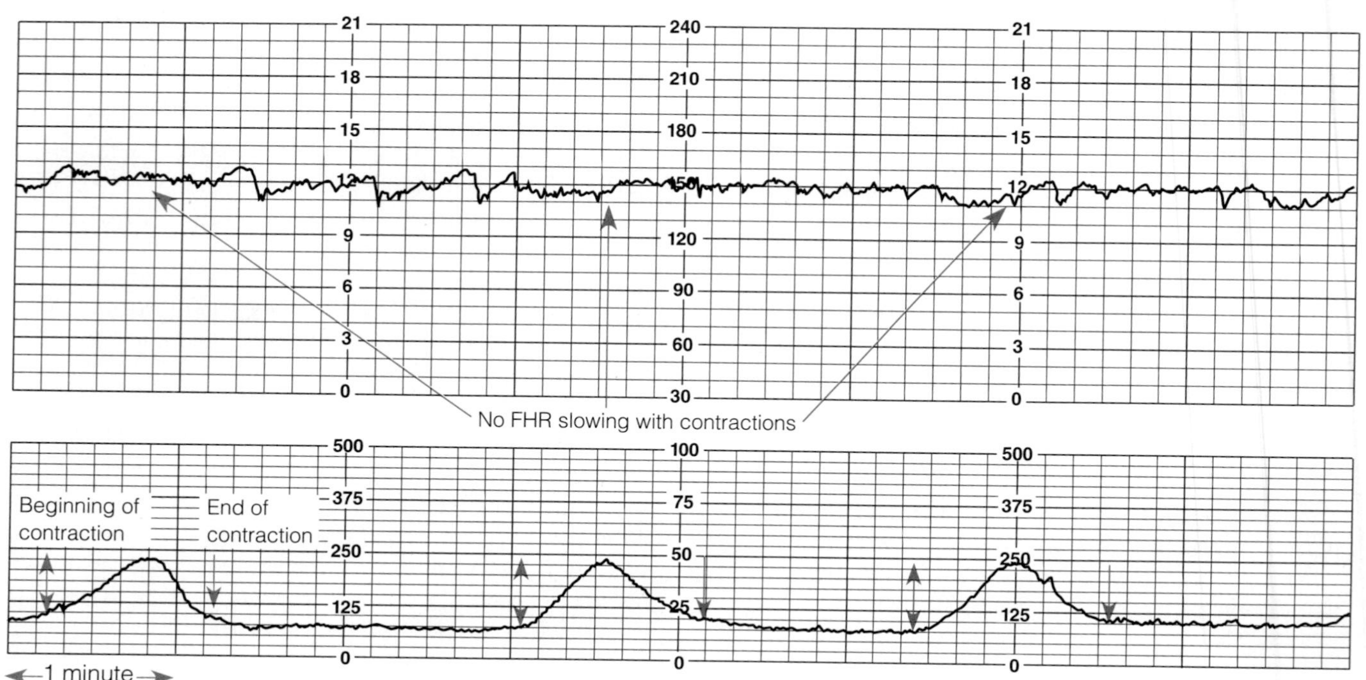

FIGURE 16–10 Normal fetal heart rate pattern obtained by internal monitoring. Note normal FHR, 140–158 beats/min, presence of long- and short-term variability, and absence of deceleration with adequate contractions. Arrows on bottom of tracing indicate beginnings of uterine contractions.

Intrauterine temperature is higher than maternal body temperature, so fetal tachycardia may be the first sign of developing intrauterine infection [Murray 1989].)

- Maternal hyperthyroidism. (Thyroid-stimulating hormones may cross the placenta and stimulate fetal heart rate.)
- Fetal anemia. (Heart rate is increased as compensatory mechanism to improve tissue perfusion.)

Tachycardia is considered an ominous sign if it is accompanied by other FHR patterns such as late deceleration, severe variable decelerations, or decreased variability (Tucker 1992). If tachycardia is associated with maternal fever, treatment may consist of antipyretics and cooling measures.

Fetal bradycardia is a rate less than 120 beats/min during a 10-minute period. Mild bradycardia ranges from 100 to 119 beats/min and is considered benign. Moderate bradycardia is less than 100 beats/min, and marked bradycardia is less than 70 beats/min. Causes of fetal bradycardia include the following (Tucker 1992, p 70):

- Late (profound) fetal hypoxia. (There is depression of myocardial activity.)
- Maternal hypotension. (Maternal hypotension results in decreased blood flow to fetus.)
- Prolonged umbilical cord compression. (Fetal baroceptors are activated by cord compression and this produces vagal stimulation, which results in decreased FHR.)
- Fetal arrhythmia, which is associated with complete heart block in the fetus.

Bradycardia may be a benign or ominous (preterminal) sign. If there is average long-term variability, the bradycardia is considered benign. When bradycardia is accompanied by decreased long-term variability and late decelerations, it is considered ominous and a sign of advanced fetal distress (Tucker 1992).

Baseline Variability Baseline variability is a measure of the interplay (the "push-pull" effect) between the sympathetic and parasympathetic nervous systems. There are two types of fetal heart variability—short term and long term. *Short-term variability* is the beat-to-beat change in FHR. It represents fluctuations of the baseline. Short-term variability is classified as either present or absent. *Long-term variability* is the waviness or rhythmic fluctuations (called cycles) of the FHR tracing, which occur from 3 to 5 cycles per minute. Variability can be classified as none, minimal, average, moderate, or marked (Figure 16–11). The most important aspect of variability is that, even in the presence of abnormal or questionable FHR patterns, if the variability is normal, the fetus is not suffering from cerebral asphyxia (Tucker 1992).

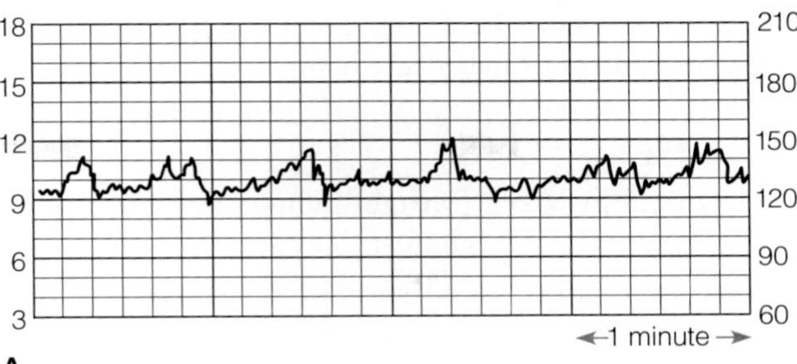

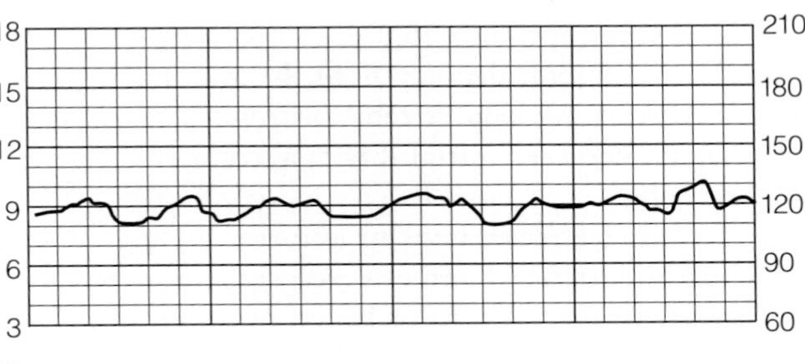

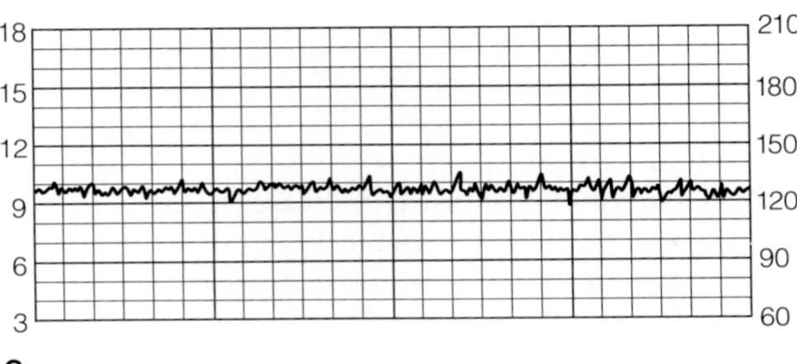

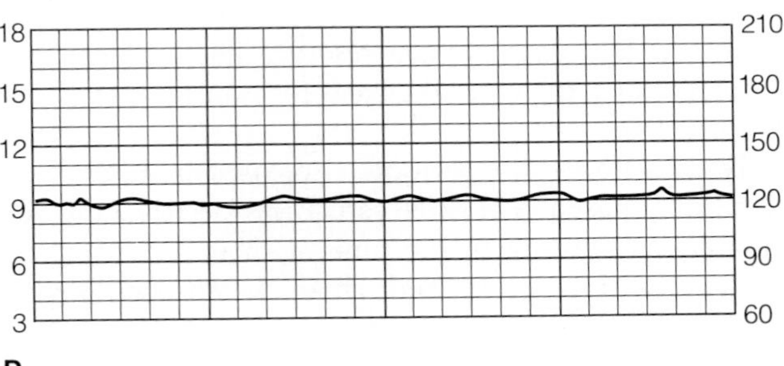

FIGURE 16–11 Short- and long-term variability. ***A*** Increased LTV; STV present. ***B*** Average LTV; STV absent. ***C*** Absent LTV; STV present. ***D*** Absent LTV; STV absent.

Causes of decreased variability include the following (Tucker 1992, p 75):

- Hypoxia and acidosis (decreased blood flow to the fetus).
- Administration of drugs such as Demerol, Valium, or Vistaril, which depress the fetal central nervous system.
- Fetal sleep cycle. (During fetal sleep, long-term variability is decreased. Fetal sleep cycles usually last for 20–30 minutes.)

- Fetus of less than 32 weeks' gestation. (Fetal neurological control of heart rate is immature.)

Causes of increased variability include the following (Tucker 1992, p 74):

- Early mild hypoxia. (Variability increases as result of compensatory mechanism.)
- Fetal stimulation (stimulation of autonomic nervous system because of abdominal palpation, maternal vaginal examination, application of spiral electrode on fetal head, or acoustic stimulation).

Decreasing variability that does not appear to be associated with a fetal sleep cycle or the administration of drugs is a warning sign of fetal distress. It is especially ominous if decreased variability is accompanied by late decelerations.

External electronic fetal monitoring is not an adequate method to assess and evaluate short-term variability. If decreased variability is noted on monitoring, application of a spiral electrode should be considered to obtain more accurate information.

Periodic Changes Periodic changes are transient decelerations or accelerations of the FHR from the baseline. They usually occur in response to uterine contractions and fetal movement.

Accelerations are transient increases in the FHR normally caused by fetal movement. When the fetus moves, its heart rate increases, just as the heart rates of adults increase during exercise. Often accelerations accompany uterine contractions, usually due to fetal movement in response to the pressure of the contractions. Accelerations of this type are thought to be a sign of fetal well-being and adequate oxygen reserve. The accelerations with fetal movement are the basis for nonstress tests (see Chapter 14).

Decelerations are periodic decreases in FHR from the normal baseline in three categories—early, late, and variable—according to the time of their occurrence in the contraction cycle and their waveform (Figure 16–12). When the fetal head is compressed, cerebral blood flow is decreased, which leads to central vagal stimulation and results in **early deceleration.** The onset of early deceleration occurs before the onset of the uterine contraction. This type of deceleration is of uniform shape, is usually considered benign, and does not require intervention (see Figure 16–13*A* on page 386).

Late deceleration is caused by uteroplacental insufficiency resulting from decreased blood flow and oxygen transfer to the fetus through the intervillous spaces during uterine contractions. The onset of the deceleration occurs after the onset of the uterine contraction and is of a uniform shape that tends to reflect associated uterine contractions. The late deceleration pattern is considered a nonreassuring sign but does not necessarily require immediate delivery (Figure 16–13*B* on page 386).

Variable decelerations occur if the umbilical cord becomes compressed, thus reducing blood flow between the placenta and fetus. The resulting increase in peripheral resistance in the fetal circulation causes fetal hypertension. The fetal hypertension stimulates the baroreceptors in the aortic arch and carotid sinuses, which slow the FHR. The onset of variable decelerations varies in timing with the onset of the contraction and they are variable in shape. This pattern requires further assessment (Figure 16–13*C* on page 387).

Nursing interventions for late and variable decelerations in FHR are presented in Table 16–2 on page 388).

Sinusoidal pattern appears similar to a wave form. The characteristics of this pattern include presence of long-term variability, absence of short-term variability, and no accelerations with fetal movement. This pattern is associated with Rh isoimmunization, fetal anemia, and a chronic fetal bleed. It may also occur with the administration of meperidine (Demerol), alphaprodine (Nisentil), and butorphanol tartrate (Stadol). When it occurs in association with medication, the pattern is usually temporary (Tucker 1992) (see Figure 16–13*D* on page 387).

Psychologic Reactions to Electronic Monitoring

Women have many different reactions to electronic monitoring. Many women have little knowledge of monitoring unless they have attended a prenatal class that dealt with this subject. Molfese, Sunshine, and Bennett (1982) found a variety of reactions to fetal monitoring. Some women react to electronic monitoring positively, viewing it as a reassurance that "the baby is OK." They may also feel that the monitor will help identify problems that develop in labor. Other women may have negative feelings about the monitor. They may think that the monitor is interfering with a natural process, and they do not want the intrusion. They may resent the time and attention that the monitor requires, time that could otherwise be spent providing nursing care. Some women may find that the equipment, wires, and sounds increase their anxiety. The discomfort of lying in one position and fear of injury to the baby are other objections (Molfese et al 1982).

Nursing Responsibilities Before applying the monitor, the nurse should fully explain the reason for its use and the information that it can provide. After the monitor is applied, basic information is recorded on a label attached to the monitor strip. The data include the date, client's name, physician/CNM, hospital number, age, gravida, para, EDB, membrane status, and maternal vital signs. As the monitor strip continues to run and care is provided, occurrences during labor should be recorded not only in the medical record but also on the monitor strip. This information helps the health care team assess current status and evaluate the tracing.

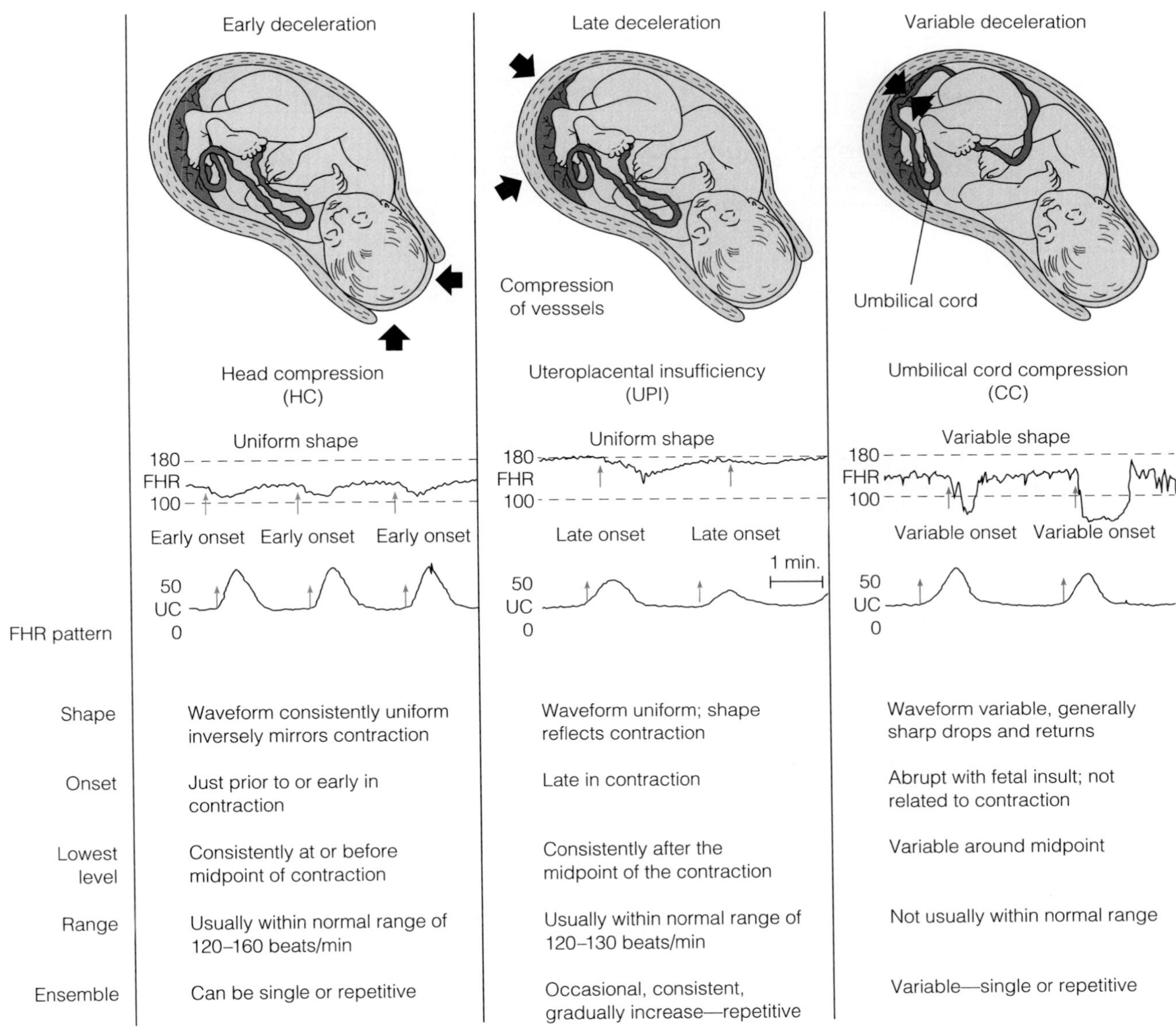

FIGURE 16–12 Types and characteristics of early, late, and variable decelerations.
Source: Hon E: *An Introduction to Fetal Heart Rate Monitoring,* 2nd ed. Los Angeles: University of Southern California School of Medicine, 1976, p 29.

The following information should be included on the tracing (AAP & ACOG 1992):

1. Vaginal examination (dilatation, effacement, station, and position)
2. Amniotomy or spontaneous rupture of membranes, color of amniotic fluid
3. Maternal vital signs
4. Maternal position in bed and changes of position
5. Application of spiral electrode or intrauterine pressure catheter
6. Medications
7. Oxygen administration
8. Maternal behaviors (emesis, coughing, hiccups)
9. Fetal scalp stimulation or fetal scalp blood sampling
10. Vomiting
11. Pushing
12. Administration of anesthesia blocks

In addition, if the monitor does not automatically add the time on the strip at specific intervals, it is important to note the time when recording any information on the strip. If more than one nurse is adding information to the monitor strip, it is wise to initial each note. The tracing is considered a legal part of the

Text continues on page 388

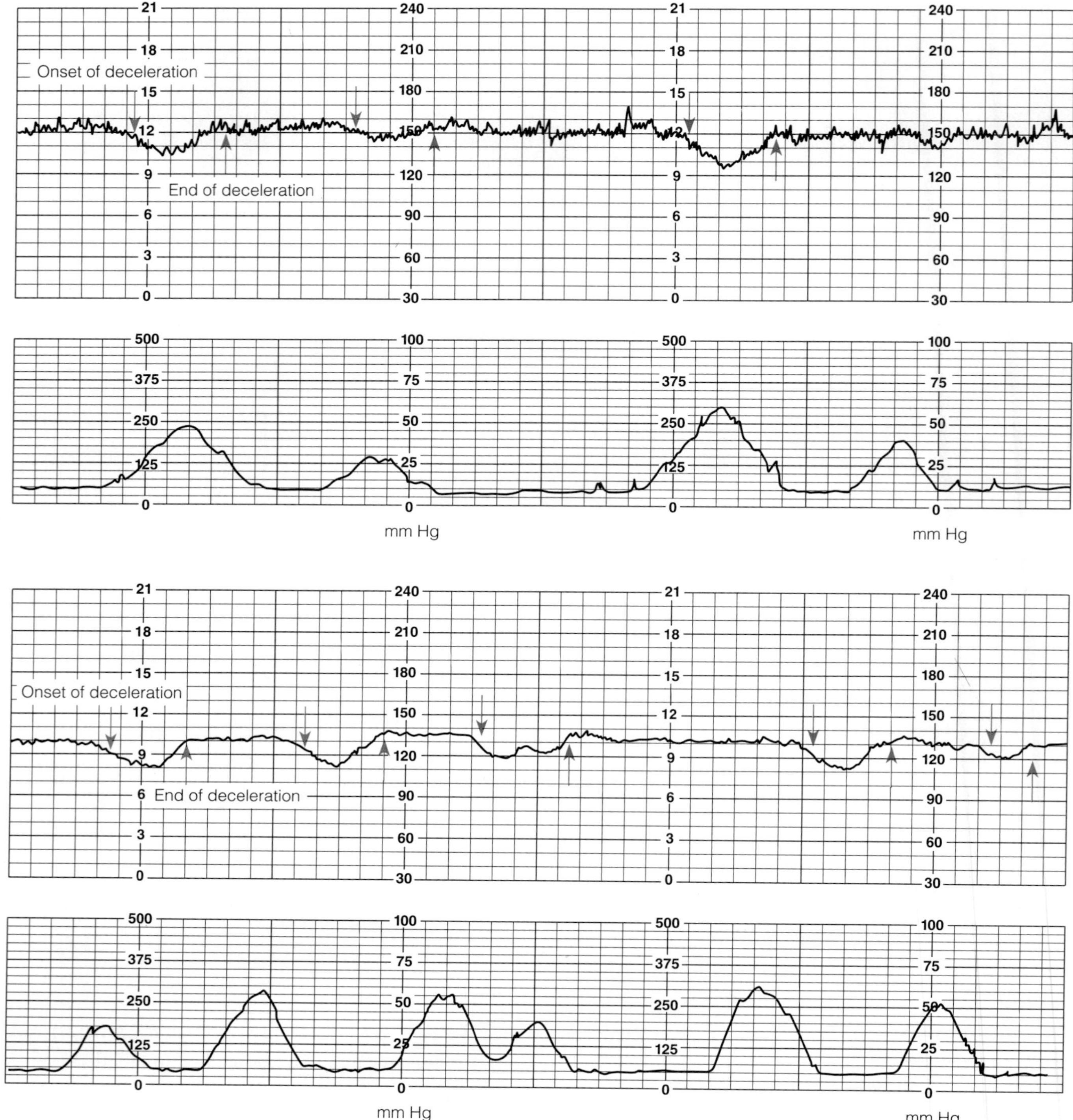

FIGURE 16–13 Types of decelerations: ***A*** Early decelerations. ***B*** Late decelerations.

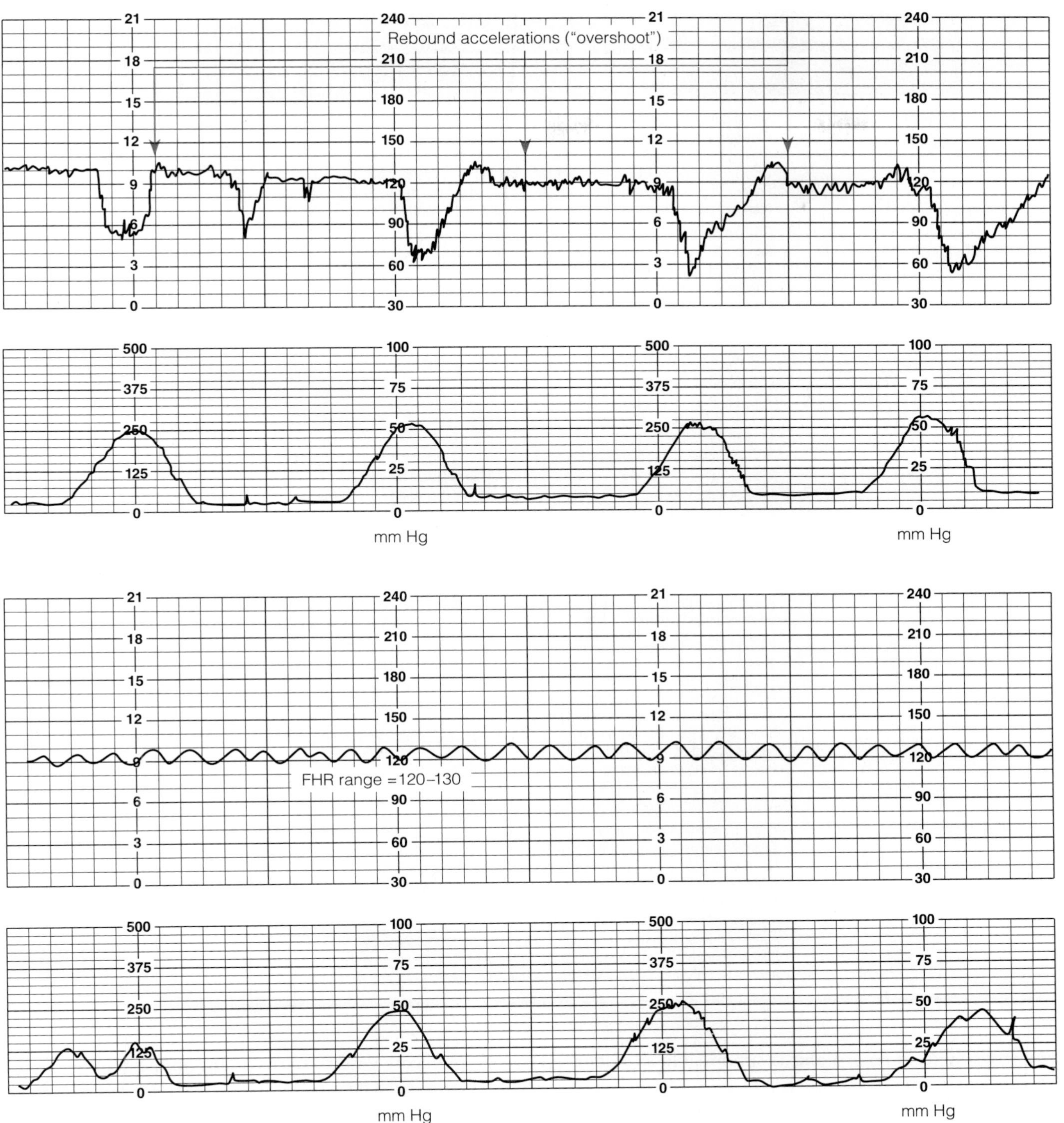

FIGURE 16–13 continued ***C*** Variable decelerations with overshoot. The timing of the decelerations is variable and most have a sharp decline. An acceleration (overshoot) occurs after most of the decelerations. ***D*** Sinusoidal pattern.

TABLE 16–2 Guidelines for Management of Variable, Late, and Prolonged Deceleration Patterns

Pattern	Nursing Interventions
Variable decelerations Isolated or occasional Moderate	Report findings to physician/CNM and document in chart. Provide explanation to woman and partner. Change maternal position to one in which FHR pattern is most improved. Discontinue oxytocin if it is being administered and other interventions are unsuccessful. Perform vaginal examination to assess for prolapsed cord or change in labor progress. Monitor FHR continuously to assess current status and for further changes in FHR pattern.
Variable decelerations Severe and uncorrectable	Give oxygen if indicated. Report findings to physician/CNM and document in chart. Provide explanation to woman and partner. Prepare for probable cesarean birth. Follow interventions listed above. Prepare for vaginal birth unless baseline variability is decreasing and/or FHR is progressively rising—then cesarean, forceps, or vacuum birth is indicated. Assist physician with fetal scalp sampling if ordered. Prepare for cesarean birth if scalp pH shows acidosis or downward trend.
Late decelerations	Give oxygen if indicated. Report findings to physician/CNM and document in chart. Provide explanation to woman and partner. Monitor for further FHR changes. Maintain maternal position on left side. Maintain good hydration with IV fluids (normal saline or lactated Ringer's). Discontinue oxytocin if it is being administered and late decelerations persist despite other interventions. Administer oxygen by face mask at 7–10 L/minute. Monitor maternal blood pressure and pulse for signs of hypotension; possibly increase flow rate of IV fluids to treat hypotension. Follow physician's orders for treatment for hypotension if present. Increase IV fluids to maintain volume and hydration (normal saline or lactated Ringer's). Assess labor progress (dilatation and station). Assist physician with fetal blood sampling: If pH stays above 7.25, physician will continue monitoring and resample; if pH shows downward trend (between 7.25 and 7.20) or is below 7.20, prepare for birth by most expeditious means.
Late decelerations with tachycardia and/or decreasing variability	Report findings to physician/CNM and document in chart. Maintain maternal position on left side. Administer oxygen by face mask at 7–10 L/minute. Discontinue oxytocin if it is being administered. Assess maternal blood pressure and pulse. Increase IV fluids (normal saline or lactated Ringer's). Assess labor progress (dilatation and station). Prepare for immediate cesarean birth. Explain plan of treatment to woman and partner. Assist physician with fetal blood sampling (if ordered).
Prolonged decelerations	Perform vaginal examination to rule out prolapsed cord or to determine progress in labor status. Change maternal position as needed to try to alleviate decelerations. Discontinue oxytocin if it is being administered. Notify physician/CNM of findings/initial interventions and document in chart. Provide explanation to woman and partner. Increase IV fluids (normal saline or lactated Ringer's). Administer tocolytic if hypertonus noted and ordered by physician/CNM. Anticipate normal FHR recovery following deceleration if FHR previously normal. Anticipate intervention if FHR previously abnormal or deceleration lasts > 3 minutes.

woman's medical record and is submissible as evidence in court.

It is important for the laboring woman to feel that what is happening to her is the central focus. The nurse can acknowledge this by always speaking to and looking at the woman when entering the room, before looking at the monitor.

Evaluation of FHR Tracings The nurse needs to use a systematic approach in evaluating FHR tracings to avoid interpreting findings on the basis of inadequate or erroneous data. With a systematic approach, the nurse can make a more accurate and rapid assessment; easily communicate data to the woman, physician/CNM, and staff; and have a systematic, universal language for documenting the woman's record.

Evaluation of the electronic monitor tracing begins by looking at the uterine contraction pattern. To evaluate the contraction pattern, the nurse should

1. Determine the uterine resting tone.
2. Assess the contractions:

   What is the frequency?

   What is the duration?

   What is the intensity (if internal monitoring)?

The next step is to evaluate the fetal heart rate tracing.

1. Determine the baseline:

    Is the baseline within normal range?

    Is there evidence of tachycardia?

    Is there evidence of bradycardia?

2. Determine FHR variability:

    Is short-term variability present or absent?

    Is long-term variability average? Minimal? Absent? Moderate? Marked?

3. Is a sinusoidal pattern present?
4. Are there periodic changes?

    Are accelerations present?

    Do they meet the criteria for a reactive NST?

    Are decelerations present?

    Are they uniform in shape? If so, determine if they are early or late decelerations.

    Are they nonuniform in shape? If so, determine whether they are variable decelerations.

After evaluating the FHR tracing for the factors just listed, the nurse may further classify the tracing as reassuring (normal) or nonreassuring (worrisome). Reassuring patterns contain normal parameters and do not require additional treatment or intervention.

Characteristics of reassuring FHR patterns include the following:

- Baseline rate is 120–160 bpm.
- Short-term variability is present.
- Long-term variability ranges from 3 to 5 cycles per minute.
- Periodic patterns consist of accelerations with fetal movement, and early decelerations may be present.

Nonreassuring patterns indicate that the fetus is becoming stressed and intervention is needed. Characteristics of nonreassuring patterns include the following:

- Severe variable decelerations. (FHR drops below 70 bpm for longer than 30–45 seconds and is accompanied by rising baseline or decreasing variability or slow return to baseline.)
- Late decelerations of any magnitude.
- Absence of variability. (No short-term or long-term variability is present.)
- Prolonged deceleration (a deceleration that lasts 60–90 seconds or more).
- Severe (marked) bradycardia (FHR baseline of 70 bpm or less).

Nonreassuring patterns may require continuous monitoring and more involved treatment and intervention (see Table 16–2).

It is important to provide information to the laboring woman regarding the FHR pattern and the interventions that will help her fetus. Most women are aware that something is happening, and sharing information with them provides reassurance that a potential or actual problem is identified and that she is an active participant in the interventions. Occasionally a problem arises that requires immediate intervention. In that case, the nurse can say something like "It is important for you to turn on your left side right now because the baby is having a little difficulty. I'll explain what is happening in just a few moments." This type of response lets the woman know that although an action needs to be accomplished rapidly, information will soon be provided. In our haste to act quickly, we must not forget that it is the woman's body and her baby.

Scalp Stimulation Test

When there is a question regarding fetal status, a scalp stimulation test can be used before the more invasive fetal blood sampling. To use this technique, the examiner applies pressure to the fetal scalp while doing a vaginal examination. The fetus who is not in any stress or distress responds with an acceleration of the FHR (Cunningham et al 1997).

Fetal Scalp Blood Sampling

When nonreassuring or confusing FHR patterns are noted, additional information about the acid-base status of the fetus is needed. This may be accomplished by **fetal blood sampling.** The physician usually draws the blood sample from the fetal scalp but may obtain it from the fetus in the breech position.

Before fetal blood can be sampled, the membranes must be ruptured, the cervix must be dilated at least 2–3 cm, and the presenting part must not be above −2 station. Sampling is not done when FHR patterns are ominous. It is contraindicated in acute emergencies and in cases of vaginal bleeding. In these instances, birth by the most expeditious means is indicated.

Normal fetal pH values during labor are at or above 7.25, with 7.20–7.24 considered preacidotic. Values below 7.20 indicate serious acidosis.

The more information is available from FHR monitoring, the less need there is for taking a fetal blood sample. Only when FHR patterns are uninterpretable, worsening, or suggestive of high risk is this adjunctive procedure indicated. Fetal blood sampling may prevent unnecessary cesarean birth. Fetal blood sampling and electronic fetal monitoring are complementary tools. They give the certified nurse-midwife/physician the knowledge to make appropriate decisions about intervention or nonintervention.

CHAPTER HIGHLIGHTS

- Intrapartal assessment includes attention to both physical and psychosociocultural parameters of the laboring woman, assessment of the fetus, and ongoing assessment for conditions that place the woman and her fetus at increased risk.
- A sterile vaginal examination determines status of fetal membranes; cervical dilatation and effacement; and fetal presentation, position, and station.
- Uterine contractions may be assessed by palpation or by an electronic monitor. The electronic monitor may be used for external or internal monitoring.
- Leopold's maneuvers provide a systematic evaluation of fetal presentation and position.
- Fetal presentation and position may also be assessed by vaginal examination or ultrasound.
- The fetal heart rate may be assessed by auscultation (with a fetoscope) or electronic monitoring.
- Electronic fetal monitoring is accomplished by indirect ultrasound or by direct methods that require the placement of a spiral electrode on the fetal presenting part.
- Indications for electronic monitoring include fetal, maternal, and uterine factors; presence of pregnancy complications; regional anesthesia; and elective monitoring.
- True variability of the FHR can be assessed only by direct electronic monitoring.
- Baseline FHR refers to the range of FHR observed between contractions, during a 10-minute period of monitoring.
- The normal range of FHR is 120–160 beats per minute.
- Baseline changes of the FHR include tachycardia, bradycardia, and variability.
- Tachycardia is defined as a rate of 160 beats per minute or more for a 10-minute segment of time.
- Bradycardia is defined as a rate of less than 120 beats per minute for a 10-minute segment of time.
- Baseline variability is an important parameter of fetal well-being. It includes both long- and short-term variability.
- Periodic changes are transient decelerations or accelerations of the FHR from the baseline. Accelerations are normally caused by fetal movement; decelerations may be termed early, late, variable, or sinusoidal.
- Early decelerations are due to compression of the fetal head during contractions and are considered reassuring.
- Late decelerations are associated with utero-placental insufficiency and are considered ominous.
- Variable decelerations are associated with compression of the umbilical cord.
- Sinusoidal patterns are characterized by an undulant sinewave.
- Psychologic reactions to monitoring vary between feelings of relief and feelings of being tied down.
- Birthing room nurses have responsibilities in recognizing and interpreting fetal monitoring patterns, notifying the physician/CNM of problems, and initiating corrective and supportive measures when needed.
- Scalp stimulation test can be used when there is a question about fetal status.
- Fetal acid-base status may be assessed by fetal blood sampling.

REFERENCES

Albers LL: Clinical issues in electronic fetal monitoring. *Birth* 1994; 21(2):108.

American Academy of Pediatrics and The American College of Obstetricians and Gynecologists: Guidelines for Perinatal Care, 2nd ed. Washington, DC, 1992.

Burian J: Helping survivors of sexual abuse through labor. *MCN* September/October 1995; 20:252.

Chez BF, Verklan MT: Documentation and electronic fetal monitoring: How, where, and what? *J Perinat Neonatol Nurs* July 1987; 1(1):22.

Cunningham FG et al: *Williams Obstetrics,* 20th ed. Stamford, CT: Appleton & Lange, 1997.

Johannsen JM: Update: Guidelines for treating hypertension. *AJN* March 1993; 93(3):42.

McFarland J, Parker B: Preventing abuse during pregnancy: An assessment and intervention protocol. *MCN* November/December 1994; 19:321.

Miller F: Fetal scalp stimulation. In: *Current Therapy in Obstetrics and Gynecology.* Quilligan EJ, Zuspan FP (editors). Philadelphia: Saunders, 1990.

Molfese V, Sunshine P, Bennett A: Reactions of women to intrapartum fetal monitoring. *Obstet Gynecol* 1982; 59(6):705.

Murray M: *Antepartal and Intrapartal Fetal Monitoring.* Washington, DC: NAACOG, 1989.

NAACOG: *Fetal Heart Rate Auscultation:* OGN Nursing Practice Resource. Washington, DC, March 1990.

NAACOG statement: *Nursing Responsibilities in Implementing Intrapartum Fetal Heart Rate Monitoring.* Washington, DC, October 1988.

Tucker SM: *Pocket Guide Fetal Monitoring.* St Louis: Mosby, 1992.

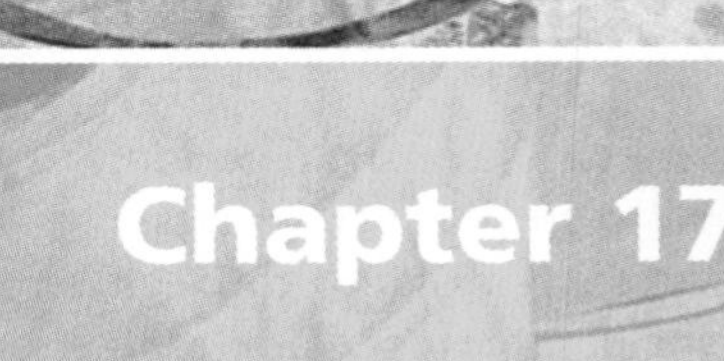

Chapter 17 The Family in Childbirth: Needs and Care

OBJECTIVES

- Identify the database to be created from information obtained when a woman is admitted to the birthing area.
- Review the nursing care that is given at admission.
- Discuss nursing interventions to meet the psychologic and physiologic needs of the woman during each stage of labor.
- Summarize the immediate needs of the newborn following birth.
- Delineate management of a precipitous birth.

KEY TERMS

Apgar score
Attachment
Birthing room
Hyperventilation
Lochia rubra
Nuchal cord
Precipitous birth
Prep

It is time for a child to be born. The waiting is over; labor has begun. The dreams and wishes of the past months fade as the expectant parents face the reality of the tasks of childbearing and childrearing that are ahead.

The parents are about to undergo one of the most meaningful and stressful events in their life together. The adequacy of their preparation for childbirth will now be tested. The coping mechanisms, communication, and support systems that they have established as a couple will be put to the test. In particular, the childbearing woman may feel that her psychologic and physical limits are about to be challenged.

The parents have also been involved in collecting information and making decisions about the setting for childbirth. Not many years ago, the only choice was an in-hospital labor unit with separate labor room, delivery room, and recovery area. This type of unit is still available in some hospitals. However, most hospitals have changed their labor and delivery units to reflect changing philosophies of family-centered childbirth. To capture this family-centered philosophy, the names of many labor and delivery departments have been changed to "birthing center" or "family birthing center."

Many birthing centers have single-purpose units, which means that the woman stays in the same room for labor, birth, recovery, and possibly the postpartal period. These rooms may be called LDR (labor, delivery, and recovery) or LDRPP (labor, delivery, recovery, and postpartum) to reflect the amount of time the woman spends in the room. When speaking to the public, birthing facility spokespersons tend to use the term **birthing room** instead of LDR or LDRPP.

The birthing room atmosphere is more relaxed and families seem to feel more comfortable. The laboring woman does not have to be transferred to another area for birth, and this increases her comfort and enhances the family's involvement in the birth. Birthing rooms usually have birthing beds that can be adapted for birth by removing a small section near the foot. Stirrups are available if needed or desired.

Maternal-newborn nursing has also kept pace with the changing philosophy of childbirth. Nurses who choose positions in a birthing area are presented with many opportunities to interact with a wide variety of situations, from a family that wants maximum participation to a single woman who enters alone. It is a challenge to provide high-level care in a relaxed atmosphere and supportive care to such a wide variety of clients and families.

The previous two chapters presented a database of information about physiologic and psychologic changes during labor and birth and needed nursing assessment. This chapter presents nursing care during labor and birth. The Intrapartal Critical Pathway starts on page 396.

Nursing Diagnosis During Labor and Birth

When a plan of care is devised for the intrapartal period, the nurse can develop a general plan that encompasses all of the process, from the beginning of labor through the fourth stage, or a plan can be developed for each stage of labor and birth. An overall plan presents an overview of the whole process, but it is usually general in nature. A plan of care that identifies nursing diagnoses for (at least) each stage provides an opportunity to identify more specific nursing care. In the first stage, nursing diagnoses that may be selected include

- Fear related to discomfort of labor and unknown labor outcome
- Ineffective individual coping related to labor process
- Pain related to uterine contractions, cervical dilatation, and fetal descent
- Knowledge deficit related to lack of information about normal labor process and comfort measures

Nursing diagnoses for the second and third stage may include

- Pain related to uterine contractions, birth process, and/or perineal trauma from birth
- Knowledge deficit related to lack of information about pushing methods before birth
- Ineffective individual coping related to birth process
- Fear related to outcome of birth process

In the fourth stage, possible nursing diagnoses include

- Pain related to perineal trauma
- Knowledge deficit related to lack of information about involutional process and self-care needs
- Alteration in family process related to incorporation of newborn into the family

Nursing Plan and Implementation During Admission

The woman is instructed during her prenatal visits to come to the birthing unit if any of the following occur:

- Rupture of membranes (ROM)
- Regular, frequent uterine contractions (nulliparas, 5–10 minutes apart for 1 hour; multiparas, 10–15 minutes apart for 1 hour)
- Any vaginal bleeding

Early admission means less discomfort for the laboring woman as she travels to the birth setting and more

COMMUNITY IN FOCUS | Midwifery Services in Rural New York

Mary Imogene Bassett Hospital (MIBH) in Cooperstown serves 10 rural counties in upstate New York. For many years the hospital served as a clinical site for obstetrical residents from Columbia University in New York City. However, census declines in the mid-1980s led to the elimination of the residency program. Without the services provided by the program, the community was faced with the problem of how best to meet the needs of childbearing women in the areas MIBH served.

The chief of obstetrics and the hospital administration recognized that certified nurse-midwives could provide needed services, and in 1986 the first CNM was hired. Currently the nurse-midwifery service is staffed by 9 CNMs. Of the 793 babies born in the Bassett Birthing Center at MIBH in 1994, 679 births were attended by nurse-midwives. This figure is especially impressive because it represents 98% of the nonsurgical births at Bassett.

The organizational model employed by the nurse-midwifery service represents a truly collaborative approach. The service is housed within the Department of Obstetrics and Gynecology; however, the director of nurse-midwifery services reports directly to both the head of the ob/gyn department and the vice-president for nursing and patient care services. Moreover, the director is a member of the nursing administration council and several staff CNMs serve on various hospital committees.

When a woman seeks prenatal care services initially, she is encouraged to attend a two-hour orientation program, New Beginnings, taught by maternity nurse educators. The program covers a variety of topics related to pregnancy and explains the Bassett system. Following the program the woman and a staff member complete a health history and routine lab tests are obtained. An appointment is then scheduled with one of the CNMs for a physical examination. CNMs complete the initial risk assessment and examination for all pregnant women. Based on the results, three methods of client management are available: (1) exclusive CNM management for women with low risk status; (2) collaborative management by CNMs and physicians for women considered high risk; and (3) physician care only for women who request it. Four of the 14 satellite clinics are managed by CNMs. For women seeking prenatal care at one of the remaining clinics, the initial plan of care is developed by the nurse-midwife; a nurse practitioner then provides ongoing management. If questions arise, CNM and physician coverage is available at Bassett around the clock.

For women considered high risk, the physician generally addresses the medical issues such as insulin requirements while the CNM addresses issues related to support and the birth process. Careful collaboration between physician and certified nurse-midwife is essential. Often the CNM attends the birth with the physician immediately available to lend assistance if necessary. No woman who wishes to have a midwife with her during labor is excluded from the midwifery service.

This incredibly collaborative model has resulted in favorable outcomes. The number of women who have given birth at Bassett have increased significantly since the program began. More importantly, the cesarean birth rate has declined from 26.2 percent to 11.2 percent with a concurrent increase in the number of VBACs (vaginal birth after cesarean). The incidence of episiotomies and lacerations has also decreased.

The program at MIBH is a striking example of the value of collaboration among nurse-midwives, physicians, nurse practitioners, staff nurses, and other health care providers.

Source: Stone SE, Brown MP, Westcott JP: Nurse-midwifery service in a rural setting. *J Nurse Midwifery* September/October 1996; 41(5):377.

time to prepare for the birth. Sometimes the labor is advanced and birth is imminent, but usually the woman is in early labor at admission. If time permits and the woman is not familiar with what will occur during her labor, the nurse can provide information. (See Teaching Guide: What to Expect During Labor.)

The woman may be facing a number of unfamiliar procedures that are routine for health care providers. It is important to remember that all women have the right to determine what happens to their bodies. *The woman's informed consent should be obtained prior to any procedure that involves touching her body.*

The manner in which the woman and her partner are greeted by the maternity nurse influences the course of her hospital stay. The sudden environmental change and the sometimes impersonal and technical aspects of admission can produce additional stress. If women are greeted in a brusque, harried manner, they are less likely to look to the nurse for support. A calm, pleasant manner indicates to the woman that she is an important person. It helps instill in the couple a sense of confidence in the staff's ability to provide quality care during this critical time.

Following the initial greeting, the woman is taken into the labor or birthing room. Some couples prefer to remain together during the admission process, and others prefer to have the partner wait outside. As the nurse helps the woman undress and get into a hospital gown, the nurse can begin conversing with her to develop rapport and establish the nursing database. The experienced labor and birth nurse can obtain essential information about the woman and her pregnancy within a few minutes after admission, initiate any immediate interventions needed, and establish individualized priorities. The nurse can then make effective nursing decisions about intrapartal care, such as the following:

- Will a "prep" and/or enema be given?
- Should ambulation or bed rest be encouraged?
- Is more frequent monitoring needed?
- What does the woman want during her labor and birth?
- Is a support person available?

A major challenge for nurses is the formulation of realistic objectives for laboring women. Each woman has different coping mechanisms and support systems.

TEACHING GUIDE What to Expect During Labor

Assessment

As each woman is admitted into the birthing area the nurse assesses the woman's knowledge regarding the childbirth experience. The woman's knowledge base will be affected by previous births, attendance at childbirth education classes, and the amount of information she has been able to gather during her pregnancy by asking questions or reading. The nurse also assesses the factors that affect communication and anxiety level. Labor progress is assessed so that decisions regarding what to teach and the time available for teaching can be ascertained. If the woman is in early labor and she needs additional information, the nurse proceeds with teaching.

Nursing Diagnosis

The key nursing diagnosis probably will be: Knowledge deficit related to lack of information about nursing care during labor.

Nursing Plan and Implementation

The teaching focuses on information regarding the assessments and support the woman will receive during labor.

Client Goals

At the completion of the teaching the woman will be able to do the following:

- Verbalize the assessments the nurse will complete during labor
- Discuss the support/comfort measures that are available

Teaching Plan

Content	Teaching Method
Aspects of the admission process include the following: • Abbreviated history • Physical assessment (maternal vital signs [VS], fetal heart rate [FHR], contraction status, status of membranes) • Assessment of uterine contractions (frequency, duration, intensity) • Orientation to surroundings • Introductions to other staff who will be assisting her • Determination of woman's and family support person's expectations of the nurse	Provide information on the basic assessment and care activities. Allow time for questions and discussion as labor progress permits.
Present aspects of ongoing physical care, such as when to expect assessment of maternal VS, FHR, and contractions.	
If electronic fetal monitor is used, orient the woman to how it works and the information it provides. Orient woman to sights and sounds of monitor. Explain what "normal" data will look like and what characteristics are being watched for.	Demonstrate fetal monitor.
Be sure to note that assessments will increase as the labor progresses; about the time the woman would like to be left alone (transition phase), the assessments increase in order to help keep the mother and baby safe by noting any changes from the normal course.	
Explain the vaginal examination and what information can be obtained.	Use cervical dilatation chart to illustrate the amount of dilatation.
Review comfort techniques that may be used in labor, and ascertain what the woman thinks will be effective in promoting comfort.	Discussion.
Review breathing techniques the woman has learned so the nurse will be able to support her technique.	Ask woman to demonstrate technique.
Review comfort/support measures such as: positioning, back rub, effleurage, touch, distraction techniques, ambulation.	Discussion.
If woman is in early labor, offer to give her a tour of the birthing area.	Provide a tour of birthing area, explaining equipment and routines. Include partner.

Evaluation

At the end of this teaching session, the woman will be able to verbalize assessments that will occur during her labor and to discuss comfort/support measures that may be used.

If indicated, the woman is assisted into bed. A side-lying or semi-Fowler's position rather than a supine position is most comfortable and avoids supine hypotensive syndrome (vena caval syndrome).

After obtaining the essential information from the woman and her records, the nurse begins the intrapartal assessment. (Chapter 16 considers intrapartal maternal assessment in depth. See also Essential Precautions for Practice: During Admission and Labor.)

The nurse auscultates the fetal heart rate (FHR). (Detailed information on monitoring FHR is presented in Chapter 16.) The nurse determines the woman's blood pressure, pulse, respirations, and oral temperature; assesses contraction frequency, duration, and intensity (possibly while gathering other data); before the sterile vaginal examination, informs the woman about the procedure and its purpose; and afterward informs the woman about the findings. If there are signs of advanced labor (frequent contractions, an urge to bear down, and so on), a vaginal examination must be done quickly. If there are signs of excessive bleeding or if the woman reports episodes of painless bleeding in the last trimester, a vaginal examination should *not* be done.

Results of FHR assessment, uterine contraction evaluation, and the vaginal examination help determine whether the rest of the admission process can proceed at a more leisurely pace or whether additional interventions have higher priority. For example, an FHR of 110 beats per minute on auscultation indicates that a fetal monitor should be applied immediately to obtain additional data. The woman's vital signs can be assessed after this is done.

After the nurse obtains admission data, a clean-voided midstream urine specimen is collected. The woman with intact membranes may collect her specimen in the bathroom. If the membranes are ruptured and the presenting part is not engaged, the woman generally remains in bed to avoid prolapse of the umbilical cord. The advisability of ambulation when membranes are ruptured depends on the woman's desires, clinician requests, or agency policy.

The nurse can test the woman's urine for the presence of protein, ketones, and glucose by using a dipstick before sending the sample to the laboratory. This procedure is especially important if edema or elevated blood pressure is noted on admission. Proteinuria of 2+ or more may be a sign of impending preeclampsia. Glycosuria is found frequently in pregnant women because of the increased glomerular filtration rate in the proximal tubules and the inability of these tubules to increase reabsorption of glucose. However, it may also be associated with latent diabetes and should not be discounted. While the woman is collecting the urine specimen, the nurse can prepare the equipment for shaving the pubic area (the shaving is referred to as the **prep**) and for the enema if one is to be given. Prep orders vary, but many certified nurse-midwives/physicians leave standing orders for prep measures. Complete preps, which involve the removal of all pubic, perineal, and rectal hair, were formerly done. But a prep now usually involves the removal of perineal hair below the vaginal orifice where an episiotomy or repair of a laceration would be done. The area can be shaved or the perineal hair clipped with a pair of sterile scissors. A miniprep is usually considered to be the removal of perineal hair from the labia parallel to the upper aspect of the vaginal orifice and downward to the rectum.

ESSENTIAL PRECAUTIONS FOR PRACTICE

During Admission and Labor

Examples of times when disposable gloves should be worn include the following:

- Assisting the woman as she removes any garments moist with bloody show and/or amniotic fluid
- Checking amniotic fluid–soaked materials with Nitrazine test tape
- Obtaining and/or handling urine specimens
- Giving an enema or a prep or handling a bedpan
- Handling chux and bedding that are moist with bloody show and/or amniotic fluid
- Placing elastic belts for the electronic monitor around a woman who has been lying in bedding moist with bloody show and/or amniotic fluid
- Assisting with fetal blood sampling and handling lab tubes

A splash apron and eye covering (such as goggles) must be worn when splashing of body fluids is possible.

REMEMBER to wash your hands prior to putting the disposable gloves on and AGAIN immediately after removing the gloves.

For further information consult OSHA and CDC guidelines.

The use of preps is controversial. Some certified nurse-midwives/physicians believe that this form of skin preparation facilitates their work during the birth, makes perineal repair easier, and prevents infection (Ganforth and Garcia 1989). Others believe that a prep is unnecessary, since hair is minimal between the vagina and rectum and shaving may actually increase the risk of infection. Many women question the need for a prep and request that it be omitted. The nurse needs to ascertain the woman's wishes in this matter. Women who do not want a prep have probably discussed this with the certified nurse-midwife/physician during the prenatal period. If the woman has not previously stated her desire not to have a prep, the nurse acts as the woman's advocate by communicating her wishes to the certified nurse-midwife/physician.

Text continues on page 398

INTRAPARTAL CRITICAL PATHWAY

Category	First Stage	Second and Third Stage	Fourth Stage Birth to 1 Hour Past Birth
Referral	Review prenatal record Advise CNM/physician of admission	Labor record for first stage	Report to recovery room nurse
Assessments	Admission assessments: ask about problems since last prenatal visit; labor status (contraction frequency and duration), membrane status (intact or ruptured); coping level; support; woman's desires during labor and birth; ability to verbalize needs; laboratory testing (blood and UA) Intrapartal assessments: Cervical assessment: from 1 to 10 cm dilatation; nullipara (1.2 cm/h), multipara (1.5 cm/h) Cervical effacement: from 0% to 100% Fetal descent: progressive descent from −4 to +4 Membrane assessment: intact or ruptured; when ruptured, Nitrazine positive, fluid clear, no foul odor Comfort level: woman states is able to cope with contractions Behavioral characteristics: facial expressions, tone of voice and verbal expressions are consistent with comfort level and ability to cope Latent Phase: • B/P, P, R q1h if in normal range (B/P 90–140/60–90 or not >30 mm Hg systolic or >15 mm Hg diastolic over baseline; pulse 60–90; respirations 12–20/min, quiet, easy) • Temp q4h unless >37.6C (99.6F) or membranes ruptured then q2h • Uterine contractions q30min (contractions q5–10min, 15–40sec, mild intensity) • FHR q60min (for low-risk women) and q30min (for high-risk women) if reassuring (reassuring FHR has: baseline 120–160, STV present, LTV average, accelerations with fetal movement, no late nor variable decelerations); if nonreassuring, position on side, start O_2, assess for hypotension, monitor continuously, notify CNM/physician Active Phase: • B/P, P, R, q1h if WNL • Temp as above • Uterine contractions q30min; contractions q2–3min, 60sec, moderate to strong • FHR q30min (for low-risk women) and q5min (for high-risk women) if reassuring; if nonreassuring institute interventions Transition: • B/P, P, R, q30min • Uterine contractions q15–30min: contractions q2min, 60–75 sec, strong • FHR q30min (for low-risk women) and q15min (for high-risk women) if reassuring; if nonreassuring, see above	Second stage assessments: • B/P, P, R q5–15min • Uterine contractions palpated continuously • FHR q15min (for low-risk women) and q5min (for high-risk women) if reassuring; if nonreassuring, monitor continuously Fetal descent: descent continues to birth Comfort level: woman states is able to cope with contractions and pushing Behavioral characteristics: response to pushing, facial expressions, verbalization Third stage assessments: • B/P, P, R q5min • Uterine contractions, palpate occasionally until placenta is delivered, fundus maintains tone and contraction pattern continues to birth of placenta Newborn assessments: • Assess Apgar score of newborn • Respirations 30–60, irregular • Apical pulse: 120–160 and somewhat irregular • Temperature: Skin temp above 36.5C (97.8F) • Umbilical cord: two arteries, one vein (if one artery, assess for anomalies and urine output) • Gestational age: 38–42 weeks	Immediate postbirth assessments of mother q15min for 1 h • B/P: 90–140/60–90; should return to prelabor level • Pulse: slightly lower than in labor; range is 60–90 • Respirations: 12–20/min; easy; quiet • Temperature: 36.2–37.6C (98–99.6F) • Fundus firm, in midline, at the umbilicus • Lochia rubra; moderate amount; <1 pad/h; no free flow or passage of clots with massage • Perineum: sutures intact; no bulging or marked swelling; minimal bruising may be present; no c/o severe pain nor rectal pain • Bladder nondistended; spontaneous void of >100 mL clear, straw-colored urine; bladder nondistended following voiding • If hemorrhoids present, no tenseness or marked engorgement; <2 cm diameter Comfort level: <3 on scale of 1 to 10 Energy level: awake and able to hold newborn Newborn assessments if newborn remains with parents: • Respirations: 30–60; irregular • Apical pulse: 120–160 and somewhat irregular • Temperature: skin temp above 36.5C (97.8F); skin feels warm to touch • Skin color noncyanotic • Mucus: small amount, clear, easily suctioned with bulb syringe without skin color change • Behavioral: newborn opens eyes widely if room is slightly darkened • Movements rhythmic; no hand tremors present

INTRAPARTAL CRITICAL PATHWAY continued

Category	First Stage	Second and Third Stage	Fourth Stage Birth to 1 Hour Past Birth
Comfort	Institute comfort measures: ambulation, frequent position change, effleurage, focal point, patterned paced breathing, visualization, therapeutic touch, back rub, moist cloths to face, holding hand, words of encouragement, changing underpad, shower, whirlpool, staying with the woman/family, warmed blanket at back, sacral pressure Offer pain medication or administer if requested Assist with administration of regional block	Institute comfort measures: • Second stage: cool cloth to forehead, encouragement, coaching, help support legs while pushing, position of comfort for pushing and birth • Third stage: cool cloth to forehead, assist parents to see newborn, position mother to hold newborn, provide encouragement	Institute comfort measures: • Perineal discomfort: gently cleanse and apply ice pack; position to decrease pressure on perineum • Uterine discomfort: palpate fundus gently • Hemorrhoids: ice pack • General fatigue: position of comfort, encourage rest • Administer pain medication ________
Teaching/ psychosocial	Establish rapport Orient to environment, expected assessments & procedures Answer questions and provide information Orient to EFM if used Teach relaxation, visualization & breathing pattern if needed Explain comfort measures available Assume advocacy role for woman/family during labor & birth	Orient to expected assessments and procedures Answer questions and provide information Explain comfort measures available Continue advocacy role	Explain immediate assessments and care after this first hour Teach self-massage of fundus and expected findings Instruct to call for assistance if mother desires to get OOB Begin newborn teaching; bulb syringe, positioning; maintaining warmth Assist parents in exploring their newborn Assist with first breastfeeding experience
Therapeutic nursing interventions and reports	Straight cath prn if bladder distended If regional block administered monitor B/P, FHR, sensation per protocol Provide continuing status reports to CNM/physician Perineal clip per woman's request Small enema per woman's request Perform sterile vaginal examination as indicated	Straight cath prn if bladder distended Continue monitoring VS, FHR and sensation if regional block has been given	Straight cath if bladder distended Monitor return of motor ability and sensation if regional block has been given Weigh perineal pads if lochia flow >1 saturated pad in 15 min, presence of boggy uterus and clots; ↓B/P, ↑P
Activity	Encourage ambulation unless contraindicated Maintain bed rest immediately after administration of IV pain medication, or following regional block Woman rests comfortably between contractions	Position comfortably for birth Woman rests comfortably between pushing efforts & while awaiting birth of placenta	Position of comfort
Nutrition	Ice chips and clear fluids Evaluate for signs of dehydration	Ice chips and clear fluids	Regular diet if assessments are WNL Encourage fluids
Elimination	Voids at least q2h; urine clear, straw-colored, negative for protein Bladder nondistended May have bowel movement Monitor I & O with IVs	May void spontaneously with pushing May pass stool with pushing	Voids spontaneously
Medications	Administer pain medication per woman's request	Local infiltration of anesthetic agent for birth by CNM/physician Pitocin 10 units IM, IVP per IV tubing, or added to IV fluids	Continue Pitocin infusion Administer pain medication ________

INTRAPARTAL CRITICAL PATHWAY continued

Category	First Stage	Second and Third Stage	Fourth Stage Birth to 1 Hour Past Birth
Discharge planning	Evaluate knowledge of labor and birth process Evaluate support system and need for referral after birth		Provide information if mother to be moved from LDR room Provide opportunity for parents to ask questions regarding newborn Evaluate knowledge of normal postpartum, newborn care
Family involvement	Identify available support person(s) Recognize possible impact of culture on responses Observe interaction between woman and partner Create moment alone with woman to identify possible abuse Assess current parenting skills	Provide opportunities for woman and support person(s) to watch newborn assessments Perform newborn assessment on mother's abdomen/chest if possible	Provide opportunity for parents to be with baby Encourage skin-to-skin contact Darken room to encourage eye-to-eye contact Provide quiet time for new family Parenting: demonstrates early culturally expected parenting behaviors

When a prep is to be done, the nurse explains the procedure to the woman. Most women feel embarrassed and vulnerable during this procedure, so the nurse needs to excercise great care to provide privacy and support. The nurse performing the prep will need to observe body substance isolation (BSI) and universal precautions by washing her hands and putting on disposable gloves. Administration of an enema is also controversial. Currently many certified nurse-midwives/physicians leave the decision up to the woman, as long as there is no vaginal bleeding present and labor is not far advanced. If the woman desires an enema, usually a small-volume enema (such as Fleets) is given. The woman may expel the enema in the bathroom unless membranes are ruptured; then she usually uses a bedpan. Before leaving the woman, the nurse must be sure that the woman knows how to operate the call system so that she can obtain help if she needs it. After the woman expels the enema, the nurse monitors the FHR again to assess any changes. If the woman's partner has been out of the birthing room, the couple is reunited as soon as possible.

Laboratory tests are also carried out during admission. Hemoglobin and hematocrit values help determine the oxygen-carrying capacity of the circulatory system and the woman's ability to withstand blood loss at birth. Elevation of the hematocrit indicates hemoconcentration of blood, which occurs with edema or dehydration. A low hemoglobin, in the absence of other evidence of bleeding, suggests anemia. Blood may be typed and crossmatched if the woman is in a high-risk category. A serology test for syphilis is obtained if one has not been done in the last 3 months or if an antepartal serology result was positive.

In many hospitals, the admission process also includes signing a delivery/birth permit, and fastening an identification bracelet to her wrist.

Depending on how rapidly labor is progressing, the nurse notifies the certified nurse-midwife/physician before or after completing the admission procedures. The report should include the following information: cervical dilatation and effacement, station, presenting part, status of the membranes, contraction pattern, FHR, vital signs that are not in the normal range, the woman's wishes, and her reaction to labor.

A nursing admission note is entered into the computer or the charting system. The admission note should include the reason for admission, the date and time of the woman's arrival, and notification of the certified nurse-midwife/physician, the condition of the woman and her baby, and labor and membrane status (AAP and ACOG 1992).

Nursing Plan and Implementation During the First Stage of Labor

After completing the nursing assessment and diagnosis steps, the nurse creates a plan of care arranged around nursing goals. Recent research provides information about which nursing actions and behaviors laboring women find most helpful. In a study by Bryanton, Fraser-Davey, and Sullivan (1994), laboring women identified the most helpful nursing behaviors as "making the woman feel cared about as an individual, giving praise, appearing calm and confident, assisting with breathing and relaxing, treating the woman with respect, explaining hospital routines, answering questions truthfully in an understandable language, providing a sense of security, and accepting what the woman said and did without judging her" (p 641).

Integration of Family Expectations

Most would agree that a family comes into the birth setting with basic expectations that they will not be harmed and that the labor and birth will be safe for the mother and baby. But what other expectations do they have? What do they want from the nurse who will be with them during this important event in their life? A study by Hodnett (1996) found that women identified five general categotries of nursing support measures that the found helpful during labor. The first area was emotional support, which included physical presence of the nurse, praise, encouragement, reassurance, and companionship. The second area focused on comfort measures such as the use of touch, providing ice chips and fluids, massage, assistance with care, and a bath or shower. Information and advice was the third area and included offering information regarding procedures, interventions as they occurred, and reports of labor progress. The fourth area concerned advocacy. The woman and her partner have goals, hopes, and dreams regarding how the labor and birth will proceed, but in reality they are not in a position of power. The nurse is able to assist the laboring couple by advocating for them with the certified nurse-midwife/physician or with other caregivers if needed. The last general area focused on support of the partner/husband by providing encouragement, praise for their efforts, and an opportunity for a break, and by role modeling, coaching, and supportive measures.

Integration of Cultural Beliefs

Knowledge of values, customs, and practices of different cultures is as important during labor as it is in the prenatal period. Without this knowledge, a nurse is less likely to understand a family's behavior and may impose personal values and beliefs on them. As cultural sensitivity increases, so does the likelihood of providing high-quality care.

The following sections briefly present a few possible cultural responses to labor. It is difficult to present even such a limited discussion in a clear, nonjudgmental way, because once a statement is made it may appear stereotypical, and of course no statement of a specific behavior can accurately reflect the preference of all people in a group. The nurse must always remain aware that an individual example of birthing practice will never be pertinent to all women in that individual's group. Within every culture, each person develops his or her own beliefs and value system. General information about any culture or belief system needs to be regarded as background knowledge in light of which we meet each individual and determine that person's own needs and desires.

Modesty

Modesty is an important consideration for women regardless of the cultural grouping; however, some women may be more uncomfortable than others with the degree of exposure needed for some procedures during labor and the birth process. Some women may be particularly uncomfortable when men are present and feel more comfortable with women; others may be uncomfortable with exposure of personal body parts regardless of the gender of the examiner or person who assists them. The nurse needs to be observant of the woman's responses to examinations and procedures and to provide the draping and privacy that the woman needs. It is more prudent to assume that embarrassment will occur with exposure and take measures to provide privacy than to assume that it will not matter to the woman if she is exposed during procedures. For example, some Asian women are not accustomed to male physicians and attendants. Modesty is of great concern, and exposure of as little of the woman's body as possible is strongly recommended.

Pain Expression

The manner in which a woman chooses to deal with the discomfort of labor varies widely. Some women seem to turn inward and remain very quiet during the whole process. They speak only to ask others to leave the room or cease conversation. Others may be very vocal, with behaviors such as counting out loud, moaning quietly, crying, or cursing loudly. They may also turn from side to side or change positions frequently. In Asian cultures it is important for individuals to act in a way that will not bring shame on the family. Therefore, the Asian woman may not express pain outwardly for fear of shaming herself and her family (Weber 1996). Women of Mexican cultural heritage, by contrast, may be vocally expressive during labor. The nurse supports a woman's individual expression, whatever it may be, in order to enhance the birthing experience for mother, baby, and family.

Cultural Beliefs: Some Examples

In looking at specific practices related to verbalization, position, food, and drink during labor, obvious differences between cultures are apparent. Differing beliefs regarding vocalizations and perception of pain during labor may be exhibited by a Chinese-American woman or a Muslim woman. Silence is valued in Chinese society, so this woman is usually quiet and stoic in order to avoid dishonor to herself or her family (Weber 1996). Muslim women may freely vocalize pain, and some believe the more loudly they vocalize during labor, the more obvious their suffering will be to their husband (Ahmad 1995). South or Central American women may tend to view pain during labor as a symbol of love toward the baby: the more intense the pain, the more intense the love (Scott-Ramos 1995).

Hmong women from Laos report that squatting during childbirth is common in their culture (LaDu 1985). During labor they may want to be active and move about. The husband is frequently present and actively involved in providing comfort. Traditionally, the woman prefers that the amniotic membranes not be ruptured until just before birth. It is thought that the escape of fluid at this time makes the birth easier. During labor the woman usually prefers only "hot" foods and warm water to drink. As soon as the baby is born, a soft-boiled egg must be given to the mother to restore her energy. During the postpartum period the mother prefers "warm" foods, such as chicken prepared with warm water and warm rice (Morrow 1986).

Vietnamese women usually maintain self-control and may smile throughout the labor. They may prefer to walk about during labor and to give birth in a squatting position. The woman may avoid drinking cold water and prefer fluids at room temperature. The newborn is protected from praise to prevent jealousy (Calhoun 1986).

Latina women have identified expectations of their partner during labor and birth such as wanting their partner to stay with them and to reassure them that everything will be all right. The women wanted the partner to show that they loved them as they went through labor and to speak to them using affectionate words (Khazoyan and Anderson 1994).

Muslim women may have their husband, a female friend or relative, or a male relative with them during childbirth. Family support may be particularly important but does not preclude the importance of the nurse's presence. The woman may want to retain her head covering (khimar), and two long-sleeved gowns can be offered. It is important to have examinations done by a female nurse, physician, or CNM whenever possible. If a male physician is involved, the woman may wish for her husband to remain in the room. After the birth Muslim fathers traditionally call praise to Allah (adhan) in the newborn's right ear and clean the newborn.

In working with women from another culture, an awareness of historical beliefs and practices helps the nurse understand and support their behavior. The maternity nurse would do well to make it a priority to become acquainted with the beliefs and practices of the various subcultures in the community. In the birthing situation, the nurse supports the family's cultural practices as long as it is safe to do so.

Support of the Adolescent During Birth

Each adolescent in labor is different. The nurse must assess what each client brings to the experience by asking the following questions:

- Has the young woman received prenatal care?
- What are her attitudes and feelings about the pregnancy?
- Who will attend the birth and what is the person's relationship to her?
- What preparation has she had for the experience?
- What are her expectations and fears regarding labor and birth?
- How has her culture influenced her?
- What are her usual coping mechanisms?
- Does she plan to keep the newborn?

Any adolescent who has not had prenatal care requires close observation during labor. Fetal well-being is established by fetal monitoring. Adolescent women are at highest risk for pregnancy and labor complications and must be monitored intensively.

The nurse should be alert to any physiologic complications of labor in the adolescent. The young woman's prenatal record is carefully reviewed for risks and the adolescent is screened for pregnancy-induced hypertension (PIH), cephalopelvic disproportion (CPD), anemia, drugs ingested during pregnancy, sexually transmitted infection, and size-date discrepancies.

The support role of the nurse depends on the woman's support system during labor. The young woman may not be accompanied by someone who will stay with her during childbirth. Whether she has a support person or not, it is important for the nurse to establish a trusting relationship with her. In this way, the nurse can help her maintain control and understand what is happening to her. Establishing rapport without recrimination for possible inappropriate behavior is essential. The adolescent who is given positive reinforcement for "work well done" will leave the experience with increased self-esteem, despite the emotional problems that may accompany her situation.

If a support person does accompany the adolescent, that person also needs the nurse's encouragement and support. The nurse must explain changes in the young woman's behavior and substantiate her wishes. The nursing staff should reinforce the adolescent's feelings that she is wanted and important.

The adolescent who has taken childbirth education classes is generally better prepared than the adolescent who has had no preparation. The nurse must keep in mind, however, that the younger the adolescent, the less she may be able to participate actively in the process.

The very young adolescent (under age 14) has fewer coping mechanisms and less experience to draw on than her older counterparts. Because her cognitive development is incomplete, the younger adolescent may have fewer problem-solving capabilities. Her ego integrity may be more threatened by the experience, and she may be more vulnerable to stress and discomfort.

The very young woman needs someone to rely on at all times during labor. She may be more childlike and dependent than older teens. The nurse must be sure that instructions and explanations are simple and concrete. During the transition phase, the young teenager may become withdrawn and unable to express her need to be nurtured. Touch, soothing encouragement, and measures to maintain her comfort help her maintain control and meet her needs for dependence. During the second stage of labor, the young adolescent may feel as if she is losing control and may reach out to those around her. By remaining calm and giving directions, the nurse helps her control feelings of helplessness (Drake 1996).

The middle adolescent (age 15 to 17 years) often attempts to remain calm and unflinching during labor. If unable to break through the teenager's stoic barrier, the nurse needs to rise above frustration and realize that a caring attitude will still help the young woman.

Many older adolescents feel that they "know it all," but they may be no more prepared for childbirth than younger counterparts. The nurse's reinforcement and nonjudgmental manner will help them save face. If the adolescent has not taken classes, she may require preparation and explanations. The older teenager's response to the stresses of labor, however, is similar to that of the adult woman (Drake 1996).

Even if the adolescent is planning to relinquish her newborn, she should be given the option of seeing and holding the infant. She may be reluctant to do this at first, but the grieving process is facilitated if the mother sees the infant. However, seeing or holding the newborn should be the young woman's choice. (See Chapter 28 for further discussion of the relinquishing mother and the adolescent parent.)

Promotion of Comfort in the First Stage

The first step in planning care is to talk with the woman and her partner to identify their goals. Usually the couple are concerned with discomfort so it is helpful to identify factors that may contribute to discomfort. These factors include uncomfortable positions, diaphoresis, continual leaking of amniotic fluid, a full bladder, a dry mouth, anxiety, and fear. Nursing interventions can minimize the effects of these factors. These interventions are described later in this section.

There are many types of responses to pain. The most frequent physiologic manifestations are increased pulse and respiratory rates, dilated pupils, increased blood pressure, and muscle tension. In labor, these reactions are transitory because the pain is intermittent. Increased muscle tension is most significant because it may impede the progress of labor. Women in labor frequently tighten skeletal muscles voluntarily during a contraction and remain motionless. As the intensity of the contraction increases with the progress of labor, the woman is less aware of the environment and may have difficulty hearing verbal instructions. The pattern of coping with labor contractions varies from the use of highly structured breathing techniques to grimacing, moaning, and loud vocalizations. Some women feel that making sounds helps them cope and do the work of labor, while others begin to make loud sounds only as they lose their ability to cope.

Some women may want physical contact during contractions. They may provide verbal and nonverbal signs such as crying, moaning, and beseeching the coach or nurse to hold their hand or rub their back. They may reach out and grasp the support person or indicate their anxiety or fear through eye contact (Weaver 1990). A woman generally wants touching and physical contact at times during the first part of labor, but when she moves into the transition phase, she usually rebuffs all efforts and pulls away. However, some women are uncomfortable with being touched at all, regardless of the phase of labor.

Many nurses like to incorporate touch into their nursing care, and they readily respond to the women's cues. Others may be more hesitant, perhaps because of previous experience with being rebuffed or their own personal values regarding touch.

As the nurse and woman or couple work together to increase comfort during contractions, a ritual of supportive measures begins to develop. The nurse watches for cues and nonverbal behaviors, and asks for feedback from the woman. As labor progresses, the nurse and couple will have their prior experience and rapport of working together to change comfort measures as needed.

A decrease in the intensity of discomfort is one of the goals of nursing support during labor. Nursing measures used to decrease pain include

- Ensuring general comfort
- Decreasing anxiety
- Providing information
- Using specific supportive relaxation techniques
- Encouraging controlled breathing
- Administering pharmacologic agents as ordered by the physician

General Comfort

General comfort measures are of utmost importance throughout labor. By relieving minor discomforts, the nurse helps the woman use her coping mechanisms to deal with pain.

The woman is encouraged to ambulate if it is not contraindicated. If she stays in bed, she may be encouraged to assume any position that she finds comfortable. A side-lying position is generally the most advantageous

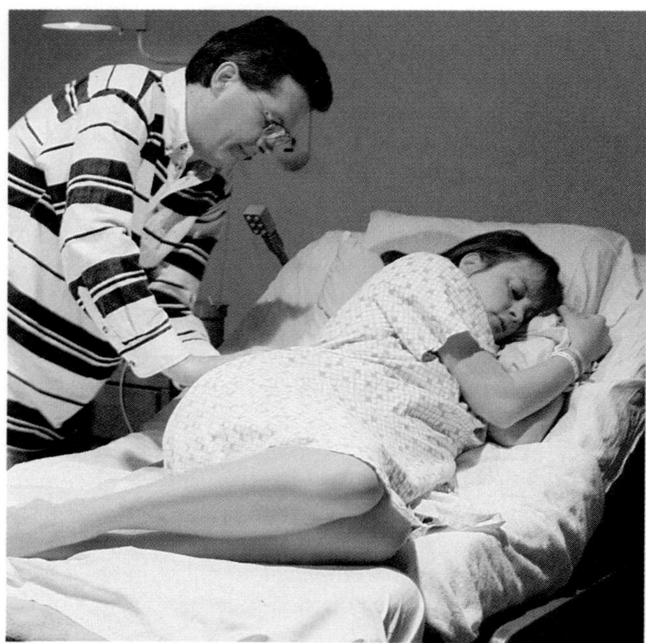

FIGURE 17–1 The partner can provide comfort and assistance during contractions.

for the laboring woman, although frequent position changes seem to achieve more efficient contractions. Care should be taken that all body parts are supported, with the joints slightly flexed. For instance, when the woman is in a side-lying position, pillows may be placed against her chest and under the uppermost arm. A pillow or folded bath blanket is placed between her knees to support the uppermost leg and relieve tension or muscle strain. A pillow placed at the woman's midback also helps provide support. If the woman is more comfortable on her back, the head of the bed should be elevated to relieve the pressure of the uterus on the vena cava. Pillows may be placed under each arm and under the knees to provide support. Since a pregnant woman is at increased risk for thrombophlebitis, excessive pressure behind the knee and calf should be avoided and the nurse needs to assess pressure points frequently. Back rubs and frequent changes of position contribute to comfort and relaxation (see Figure 17–1).

Diaphoresis and the constant leaking of amniotic fluid can dampen the woman's gown and bed linen. Fresh, smooth, dry bed linen promotes comfort. To avoid having to change the bottom sheet following rupture of the membranes, the nurse may replace chux at frequent intervals (BSI precautions need to be followed). The perineal area should be kept as clean and dry as possible to promote comfort as well as to prevent infection. A full bladder adds to the discomfort during a contraction and may prolong labor by interfering with the descent of the fetus. The bladder should be kept as empty as possible. Even if the woman is voiding, urine may be retained because of the pressure of the fetal presenting part. A full bladder can be detected by palpation directly over the symphysis pubis. Some of the regional procedures for analgesia during labor contribute to the inability to void, and catheterization may be necessary. The woman should be encouraged to empty her bladder every 2–3 hours.

The woman may experience dryness of the oral mucous membranes. A lemon glycerine swab, popsicles, ice chips, or a wet 4 × 4 sponge may relieve the discomfort. Some prepared childbirth programs advise the woman to bring lollipops to help combat the dryness that occurs with some of the breathing patterns.

Some women feel discomfort from cold feet. Wearing socks or slippers may increase their comfort.

Family members also need to be encouraged to maintain their own comfort. As their attention is directed toward the laboring woman, they may forget their own needs. The nurse may have to encourage them to take breaks, to maintain food and fluid intake, and to rest.

Handling Anxiety

The anxiety experienced by women entering labor is related to a combination of factors inherent to the process. A moderate amount of anxiety about the pain enhances the woman's ability to deal with the pain. An excessive degree of anxiety decreases her ability to cope with the pain. Wuitchik et al (1989) found that women in the latent phase of labor who were experiencing increased levels of anxiety about safety and their ability to cope were much more likely to describe their pain as "horrible" or "excruciating." They were more likely to have FHR decelerations in labor, a slow second stage, and/or a cesarean birth, and more likely to need pediatric assistance for neonatal resuscitation at birth.

Ways to decrease anxiety not related to pain are to give information (which eases fear of the unknown), establish rapport with the couple (which helps them preserve their personal integrity), and express confidence in the couple's ability to work with the labor process. In addition to being a good listener, the nurse must demonstrate genuine concern for the laboring woman. Remaining with the woman as much as possible conveys a caring attitude and dispels fears of abandonment. Praise for breathing, relaxation, and pushing efforts not only encourages repetition of the behavior but also decreases anxiety about the ability to cope with labor (Hodnett 1996). Incorporating each individual in the family as a unique person is also essential to decreasing anxiety (Tomlinson and Bryan 1996).

Client Teaching

Providing information about the nature of the discomfort that will occur during labor is important. Stressing the intermittent nature and maximum duration of the contractions can be most helpful. The woman can cope with pain better when she knows that a period of relief will follow. Describing the type of discomfort and specific sensations that will occur as labor progresses helps the woman recognize these sensations as normal and expected when she does experience them.

During the second stage, the woman may interpret rectal pressure as a need to move her bowels. The instinctive response is to tighten muscles rather than bear down (push). A sensation of splitting apart also occurs in the latter part of the second stage, and the woman may be afraid to bear down. The woman who expects these sensations and understands that bearing down contributes to progress at this stage is more likely to do so.

Descriptions of sensations should be accompanied with information on specific comfort measures. Some women experience the urge to push during transition when the cervix is not fully dilated and effaced. This sensation can be controlled by panting (it is very difficult to pant and bear down at the same time), and instructions should be given before the time that panting is required.

A thorough explanation of surroundings, procedures, and equipment being used also decreases anxiety, thereby reducing pain. Attachment to an electronic monitor can produce fear because equipment of this type is associated with critically ill people. The beeps, clicks, and other strange noises should be explained, and a simplified explanation of the monitor strip should be given. The nurse can emphasize that the use of the monitor provides a more accurate way to assess the well-being of the fetus during the course of labor. In addition, the nurse can show the woman and her coach how the monitor can help them use controlled breathing techniques to relieve pain. The monitor may indicate the beginning of a contraction just seconds before the woman feels it. The woman and coach can learn how to read the tracing to identify the beginning of the contraction.

Supportive Relaxation Techniques

Tense muscles increase resistance to the descent of the fetus and contribute to maternal fatigue. This fatigue increases pain perception and decreases the woman's ability to cope with the pain. Comfort measures, massage, techniques for decreasing anxiety, and client teaching can contribute to relaxation. Adequate sleep and rest are also important. The laboring woman needs to be encouraged to use the periods between contractions for rest and relaxation. A prolonged prodromal phase of labor may have prohibited sleeping. An aura of excitement naturally accompanies the onset of labor, making it difficult for the woman to sleep even though the contractions are mild and infrequent.

Distraction is another method of increasing relaxation and coping with discomfort. During early labor, conversation or activities such as light reading, cards, or other games serve as distractions. One technique that is effective for relieving moderate pain is to have the woman concentrate on a pleasant experience she has had in the past.

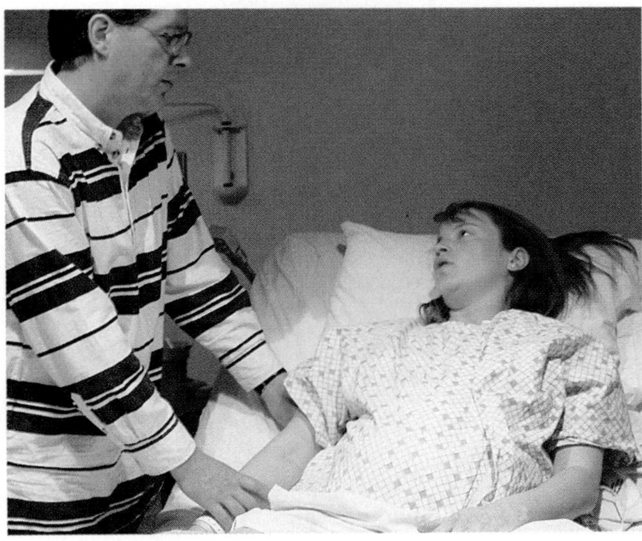

FIGURE 17–2 The woman's partner provides support and encouragement during labor.

Touch is another type of distraction (Figure 17–2). Although some women regard touching as an invasion of privacy or threat to their independence, others want to touch and be touched during a painful experience. Nurses can make themselves available to the woman who desires touch. The nurse can place a hand on the side of the bed within the woman's reach. The person who needs touch will reach out for contact, and the nurse can pick up and follow through with this behavioral cue.

Visualization techniques enhance relaxation; with this method the woman visualizes her body relaxing, or the perineum relaxing (Nichols and Humenick 1988). Mild to moderate abdominal discomfort during contractions may be relieved or lessened by effleurage. Back pain associated with labor may be relieved more effectively by firm pressure on the lower back or sacral area. To apply firm pressure, the nurse places her hand or a rolled, warmed towel or blanket in the small of the woman's back.

In addition to the measures just described, the nurse can enhance the woman's relaxation by providing encouragement and support for her controlled breathing techniques.

Breathing Techniques

Breathing techniques may help the laboring woman. Used correctly, they increase the woman's pain threshold, permit relaxation, enhance the woman's ability to cope with the uterine contractions, and allow the uterus to function more efficiently.

TABLE 17–1 Nursing Support of Patterned-Paced Breathing

Determine which breathing method the woman (couple) has learned. Provide encouragement as needed in maintaining breathing pattern. Provide support to the labor coach and assist as needed.

Lamaze Breathing Pattern Levels

First level (slow paced)

Pattern begins and ends with a cleansing breath (in through the nose and out through pursed lips as if cooling a spoonful of hot food). While inhaling through the nose and exhaling through pursed lips, slow breaths are taken, moving only the chest. The rate should be approximately 6–9/minute or 2 breaths/15 seconds. The coach or nurse may assist by reminding the woman to take a cleansing breath, and then the breaths could be counted out if needed to maintain pacing. The woman inhales as someone counts "one one thousand, two one thousand, three one thousand, four one thousand." Exhalation begins and continues through the same count.

First level for use during uterine contractions (The level begins and ends with a cleansing breath [CB].)

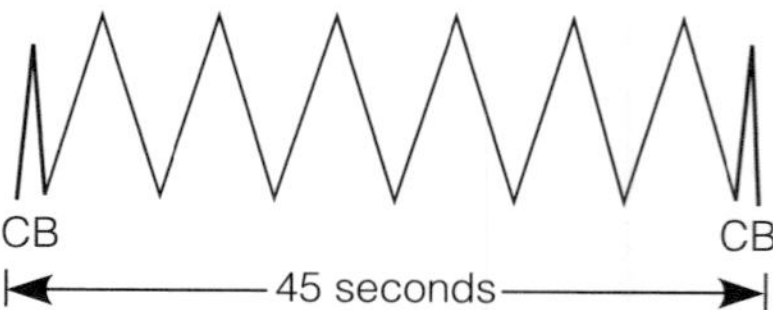

Second level (modified paced)

Pattern begins and ends with a cleansing breath. Breaths are then taken in and out silently through the mouth at approximately 4 breaths/5 seconds. The jaw and entire body need to be relaxed. The rate can be accelerated to 2–2 1/2 breaths/second. The rhythm for the breaths can be counted out as "one and two and one and two and. . ." with the woman exhaling on the numbers and inhaling on *and.*

Second level

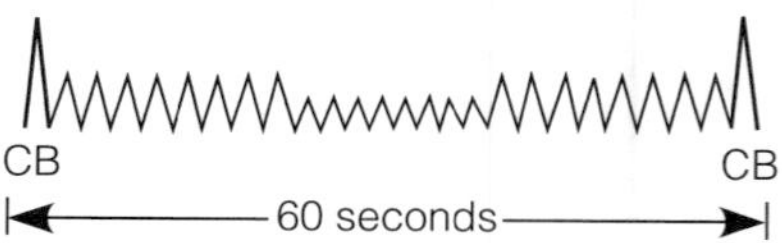

Third level (pattern paced)

Pattern begins and ends with a cleansing breath. All breaths are rhythmical, in and out through the mouth. Exhalations are accompanied by a "hee" or "hoo" sound in a varying pattern, 2:1, which begins as 3:1 (hee hee hee hoo) and can change to 2:1 (hee hee hoo) or 1:1 (hee hoo) as the intensity of the contraction changes. The rate should not be more rapid than 2–2 1/2 breaths/seconds. The rhythm of the breaths would match a "one and two and. . ." count.

Third level (Darkened spike represents "hoo.")

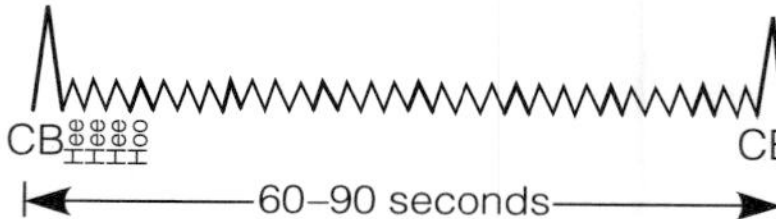

Abdominal Breathing Pattern Cues

The abdomen moves outward during inhalation and downward during exhalation. The rate remains slow with approximately 6–9 breaths/minute.

Breathing sequence for abdominal breathing

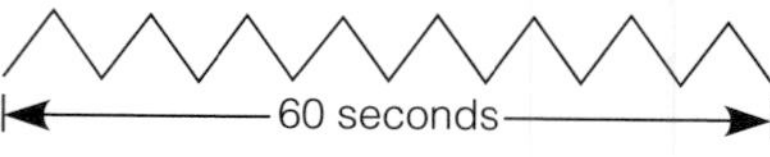

Quick Method

When the woman has not learned a particular method and is in active phase of labor, the nurse may teach her a combination of two patterns. Abdominal breathing may be used until labor is more advanced. Then a more rapid pattern consisting of two short blows from the mouth followed by a longer blow can be used. (This pattern is called "pant-pant-blow" even though all exhalations are a blowing motion.)

Pant-pant-blow breathing pattern

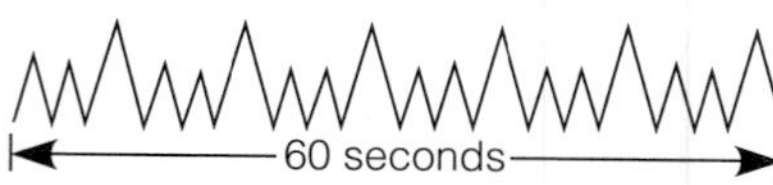

Many women learn Lamaze breathing during prenatal education classes. This type of controlled breathing has three levels. The woman tends to begin with the first level and then proceed to the next when she feels the need. Regardless of the level of breathing used, a cleansing breath begins and ends each pattern. A cleansing breath involves only the chest. It consists of inhaling through the nose and exhaling through pursed lips (see Table 17–1).

First Pattern This pattern may also be called *slow, deep breathing* or *slow-paced breathing.* During the breathing movements only the chest moves. The woman inhales slowly through her nose. She moves her chest up and out during the inhalation. She exhales through pursed lips. The breathing rate is 6–9 breaths a minute.

Second Pattern This pattern may also be called *shallow* or *modified-paced breathing.* The woman begins with a cleansing breath and at the end of the cleansing breath she pushes out a short breath. She then inhales and exhales through the mouth at a rate of about four breaths every 5 seconds. This pattern can be altered into a more rapid rate that does not exceed 2–2.5 breaths every second.

Third Pattern This is also called *pant-blow* or *pattern-paced breathing.* It is similar to modified-paced breathing except the breathing is punctuated every few breaths by a forceful exhalation through pursed lips. A pattern of four breaths may be used to begin. All breaths are kept equal and rhythmical. As the contraction becomes more intense, the woman may adjust the pattern as needed to 3:1, 2:1, and finally 1:1.

If the woman has not learned Lamaze or another controlled breathing technique, teaching her may be difficult when she is admitted in active labor. In this instance, the nurse can teach abdominal and pant-pant-blow breathing (see Table 17–1). In *abdominal breathing,* the woman moves the abdominal wall upward as she inhales and downward as she exhales. This method tends to lift the abdominal wall off the contracting uterus and thus may provide some pain relief. The breathing is deep and rhythmical. As transition approaches, the woman may feel the need to breathe more rapidly. To avoid breathing too rapidly, which may occur with deep abdominal breathing, the woman can use the *pant-pant-blow breathing pattern.*

As the woman uses her breathing technique, the nurse can assess and support the interaction between the woman and her coach or support person. In the absence of a coach, the nurse supports the laboring woman by helping to identify the beginning of each contraction and encouraging her as she breathes through it. Continued encouragement and support with each contraction throughout labor have immeasurable benefits.

Hyperventilation may occur when a woman breathes very rapidly over a prolonged period of time. Hyperventilation is the result of an imbalance of oxygen and carbon dioxide (that is, too much carbon dioxide is exhaled, and too much oxygen remains in the body). The signs and symptoms of hyperventilation are tingling or numbness in the tip of nose, lips, fingers, or toes; dizziness; spots before the eyes; or spasms of the hands or feet (carpal-pedal spasms). If hyperventilation occurs, the woman should be encouraged to slow her breathing rate and take shallow breaths. With instruction and encouragement, many women are able to change their breathing to correct the problem. Encouraging the woman to relax and counting out loud for her so she can pace her breathing during contractions are also helpful. If the signs and symptoms continue or become more severe (they progress from numbness to spasms), the woman can breathe into a paper surgical mask or a paper bag until symptoms abate. Breathing into a mask or bag causes rebreathing of carbon dioxide. The nurse should remain with the woman to reassure her.

In some instances, analgesics or regional anesthetic blocks may be used to enhance comfort and relaxation during labor. See Chapter 18 for a discussion of analgesia and anesthesia. Table 17–2 summarizes labor progress, possible responses of the laboring woman, and support measures.

Provision of Care in the First Stage of Labor

After the admission process is completed, the nurse helps the laboring woman and her partner become comfortable with the surroundings. The nurse assesses their individual needs and plans for this experience. As long as there are no contraindications (such as vaginal bleeding or ROM with the fetus unengaged), the woman may be encouraged to ambulate. Many women feel much more at ease and comfortable if they can move around and do not have to remain in bed.

The nurse needs to evaluate physical parameters of the woman and her fetus. Maternal temperature is monitored every 4 hours unless the temperature is over 37.5C (99.6F); if it is, it must be taken every hour. Blood pressure, pulse, and respirations are monitored every hour. If the woman's blood pressure is over 140/90 mm Hg or her pulse is more than 100, the nurse must notify the certified nurse-midwife/physician and reevaluate the blood pressure and pulse more frequently. The nurse palpates uterine contractions for frequency, intensity, and duration and auscultates the FHR every 60 minutes for low-risk women and every 30 minutes for high-risk women as long as it remains between 120 and 160 beats/min and is reassuring. The FHR should be auscultated throughout one contraction and for about 15 seconds after the contraction to assure that there are no decelerations. If the FHR is not in the 120–160 range or decelerations are heard, continuous electronic monitoring is recommended (Table 17–3).

The laboring woman may be feeling some discomfort during contractions. The nurse can assist with diversions or by repositioning the woman. The woman may begin to use her breathing method during contractions (see the preceding discussion of pain management).

The nurse should offer fluids in the form of clear liquids or ice chips at frequent intervals. Because gastric emptying time is prolonged during labor, solid foods are usually avoided. However, fasting during labor is becoming a controversial practice. Some providers believe that eating and drinking during labor should be an option. Many nurse-midwifery practices are now encouraging mothers to eat and drink to toleration, based on the current literature (Ludka and Roberts 1993).

Active Phase

During this phase, the contractions have a frequency of 2–3 minutes, a duration of 50–60 seconds, and a moderate intensity. Contractions need to be palpated every 15–30 minutes. As the contractions become more frequent and intense, vaginal exams are done to assess cervical dilatation and effacement and fetal station and position. During the active phase, the cervix dilates from 4 to 7 cm, and vaginal discharge and bloody show increase. Maternal blood pressure, pulse, and respirations should be monitored every hour for low-risk women

TABLE 17–2 Normal Progress, Psychologic Characteristics, and Nursing Support During First and Second Stages of Labor

Phase	Cervical Dilatation	Urine Contractions	Woman's Response	Support Measures
Stage 1				
Latent phase	1–4 cm	Every 10–20 minutes, 15–20 seconds duration Mild intensity *progressing to* Every 5–7 minutes, 30–40 seconds duration Moderate intensity	Usually happy, talkative, and eager to be in labor Exhibits need for independence by taking care of own bodily needs and seeking information	Establish rapport on admission and continue to build during care. Assess information base and learning needs. Be available to consult regarding breathing technique if needed; teach breathing technique if needed and in early labor. Orient family to room, equipment, monitors, and procedures. Encourage woman and partner to participate in care as desired. Provide needed information. Assist woman into position of comfort; encourage frequent change of position; encourage ambulation during early labor. Offer fluids/ice chips. Keep couple informed of progress. Encourage woman to void every 1 to 2 hours. Assess need for an interest in using visualization to enhance relaxation and teach if appropriate.
Active phase	4–7 cm	Every 2–3 minutes, 40–60 seconds duration Moderate to strong intensity	May experience feelings of helplessness Exhibits increased fatigue and may begin to feel restless and anxious as contractions become stronger Expresses fear of abandonment Becomes more dependent as she is less able to meet her needs	Encourage woman to maintain breathing patterns. Provide quiet environment to reduce external stimuli. Provide reassurance, encouragement, support; keep couple informed of progress. Promote comfort by giving back rubs, sacral pressure, cool cloth on forehead, assistance with position changes, support with pillows, effleurage. Provide ice chips, ointment for dry mouth and lips. Encourage to void every 1 to 2 hours. Offer shower/whirlpool/warm bath if available.
Transition phase	8–10 cm	Every 2 minutes, 60–75 seconds duration Strong intensity	Tires and may exhibit increased restlessness and irritability May feel she cannot keep up with labor process and is out of control Physical discomforts Fear of being left alone May fear tearing open or splitting apart with contractions	Encourage woman to rest between contractions. If she sleeps between contractions, wake her at beginning of contraction so she can begin breathing pattern (increases feeling of control). Provide support, encouragement, and praise for efforts. Keep couple informed of progress; encourage continued participation of support persons. Promote comfort as listed above but recognize many women do not want to be touched when in transition. Provide privacy. Provide ice chips, ointment for lips. Encourage to void every 1–2 hours.
Stage 2	Complete	Every 2 minutes	May feel out of control, helpless, panicky	Assist woman in pushing efforts. Encourage woman to assume position of comfort. Provide encouragement and praise for efforts. Keep couple informed of progress. Provide ice chips. Maintain privacy as woman desires.

(unless elevated, as previously noted) and every 30 minutes for high-risk women. The FHR is auscultated and evaluated every 30 minutes for low-risk women and every 15 minutes for high-risk women (NAACOG 1990).

A woman who has been ambulatory up to this point may now wish to sit in a chair or on a bed (Figure 17–3). If the woman wants to lie on the bed, she is encouraged to assume a side-lying position. The nurse can assist her to a position of comfort and may place pillows to support her body. To increase comfort, the nurse can give back rubs or effleurage, or place a cool cloth on the woman's forehead or across her neck. Because vaginal discharge increases, the nurse needs to change the chux frequently. Washing the perineum with warm soap and water removes secretions and increases comfort. The nurse needs to wear disposable gloves to avoid exposure to vaginal discharge.

If the amniotic membranes have not ruptured previously, they may during this phase. When the membranes rupture, the nurse notes the color and odor of the amniotic fluid and the time of rupture and immediately auscultates the FHR. The fluid should be clear with no odor. Fetal stress leads to intestinal and anal sphincter relaxation, and meconium may be released into the amniotic fluid. Meconium turns the fluid greenish-brown. Whenever the nurse notes meconium-stained fluid, an

TABLE 17–3 Nursing Assessments in the First Stage

Phase	*Mother*	*Fetus*
Latent	Blood pressure, respirations each hour if in normal range Temperature every 4 hours unless over 37.5C (99.6F) or membranes ruptured, then every hour Uterine contractions every 30 minutes	FHR every 60 minutes for low-risk women and every 30 minutes for high-risk women if normal characteristics present (average variability, baseline in the 120–160 bpm range, without late or variable decelerations) (NAACOG 1990). Note fetal activity. If electronic fetal monitor in place, assess for reactive NST.
Active	Blood pressure, pulse, respirations every hour if in normal range Uterine contractions every 30 minutes	FHR every 30 minutes for low-risk women and every 15 minutes for high-risk women if normal characteristics are present (NAACOG 1990).
Transition	Blood pressure, pulse, respiration every 30 minutes	FHR every 30 minutes for low-risk women and every 15 minutes for high-risk women if normal characteristics are present (NAACOG 1990).

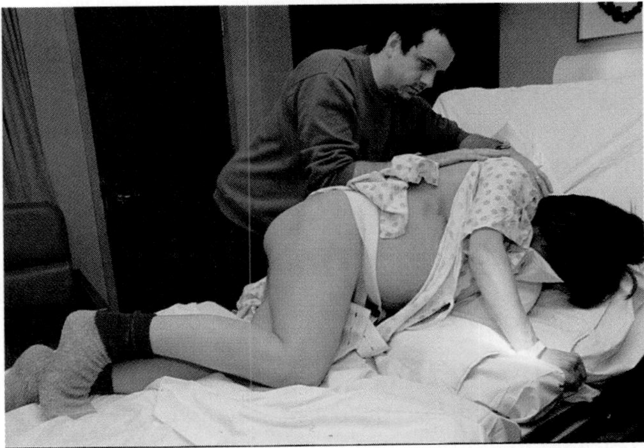

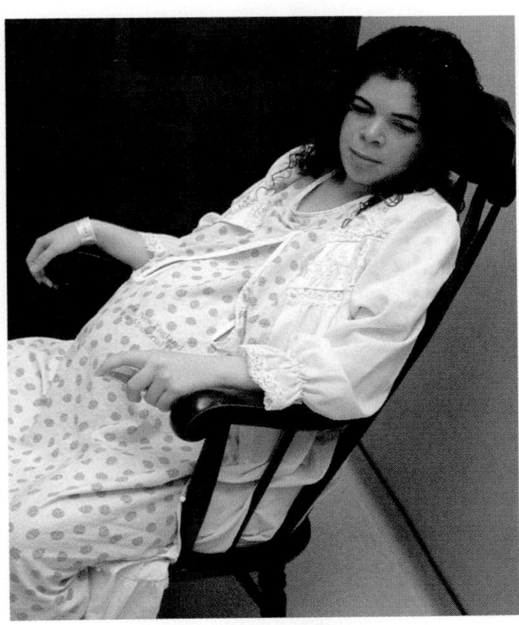

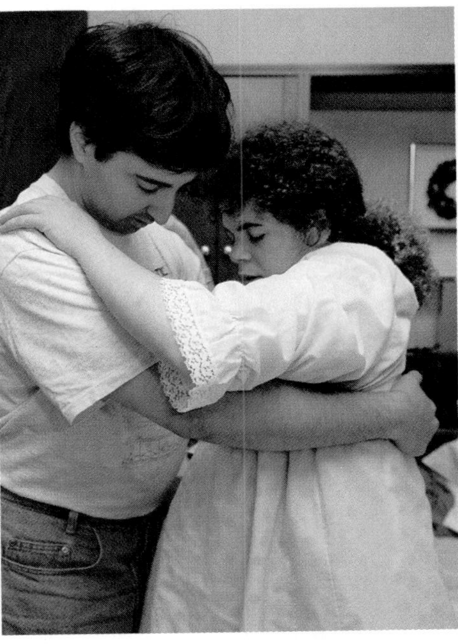

FIGURE 17–3 The laboring woman is encouraged to choose a position of comfort. The nurse modifies assessments and intervention as necessary.

TABLE 17–4 Deviations from Normal Labor Process Requiring Immediate Intervention

Problem	Immediate Action
Woman admitted with vaginal bleeding or history of painless vaginal bleeding	Do not perform vaginal examination. Assess FHR. Evaluate amount of blood loss. Evaluate labor pattern. Notify physician/CNM immediately.
Presence of greenish or brownish amniotic fluid	Continuously monitor FHR. Evaluate dilatation of cervix and determine if umbilical cord is prolapsed. Evaluate presentation (vertex or breech). Maintain woman on complete bed rest on left side. Notify physician/CNM immediately.
Absence of FHR and fetal movement	Notify physician/CNM. Provide truthful information and emotional support to laboring couple. Remain with the couple.
Prolapse of umbilical cord	Relieve pressure on cord manually. Continuously monitor FHR; watch for changes in FHR pattern. Notify physician/CNM. Assist woman into knee-chest position. Administer oxygen.
Woman admitted in advanced labor; birth imminent	Prepare for immediate birth. Obtain critical information: EDB History of bleeding problems History of medical or obstetric problems Past and/or present use/abuse of prescription/OTC/illicit drugs Problems with this pregnancy FHR and maternal vital signs Whether membranes are ruptured and how long since rupture Blood type and Rh Direct another person to contact physician/CNM. Do not leave woman alone. Provide support to couple. Put on gloves.

electronic monitor is applied to assess the FHR continuously. The time of rupture is noted, because current practice suggests that birth should occur within 24 hours of ROM. An additional concern is prolapse of the umbilical cord, which may occur when membranes rupture and the fetus is not engaged. The concern is that the amniotic fluid coming through the cervix will propel the umbilical cord through the cervix (prolapsed cord). The FHR is auscultated because a drop in the rate might indicate an undetected prolapsed cord. Immediate intervention is necessary to remove pressure on a prolapsed umbilical cord (see Chapter 19). See Table 17–4 for additional deviations from normal.

Transition

During transition, the contraction frequency is every 2–3 minutes, duration is 60–75 seconds, and intensity is strong. Cervical dilatation increases from 8 to 10 cm, effacement is complete (100%), and there is usually a heavy amount of bloody show. Contractions are palpated at least every 15 minutes. Sterile vaginal examinations may be done more frequently because this stage of labor usually is accompanied by rapid change. Maternal blood pressure, pulse, and respirations are taken at least every 30 minutes, and FHR is auscultated every 15 minutes.

Comfort measures become very important in this phase of labor, but continual assessment is required to intervene appropriately. The woman may rapidly change from wanting a back rub and other "hands-on" care to wanting to be left completely alone. The support person and the nurse need to follow her cues and change interventions as needed. Because the woman is breathing more rapidly, the nurse can increase her comfort by offering small spoons of ice chips to moisten her mouth or applying petroleum jelly to dry lips. The nurse can encourage the woman to rest between contractions. If analgesics have been administered, a quiet environment enhances the quality of rest between contractions. The nurse can awaken the woman just before another contraction begins so that she can begin controlled breathing.

Some women have difficulty coping during this time and need help with their breathing. Either the support person or the nurse can breathe along with the woman during each contraction to help her maintain her pattern. It is helpful to encourage her and assure her that she is doing a good job. The woman will begin to feel increased rectal pressure as the fetal presenting part moves down the birth canal. The nurse encourages the woman to refrain from pushing until the cervix is completely dilated. This measure helps prevent cervical edema.

The end of transition and beginning of second stage may be indicated by a change in the woman's voice or the sounds she is making. As the fetus moves down and she feels increased pressure and a bearing-down sensation, her voice tends to deepen. A moan during a contraction takes on a more guttural quality. Expert nurses recognize this sound as a sign of changes in the woman.

Nursing Plan and Implementation During the Second Stage of Labor

Provision of Care in the Second Stage

The second stage is reached when the cervix is completely dilated (10 cm). The uterine contractions continue as in the transition phase. Maternal pulse, blood

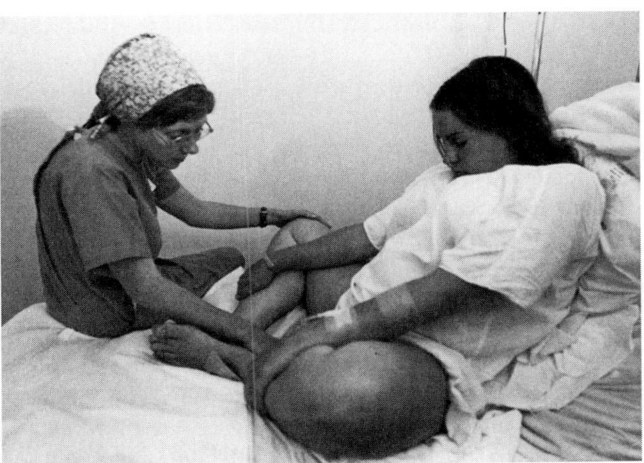

FIGURE 17–4 The nurse provides support during pushing efforts.

KEY FACTS TO REMEMBER

Indications of Imminent Birth

Birth is imminent if the woman shows the following changes:

- Bulging of the perineum
- Uncontrollable urge to bear down
- Increased bloody show

pressure, and FHR are assessed every 5–15 minutes; some protocols recommend assessment after each contraction. As the woman pushes during the second stage, she may make a variety of sounds. A low-pitched, grunting sound ("uhhh") usually indicates the woman is working with the pushing (McKay and Roberts 1990). If she begins to feel she is going to lose control, her sound may change to a high-pitched cry or whimper. A woman who has lost control may shout and yell (McKay and Roberts 1990).

Nursing responses to the woman may vary. At times the sounds are disturbing for nurses and physicians, and they feel the need to help or encourage her to be more quiet. Other nurses feel more comfortable with maternal sounds and use the sounds as cues. The nurse provides support during the woman's pushing effort and stays sensitive to changes in the sounds for clues that the woman is losing control. The nurse may encourage her to push harder and not let any breath out, or to put all her effort into the push and not into making noise. Nurses and physicians seem to value staying in control—but, more important, childbearing women indicate they do not want to lose control (McKay and Roberts 1990).

When the woman feels an uncontrollable urge to push (bear down), the nurse can help by encouraging her and by assisting with positioning (Figure 17–4). The woman may want to be supported with pillows in a semi-reclining position, be side-lying, position herself on her hands and knees, use a squatting bar, or sit on the toilet. Most women spontaneously push in a very effective manner. (Roberts and Woolley 1996). However, in many settings, nurses feel that coaching is necessary. In that case, when the contraction begins, the nurse tells the woman to take two short breaths, in and out, then to take a third breath and hold it while pushing down with her abdominal muscles. Some women prefer to exhale slightly *(exhale breathing)* while pushing to avoid the physiologic effects of the Valsalva maneuver. With this method, the woman takes several deep breaths and then holds her breath for 5–6 seconds. Then, through slightly pursed lips, she exhales slowly every 5–6 seconds while continuing to hold her breath. The woman takes another breath and continues exhale breathing and pushing during the contraction (McKay 1981).

A nullipara is usually prepared for birth when perineal bulging is noted. A multipara usually progresses much more quickly, so she may be prepared for the birth when the cervix is dilated 7–8 cm. As the birth approaches, the woman's partner or support person also prepares for the birth. (See Key Facts to Remember: Indications of Imminent Birth.)

The woman's blood pressure and the FHR are monitored between contractions, and the contractions are palpated until the birth. The nurse continues to assist the woman in her pushing efforts, to keep both the woman and the coach informed of procedures and progress, and to support them both throughout the birth.

In addition to assisting the woman and her partner, the nurse also assists the physician or certified nurse-midwife in preparing for the birth. The physician/CNM dons a sterile gown and gloves and places sterile drapes over the woman's abdomen and legs (see Essential Precautions for Practice: During Birth). An episiotomy may be done just before birth if there is a need for one. See the discussion of episiotomy in Chapter 20.

Promotion of Comfort in the Second Stage

Most of the comfort measures that have been used during the first stage remain appropriate at this time. Cool cloths to the face and forehead may help provide cooling as the woman is involved in the intense physical exertion of pushing. The woman may feel hot and want to remove some of the covering. Care still needs to be taken

ESSENTIAL PRECAUTIONS FOR PRACTICE

During Birth

- The labor nurse who continues to provide support for the woman dons disposable gloves and adds further protection by wearing goggles or her own glasses.
- The physician/certified nurse-midwife wears sterile gloves, a protective gown with a splash apron, or a protective plastic apron, glasses or goggles. The nurse also wears a splash apron and eye covering if splashing of fluids is possible.
- The nurse who provides care for the newborn wears disposable gloves when handling the newborn or any objects or bedding that have been used for the newborn.
- All nurses and physicians/CNMs need to avoid exposure to blood, amniotic fluid, urine, feces, and tracheal, esophageal, or gastric aspirate from the baby.
- Immediately after the birth disposable gloves need to be worn when assessing the perineum and lochial flow, changing perineal pads and chux, placing cold packs, and cleansing the perineum.
- Examples of times when disposable gloves should be worn include changing any garments, chux, bedding, pads, or cold packs that have bloody discharge on them.

A splash apron and eye covering (such as goggles) must be worn when splashing of body fluids is possible.

REMEMBER to wash your hands prior to putting the disposable gloves on and AGAIN immediately after removing the gloves.

For further information consult OSHA and CDC guidelines.

to provide privacy even though covers are removed. The woman can be encouraged to rest and "let all muscles go" during the period between contractions. The nurse and support person(s) can assist the woman into a pushing position with each contraction to further conserve energy. Sips of fluids or ice chips may be used to provide moisture and relieve dryness of the mouth.

Assisting During Birth

Shortly before the birth, the birthing room or delivery room is prepared with equipment and materials that may be needed. Family members do not need to change into other clothing if the birth occurs in a birthing room; they don a disposable scrub suit if the birth is to occur in a delivery room or surgery suite. Good handwashing is required of the nurses and certified nurse-midwife/physician. Nurses who will be in direct contact with the mother at the time of birth need to wear protective clothing such as an apron or gown with a splash apron, disposable gloves, and eye covering (see Essential Precautions for Practice: During Birth). The certified nurse-midwife/physician also needs to wear a gown with a splash apron, or plastic apron, eye covering, and sterile gloves.

If the laboring woman is to give birth in a delivery room, she is moved shortly before birth on her bed or a cart. It is important to preserve her privacy during the transfer, and safety must be provided by raising the side rails into a locked position. In the delivery room, the labor bed or transfer cart must be carefully braced against the delivery table; this ensures the woman's safety during the transfer.

It is important that the woman move from one bed to another between contractions. During the contraction, the woman feels increased discomfort and may be involved in pushing efforts. Perineal bulging may be occurring, which adds to the discomfort and difficulty in moving. All of these factors make moving very uncomfortable.

If birth seems imminent (within the next minute), it is safer for the woman to give birth in her labor bed or on the cart. She is transferred to the delivery table after the baby is born and the cord has been clamped and cut.

Even though there are differences in the delivery room setting, the family can still be together during the birth. It is important to provide encouragement for family members to participate, as the delivery room environment may be unfamiliar and seem less relaxed. The family member may hesitate to continue providing support for fear of interfering or being in the way.

Maternal Birthing Positions

The woman is usually positioned for birth on a bed, in a squatting position, or perhaps on her hands and knees. The position the woman assumes is determined not only by her individual wishes but also by the certified nurse-midwife/physician.

Stirrups, if used, are padded to alleviate pressure, and both legs should be lifted simultaneously to avoid strain on abdominal, back, and perineal muscles. The stirrups should be adjusted to fit the woman's legs. The feet are supported in the stirrup holders. The height and angle of the stirrups are adjusted so there is no pressure on the back of the knees or the calf, which might cause discomfort and postpartal vascular problems. If a birthing bed is used the back is elevated 30 to 60 degrees to help the woman bear down.

The upright posture for birth was considered normal in most societies until modern times. Squatting, kneeling, standing, and sitting were variously selected by women for birth. Only within the last two hundred years has the recumbent position become more usual in the Western world. Its use in this century has been reinforced because of the convenience it offers in applying new technology. The lithotomy position has thus become the conventional manner in which North American women give birth in hospitals. In searching for alternative positions, consumers and professionals alike are refocusing on the comfort of the laboring woman

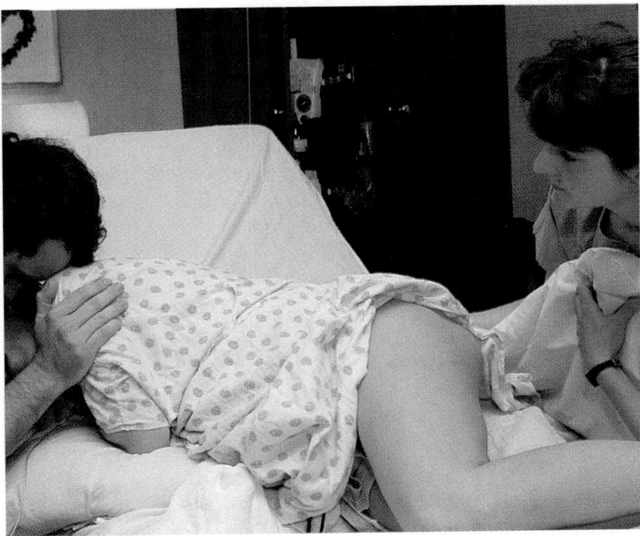

A

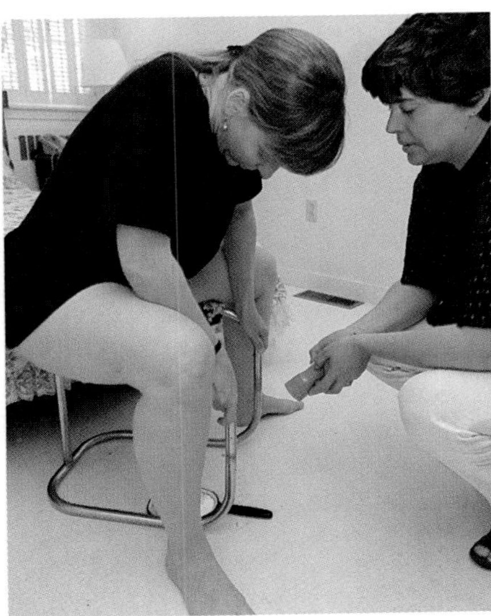

B

FIGURE 17–5 Birthing positions. ***A*** Side-lying position ***B*** Using a birthing stool

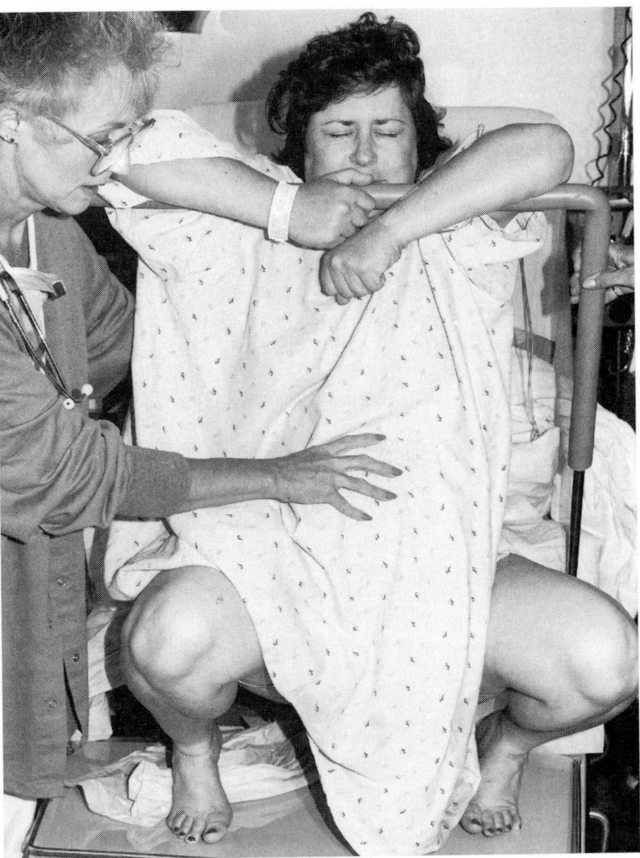

FIGURE 17–6 Use of a birthing bar.

rather than on the convenience of the certified nurse-midwife/physician (Figures 17–5 and 17–6 and Table 17–5).

Cleansing the Perineum

After the woman has been positioned for the birth, her vulvar and perineal area is cleansed to increase her comfort and to remove the bloody discharge that is present prior to the actual birth. An aseptic technique such as the one that follows is recommended.

After a thorough hand washing, the nurse opens the sterile prep tray, dons sterile gloves, and cleanses the woman's vulva and perineum with the cleansing solution (Figure 17–7). Some agency policies dictate the area be rinsed with sterile water. Beginning with the mons, the area is cleansed up to the lower abdomen. The second sponge is used to cleanse the inner groin and thigh of one leg, and the third one is used to cleanse the other leg, moving outward to avoid carrying material from surrounding areas to the vaginal outlet. The last three sponges are used to cleanse the labia and vestibule with one downward sweep each. The used sponges are then discarded. Once the cleansing is completed, the woman returns to the desired birthing position.

Both the woman's partner and the nurse who has been with the laboring woman during the labor continue to provide support during contractions. The woman is encouraged to push with each contraction and, as the fetal head emerges, she is asked to take shallow breaths or pant to prevent pushing. While supporting the fetal head, the physician/certified nurse-midwife assesses whether the umbilical cord is around the fetal neck and removes it if it is, then suctions the mouth and nose with a bulb syringe. The mouth is suctioned first to prevent reflex inhalation of mucus when the sensitive nares are touched with the bulb syringe tip. The woman is encouraged to push again as the rest of the body is born. Figure 17–8 depicts an entire birthing experience.

Text continues on page 414

TABLE 17–5 Comparison of Birthing Positions

Position	Advantages	Disadvantages	Nursing Actions
Sitting on birthing stool	Gravity aids descent and expulsion of infant. Does not compromise venous return from lower extremities. Woman can view birth process.	It is difficult to provide support for the woman's back	Encourage woman to sit in a position that increases her comfort.
Semi-Fowler's	Does not compromise venous return from lower extremities. Woman can view birth process.	If legs are positioned wide apart, relaxation of perineal tissues is decreased.	Assess that upper torso is evenly supported. Increase support of body by changing position of bed or using pillows as props.
Left lateral Sims'	Does not compromise venous return from lower extremities. Increases perineal relaxation and decreases need for episiotomy. Appears to prevent rapid descent.	It is difficult for the woman to see the birth.	Adjust position so that the upper leg lies on the bed (scissor fashion) or is supported by the partner or on pillows.
Squatting	Size of pelvic outlet is increased. Gravity aids descent and expulsion of newborn. Second stage may be shortened (Sleep et al 1989).	It may be difficult to maintain balance while squatting.	Help woman maintain balance. Use a squatting bar if available.
Sitting in birthing bed	Gravity aids descent and expulsion of the fetus. Does not compromise venous return from lower extremities. Woman can view the birth process. Leg position may be changed at will.		Ensure that legs and feet have adequate support.
Hands and knees	Increases perineal relaxation and decreases need for episiotomy. Increases placental and umbilical blood flow and decreases fetal distress. Improves fetal rotation. Nurse is better able to assess perineum. Nurse has better access to fetal nose and mouth for suctioning at birth. Facilitates birth of infant with shoulder dystocia.	Woman cannot view birth. There is decreased contact with birth attendant. Caregivers cannot use instruments. There may be increased maternal fatigue.	Adjust birthing bed by dropping the foot down. Supply extra pillows for increased support.

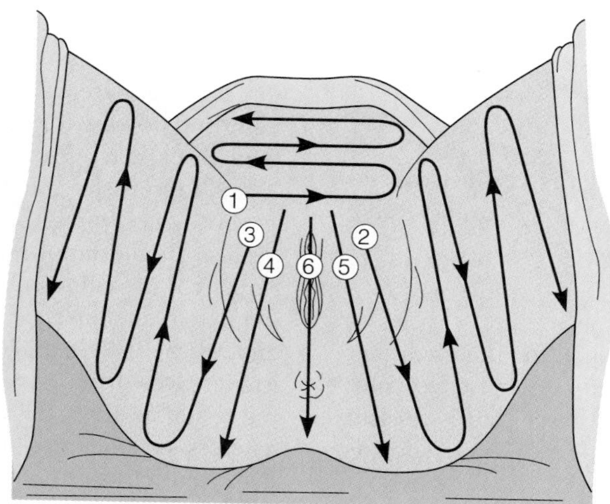

FIGURE 17–7 Cleansing the perineum before birth. The nurse follows the numbered diagram, using a new sponge for each area.

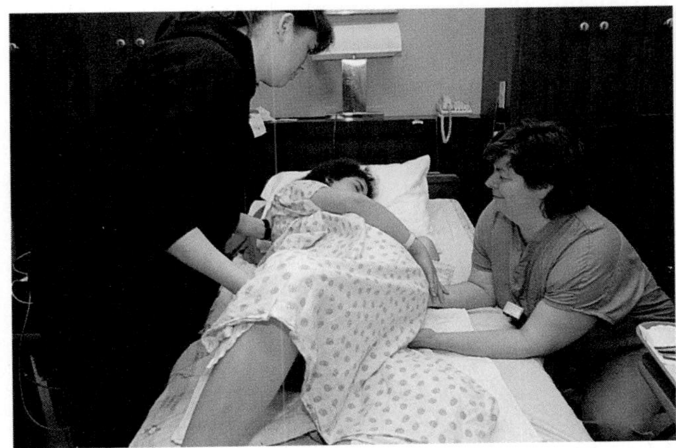

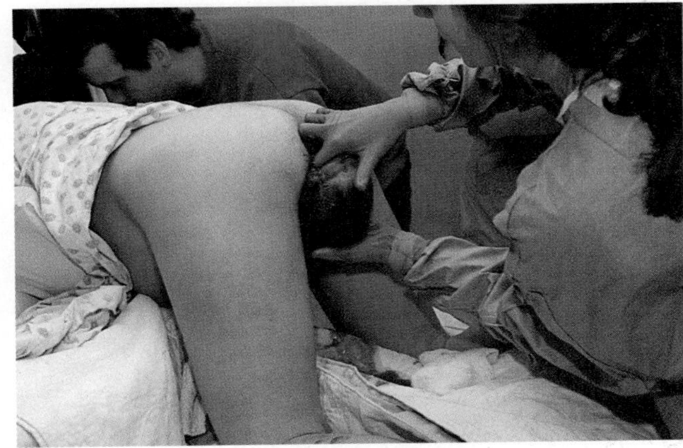

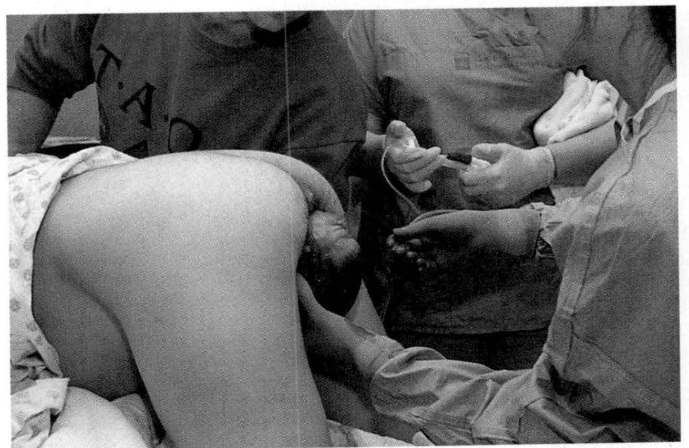

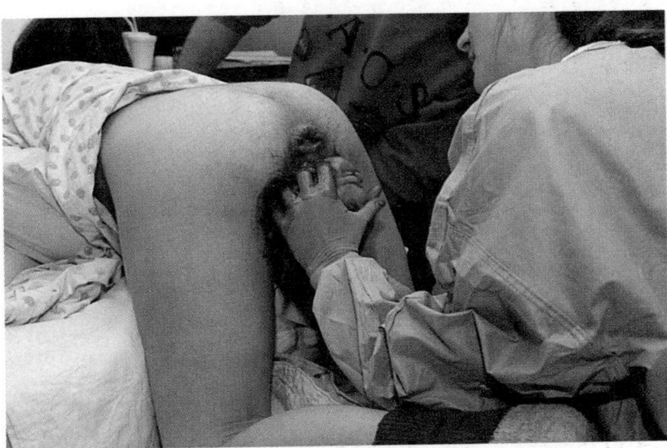

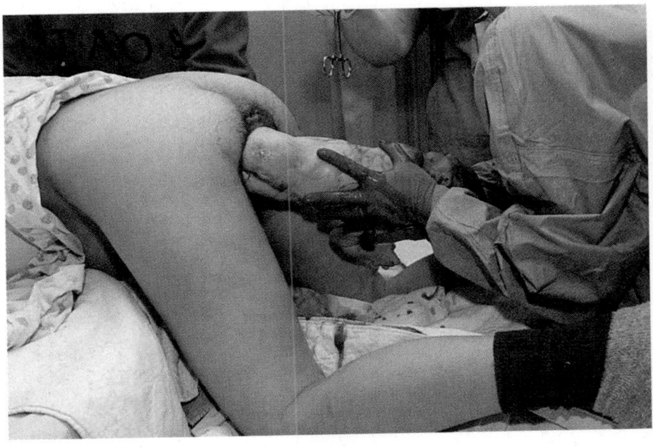

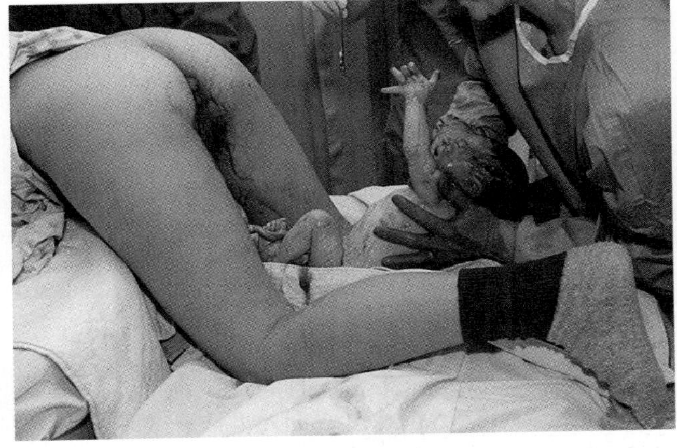

FIGURE 17–8 A birthing sequence.

TABLE 17–6 The Apgar Scoring System

Sign	Score 0	1	2
Heart rate	Absent	Slow—below 100	Above 100
Respiratory effort	Absent	Slow—irregular	Good crying
Muscle tone	Flaccid	Some flexion of extremities	Active motion
Reflex irritability	None	Grimace	Vigorous cry
Color	Pale blue	Body pink, blue extremities	Completely pink

Source: Apgar V: The newborn (Apgar) scoring system, reflections and advice. *Pediatr Clin North Am* August 1966; 13:645.

Nursing Plan and Implementation During the Third and Fourth Stages

Provision of Initial Care to the Newborn

The certified nurse-midwife/physician places the newborn on the mother's abdomen or in the radiant-heated unit. The newborn is maintained in a modified Trendelenburg position. This position aids drainage of mucus from the nasopharynx and trachea by gravity. The newborn is dried immediately. Warmth can be maintained by placing warmed blankets over the newborn or placing the newborn in skin-to-skin contact with the mother. If the newborn is in a radiant-heated unit, he or she is dried, placed on a dry blanket, and left uncovered under the radiant heat. Because radiant heat warms the outer surface of objects, a newborn wrapped in blankets will receive no benefit from radiant heat.

The newborn's nose and mouth are suctioned with a bulb syringe as needed. Most immediate care of the newborn can be accomplished while the newborn is in the parent's arms or in the radiant-heated unit.

Apgar Scoring System

The Apgar scoring system (Table 17–6) was designed in 1952 by Dr. Virginia Apgar. The purpose of the **Apgar score** is to evaluate the physical condition of the newborn at birth. The newborn is rated 1 minute after birth and again at 5 minutes, and receives a total score ranging from 0 to 10 based on the following assessments:

1. The *heart rate* is auscultated or palpated at the junction of the umbilical cord and skin. This is the most important assessment. A newborn heart rate of less than 100 beats/min indicates the need for immediate resuscitation.
2. The *respiratory effort* is the second most important Apgar assessment. Complete absence of respirations is termed apnea. A vigorous cry indicates adequate respirations.
3. The *muscle tone* is determined by evaluating the degree of flexion and resistance to straightening of the extremities. A normal newborn's elbows and hips are flexed, with the knees positioned up toward the abdomen.
4. The *reflex irritability* is evaluated by stroking the baby's back along the spine, or by flicking the soles of the feet. A cry merits a full score of 2. A grimace is 1 point, and no response is 0.
5. The *skin color* is inspected for cyanosis and pallor. Generally, newborns have blue extremities, and the rest of the body is pink, which merits a score of 1. This condition is termed acrocyanosis and is present in 85 percent of normal newborns at 1 minute after birth. A completely pink newborn scores a 2, and a totally cyanotic, pale infant scores 0. Newborns with darker skin pigmentation will not be pink in color. Their skin color is assessed for pallor and acrocyanosis, and a score is selected based on the assessment.

A score of 8–10 indicates a newborn in good condition who requires only nasopharyngeal suctioning and perhaps some oxygen near the face (called "blow-by" oxygen). If the Apgar score is below 8, resuscitative measures may need to be instituted. See the discussion in Chapter 25.

Care of Umbilical Cord

If the clinician has not placed some type of cord clamp on the newborn's umbilical cord, the nurse must do so. Before applying the cord clamp, the nurse examines the cut end for the presence of two arteries and one vein. The umbilical vein is the largest vessel, and the arteries are seen as smaller vessels. The number of vessels is recorded on the birth and newborn records. The cord is clamped approximately ½ to 1 inch from the abdomen to allow room between the abdomen and clamp as the cord dries. Abdominal skin must not be clamped, as this will cause necrosis of the tissue. The most common types of cord clamps are the plastic Hollister cord clamp (Figure 17–9), the metal Hesseltine clamp, and the cord bander. The Hollister or Hesseltine clamp is removed in the newborn nursery approximately 24 hours after the cord has dried. The rubber band that remains on the umbilical cord stump if a cord bander is used will remain in place until the cord falls off.

Cord Blood Collection for Banking

A growing number of parents are arranging for cord blood banking (see discussion in Chapter 1). Immediately after the newborn's umbilical cord is clamped and cut and the placenta is expelled, the certified nurse-midwife/physician withdraws blood from the remaining umbilical cord and the placenta. The blood is placed in

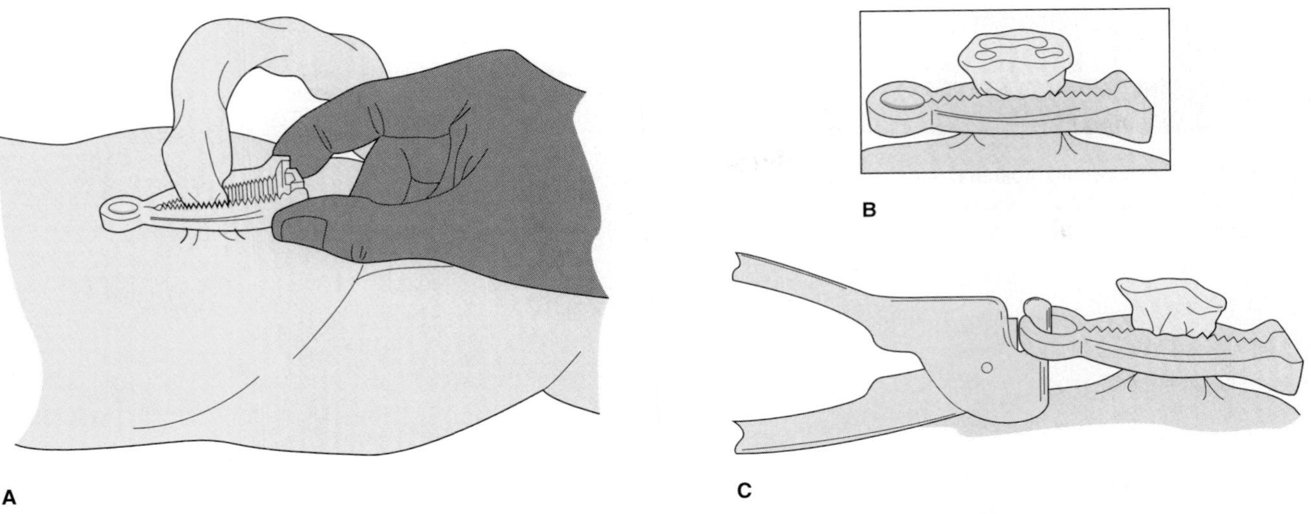

FIGURE 17–9 Hollister cord clamp. ***A*** Clamp is positioned ½ to 1 inch from the abdomen and then secured. ***B*** Cut cord. The one vein and two arteries can be seen. ***C*** Plastic device for removing clamp after cord has dried. After the cord is cut, the nurse grasps the Hollister clamp on either side of the cut area and gently separates it.

a special container that parents receive from the Cord Blood Registry and bring with them for the birth. The parents will also have any special directions that are required for storage and care of the container.

Physical Assessment of Newborn by Nurse

The nurse performs an abbreviated systematic physical assessment in the birthing area to detect any abnormalities (Table 17–7). First, the nurse notes the size of the newborn and the contour and size of the head in relationship to the rest of the body. The newborn's posture and movements indicate tone and neurologic functioning.

The nurse inspects skin for discoloration, presence of vernix caseosa and lanugo, and evidence of trauma and desquamation (peeling of skin). Vernix caseosa is a white, cheesy substance found normally on newborns. It is absorbed within 24 hours after birth. Vernix is abundant on preterm infants and absent on postterm newborns. A large quantity of fine hair (lanugo) is often seen on preterm newborns, especially on their shoulders, foreheads, backs, and cheeks. Desquamation of the skin is seen in postterm newborns.

The nurse observes the nares for flaring and, as the newborn cries, inspects the palate for cleft palate. The nurse looks for mucus in the nose and mouth and removes it with a bulb syringe as needed. The nurse inspects the chest for respiratory rate and the presence of retractions. If retractions are present, the nurse assesses the newborn for grunting or stridor. A normal respiratory rate is 30–40 per minute. The lungs may be auscultated bilaterally for breath sounds. Absence of breath sounds on one side could mean pneumothorax. Rales may be heard immediately after birth because a small amount of fluid may remain in the lungs; this fluid will be absorbed. Rhonchi indicate aspiration of oral secretions. If there is excessive mucus or respiratory distress, the nurse suctions the newborn with a mucus trap. See Procedure 17–1: Performing Nasal Pharyngeal Suctioning, and Figure 17–10 (p 416).

TABLE 17–7 Initial Newborn Evaluation

Assess	*Normal Findings*
Respirations	Rate 36–60, irregular No retractions, no grunting
Apical pulse	Rate 120–160 and somewhat irregular
Temperature	Skin temp above 36.5C (97.8F)
Skin color	Body pink with bluish extremities
Umbilical cord	Two arteries and one vein
Gestational age	Should be 38–42 weeks to remain with parents for extended time
Sole creases	Sole creases that involve the heel

In general expect scant amount of vernix on upper back, axilla, groin; lanugo only on upper back; ears with incurving of upper 2/3 of pinnae and thin cartilage that springs back from folding; male genitalia—testes palpated in upper or lower scrotum; female genitalia—labia majora larger; clitoris nearly covered

In the following situations newborns should generally be stabilized rather than remaining with parents in the birth area for an extended period of time:

- Apgar less than 8 at 1 minute and less than 9 at 5 minutes or baby requires resuscitation measures (other than whiffs of oxygen)
- Respirations below 30 or above 60, with retractions and/or grunting
- Apical pulse below 120 or above 160 with marked irregularities
- Skin temperature below 36.5C (97.8F)
- Skin color pale blue or circumoral pallor
- Baby less than 38 or more than 42 weeks' gestation
- Baby very small or very large for gestational age
- Congenital anomalies involving open areas in the skin (meningomyelocele)

PROCEDURE 17–1 Performing Nasal Pharyngeal Suctioning

Nursing Action	Rationale
Objective: Clear secretions from the newborn's nose and/or oropharynx if respirations are depressed and/or if amniotic fluid was meconium-stained.	
• Tighten the lid on the DeLee mucus trap or other suction device collection bottle.	This avoids spillage of secretions and prevents air from leaking out of the lid.
• Connect one end of the DeLee tubing to low suction.	
• Insert the other end of the tubing 3 to 5 inches in the newborn's nose or mouth (Figure 17–10).	
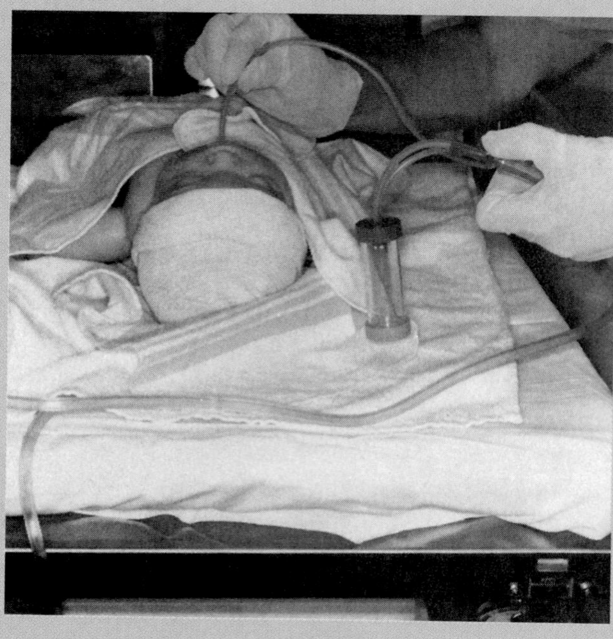 **FIGURE 17–10** DeLee mucus trap.	
• Continue suction as you remove the tube.	This avoids redepositing secretions in the newborn's nasopharynx.
• Continue to reinsert the tube and provide suction for as long as fluid is aspirated. *Note: Excessive suctioning can cause vagal stimulation, which causes decreased heart rate.*	
• If it is necessary to pass the tube into the newborn's stomach to remove meconium secretions that the newborn swallowed before birth, insert the tube into the newborn's mouth and then into the stomach. Provide suction and continue suction as you remove the tube.	
Objective: Record relevant information on the newborn's chart.	
• Document completion of the procedure and the amount and type of secretions.	This provides documentation of intervention and status at birth.

The nurse notes and records elimination of urine or meconium on the newborn record.

Newborn Identification

To ensure correct identification, the nurse gives the mother and the newborn matching identification bands in the birthing or delivery room. One bracelet is placed on the mother's wrist. Two bracelets are placed on the newborn—one on the wrist and one on the ankle. The newborn bands must fit snugly to prevent their loss.

Most hospitals also footprint the newborn and fingerprint the mother. To prepare the newborn for footprinting, the nurse wipes the soles of both the newborn's feet to remove any vernix caseosa.

Provision of Care in the Third Stage

After birth, the certified nurse-midwife/physician prepares for the delivery of the placenta (see Chapter 15). The following signs suggest placental separation:

1. The uterus rises upward in the abdomen.
2. As the placenta moves downward, the umbilical cord lengthens.
3. A sudden trickle or spurt of blood appears.
4. The shape of the uterus changes from a disk to a globe.

While waiting for these signs, the nurse palpates the uterus to check for ballooning caused by uterine relaxation and subsequent bleeding into the uterine cavity. After the placenta has separated, the woman may be asked to bear down to aid delivery of the placenta.

Oxytocics are frequently given at the time of the delivery of the placenta, so the uterus will contract and bleeding will be minimized. Oxytocin (Pitocin), 10 units, may be added to an intravenous infusion or given by slow intravenous push. Some physicians order methylergonovine maleate (Methergine), 0.2 mg, intramuscularly. In addition to administering the ordered medications, the nurse assesses and records maternal blood pressure before and after administration of oxytocics. For further information, refer to the Drug Guides: Oxytocin in Chapter 20 and Methylergonovine Maleate in Chapter 28.

Provision of Care in the Fourth Stage

After the delivery of the placenta, the certified nurse-midwife/physician inspects the placental membranes to make sure they are intact and that all cotyledons are present. This inspection is especially important with Duncan placentas because there is an increased risk that placental fragments are left in the uterus. If there is a defect or a part missing from the placenta, a manual uterine examination is done. The nurse notes on the birth record the time and mechanism (Schultze or Duncan) of delivery of the placenta.

The vagina and cervix are inspected for lacerations, and any necessary repairs are made. The episiotomy may be repaired now if it has not been done previously (see Chapter 20). The fundus of the uterus is palpated; normal position is at the midline and below the umbilicus. A displaced fundus may be caused by a full bladder or blood collected in the uterus. The uterus may be emptied of blood by grasping it with one hand anteriorly and posteriorly and squeezing.

The uterine fundus is palpated at frequent intervals to ensure that it remains firmly contracted. The maternal blood pressure is monitored at 5- to 15-minute intervals to detect any changes. An increase in blood pressure may be due to oxytocic drugs. A decrease may be associated with excessive blood loss.

The nurse washes the woman's perineum with gauze squares and warmed solution and dries the area with a sterile towel before placing the maternity pads. If stirrups have been used the woman's legs are removed from the stirrups at the same time to avoid muscle strain. The legs may be bicycled to help circulation return. The woman remains in the same bed or is transferred to a recovery room bed, and the nurse helps her don a clean gown. The mother may feel cold and begin shivering. She can be covered with a warmed bath blanket and a second blanket. The nurse ensures that the mother, father or her partner, and newborn are provided with time to begin the attachment process. See Chapter 27 for further discussion of attachment. Also see Essential Precautions for Practice: During the Fourth Stage.

ESSENTIAL PRECAUTIONS FOR PRACTICE

During the Fourth Stage

Examples of times when disposable gloves should be worn include the following:

- Changing any garments, chux, bedding, pads, or cold packs that have bloody discharge on them
- Assessing the perineum and amount of lochia
- Assisting the woman with urination, emptying bedpans, and so forth
- Cleansing the perineal area
- Handling the newborn (Disposable gloves are required until the newborn has received the first bath.)

REMEMBER to wash your hands prior to putting the disposable gloves on and AGAIN immediately after removing the gloves.

For further information consult OSHA and CDC guidelines.

TABLE 17–8 Maternal Adaptations Following Birth

Characteristic	Normal Finding
Blood pressure	Returns to prelabor level
Pulse	Slightly lower than in labor
Uterine fundus	In the midline at the umbilicus or 1–2 fingerbreadths below the umbilicus
Lochia	Red (rubra), small to moderate amount (from spotting on pads to 1/4 – 1/2 of pad covered in 15 minutes) Doesn't exceed saturation of one pad in first hour
Bladder	Nonpalpable
Perineum	Smooth, pink, without bruising or edema
Emotional state	Wide variation, including excited, exhilarated, smiling, crying, fatigued, verbal, quiet, pensive, and sleepy

KEY FACTS TO REMEMBER

Immediate Postbirth Danger Signs

In the immediate postbirth recovery period, the following conditions should be reported to the CNM or physician:

- Hypotension
- Tachycardia
- Uterine atony
- Excessive bleeding
- Hematoma

During the recovery period (1–4 hours) the woman is monitored closely. Deviations from normal in vital signs require frequent checking. Blood pressure should return to the prelabor level due to an increased volume of blood returning to the maternal circulation from the uteroplacental shunt. Pulse rate should be slightly lower than it was during labor. Baroreceptors cause a vagal response, which slows the pulse. A rise in blood pressure may be a response to oxytocic drugs or may be caused by PIH. Blood loss may be reflected by a lowered blood pressure and a rising pulse rate (Table 17–8).

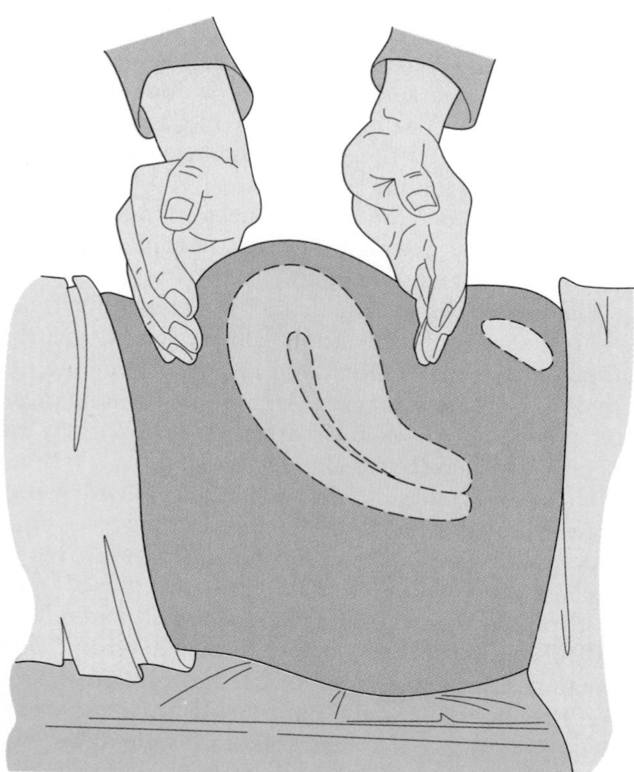

FIGURE 17–11 Suggested method of palpating the fundus of the uterus during the fourth stage. The left hand is placed just above the symphysis pubis, and gentle downward pressure is exerted. The right hand is cupped around the uterine fundus.

The fundus should be firm, at the umbilicus or lower, and in the midline. It is palpated (Figure 17–11) but not massaged unless it is soft (boggy). If it becomes boggy or appears to rise in the abdomen, the fundus is massaged until firm; then the nurse exerts firm pressure on the fundus in an attempt to express retained clots. During all aspects of fundal massage, the nurse uses one hand to provide support for the lower portion of the uterus.

The nurse inspects the bloody vaginal discharge for amount and charts it as minimal, moderate, or heavy and with or without clots. This discharge, or **lochia rubra,** should be bright red. A soaked perineal pad contains approximately 100 mL of blood. If the perineal pad becomes soaked in a 15-minute period or if blood pools under the buttocks, continuous observation is necessary. (See Procedure 17–2: Evaluating Lochia After Birth.) When the fundus is firm, a continuous trickle of blood may signal laceration of the vagina or cervix or an unligated vessel in the episiotomy. See Key Facts to Remember: Immediate Postbirth Danger Signs.

If the fundus rises and displaces to the right, the nurse must be concerned about two factors:

1. As the uterus rises, the uterine contractions become less effective and increased bleeding may occur.
2. The most common cause of uterine displacement is bladder distention.

The nurse palpates the bladder to determine whether it is distended. The bladder fills rapidly with the extra fluid volume returned from the uteroplacental circulation (and with any fluid received intravenously during labor and birth). The postpartal woman may not realize that her bladder is full because trauma to the bladder and urethra during childbirth and the use of regional anesthesia decreases bladder tone and the urge to void.

All measures should be taken to enable the mother to void. A warm towel placed across the lower abdomen or

PROCEDURE 17–2 Evaluating Lochia After Birth

Nursing Action	Rationale
Objective: Prepare the woman.	
• Explain the procedure, the reason for performing the procedure, and the information that will be obtained.	Explanation of the procedure decreases anxiety and increases relaxation.
Objective: Obtain and evaluate maternal vital signs.	
• Assess maternal temperature, blood pressure, and pulse.	This provides information regarding the woman's physiologic status.
Objective: Accurately evaluate the amount of lochia after birth.	
• Don disposable gloves.	Universal precautions and body substance isolation require use of gloves when exposed to body secretions.
• Lower the perineal pad so that you can visualize the amount of lochia.	
• Palpate the uterine fundus, located in the midlines at the umbilicus or one to two fingerbreadths below the umbilicus, by placing one hand on the fundus and the other hand just over the symphysis pubis and press downward. Use your other hand to palpate the fundus.	Downward pressure exerted just above the symphysis pubis will prevent excessive downward movement of the uterus during assessment.
• Determine the firmness of the fundus.	The uterus must remain firmly contracted to prevent excessive blood loss.
• If the fundus is boggy, massage by rubbing in a circular motion.	Manual pressure stimulates uterine contractions.
• Evaluate the color and amount of lochia, and observe for clots.	
Lochia Evaluation Guidelines	
Small: Smaller than a 4 inch stain on the pad; 10 to 25 mL	
Moderate: Smaller than a 6 inch stain; 25 to 50 mL	
Large: Larger than a 6 inch stain; 50 to 80 mL (Leugenbiehl et al 1990)	
• If blood loss exceeds the above guidelines, you weigh the perineal pads and the chux to estimate the blood loss more accurately. 1 g of weight = 1 mL	Weighing the pads and chux can provide important information as amounts of blood loss may be underestimated due to the expectation that some blood will be lost normally.

warm water poured over the perineum may relax the urinary sphincter and facilitate voiding. If the woman is unable to void, catheterization is necessary. The perineum is inspected for edema and hematoma formation. An ice pack often reduces the swelling and alleviates the discomfort of an episiotomy.

Frequently women have tremors in the immediate postpartal period. This shivering response may be caused by a difference in internal and external body temperatures (higher temperature inside the body than on the outside). Another theory is that the woman is reacting to the fetal cells that have entered the maternal circulation at the placental site. A heated bath blanket placed next to the woman tends to alleviate the problem.

The couple may be tired, hungry, and thirsty. Some agencies serve the couple a meal. The tired mother will probably drift off into a welcome sleep. The partner can also be encouraged to rest, since his supporting role is physically and mentally tiring. If the mother is not in a birthing room, she is usually transferred from the birthing unit to the postpartal or mother-baby area after 2 hours or more, depending on agency policy and whether the following criteria are met:

- Stable vital signs
- No bleeding
- Undistended bladder
- Firm fundus
- Sensations fully recovered from any anesthetic agent received during birth

Enhancing Attachment

Dramatic evidence indicates that the first few hours and even minutes after birth are an important period for the **attachment** of mother and infant (Klaus and Kennell 1982). Separation during this period not only delays attachment but also may affect maternal and child behavior over a much longer period.

Klaus and Kennell (1982) believe the bonding experience can be enhanced by at least 30–60 minutes of early contact in privacy. If this period of contact can occur during the first hour after birth, the newborn will be in the quiet state and able to interact with parents by looking at them. Newborns also turn their heads in

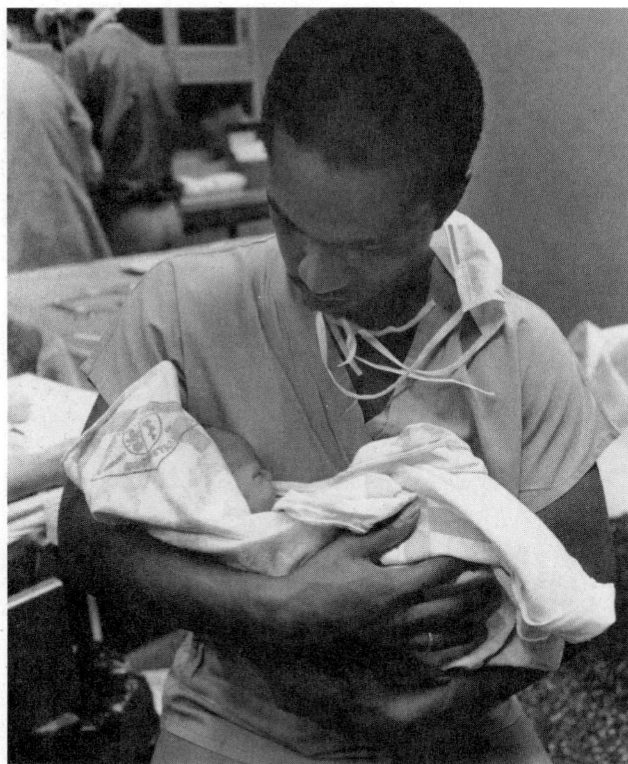

FIGURE 17–12 A father holds his newborn.

response to a spoken voice. See Chapter 21 for further discussion of newborn states.

The first parent-newborn contact may be brief (a few minutes) to be followed by a more extended contact after uncomfortable procedures (delivery of the placenta and suturing of the episiotomy) are completed. When the newborn is returned to the mother, she can be assisted to begin breastfeeding if she so desires. Various researchers emphasize that the baby will seek out the mother's breast and that early contact between the two can greatly affect breastfeeding success (Kennell 1994; Richard and Alade 1990). Even if the newborn does not actively nurse, he or she can lick, taste, and smell the mother's skin. This activity by the newborn stimulates the maternal release of prolactin, which promotes the onset of lactation.

Darkening the birthing room by turning out most of the lights causes newborns to open their eyes and gaze around. This in turn enhances eye-to-eye contact with the parents. (*Note:* If the physician or CNM needs a light source, the spotlight can be left on.) Treatment of the newborn's eyes may also be delayed. Many parents who establish eye contact with the newborn are content to quietly gaze at their infant. Others may show more active involvement by touching or inspecting the newborn. Some mothers talk to their babies in a high-pitched voice, which seems to be soothing to newborns. Some couples verbally express amazement and pride when they see they have produced a beautiful, healthy baby. Their verbalization enhances feelings of accomplishment and ecstasy. Figure 17–12 shows a new parent establishing bonds with his newborn son.

Both parents need to be encouraged to do whatever they feel most comfortable doing. Some parents prefer only limited contact with the newborn immediately after birth and instead desire private time together in a quiet environment. In spite of the current zeal for providing immediate attachment opportunities, nursing personnel need to be aware of parents' wishes. The desire to delay interaction with the newborn does not necessarily imply a decreased ability of the parents to bond to their newborn. See Chapter 26 for further discussion of parent-newborn attachment.

Nursing Plan and Implementation During Nurse-Attended Birth

Occasionally labor progresses so rapidly that the maternity nurse is faced with the task of assisting in the actual birth of the baby. This is called a **precipitous birth.** The attending maternity nurse has the primary responsibility for providing a physically and psychologically safe experience for the woman and her baby.

A woman whose certified nurse-midwife/physician is not present may feel disappointed, frightened, abandoned, angry, and cheated. She may fear what is going to happen and feel that everything is out of control. In working with the woman, the nurse provides support by keeping her informed about the labor progress and assuring her that the nurse will stay with her. If birth is imminent, the nurse must not leave the mother alone. Auxiliary personnel can be directed to contact the certified nurse-midwife/physician and retrieve the emergency birth pack ("precip pack"). An emergency birth pack should be readily accessible to birthing rooms. A typical pack contains

1. A small drape that can be placed under the woman's buttocks to provide a sterile field
2. A bulb syringe to clear mucus from the newborn's mouth
3. Two sterile clamps (Kelly or Rochester) to clamp the umbilical cord before applying a cord clamp
4. Sterile scissors to cut the umbilical cord
5. A sterile umbilical cord clamp, either Hesseltine or Hollister
6. A baby blanket to wrap the newborn in after birth
7. A package of sterile gloves

As the materials are being gathered, the nurse must remain calm. The woman is reassured by the composure of the nurse and feels that the nurse is competent.

The nurse assists in the precipitous birth as follows. The woman is encouraged to assume a comfortable position. If time permits, the nurse scrubs her hands with soap and water and puts on sterile gloves. Sterile drapes are placed under the woman's buttocks.

At all times during the birth, the nurse provides suggestions such as when to maintain a controlled breathing pattern and when to push, supports the woman's efforts, and provides reassurance.

The nurse may place an index finger inside the lower portion of the vagina and the thumb on the outer portion of the perineum and gently massage the area to help stretch perineal tissues and prevent perineal lacerations. This is called "ironing the perineum."

When the infant's head crowns, the nurse instructs the woman to pant, which decreases her urge to push. The nurse checks whether the amniotic sac is intact. If it is, the nurse tears the sac so the newborn will not breathe in amniotic fluid with the first breath.

With one hand, the nurse applies gentle pressure against the fetal head to prevent it from popping out rapidly. *The nurse does not hold the head back forcibly.* Rapid birth of the head may result in tears in the woman's perineal tissues. In the fetus the rapid change in pressure within the fetal head may cause subdural or dural tears. The nurse supports the perineum with the other hand and allows the head to be born between contractions.

As the woman continues to pant, the nurse inserts one or two fingers along the back of the fetal head to check for the umbilical cord. If there is a **nuchal cord** (umbilical cord around the neck), the nurse bends her fingers like a fish hook, grasps the cord, and pulls it over the baby's head. It is important to check that the cord is not wrapped around more than one time. If the cord is tightly looped and cannot be slipped over the baby's head, two clamps are placed on the cord, the cord is cut between the clamps, and the cord is unwound.

Immediately after birth of the head, the nurse suctions the mouth, throat, and nasal passages. The nurse then places one hand on each side of the head and exerts gentle downward traction until the anterior shoulder passes under the symphysis pubis. Then gentle upward traction aids the birth of the posterior shoulder. The nurse then instructs the woman to push gently so that the rest of the body can be born quickly. The newborn must be supported as she or he emerges.

The newborn is held at the level of the uterus to facilitate blood flow through the umbilical cord. The combination of amniotic fluid and vernix makes the newborn very slippery, so the nurse must be careful to avoid dropping the baby. The nose and mouth of the newborn are suctioned again, using a bulb syringe. The nurse then dries the newborn to prevent heat loss.

As soon as the nurse determines that the newborn's respirations are adequate, the infant can be placed on the mother's abdomen. The newborn's head should be slightly lower than the body to aid drainage of fluid and mucus. The weight of the newborn on the mother's abdomen stimulates uterine contractions, which aid in placental separation. The umbilical cord should not be pulled.

The nurse is alert for signs of placental separation (slight gush of dark blood from the vagina, lengthening of the cord, or a change in uterine shape from discoid to globular). When these signs are present, the mother is instructed to push so that the placenta can be delivered. The nurse inspects the placenta to determine whether it is intact.

The nurse checks the firmness of the uterus. The fundus may be gently massaged to stimulate contractions and decrease bleeding. Putting the newborn to breast also stimulates uterine contractions through release of oxytocin from the pituitary gland.

The umbilical cord may now be cut. The nurse places two sterile Kelly clamps approximately 1–3 inches from the newborn's abdomen. The cord is cut between the Kelly clamps with sterile scissors. The nurse places a sterile umbilical cord clamp (Hollister or Hesseltine) adjacent to the clamp on the newborn's cord, between the clamp and the newborn's abdomen. The clamp *must not* be placed snugly against the abdomen, because the cord will dry and shrink.

The nurse cleanses the area under the mother's buttocks and inspects her perineum for lacerations. Bleeding from lacerations may be controlled by pressing a clean perineal pad against the perineum and instructing the woman to keep her thighs together.

If the certified nurse-midwife/physician's arrival is delayed or if the newborn is having respiratory distress, the newborn should be transported immediately to the nursery. *The newborn must be properly identified before he or she leaves the birth area.*

The nurse notes and places on a birth record the following information:

1. Position of fetus at birth
2. Presence of cord around neck or shoulder (nuchal cord)
3. Time of birth
4. Apgar scores at 1 and 5 minutes after birth
5. Gender of newborn
6. Time of expulsion of placenta
7. Method of placental expulsion
8. Appearance and intactness of placenta
9. Mother's condition
10. Any medications that were given to mother or newborn (per agency protocol)

Evaluation

Evaluation provides an opportunity to determine the effectiveness of nursing care. As a result of comprehensive nursing care during the intrapartal period, the following outcomes may be anticipated:

- The mother's physical and psychologic well-being has been maintained and supported.
- The baby's physical and psychologic well-being has been protected and supported.
- The couple have had input into the birth process and have participated as much as they desired.
- The mother and her baby have had a safe birth.

CHAPTER HIGHLIGHTS

- Before care is begun it is important to explain what will be done, the reasons, potential benefits and risks, and possible alternatives if appropriate. This helps the woman determine what happens to her body.
- Behavioral responses to labor vary with the phase of labor, the preparation the woman has had, and her previous experience, cultural beliefs, and developmental level.
- The childbearing family may have a variety of expectations of the nurse during labor and birth. Some families want to make all decisions themselves with limited nursing contact; others want a moderate amount of contact and see the relationship as a cooperative venture; and some families want a lot of involvement, looking to the nurse to make decisions and instill confidence in them that everything will be all right.
- Each woman's cultural beliefs affect her needs for privacy, expression of discomfort, and expectations for the birth and the role she wishes the father to play in the birth event.
- The adolescent mother has special needs in the birth setting. Her developmental needs require specialized nursing care.
- The laboring woman's comfort may be increased by general comfort measures, supportive relaxation techniques, methods of handling anxiety, controlled breathing, and support by a caring person.
- Maternal birthing positions include a wide variety of possibilities, from side-lying to sitting, squatting, and semi-Fowler's.
- Immediate assessments of the newborn include evaluation of the Apgar score and an abbreviated physical assessment. These early assessments help determine the need for resuscitation and whether the newborn's adaptation to extrauterine life is progressing normally. The newborn who is not experiencing problems may remain with the parents for an extended period of time after birth.
- Immediate care of the newborn also includes maintenance of respirations, promotion of warmth, prevention of infection, and accurate identification.
- The placenta separates from the uterine wall and is expelled with either the maternal or fetal side emerging from the vagina. The maternal side contains the cotyledons, appears rough in texture, and may be associated with retention of placental fragments.
- The fourth stage includes the first 1 to 4 hours following birth. Many physiologic and psychologic changes occur during this period.
- At times a baby is born rapidly without the physician/certified nurse-midwife present. This instance is referred to as a precipitous birth. The nurse in the birthing area remains with the woman and attends her during the birth until a certified nurse-midwife/physician can be present.

REFERENCES

Ahmad S: Culturally sensitive caregiving for the Pakistani woman. Lecture presented at the Medical College of Virginia Hospitals, Richmond, VA. (November 1994.) In Weber SE: Cultural aspects of pain in childbearing women. *JOGNN* January 1996; 25:67.

American Academy of Pediatrics and The American College of Obstetrician and Gynecologists: *Guidelines for Perinatal Care,* 2nd ed, Washington, DC, 1992.

Bryanton J, Fraser-Davey H, Sullivan P: Women's perceptions of nursing support during labor. *JOGNN* 1994; 23(8):638.

Calhoun MA: The Vietnamese woman: Health/illness attitudes and behaviors. In: *Women, Health and Culture.* Stern PN (editor). Washington, DC: Hemisphere, 1986.

Drake P: Addressing developmental needs of pregnant adolescents. *JOGNN* July/August 1996; 25:518.

Ganforth S, Garcia J: Hospital admission practices. In: *Effective Care in Pregnancy and Childbirth, Vol. 2: Childbirth.* Chalmers I et al (editors). New York: Oxford University Press, 1989.

Higgins PG, Wayland JR: Labour and delivery in North America. *Nurs Times* September 1981 (Midwifery Suppl): 77.

Hodnett E: Nursing support of the laboring woman. *JOGNN* March/April 1996; 25:257.

Hutchinson MK, Baqi-Aziz M: Nursing care of the childbearing Muslim family. *JOGNN* 1994; 23(9):767.

Kennell JH: The time has come to reassess delivery room routines. *Birth* March 1994; 21(1):49.

Khazoyan CM, Anderson NLR: Latinas' expectations for their partners during childbirth. *MCN* 1994; 19:226.

Klaus MH, Kennell JH: *Parent-Infant Bonding,* 2nd ed. St Louis: Mosby, 1982.

LaDu EB: Childbirth care for Hmong families. *MCN* November/December 1985; 10:382.

Leugenbiehl DL et al: Standardized assessment of blood loss. *MCN* July/August 1990; 15:241.

Ludka LM, Roberts CC: Eating and drinking in labor: A literature review. *J Nurse-Midwifery* 1993; 38:199.

McKay S, Roberts J: Obstetrics by ear: Maternal and caregiver perceptions of the meaning of maternal sounds during second stage of labor. *J Nurse-Midwifery* September/October 1990; 35(5):266.

NAACOG OGN Nursing Practice Resource: *Fetal Heart Rate Auscultation.* Washington, DC, March 1990.

Nichols FH, Humenick SS: *Childbirth Education: Practice, Research and Theory.* Philadelphia: Saunders, 1988.

Richard L, Alade MO: Effect of delivery room routines on success of first breastfeed. *Lancet* 1990; 336:1105.

Roberts JE et al: The effects of maternal position on uterine contractility and efficiency. *Birth* Winter 1983; 10(4):243.

Roberts J, Woolley D: A second look at the second stage of labor. *JOGNN* June 1996; 25:415.

Scott-Ramos I: Culturally sensitive care giving for the Latino woman. In Weber SE: Cultural aspects of pain in childbearing women. *JOGNN* January 1996; 25:67.

Sleep J, Roberts S, Chalmers I: Care during the second stage of labor. In: *Effective Care in Pregnancy and Childbirth, Vol 2: Childbirth.* Chalmers I, Enkin M, Keirse MJNC (editors). New York: Oxford University Press, 1989.

Tomlinson PS, Bryan A: Family centered intrapartum care: Revisiting an old concept. *JOGNN* May 1996; 25:331.

Weaver DF: Nurses' views on the meaning of touch in obstetrical nursing practice. *JOGNN* March/April 1990; 19(2):157.

Weber SE: Cultural aspects of pain in childbearing women. *JOGNN* January 1996; 25:67.

Wuitchik M et al: The clinical significance of pain and cognitive activity in latent labor. *Obstet Gynecol* January 1989; 73(1):35.

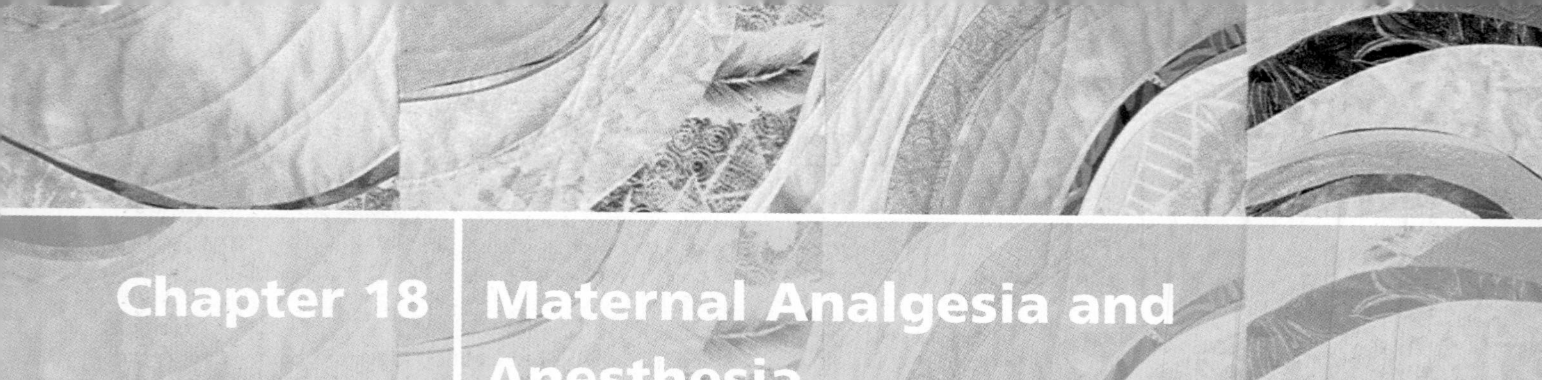

Chapter 18 Maternal Analgesia and Anesthesia

OBJECTIVES

- Describe the use of systemic drugs to promote pain relief during labor.
- Compare the major types of regional analgesia and anesthesia, including area affected, advantages, disadvantages, techniques, and nursing implications.
- Discuss the possible complications of regional anesthesia.
- Describe the major inhalation and intravenous anesthetics used to provide general anesthesia.
- Delineate the major complications of general anesthesia.

KEY TERMS

Epidural block
Local anesthesia
Pudendal block
Regional analgesia
Regional anesthesia
Spinal block

The childbearing woman experiences many demanding sensations and discomforts during labor and birth. The nurse can help her have a positive childbirth experience by providing effective comfort measures. Nursing interventions directed toward pain relief begin with nonpharmacologic measures such as providing information, support, and physical comfort. Back rubs, the application of cool cloths to her forehead, and encouragement as the woman practices breathing techniques are examples of comfort measures. Some laboring women need no further interventions. For other women, the progression of labor brings increasing discomfort that interferes with their ability to perform breathing techniques and maintain a sense of control. Pharmacologic analgesics may be used to decrease this discomfort, increase relaxation, and reestablish the woman's sense of control. The nurse may need to remind her that there is medication to take the edge off her pain and to reassure her that it is all right to take pain medication.

Methods of Pain Relief

Pain and discomfort during labor may be relieved by several different methods. In addition to the nursing measures and patterned-paced breathing discussed in Chapter 17, systemic drugs, epidural analgesics, intrathecal narcotics, and regional nerve blocks are available.

The methods are not all mutually exclusive, and any of them may be used in combination with other comfort measures. Systemic drugs such as meperidine (Demerol) may help the laboring woman rest and cope with her labor contractions. Regional nerve blocks such as an epidural may be used to relieve the discomfort of labor contractions and still make it possible for the expectant couple to be involved in the labor and birth process.

Although systemic analgesics and regional local anesthetic blocks may affect the fetus, so do the pain and stress experienced by the laboring woman. During the pain and stress of labor there is an increase in maternal ventilation and oxygen consumption, which decreases the amount of oxygen available to the fetus.

Many couples who have had childbirth education approach childbirth confident that the psychoprophylactic techniques they have learned will enable them to cope with the discomforts of labor. There is a good deal of peer pressure on expectant parents to have the "ideal" birth experience. They may plan a natural childbirth with perhaps local infiltration anesthesia for episiotomy repair. A need for analgesia may make them feel inadequate and guilty. The nurse has a very special role in helping a woman and her partner accept alterations in their original plan. Reassurance that accepting analgesia for discomfort is not a failure is important in maintaining the woman's self-esteem. The emphasis should be placed on the goal of a healthy, satisfying outcome for the family.

Systemic Drugs

The goal of pharmacologic pain relief during labor is to provide maximum analgesia at minimum risk for the mother and fetus. To reach this goal, clinicians must consider a number of factors, including the following:

- All systemic drugs used for pain relief during labor cross the placental barrier by simple diffusion, but some drugs cross more readily than others.
- Drug action in the body depends on the rate at which the substance is metabolized by liver enzymes and excreted by the kidneys.
- High drug doses remain in the fetus for long periods because fetal liver enzymes and kidney excretion are inadequate for metabolizing analgesic agents.

Nursing Care

Analgesic drugs provide pain relief for the laboring woman, but also affect the fetus and the labor process. The nurse assesses the mother and fetus and also evaluates the contraction pattern before administering systemic medications.

Maternal Assessment

- The woman is willing to receive medication after being advised about it.
- Vital signs are stable.

Fetal Assessment

- The fetal heart rate (FHR) is between 120 and 160 beats per minute, and no late or variable decelerations are present.
- Short-term variability is present and long-term variability is average.
- The fetus exhibits normal movement, and accelerations are present with fetal movement.
- The fetus is at term.
- Meconium staining is not present.

Assessment of Labor

- Contraction pattern is well established.
- The cervix is dilated at least 4–5 cm in nulliparas and 3–4 cm in multiparas.

KEY FACTS TO REMEMBER

What Women Need to Know About Pain Relief Medications

Before receiving medications, the woman should understand the following:

- Type of medication administered
- Route of administration
- Expected effects of medication
- Implications for fetus/neonate
- Safety measures needed (for example, remain in bed with side rails up)

- The fetal presenting part is engaged.
- There is progressive descent of the fetal presenting part. No complications are present.

If normal parameters are not present, the nurse may need to complete further assessments with the physician/certified nurse-midwife.

Before administering the medication, the nurse once again validates whether the woman has a history of any drug reactions or allergies and provides information about the medication. See Key Facts to Remember: What Women Need to Know About Pain Relief Medications. After giving the medication, the nurse records the drug name, dose, route, and site, and the woman's B/P and pulse, on the FHR monitor strip and on the woman's records. If the woman is alone, side rails should be raised to provide safety. The nurse assesses the FHR for possible effects of the medication. See Essential Precautions for Practice: During Administration of Analgesic and Anesthesia.

When an analgesic medication is administered by intramuscular or subcutaneous route, it takes a few minutes for the effect to be felt. The nurse can continue with other supportive measures to enhance comfort, such as ensuring a quiet environment, providing a back rub or cool cloth, assisting with relaxation exercises and visualizations, or providing therapeutic touch until the effect of the medication is felt. When the medication is felt, the woman may sleep between contractions. This short period of rest helps her relax and can restore her energy. When an intravenous route is ordered by the certified nurse-midwife/physician, the effect of the drug will be felt within a couple of minutes, so if any change of position is necessary or if the woman needs to void, the nurse may suggest that these activities be completed before the drug administration. Some women may be so uncomfortable that they do not want anything except the medication. In this case, administering the medication first would be more helpful for the woman.

ESSENTIAL PRECAUTIONS FOR PRACTICE

During Administration of Analgesia and Anesthesia

Examples of times when disposable gloves should be worn include:

- Administering intravenous medications for analgesia to prevent exposure to blood.
- Starting intravenous fluids prior to regional blocks.
- Assisting the woman into position for an epidural or spinal. While the nurse assists the woman into position, the nurse may inadvertently be exposed to vaginal fluids or amniotic fluid.

REMEMBER to wash your hands prior to putting on the disposable gloves and AGAIN immediately after you remove the gloves.

For further information consult OSHA and CDC guidelines.

Narcotic Analgesics

Meperidine Hydrochloride (Demerol)

Meperidine hydrochloride (Demerol) is a narcotic analgesic that is effective for alleviating pain during the first stage of labor. It may be given by the intravenous or intramuscular route. The IV route provides effective analgesia within 5 to 10 minutes and has a duration of about 3 hours; the usual IV dose is 25 mg. When Demerol is given intramuscularly, the dose is usually between 50 and 75 mg; the duration of the effect is 2–4 hours.

Neonatal depression can occur, particularly when Demerol has been administered IM 1–2 hours before birth (Cunningham et al 1997). If maternal or fetal depression occurs, naloxone may be ordered to reverse the effects. See Drug Guide: Meperidine Hydrochloride for further discussion and nursing implications.

Butorphanol Tartrate (Stadol)

Butorphanol tartrate (Stadol) is a synthetic parenteral analgesic agent that can be given by the intramuscular or intravenous route. Its onset of action occurs 10 minutes after IV injection and the duration is from 3 to 4 hours (McDonald 1992). The recommended initial dose is 2 mg IM every 3–4 hours. If it is given IV, the dosage is reduced. Respiratory depression of both the mother and fetus/neonate can occur. The effects of Stadol can also be reversed with naloxone. Stadol should not be used for women with a known opiate dependency and should be used with caution if drug dependence is suspected because it may precipitate withdrawal.

Urinary retention following administration of this drug is rare. The nurse should, however, be alert for

DRUG GUIDE Meperidine Hydrochloride (Demerol)

Overview of Action

Meperidine hydrochloride is a narcotic analgesic that interferes with pain impulses at the subcortical level of the brain. In addition it enhances analgesia by altering the physiologic response to pain, suppressing anxiety and apprehension, and creating a euphoric feeling. Meperidine hydrochloride is used during labor to provide analgesia. Peak analgesia occurs in 40–60 minutes with intramuscular and in 5 minutes with intravenous administration. Duration is 2–4 hours (Skidmore-Roth 1994). Administration after labor has reached the active phase does not appear to delay labor or decrease uterine contraction frequency or duration. Meperidine HCl crosses the placental barrier and appears in cord blood within 2 minutes and after maternal intravenous injection can be detected in amniotic fluid 30 minutes after IM injection (Briggs et al 1994).

Route, Dosage, Frequency

IM: 50–100 mg every 3–4 hours

IV: 25 mg by slow intravenous push every 3–4 hours

Maternal Contraindications

Hypersensitivity to meperidine, asthma

CNS depression

Respiratory depression

Fetal distress

Preterm labor if birth is imminent

Hypotension

Respirations <12 per minute

Concurrent use with anticonvulsants may increase depressant effects

Maternal Side Effects

Respiratory depression

Nausea and vomiting, dry mouth

Drowsiness, dizziness, flushing

Transient hypotension

Increased intracranial pressure (Skidmore-Roth 1994)

Effect on Fetus/Neonate

Possible neonatal respiratory depression if birth occurs 60 minutes or longer after administration of the drug to the mother; incidence of respiratory depression peaks at 2–3 hours after IM administration (Briggs et al 1994)

Neonatal hypotonia, lethargy, interference of thermoregulatory response

Neurologic and behavioral alterations for several days after birth; presence of meperidine in neonatal saliva up to 48 hours following birth (Briggs et al 1994)

May have depressed attention and social responsiveness for first 6 weeks of life (Briggs et al 1994)

Nursing Considerations

Assess the woman's history, labor and fetal status, maternal blood pressure, and respirations to identify contraindications to administration.

Intramuscular doses should be injected deeply to avoid irritation to subcutaneous tissue.

Intravenous doses should be diluted and administered slowly.

Provide for the woman's safety by instructing her to remain on bed rest, by keeping side rails up, and placing call bell within reach.

Evaluate effect of drug.

Observe for maternal side effects.

Assess for respiratory depression, notify physician/CNM if respirations are <12/minute (Skidmore-Roth 1994).

Observe newborn for respiratory depression; be prepared to initiate resuscitative measures and administer antagonist naloxone if needed.

bladder distention when a woman has received butorphanol for analgesia during labor, has intravenous fluids infusing, and receives regional anesthesia for the birth. Butorphanol should be protected from light and stored at room temperature. This agent is not federally controlled and has been placed in the nonscheduled category. Hospitals vary in their own control of the drug.

Opiate Antagonists: Naloxone (Narcan)

Since naloxone is an antagonist with little or no agonistic effect, it exhibits little pharmacologic activity in the absence of narcotics. Naloxone can be used to reverse the mild respiratory depression following small doses of opiates. The drug is useful for respiratory depression caused by fentanyl, alpha-prodine, morphine, and meperidine as well as pentazocine and butorphanol. *Naloxone is the drug of choice when the depressant is unknown because it will cause no further depression.* An initial dose of 0.4 mg to 2.0 mg may be administered intravenously to the laboring woman. The dose of naloxone for the newborn if needed after birth is 0.1 mg/kg (Cunningham et al 1997) given intravenously, intramuscularly, subcutaneously, or via the endotracheal tube (Ostheimer 1992). See Drug Guide: Naloxone Hydrochloride: Narcan, in Chapter 26. After naloxone administration the newborn should be observed for at least 4–6 hours.

When naloxone is given, other resuscitative measures may be indicated and trained personnel should be readily available. The duration of the drug is shorter than the analgesic drug it is acting as an antagonist for, so the nurse must be alert to the return of respiratory depression and the need for repeated doses. Naloxone should be given with caution in women with known or

TABLE 18–1 Summary of Commonly Used Regional Blocks

Type of Block	Areas Affected	Use During Labor and Birth	Nursing Actions
Lumbar epidural	Vagina and perineum	Given in first stage and second stage of labor	Assess woman's knowledge regarding the block. Act as advocate to help her obtain further information if needed. Monitor maternal blood pressure to detect the major side effect, which is hypotension. Provide support and comfort. See Regional Anesthesia—Lumbar Epidural Critical Pathway for further nursing actions.
Pudendal	Perineum and lower vagina	Given in the second stage just prior to birth to provide anesthesia for episiotomy or for low forceps birth	Assess woman's knowledge regarding the block. Act as advocate to help her obtain further information if needed.
Local infiltration	Perineum	Administered just before birth to provide anesthesia for episiotomy	Assess woman's knowledge regarding the block. Provide information as needed. Provide comfort and support. Observe perineum for bruising or other discoloration in the recovery period.

suspected opiate dependency because it may precipitate severe withdrawal.

Sedatives

The principal use of barbiturates in current obstetric practice is false labor or in the early stages of beginning labor. An oral dose of secobarbital (Seconal) or pentobarbital (Nembutal) promotes relaxation and allows the woman to sleep for a few hours. The woman can then enter the active phase of labor in a more relaxed and rested state.

Regional Analgesia for Labor

Controversy and some confusion has surrounded the concept of regional analgesia and anesthesia during labor for many years. Until fairly recently, regional blocks, such as an epidural, have relied on injecting only a local anesthetic agent. The resulting effects on the woman have been to induce an analgesic effect (through relief of pain and discomfort), but, in addition, the use of the anesthetic agent produces some anesthesia and this alters transmission of impulses to the bladder, affects the maintenance of blood pressure, ability to move extremities, descent of the fetus, and ability to push during the second stage (Thorpe and Breedlove 1996; Youngstrom and Miller 1996).

Regional analgesia differs from a regional anesthesia block in that to obtain epidural analgesia, a narcotic agent such as Fentanyl is injected along with a very small amount of local anesthetic agent. Effective analgesia is obtained and the troublesome side effects of regional anesthesia are usually avoided. The woman has pain relief, her blood pressure remains stable, and without motor blockage she is able to move about freely and ambulate. At times she has difficulty urinating, and that can be relieved by a straight catheterization (Youngstrom and Baker 1996).

Another type of analgesia is obtained through the use of intrathecal narcotics. "With intrathecal narcotics, the drug is injected into the subarachnoid space, not the epidural space." (Manning 1996, p 221.) Fentanyl citrate, sufentanil citrate, and preservative-free morphine are the most frequently used narcotic agents. The woman usually has good pain relief but may experience side effects such as pruritus, nausea and vomiting, and urinary retention. Delayed respiratory depression may also occur and seems to be more frequent with the use of morphine (Manning 1996).

Nursing care is directed toward assisting the woman during the intrathecal injection by having her void prior to the injection, assisting with positioning, monitoring and assessing vital signs and respiratory status, monitoring analgesic effect, and assisting with ambulation if needed. Additional measures may be needed to address pruritus, nausea and vomiting, and urinary retention (Manning 1996).

Regional Anesthesia

Regional anesthesia refers to relief of pain in a particular portion of the body. It is achieved by injecting local anesthetic agents so they come into direct contact with nervous tissue. The methods most commonly used in labor are epidural block, spinal block, pudendal block, and local infiltration (Table 18–1).

Essential prerequisites for the administration of regional analgesia and anesthesia are knowledge of the anatomy and physiology of pertinent structures, techniques for administration, the pharmacology of local anesthetics, and potential complications. With the exception of nurse anesthetists and certified nurse-midwifes, who may perform procedures for which they have been trained, nurses in the United States may not legally administer these anesthetic blocks. However, the nurse

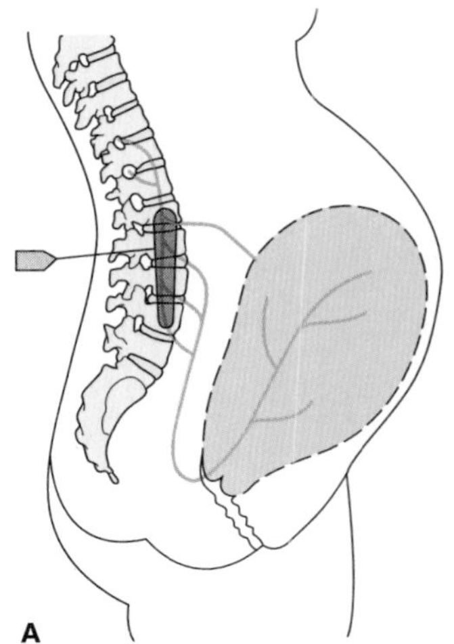

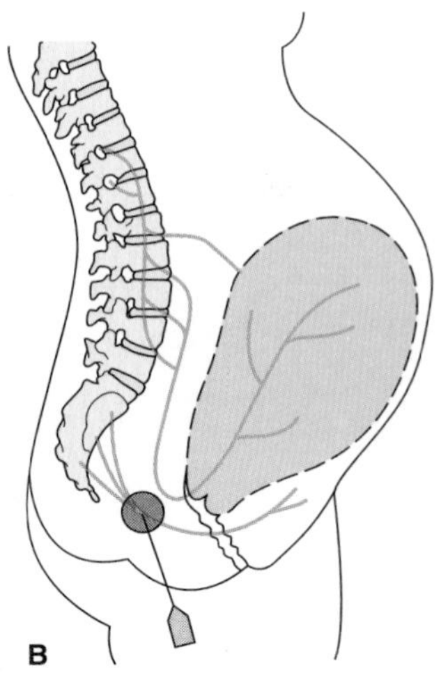

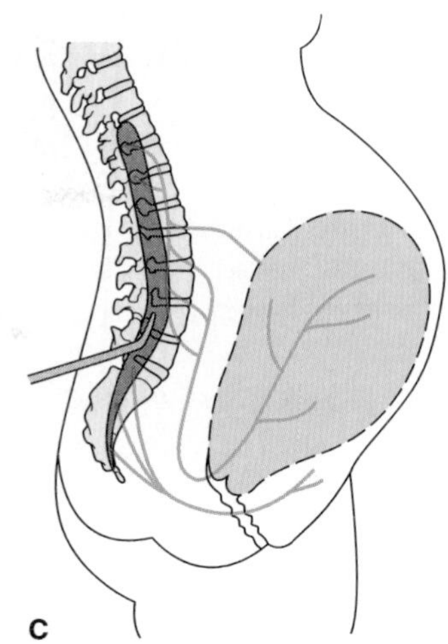

FIGURE 18–1 Schematic diagram showing pain pathways and sites of interruption. ***A*** Lumbar sympathetic (spinal) block: relief of uterine pain only. ***B*** Pudendal block: relief of perineal pain. ***C*** Lumbar epidural block: dark area demonstrates peridural (epidural) space and nerves affected, and the gray tube represents a continuous plastic catheter.

Source: Bonica JJ: *Principles and Practice of Obstetric Analgesia and Anesthesia.* Philadelphia: Davis, 1972, pp 492, 512, 521, 614.

must have an adequate knowledge of aspects of regional anesthesia to provide support and give appropriate reinforcement of the administrator's explanation to the woman. The nurse who has a thorough understanding of the techniques and agents can also recognize complications and immediately initiate appropriate intervention.

The relief of pain associated with the first stage of labor can be accomplished by blocking the sensory nerves that supply the uterus with an epidural block. Pain associated with the second stage and with vaginal birth can be alleviated with pudendal and epidural blocks (Figure 18–1).

It is important for the laboring woman to have information about the regional block that is to be administered. As with other procedures, the woman needs to know how the block is given, the expected effect on her and the fetus, advantages and disadvantages, and possible complications. Many women discuss possible anesthetic blocks with their care provider at some point in the pregnancy. If they have not, it is important to give them an opportunity to ask questions and obtain information before receiving the block while in labor.

Anesthetic Agents for Regional Blocks

Local anesthetic agents block the conduction of nerve impulses from the periphery to the central nervous system by preventing the propagation of an action potential from the source of pain (Firestone et al 1993). The types of nerve fibers are differentially sensitive to the various anesthetic agents. In general, the smaller the fiber, the more sensitive it is to local agents. For example, it is possible to block the small C and A delta fibers, which transmit pain and temperature, without blocking the larger A alpha, A beta, and A gamma fibers, which continue to maintain a sense of pressure, muscle tone, position sense, and motor function.

Absorption of local anesthetics depends primarily on the vascularity of the area of injection. The agents also contribute to increased blood flow by causing vasodilation. High concentrations of drugs cause greater vasodilation. Good maternal physical condition or a high metabolic rate aids absorption. Malnutrition, dehydration, electrolyte imbalance, and cardiovascular and pulmonary problems increase the potential for toxic effects. The pH of tissues affects the rate of absorption, which has implications for fetal complications such as acidosis. The addition of vasoconstrictors such as epinephrine delays absorption and prolongs the anesthetic effect. Recent studies have demonstrated that epinephrine decreases uteroplacental blood flow, making it an undesirable additive in many situations. The breakdown of local anesthetics in the body is accomplished by the liver and plasma esterase, and the resulting substance is eliminated by the kidneys.

It is important to use the weakest concentration and the smallest amount necessary to produce the desired results.

Types of Local Anesthetic Agents

Three types of local anesthetic agents are currently available: esters, amides, and opiates. The ester type includes procaine hydrochloride (Novocain), chloroprocaine hydrochloride (Nesacaine), and tetracaine hydrochloride (Pontocaine). Esters are rapidly metabolized; therefore, toxic maternal levels are not as likely to

CRITICAL THINKING IN ACTION

Luisa Silva, a 33-year-old G1 P0, is 32 weeks pregnant. She is trying to decide if she should accept any analgesia during her labor. She has finished childbirth education classes and wants an unmedicated labor and birth. She says, "I want to do this on my own but I'm afraid it may be too much. Will it be OK if I need to take something?" What will you tell her?

Answers can be found in Appendix H.

be reached, and placental transfer to the fetus is prevented. Amide types include lidocaine hydrochloride (Xylocaine), mepivacaine hydrochloride (Carbocaine), and bupivacaine hydrochloride (Marcaine). Amide types are more powerful and longer-acting agents. They readily cross the placenta, can be measured in the fetal circulation, and affect the fetus for a prolonged period.

Adverse Maternal Reactions to Local Anesthetic Agents

Reactions to local anesthetic agents range from mild symptoms to cardiovascular collapse. Mild reactions include palpitations, vertigo, tinnitus, apprehension, confusion, headache, and a metallic taste in the mouth. Moderate reactions include more severe degrees of mild symptoms plus nausea and vomiting, hypotension, and muscle twitching, which may progress to convulsions and loss of consciousness. The severe reactions are sudden loss of consciousness, coma, severe hypotension, bradycardia, respiratory depression, and cardiac arrest. High concentrations of the agents may also cause local toxic effects on tissues. Anesthetic agents should not be used unless an intravenous line is in place.

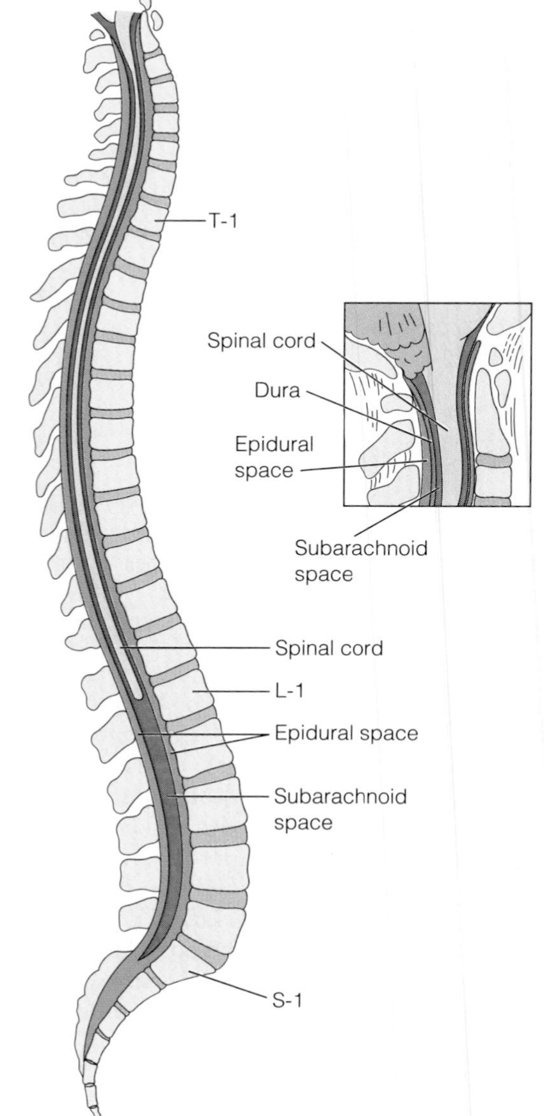

FIGURE 18–2 The epidural space is between the dura mater and the ligamentum flavum, extending from the base of the skull to the end of the sacral canal.

Epidural Block

An **epidural block** can provide pain relief throughout the course of labor. The *epidural space* is a potential space between the dura mater and the ligamentum flavum extending from the base of the skull to the end of the sacral canal (Figure 18–2). It contains areolar tissue, fat lymphatics, and internal vertebral venous plexus. Access to the space is through the lumbar area. The technique is most frequently used as a continuous block to provide analgesia and anesthesia from active labor through episiotomy repair.

Considerable skill is required for epidural blocks, and the incidence of success correlates highly with the skill and experience of the administrator. Pain relief is slower than with other methods, and a higher volume of anesthetic agent is required than for spinal anesthesia.

Fewer bony abnormalities occur in the lumbar vertebras than in the sacrum. The administrator must guard against accidental perforation of the dura mater, particularly with the lumbar epidural methods, and against the injection of an epidural dose into the spinal canal, with resultant high spinal anesthesia (Figure 18–3).

Epidurals have become a relatively common method of analgesia and anesthesia during labor and birth in the United States. An epidural can be given as soon as active labor is established.

Advantages

The epidural block produces good relief from discomfort during labor and birth, and the woman is fully awake and a part of the birth process. The continuous

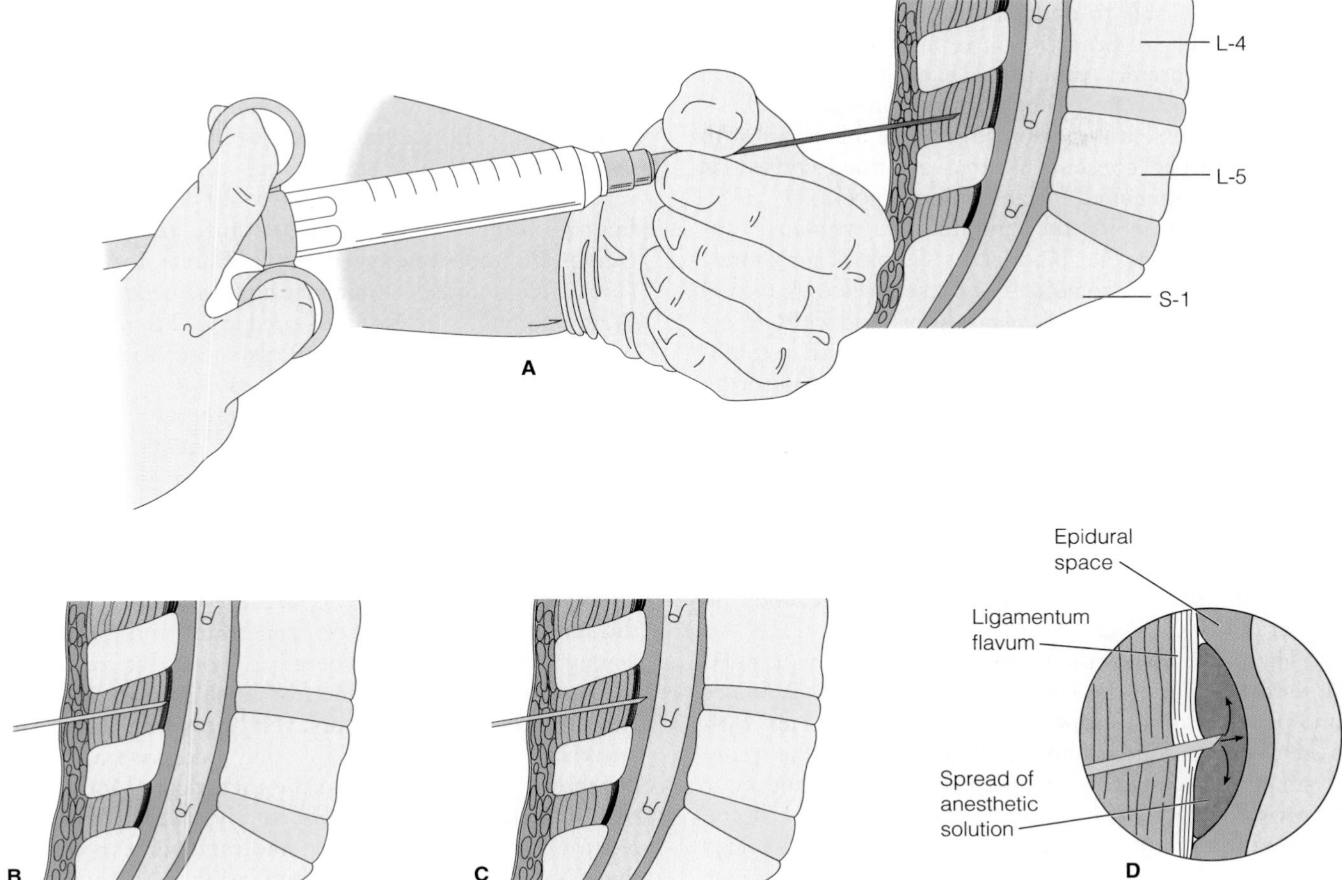

FIGURE 18–3 Technique for lumbar epidural block. ***A*** Proper position of insertion. ***B*** Needle in the ligamentum flavum. ***C*** Tip of needle in epidural space. ***D*** Force of injection pushing dura away from tip of needle.

Source: Bonica JJ: *Principles and Practice of Obstetric Analgesia and Anesthesia.* Philadelphia: Davis, 1972, p 631.

epidural allows different blocking for each stage of labor so that the fetus is able to descend and rotate, and many times the woman's urge to bear down is preserved.

Disadvantages

The most common complication of an epidural block is maternal hypotension, and this is generally prevented through intravenous fluid administration, left uterine displacement, and maternal positioning on her side. In some instances, labor progress and fetal descent may be slowed, pushing efforts in the second stage may be less effective, and the use of forceps or a vacuum extractor is more common (Thorp and Breedlove 1996). Delay in return of bladder sensation may result in the need for catheterization during labor and in the fourth stage.

Contraindications

The absolute contraindications for epidural block are client refusal, infection at the site of the needle puncture, maternal problems with coagulation (coagulopathies), and hypovolemic shock (Shnider and Levinson 1993).

The use of epidural (or spinal) block for cesarean birth in a woman with herpetic lesions is controversial. Some feel that the virus may be present on the skin and the skin puncture may allow for dissemination of the virus into the epidural or subarachnoid space. Shnider and Levinson (1993) note that generalized dissemination is very unlikely. Reactivation of herpes labialis has occasionally been associated with the administration of opiates into the epidural space (during an epidural) or the intrathecal space (during a spinal block).

Nursing Care

Assessment of the woman's knowledge level about an epidural block is essential. Before providing information, the nurse determines current knowledge about the epidural and evaluates factors related to learning, such as primary language spoken, ability to hear and interpret information, and the presence of anxiety. If the woman is not able to understand due to language barrier or inability to hear, the nurse must locate and provide an interpreter. Although the nurse is an integral person involved in providing information, the anesthesiologist is the essential person to provide information to obtain informed consent. Written informed consent is strongly recommended for an epidural block.

In preparation for the epidural, the woman is encouraged to empty her bladder, as the block may interfere with her ability to void. The nurse assesses maternal blood pressure, pulse and respirations, and FHR to establish that normal parameters are present and to establish a baseline. Continuous electronic fetal monitoring to assess fetal status and frequent monitoring of maternal blood pressure and pulse for hypotension will be required. An intravenous infusion is ordered and the nurse starts the IV with an 18-gauge plastic indwelling catheter. A large-gauge catheter is used so that IV fluids can be administered quickly if hypotension occurs. A bolus of 500–1000 mL of IV fluid is given before beginning the epidural block.

The nurse assists the woman into a side-lying position at the edge of the bed, where the mattress is firmer and provides more support. Her head is supported with a small pillow so it remains in alignment with the spine. A small pillow may also be placed in front of her chest to provide support for her upper arms. Her back needs to remain straight with the shoulders square. Her legs are bent and her knees kept together so that the upper hip does not roll forward and cause the spine to twist (Shnider and Levinson 1993). The block may also be given with the woman in a sitting position, with her back arched and her feet supported on a stool. After positioning, the nurse continues to provide support and encouragement and tries to ensure that the woman does not move during the procedure. After the block, maternal vital signs are assessed every 1–2 minutes for approximately 20 minutes or until stable, and then every 5 minutes. The blood pressure can be monitored by a mechanical blood pressure device or by the nurse directly. The vital signs are recorded on the fetal monitor strip and on the client record. The nurse maintains the woman in a side-lying position to maximize uteroplacental blood flow and changes her position at least once every hour to increase circulation, promote comfort, and avoid a one-sided block (Shnider and Levinson 1993). The nurse should assess the woman's ability to lift her legs every 30 minutes to monitor the effects of the nerve block.

The nurse assesses the woman's bladder at frequent intervals because the epidural block lessens the urge to urinate. During the second stage of labor, the woman with an epidural block may need more assistance with pushing. The nurse may need to tell the woman when contractions begin and give extra assistance by holding her legs during pushing efforts. The woman's legs need to be protected from pressure applied to them while sensation is diminished.

The most common side effect of epidural regional block is hypotension. If hypotension occurs (systolic below 100 mm Hg) the nurse increases the IV flow rate (to increase intravascular volume and raise the blood pressure), places the woman in a 10- to 20-degree Trendelenburg position (to increase circulation), and administers oxygen (to improve oxygenation). Shnider and Levinson (1993) recommend administering ephedrine, 5–15 mg IV, if blood pressure is not restored in 1–2 minutes (given per physician order). The FHR also needs to be assessed continuously to monitor fetal effects.

Elevation of maternal temperature may occur as an effect of the epidural (Cunningham et al 1997). The pyrexia may be confused with maternal infection and frequently results in additional testing for the newborn to rule out infection.

Headache (as occurs with spinal blocks) is not a side effect of epidural anesthesia, because the dura mater of the spinal canal has not been penetrated and there is no leakage of spinal fluid. Therefore, lying flat for a prescribed number of hours after birth is not required. Ambulation should be delayed, however, until the anesthesia has worn off. This may take several hours, depending on the agent and the total dose. Motor control of the legs is weak but not totally absent after birth. Return of complete sensation and the ability to control the legs are essential before ambulation is attempted.

To assess sensation the nurse can touch various parts of the woman's legs to determine if the touch can be felt. The nurse can evaluate motor control by asking the woman to raise her knees, to lift her feet (one at a time) off the bed, or to dorsiflex her foot. Even though assessments may indicate that sensation and motor control have returned, care should be taken to support the woman as she stands. The nurse needs to be ready to support the woman's weight and quickly return her to bed if motor control is inadequate. In addition, blood pressure assessments help the nurse determine the safety of ambulation. The nurse assesses blood pressure while the woman is lying down, then sitting in the bed. As long as the blood pressure values remain stable (no evidence of orthostatic hypotension), a standing blood pressure is assessed. It is advisable to have additional assistance when the woman stands for the first time, to maintain safety (Vender and Spiess 1992). (See the Regional Anesthesia—Lumbar Epidural Critical Pathway).

Continuous Epidural Infusion Pumps

Epidural anesthesia may be given with a continuous infusion pump. Some of the benefits (Cohen 1990) include: good to excellent analgesia; infrequent nausea; minimal sedation; decreased anxiety; earlier mobiliza-

Text continues on page 436

CRITICAL PATHWAY FOR REGIONAL ANESTHESIA—LUMBAR EPIDURAL

Category	First Stage	Second and Third Stage	Fourth Stage—Birth to One Hour Past Birth
Referral	Review Prenatal Record Advise CNM/physician of admission	Labor record for first stage	Report to Recovery Room nurse
Assessment	• Admission assessments: ask about problems since last prenatal visit; labor status (contraction frequency and duration cervical dilatation and effacement), membrane status; coping level; support; woman's desires during labor and birth, ability to verbalize needs, laboratory testing (blood and UA) • Woman's request for epidural • Intrapartal assessment: timing • *Latent Phase:* a. B/P, P, R, q1h if in normal range (B/P 90–140/60–90 or no increase >30 mm Hg systolic or 15 mm Hg diastolic over baseline; pulse 60–90; respirations 12–20/min, quiet, easy) b. Temp q4h unless >37.6C (99.6F) or membranes ruptured; then q2h. Uterine contractions q30min: contractions q5–10min, 15–40sec, mild intensity) c. FHR q60min (for low-risk women) and q30min for high-risk women if reassuring (FHR baseline 120-160, STV present, LTV average, accelerations with fetal movement, no late nor variable decelerations); if nonreassuring, position on side, start O_2, assess for hypotension, monitor continuously, notify CNM/physician • *Active Phase:* a. B/P, P, R, q1h if WNL b. Temp as above c. Uterine contractions assessed continuously d. FHR assessed continuously per EFM e. Pulse ox >90% • *Transition:* a. B/P, P, R, q30min if in normal range b. Uterine contractions q15–30min c. FHR q30min (for low-risk women) and q15min (for high-risk women) if reassuring: if nonreassuring, see above d. Pulse ox >90% • Cervical assessment: from 1–10 cm dilatation; nullipara (1.2 cm/h), multipara (1.5 cm/h) • Cervical effacement: from 0% to 100% • Fetal descent: progressive descent from −4 to ÷4 • Membrane assessment: when ruptured, Nitrazine positive, fluid clear, no foul odor • Behavioral characteristics: response to labor process, facial expressions, verbalizations, tone of voice, changes in behavior during contractions, body movement	• Second stage assessments: a. B/P, P, R q5–15min b. Uterine contractions palpated continuously c. FHR q15min (for low-risk women) and q5min (for high-risk women) if reassuring; if nonreassuring, monitor continuously • Fetal descent: descent continues to birth • Behavioral characteristics: response to pushing, facial expressions, verbalization • Third stage assessments: a. B/P, P, R q5min b. Uterine contractions, palpate occasionally until placenta is delivered, fundus maintains tone and contraction pattern continues to birth of placenta • Newborn assessments: a. Assess Apgar score of newborn b. Respirations: 30–60, irregular c. Apical pulse:120–160 and somewhat irregular d. Temperature: skin temp above 36.5C (97.8F) e. Umbilical cord: 2 arteries, 1 vein (if 1 artery, assess for anomalies and urine output) f. Gestational age: 38 to 42 weeks	• Immediate post-birth assessments q15 min for one hour a. B/P: 90–140/60–90; should return to prelabor level b. Pulse: slightly lower than in labor; range is 60–90 c. Respirations: 12–20/min; easy; quiet d. Temperature: 36.2–37.6C (98-99.6F) e. Fundus firm, in midline, at the umbilicus or 1–2 fingerbreadths below the umbilicus f. Lochia rubra; moderate amount; <1 pad/h; no free flow or passage of clots with massage g. Perineum: sutures intact; no bulging or marked swelling; minimal bruising may be present; no c/o severe pain nor rectal pain h. Bladder nondistended; spontaneous void of >100 mL clear, straw-colored urine; bladder nondistended following voiding (catheterize if necessary) i. If hemorrhoids present, no tenseness or marked engorgement; <2 cm diameter • Comfort level: <3 on scale of 1 to 10 • Energy level: awake and able to hold newborn • Newborn assessments if newborn remains with parents: a. Respirations: 30–60; irregular b. Apical pulse: 120–160 and somewhat irregular c. Temperature: skin temp above 36.5C (97.8F); skin feels warm to touch d. Skin color noncyanotic e. Mucus: small amount, clear, easily suctioned with bulb syringe without skin color change f. Behavioral: newborn opens eyes widely if room is slightly darkened g. Movements rhythmic; no hand tremors present

CRITICAL PATHWAY FOR REGIONAL ANESTHESIA—LUMBAR EPIDURAL continued

Category	First Stage	Second and Third Stage	Fourth Stage—Birth to One Hour Past Birth
Comfort	• Woman states that she desires regional anesthesia • Assist with administration of regional block	a. Second stage: assess and inform woman of progress of labor. Provide reassurance throughout labor. Assist with "sitting dose" reinjection for birth. Encouragement, coaching, help support legs while pushing, position of comfort for pushing and birth. b. Third stage: cool cloth to forehead, assist parents to see newborn, position mother to hold newborn, provide encouragement	• Institute comfort measures: a. Perineal discomfort: gently cleanse and apply ice pack; position to decrease pressure on perineum b. Uterine discomfort: palpate fundus gently c. Henorrhoids: ice pack d. General fatigue: position of comfort, encourage rest e. Administer pain medication
Teaching/ psychosocial	a. Establish rapport b. Orient to environment, expected assessments and procedures c. Answer questions and provide information/give emotional support d. Orient to EFM if used e. Teach relaxation, visualization and breathing pattern if needed f. Explain comfort measures available. Provide information regarding the reason for the block, possible side effects and nursing care that may be expected g. Assume advocacy role for woman/family during labor and birth h. Explain possible delayed effects of anesthetic agents on fetus	a. Orient to expected assessments and procedures b. Answer questions and provide information c. Continue advocacy role d. Instruct woman to maintain bed rest until full function of lower extremities returns	a. Explain immediate assessments and care after this first hour b. Teach self-massage of fundus and expected findings c. Instruct to call for assistance if mother desires to get OOB d. Begin newborn teaching; bulb syringe, positioning, maintaining warmth e. Assist with first breastfeeding experience
Therapeutic nursing interventions and reports	a. Straight cath PRN if bladder distended b. If regional block administered monitor B/P, FHR, sensation per protocol and obtain consent for procedure c. Provide continuing status reports d. Perineal clip per woman's request e. Small enema per woman's request f. Perform sterile vaginal examination as indicated g. Position woman correctly for regional block • Assess maternal status: a. Obtain baseline vital signs before any anesthetic agent is given b. Monitor blood pressure q1–2min for 10 min and then q5–15min following administration of anesthetic agent c. Monitor pulse and respiration d. Monitor FHR continuously • Observe, record, and report complications of anesthesia, including hypotension, fetal stress, respiratory paralysis, changes in uterine contractility, decrease in voluntary muscle effort, trauma to extremities, nausea and vomiting, and loss of bladder tone • Observe, record, and report symptoms of hypotension, including systolic pressure <100 mm Hg or a 20–30% fall in systolic pressure, apprehension, restlessness, dizziness, tinnitus, headache • Initiate treatment measures: a. Place woman in left lateral position with the foot of the bed elevated	a. Straight cath PRN if bladder distended b. Continue monitoring VS, FHR, and sensation c. Assess for potential problems of epidural infusion: sedation, nausea, vomiting, pruritus, hypotension, and "breakthrough pain"	a. Straight cath if bladder distended b. Monitor return of motor ability and sensation if regional block has been given c. Weigh perineal pads if lochia flow >1 saturated pad in 1 h; presence of boggy uterus and clots; decreased B/P, increased P

CRITICAL PATHWAY continued

Category	First Stage	Second and Third Stage	Fourth Stage—Birth to One Hour Past Birth
Therapeutic nursing interventions and reports *continued*	b. Increase IV fluid rate c. Administer oxygen by face mask at 7–10 L/min d. Administer vasopressors as ordered (usually ephedrine 5–15 mg IV) e. Manually displace uterus laterally to left f. Keep woman supine (semireclining) for 5–10 min following administration of block to allow drug to diffuse bilaterally. After 5–10 min position woman on side • Observe, record, and report fetal bradycardia (FHR <120 bpm) and loss of beat-to-beat variability		
Activity	a. Encourage ambulation unless contraindicated b. Maintain bed rest immediately after administration of IV pain medication, or following regional block c. Woman rests comfortably between contractions	a. Position comfortably for birth b. Woman rests comfortably between pushing efforts, and while awaiting birth of placenta	a. Position of comfort
Nutrition	a. Ice chips and clear fluids b. Evaluate for signs of dehydration	a. Ice chips and clear fluids	a. Regular diet if assessments are WNL b. Encourage fluids
Elimination	a. Voids at least q2h; urine clear, straw colored, negative for protein b. Bladder nondistended; empty before regional block administered c. May have bowel movement d. Monitor I & O with IVs	a. Monitor bladder at frequent intervals	a. Monitor bladder status with each assessment
Medications	a. Hydrate the woman receiving an epidural block with 500–1000 mL fluid prior to procedure (dextrose-free solution is recommended)	a. Local infiltration of anesthetic agent for birth by CNM/physician b. Pitocin 10 units IM, IVP per IV tubing, or added to IV fluids	a. Continue Pitocin infusion b. Administer pain medication
Discharge planning/ home care	a. Evaluate knowledge of labor and birth process b. Evaluate support system and need for referral after birth		a. Provide information if mother to be moved from LDR room b. Provide opportunity for parents to ask questions regarding newborn c. Evaluate knowledge of normal postpartum, newborn care
Family involvement	a. Identify available support person(s) b. Recognize possible impact of culture on responses c. Observe interaction between woman and partner d. Create moment alone with woman to identify possible abuse e. Assess current parenting skills	a. Provide opportunities for woman and support person(s) to watch newborn assessments b. Perform newborn assessment on mother's abdomen/chest if possible	a. Provide opportunity for parents to be with baby b. Encourage skin-to-skin contact c. Darken room to encourage eye-to-eye contact d. Provide quiet time for new family e. Parenting: demonstrates early culturally expected parenting behaviors
Date			

DRUG GUIDE | Postbirth Epidural Morphine

Overview of Action
Epidural morphine is used to provide relief of pain associated with cesarean birth, extensive episiostomies (mediolaterals), or third- and fourth-degree lacerations. Epidural morphine pain relief results directly from its effect on the opiate receptors in the spinal cord (it depresses pain impulse transmission). Morphine binds opiate receptors, thereby altering both the perception of and the emotional response to pain. Women experience little or no discomfort or pain during recovery and for up to 24 hours afterward. There is no motor or sympathetic block or associated hypotension. Onset of analgesia is slower, but duration is longer.

Dosage, Route
5–10 mg of morphine is injected through a catheter into the epidural space, providing relief for about 24 hours (Wilson, Shannon, and Strang 1997).

Maternal Contraindications
Hypersensitivity to opiates
Narcotic addiction
Chronic debilitating respiratory disease
Reduced blood volume

Maternal Side Effects
Late onset respiratory depression (rare but may occur 8–12 hours after administration)
Nausea and vomiting (occurring between 4 and 7 hours after injection)
Itching (begins within 3 hours and lasts up to 10 hours)
Urinary retention
Somnolence (rarely)
Side effects can be managed with naloxone (Cunningham et al 1997)

Effect on Fetus/Neonate
No adverse effects since medication is injected after birth of baby

Nursing Considerations
Assess client's sensitivity to narcotics on admission.
Monitor and evaluate analgesic effect. Ask client about comfort level and notify anesthesiologist of inadequate pain relief.
Check epidural catheter for obvious knots, breaks, and leakage at insertion site and catheter hub.
Assess for pruritus (scratching and rubbing, especially around the face and neck).
Administer comfort measures for narcotic-induced pruritus, such as lotion, back rubs, cool/warm packs, or diversional activities. If the itching can be tolerated, naloxone should be avoided, especially since it counteracts the pain relief.
If allergic reaction (urticaria, edema, or respiratory difficulties) occurs, administer naloxone or diphenhydramine per physician order.
Provide comfort measures for nausea/vomiting, such as frequent oral hygiene or gradual increase in activity; administration of naloxone, trimethobenzamide, or metoclopramide HCl per physician order.
Assess postural blood pressure and heart rate before ambulation.
Assist client with her first ambulation and then as needed.
Assess respiratory function every 24 hours, then every 2–8 hours as needed. Also assess level of consciousness and mucous membrane color.
May need to monitor client via apnea monitor for 24 hours.
Monitor urinary output and assess bladder for distention. Assist client to void.

tion; retained cough reflex; decreased risk of deep vein thrombosis; decreased myocardial oxygen demand; and ease of administration.

Obviously, ease of administration does not indicate lack of need for close observation. Malfunctioning equipment with subsequent overdose is always a possibility. Infusion pumps specifically designed for use in epidural anesthesia have safety factors incorporated. Continuous epidural infusions should be administered with the same precautions used for intermittent injections.

Some of the potential problems of epidural infusions include "breakthrough pain," sedation, nausea and vomiting, pruritus, and hypotension. Breakthrough pain may occur at any time during the epidural infusion. It usually occurs when the infusion rate of the agent is below the recommended rate for therapeutic dose. It may also occur when the infusion pump rate is altered or the integrity of the epidural line is broken. When breakthrough pain occurs, the nurse should check the integrity of the epidural infusion line and notify the anesthesiologist. There may be standing orders for treatment of breakthrough pain, but it is best to inform the anesthesiologist of any problems that do occur.

Sedation may occur from the systemic effect of the narcotic. The epidural agents are absorbed into the circulation and can cause enough general sedation that the treatment is prevention. The respiratory rate, along with the quality of respirations, should be assessed no less than every 15–30 minutes. The nurse should notify the anesthetist of any significant decreases in respiratory rate or respiratory pattern change. If respiratory rate decreases below 14 respirations per minute, naloxone may be given to remove the effect of the anesthetic agent; respirations will then return to a normal rate.

Nausea and vomiting can occur at any time during or after epidural infusion. The nurse should give an antiemetic if one is ordered and notify the anesthesiologist. The nausea and vomiting can make the woman very uncomfortable, and the infusion rate of the epidural may need to be decreased or terminated to alleviate this discomfort.

Pruritus (rash) may occur at any time during the epidural infusion. It usually appears first on the face, neck, or torso and is usually the result of the agent in the epidural infusion. Treatment involves administration of Benadryl. The usual dose is 50 mg given intramuscu-

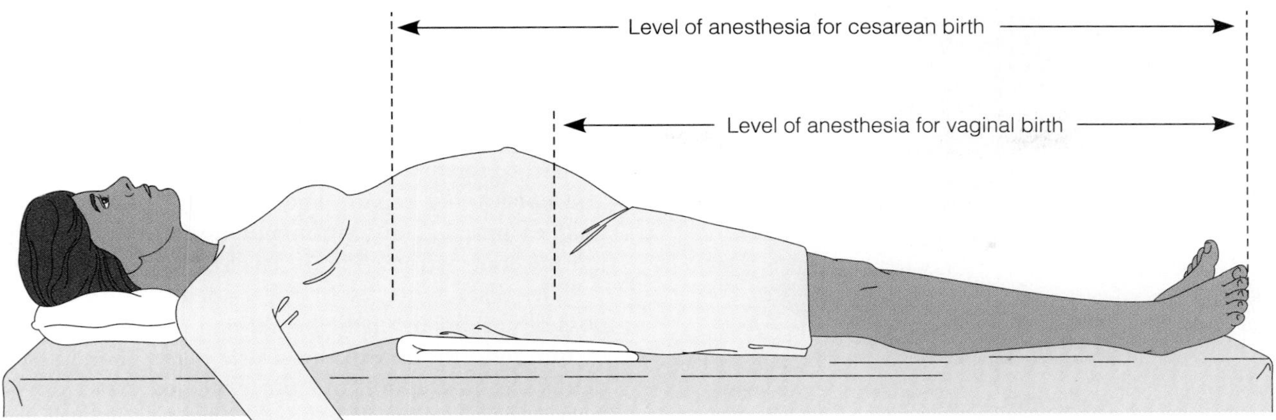

FIGURE 18–4 Levels of anesthesia for vaginal and cesarean births.
Source: Reprinted with permission of Ross Laboratories, Columbus, OH. From *Clinical Education Aid No. 17.*

larly. Should no standing order exist, the nurse notifies the anesthetist and identifies the problem. The epidural infusion may need to be terminated or decreased. The nurse assesses the woman for any signs of pruritus at regular intervals or when assessing respirations.

Hypotension may occur from hypovolemia or from the effect of the epidural agent. Treatment involves administering oxygen by mask, administering a bolus of crystalloid (usually 200–400 mL), and notifying the anesthetist. Usually there are standing orders for treatment of hypotension that are graded in terms of the degree of hypotension. The epidural infusion may have to be terminated and the woman placed in the Trendelenburg position.

Epidural Narcotic Analgesia After Birth

To provide analgesia for approximately 24 hours after the birth, the anesthesiologist may inject morphine, 5.0 mg or 7.5 mg, into the epidural space immediately after the birth. The analgesic effect begins approximately 30 to 60 minutes after the injection. The side effects include pruritus, which occurs in 11 to 90 percent of clients. The onset seems to occur early, and it resolves within 14 to 16 hours after the birth. (See Drug Guide: Postbirth Epidural Morphine.)

Spinal Block

In a **spinal block,** a local anesthetic agent is injected directly into the spinal fluid in the spinal canal to provide anesthesia for cesarean birth and occasionally for vaginal birth. The technique of administration varies depending on whether the spinal block is being given for a cesarean or vaginal birth. With a cesarean birth, the level of anesthesia needs to be higher up on the maternal abdomen (Figure 18–4).

Advantages

The advantages are immediate onset of anesthesia, relative ease of administration, a smaller drug volume, and maternal compartmentalization of the drug.

Disadvantages

The disadvantages include a fairly high incidence of hypotension after the block, inability to move lower legs, inability to void, the need for the woman to remain flat for 6–12 hours after the block, and possible headache afterward.

Contraindications

Contraindications for spinal block include hypotension, infection at the site of puncture, coagulation problems, and client refusal (Shnider and Levinson 1993).

Nursing Care

If an intravenous infusion is not already in place, it is started with a 16- to 18-gauge plastic catheter, and a bolus of 500–1000 mL is infused rapidly. The nurse assesses maternal vital signs and the FHR to establish a baseline and then positions the woman in a sitting position (a side-lying position may also be used). The woman sits on the side of the bed or operating room table, and places her feet on a stool. The woman places her arms between her knees or up around the nurse's shoulders, bows her head, and arches her back to widen the intervertebral spaces. The nurse supports the woman in this position and palpates the uterus to identify the beginning of uterine contractions (if labor is present). The physician injects the anesthetic agent between contractions. If the anesthetic agent is injected during a contraction, the level of anesthesia is higher and may compromise respirations.

The woman remains in a sitting position for 30 seconds and then returns to a lying position with a rolled

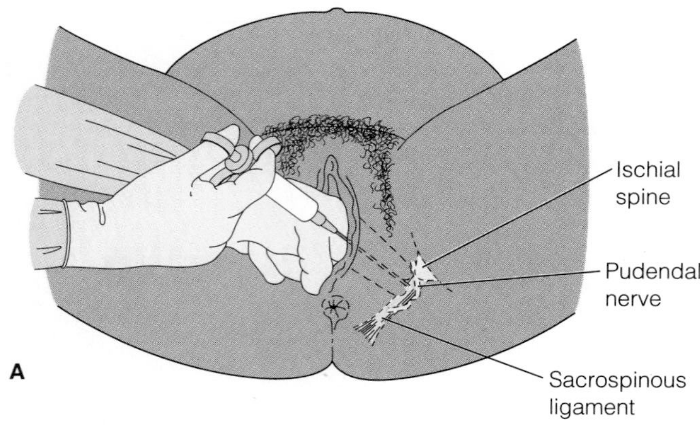

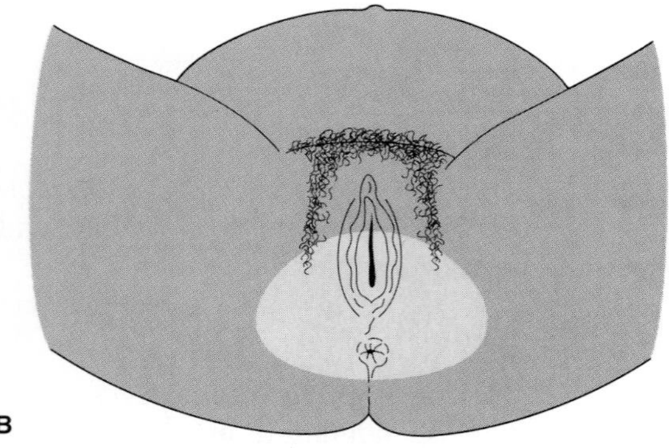

FIGURE 18–5 ***A*** Pudendal block by the transvaginal approach. ***B*** Area of perineum affected by pudendal block.

towel or blanket under her right hip, to displace the uterus from the vena cava. Maternal blood pressure and pulse are monitored every 1–2 minutes for the first 20 minutes after the injection of local anesthetic agent, and then every 5–10 minutes (Cunningham et al 1997). The blood pressure needs to be reassessed when the woman is moved after birth, or when her legs are removed from stirrups after vaginal birth (movement affects the blood pressure).

If the spinal is being used during vaginal birth, the nurse continues to monitor uterine contractions and instructs the woman to bear down during a contraction. The block usually takes away the woman's ability to push effectively, and the birth may be assisted with forceps or vacuum extractor (see Chapter 20).

After birth, the temporary motor paralysis of the woman's legs continues. The nurse needs to exercise caution when moving the woman from the birthing bed (or operating room table) to protect her from injury. The woman remains flat in bed for 6–12 hours following the block. The woman may not regain sensation and control of her bladder for 8–12 hours and may need to be catheterized. Women who have a cesarean birth usually have an indwelling bladder catheter inserted before surgery.

Pudendal Block

A **pudendal block,** administered by a transvaginal method, intercepts signals to the pudendal nerve. The pudendal block provides perineal anesthesia for the latter part of the first stage of labor, the second stage, birth, and episiotomy repair. The pudendal block stops the pain of perineal distention but not the discomfort of uterine contractions (Figure 18–5).

The disadvantages of the pudendal block include possible broad ligament hematoma, perforation of the rectum, and trauma to the sciatic nerve. The nurse explains the procedure and the expected effect and answers any questions. Because a pudendal block does not alter maternal vital signs or FHR, additional assessments are not necessary.

Local Infiltration Anesthesia

Local anesthesia is accomplished by injection of an anesthetic agent into the intracutaneous, subcutaneous, and intramuscular areas of the perineum (Figure 18–6). It is generally used at the time of birth, both in preparation for making an episiotomy and for the episiotomy repair. Women who have followed some type of prepared childbirth method and want minimal analgesia/anesthesia usually do not object to local anesthesia for the episiotomy. The administration procedure is technically uncomplicated and is practically free from complications.

A disadvantage of local infiltration is that large amounts of local anesthetic must be used to infuse the tissues. The nurse explains the procedure and the expected effect and answers any questions. Because local anesthetic agents have no effect on maternal vital signs or FHR, additional assessments are unnecessary.

General Anesthesia

A general anesthesia may be needed for cesarean birth and for surgical intervention with some complications. The method used to achieve general anesthesia may be intravenous injection, inhalation of anesthetic agents, or a combination of both.

Intravenous Anesthetics

Thiopental sodium (Pentothal) is an ultrashort-acting barbiturate, which means that it exerts its effect rapidly and has a brief duration of action. Thiopental sodium produces narcosis within 30 seconds after intravenous administration. Induction and emergence from its effects are smooth and pleasant, with little incidence of nausea and vomiting. Thiopental sodium is most frequently used for induction and as an adjunct to other more potent anesthetics.

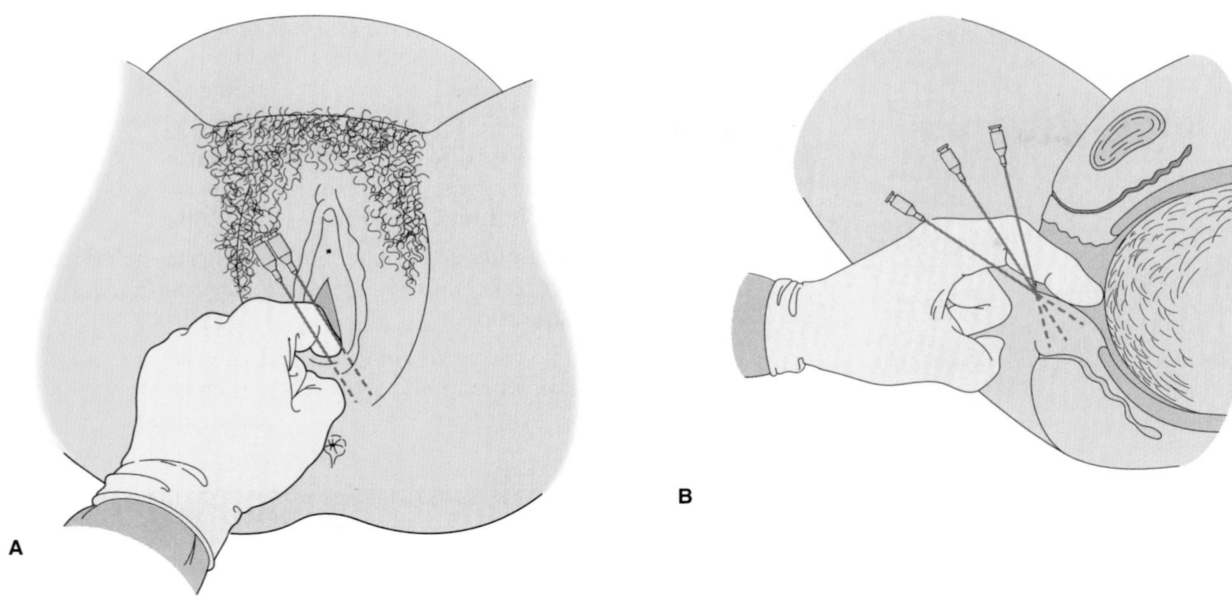

FIGURE 18–6 Local infiltration anesthesia. ***A*** Technique of local infiltration for episiotomy and repair. ***B*** Technique of local infiltration showing fan pattern for fascial planes.

Source: Bonica JJ: *Principles and Practice of Obstetric Analgesia and Anesthesia.* Philadelphia: Davis, 1972, p 505.

Complications of General Anesthesia

A primary danger of general anesthesia is fetal depression. Most general anesthetic agents reach the fetus in about 2 minutes. The depression in the fetus is directly proportional to the depth and duration of the anesthesia. The long-term significance of fetal depression in a normal delivery has not been determined. The poor fetal metabolism of general anesthetic agents is similar to that of analgesic agents administered during labor. General anesthesia is not advocated when the fetus is considered to be at high risk, particularly in premature delivery.

The majority of general anesthetic agents cause some degree of uterine relaxation. They may also cause vomiting and aspiration.

Pregnancy results in decreased gastric motility, and the onset of labor halts the process almost entirely. Food eaten hours earlier may remain undigested in the stomach. The nurse must find out when the laboring woman last ate and record this information on the client's chart and on her anesthesia record.

Even when food and fluids have been withheld, the gastric juice produced during fasting is highly acidic and can produce chemical pneumonitis if aspirated. Such pneumonitis is known as Mendelson's syndrome. The signs and symptoms are chest pain, respiratory embarrassment, cyanosis, fever, and tachycardia.

Care During General Anesthesia

Prophylactic antacid therapy to reduce the acidic content of the stomach before general anesthesia has become common practice. Administration of a nonparticulate antacid (such as polycitra or bicitra) may be used. Cimetidine (Tagamet) has been suggested by some anesthesiologists (Cunningham et al 1997).

Before induction to anesthesia, the woman should have a wedge placed under her right hip to displace the uterus and avoid vena caval compression in the supine position. She should also be preoxygenated with 3–5 minutes of 100 percent oxygen. Intravenous fluids should be started so that access to the intravascular system is immediately available.

During the process of rapid induction of anesthesia, the nurse applies cricoid pressure. This is accomplished by depressing the cricoid cartilage 2–3 cm posteriorly so that the esophagus is occluded. Cricoid pressure is continued until the anesthesiologist has placed the endotracheal tube and indicates that the pressure can be released. Figure 18–7 shows the appropriate technique. Cheek and Gutsche (1993) suggest that the woman's head be supported with a small pillow and that the nurse support the woman's neck with her other hand.

Neonatal Neurobehavioral Effects of Anesthesia and Analgesia

Many studies have focused on the neurobehavioral effects on the newborn of pharmacologic agents used during labor and birth. Although analgesic and anesthetic agents may alter the behavioral and adapative function of the newborn, physiologic factors such as hunger, degree of hydration, and time within the sleep-wake cycle

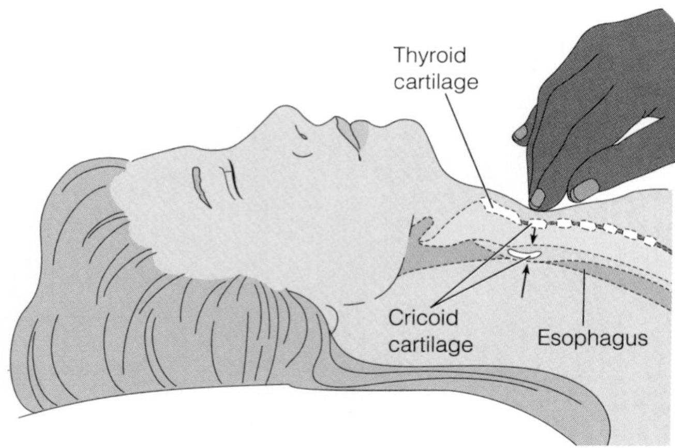

FIGURE 18–7 Proper position for fingers in applying cricoid pressure until a cuffed endotracheal tube is placed by the anesthesiologist or certified nurse-anesthetist. The cricoid cartilage is depressed 2–3 cm posteriorly so that the esophagus is occluded.

may also exert an influence (Capogna and Celleno 1993). The long-range importance of these findings has not been well established.

CHAPTER HIGHLIGHTS

- Pain relief during labor may be enhanced by childbirth preparation methods and administration of analgesics and regional anesthesia blocks.
- The goal of pharmacologic pain relief during labor is to provide maximum analgesia with minimum risk for the mother and fetus.
- The best time for administering analgesia is determined after making a complete assessment of many factors. An analgesic agent is generally administered to nulliparas when the cervix has dilated 5 to 6 cm and to multiparas when the cervix has dilatation 3 to 4 cm.
- Analgesic agents include meperidine and butorphanol.
- Narcotic antagonists (such as naloxone) counteract the respiratory depressant effect of the opiate narcotics by acting at specific receptor sites in the CNS.
- Regional analgesia and anesthesia are achieved by injecting local anesthetic agents into an area that will bring the agent into direct contact with nerve tissue. Methods most commonly used in childbearing include epidural block, spinal block, pudendal block, and local infiltration.
- Two types of local anesthetic agents used in regional blocks are the amide and ester groups. The amides are absorbed quickly and can be found in maternal blood within minutes after administration, while the esters are metabolized more rapidly and have only limited placental transfer.
- Untoward reactions of the woman to local anesthetic agents range from mild symptoms, such as palpitations, to cardiovascular collapse.
- Complications of general anesthesia include fetal depression, uterine relaxation, vomiting, and aspiration.
- The choice of analgesia and anesthesia for the high-risk woman and fetus requires careful evaluation.

REFERENCES

Briggs GG et al: *Drugs in Pregnancy and Lactation,* 4th ed. Baltimore: Williams & Wilkins, 1994.

Capogna G, Celleno D: The effects of anesthetic agents on the newborn. In: *The Effects on the Baby of Maternal Analgesia and Anesthesia.* Reynolds F (editor). London: Saunders, 1993.

Cheek TG, Gutsche BR: Pulmonary aspiration of gastric contents. Chapter 23 in: *Anesthesia for Obstetrics.* Shnider SM, Levinson G (editors). Baltimore: Williams & Wilkins, 1993.

Cohen M: Continuous epidural infusions for acute postoperative pain: Part II. *Curr Rev Nurs Anesthetists* 1990; 22:181.

Cunningham FG et al: *Williams Obstetrics,* 20th ed. Stamford, CT: Appleton & Lange, 1997.

Firestone L et al: *Clinical Anesthesia Procedures by the Massachusetts General Hospital,* 4th ed. Boston: Little, Brown, 1993.

Giacoia GP, Yaffee S: Perinatal pharmacology. In: *Gynecology and Obstetrics,* Vol. 3. Sciarra JJ (editor). Philadelphia: Harper & Row, 1982.

Manning J: Intrathecal narcotics: New approach for labor analgesia. *JOGNN* March/April 1996; 25:221.

Ostheimer G: *Manual of Obstetric Anesthesia,* 2nd ed. New York: Churchill-Livingstone, 1992.

Paradise NF: Personal communication. Biology Department, University of Akron, Akron, OH, 1990.

Shnider SM, Levinson G: *Anesthesia for Obstetrics,* 3rd ed. Baltimore: Williams & Wilkins, 1993.

Skidmore-Roth L: *Mosby's 1994 Nursing Drug Reference.* St Louis: Mosby-Year Book, 1994.

Thorp J, Breedlove G: Epidural analgesia in labor: An evaluation of risks and benefits. *Birth* June 1996; 23:63.

Vender JS, Spiess BD: *Post Anesthesia Care.* Philadelphia: Saunders, 1992.

Wilson BA, Shannon MT, Stang CL: *Nurses Drug Guide 1997.* Stamford, CT: Appleton & Lange, 1997.

Youngstrom P, Baker SW, Miller JL: Epidurals redefined in analgesia and anesthesia: A distinction with a difference. *JOGNN* May 1996; 25:350.

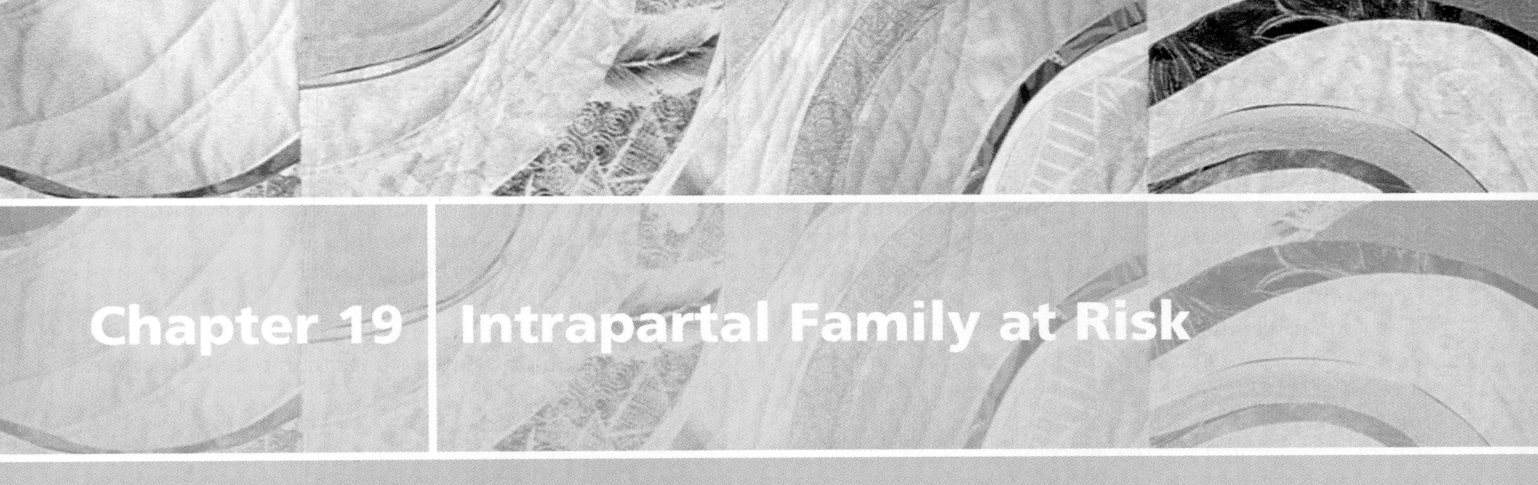

Chapter 19 Intrapartal Family at Risk

OBJECTIVES

- Describe the psychologic factors that may contribute to complications during labor and birth.
- Discuss dysfunctional labor patterns.
- Describe the impact of postterm pregnancy on the childbearing family.
- Explore the causes and management of uterine rupture.
- Summarize various types of fetal malposition and malpresentation and possible associated problems.
- Discuss the identification, management, and care of fetal developmental abnormalities such as macrosomia and hydrocephalus.
- Discuss the nursing care that is indicated in the event of fetal distress.
- Discuss intrauterine fetal death including etiology, diagnosis, management, and the nurse's role in assisting the family.
- Compare abruptio placentae and placenta previa.
- Identify variations that may occur in the umbilical cord and insertion into the placenta.
- Discuss the identification, management, and nursing care of women with amniotic fluid embolus, hydramnios, and oligohydramnios.
- Delineate the effects of pelvic contractures on labor and birth.
- Discuss complications of the third and fourth stages.

KEY TERMS

Abruptio placentae
Amniotic fluid embolism
Cephalopelvic disproportion (CPD)
Dystocia
Hydramnios
Macrosomia
Oligohydramnios
Persistent occiput-posterior (OP) position
Placenta previa
Postterm pregnancy
Precipitous labor
Uterine inversion

The successful completion of the 40-week gestational period requires the harmonious functioning of four components: emotional factors, contractile forces, fetus, and pelvis. (These components are described in depth in Chapter 15.) The emotional factors are the intellectual and emotional processes of the pregnant woman as influenced by heredity and environment; they include her feelings about pregnancy and motherhood. The contractile forces are the myometrial forces of the contracting uterus. The fetus includes all the products of conception: the fetus, placenta, cord, membranes, and amniotic fluid. The pelvis comprises the vagina, introitus, and bony pelvis. Disruptions in any of the four components may affect the others and cause **dystocia** (abnormal or difficult labor). Some of the most common of these disruptions are discussed in this chapter.

Care of the Woman at Risk Due to Anxiety and Fear

The anxiety, fear, and pain associated with labor may lead to a vicious cycle of increased fear and anxiety because of continued central pain perception. This enhances catecholamine release, which in turn increases physical distress and results in myometrial dysfunction and possibly ineffectual labor.

Medical Therapy

The medical therapy for anxiety and fear is directed by the individual circumstances of each laboring woman. The physician/certified nurse-midwife may first attempt to use communication and sharing of information to allay anxiety. When needed, pharmacologic measures such as ataractics or sedatives may be ordered to help the woman feel calmer.

APPLYING THE NURSING PROCESS

Nursing Assessment

Unless birth is imminent or severe complications exist, the nurse begins the assessment by reviewing the woman's background. Factors such as age, parity, marital and socioeconomic status, culture, and knowledge and understanding of the labor process contribute to the woman's psychologic response to labor. As labor progresses, the nurse is alert to the woman's verbal and nonverbal behavioral responses to the pain and anxiety of labor. The woman who is agitated and seems uncooperative or is too quiet and compliant may require further appraisal for anxiety. Verbal statements such as "Is everything okay?" "I'm really nervous," or "What's going on?" usually indicate some degree of anxiety and concern. Other women may be irritable, require frequent explanations, or repeat questions. The nurse further observes for nonverbal cues, including a tense posture, clenched hands, or pain out of proportion to the stage of labor. Recognizing the impact of fatigue on pain and anxiety is another important nursing function.

Nursing Diagnosis

Nursing diagnoses that may apply to the woman with excessive fear or anxiety include the following:

- Anxiety related to stress of the labor process
- Fear related to unknown outcome of labor
- Ineffective individual coping related to inability to use relaxation techniques during labor

Nursing Plan and Implementation

Nursing research demonstrates that anticipatory education during the prenatal period is effective in minimizing the stress accompanying labor. Research findings indicate that women who participate in prenatal classes benefit by maintaining more positive attitudes, experiencing feelings of anticipation rather than fear, and developing a heightened awareness that fosters early maternal attachment (Lowe 1996).

Prenatal classes provide relevant information about the developmental and psychologic changes that can be expected during childbirth and teach relaxation strategies to reduce the anxiety and pain of labor. Couples learn coping mechanisms in the form of physical and emotional comfort measures, controlled breathing exercises, and relaxation techniques.

During labor and birth, the nurse should offer support and encouragement to prepared couples as they employ the techniques they have learned. If the woman begins to lose control, the nurse can often assist the partner in helping her regain control. If anxiety is evident, the nurse should acknowledge and alleviate it, if possible, through comfort measures (see Chapters 17 and 18).

Unprepared couples can be taught many of these activities at the time of admission, especially if active labor has not begun. The nurse can give clear but succinct information about the labor process, medical procedures, the environment, simple breathing exercises, and relaxation techniques, thereby preventing or relieving some apprehension and fear. Even a woman in active labor who has had no prior preparation can achieve a great deal of relaxation from physical comfort measures, touch, frequent attention, therapeutic interaction, and, possibly, analgesics.

The nurse's ability to help the woman and her partner cope with the stress of labor is directly related to the

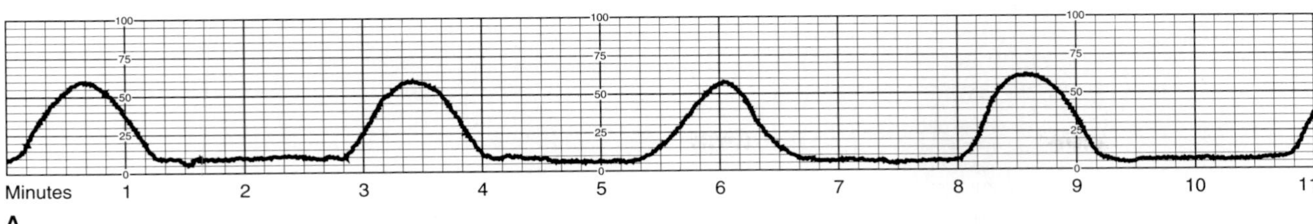

A

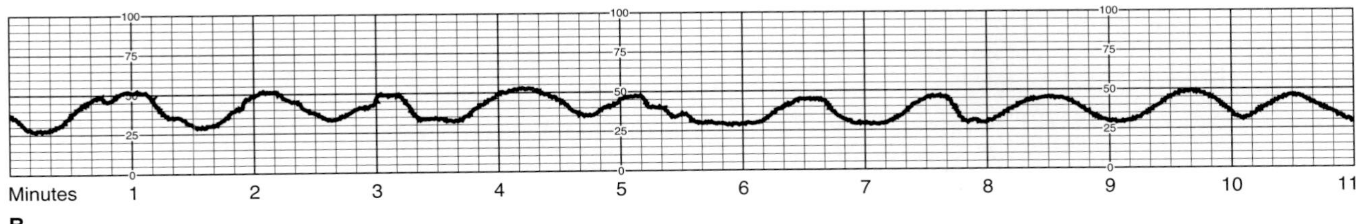

B

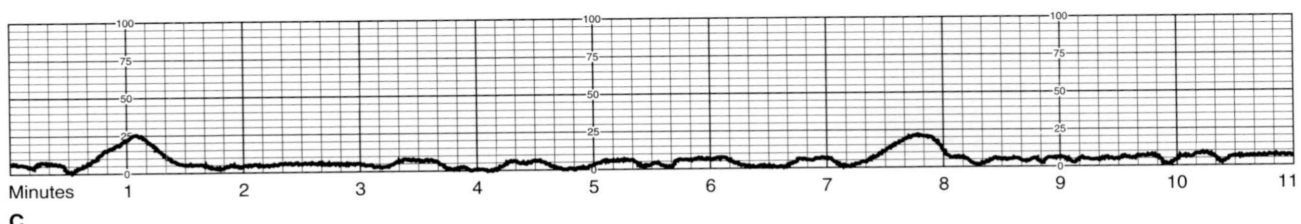

C

FIGURE 19–1 Comparison of labor patterns. ***A*** Normal uterine contraction pattern. In this example contraction frequency is every 3 minutes; duration is 60 seconds. The baseline resting tone is below 10 mm. Hg. ***B*** Hypertonic uterine pattern. In this example the contraction frequency is every minute, duration is 50 seconds (which allows only a 10-second rest between contractions), intensity increases approximately 25 mm Hg during the contraction, and the resting tone of the uterus is increased. ***C*** Hypotonic uterine contraction pattern. In this example the contraction frequency is every 7 minutes with some uterine activity between contractions, duration is 50 seconds, and intensity increases approximately 25 mm Hg during contractions.

rapport they have established. By employing a calm, caring, confident, nonjudgmental approach, the nurse is able not only to acknowledge the anxiety, but also is often able to identify the source of the distress. Once the causative factors are known, the nurse can implement appropriate interventions such as information, comfort measures, touch, or therapeutic communication.

Evaluation

Anticipated outcomes of nursing care include

- The woman experiences a decrease in physiologic signs of stress and an increase in psychologic comfort.
- The woman is able to use effective coping mechanisms to manage her anxiety during labor.
- The woman's fear decreases.
- The woman is able to verbalize feelings about her labor.

Care of the Woman with Dysfunctional Labor

Complications of the contractile forces involve problems with the frequency, duration, and intensity of contractions, or the resting tone of the uterus between contractions. These problems lead to dysfunctional labor and can be associated with additional complications, such as maternal exhaustion, dehydration, increased risk of infection, and fetal complications.

Hypertonic Labor Patterns

In hypertonic labor patterns, ineffectual uterine contractions of poor quality occur in the latent phase of labor, and the resting tone of the myometrium increases. Contractions usually become more frequent, but their intensity may decrease (Figure 19–1*B*). The contractions are painful but ineffective in dilating and effacing the cervix, and a prolonged latent phase may result.

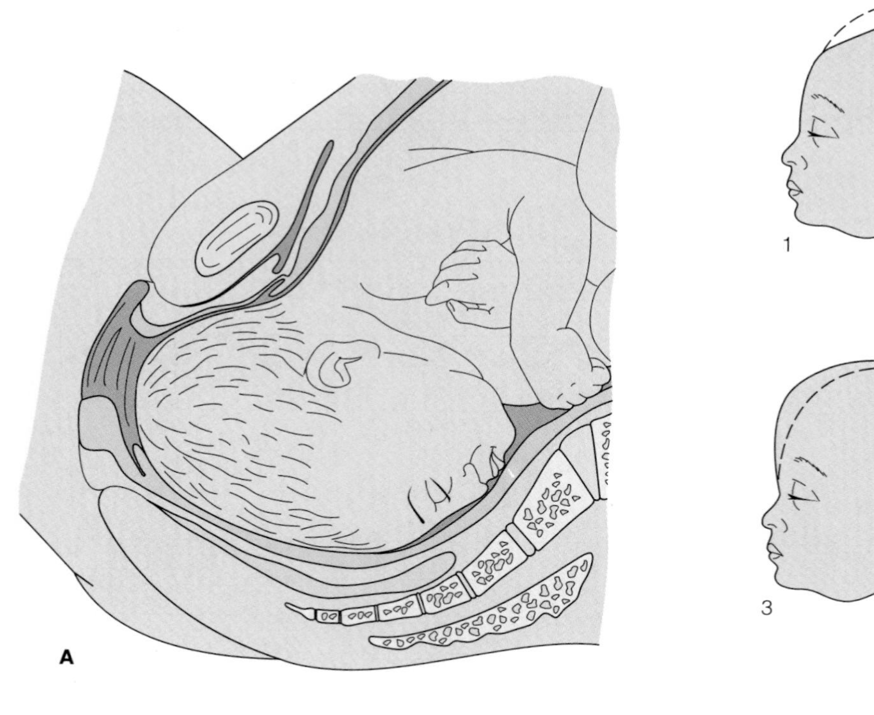

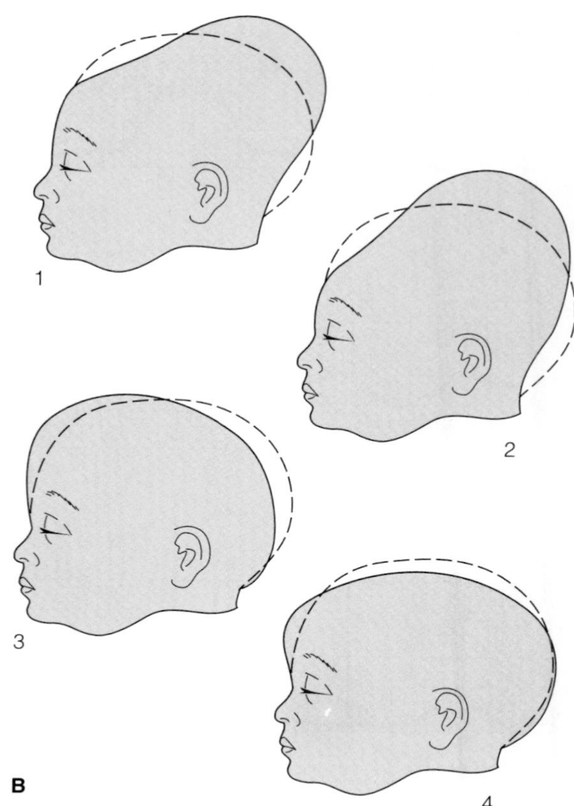

FIGURE 19–2 Effects of labor on the fetal head. ***A*** Caput succedaneum formation. The presenting portion of the scalp area is encircled by the cervix during labor, causing swelling of the soft tissue. ***B*** Molding of the fetal head in cephalic presentations: (1) occiput anterior, (2) occiput posterior, (3) brow, (4) face.

Maternal implications of hypertonic labor include

- Increased discomfort due to uterine muscle cell anoxia
- Fatigue as the pattern continues and no labor progress results
- Dehydration and increased incidence of infection if labor is prolonged
- Stress on coping abilities

Fetal-neonatal implications include

- Early fetal distress because contractions and increased resting tone interfere with the uteroplacental exchange
- Prolonged pressure on the fetal head, which may result in cephalhematoma, caput succedaneum, or excessive molding (Figure 19–2)

Medical Therapy

Management of hypertonic labor may include bed rest and sedation to promote relaxation and reduce pain. Oxytocin is not administered to a woman suffering from hypertonic uterine activity because it is likely to accentuate the abnormal labor pattern (Cunningham et al 1997). If the hypertonic pattern continues and develops into a prolonged latent phase, oxytocin infusion or amniotomy may be used as treatment methods (see Chapter 20). These methods are instituted only after cephalopelvic disproportion (CPD) and fetal malpresentation have been ruled out. When an oxytocin infusion is used to stimulate uterine contractions, the physician/certified nurse-midwife needs to assess whether vaginal birth is possible; in other words, whether the maternal pelvis is large enough for the fetus to pass through. If the maternal pelvic diameters are less than average, or if the fetus is particularly large or is in a malpresentation or malposition, **cephalopelvic disproportion (CPD)** is said to be present. In the presence of CPD, labor is not stimulated because vaginal birth is not possible.

APPLYING THE NURSING PROCESS

Nursing Assessment

As part of the labor assessment, the nurse should evaluate the relationship between the intensity of the pain being experienced and the degree to which the cervix is dilating and effacing. The nurse should also note whether anxiety is having a deleterious effect on labor progress, especially if the mother is a primigravida or is postterm. Evidence of increasing frustration and discouragement on the part of the mother and her partner may become apparent as labor ensues and their birth plan cannot be followed.

Nursing Diagnosis

Nursing diagnoses that may apply to the woman in hypertonic labor include the following:

- Pain related to the woman's inability to relax secondary to hypertonic uterine contractions
- Ineffective individual coping related to ineffectiveness of breathing techniques to relieve discomfort
- Anxiety related to slow labor progress
- Knowledge deficit related to lack of information about dysfunctional labor patterns

Nursing Plan and Implementation

A key nursing role is to provide comfort and support to the laboring woman and her partner. The woman experiencing a hypertonic labor pattern will probably be very uncomfortable because of the increased force of contractions. Her anxiety level and that of her partner may be high. The nurse attempts to reduce the woman's discomfort and promote a more effective labor pattern.

The nurse may suggest supportive measures such as a change of position: left lateral side-lying, high Fowler's, on her knees in the bed with her arms up around the top of the bed while it is in high Fowler's, rocking in a rocking chair, sitting up, and walking. Soothing measures such as a warm shower, Jacuzzi, quiet environment, use of music the woman finds soothing, back rub, therapeutic touch, and visualization may also be helpful. Comfort measures may also be used: mouth care, change of linens, effleurage, and relaxation exercises may provide more comfort. If sedation is ordered, the nurse ensures that the environment is conducive to relaxation. The labor coach may also need assistance in helping the woman cope. A calm, understanding approach by the nurse offers the woman and her partner further support. Provision of information about the cause of the hypertonic labor pattern and assurances that the woman is not overreacting to the situation are also important nursing actions.

To promote maternal-fetal physical well-being, the nurse maintains the woman's fluid balance through adequate hydration. Urine ketones should be monitored hourly. If possible, the couple should be informed of labor progress.

Client education is key for the woman experiencing hypertonic labor. She needs to have information about the dysfunctional labor pattern and the possible implications for her and her baby. Information will help relieve anxiety and thereby increase relaxation and comfort. The nurse needs to explain treatment methods and offer opportunities for questions.

Evaluation

Anticipated outcomes of nursing care include

- The woman experiences a more effective labor pattern.
- The woman has increased comfort and decreased anxiety.
- The woman and her partner are able to cope with the labor.
- The woman and her partner understand the labor pattern and its possible implications.

Hypotonic Labor Patterns

A hypotonic labor pattern usually occurs in the active phase of labor, although it may occur in the latent phase. When this pattern occurs in the active phase, it usually develops after labor has been well established. Hypotonic labor is characterized by fewer than 2–3 contractions in a 10-minute period (Figure 19–1C, p 443).

Hypotonic labor may occur when the uterus is overstretched from a twin gestation, or in the presence of a large fetus, hydramnios, or grandmultiparity. Bladder or bowel distention and CPD may also be associated with this pattern. Maternal implications of hypotonic labor patterns include

- Risk of intrauterine infection if labor is prolonged
- Risk of postpartal hemorrhage from insufficient uterine contractions following delivery
- Maternal exhaustion
- Stress on coping abilities

Fetal-neonatal implications include

- Fetal distress, due to prolonged labor pattern
- Fetal sepsis from maternal pathogens that ascend from the birth canal

Medical Therapy

Improving the quality of the uterine contractions while ensuring a safe outcome for the woman and her baby are the goals of therapy.

Before initiating treatment for hypotonic labor, the physician validates the adequacy of pelvic measurements and completes tests to establish gestational age if there is any question about fetal maturity. After CPD, fetal malpresentation, and fetal immaturity have been

CRITICAL THINKING IN ACTION

A fetal heart tracing demonstrates the following: A baseline heart rate of 140 with variability of 6–10 bpm. When you compare the FHR with the uterine contractions, you note that there is a slowing of the FHR at the time of the contraction and that the FHR tracing looks like the contraction curve but is upside down.

Based on this tracing, what would you do?

Answers can be found in Appendix H.

ruled out, oxytocin (Pitocin) may be given intravenously via an infusion pump to improve the quality of uterine contractions. Intravenous fluid is useful to maintain adequate hydration and prevent maternal exhaustion. Amniotomy may be done to stimulate the labor process.

An improvement in the quality of uterine contractions is demonstrated by noticeable progress in the labor process. If the labor pattern does not become effective, or if other complications develop, further interventions, including cesarean birth, may be necessary.

APPLYING THE NURSING PROCESS

Nursing Assessment

Assessing contractions (for frequency and intensity), maternal vital signs, and fetal heart rate (FHR) provides the nurse with data to evaluate maternal-fetal status. The nurse is also alert for signs and symptoms of infection and dehydration. Because of the stress associated with a prolonged labor, observing the woman and her partner's degree of success with their coping mechanisms is also important.

Nursing Diagnosis

Nursing diagnoses that may apply to the woman in hypotonic labor include the following:

- Pain related to inability to cope with uterine contractions secondary to dysfunctional labor
- Knowledge deficit related to lack of information about dysfunctional labor

Nursing Plan and Implementation

Nursing measures to promote maternal-fetal physical well-being include frequent monitoring of contractions, maternal vital signs, and FHR. If meconium (dark green or black stool present in the fetal large intestine) is present in the amniotic fluid, observing fetal status closely becomes more critical. Maintaining an intake and output record provides a way of determining maternal hydration or dehydration. The woman should be encouraged to void every 2 hours, and her bladder should be checked for distention. Because her labor may be prolonged, the woman must continue to be monitored for signs of infection (elevated temperature, chills, changes in characteristics of amniotic fluid). Vaginal examinations should be kept to a minimum. The nursing implications of oxytocin infusion are presented in Drug Guide: Oxytocin in Chapter 20. See Essential Precautions for Practice: During Care of the Woman at Risk for Intrapartal Complication.

Provision of emotional support is a key measure for clients experiencing a hypotonic labor pattern. The nurse assists the woman and her partner to cope with the frustration of a lengthy labor process. A warm, caring approach is coupled with techniques to reduce anxiety.

The teaching plan must include information regarding the dysfunctional labor process and implications for the mother and baby. Disadvantages of and alternatives to treatment also need to be discussed and understood.

Evaluation

Anticipated outcomes of nursing care include

- The woman maintains comfort during labor.
- The woman understands the type of labor pattern that is occurring and the treatment plan.

Precipitous Labor

Precipitous labor is labor that lasts for less than three hours. Contributing factors in precipitous labor are (a) multiparity, (b) large pelvis, (c) previous precipitous labor, and (d) a small fetus in a favorable position. One or more of these factors, plus strong contractions, result in a rapid transit of the infant through the birth canal (Cunningham et al 1997).

Precipitous labor and precipitous birth are not the same. A *precipitous birth* is an unexpected, sudden, and often unattended birth. See Chapter 17 for discussion of emergency delivery.

Maternal implications of precipitous labor include

- Increased risk of uterine rupture from intense contractions
- Loss of coping abilities
- Lacerations of the cervix, vagina, and perineum due to rapid descent and birth of the fetus
- Postpartal hemorrhage due to undetected lacerations or inadequate uterine contractions after birth

Fetal-neonatal implications include

- Fetal distress or hypoxia from decreased uteroplacental circulation due to intense uterine contractions
- Cerebral trauma from rapid descent through birth canal

Medical Therapy

Any woman with a history of precipitous labor requires close medical monitoring and preparation for an emergency delivery to facilitate a safe outcome for the mother and fetus (Cunningham et al 1997).

APPLYING THE NURSING PROCESS

Nursing Assessment

During the intrapartal nursing assessment, the nurse can identify a woman at increased risk of precipitous labor (for example, a previous history of precipitous or short labor places a woman at risk). During the labor the presence of one or both of the following factors may indicate potential problems:

- Accelerated cervical dilatation and fetal descent
- Intense uterine contractions with little uterine relaxation between contractions

Nursing Diagnosis

Nursing diagnoses that may apply to the woman with precipitous labor include the following:

- Potential for injury related to rapid labor and birth
- Pain related to rapid labor process

Nursing Plan and Implementation

If the woman has a history of precipitous labor, she is closely monitored, and an emergency birth pack is kept at hand. The nurse stays in constant attendance if at all possible and promotes comfort and rest by assisting the woman to a comfortable position, providing a quiet environment, and administering sedatives as needed. The nurse provides information and support before and after the birth.

To avoid hyperstimulation of the uterus and possible precipitous labor during oxytocin administration, the nurse should be alert to the dangers of oxytocin overdosage (see Drug Guide: Oxytocin, Chapter 20). If the woman who is receiving oxytocin develops an accelerated labor pattern, the oxytocin is discontinued immediately, and the woman is turned on her left side to improve uterine perfusion. Oxygen may be started to increase the available oxygen in the maternal circulating blood; this increases the amount available for exchange at the placental site.

The fetus is monitored for signs of hypoxia and other indications of fetal distress. Nursing interventions to relieve fetal distress are discussed in the critical pathway on page 461.

ESSENTIAL PRECAUTIONS FOR PRACTICE

During Care of the Woman at Risk for Intrapartal Complications

Examples of times when disposable gloves should be worn include the following:

- Handling chux and bedding that are moist with bloody show or amniotic fluid
- Cleansing the perineum
- Assessing the perineum

REMEMBER to wash your hands before putting on the disposable gloves and AGAIN immediately after you remove the gloves.

For further information consult OSHA and CDC guidelines.

Evaluation

Anticipated outcomes of nursing care include

- The woman and her baby remain free of injury during birth.
- The woman is supported during the birth process.

Care of the Woman with Postterm Pregnancy

A **postterm pregnancy** is one that extends more than 294 days or 42 weeks past the first day of the last menstrual period. The incidence is approximately 10 percent of all pregnancies, and about 5 percent continue beyond 43 weeks (Lake 1992; Resnik 1994). Some of the 10 percent are not truly postterm but occur in women who have variable menstrual cycles (Kochenour 1992). While many pregnancies extend beyond the anticipated due date, the true postterm pregnancy is associated with increased risk for asphyxia and trauma in the fetus.

The cause of postterm pregnancy is unknown. It does seem to occur more frequently in nulliparas between ages 15 and 20, in multigravidas over age 35, and when an anencephalic fetus is present (Lake 1992).

Maternal implications of postterm pregnancy include the following:

- Minimal physiologic risks
- Increased psychologic stress as the due date passes and concern for the baby increases

Fetal implications include

- Decreased perfusion from the placenta
- **Oligohydramnios** (decreased amount of amniotic fluid), which increases the risk of cord compression
- Meconium aspiration (aspiration of meconium-stained amniotic fluid by the fetus at the time of birth), which is more likely if oligohydramnios and thick meconium are present (Kochenour 1992).
- Varying growth rates.

Some fetuses continue to grow throughout the pregnancy and can even be excessively large at birth (**macrosomia**). In other cases, the intrauterine environment is unfavorable for growth, and at birth the infant has lost muscle mass and subcutaneous fat (Kochenour 1992). The macrosomic fetus is at risk for birth trauma and the SGA fetus is at greatest risk for fetal distress during labor because there is frequently an associated oligohydramnios (Kochenour 1992).

Perinatal mortality doubles by 43 weeks' gestation and triples by 44 weeks (Kochenour 1992).

Medical Therapy

When the 40th week of gestation is completed and birth has not occurred, most obstetricians begin using the nonstress test (NST) and biophysical profile (BPP) (especially the amniotic fluid volume portion of the BPP) as assessment tools. The tests may be done two to three times a week and some physicians advise a contraction stress test (CST) once a week (Resnik 1994). If at any time the fetal assessment tests indicate a problem, interventions are taken to accomplish the birth. Hannah and colleagues (1996) have suggested that induction of labor at 41 weeks' gestation would decrease the number of cesarean births and decrease neonatal morbidity and mortality.

APPLYING THE NURSING PROCESS

Nursing Assessment

Assessment of the woman with postterm pregnancy usually occurs in the birth setting. The nurse needs to stay alert for evidence of variable decelerations of the FHR, which are associated with cord compression due to the oligohydramnios. Meconium may be present and become evident when the amniotic membranes rupture. The nurse needs to assess the woman's knowledge base about the condition, implications for her baby, risks, and possible interventions.

Nursing Diagnosis

Nursing diagnoses that may apply to the woman with postterm pregnancy include the following:

- Knowledge deficit related to lack of information about postterm pregnancy
- Fear related to the unknown outcome for the baby
- Ineffective individual coping related to anxiety about the status of the baby

Nursing Plan and Implementation

Promotion of fetal well-being requires careful assessment of the response of the fetus during labor. If oligohydramnios exists, a continuous FHR tracing is obtained and evaluated frequently. Variable decelerations are often associated with oligohydramnios, because the decreased amount of fluid allows the umbilical cord to be compressed. If the fetus is macrosomic, careful assessment of labor progress (contraction characteristics, progressive cervical dilatation, and fetal descent) is also needed.

Research indicates that provision of emotional support is a key nursing intervention for women with pregnancies that extend past the due date. Women frequently report that they feel increased stress and anxiety and have more difficulty coping. Encouragement, support, and recognition of the woman's anxiety were all identified as helpful strategies by health personnel.

Client education is another important nursing responsibility. The woman needs to have information about the postterm pregnancy. The nurse should address the implications and associated risks for the baby, as well as possible treatment plans. The woman and her partner need opportunities to ask questions and clarify information.

Evaluation

Anticipated outcomes of nursing care include

- The woman has knowledge about the postterm pregnancy.
- The woman and her partner feel supported and able to cope with the postterm pregnancy.
- Fetal status is maintained, any abnormalities are quickly identified, and supportive measures are initiated.

Care of the Woman with a Ruptured Uterus

A ruptured uterus is the tearing of previously intact uterine muscles or of an old uterine scar. The rupture can be caused by a weakened cesarean scar, usually from a "classic" incision; obstetric trauma; mismanagement of oxytocin induction or augmentation; CPD; and congenital defects of the birth canal.

The signs and symptoms of a complete rupture include excruciating pain and cessation of contractions. Vaginal hemorrhage may occur, but vaginal bleeding is usually not profuse. Massive intraperitoneal hemorrhage and hematomas of the broad ligament are hidden sources of bleeding and may account for the scant vaginal bleeding. The woman exhibits signs of hypovolemic shock, and the fetal heart stops beating.

Maternal implications of ruptured uterus include

- Development of profound shock and risk of maternal death
- Abdominal surgery and possible hysterectomy
- Prolonged hospitalization for intensive care and recuperation
- Loss of the expected baby

Fetal-neonatal implications are fetal asphyxia and death.

Medical Therapy

In the presence of a threatened or actual rupture, emergency surgical intervention is done to save the mother and her baby. Delivery is by cesarean birth. If the rupture (uterine tear) is small, the physician may be able to repair it. If the rupture is large, the physician may do a hysterectomy.

Nursing Care

The nurse may be the one to identify the signs of uterine rupture. The nurse monitors vital signs, evaluates maternal hemorrhage, and quickly mobilizes the team for an emergency laparotomy or cesarean birth. When the physiologic needs of the woman are met, the nurse can focus on the emotional needs of the family. The family must have a clear understanding of the procedure and its implications for future childbearing. In addition, if fetal death has occurred, the couple should be given an opportunity to grieve and be allowed to see their infant if they desire. (See p 462 for further discussion.)

Care of the Woman and Fetus at Risk Due to Fetal Malposition

Persistent occiput-posterior (OP) position of the fetus is probably one of the most common complications encountered during childbirth. If the fetus is in this position, the occiput of the fetal head is directed toward the back of the maternal pelvis. The fetus may remain in this position throughout labor and birth, or it may rotate (or change) to an occiput-anterior (OA) position during birth.

Maternal implications of persistent occiput-posterior position include

- Risk of third- or fourth-degree perineal lacerations during birth
- Risk of extension of a midline episiotomy

Fetal implications include no increased risk of fetal mortality unless labor is prolonged or additional interventions such as forceps-assisted birth, vacuum extraction, or cesarean birth are required.

Medical Therapy

Medical treatment focuses on close monitoring of maternal and fetal status and labor progress to determine whether vaginal or cesarean birth is the safer birth method. A cesarean birth is chosen if maternal or fetal problems make a vaginal birth unwise or if CPD is present. Most persistent occiput-posterior fetuses are born vaginally; however, the birth may need to be assisted with forceps. The forceps can be used to deliver the fetus while it is still in the occiput-posterior position, or to rotate the occiput to an anterior position (called Scanzoni's maneuver). A manual rotation from LOP or ROP to an anterior position may be possible. A vacuum extractor may also be used. See Chapter 20 for further discussion of forceps and vacuum extraction.

APPLYING THE NURSING PROCESS

Nursing Assessment

Signs and symptoms of a persistent occiput-posterior position are a dysfunctional labor pattern, a prolonged active phase, secondary arrest of dilatation or arrest of descent, and complaints of intense back pain by the laboring woman. The back pain is caused by the fetal occiput compressing the sacral nerves. Further assessment may reveal a depression in the maternal abdomen above the symphysis. Fetal heart rates will be heard far laterally on the abdomen, and on vaginal examination the certified nurse-midwife/physician will find the wide diamond-shaped anterior fontanelle in the anterior portion of the pelvis. This fontanelle may be difficult to feel because of molding of the fetal head.

Nursing Diagnosis

Nursing diagnoses that may apply to women with persistent occiput posterior include the following:

- Pain related to back discomfort secondary to occiput-posterior position
- Ineffective individual coping related to unanticipated discomfort and slow progress in labor

Nursing Plan and Implementation

Changing maternal posture has been used for many years to enhance rotation of OP or occiput-transverse (OT) to OA. The woman may be placed on one side and then asked to move to the other side as the fetus begins to rotate. This side-lying position may promote rotation; it also enables the support persons to apply counterpressure on the sacral area to decrease discomfort. A knee-chest position provides a downward slant to the vaginal canal, directing the fetal head downward on descent. A hands-and-knees position is often effective in rotating the fetus. In addition to maintaining a hands-and-knees position on the bed, the woman may do pelvic rocking, and the support person may perform firm stroking motions on the abdomen. The stroking begins over the fetal back and swings around to the other side of the abdomen. After the fetus has rotated, the woman lies in a Sims' position on the side opposite the fetal back (Andrews and Andrews 1983).

Evaluation

Anticipated outcomes of nursing care include

- The woman's discomfort is decreased.
- The woman and her partner understand comfort measures and position changes that may assist her.
- The woman's coping abilities are strengthened.
- The woman and her partner feel supported and encouraged.

Care of the Woman and Fetus at Risk Due to Fetal Malpresentation

Fetal malpresentations include brow, face, breech, shoulder (transverse lie), and compound presentation.

Brow Presentation

In a brow presentation, the forehead of the fetus becomes the presenting part. The fetal neck is hyperextended instead of flexed, with the result that the fetal head enters the birth canal with the widest diameter of the head (occipitomental) foremost (Figure 19–3). The incidence is 1:1500 births (Seeds and Walsh 1996).

The brow presentation occurs more often in the multipara than the nullipara and is thought to be due to lax abdominal and pelvic musculature. Some brow presentations will spontaneously convert to face or occipital presentation (Seeds and Walsh 1996).

Maternal implications of brow presentation include

- Longer labor due to ineffective contractions and slow or arrested fetal descent
- Cesarean birth if brow presentation persists (Seeds and Walsh 1996)

Fetal-neonatal implications include cephalhematoma of the forehead.

Medical Therapy

Once brow presentation is identified, most obstetricians plan a cesarean birth.

APPLYING THE NURSING PROCESS

Nursing Assessment

A brow presentation can be detected on vaginal examination by palpation of the diamond-shaped anterior fontanelle on one side and orbital ridges and root of the nose on the other side. If a large cephalhematoma is present, it will be difficult to identify fetal structures while doing a vaginal examination.

Nursing Diagnosis

Nursing diagnoses that may apply to a woman with a brow presentation include the following:

- Knowledge deficit related to lack of information about the possible maternal-fetal effects of brow presentation
- Injury: high risk for fetus related to pressure on fetal structures secondary to brow presentation

Nursing Plan and Implementation

To promote maternal-fetal physical well-being, the nurse closely observes the woman for labor aberrations and the fetus for signs of distress. The fetus should be observed closely during labor for signs of hypoxia as evidenced by late decelerations and bradycardia.

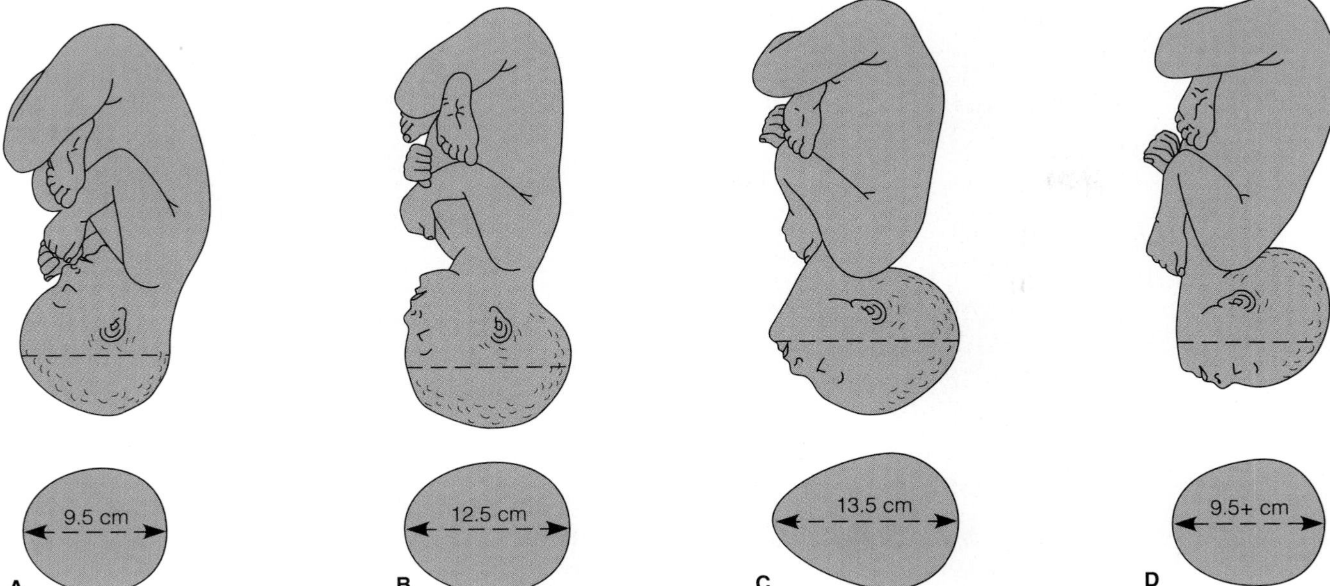

FIGURE 19–3 Types of cephalic presentations. ***A*** The occiput is the presenting part because the head is flexed and the fetal chin is against the chest. The largest anteroposterior (AP) diameter that presents and passes through the pelvis is approximately 9.5 cm. ***B*** Military presentation. The head is neither flexed nor extended. The presenting AP diameter is approximately 12.5 cm. ***C*** Brow presentation. The largest diameter of the fetal head (approximately 13.5 cm) presents in this situation. ***D*** Face presentation. The AP diameter is 9.5 cm.
Source: Danforth DN, Scott JR (editors): *Obstetrics and Gynecology,* 5th ed. New York: Lippincott, 1990, Fig 8–9, p 170.

The nurse also provides emotional support to the family. This may require the nurse to explain the position to the laboring couple or to interpret what the certified nurse-midwife/physician has told them. The nurse should stay close at hand to reassure the couple, inform them of any changes, and assist them with labor-coping techniques. In face and brow presentations, the appearance of the newborn may be affected. The couple may need help in beginning the attachment process because of the newborn's facial appearance. After the infant is inspected for gross abnormalities, the pediatrician and nurse can assure the couple that the facial edema and excessive molding are only temporary and will subside in 3 or 4 days.

Evaluation

Anticipated outcomes of nursing care include

- The woman and her partner understand the implications and associated problems of brow presentation.
- The mother and her baby have a safe labor and birth.

Face Presentation

In a face presentation, the face of the fetus is the presenting part (Figure 19–4; also see Figure 19–3*D*). The fetal head is hyperextended even more than in the brow presentation. Face presentation occurs most frequently in multiparas, in preterm birth, and in the presence of anencephaly. The incidence of face presentation is about 1 in 500 deliveries (Seeds and Walsh 1996).

Maternal implications of face presentation include

- Increased risk of CPD and prolongation of labor
- With prolongation of labor, an increased risk of infection
- Difficulty bonding with the newborn if cephalhematoma of the face is present
- Cesarean birth if fetal chin is posterior (mentum posterior)

Fetal-neonatal implications include

- Cephalhematoma of the face
- Edema of the face and throat if the fetal chin is anterior (mentum anterior) and a vaginal birth occurs (may also occur during fetal descent)

Medical Therapy

A vaginal birth may be anticipated if no CPD is present, the chin (mentum) is anterior, the labor pattern is effective, and no fetal stress or distress is present. If the mentum is posterior, a cesarean birth is planned (Figure 19–5).

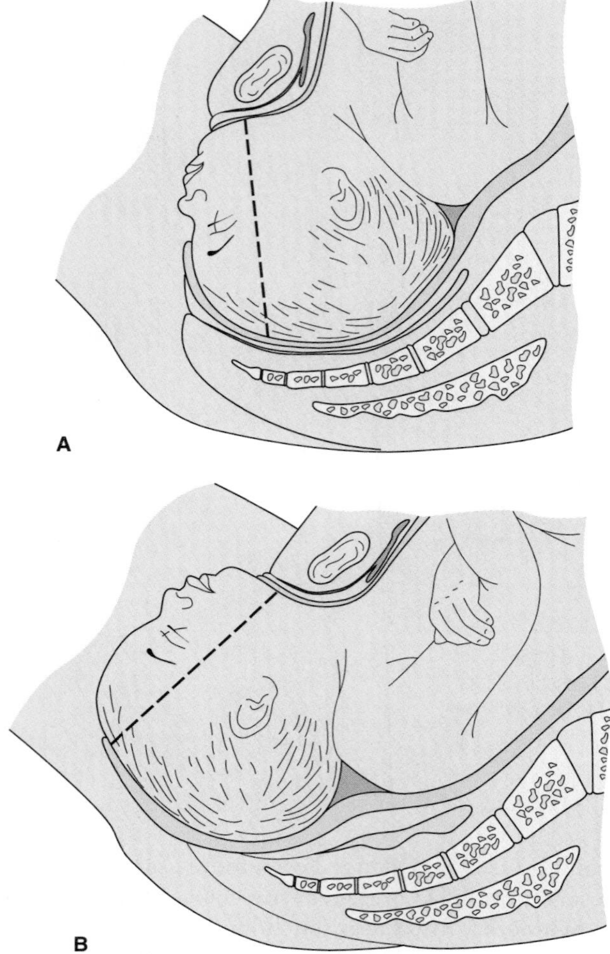

FIGURE 19–4 Mechanism of birth in face (mentoanterior) position. *A* The submentobregmatic diameter at the outlet. *B* The fetal head is born by the movement of flexion.

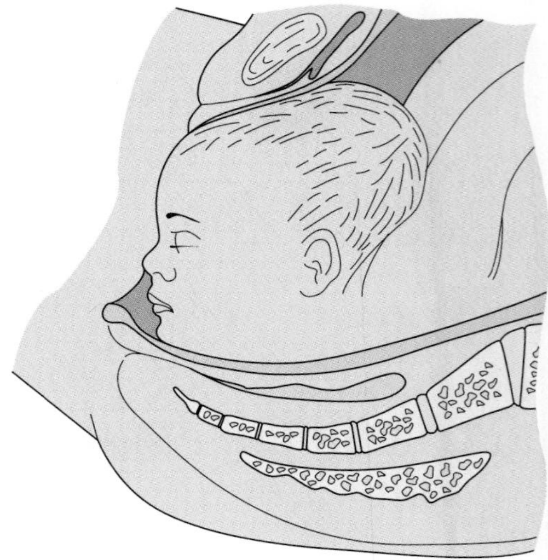

FIGURE 19–5 Face presentation. Mechanism of birth in mentoposterior position. Fetal head is unable to extend farther. The face becomes impacted.

APPLYING THE NURSING PROCESS

Nursing Assessment

When performing Leopold's maneuvers, the nurse finds that the back of the fetus is difficult to outline, and a deep furrow can be palpated between the hard occiput and the fetal back (Figure 19–6). Fetal heart tones are audible on the side where the fetal feet are palpated. It may be difficult to determine by vaginal examination whether a breech or face is presenting, especially if facial edema is already present. During the vaginal examination, palpation of the saddle of the nose and the gums should be attempted. When assessing engagement, the nurse must remember that the face has to be deep within the pelvis before the biparietal diameters have entered the inlet.

Nursing Diagnosis

Nursing diagnoses that may apply to the woman with a fetus in face presentation include the following:

- Fear related to unknown outcome of the labor
- Potential for injury to the newborn's face related to edema secondary to the birth process

Nursing Plan and Implementation

Nursing interventions are the same as those indicated for the brow presentation.

Evaluation

Anticipated outcomes of nursing care include

- The woman and her partner understand the implications and associated problems of face presentation.
- The mother and her baby have a safe labor and birth.

Breech Presentation

The exact cause of breech presentation (Figure 19–7) is unknown. This malpresentation occurs in 3 to 4 percent of labors and perinatal mortality is 3 to 5 times that of cephalic presentation (Seeds and Walsh 1996). Breech presentation is frequently associated with preterm birth, placenta previa, hydramnios, multiple gestation, uterine anomalies (such as bicornuate uterus), and fetal anom-

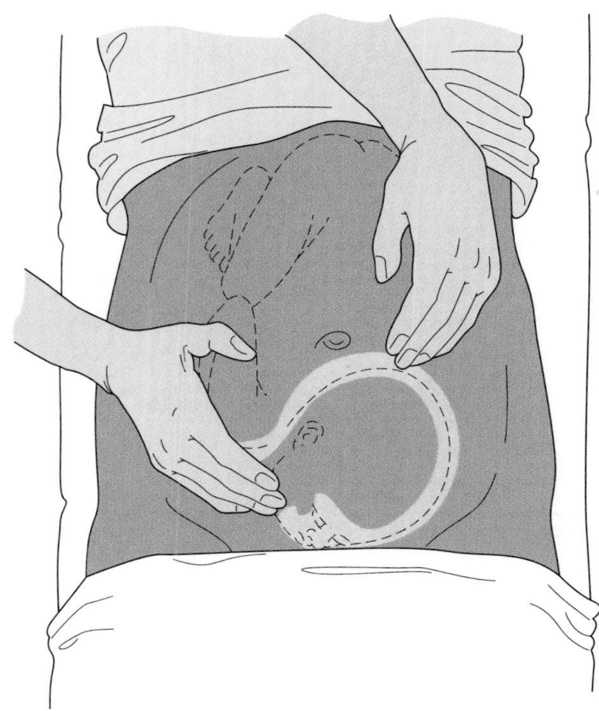

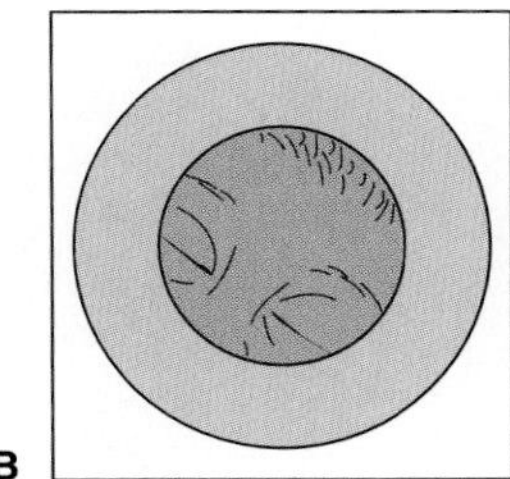

FIGURE 19–6 Face presentation. ***A*** Palpation of the maternal abdomen with the fetus in right mentum posterior (RMP). ***B*** Vaginal examination may permit palpation of facial features of the fetus.

alies (especially anencephly and hydrocephaly). The incidence of hydrocephalus is ten times greater and of anencephalus five times greater than in vertex presentations. In 50 percent of breech presentations no cause is found (Cruikshank 1990).

The maternal implication of breech presentation is a likelihood of cesarean birth.

Fetal-neonatal implications include

- Higher perinatal mortality rate (four times greater for breech infants than for cephalic infants)
- Increased risk of prolapsed cord, especially in incomplete breeches, because space is available between the cervix and presenting part
- Increased risk of cervical cord injuries due to hyperextension of the fetal head during vaginal birth
- Increased risk of birth trauma (especially of the head) during either vaginal or cesarean breech birth

Medical Therapy

An external version may be done at 38–40 weeks of gestation as long as the woman is not in labor. (See Chapter 20 for discussion of external version.) There are differing opinions about the best method of birth for the fetus in a breech presentation. When the fetus is still in breech presentation and labor occurs, the method of birth may vary depending on gestational age, estimated fetal weight, type of breech, and physician preference. If the fetus is at less than 36 weeks of gestation and active labor cannot be stopped, a cesarean birth is planned to decrease the birth stress for the preterm baby. When the fetus is at 38 weeks of gestation or more and the fetus is between 2500 and 3800 g, the head is flexed, and there are normal pelvic diameters, a vaginal birth may be the method of choice. At the time of vaginal birth, an additional obstetrician is usually in attendance, as well as an anesthesiologist, in case a cesarean needs to be done (Quilligan 1990).

APPLYING THE NURSING PROCESS

Nursing Assessment

Frequently it is the nurse who first recognizes a breech presentation. On palpation the hard vertex is felt in the fundus and ballottement of the head can be done independently of the fetal body. The wider sacrum is palpated in the lower part of the abdomen. If the sacrum has not descended, on ballottement the entire fetal body will move. Furthermore, fetal heart rate (FHR) is usually auscultated above the umbilicus. Passage of meconium from compression of the infant's intestinal tract on descent is common.

The nurse is particularly alert for a prolapsed umbilical cord, especially in footling breeches, because there is space between the cervix and presenting part through which the cord can slip. If the infant is small and the membranes rupture, the danger is even greater. This is one reason why any woman admitted to the birthing

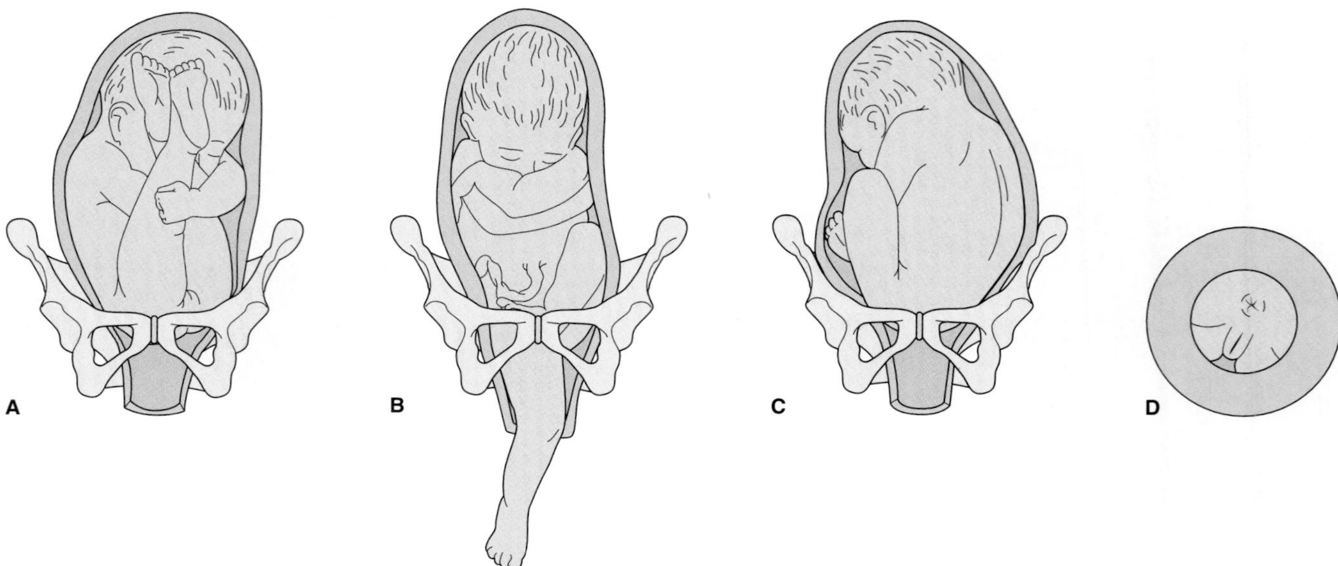

FIGURE 19–7 Breech presentation. ***A*** Frank breech. ***B*** Incomplete (footling) breech. ***C*** Complete breech in left sacral anterior (LSA) position. ***D*** On vaginal examination the nurse may feel the anal sphincter. The tissue of the fetal buttocks feels soft.

area with a history of ruptured membranes should not be ambulated until a full assessment, including vaginal examination, has been performed.

Nursing Diagnosis

Nursing diagnoses that may apply to a woman with a breech presentation include the following:

- Impaired gas exchange in the fetus related to interruption in umbilical blood flow secondary to compression of the cord
- Knowledge deficit related to lack of information about the implications and associated complications of breech presentation on the mother and fetus

Nursing Plan and Implementation

Promotion of Maternal-Fetal Physical Well-Being

During labor, the nurse promotes maternal-fetal physical well-being by making frequent assessments to evaluate fetal and maternal status. The nurse needs to be aware of the associated problems of breech presentation and look for subtle clues of beginning problems. The nurse provides teaching and information about the breech presentation and the nursing care needed.

Although many infants in breech presentations are born by cesarean birth, a few are born vaginally. The nurse assists the vaginal birth by including Piper forceps (used to guide the aftercoming fetal head) in the birth table setup. During the birth process, the nurse may have to help support the infant's body if the physician elects to use forceps. An additional nurse then monitors the FHR closely during the birth.

If the family and certified nurse-midwife/physician elect a cesarean birth, the nurse intervenes as with any cesarean birth.

Evaluation

Anticipated outcomes of nursing care include

- The woman and her partner understand the implications and associated problems of breech presentation.
- Major complications are recognized early and corrective measures are instituted.
- The mother and baby have a safe labor and birth.

Transverse Lie (Shoulder Presentation)

A transverse lie occurs in approximately 3 to 4 per 1000 term births (King 1994). Maternal conditions associated with a transverse lie are grandmultiparity with relaxed uterine muscles, and placenta previa (Cruikshank 1990) (Figure 19–8).

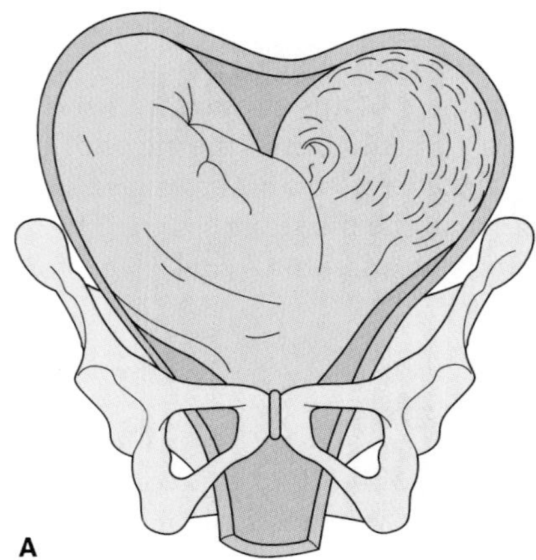

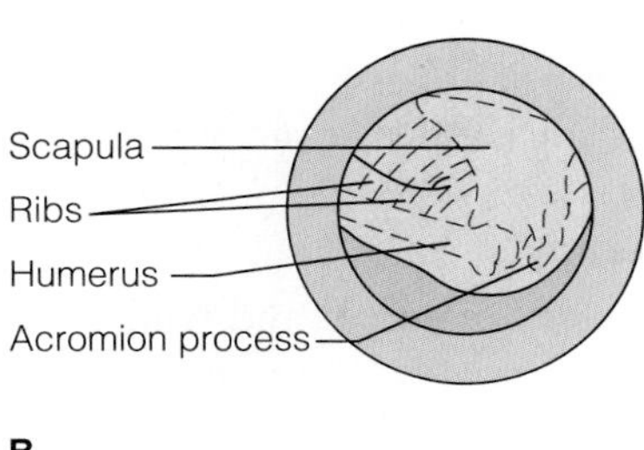

FIGURE 19–8 Transverse lie. ***A*** Shoulder presentation. ***B*** On vaginal examination the nurse may feel the acromion process as the fetal presenting part.

Maternal implications of transverse lie include

- Dysfunctional labor
- Uterine rupture, if labor is allowed to occur (King 1994)
- Cesarean birth

Fetal-neonatal implications include

- Increased risk of prolapsed cord
- Increased risk of stillbirth (King 1994)

Medical Therapy

The management of shoulder presentation depends on the gestational age. If discovered before term, the management is expectant (watchful), as many fetuses change into another presentation without any intervention. When a shoulder presentation is still evident at 38 completed weeks of gestation, an external version may be done, followed immediately by induction of labor. If the woman is in active labor, cesarean birth is selected (Cruikshank 1990).

Nursing Care

The nurse can identify a transverse lie by inspection and palpation of the abdomen, by auscultation of FHR in the midline of the abdomen (not conclusive), and by vaginal examination.

On palpation no fetal part is felt in the fundal portion of the uterus or above the symphysis. The head may be palpated on one side and the breech on the other. Fetal heart rate is usually auscultated just below the midline of the umbilicus. On vaginal examination, if a presenting part is palpated, it is the ridged thorax or possibly an arm that is compressed against the chest.

The primary nursing actions are to assist in the interpretation of the fetal presentation and to provide information and support to the couple. The nurse assesses maternal and fetal status frequently and prepares the woman for an operative birth. The nurse explains to the couple the need for cesarean and the assessments and care surrounding a cesarean. (See Chapter 20 for further information about teaching with cesarean birth.)

Compound Presentation

A compound presentation is one in which there are two presenting parts such as occiput and fetal hand, occiput and fetal foot, or breech and fetal hand. Some compound presentations resolve themselves spontaneously, but others require additional manipulation at birth.

Care of the Woman and Fetus at Risk Due to Developmental Abnormalities

Macrosomia

Fetal macrosomia occurs when a newborn weighs more than 4000 g at birth. This condition is more common among offspring of large parents and diabetic women and in cases of grandmultiparity and postterm gestation.

Maternal implications of macrosomia include

- Risk of CPD
- Risk of dysfunctional labor
- Soft tissue laceration during vaginal birth
- Increased incidence of postpartal hemorrhage

Fetal-neonatal implications include

- Meconium aspiration
- Asphyxia

- Shoulder dystocia, in which, after delivery of the head, the anterior shoulder fails to deliver either spontaneously or with gentle traction (Bowes 1994)
- Increased risk of upper brachial plexus injury and fractured clavicles (Seeds and Walsh 1996)

Medical Therapy

The occurrence of maternal and fetal problems associated with excessively large infants may be somewhat lessened by identifying macrosomia before the onset of labor. If a large fetus is suspected, the maternal pelvis should be evaluated carefully. An estimation of fetal size can be made by palpating the crown–rump length of the fetus in utero, but the greatest errors in estimation occur on both ends of the spectrum–the macrosomic fetus and the very small fetus. Fundal height can give some clue. Ultrasound or x-ray pelvimetry may give further information about fetal size. Whenever the uterus appears excessively large, hydramnios, an oversized fetus, or multiple pregnancies must be considered as possible causes.

When fetal weight is estimated to be 4500 g or more, a cesarean birth is usually planned (Seeds and Walsh 1996). Controversy exists about the best method of birth for estimated fetal weight of 4000–4500 g. The discussion centers primarily around the incidence of shoulder dystocia and the difficulty in accurately estimating the fetal weight. When shoulder dystocia unexpectedly occurs at the time of vaginal birth it can be a grave problem, and the physician/CNM may find it necessary to fracture the clavicles to save the fetus's life. As an emergency measure the CNM/physician may ask the nurse to apply suprapubic or fundal pressure in an attempt to aid the delivery of the fetal shoulders (Kline-Kaye and Miller-Slade 1990).

Nursing Care

The nurse assists in identifying women who are at risk for a large fetus or those who exhibit signs of macrosomia. Because these women are prime candidates for dystocia and its complications, the nurse frequently assesses the FHR for indications of fetal distress and evaluates the rate of cervical dilatation and fetal descent.

The fetal monitor is applied for continuous fetal evaluation. Early decelerations could mean disproportion at the bony inlet. Any sign of labor dysfunction or fetal distress should be reported to the physician.

The nurse provides support for the laboring woman and her partner and information about the implications and possible associated problems. During the birth, the nurse continues to provide support and encouragement to the couple. If asked to apply fundal pressure, the nurse needs to follow protocols developed by the facility (Kline-Kaye and Miller-Slade 1990).

The nurse inspects macrosomic newborns after birth for skull fractures, cephalhematoma, and Erb palsy, and informs the nursery of any problems. If the nursery staff is aware of a difficult birth, the newborn will be observed more closely for cerebral and neurologic damage.

After the birth the nurse checks the uterus for potential atony and the maternal vital signs for deviations suggesting shock.

Hydrocephalus

In hydrocephalus, 500–1000 mL of cerebrospinal fluid accumulates in the ventricles of the fetal brain. When this occurs before birth, severe CPD results because of the enlarged cranium of the fetus.

With the use of ultrasound during pregnancy, diagnosis of this fetal abnormality is more likely. Once the woman is in labor, hydrocephalus should be suspected if labor contractions progress yet the fetal head does not enter the birth canal. If a hydrocephalic fetus is in vertex presentation, the person doing a vaginal examination will feel wide suture lines.

Maternal implications of hydrocephalus include emotional responses related to the implications of hydrocephalus for the baby and the family. Additional implications may include obstruction of labor.

The outlook for the fetus is questionable. If hydrocephalus is identified early in the gestation, intrauterine surgery may be performed to place a shunt, thereby preventing excessive accumulation of fluid in the fetal head. However, this surgery is not currently available to all mothers in all parts of the country.

Medical Therapy

Medical intervention is directed toward delivering the fetus by the least traumatic means. It is important to know the degree of hydrocephalus and whether other anomalies or abnormalities are present that would make it very unlikely that the baby could live after the birth. A cesarean birth may give the newborn the best chance, and a vaginal birth may be very traumatic. If the predicted chance of survival is very small, or if the fetus is already dead, a cesarean birth unnecessarily increases the risk to the mother, so a vaginal birth might be the best choice. The decisions about method of birth are not easy; they are best made by the parents and health care providers together.

Nursing Care

Nursing assessments focus on the information needs of the woman and her partner. It is also important to assess their emotional state to provide support.

The nurse helps the couple cope with the crisis and to deal with their grief (see discussion on page 462).

The nurse assists with diagnostic procedures and interprets the findings if the couple has questions after conversations with the physician. The type of assistance at birth depends on the method chosen.

Care of the Woman with a Twin Pregnancy

The incidence of naturally occurring twins in the United States is 1 per 94 pregnancies (Cunningham et al 1997). Twins can develop from either the fertilization of two separate ova or from the division of one fertilized ovum. Twins that occur from two separate ova are called *dizygotic* and may be of the same or different sexes. In this type of twinning, there are two amnions (diamniotic) and two chorions (dichorionic). The incidence of twins varies and is highest in African Americans, women of higher age and parity, and women who are tall and tend to be heavier. The incidence is low in the Asian population.

Twins from one fertilized ovum are called *monozygotic* and are always of the same sex. If the fertilized ovum (zygote) divides within the first 72 hours after fertilization, the twins will be diamniotic and dichorionic. If the division occurs from the 4th to the 8th day after fertilization, the embryos will develop with two separate amnions (diamniotic) and one chorion (monochorionic). If the division happens after the 8th day, the two fetuses will share both a common amniotic sac and chorion (monoamniotic, monochorionic). The terminology is important because the perinatal morbidity and mortality rates differ greatly between different types of twins (Chitkara and Berkowitz 1996).

During the prenatal period, a fundal height greater than expected for the weeks of gestation, and auscultation of two heartbeats that differ by at least 10 bpm, are the most likely clues to twins. Some women experience severe nausea and vomiting and develop severe anemia despite multiple vitamin therapy. The α-fetoprotein level may be elevated (Chitkara and Berkowitz 1996).

Maternal Implications

During her pregnancy, the woman may experience physical discomfort such as shortness of breath, dyspnea on exertion, backaches, and pedal edema. Other associated problems include urinary tract infections, PIH, preterm labor, and placenta previa (Cunningham et al 1997).

Complications during labor include abnormal fetal presentations, abruptio placentae, prolapsed cord, and hemorrhage immediately, or in the first few hours after the birth (Chitkara and Berkowitz 1996).

Fetal-Neonatal Implications

The perinatal mortality rate is approximately four times greater for twins than for a single fetus. The perinatal mortality rate for monoamniotic, monochorionic twins has been estimated as high as 50 percent (D'Alton and Simpson 1995). Fetal problems include decreased intrauterine growth rate for each fetus, increased incidence of fetal anomalies, increased risk of prematurity and the associated problems of being a preterm baby, and abnormal presentations.

Monochorionic, monoamniotic twins may develop artery-to-artery anastomosis, which compromises fetoplacental circulation. In such cases, one twin is overperfused, is born with polycythemia and hypervolemia, and may have hypertension with an enlarged heart. This twin's amniotic sac exhibits hydramnios because of the increased renal perfusion and excessive voiding. The other twin has hypovolemia and exhibits intrauterine growth retardation (IUGR) (Chitkara and Berkowitz 1996).

Medical Therapy

The goals of medical care are the promotion of normal fetal development for both fetuses, preventing the birth of preterm fetuses, and diminishing fetal trauma during labor.

Once the presence of twins has been detected, preventing and treating problems that infringe on the development and birth of normal fetuses is a significant medical activity. Prenatal care is comprehensive. The woman's visits are more frequent than those of the woman with one fetus. The woman needs to understand nutritional implications, assessment of fetal activity, signs of preterm labor, and danger signs of pregnancy.

Serial ultrasounds are done to assess the growth of each fetus and to provide early recognition of IUGR. A program of restricted activity should begin as early as 20 weeks, and modified bed rest at home should start at 20 to 24 weeks (Cunningham et al 1997). Some physicians believe that bed rest in the lateral position enhances uterine-placental-fetal blood flow and decreases the risk of preterm labor. Others question the value of bed rest, especially for the prevention of uterine contractions, which seem to precede preterm labor (Cunningham et al 1997).

Testing usually begins at 30 to 34 weeks' gestation and may include NST, FBPP, and Doppler ultrasound to assess umbilical blood waveforms. A reactive NST is associated with good fetal outcome if birth occurs within one week of the testing. The NST is done every 3–7 days until birth or until results become nonreactive (Hunter 1989). The BPP is also accurate in assessing fetal status with twin pregnancies. A biophysical profile of 8 or better for each fetus is considered reassuring, and weekly or biweekly BPPs and NSTs continue until birth.

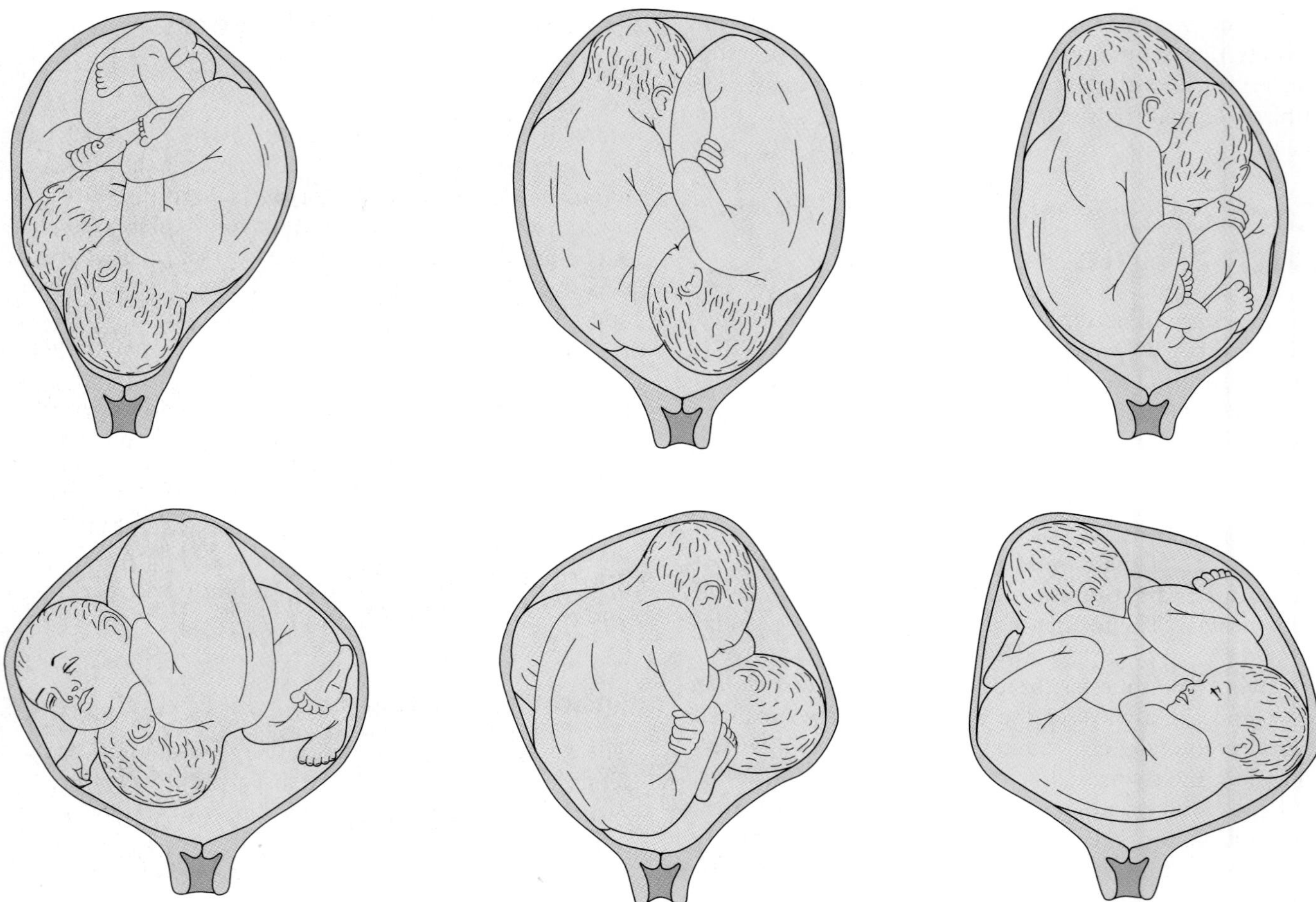

FIGURE 19–9 Twins may be in any of these presentations while in utero.

Intrapartal management and assessment require careful attention to maternal and fetal status. The mother should have an IV in place with a large bore needle. Anesthesia and crossmatched blood should be readily available. The twins are monitored by dual electronic fetal monitoring. The labor may progress very slowly or very quickly.

The decision about method of birth may not be made until labor occurs, and the method depends on a variety of factors. The presence of maternal complications such as placenta previa, abruptio placentae, or severe PIH usually indicates the need for cesarean birth. Fetal factors such as severe IUGR, preterm birth, fetal anomalies, fetal distress, or unfavorable fetal position or presentation also require cesarean birth.

Any combination of presentations and positions can occur with twins (Figure 19–9). The majority of twins are born by cesarean when the presenting twin is in a non-vertex position (Chitkara and Berkowitz 1996).

Nursing Care

During pregnancy the woman may need counseling about diet and daily activities. The nurse can help her plan meals to meet her increased needs. A daily intake of 4000 kcal (minimum) and 135 g of protein is recommended for optimal weight gain and fetal growth. A prenatal vitamin and 1 mg of folic acid should also be taken daily. A weight gain of 40–60 pounds has been recommended with a 15–20-pound weight gain by 20 weeks (Hunter 1989).

Counseling about daily activities may include encouraging the woman to plan frequent rest periods during the day. The rest period will have optimal effects if the woman rests in a side-lying position (which increases uteroplacental blood flow) and elevates her lower legs and feet to reduce edema. Back discomfort may be relieved by pelvic rocking, maintaining good posture, and using good body mechanics when lifting objects or moving about.

During labor, the FHR of the twins is monitored continuously by EFM. Recent developments in electronic monitoring equipment now make it possible to monitor both twins simultaneously, whether by external or internal means. The twins are monitored throughout labor and vaginal birth or up to the time of abdominal incision if a cesarean is done (Eganhouse 1992).

After birth the nurse must prepare to receive two newborns instead of one. This means duplicating everything, including resuscitation equipment, radiant warmers, and newborn identification papers and bracelets. Two physicians or nurses should be available for newborn resuscitation.

Care of the Woman and Fetus in the Presence of Fetal Distress

Fetal distress is defined as "a precarious fetal condition that, if allowed to persist, may lead to permanent damage or perinatal death" (Huddleston and Freeman 1992, p 100). This definition implies awareness that, although fetal distress is precarious, if it is recognized and treated appropriately, the fetus may be spared any permanent damage. Fetal distress is associated with decreased blood flow to the fetus, which can occur with maternal supine position, decreased maternal blood pressure, compression of the umbilical cord, and contraction frequency and intensity that does not allow recovery from the decreased blood flow that normally occurs during contractions and maternal hyperventilation.

Fetal stress is indicated by persistent late decelerations (regardless of the depth of deceleration), persistent severe variable decelerations, especially if the return to the baseline is prolonged, and prolonged decelerations (Huddleston and Freeman 1992). When fetal distress is indicated, intrauterine resuscitation (corrective measures) should be taken without delay. Treatment of maternal hypotension involves having the woman turn to a left lateral decubitus position (right lateral decubitus may also be tried), beginning an intravenous infusion or increasing the flow rate if an infusion is already in place, or, if cord prolapse is suspected, having the woman assume a knee-chest position. Uterine activity can be decreased by discontinuing intravenous oxytocin, or administering a tocolytic agent (Ritodrine or Terbutaline) to decrease contraction frequency and intensity. Oxygen is administered to the woman.

Caregivers can obtain additional information about the condition of the fetus by fetal scalp blood sampling, fetal scalp stimulation, or fetal acoustical stimulation (see Chapter 14). The management scheme for fetal distress is illustrated in Figure 19–10.

Maternal Implications

Indications of fetal distress greatly increase the psychologic stress a laboring woman must face. The professional staff may become so involved in assessing fetal status and initiating corrective measures that they fail to give explanations and emotional support to the woman and her partner. It is imperative to provide both. In many instances, if birth is not imminent, the woman must undergo cesarean birth. This method of birth may be a source of fear for the couple, and of frustration, too, if they prepared for a shared vaginal birth experience.

Medical Therapy

When there is evidence of possible fetal distress, treatment is centered on improving the blood flow to the fetus by correcting maternal hypotension, decreasing the intensity and frequency of contractions if present, administering oxygen, and gathering further information about fetal status. The fetal response to the intrauterine resuscitation measures will dictate subsequent actions.

Nursing Care

The nurse reviews the woman's prenatal history and notes the presence of any conditions (such as PIH, diabetes, renal disease, IUGR) that may be associated with decreased utero-placental-fetal blood flow. When the membranes rupture, the nurse assesses the FHR immediately and notes the characteristics of the amniotic fluid. As labor progresses, the nurse is especially alert to suspicious changes in the FHR. At all times, the nurse encourages and supports maternal positioning that maximizes the uterine-placental-fetal blood flow. Refer to the Critical Pathway for Fetal Stress (p 461) for additional nursing interventions.

Care of the Family at Risk Due to Intrauterine Fetal Death

Fetal death, often referred to as fetal demise, accounts for one-half of perinatal mortality after 20 weeks' gestation. Intrauterine fetal death (IUFD) results from unknown causes or from a number of physiologic maladaptations including preeclampsia-eclampsia, abruptio placentae, placenta previa, diabetes, infection, congenital anomalies, and isoimmune disease.

Prolonged retention of the fetus may lead to the development of disseminated intravascular coagulation

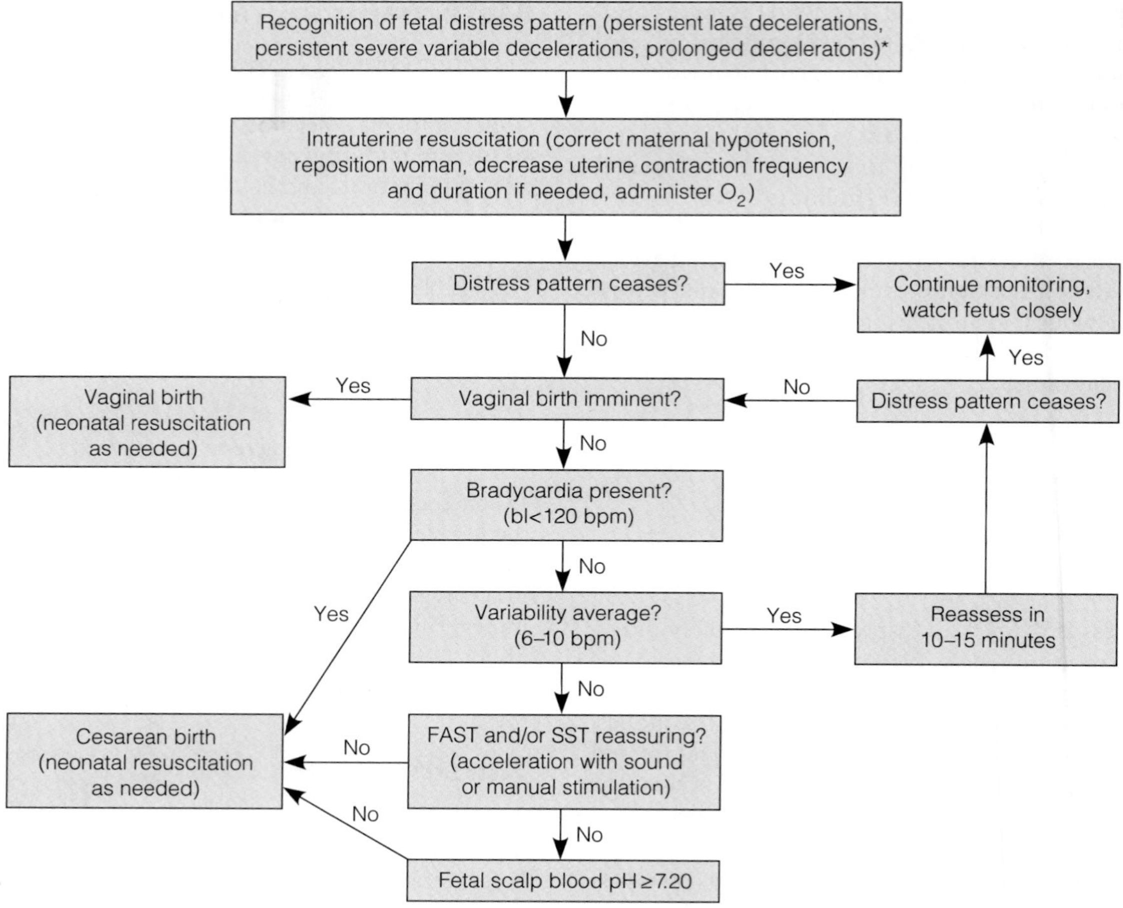

FIGURE 19–10 Intrapartum fetal distress management. Note: Bl = baseline; FAST = fetal acoustic stimulation test; SST = scalp stimulation test.

Sources: Based on information from Strong TH: Fetal distress in the intrapartum period. In: *Current Therapy in Obstetrics and Gynecology,* 3rd ed. Quilligan EJ, Zuspan FP (editors). Philadelphia: Saunders, 1990; *Huddleston JF, Freeman RK: Estimation of fetal well-being. In: *Neonatal-Perinatal Medicine: Diseases of the Fetus and Newborn,* 5th ed. Fanroff AA, Martin RS (editors). St Louis: Mosby-Year Book, 1992.

(DIC) in the mother, also called consumption coagulopathy. After the release of thromboplastin from the degenerating fetal tissues into the maternal bloodstream, the extrinsic clotting system is activated, triggering the formation of multiple tiny blood clots. Fibrinogen and factors V and VII are subsequently depleted, and the woman begins to display symptoms of DIC. Fibrinogen levels begin a linear descent 3 to 4 weeks after the death of the fetus and continue to decrease without appropriate medical intervention.

Medical Therapy

Abdominal x-ray examination may reveal Spalding's sign, an overriding of the fetal cranial bones. In addition, maternal estriol levels fall. Diagnosis of IUFD is confirmed by absence of heart action on ultrasound. Most women have spontaneous labor within 2 weeks of fetal death and if other complications are not present, some physicians wait for labor to begin spontaneously (Cunningham et al 1997).

APPLYING THE NURSING PROCESS

Nursing Assessment

Cessation of fetal movement reported by the mother to the nurse is frequently the first indication of fetal death. It is followed by a gradual decrease in the signs and symptoms of pregnancy. Fetal heart tones are absent, and fetal movement is no longer palpable. Once fetal demise is established, the nurse assesses the family's ability to adapt to their loss. Open communication between

CRITICAL PATHWAY FOR FETAL STRESS

Category	
Referral	• Physician • Neonatologist
Assessment	• Preexisting maternal diseases • Maternal hypotension, bleeding • Placental abnormalities • Diagnostic studies 1. Maternal hemoglobin and hematocrit 2. Urinalysis • Nursing assessment: • Determine FHR baseline • Assess variability • Monitor decelerations • Monitor accelerations • Evaluate contraction pattern • Monitor uterine resting tone • Take maternal vital signs • Evaluate amniotic fluid
Comfort	• Assess comfort level
Nursing interventions and report	• Decreased variability of fetal heart rate • Late decelerations in FHR • Fetal hyperactivity • Presence of meconium in the amniotic fluid If any of the above are found, initiate the following interventions: 1. Administer oxygen to the woman with tight face mask at 7–10 L/minute, per physician order 2. Notify physician of maternal and fetal assessment findings. Document assessment and specific information relayed to physician 3. Assess maternal vital signs 4. Institute emergency measures for prolapse of cord: • Manually exert pressure on the presenting part. This must be done continuously. Woman may be maintained in supine position, Trendelenburg position, knee-chest position, or on her side with a pillow to elevate her hips • If occult prolapse is suspected, change maternal position to side-lying • Notify physician/certified nurse-midwife immediately • Potential fetal stress if: • Tachycardia > 160 bpm; bradycardia < 110 bpm • Decreased long-term variability; short-term variability absent • Persistent late decelerations; prolonged variable decelerations • Absence of accelerations with fetal movement or scalp stimulation • Temperature 100.4F or >; hypotension • Meconium stained amniotic fluid • Contractions closer than every 2 minutes lasting > 90 seconds • Inadequate resting tone between contractions • Ripe cervix feels soft to the examining finger, is located in a medial to anterior position, is more than 50% effaced, and is 2–3 cm dilated • Unripe cervix feels firm to the examining finger, is long and thick, is perhaps in a posterior position, and is dilated little or not at all
Activity	• Change maternal position (lateral, left side preference)
Nutrition	• IV infusion • Ice chips
Elimination	• Encourage voiding q2h • Monitor and record I/O
Medications	• Increase IV fluid (as per institutional protocol) • Discontinue oxytocin if infusing
Discharge planning/ home care	• Plan for home care visits after discharge from birthing facility • Introduce the home care nurse to the family before discharge

CRITICAL PATHWAY FOR FETAL STRESS continued

Category	
Family involvement	• Keep woman and family well informed through factual information
Teaching/ psychosocial	• Inform woman of fetal status • Explain treatment plan. Provide accurate information. • Assess the emotional status of patient and family • Reassure woman and family
Date	

the mother, her partner, and the health team members contributes to a more realistic understanding of the medical condition and its associated treatments. The nurse may discuss prior experiences the family has had with stress and what they feel were their coping abilities at that time. Identifying the family's social supports and resources is also important.

Nursing Diagnosis

Nursing diagnoses that may apply include the following:

- Grief related to an actual loss
- Alteration in family process related to loss of a family member
- Ineffective individual and family coping related to depression in response to loss of a child
- Ineffective family coping related to death of a child
- Anxiety related to death of a child

Nursing Plan and Implementation

The parents of a stillborn infant suffer a devastating experience, precipitating an intense emotional trauma. During the pregnancy, the couple has already begun the attachment process, which now must be terminated through the grieving process. The behaviors that couples exhibit while mourning may be associated with the five stages of grieving described by Elizabeth Kübler-Ross (1969). Often the first stage is *denial* of the death of the fetus. Even when the initial health care provider suspects fetal demise, the couple is hoping that a second opinion will be different. Some couples may not be convinced of the death until they view and hold the stillborn infant. The second stage is *anger,* resulting from the feelings of loss, loneliness, and perhaps guilt. The anger may be projected at significant others and health team members, or it may be omitted when the death of the fetus is sudden and unexpected. *Bargaining,* the third stage, may or may not be present depending on the couple's preparation for the death of the fetus. If the death is unanticipated, the couple may have no time for bargaining. In the fourth stage, *depression* is evidenced by preoccupation, weeping, and withdrawal. Physiologic postpartal depression appearing 24–48 hours after birth may compound the depression of grief. The final stage is *acceptance,* which involves the process of resolution. This is a highly individualized process that may take months to complete.

Some facilities use a checklist to ensure that caregivers address important aspects of working with the parents. The checklist becomes a communication tool between staff members to share information particular to this couple (Brown 1992). Such a checklist might include the following items:

- When the fetal death is known before admission, inform the admission department and nursing staff so they can avoid making inappropriate remarks.
- Allow the woman and her partner to remain together as much as they wish. Provide privacy by assigning them a private room.
- Stay with the couple; do not leave them alone and isolated.
- As much as possible, have the same nurse provide care to increase the support for the couple. Develop a care plan to provide for continuity of care. Encourage family members to visit support persons.
- Have the most experienced labor and birth nurse auscultate for fetal heart tones. This avoids the searching that a more inexperienced nurse might feel compelled to do. Avoid the temptation to listen again "to make sure."
- Listen to the couple; do not offer explanations. They require solace without minimizing the situation.
- Facilitate the woman and her partner's participation in the labor and birth process. When possible, allow them to make decisions about who will be present and what ritual will occur during the birth process. Allow the woman to make the decision whether to have sedation during labor and birth. Provide a

quiet, supportive environment; ideally labor and birth should occur in a labor or birthing room rather than a delivery room.

- Give parents accurate information about plans for labor and birth.
- Provide ongoing opportunities for the couple to ask questions.
- Arrange for the woman to be assigned to a room that is away from new mothers and babies if she requests it. It is important to let the woman decide if she wants to be on another unit. If early discharge is an option, allow the family to make that selection.
- Encourage the couple to experience the grief that they feel. Accept the weeping and depression. A couple may have intense feelings that they are unable to share with each other. Encourage them to talk together and allow emotions to show freely. Help them understand that they may each experience different feelings (Wallerstedt and Higgins 1996).
- Give the couple an opportunity to see and hold the stillborn infant in a private, quiet location. (Advocates of seeing the stillborn believe that viewing assists in dispelling denial and enables the couple to progress to the next step in the grieving process.) If they choose to see their stillborn infant, prepare the couple for what they will see by saying "the baby is cold," "the baby is blue," "the baby is bruised," or other appropriate statements (Furrh and Copley 1989).
- Some families may elect to bathe or dress their stillborn; support them in their choice.
- Take a photograph of the infant, and let the family know it is available if they want it now or some time in the future.
- Offer a card with footprints, crib card, ID band, and possibly a lock of hair to the parents. These items may be kept with the photo if the parents do not want them at this time (Beckey et al 1985).
- Prepare the couple to return home. If there are siblings, each will usually progress through age-appropriate grieving. Provide the parents with information about normal mourning reactions, both psychologic and physiologic.
- Furnish the mother with educational materials that discuss the changes she will experience in returning to a nonpregnant state.
- Provide information about community support groups, including group name, contact person if possible, and phone number. Use materials such as the book *When Hello Means Goodbye* by Schwiebert and Kirk (1985).
- Contact religious support systems if the parents desire.
- Discuss further care of the stillborn baby (dress, rituals).

The nurse experiences many of the same grief reactions as the parents of a stillborn infant. It is important to have support persons and colleagues available for counseling and support.

Evaluation

Anticipated outcomes of nursing care include

- The family members express their feelings about the death of their baby.
- The family participates in the decision whether to see their baby and other decisions about the baby.
- The family has resources available for continued support.
- The family knows the community resources available and has names and phone numbers to use if they choose.
- The family is moving into and through the grieving process.

Care of the Woman and Fetus at Risk Due to Placental Problems

The most common types of placental problems are abruptio placentae, placenta previa, and abnormalities in placental formation and structure. Because the placenta is very vascular, problems are usually associated with maternal and possibly fetal hemorrhage. Abruptio placentae is a major emergency in labor and birth and requires rapid, effective interventions. Although placenta previa is primarily an antepartal problem, it is presented here for the sake of comparison. Causes and sources of hemorrhage are highlighted in Key Facts to Remember: Causes and Sources of Hemorrhage.

Abruptio Placentae

Abruptio placentae is the premature separation of a normally implanted placenta from the uterine wall. Premature separation is considered a catastrophic event because of the severity of the resulting hemorrhage. The incidence of abruptio placentae is 1 in 120 births (Benedetti 1996) and is more frequent in pregnancies complicated by cocaine abuse (Dombrowski et al 1991). The risk of recurrence is much higher than for the general population.

The cause of abruptio placentae is largely unknown. Theories have been proposed relating its occurrence to decreased blood flow to the placenta through the sinuses

KEY FACTS TO REMEMBER

Causes and Sources of Hemorrhage

Causes and Sources	Signs and Symptoms
Antepartal Period	
Abortion	Vaginal bleeding Intermittent uterine contractions Rupture of membranes
Placenta previa	Painless vaginal bleeding after seventh month
Abruptio placentae	
Marginal (partial)	Vaginal bleeding; no increase in uterine pain
Central (severe)	No vaginal bleeding Extreme tenderness of abdominal area Rigid, boardlike abdomen Increase in size of abdomen
Intrapartal Period	
Placenta previa	Bright red vaginal bleeding
Abruptio placentae	Same signs and symptoms as listed for the types of abruptio placentae
Uterine atony in stage 3	Bright red vaginal bleeding, ineffectual contractility
Postpartal Period	
Uterine atony	Boggy uterus Dark vaginal bleeding Presence of clots
Retained placental fragments	Boggy uterus Dark vaginal bleeding Presence of clots
Lacerations of cervix or vagina	Firm uterus Bright red vaginal bleeding

during the last trimester. Excessive intrauterine pressure caused by hydramnios or multiple pregnancy, maternal hypertension, cigarette smoking, alcohol ingestion, increased maternal age and parity, trauma, and sudden changes in intrauterine pressure (as with amniotomy) have been suggested as contributing factors.

Abruptio placentae is subdivided into three types (Figure 19–11):

- *Marginal.* In this case, the blood passes between the fetal membranes and the uterine wall and escapes vaginally (also called marginal sinus rupture).
- *Central.* In this situation, the placenta separates centrally, and the blood is trapped between the placenta and the uterine wall. Entrapment of the blood results in concealed bleeding.
- *Complete.* Massive vaginal bleeding is seen in the presence of total separation.

The signs and symptoms of these three types of placental abruption are given in Key Facts to Remember: Differential Signs and Symptoms of Placenta Previa and Abruptio Placentae. In severe cases of central abruptio placentae, the blood invades the myometrial tissues between the muscle fibers. This occurrence accounts for the uterine irritability that is a significant sign of abruptio placentae. If hemorrhage continues, eventually the uterus turns entirely blue. After birth the uterus contracts poorly. This condition is known as Couvelaire uterus and frequently necessitates hysterectomy.

As a result of the damage to the uterine wall and the retroplacental clotting with central abruption, large amounts of thromboplastin are released into the maternal blood supply. This in turn triggers the development of DIC and resultant hypofibrinogenemia. Fibrinogen levels, which are ordinarily elevated in pregnancy, may drop in minutes to the point at which blood will no longer coagulate.

Maternal Implications

Maternal mortality is now uncommon, but maternal morbidity is common (Cunningham et al 1997). Problems following birth depend in large part on the severity of the intrapartal bleeding, coagulation defects (DIC), hypofibrinogenemia, and time between separation and birth. Moderate to severe hemorrhage results in hemorrhagic shock, which may prove fatal to the mother if it is not reversed. In the postpartal period, women who have suffered this disorder are at risk for hemorrhage and renal failure due to shock, vascular spasm, intravascular clotting, or a combination of the three.

Fetal-Neonatal Implications

Perinatal mortality associated with abruptio placenta ranges from 20 to 30 percent (Benedetti 1996). In severe cases, in which most of the placenta has separated, infant mortality is 100 percent. In less severe separation, fetal outcome depends on the level of maturity. The most serious complications in the newborn arise from preterm labor, anemia, and hypoxia. If fetal hypoxia progresses unchecked, irreversible brain damage or fetal demise may result. Thorough assessment and prompt action on the part of the health team can improve both fetal and maternal outcomes.

Medical Therapy

Because of the risk of DIC, evaluating the results of coagulation tests is imperative. In DIC, fibrinogen levels

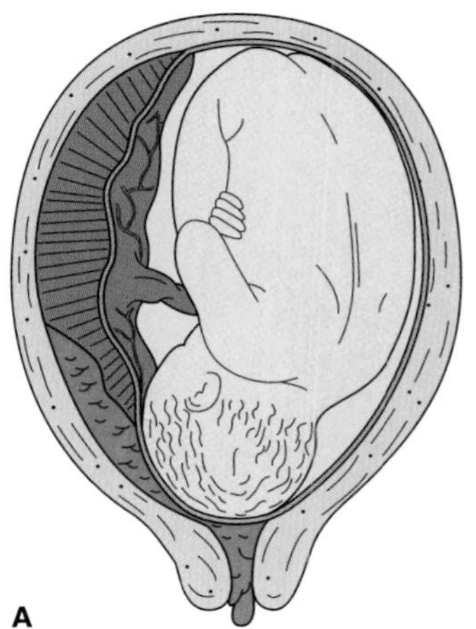

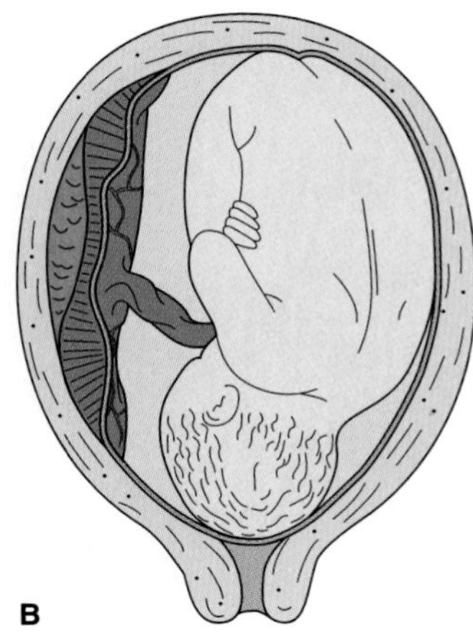

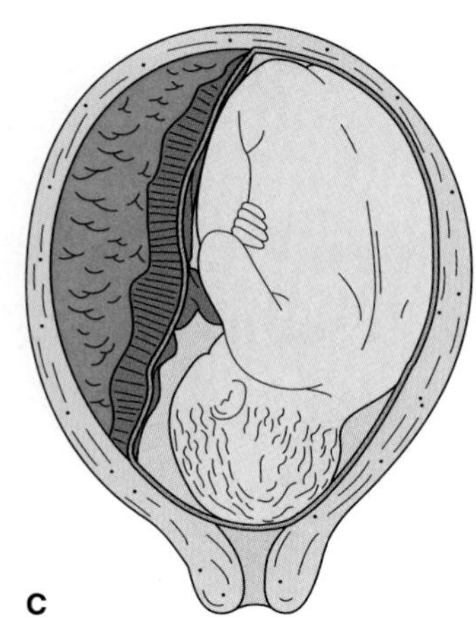

FIGURE 19–11 Abruptio placentae. ***A*** Marginal abruption with external hemorrhage. ***B*** Central abruption with concealed hemorrhage. ***C*** Complete separation.

and platelet counts usually decrease; prothrombin times and partial thromboplastin times are normal to prolonged. If the values are not markedly abnormal, serial testing may be helpful in establishing an abnormal trend that is indicative of coagulopathy. Another very sensitive test determines levels of fibrin-degradation products; these values rise with DIC.

After establishing the diagnosis, emphasis is placed on maintaining the cardiovascular status of the mother and developing a plan for effecting the birth of the fetus. Which birth method is selected depends on the condition of the woman and fetus; in many circumstances, cesarean birth may be the safest option.

If the separation is mild and gestation is near term, labor may be induced and the fetus born vaginally with as little trauma as possible. If the induction of labor by rupture of membranes and oxytocin infusion by pump does not initiate labor within 8 hours, a cesarean birth is usually done. A longer delay would raise the risk of increased hemorrhage, with resulting hypofibrinogenemia. Supportive treatment to decrease risk of DIC includes typing and crossmatching for blood transfusions (at least 3 units), clotting mechanism evaluation, and intravenous fluids.

In cases of moderate to severe placental separation, a cesarean birth is done after hypofibrinogenemia has been treated by intravenous infusion of cryoprecipitate or plasma. Vaginal birth is impossible in the event of a Couvelaire uterus, because the uterus would not contract properly in labor. Cesarean birth is necessary in the face of severe hemorrhage to allow an immediate hysterectomy to save both woman and fetus.

The hypovolemia that accompanies severe abruptio placentae is life threatening and must be combated with whole blood. If the fetus is alive but in distress, emergency cesarean birth is the method of choice. With a stillborn fetus, vaginal birth is preferable unless shock from hemorrhage is uncontrollable. Intravenous fluids of a balanced salt solution such as lactated Ringer's are given through a 16- or 18-gauge cannula (Cunningham et al 1997). Central venous pressure (CVP) monitoring may be needed to evaluate intravenous fluid replacement. A normal CVP of 10 cm H_2O is the goal. The CVP is evaluated hourly, and results are communicated to the physician. Elevations of CVP may indicate fluid overload and pulmonary edema. The hematocrit is

KEY FACTS TO REMEMBER

Differential Signs and Symptoms of Placenta Previa and Abruptio Placentae

	Placenta Previa	Abruptio Placentae
Onset	Quiet and sneaky	Sudden and stormy
Bleeding	External	External or concealed
Color of blood	Bright red	Dark venous
Anemia	= Blood loss	> Apparent blood loss
Shock	= Blood loss	> Apparent blood loss
Toxemia	Absent	May be present
Pain	Only labor	Severe and steady
Uterine tenderness	Absent	Present
Uterine tone	Soft and relaxed	Firm to stony hard
Uterine contour	Normal	May enlarge and change shape
Fetal heart tones	Usually present	Present or absent
Engagement	Absent	May be present
Presentation	May be abnormal	No relationship

Source: Oxom H: *Human Labor and Birth,* 5th ed. Norwalk, CT: Appleton & Lange, 1986, p 507.

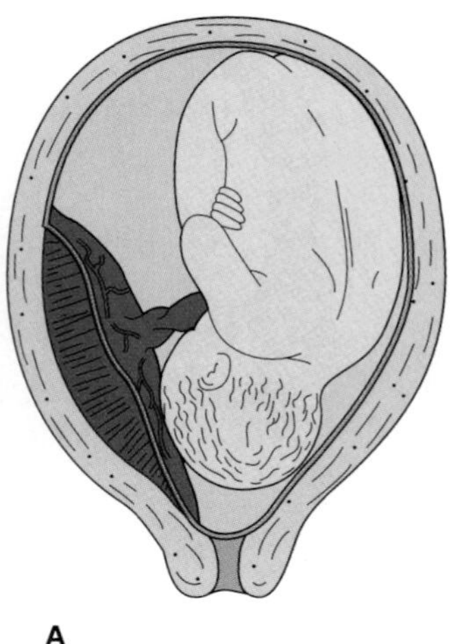

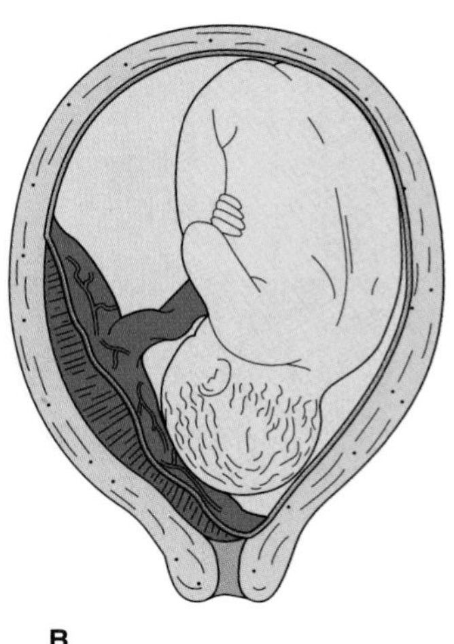

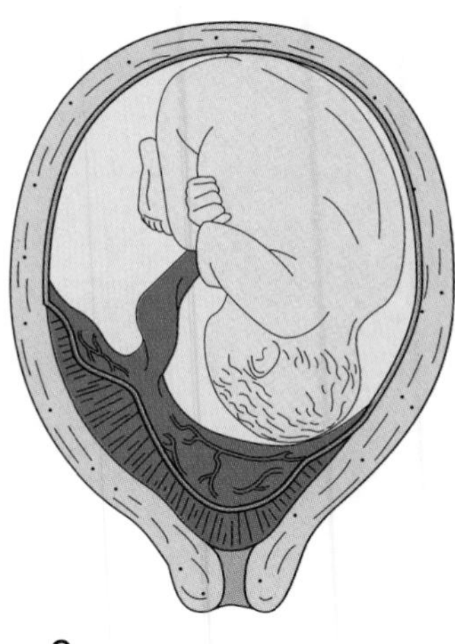

FIGURE 19–12 Placenta previa. ***A*** Low placental implantation. ***B*** Partial placenta previa. ***C*** Total placenta previa.

maintained at 30 percent through the administration of packed red cells or whole blood (Cunningham et al 1997).

Laboratory testing is ordered to provide ongoing data regarding hemoglobin, hematocrit, and coagulation status. Measures are taken to stimulate labor to prevent DIC. An amniotomy may be performed and oxytocin stimulation is given to hasten delivery. Progressive dilatation and effacement usually occur (Cunningham et al 1997).

Nursing Care

Electronic monitoring of the uterine contractions and resting tone between contractions provides information about the labor pattern and effectiveness of the oxytocin induction. Since uterine resting tone is frequently increased with abruptio placentae, it must be evaluated frequently for further increase. Abdominal girth measurements may be ordered hourly and are obtained by placing a tape measure around the maternal abdomen at the level of the umbilicus. Another method of evaluating uterine size, which increases as more bleeding occurs at the site of abruption, is to place a mark at the top of the uterine fundus. The distance from the symphysis pubis to the mark may be evaluated hourly. For further information on nursing care, see the Critical Pathway for Hemorrhage in Third Trimester and at Birth on p 468.

Placenta Previa

In **placenta previa,** the placenta is implanted in the lower uterine segment rather than the upper portion of the uterus. This implantation may be on a portion of the lower segment or over the internal cervical os. As the lower uterine segment contracts and dilates in the later weeks of pregnancy, the placental villi are torn from the uterine wall, thus exposing the uterine sinuses at the placental site. Bleeding begins, but because its amount depends on the number of sinuses exposed, initially it may be either scanty or profuse (Figure 19–12).

The cause of placenta previa is unknown. Statistically it occurs in about 1 in every 250 births. Women with a previous history of placenta previa have a recurrence rate of 4 to 8 percent (Lavery 1990). Other factors associated with placenta previa are multiparity, increasing age, placenta accreta, defective development of blood vessels in the decidua, and a large placenta (Cunningham et al 1997).

Fetal-Neonatal Implications

The prognosis for the fetus depends on the extent of placenta previa. Changes in the FHR and meconium staining of the amniotic fluid may be apparent. In a profuse

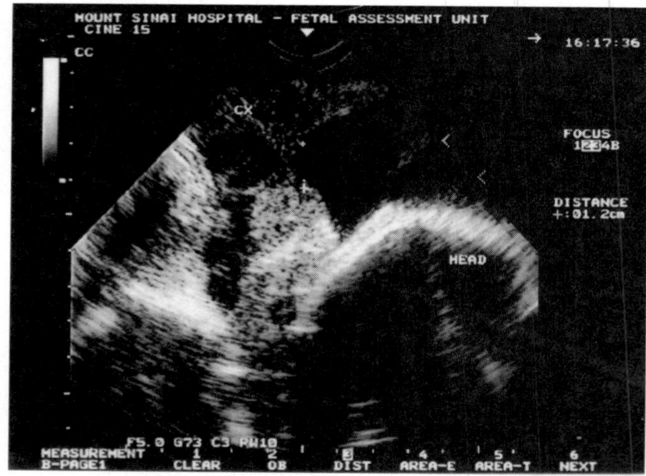

FIGURE 19–13 Ultrasound of placenta previa.

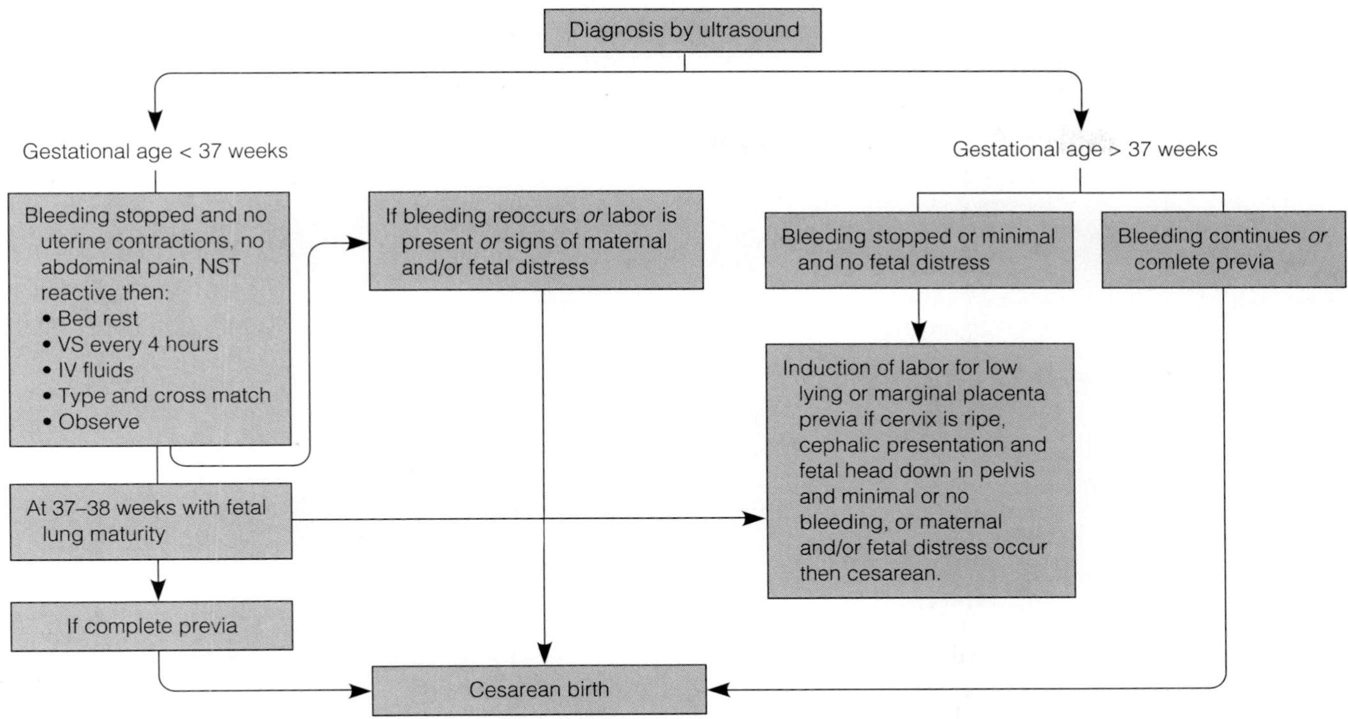

FIGURE 19–14 Management of placenta previa.
Source: Based on information from Barker, RK, Fields DH, Kaufman SA: *Quick Reference to OB-GYN Procedures,* 3rd ed. New York: Lippincott/Harper & Row, 1990.

bleeding episode, the fetus is compromised and does suffer some hypoxia. FHR monitoring is imperative when the woman is admitted, particularly if a vaginal birth is anticipated. This is important because the presenting part of the fetus may obstruct the flow of blood from the placenta or umbilical cord. If fetal distress occurs, cesarean birth is indicated.

After birth, blood sampling should be done to determine whether the intrauterine bleeding episodes of the woman have caused anemia in the newborn.

Medical Therapy

The goal of medical care is to identify the cause of bleeding and to provide treatment that will ensure birth of a mature newborn. Indirect diagnosis is made by localizing the placenta through tests that require no vaginal examination. The most commonly employed diagnostic test is the ultrasound scan (Figure 19–13). If placenta previa is ruled out, a vaginal examination can be performed with a speculum to determine the cause of bleeding (such as cervical lesions).

Direct diagnosis of placenta previa can be made only by feeling the placenta inside the cervical os. However, such an examination may cause profuse bleeding due to tearing of tissue in the cotyledons of the placenta. *Because of the danger of bleeding, a vaginal examination should be performed only if ultrasound is not available, the pregnancy is near term, and there is profuse vaginal bleeding.* The examination may be done using a double setup procedure. In this situation, it must be determined whether the cause of the bleeding is placenta previa or advanced labor with copious bloody show (which is normal). *Double setup* means that the delivery room is set up for the vaginal examination and normal vaginal birth and for a cesarean birth should placenta previa be present and the examination precipitate brisk bleeding. Adequate personnel must be present to respond to treatment decisions.

The differential diagnosis of placental or cervical bleeding takes careful consideration. Partial separation of the placenta may also present with painless bleeding, and a true placenta previa may not demonstrate overt bleeding until labor begins, thus confusing the diagnosis. Another important fact to note is that the causes of slight-to-moderate antepartal bleeding episodes in 20 to 25 percent of women are never accurately diagnosed.

Care of the woman with painless late gestational bleeding depends on (a) the week of gestation during which the first bleeding episode occurs, and (b) the amount of bleeding (Figure 19–14). If the pregnancy is less than 37 weeks' gestation, expectant management is employed to delay birth until about 37 weeks' gestation to allow the fetus to mature. Expectant management involves stringent regulation of the following:

1. Bed rest with bathroom privileges only as long as the woman is not bleeding
2. No rectal or vaginal exams

CRITICAL PATHWAY FOR HEMORRHAGE IN THIRD TRIMESTER AND AT BIRTH

Category	
Referral	• Perinatologist • Neonatologist • Psychiatric Clinical Nurse Practitioner
Assessment	• Obtain history to identify if any factors are present predisposing to hemorrhage: a. Presence of preeclampsia-eclampsia (PIH) b. Overdistension of the uterus; multiple pregnancy; hydramnios c. Grandmultiparity d. Advanced age e. Uterine contractile problems: hypotonicity; hypertonicity f. Painless vaginal bleeding after seventh month g. Presence of hypertension h. Presence of diabetes i. History of previous hemorrhage or bleeding problems, blood coagulation defects, abortion j. Retention of placental fragments k. Cervical and/or vaginal lacerations • Determine religious preference to establish whether client will permit a blood transfusion
Comfort	• Assess comfort of woman
Nursing interventions and report	• Observe, record, and report blood loss. • Evaluate using the following parameters: a. Monitor rate and quality of respirations frequently b. Measure pulse rate c. Assess pulse quality by direct palpation d. Determine pulse deficit by comparing apical-radial rates e. Compare present BP with woman's baseline BP; note pulse pressure f. Inspect skin for presence of pallor and cyanosis, coldness, and clamminess g. Evaluate state of consciousness frequently h. Measure CVP: normal CVP is 5–10 cm H_2O i. Assess amount of blood loss: • Count pads • Weigh pads and chux (1 g = approximately 1 mL blood) • Record amount in a specific amount of time (eg, 50 mL bright red blood on pad in 20 min) • Relieve decreased blood pressure by administering whole blood per physician order • While waiting for whole blood to be available, infuse isotonic fluids, plasma, plasma expanders, or serum albumin, per physician order If marginal abruptio placentae is present: a. Evaluate blood loss b. Assess uterine contractile pattern, tenderness, and height c. Start continuous monitoring of uterine contractions by EFM d. Monitor maternal vital signs e. Assess fetal status per continuous EFM f. Assess cervical dilatation and effacement to determine labor progress if uterine contractions are present g. Rule out placenta previa h. Assist with amniotomy, and begin oxytocin infusion per physician order if labor does not start immediately or is ineffective i. Review and evaluate diagnostic lab tests (hemoglobin, hematocrit, PT, APPT, fibrin split products, fibrinogen, platelets)

3. Monitoring blood loss, pain, and uterine contractility
4. Evaluating FHTs with external monitor
5. Monitoring vital signs
6. Complete laboratory evaluation: hemoglobin, hematocrit, Rh factor, and urinalysis
7. Intravenous fluid (lactated Ringer's) with drip rate monitored
8. Two units of crossmatched blood available for transfusion

If frequent, recurrent, or profuse bleeding persists, or if fetal well-being appears threatened, a cesarean birth may be performed before 37 weeks.

APPLYING THE NURSING PROCESS

Nursing Assessment

Assessment of the woman with placenta previa must be ongoing to prevent or treat complications that are po-

CRITICAL PATHWAY continued

Category	
Nursing interventions and report *continued*	If central abrutio placentae with severe blood loss is present: a. Perform same assessments as for marginal abruptio placentae b. Monitor CVP c. Replace blood loss d. Effect immediate birth e. Observe for signs and symptoms of disseminated intravascular coagulation (DIC) • Woman is at risk for uterine atony following birth: a. Assess contractility of uterus and amount of vaginal bleeding b. Assess uterus q15min × 4, q30min × 2, q60min × 2–4. Evaluate more frequently if uterus is boggy or not in the midline. Administer oxytocin per protocol or physician order.
Activity	• Complete bed rest • Diversional activity
Nutrition	• IV fluids infusing • NPO
Elimination	• Monitor urine output (decrease to less than 30 mL/h is sign of shock): a. Insert Foley catheter b. Measure output hourly c. Measure specific gravity to determine concentration of urine
Medications	• IV—lactated Ringer's at 150 mL/h • If premature—Betamethasone • O_2 as indicated
Discharge planning/ home care	• Determine need for assistance in the home • Provide information regarding community resources
Family involvement	• Establish a trusting relationship with family
Teaching/ psychosocial	• Keep woman informed of present status • Provide accurate information • Provide opportunities for questions • Establish a trusing relationship with client • Encourage the woman to participate in decision making if at all possible • Instruct patient to keep bladder empty • Notify RN if vag bleeding or leaking noted, decrease FM, abd pain/discomfort or uterine contractions • Report saturation > 1 pad within 1 h or less
Date	

tentially lethal to the mother and fetus. Painless, bright red vaginal bleeding is the best diagnostic sign of placenta previa. If this sign should develop during the last 3 months of a pregnancy, placenta previa should always be considered until ruled out by examination. The first bleeding episode is generally scanty. If no rectal or vaginal examinations are performed, it often subsides spontaneously. However, each subsequent hemorrhage is more profuse.

The uterus remains soft, and if labor begins, it relaxes fully between contractions. The FHR usually remains stable unless profuse hemorrhage and maternal shock occur. As a result of the placement of the placenta, the fetal presenting part is often unengaged, and transverse lie is common.

Blood loss, pain, and uterine contractility are appraised by the nurse from both subjective and objective perspectives. Maternal vital signs and the results of blood and urine tests provide the nurse with additional data about the woman's condition. FHR is evaluated with an external fetal monitor. Another pressing nursing responsibility is observing and verifying the family's ability to cope with the anxiety associated with an unknown outcome.

Nursing Diagnosis

Nursing diagnoses that may apply include the following:

- Fluid volume deficit related to hypovolemia secondary to excessive blood loss
- Risk for impaired fetal gas exchange related to decreased blood volume and maternal hypotension
- Anxiety related to concern for own personal status and the baby's safety
- Risk for altered tissue perfusion related to blood loss secondary to uterine atony following birth

Nursing Plan and Implementation

Before a double setup procedure is performed, the laboring couple should be physiologically and psychologically prepared for possible surgery (Chapter 20). A whole-blood setup should be ready for intravenous infusion and a patent intravenous line established before caregivers undertake any intrusive procedures. Maternal vital signs should be monitored every 15 minutes in the absence of hemorrhage and every 5 minutes with active hemorrhage. The external tocodynamometer should be connected to the maternal abdomen to monitor uterine activity continuously.

To promote maternal-fetal physical well-being, the nurse monitors the woman and her fetus to determine the status of the bleeding and the mother's and baby's responses. Vital signs, intake and output, and other pertinent assessments must be made frequently. The nurse evaluates the electronic monitor tracing to evaluate the fetal status.

Provision of emotional support for the family is an important nursing care goal. When active bleeding is occurring, the assessments and management must be directed toward physical support. However, emotional aspects need to be addressed simultaneously. The nurse can explain the assessments being completed and the treatment measures that need to be done. Time can be provided for questions, and the nurse can act as an advocate in obtaining information for the family. Emotional support can also be offered by staying with the family and the use of touch.

Promotion of neonatal physiologic adaptation is another important nursing responsibility. The newborn's hemoglobin, cell volume, and erythrocyte count should be checked immediately and then monitored closely. The newborn may require oxygen and administration of blood. Nursing care of the woman with bleeding is addressed fully in the Critical Pathway for Hemorrhage in Third Trimester and at Birth on p 468.

Evaluation

Anticipated outcomes of nursing care include

- The cause of hemorrhage is recognized promptly and corrective measures are taken.
- The woman's vital signs remain in the normal range.
- Any other complications are recognized and treated early.
- The family understands what has happened and the implications and associated problems of placenta previa.
- The woman and her baby have a safe labor and birth.

Other Placental Problems

Other problems of the placenta are presented in Table 19–1.

Care of the Woman and Fetus with a Prolapsed Umbilical Cord

A prolapsed umbilical cord results when the umbilical cord precedes the fetal presenting part. When this occurs, pressure is placed on the umbilical cord as it is trapped between the presenting part and the maternal pelvis. Consequently the vessels carrying blood to and from the fetus are compressed (Figure 19–15). Prolapse of the cord may occur with rupture of the membranes if the presenting part is not well engaged in the pelvis.

Maternal Implications

Although a prolapsed cord does not directly precipitate physical alterations in the woman, her immediate concern for the baby creates enormous stress. The woman may need to deal with some unusual interventions; a cesarean birth; and, in some circumstances, the death of her baby.

Fetal-Neonatal Implications

Compression of the cord results in decreased blood flow and leads to fetal distress. If labor is underway, the cord is compressed further with each contraction. If the pressure on the cord is not relieved, the fetus will die.

Medical Therapy

Preventing the occurrence of prolapse of the cord is the preferred medical approach. If the prolapse does happen, relieving the compression on the cord is critical to fetal outcome. The medical and nursing team must work together to facilitate birth.

Bed rest is indicated for all laboring women with a history of ruptured membranes, until engagement with

TABLE 19–1 Placental and Umbilical Cord Variations

Placental Variation	Maternal Implications	Fetal-Neonatal Implications	
Succenturiate Placenta One or more accessory lobes of fetal villi will develop on the placenta.	Postpartal hemorrhage from retained lobe	None, as long as all parts of the placenta remain attached until after birth of the fetus	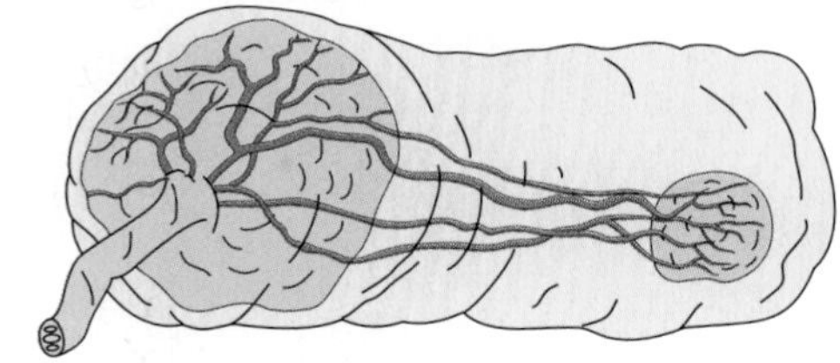
Circumvallate Placenta A double fold of chorion and amnion form a ring around the umbilical cord, on the fetal side of the placenta.	Increased incidence of late abortion, antepartal hemorrhage, and preterm labor	Fetal death	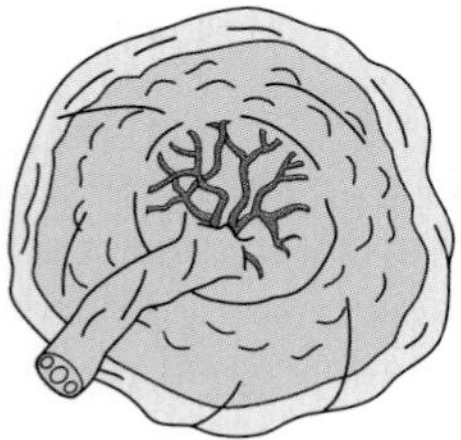
Battledore Placenta The umbilical cord is inserted at or near the placental margin.	Increased incidence of preterm labor and bleeding	Prematurity, fetal distress	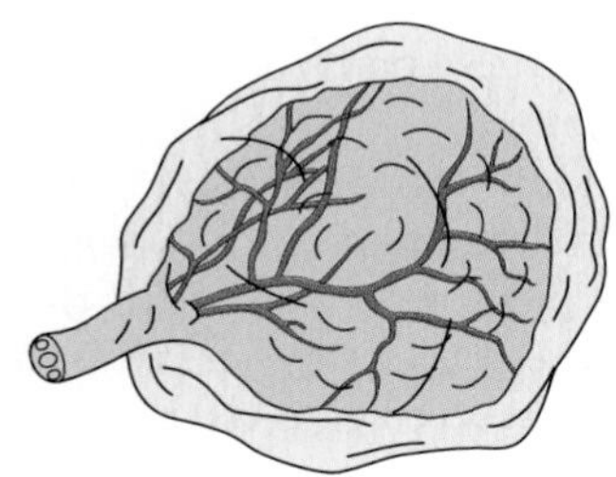
Velamentous Insertion of the Umbilical Cord The vessels of the umbilical cord divide some distance from the placenta in the placental membranes.	Hemorrhage if one of the vessels is torn	Fetal distress, hemorrhage	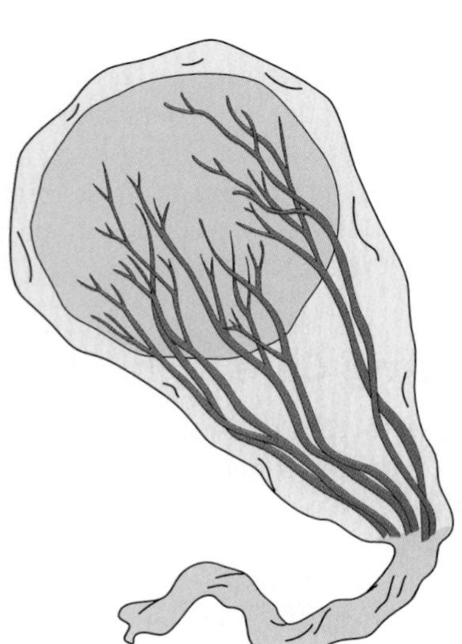

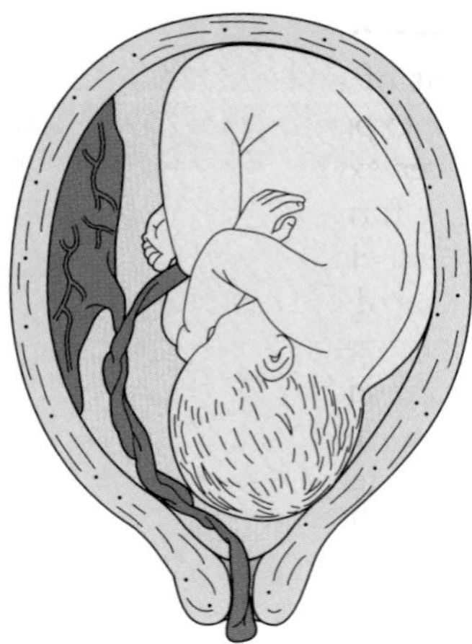

FIGURE 19–15 Prolapse of the umbilical cord.

no cord prolapse has been documented. Furthermore, at the time of spontaneous rupture of membranes or amniotomy, the FHR should be auscultated for at least a full minute and again at the end of a contraction and after a few contractions. If fetal bradycardia is detected on the auscultation, the woman should be examined to rule out a cord prolapse. In the presence of cord prolapse, electronic monitor tracings show severe, moderate, or prolonged variable decelerations with baseline bradycardia. If these patterns are found, the woman is examined vaginally.

If a loop of cord is discovered, the examiner's gloved fingers must remain in the vagina and attempts must be made to lift the fetal head off the cord (to relieve compression) until the physician/CNM arrives. This is a lifesaving measure. Begin oxygen and monitor FHR to see if cord compression is adequately relieved.

The force of gravity can be employed to relieve the compression. The woman assumes the knee-chest position or the bed is adjusted to the Trendelenburg position and the woman is transported to the delivery or operating room in this position. The nurse must remember that the cord may be occultly prolapsed with an actual loop extending into the vagina or lying alongside the presenting part. It may be pulsating strongly or so weakly that it is difficult to determine on palpation of the cord whether the fetus is alive.

Nursing Care

Because there are few outward signs of cord prolapse, each pregnant woman is advised to call her physician or certified nurse-midwife when the membranes rupture and to go to the office, clinic, or birthing facility. A sterile vaginal examination determines if there is danger of cord prolapse. If the presenting part is well engaged, the risk of cord prolapse is minimal, and ambulation may be encouraged. If the presenting part is not well engaged, bed rest is recommended to prevent cord prolapse.

Because cord prolapse can be associated with fetal death, some physicians and certified nurse-midwives may insist that bed rest be maintained after rupture of membranes regardless of fetal engagement. This can lead to conflict if the laboring woman and her partner do not hold the same opinions. The nurse can ease this situation by assisting communication between the physician/CNM and the couple.

During labor, any alteration of FHR or presence of meconium in the amniotic fluid indicates the need to assess for the presence of cord prolapse. Vaginal birth is possible with prolapsed cord if the cervix is completely dilated and pelvic measurements are adequate.

If these conditions are not present, cesarean birth is the method of choice. The woman is taken to the delivery room while the examiner continues to relieve the pressure on the cord until the infant has been born.

Care of the Woman and Fetus at Risk Due to Amniotic Fluid–Related Complications

Amniotic Fluid Embolism

In the presence of a small tear in the amnion or chorion high in the uterus, a small amount of amniotic fluid may leak into the chorionic plate and enter the maternal circulation as an **amniotic fluid embolism.** The fluid can also enter at areas of placental separation or cervical tears. Under pressure from the contracting uterus, the fluid is driven into the maternal system. The more debris in the amniotic fluid (such as meconium), the greater the maternal problems. The incidence is 1 in 8,000 to 80,000 pregnancies with a mortality rate of 50–60 percent (Benedetti 1996).

Maternal Implications

This condition frequently occurs during or after the birth when the woman has had a difficult, rapid labor. Suddenly she experiences respiratory distress, circulatory collapse, acute hemorrhage, and cor pulmonale as the embolism blocks the vessels of the lungs. The woman exhibits a sudden onset of dyspnea, cyanosis, cardiovascular collapse, shock, and coma. If she survives for more than 1 hour, she has a 50 percent chance of developing DIC caused by thromboplastin-like material in the amniotic fluid. This results in massive hemorrhage.

Fetal-Neonatal Implications

Birth must be facilitated immediately to obtain a live fetus. If labor has been tumultuous (very strong, frequent contractions), the fetus may suffer problems associated with dysfunctional labor.

Medical Therapy

The goals of medical therapy are to maintain oxygenation, support the cardiovascular system and blood pressure, and assess coagulopathy (Clark et al 1986).

Any woman exhibiting chest pain, dyspnea, cyanosis, frothy sputum, tachycardia, hypotension, and massive hemorrhage needs the cooperation of every member of the health team if her life is to be saved. Medical interventions are supportive. Recovery is contingent on the return of the mother's cardiovascular and respiratory stability. If necessary, the birth is assisted to enhance the health of the newborn.

Nursing Care

In the absence of the physician/CNM, the nurse administers oxygen under positive pressure until medical help arrives. An intravenous line is quickly established. If respiratory and cardiac arrest occurs, cardiopulmonary resuscitation (CPR) is initiated immediately.

The nurse readies the equipment necessary for blood transfusion and for the insertion of the CVP line. As the blood volume is replaced, using fresh whole blood to provide clotting factors, the CVP is monitored frequently. In the presence of cor pulmonale, fluid overload could easily occur.

Hydramnios

Hydramnios (also called *polyhydramnios*) occurs when there is more than 2000 mL of amniotic fluid. The exact cause of hydramnios is unknown; however, it often occurs in cases of major congenital anomalies.

During the second half of the pregnancy, the fetus begins to swallow and inspire amniotic fluid and to urinate, which contributes to the amount present. In cases of hydramnios, no pathology has been found in the amniotic epithelium. However, hydramnios is associated with fetal malformations that affect the fetal swallowing mechanism and neurologic disorders in which the fetal meninges are exposed in the amniotic cavity. This condition is also found in cases of anencephaly, in which the fetus is thought to urinate excessively due to overstimulation of the cerebrospinal centers. When monozygotic twins manifest hydramnios, it is because the twin with the increased blood volume urinates excessively. The weight of the placenta has been found to be increased in some cases of hydramnios, indicating that increased functioning of the placental tissue may be a factor.

There are two types of hydramnios: chronic and acute. In the chronic type, the fluid volume gradually increases and is a problem of the third trimester. Most cases are of this variety. In acute cases, the volume increases rapidly over a period of a few days. The acute type is usually diagnosed between 20 and 24 weeks' gestation (Queenan 1992).

Maternal Implications

When the amount of amniotic fluid is more than 3000 mL, the woman experiences shortness of breath and edema in the lower extremities from compression of the vena cava. Milder forms of hydramnios occur more frequently and are associated with minimal symptoms. Hydramnios is associated with such maternal disorders as diabetes and Rh sensitization and with multiple gestations.

If the amniotic fluid is removed rapidly before birth, abruptio placentae can result from too sudden a change in the size of the uterus. Because of overdistention of uterine muscles, uterine dysfunction can occur in the intrapartal period, and the incidence of postpartal hemorrhage increases.

Fetal-Neonatal Implications

Fetal malformations and preterm birth are common with hydramnios; thus perinatal mortality is 35 to 40 percent (Queenan 1992). Prolapsed cord can occur when the membranes rupture, a further complication for the fetus. The incidence of malpresentations also increases.

Medical Therapy

Hydramnios is managed with supportive treatment unless the intensity of the woman's distress and symptoms dictates otherwise.

If the accumulation of amniotic fluid is severe enough to cause maternal dyspnea and pain, hospitalization and removal of the excessive fluid are required. Fluid can be removed vaginally or by amniocentesis. The dangers of performing the technique vaginally are prolapsed cord and the inability to remove the fluid slowly. If amniocentesis is performed, it should be done with the aid of sonography to prevent inadvertent damage to the fetus and placenta. The fluid should be removed slowly to prevent abruption (Cunningham et al 1997).

Nursing Care

Hydramnios should be suspected when the fundal height increases out of proportion to the gestational age. As the amount of fluid increases, the nurse may have difficulty palpating the fetus and auscultating the FHR. In more severe cases, the maternal abdomen appears extremely tense and tight on inspection. On sonography, large spaces can be identified between the fetus and the uterine wall. When amniocentesis is performed, it is vital to maintain sterile technique to prevent infection. The nurse can offer support to the couple by explaining the procedure to them. The nurse also assists the clinician in interpreting sonographic findings.

If the fetus has been diagnosed with a congenital defect in utero or is born with the defect, psychologic support is needed to assist the family. Often the nurse collaborates with social services to offer the family this additional help.

Oligohydramnios

Oligohydramnios, in which the amount of amniotic fluid is severely reduced and concentrated, is a rare maternal finding. The exact cause of this condition is unknown. It is found in cases of postmaturity, with IUGR secondary to placental insufficiency, and in fetal conditions associated with major renal malformations, including renal aplasia with dysplastic kidneys and obstructive lesions of the lower urinary tract (Cunningham et al 1997). If oligohydramnios occurs in the first part of pregnancy, there is a danger of fetal adhesions (one part of the fetus may adhere to another part).

Maternal Implications

Labor can be dysfunctional, and progress is slow.

Fetal-Neonatal Implications

During the gestational period, fetal skin and skeletal abnormalities may occur because fetal movement is impaired as a result of reduced amniotic fluid volume. Because there is less fluid available for the fetus to use during fetal breathing movements, pulmonary hypoplasia may develop. During the labor and birth, the lessened amounts of fluid reduce the cushioning effect for the umbilical cord, and cord compression is more likely to occur.

Medical Therapy

During the antepartum period oligohydramnios may be suspected when the uterus does not increase in size according to the dates, the fetus is easily palpated and outlined by the examiner, and the fetus is not ballotable. The fetus can be assessed by biophysical profiles, nonstress tests, and serial ultrasound. During labor, the fetus will be monitored by continuous electronic fetal monitoring (EFM) to detect cord compression, which will be indicated by variable decelerations. Some clinicians advocate the use of an amnioinfusion (a transcervical instillation of 200–300 mL of sterile saline after membranes have ruptured) to decrease the frequency and severity of variable decelerations in the FHR during labor. The infusion of saline provides more fluid for the umbilical cord to float in and thereby lessens or prevents cord compression.

Nursing Care

Continuous electronic fetal monitoring is an important part of the assessment during the labor and birth. The nurse evaluates the EFM tracing for presence of variable decelerations or other nonreassuring signs (such as increasing or decreasing baseline, decreased variability, or presence of late decelerations). If variable decelerations are noted, the woman's position can be changed (to relieve pressure on the umbilical cord), and the certified nurse-midwife/physician needs to be notified. After the birth, the newborn is evaluated for signs of congenital anomalies, pulmonary hypoplasia, and postmaturity.

Care of the Woman with Cephalopelvic Disproportion (CPD)

The birth passage includes the maternal bony pelvis, beginning at the pelvic inlet and ending at the pelvic outlet, and the maternal soft tissues within these anatomic areas. A contracture (narrowed diameter) in any of the described areas can result in cephalopelvic disproportion (CPD) if the fetus is larger than the pelvic diameters. Abnormal fetal presentations and positions occur in CPD as the fetus moves to accommodate its passage through the maternal pelvis.

The gynecoid and anthropoid pelvic types are usually adequate for vertex birth, but the android and platypelloid types predispose to CPD. Certain combinations of types also can result in pelvic diameters inadequate for vertex birth. (See Chapter 15 for a description of pelvic types and their implications for childbirth.)

Types of Contractures

The pelvic inlet is contracted if the shortest anterior-posterior diameter is less than 10 cm or the greatest transverse diameter is less than 12 cm. The anterior-posterior diameter may be approximated by measuring the diagonal conjugate, which in the contracted inlet is less than 11.5 cm. Clinical and x-ray pelvimetry are used to determine the smallest anterior-posterior diameter through which the fetal head must pass.

The treatment goal is to allow the natural forces of labor to push the biparietal diameter of the fetal head beyond the potential interspinous obstruction. Although forceps may be used, they cause difficulty because pulling on the head destroys flexion, and the space is further diminished. A bulging perineum and crowning indicate that the obstruction has been passed.

An interischial tuberous diameter of less than 8 cm constitutes an outlet contracture. Outlet and midpelvic contractures frequently occur simultaneously. Whether vaginal birth can occur depends on the woman's interischial tuberous diameters and the fetal posterosagittal diameter.

Implications of Pelvic Contractures

Maternal Implications

Labor is prolonged in the presence of CPD. Membrane rupture can result from the force of the unequally distributed contractions being exerted on the fetal membranes. In obstructed labor, where the fetus cannot descend, uterine rupture can occur. With delayed descent, necrosis of maternal soft tissues can result from pressure exerted by the fetal head. Eventually, necrosis can cause fistulas from the vagina to other nearby structures. Difficult forceps deliveries can also result in damage to maternal soft tissue.

Fetal-Neonatal Implications

If the membranes rupture and the fetal head has not entered the inlet, there is a danger of cord prolapse. Excessive molding of the fetal head can result. Traumatic forceps-assisted birth can damage the fetal skull and central nervous system.

Medical Therapy

Fetopelvic relationships can be assessed by comparing pelvic measurements obtained by a manual exam before labor and by computed tomography (CT) with estimated weight of the fetus as obtained by ultrasound measurements.

When the pelvic diameters are borderline or questionable, a trial of labor (TOL) may be advised. In this process, the woman continues to labor and careful, frequent assessments of cervical dilatation and fetal descent are made by the physician/certified nurse-midwife. As long as there is continued progress, the TOL continues. If progress ceases, the decision for a cesarean birth is made.

Nursing Care

The adequacy of the maternal pelvis for a vaginal birth should be assessed during as well as before labor. During the intrapartal assessment, the size of the fetus and its presentation, position, and lie must also be considered. (See Chapter 16 for intrapartal assessment techniques.)

The nurse should suspect CPD when labor is prolonged, cervical dilatation and effacement are slow, and engagement of the presenting part is delayed. The couple may need support in coping with the stresses of this complicated labor. The nurse should keep the couple informed of what is happening and explain the procedures that are being used. This knowledge reassures the couple that measures are being taken to resolve the problem.

Nursing actions during the TOL are similar to care during any labor with the exception that the assessments of cervical dilatation and fetal descent are more frequent. Contractions should be monitored continuously. The fetus should also be monitored continuously. Any signs of fetal distress are reported to the certified nurse-midwife/physician immediately.

The mother may be positioned in a variety of ways to increase the pelvic diameters. Sitting or squatting increases the outlet diameters and may be effective in instances where there is failure of, or slow, fetal descent. Changing from one side to the other or maintaining a hands-and-knees position may assist the fetus in occiput posterior position to change to an occiput anterior. The mother may instinctively want to assume one of these positions. If not, the nurse may encourage a change of position.

Care of the Woman at Risk Due to Complications of Third and Fourth Stages

Lacerations

Lacerations of the cervix or vagina may be indicated when bright red vaginal bleeding persists in the presence of a well-contracted uterus. The incidence of lacerations is higher when the childbearing woman is young or a nullipara, has an epidural, has forceps-assisted birth and an episiotomy, and has not done perineal massage or preparation during pregnancy. Vaginal and perineal lacerations are often categorized in terms of degree, as follows:

- First-degree laceration is limited to the fourchet, perineal skin, and vaginal mucous membrane.
- Second-degree laceration involves the perineal skin, vaginal mucous membrane, underlying fascia, and muscles of the perineal body; it may extend upward on one or both sides of the vagina.
- Third-degree laceration extends through the perineal skin, vaginal mucous membranes, and perineal body and involves the anal sphincter; it may extend up the anterior wall of the rectum.
- Fourth-degree laceration is the same as third degree but extends through the rectal mucosa to the lumen of the rectum; it may be called a third-degree laceration with a rectal wall extension.

Placenta Accreta

The chorionic villi attach directly to the myometrium of the uterus in *placenta accreta.* Two other types of placental adherence are *placenta increta,* in which the myometrium is invaded, and *placenta percreta,* in which the myometrium is penetrated. The adherence itself may be total, partial, or focal, depending on the amount of placental involvement. The incidence of placenta accreta is 1 in 2000–3570 births (Zahn and Yeomans 1990). Placenta accreta is the most common type and accounts for 80 percent of adherent placentas, while 15 percent of adherent placentas are placenta increta, and 5 percent are placenta percreta (Zahn and Yeomans 1990).

The primary complication with placenta accreta is maternal hemorrhage and failure of the placenta to separate following birth of the infant. An abdominal hysterectomy may be the necessary treatment, depending on the amount and depth of involvement.

Inversion of Uterus

Uterine inversion occurs when the fundus of the uterus is prolapsed, inside out, through the cervix (Barber et al 1990). The incidence of uterine inversion is approximately 1 in 2500 births (Zahn and Yeomans 1990). It can be caused by a lax uterine wall coupled with undue tension on an umbilical cord when the placenta has not separated. Forceful pressure on the fundus with a dilated cervix and sudden emptying of the uterine contents may be contributing factors. Maternal bleeding occurs in 94 percent of women with uterine inversion, and blood loss ranges from 800 to 1800 mL (Zahn and Yeomans 1990).

Restoration of the uterus to its normal position manually or by surgical intervention is the goal of medical treatment. The uterus is replaced manually by grasping the vaginal mass, spreading the cervical ring with the fingers and thumb, and steadily forcing the fundus upward. The woman is often placed under deep anesthesia for this procedure.

CHAPTER HIGHLIGHTS

- Stress, anxiety, and fear have a profound effect on labor, particularly when complications occur that imply maternal or fetal jeopardy.
- A hypertonic labor pattern is characterized by painful contractions that are not effective in effacing and dilating the cervix. It usually leads to a prolonged latent phase.
- Hypotonic labor patterns begin normally and then progress to infrequent, less intense contractions. If there are no contraindications, IV oxytocin is used as treatment.
- Precipitous labor is extremely rapid labor that lasts less than 3 hours. It is associated with an increased risk to the mother and newborn infant.
- Postterm pregnancy is one that extends more than 294 days, or 42 weeks past the first day of the last menstrual period.
- Ruptured uterus is the tearing of previously intact uterine muscles or of an old uterine scar. The rupture can be caused by a weakened cesarean scar, obstetric trauma, CPD, and congenital defects of the birth canal.
- The occiput posterior position of the fetus during labor prolongs the labor process, causes severe back discomfort in the laboring woman, and predisposes her to vaginal and perineal trauma and lacerations during birth.
- The types of fetal malpresentations include face, brow, breech, and shoulder.
- A fetus or newborn weighing more than 4000 g is termed macrosomic. Problems may occur during labor, birth, and in the early neonatal period.
- Preventing and treating problems that infringe on the development and birth of normal fetuses are significant medical-nursing activities once the presence of twins has been detected.
- Fetal distress is indicated by persistent late decelerations, persistent severe variable decelerations, and prolonged decelerations. If fetal distress is recognized and treated appropriately, the fetus may be spared any permanent damage.
- Intrauterine fetal death poses a major nursing challenge to provide support and care for the parents.
- Major bleeding problems in the intrapartal period are abruptio placentae and placenta previa.
- Abruptio placentae is the separation of the placenta from the side of the uterus prior to birth of the infant. Abruptio placentae may be central, marginal, or complete.
- Placenta previa occurs when the placenta implants low in the uterus near or over the cervix. A low-lying or marginal placenta is one that lies near the cervix. In partial placenta previa, part of the placenta lies over the cervix. In complete placenta previa the cervix is completely covered.
- Prolapsed umbilical cord results when the umbilical cord precedes the fetal presenting part. This places pressure on the umbilical cord and diminishes blood flow to the fetus.
- Amniotic fluid embolism occurs when a bolus of amniotic fluid enters the maternal circulation and then the maternal lungs. Maternal mortality is very high with this complication.
- Hydramnios (also called polyhydramnios) occurs when there is more than 2000 mL of amniotic fluid contained within the amniotic membranes. Hydramnios is associated with fetal malformations that affect fetal swallowing, and with maternal diabetes mellitus, Rh sensitization, and multiple gestations.
- Oligohydramnios is present when there is a severely reduced volume of amniotic fluid. Oligohydramnios is associated with IUGR, with postmaturity, and with fetal renal or urinary malfunctions. The fetus is more likely to experience variable decelerations because the amniotic fluid is insufficient to keep pressure off the umbilical cord.
- Cephalopelvic disproportion (CPD) occurs when there is a narrowed diameter in the maternal pelvis. The narrowed diameter is called a contracture and may occur in the pelvic inlet, the midpelvis, or the outlet. If pelvic measurements are borderline, a trial

of labor (TOL) may be attempted. Failure of cervical dilatation or fetal descent necessitates a cesarean birth.

- Third- and fourth-stage complications usually involve a hemorrhage. The causes of hemorrhage include lacerations of the birth canal or cervix, placenta accreta, and uterine inversion.

REFERENCES

Andrews CM, Andrews EC: Nursing, maternal postures, and fetal positions. *Nurs Res* 1983; 32:6.

Barber KRK, Fields DH, Kaufman SA: *Quick Reference to OB-GYN Procedures,* 3rd ed. Philadelphia: Lippincott, 1990.

Beckey RD et al: Development of a perinatal grief checklist. *JOGNN* May/June 1985; 14:194.

Benedetti TJ: Obstetric hemorrhage. In: *Obstetrics: Normal and Problem Pregnancies,* 3rd ed. Gabbe SG, Niebyl JR, Simpson JL (editors). New York: Churchill Livingstone, 1996.

Bowes WA: Clinical aspects of normal and abnormal labor. In: *Maternal-Fetal Medicine.* Creasy RK, Resnik R (editors). Philadelphia: Saunders, 1994.

Brown Y: The crisis of pregnancy loss: A team approach to support. *Birth* June 1992; p 82.

Chitkara U, Berkowitz RL: Multiple gestation. Chapter 24 in: *Obstetrics: Normal and Problem Pregnancies,* 3rd ed. Gabbe SG, Niebyl JR, Simpson JL (editors). New York: Churchill Livingstone, 1996.

Clark SL: Care of the critically ill obstetric patient. In: *Danforth's Obstetrics and Gynecology,* 7th ed. Scott JR et al (editors). Philadelphia: Lippincott, 1994.

Cordell AS, Thomas N: Fathers and grieving: Coping with infant death. *J Perinatol* 1989; 10:75.

Cruikshank DP: Malpresentations and umbilical cord complications. In: *Danforth's Obstetrics and Gynecology,* 6th ed. Scott JR et al (editors). Philadelphia: Lippincott, 1990.

Cunningham FG et al: *Williams Obstetrics,* 20th ed. Stamford, CT: Appleton & Lange, 1997.

D'Alton ME, Simpson LL: Syndromes in twins. *Semin Perinatol* 1995; 19:375.

Dombrowski MP et al: Cocaine abuse is associated with abruptio placentae and decreased birth weight, but not shorter labor. *Obstet Gynecol* January 1991; 77(1):139.

Eganhouse DJ: Fetal monitoring of twins. *J Obstet Gynecol Neonatal Nurs* January/February 1992; 21(1):17.

Furrh CB, Copley R: One precious moment. *Nursing 89* September 1989; 52.

Gillogley K: Abnormal labor and delivery. Chapter 30 in: *Manual of Obstetrics.* Niswander KR (editor). Boston: Little, Brown, 1991.

Gimovsky ML, Shifrin BS: Breech management. *J Perinatol* 1992; 11:143.

Hannah ME et al: Postterm pregnancy: Putting the merits of a policy of induction of labor into perspective. *Birth* March 1996; 23:13.

Huddleston JF, Freeman RK: Estimations of fetal well-being. Chapter 8 in: *Neonatal-Perinatal Medicine: Diseases of the Fetus and Newborn,* 5th ed. Fanaroff AA, Martin RJ (editors). St Louis: Mosby-Year Book, 1992.

Hunter LP: Twin gestation: Antepartum management. *J Perinat Neonatal Nurs* 1989; 3:1.

King JC: Transverse and oblique lie. In: *Gynecology and Obstetrics, Vol 2.* Dilts PV, Sciarri JJ (editors). Philadelphia: Lippincott, 1994.

Kline-Kaye V, Miller-Slade D: The use of fundal pressure during the second stage of labor. *JOGNN* November/December 1990; 19(6):511.

Knuppel RA, Drukker JE: Twins and other multiple gestations. In: *High-Risk Pregnancy: A Team Approach,* 2nd ed. Knuppel RA, Drukker JE (editors). Philadelphia: Saunders, 1993.

Kochenour NK: Postterm pregnancy. In: *Neonatal-Perinatal Medicine: Diseases of the Fetus and Newborn,* 5th ed. Fanaroff AA, Martin RJ (editors). St Louis: Mosby-Year Book, 1992.

Kübler-Ross E: *On Death and Dying.* New York: Macmillan, 1969.

Lake M: Prolonged pregnancy. Chapter 6 in: *High-Risk Intrapartum Nursing.* Mandeville LK, Troiano NH (editors). Philadelphia: Lippincott, 1992.

Lavery JP: Placenta previa. *Clin Obstet Gynecol* September 1990; 33:414.

Lowe NK: The pain and discomfort of labor and birth. *JOGNN* 1996; 25:82

Queenan JT: Polyhydramnios, oligohydramnios, and hydrops fetalis. Chapter 18 in: *Neonatal-Perinatal Medicine,* 5th ed. Fanaroff AA, Martin RJ (editors). St Louis: Mosby-Year Book, 1992.

Quilligan EJ: Breech delivery. In: *Current Therapy in Obstetrics and Gynecology,* 3rd ed. Quilligan EJ, Zuspan FP (editors). Philadelphia: Saunders, 1990.

Resnik R: Post-term pregnancy. In: *Maternal-Fetal Medicine: Principles and Practice,* 3rd ed. Creasy RK, Resnik R (editors). Philadelphia: Saunders, 1994.

Schwiebert P, Kirk P: *When Hello Means Goodbye.* Eugene: Oregon Health Sciences University, 1985.

Seeds JW, Walsh M: Malpresentations. In: *Obstetrics: Normal and Problem Pregnancies,* 3rd ed. Gabbe SG, Niebyl JR, Simpson JL (editors). New York: Churchill Livingstone, 1996.

Taipale P, Hiilesmaa V, Ylostalo P: Diagnosis of placenta previa by transvaginal sonographic screening at 12–16 weeks in a nonselected population. *Obstet Gynecol* 1997; 89:364.

Tomlinson PS, Bryan AA: Family-centered intrapartum care: Revisiting and old concept. *JOGNN* 1996; 25:331.

Wallerstedt C, Higgins P: Facilitating perinatal grieving between the mother and the father. *JOGNN* 1996; 25:389.

Zahn CN, Yeomans ER: Postpartum hemorrhage: Placenta accreta, uterine inversion, and puerperal hematomas. *Clin Obstet Gynecol* September 1990; 33(3):422.

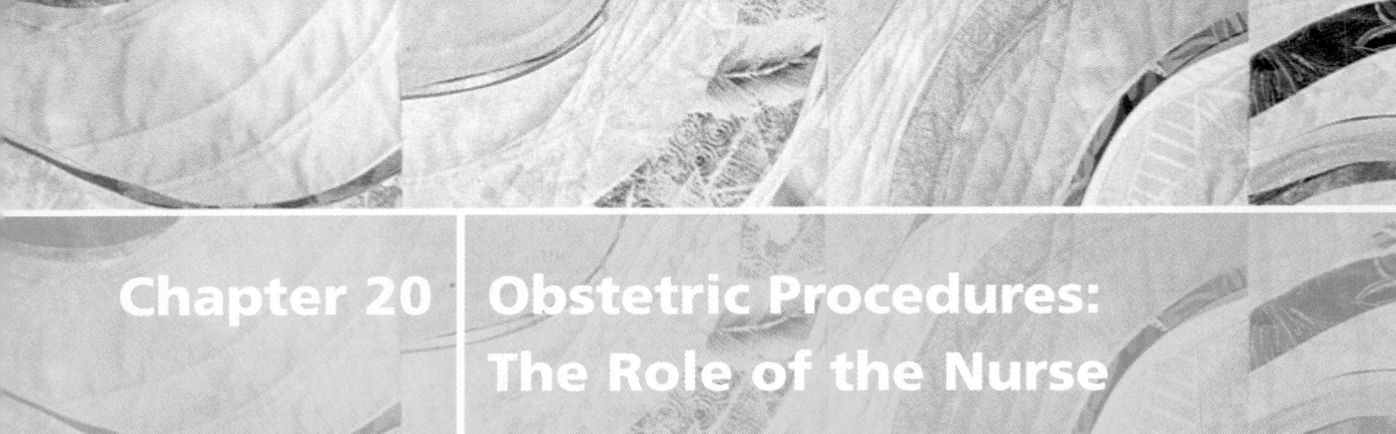

Chapter 20 Obstetric Procedures: The Role of the Nurse

OBJECTIVES

- Delineate the nursing interventions indicated for external version.
- Discuss the use of amniotomy in current maternity care.
- Briefly discuss the use of prostaglandin E vaginal suppositories for women with intrauterine fetal death.
- Compare methods for inducing labor, explaining their advantages and disadvantages.
- Describe the types of episiotomies performed, the rationale for each, and the associated nursing interventions.
- Summarize the indications for forceps assisted birth and types of forceps that may be used.
- Discuss the use of vacuum extraction, including indications, procedure, complications, and related nursing interventions.
- Explain the indications for cesarean birth, impact on the family unit, preparation and teaching needs, and associated nursing interventions.

KEY TERMS

Amniotomy
Elective induction
Episiotomy
External version
Forceps
Indicated induction
Induction of labor
Internal version
Vaginal birth after cesarean (VBAC)
Version

Most births occur without the need for operative obstetric intervention. In some instances, however, obstetric procedures are necessary to maintain safety for the woman and the fetus. The most common obstetric procedures are induction of labor, episiotomy, cesarean birth, and vaginal birth following a previous cesarean birth.

Most women are aware of the possible need for an obstetric procedure during their birth; however, some women expect to have a natural labor and birth and do not anticipate the need for any medical intervention. This conflict between expectation and the need for intervention presents a challenge to maternity nurses. To make sure the woman and her partner understand what is proposed, the nurse can provide information about a procedure, the anticipated benefits and possible risks, and any possible alternative treatments.

Care of the Woman During Version

Procedure

Version, or turning the fetus, is a procedure used to change the fetal presentation by abdominal or intrauterine manipulation. The most common type of version is **external** (or cephalic) **version,** in which the physician attempts to rotate the fetus from a breech to cephalic presentation by external manipulation of the maternal abdomen (Figure 20–1). A less common type of version, called **internal** (or podalic) **version,** is used only with the second twin during a vaginal birth if that twin is breech or if the twin is cephalic but does not descend readily or shows signs of fetal distress. In such cases, an anesthesiologist administers an agent that produces uterine relaxation. The obstetrician then reaches into the uterus, grasps one or both feet of the second twin, and draws them through the cervix (Seeds and Walsh 1996).

External Version

Before attempting external version, the placenta is localized using ultrasound. The following criteria should be met before performing external version (Kochenour 1994):

- A single fetus (also called a singleton). If a multiple gestation exists, a variety of concerns preclude external version. For example, a cesarean rather than vaginal birth may need to be considered, and the fetuses might become entangled during a version.
- The fetal breech is not engaged. Once the presenting part is engaged, it is difficult to do a version.
- There must be an adequate amount of amniotic fluid. The amniotic fluid helps ease movement of the fetus and provides adequate room for the umbilical cord to float without being compressed.
- A reactive nonstress test (NST) should be obtained immediately before performing the version. A reactive NST indicates fetal well-being.
- The fetus must be at 38 or more weeks' gestation. A version may be accompanied by complications that require immediate birth by cesarean. If gestation is less than 38 weeks, a preterm birth would result.

Absolute contraindications include the following (Kochenour 1994):

- Marked or severe oligohydramnios. The decreased amount of amniotic fluid would increase the risk of cord compression and make it difficult to move the fetus within the uterus.
- Premature rupture of the membranes. Rupture of the membranes would result in an inadequate amount of amniotic fluid.
- Placenta previa. If a complete placenta previa is present, birth will be by cesarean. If a marginal previa or low-lying placenta is present, the manipulation during the version may precipitate bleeding.
- Previous third trimester bleeding. Previous bleeding may indicate placenta previa or abruption.

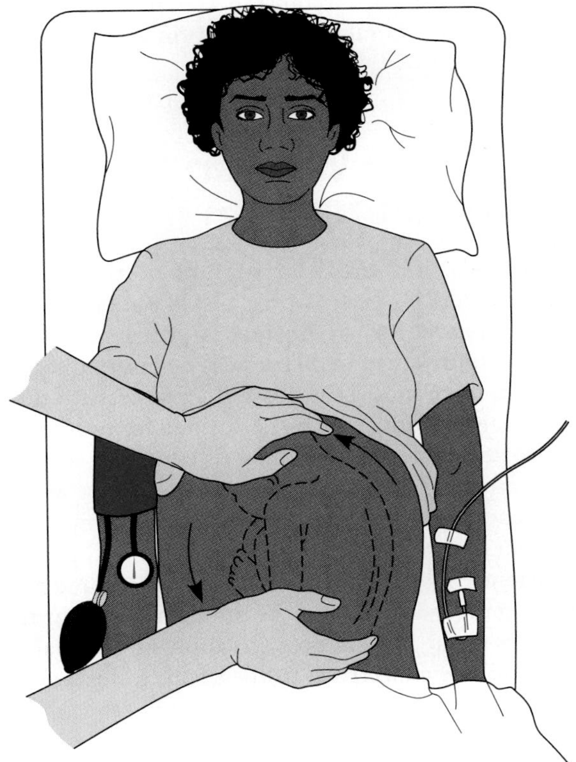

FIGURE 20–1 External (or cephalic) version of the fetus. A new technique involves pressure on the fetal head and buttocks so that the fetus completes a "backward flip" or "forward roll."

Before an external version, the woman receives an intravenous or subcutaneous dose of terbutaline to relax the uterus. While being assessed with ultrasound or external fetal monitoring, the fetus is turned from breech to vertex presentation (Figure 20–1).

Nursing Care

As the woman is admitted, the nurse begins assessment by validating that there are no contraindications to the version. Maternal vital signs and fetal heart rate (FHR) are assessed and an NST is done to ascertain reactivity of the FHR. The nurse assesses maternal vital signs before the version, every 5 minutes throughout the procedure, and for 30 minutes following it. In addition, the fetus is monitored before the version, intermittently during the procedure, and for 30 minutes following it. Assessments of the maternal-fetal response to the β-mimetic are also done (see Drug Guide: Terbutaline, in Chapter 13). The admission period and time when the initial NST is performed are excellent opportunities for educating the woman and her support person. They should be encouraged to express their understanding and expectations of the procedure, verbalize their fears, and ask questions. The possibility of failure of the procedure and operative intervention if the fetus becomes distressed should be discussed. Explaining what will occur in either of these circumstances will better prepare the childbearing family if intervention becomes necessary.

Care of the Woman During an Amniotomy

Amniotomy is the artificial rupture of the amniotic membranes (AROM). It is probably the most common operative procedure in obstetrics. Because the amniotomy requires that an instrument be inserted through the cervix, there must be at least 2 cm of cervical dilatation. The amniotomy may be performed for **induction of labor** (to stimulate the beginning of labor), or it may be done at any time during the first stage of labor with the goal of accelerating the labor. If an amniotomy is done after 3 cm of cervical dilatation, the labor will probably be shortened by 90 to 120 minutes (Fraser and Sokol 1992). Amniotomy may also be done during labor to allow access to the fetus in order to apply an internal fetal heart monitoring electrode to the scalp, to insert an intrauterine pressure catheter, or to obtain a fetal scalp blood sample for acid-base determination.

Amniotomy as a method of labor induction has the following advantages:

- The contractions elicited are similar to those of spontaneous labor.
- There is usually no risk of hypertonus or rupture of the uterus, as there is with intravenous oxytocin induction.
- The woman does not require the same intensive monitoring as with intravenous oxytocin induction.
- Electronic fetal monitoring (EFM) is facilitated because, once the membranes are ruptured, a fetal scalp electrode may be applied, an intrauterine catheter may be inserted, and scalp blood sampling for pH determinations may be done to assist in evaluating a fetal heart rate pattern.
- The color and composition of amniotic fluid can be evaluated.

Amniotomy has the following disadvantages:

- Once an amniotomy is done, birth must occur because microorganisms can now invade the intrauterine cavity and cause amnionitis.
- The danger of a prolapsed cord is increased once the membranes have ruptured, especially if the fetal presenting part is not firmly pressed down against the cervix.
- Compression and molding of the fetal head are increased due to loss of the cushioning effect of the amniotic fluid for the fetal head during uterine contractions.

AROM Procedure

While performing a sterile vaginal examination, the physician/CNM introduces an amnihook (or other rupturing device) into the vagina and makes a small tear in the amniotic membrane to allow amniotic fluid to escape.

Nursing Care

The nurse explains the AROM procedure to the woman. The fetal presentation, position, and station are assessed because amniotomy is usually delayed until engagement has occurred. The woman is positioned in a semireclining position and draped to provide privacy. The FHR is assessed just before and immediately after the amniotomy, and the two FHR assessments are compared. If there are marked changes, the nurse should check for prolapse of the cord. The amniotic fluid is inspected for amount, color, odor, and the presence of meconium or blood. While wearing disposable gloves, the nurse cleanses and dries the perineal area and changes the chux pads. Because there is now an open pathway for organisms to ascend into the uterus, strict sterile technique must be observed during vaginal examinations (see Essential Precautions for Practice: During Procedures). In addition, the number of vaginal examinations must be kept to a minimum to reduce the chance of introducing an infection, and the woman's temperature should be monitored every 2 hours.

ESSENTIAL PRECAUTIONS FOR PRACTICE

During Procedures

Examples of times when disposable gloves should be worn include the following:

- Handling amniotic fluid–soaked chux pads and bedding at the time of an amniotomy and the cleansing of the perineum afterward.
- Insertion of the intravenous catheter for induction of labor with oxytocin.
- During the abdominal-perineal preparation of the woman for cesarean birth. Note: sterile gloves are also worn during insertion of an indwelling bladder catheter. This provides asepsis for the woman and also protects the nurse from exposure to the perineal area and to urine.

REMEMBER to wash your hands before putting on the disposable gloves and AGAIN immediately after you remove the gloves.

For further information consult OSHA and CDC guidelines.

Care of the Woman During Prostaglandin Administration at Term

Prostaglandin (PGE) gel for cervical ripening (softening the cervix) may be used for pregnant women at or near term when there is a medical or obstetric indication for induction of labor. The gel contains 0.5 mg of dinoprostone (a form of prostaglandin E_2) per 3 g of gel. Although the gel has been demonstrated to cause cervical ripening, shorter labor, and lower requirements for oxytocin during labor induction, most research has not found an improvement in the failed induction rate or a decrease in the overall cesarean birth rate when the gel is used (ACOG 1993).

Contraindications to the use of PGE gel include evidence of cephalopelvic disproportion (CPD), placenta previa, vasa previa, unexplained vaginal bleeding, and obstetric emergencies that may require surgical intervention (ACOG 1993). Possible maternal side effects include hyperstimulation of uterine contractions (more than five contractions in 10 minutes or two or more contractions lasting more than 2 minutes [Arias 1993]), nausea, and vomiting (Day and Snell 1993; Trofatter 1992). At this time it is recommended that prostaglandin gel be used only in a hospital birthing unit and that an obstetrician be readily available in case an emergency cesarean birth is needed.

Physicians, certified nurse-midwives, and birthing room nurses who have had special education and training may administer PGE gel or other PGE products such as Cervidil or Prepidil (see Drug Guide: Dinoprostone [Cervidil] on p 482). Maternal vital signs are assessed for a baseline, and an electronic fetal monitor is applied to obtain an external tracing of uterine activity and FHR. If a gel is used, after insertion the woman is instructed to remain supine (with a rolled blanket under her right hip to tip the uterus slightly to the left) for 15–30 minutes to minimize leakage of the gel from the endocervix (AWHONN 1993). If Prepidil or Cervidil is used, the woman is able to assume any position of comfort. The nurse monitors the woman for uterine hyperstimulation and FHR abnormalities for about 1–2 hours past insertion.

Care of the Woman During Labor Induction

The American College of Obstetricians and Gynecologists (ACOG) defines induction of labor as the stimulation of uterine contractions before the spontaneous onset of labor, with or without ruptured fetal membranes, for the purpose of accomplishing birth (ACOG 1991). The procedure may be either elective or indicated.

Elective induction is defined as the initiation of labor for convenience. ACOG guidelines do not recommend elective induction (ACOG 1991).

Indicated induction may be considered in the presence of a preexisting maternal disease (such as diabetes mellitus or renal disease), PIH, premature rupture of the membranes (PROM), chorioamnionitis, fetal demise, postterm gestation, and logistic factors (such as risk of rapid labor or distance from the hospital) (ACOG 1991). Additional indications include severe fetal hemolytic disease, IUGR, and mild abruptio placentae with no fetal distress (Dunn 1990).

Contraindications

All contraindications to spontaneous labor and vaginal birth are contraindications to the induction of labor (Dunn 1990).

CRITICAL THINKING IN ACTION

You are a birthing center nurse caring for Mary Johnson, gravida 2, para 1, during an oxytocin infusion to induce her labor. Mary has been receiving the medication via infusion pump for 4 hours and currently is receiving 6 mU/minute (36 mL/hour). You have just completed your assessments and found the following: BP 120/80, pulse 80, respirations 16; contractions every 3 minutes lasting 60 seconds and of strong intensity; the FHR baseline is 144–150 with average long-term variability; and cervical dilatation is 6 cm. Will you continue the same infusion rate, increase the rate, or decrease the rate?

Answers can be found in Appendix H.

DRUG GUIDE | Dinoprostone (Cervidil) Vaginal Insert

Pregnancy Risk Category: C

Overview of Maternal-Fetal Action

Dinoprostone is a naturally occurring form of prostaglandin E_2. Dinoprostone can be used at term to ripen the cervix and can stimulate the smooth muscle of the uterus to enhance uterine contractions. A single vaginal insert may be used to ripen the cervix and then oxytocin can be administered 30 minutes later (Zatuchni and Slupik 1996; Forest Pharmaceuticals, Inc. Drug Insert 1995).

Route, Dosage, Frequency

The vaginal insert contains 10 mg of Dinoprostone. The insert is placed transversely in the posterior fornix of the vagina and the patient is kept supine for two hours but then may ambulate. The Dinoprostone is released at approximately 0.3 mg/hour over a 12 hour period. The vaginal insert should be removed by pulling on the retrieval string upon onset of uterine contractions or after 12 hours (Forest Pharmaceuticals, Inc. Drug Insert 1995).

Contraindications

Patient with known sensitivity to prostaglandins.

Presence of fetal distress.

Patient who has had unexplained bleeding during pregnancy.

Patient with strong suspicion of cephalopelvic disproportion.

Patient already receiving oxytocin.

Patient with 6 or more previous term pregnancies.

Patient who is not anticipated to be able to give birth vaginally.

Dinoprostone Vaginal Insert should be used with CAUTION in patients with ruptured membranes, a fetus in breech presentation, presence of glaucoma or history of asthma (Forrest Pharmaceuticals, Inc. 1995).

Maternal Side Effects

Uterine hyperstimulation with or without fetal distress has occurred in a very small number (2.8–4.7%) of patients. Less than 1% of patients have experienced fever, nausea, vomiting, diarrhea, or abdominal pain (Forest Pharmaceuticals, Inc. 1995).

Effects on Fetus/Neonate

Fetal distress (Zatuchni and Slupik 1996).

Nursing Considerations

Assess for presence of contraindications.

Monitor maternal vital signs, cervical dilatation and effacement carefully.

Monitor fetal status for presence of reassuring fetal heart rate pattern (baseline 120–160 bpm, presence of short-term variability, average variability, presence of accelerations with fetal movement, absence of late or variable decelerations).

Remove vaginal insert if uterine hyperstimulation, sustained uterine contractions, fetal distress, or any other maternal adverse actions occur.

Relative maternal contraindications include but are not limited to the following (ACOG 1991):

- Client refusal
- Placenta previa or vasa previa
- Abnormal fetal presentation
- Cord presentation
- Presenting part above the pelvic inlet
- Prior classic uterine incision
- Active genital herpes infection
- Pelvic structural deformities or cephalopelvic disproportion (CPD)
- Invasive cervical carcinoma

Before an induction is attempted, assessment must indicate that both the woman and the unborn child are ready for labor. This assessment includes evaluation of fetal maturity and cervical readiness.

Labor Readiness

Fetal Maturity

Gestational age of the fetus can be determined throughout the gestational period by ultrasound examination. Amniotic fluid studies also provide important information on fetal maturity. (See Chapter 14 for a discussion of methods to assess fetal maturity.)

Cervical Readiness

The findings of vaginal examinations help determine whether cervical changes favorable to induction have occurred. Bishop (1964) developed a prelabor scoring system that has proved helpful in predicting the inducibility of women (Table 20–1). Components evaluated are cervical dilatation, effacement, consistency, and position, as well as the station of the fetal presenting part. A score of 0, 1, 2, or 3 is given to each assessed characteristic. The higher the total score for all the criteria, the more likely it is that labor will ensue. The lower the total score, the higher the failure rate. A favorable cervix is the most important criterion for a successful induction.

The presence of a cervix that is anterior, soft, more than 50 percent effaced, and dilated at least 3 cm, with the fetal head at +1 station or lower is favorable for a successful induction (Dunn 1990).

Procedure for Oxytocin Infusion

The most frequently used methods of induction are amniotomy, described earlier, and intravenous oxytocin infusion, or both.

Intravenous administration of oxytocin is an effective method of initiating uterine contractions (inducing

TABLE 20–1 Prelabor Status Evaluation Scoring System

Factor	Assigned Value 0	1	2	3
Cervical dilatation	Closed	1–2 cm	3–4 cm	5 cm or more
Cervical effacement	0% to 30%	40% to 50%	60% to 70%	80% or more
Fetal station	−3	−2	−1, 0	+1, or lower
Cervical consistency	Firm	Moderate	Soft	
Cervical position	Posterior	Midposition	Anterior	

Source: Bishop EH: Pelvic scoring for elective inductions. *Obstet Gynecol* 1964; 24:266.

labor). It may also be used to augment labor (enhance contractions that are ineffective). A primary line of 1000 mL electrolyte solution (lactated Ringer's, for example) is started intravenously. To prepare the secondary line, 1000 mL of matching solution is prepared with 10 units of Pitocin. The secondary line is regulated by an infusion pump and is connected as closely as possible to the primary venipuncture site (see Drug Guide: Oxytocin on p 484). During administration, the goal is to achieve contractions of good intensity every 2–3 minutes, each of which lasts 40–50 seconds. The uterus should relax to normal baseline tone between contractions.

Oxytocin induction is not without some risks. Rapid progression of infusion rates or continuance of a particular rate without adequate assessment of the uterine contractions may lead to hyperstimulation of the uterus, fetal distress due to decreased placental perfusion, a rapid labor and birth with the danger of cervical or perineal lacerations, or uterine rupture. Water intoxication may occur if large doses are given in electrolyte-free solution over a prolonged period of time.

Nursing Care

Close observation and accurate assessments are mandatory to provide safe, optimal care for both woman and fetus. Baseline data (maternal temperature, pulse, respiration, blood pressure, and FHR) should be obtained before beginning the infusion. A fetal monitor is used to provide continuous data. Many institutions recommend obtaining a 15-minute recording before the infusion is started to obtain baseline data on uterine contractions and FHR. Before each advancement of the infusion rate, assessments of the following should be made:

- Maternal blood pressure and pulse
- Rate and reactivity of the FHR tracing (any bradycardia or decelerations are noted)
- Contraction status, frequency, intensity, duration, and resting tone between contractions

During the induction, urinary output is assessed to identify any problems with retention, fluid deficit, and possibility of the development of water intoxication. As contractions are established, vaginal examinations are done to evaluate cervical dilatation, effacement, and station. The frequency of vaginal examinations primarily depends on the number of pregnancies and on characteristics of the contractions. For example, a nullipara who has contractions every 5–7 minutes, each lasting 30 seconds, and who does not perceive her contractions does not usually require a vaginal examination. When her contractions are every 2–3 minutes, lasting 50–60 seconds with good intensity, a vaginal examination will be needed to evaluate her progress.

For additional information on nursing interventions, see Drug Guide: Oxytocin, and Critical Pathway for Induction of Labor, which begins on p 487.

Aspects to address during client teaching include the purpose and procedure for the induction, nursing care that will be provided, assessments during the induction procedure, comfort measures, and a review of breathing techniques that may be used during labor.

Augmentation of Labor

At times, labor begins spontaneously and then slows dramatically and little progress is made. When this happens, the physician/CNM may decide to augment (or stimulate) the labor. Note that while induction is used to initiate uterine contractions, augmentation is used to stimulate uterine contractions that are already present. Augmentation is accomplished through administration of intravenous oxytocin, in the same manner as an induction procedure.

Care of the Woman During Amnioinfusion

Amnioinfusion is a technique by which approximately 250–300 mL of warmed, sterile, normal saline is introduced into the uterus. The normal saline is infused through an intrauterine catheter under the control of an infusion pump. Amnioinfusion is used in cases of oligohydramnios or thick, meconium-stained amniotic fluid

DRUG GUIDE Oxytocin (Pitocin)

Overview of Obstetric Action

Oxytocin (Pitocin) exerts a selective stimulatory effect on the smooth muscle of the uterus and blood vessels. Oxytocin affects the myometrial cells of the uterus by increasing the excitability of the muscle cell, increasing the strength of the muscle contraction, and supporting propagation of the contraction (movement of the contraction from one myometrial cell to the next). Its effect on the uterine contraction depends on the dosage used and on the excitability of the myometrial cells. During the first half of gestation little excitability of the myometrium occurs, and the uterus is fairly resistant to the effects of oxytocin. However, from midgestation on, the uterus responds increasingly to exogenous intravenous oxytocin. Cautious use of diluted oxytocin administered intravenously at term results in a slow rise of uterine activity.

The circulatory half-life of oxytocin is 3–5 minutes. It takes approximately 40 minutes for a particular dose of oxytocin to reach a steady-state plasma concentration (Arias 1993; ACOG 1991).

The effects of oxytocin on the cardiovascular system can be pronounced. There may be an initial decrease in the blood pressure, but with prolonged administration a 30% increase in the baseline blood pressure may be noted. Cardiac output and stroke volume are increased. With doses of 20 mU/minute or above, the antidiuretic effect of oxytocin results in a decrease of free water exchange in the kidney and a marked decrease in urine output (Marshall 1985).

Oxytocin is used to **induce** labor at term and to **augment** uterine contractions in the first and second stages of labor. Oxytocin may also be used **immediately after birth to stimulate uterine contraction** and thereby control uterine atony.

Route, Dosage, Frequency

For induction of labor: Add 10 units Pitocin (1 mL) to 1000 mL of intravenous solution. (The resulting concentration is 10 mU oxytocin per 1 mL of intravenous fluid.) Using an infusion pump, administer IV, starting at 0.5–1 mU/minute and increase by 1–2 mU/minute every 40–60 minutes. Or start at 1–2 mU/minute and increase by 1 mU/minute every 15 minutes until a good contraction pattern (every 2–3 minutes and lasting 40–60 seconds) is achieved (ACOG 1991).

Maternal Contraindications

- Severe preeclampsia-eclampsia (PIH)
- Predisposition to uterine rupture (in nullipara over 35 years of age, multigravida 4 or more, overdistention of the uterus, previous major surgery of the cervix or uterus)
- Cephalopelvic disproportion
- Malpresentation or malposition of the fetus, cord prolapse
- Preterm infant
- Rigid, unripe cervix; total placenta previa
- Presence of fetal distress

Maternal Side Effects

Hyperstimulation of the uterus results in hypercontractility, which in turn may cause the following:

- Abruptio placentae
- Impaired uterine blood flow → fetal hypoxia
- Rapid labor → cervical lacerations
- Rapid labor and birth → lacerations of cervix, vagina, perineum, uterine atony, fetal trauma
- Uterine rupture
- Water intoxication (nausea, vomiting, hypotension, tachycardia, cardiac arrhythmia) if oxytocin is given in electrolyte-free solution or at a rate exceeding 20 mU/minute; hypotension with rapid IV bolus administration postpartum

Effect on Fetus-Neonate

- Fetal effects are primarily associated with the presence of hypercontractility of the maternal uterus. Hypercontractility causes a decrease in the oxygen supply to the fetus, which is reflected by irregularities and/or decrease in FHR.
- Hyperbilirubinemia (Bachman and Kendrick 1996).
- Trauma from rapid birth.

and for intrauterine administration of antibiotics (Wenstrom et al 1995). When oligohydramnios is present, there is not enough fluid to allow the umbilical cord to float freely, so it can become compressed against various parts of the fetus. When cord compression occurs, the blood supply to the fetus diminishes, and FHR bradycardia, variable decelerations, or both develop. Increasing the fluid volume of the uterus allows the cord to float and decreases the incidence and severity of variable decelerations.

If stressed, the fetus may release meconium into the amniotic fluid. If a small amount of meconium is released, light meconium staining of the amniotic fluid (light blackish-green discoloration) may occur. Release of a large amount of meconium results in amniotic fluid that is more discolored and contains a high concentration of meconium. This concentrated fluid, if not expelled from the fetal mouth and throat during chest compression at birth, may be inspired by the fetus. Meconium aspiration or pneumonitis may occur. When thick, meconium-stained amniotic fluid is present during labor, amnioinfusion may be used to dilute the amniotic fluid and decrease the newborn's chances of inspiring meconium. If chorioamnionitis (infection within the uterus) is present, an amnioinfusion may be used to instill antibiotics directly into the uterus.

The nurse helps with the amnioinfusion and monitors the woman's vital signs and contraction status, and the FHR. It is very important to provide ongoing information to the laboring woman and her partner and to answer questions as they arise. Comfort measures and positioning will be very important because the woman will now be on bed rest.

DRUG GUIDE continued

Nursing Considerations

- Explain induction or augmentation procedure to client.
- Apply fetal monitor and obtain 15- to 20-minute tracing and NST to assess FHR before starting IV oxytocin.
- For induction or augmentation of labor, start with primary IV and piggyback secondary IV with oxytocin and infusion pump.
- Ensure continuous fetal and uterine contraction monitoring.
- The maximum rate is 40 mU/minute (ACOG 1988). Not all protocols recommend a maximum dose. When indicated, it is generally between 16 and 40 mU/minute (Owen and Hauth 1992). Decrease oxytocin by similar increments once labor has progressed to 5–6 cm dilatation (ACOG 1988; Arias 1993).

0.5 mU/minute	= 3 mL/hour	8 mU/minute	= 48 mL/hour
1.0 mU/minute	= 6 mL/hour	10 mU/minute	= 60 mL/hour
1.5 mU/minute	= 9 mL/hour	12 mU/minute	= 72 mL/hour
2 mU/minute	= 12 mL/hour	15 mU/minute	= 90 mL/hour
4 mU/minute	= 24 mL/hour	18 mU/minute	= 108 mL/hour
6 mU/minute	= 36 mL/hour	20 mU/minute	= 120 mL/hour

Protocols may vary from one agency to another.

- Assess FHR, maternal blood pressure, pulse, and uterine contraction frequency, duration, and resting tone before each increase in oxytocin infusion rate.
- Record all assessments and IV rate on monitor strip and on client's chart.
- Record oxytocin infusion rate in mU/minute and mL/hour (eg, 0.5 mU/minute [3 mL/hour]).
- Record all client activities (such as change of position, vomiting), procedures done (amniotomy, sterile vaginal examination), and

Nursing Considerations *continued*

administration of analgesics on monitor strip to allow for interpretation and evaluation of tracing.

- Assess cervical dilatation as needed.
- Apply nursing comfort measures.
- Discontinue IV oxytocin infusion and infuse primary solution when (1) fetal distress is noted (bradycardia, late or variable decelerations; (2) uterine contractions are more frequent than every 2 minutes; (3) duration of contractions exceeds more than 60 seconds; or (4) insufficient relaxation of the uterus between contractions or a steady increase in resting tone are noted (ACOG 1991); in addition to discontinuing IV oxytocin infusion, turn client to side, and if fetal distress is present, administer oxygen by tight face mask at 7–10 L/minute; notify physician.
- Maintain intake and output record.

For augmentation of labor: Prepare and administer IV Pitocin as for labor induction. Increase rate until labor contractions are of good quality. The flow rate is gradually increased at no less than every 30 minutes to a maximum of 10 mU/minute (Cunningham et al 1997). In some settings or in a situation when limited fluids may be administered, a more concentrated solution may be used. When 10 U Pitocin is added to 500 mL IV solution, the resulting concentration is 1 mU/minute = 3 mL/hour. If 10 U Pitocin is added to 250 mL IV solution, the concentration is 1 mU/minute = 1.5 mL/hour.

For administration after delivery of placenta: One dose of 10 units Pitocin (1 mL) is given intramuscularly or by slow intravenous push or added to IV fluids for continuous infusion.

Care of the Woman During an Episiotomy

An episiotomy is a surgical incision into the perineal body that is done to enlarge the area of the outlet (O'Brien and Cefalo 1996).

An episiotomy is one of the most common procedures in maternal-child care. Researchers estimate the rate of episiotomies in all births is 50 percent (Albers et al 1996). Even though the procedure is very common, its routine use has been questioned (Woolley 1995). Current research suggests that rather than protecting the perineum from lacerations, the presence of an episiotomy makes it more likely that the woman will have a deep perineal tear. Additional complications associated with an episiotomy may be infection, blood loss, and pain and perineal discomfort that may continue for days or weeks past birth, including dyspareunia (Woolley 1995).

Procedure

The episiotomy is performed with sharp scissors with rounded points, just before birth, when approximately 3 to 4 cm of the fetal head is visible during a contraction (Cunningham et al 1997). The incision begins at the midline and may be extended down the midline through the perineal body, or it may extend at a 45-degree angle in a mediolateral direction to the right or left (Figure 20–2). A midline episiotomy is preferred if the perineum is of adequate length and no difficulty during birth is anticipated, because blood loss is less, the incision is easy to repair, and it heals with less discomfort. The major

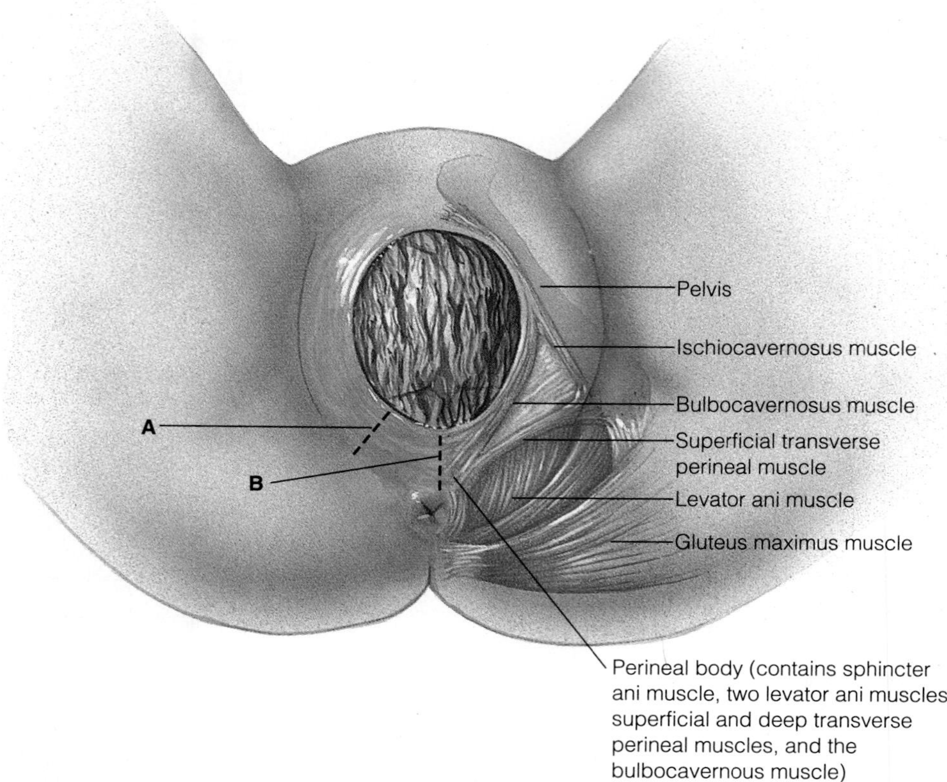

FIGURE 20–2 The two most common types of episiotomies are midline and mediolateral. ***A*** Right mediolateral. ***B*** Midline.

disadvantage is that the midline incision frequently extends through the anal sphincter and rectum. In the presence of a short perineum or an anticipated difficult birth, a mediolateral episiotomy provides more room for the birth and decreases the possibility of a traumatic extension into the rectum (Crawford et al 1993). The mediolateral episiotomy may be complicated by greater blood loss, a longer healing period, and more discomfort postpartally.

The episiotomy is usually performed with regional or local anesthesia but may be performed without anesthesia in emergency situations. It is generally proposed that as crowning occurs, the distention of the tissues causes numbing.

Repair of the episiotomy (episiorrhaphy) and any lacerations is accomplished either during the period between birth of the newborn and delivery of the placenta, or after the delivery of the placenta. Adequate anesthesia must be given for the repair.

Nursing Care

The woman needs to be supported during the repair, as she may feel some pressure sensations. In the absence of adequate anesthesia, she may feel pain. Placing a hand on her shoulder and talking with her can provide comfort and distraction from the repair process. If the woman is having more discomfort than she can comfortably handle, the nurse needs to act as an advocate in communicating the woman's needs to the physician/certified nurse-midwife. At all times the woman needs to be the one who decides whether the amount of discomfort is tolerable, and she should never be told "This doesn't hurt." She is the person experiencing the discomfort, and her evaluation must be respected. If there are just a few (3–5) stitches left, she may choose to forego more local anesthesia, but she should be given the choice.

The type of episiotomy is recorded on the birth record. This information should also be included in a report to the nurse who will care for her after birth, so that adequate assessments can be made and relief measures instituted if necessary.

Pain relief measures may begin immediately after birth with application of an ice pack to the perineum. For optimal effect the ice pack should be applied for 20 to 30 minutes and removed for at least 20 minutes before being reapplied. The perineal tissues should be assessed frequently to prevent injury from the ice pack.

The nurse provides information about possible comfort measures. After the fourth stage is completed, warm sitz baths (101F to 105F) are recommended to increase circulation to the area and promote healing. The use of cool sitz baths is currently being investigated; some women report increased pain relief from using a lukewarm sitz bath to which ice chips have been added. The

CRITICAL PATHWAY FOR INDUCTION OF LABOR

Category	
Referral	• Review prenatal record • Advise CNM/physician of admission • Anesthesia
Assessment	• Previous pregnancies, present pregnancy, and childbirth preparation • Estimated gestational age of the fetus • Assess woman's feelings regarding induction as well as knowledge base regarding the induction process • Assess knowledge of breathing techniques. If woman does not have a method to use, teach breathing techniques before starting oxytocin infusion
Comfort	• Provide support to woman as she uses breathing techniques • Encourage use of effluerage, back rub, and other supportive measures • Assess need for analgesia or anesthesia
Nursing interventions and report	• Examination of pregnant uterus (Leopold's maneuvers to determine fetal size and position) • Vaginal examination to evaluate cervical readiness: a. Ripe cervix feels soft to the examining finger, is located in a medial to anterior position, is more than 50% effaced, and is 2–3 cm dilated b. Unripe cervix feels firm to the examining finger, is long and thick, is perhaps in a posterior position, and is dilated little or not at all • Presence of contractions • Membranes intact or ruptured • Maternal vital signs and a 20 min baseline fetal monitoring strip prior to induction to determine fetal well-being • Diagnostic studies: a. Fetal maturity tests (L/S ratio, creatinine concentrations, ultrasonography), NST, CST, BPP b. Maternal blood studies (CBC, hemoglobin, hematocrit, blood type, Rh factor) c. Urinalysis • Monitor for nausea, vomiting, hypotension, tachycardia, cardiac arrhythmias, headache, mental confusion, decreased. urinary output • Monitor FHR by continuous electronic fetal monitoring. Do not start infusion or advance rate (if induction has already begun) if FHR is not in range of 120–160 bpm, if decelerations are present, or if variability decreases • Evaluate and document maternal BP and pulse before beginning induction and then before each increase in infusion rate. Do not advance infusion rate in presence of maternal hypertension or hypotension or radical changes in pulse rate • If the woman becomes hypotensive: a. Keep her on her side. May change to other side. b. Discontinue oxytocin infusion c. Increase rate of primary IV d. Monitor FHR e. Notify physician f. Assess for cause of hypotension • Evaluate and document contraction frequency, duration, and intensity prior to each increase in infusion rate • Discontinue oxytocin infusion if: a. Contractions are more frequent than q2min b. Contraction duration exceeds 90 sec c. Uterus does not relax between contractions

›

episiotomy site should be inspected every 15 minutes during the first hour after delivery and thereafter daily for redness, swelling, tenderness, and hematomas. Mild analgesic sprays and oral analgesics are ordered as needed. The mother will need instruction in perineal hygiene care and may need instructions about use of the analgesic spray. (See Chapter 29 for additional discussion of relief measures.)

Care of the Woman During Forceps-Assisted Birth

Forceps are designed to assist the birth of a fetus by providing traction or by providing the means to rotate the fetal head to an occiput-anterior position. Forceps are used with vaginal birth, and occasionally during a cesarean birth to assist in the removal of the fetal head

CRITICAL PATHWAY FOR INDUCTION OF LABOR continued

Category	
Nursing interventions and report ***continued***	• Increase oxytocin IV infusion rate q20min until adequate contractions are achieved. Do not exceed an infusion rate of 20–40 mL/min. (Note: Protocols directing how often oxytocin is increased may vary from 15–60 min. See ACOG 1991 guidelines and institutional protocol.) • Check infusion pump to assure oxytocin is infusing. Check whether pump is on, chamber refills and empties, level of fluid in IV bottle becomes lower. If problem is found, correct and restart infusion at beginning dose. Check main IV site frequently. Check piggyback connection to primary tubing to assure solution is not leaking. • Evaluate cervical dilatation by vaginal examination with each oxytocin dosage increase after labor is established • Monitor FHR continuously (normal range is 120–160 bpm). In episodes of bradycardia (<120 bpm) lasting for more than 30 sec, administer oxygen by face mask at 7–10 L/min. Stop oxytocin infusion. Position woman on left side if quick recovery of FHR does not occur. • Carefully evaluate fetal tachycardia (>160 bpm). Sustained tachycardia may necessitate discontinuation of oxytocin infusion. Assess for presence of meconium staining. Notify physician.
Activity	• Ambulate until 5–10 cm then bed • Position woman in left lateral or semi-Fowler's position • Encourage her to avoid supine position
Nutrition	• IV/lactated Ringer's • Ice chips, clear fluids
Elimination	• Encourage voiding q2 h. Monitor and record I/O.
Medications	• Start primary IV of lactated Ringer's • Administer oxytocin in electrolyte solution (Piggyback oxytocin onto primary IV at closest site to IV needle insertion.) • Pain meds prn
Discharge planning/ home care	• Photo packet • Birth certificate worksheet • Sibling visitation • Car seat
Family involvement	• Family visitation policy per institutional protocol • Encourage significant other to stay close and assist with breathing of woman
Teaching/ psychosocial	• Provide emotional support through teaching and answering all questions
Date	

from the uterus. There are three categories of forceps applications:

1. *Outlet forceps* are applied when the fetal skull has reached the perineum, the scalp is visible between contractions, and the sagittal suture is not more than 45 degrees from the midline.
2. *Low forceps* application is used when the leading edge of the fetal skull is at a station of +2 or more.
3. *Midforceps* application is used when the fetal head is engaged but the leading edge of the fetal skull is above +2 station.

In addition, a special type of forceps is designed to be used with a breech presentation, in which forceps are applied to the aftercoming fetal head (called *aftercoming* because the head is born after the body).

Types of forceps are illustrated in Figure 20–3.

Indications

Indications for the use of forceps include the presence of any condition that threatens the mother or fetus and can be relieved by birth. Conditions that put the woman at risk include heart disease and exhaustion. Fetal conditions include fetal distress. Low forceps may be used electively to shorten the second stage of labor and spare the woman's pushing effort (when exhaustion or heart disease is present), or when regional anesthesia has af-

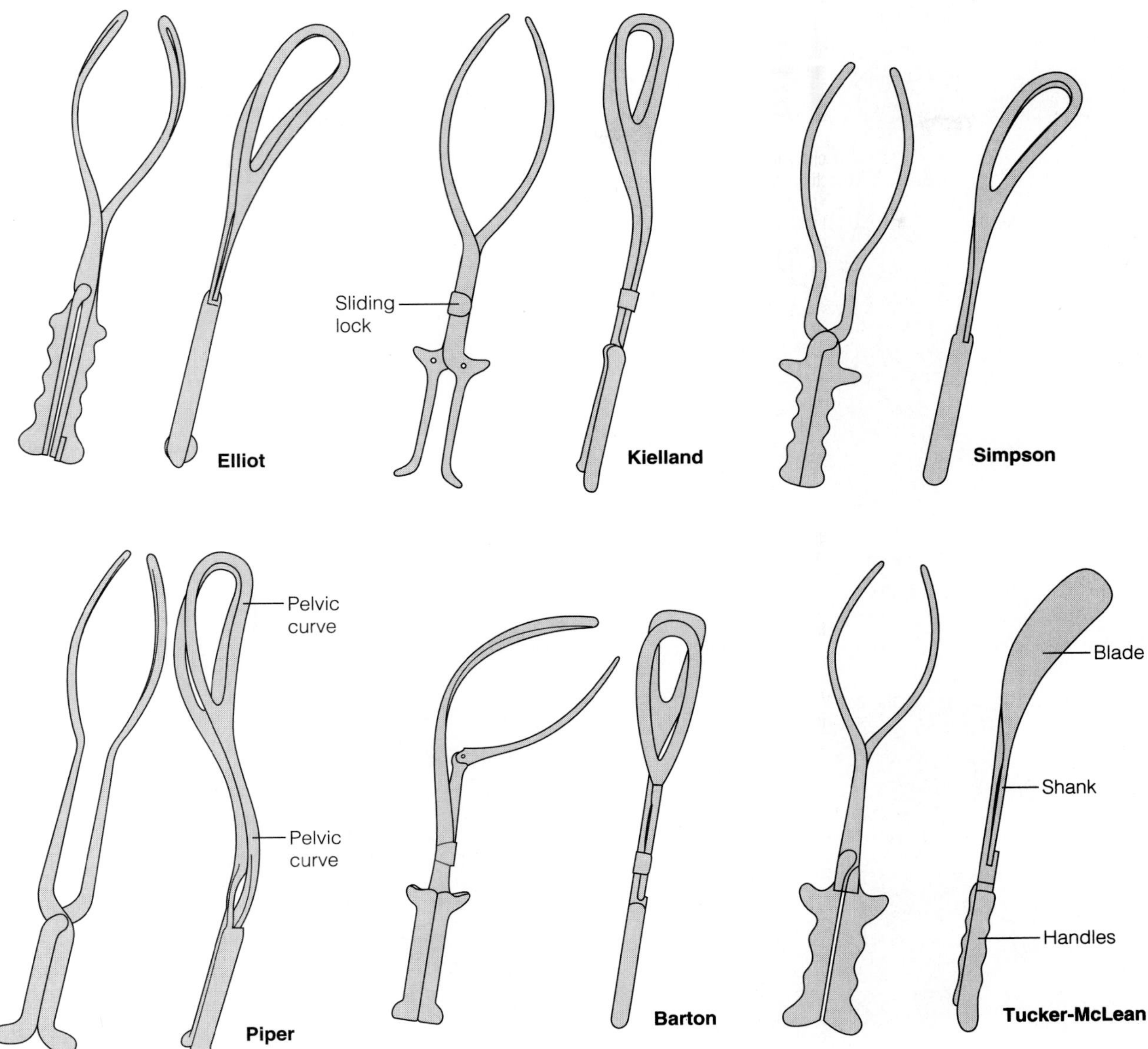

FIGURE 20–3 Forceps are composed of a blade, shank, and handle and may have a cephalic and pelvic curve. (Note labels on Piper and Tucker-McLean forceps.) The blades may be fenestrated (open) or solid. The front and lateral views of these forceps illustrate differences in blades, open and closed shanks, and cephalic and pelvic curves. Elliot, Simpson, and Tucker-McLean forceps are used as outlet forceps. Kielland and Barton forceps are used for midforceps rotations. Piper forceps are used to provide traction and flexion of the after-coming head (the head comes after the body) of a fetus in breech presentation.

fected the woman's motor innervation and she cannot push effectively (Laufe et al 1990). In the past, outlet forceps have been used to protect the head of a preterm infant during birth; however, the advantages of this practice are now being questioned (ACOG 1991; Cunningham et al 1997).

Maternal-Neonatal Risks

Maternal risks may include lacerations of the birth canal and perineum and increased bleeding. Some newborns may develop a small area of ecchymosis or edema along the sides of the face as a result of forceps application. Caput succedaneum or cephalhematoma (and possible subsequent hyperbilirubinemia) may occur as well as transient facial paralysis.

Prerequisites for Forceps Application

Use of forceps requires complete dilatation of the cervix and knowledge of the exact position and station of the fetal head. The membranes must be ruptured to allow a

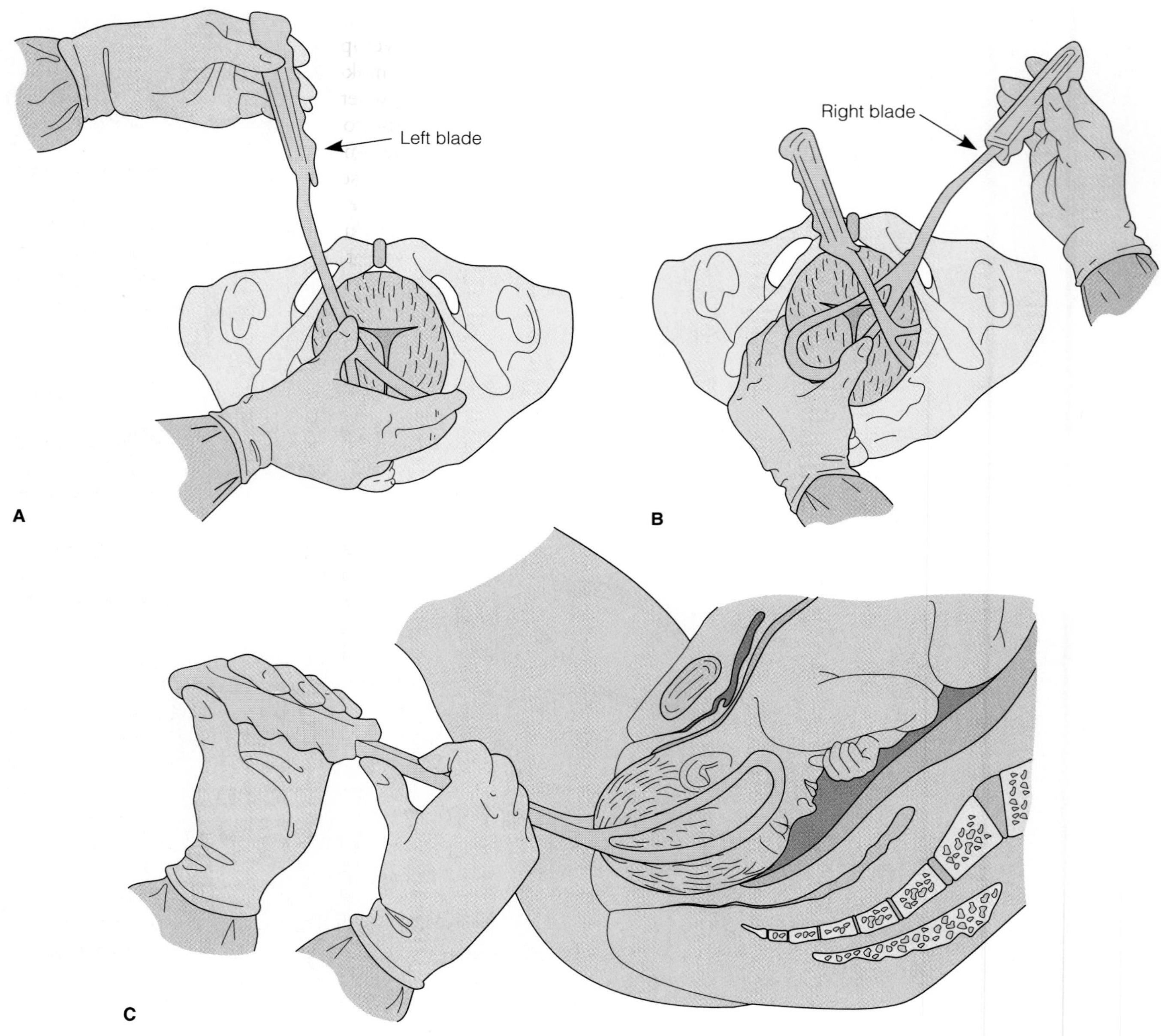

FIGURE 20–4 Application of forceps in occiput anterior (OA) position. ***A*** The left blade is inserted along the left side wall of the pelvis over the parietal bone. ***B*** The right blade is inserted along the right side wall of the pelvis over the parietal bone. ***C*** With correct placement of the blades, the handles lock easily. During uterine contractions, traction is applied to the forceps in a downward and outward direction to follow the birth canal.

firm grasp on the fetal head. The presentation must be vertex or face with the chin anterior, and the head must be engaged, preferably on the perineum. Under no circumstances should there be any disproportion between the fetal head and the maternal pelvis (Cunningham et al 1997).

Nursing Care

The nurse can explain the procedure briefly to the woman if she is awake. With adequate regional anesthesia, she should feel some pressure but no pain. The woman is encouraged to maintain breathing techniques to prevent her from pushing during application of the forceps (Figure 20–4). The nurse monitors contractions and with each contraction the physician/CNM provides traction as the woman pushes. The nurse should monitor the FHR continuously until the birth. It is not uncommon to observe bradycardia as traction is being applied to the forceps. Bradycardia results from head compression and is transient in nature.

The newborn is assessed for facial edema, bruising, caput succedaneum, cephalhematoma, or any sign of cerebral edema. In the fourth stage, the nurse assesses the woman for perineal swelling or bruising, hematoma, and hemorrhage.

The nurse answers questions and reiterates explanations provided, reviews nursing assessments of the woman and her newborn, and provides opportunities for questions.

Care of the Woman During Vacuum Extraction

Procedure

In vacuum extraction, suction is used to help deliver the fetal head. The vacuum extractor is composed of a soft silicone cup attached by tubes to a suction bottle (pump). The suction cup, which comes in various sizes, is placed against the fetal occiput. The pump is used to create negative pressure (suction) inside the cup. Traction is applied in coordination with uterine contractions to help deliver the fetal head (Figure 20–5).

The indications for use of the vacuum extractor are much the same as for forceps: for the elective shortening of the second stage of labor and relieving the woman of the pushing effort or when anesthesia or fatigue interfere with the woman's ability to push effectively (O'Brien and Cefalo 1996).

Risks of vacuum extraction for the fetus include cephalhematoma, brachial plexus palsy, hyperbilirubinemia, and retinal and intracranial hemorrhage. Maternal risks involve vaginal and rectal lacerations (O'Brien and Cefalo 1996).

Nursing Care

During the procedure, the nurse keeps the woman informed about what is happening. If adequate regional anesthesia has been administered, the woman feels only pressure during the procedure. The FHR should be auscultated every 5 minutes or more frequently. Parents need to be informed that the caput on the baby's head will disappear in a few hours.

Assessment of the newborn should include inspection and continued observation for cerebral trauma and soft tissue necrosis.

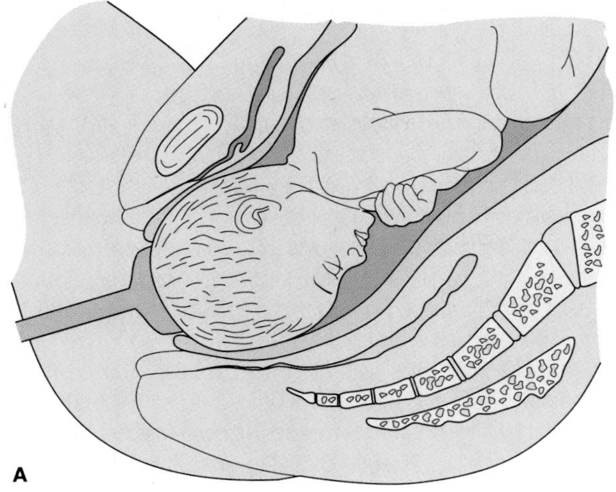

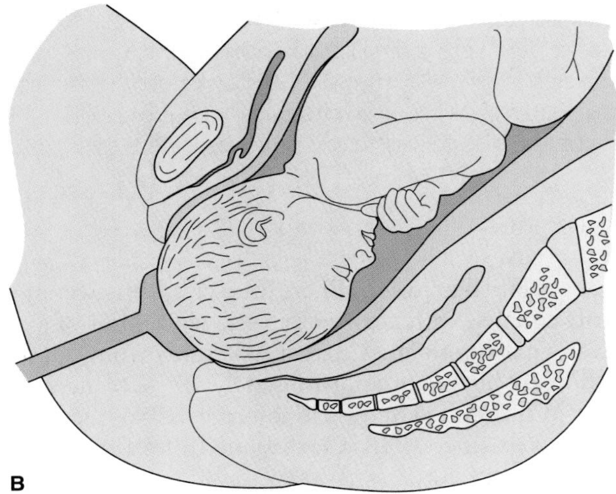

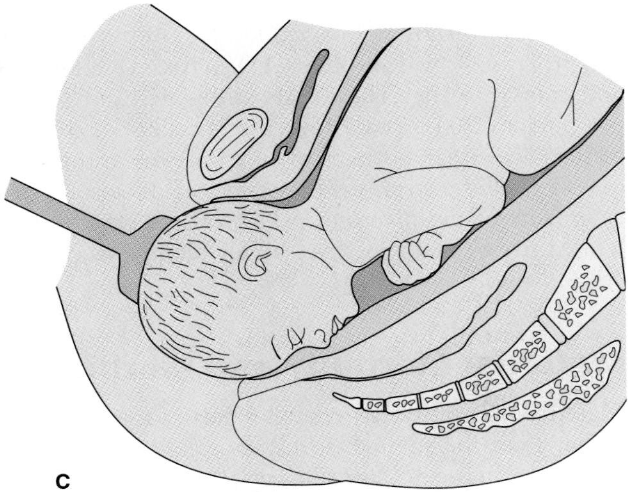

FIGURE 20–5 Vacuum extractor traction. ***A*** The cup is placed on the fetal occiput and suction is created. Traction is applied in a downward and outward direction. ***B*** Traction continues in a downward direction as the fetal head begins to emerge from the vagina. ***C*** Traction is maintained to lift the fetal head out of the vagina.

Care of the Family During Cesarean Birth

Cesarean birth is the birth of the infant through an abdominal and uterine incision. The word *cesarean* is derived from the Latin word *caedere,* meaning "to cut." Cesarean birth is one of the oldest surgical procedures

COMMUNITY IN FOCUS | ICAN (International Cesarean Awareness Network)

The International Cesarean Awareness Network (ICAN) is a volunteer organization committed to three broad goals: (1) to lower the high cesarean birth rate through education; (2) to provide a forum through which individuals can express their thoughts and concerns about the birth experience; and (3) to provide a support network for women who are healing from past birth experiences and those who are preparing for future births. With headquarters in Redondo Beach, California, the organization currently has approximately thirty-two chapters throughout the United States including ICAN of Southeast Minnesota, New York City, Los Angeles, Northeast Ohio, Houston, Washington DC, and Denver, to name a few.

ICAN was founded in 1982 by Esther Zorn, a woman who had a traumatic cesarean birth experience and wanted to have a vaginal birth in a subsequent pregnancy. At the time, VBAC (vaginal birth after cesarean) was extremely rare, but Ms Zorn persevered and was able to find a like-minded caregiver to enable her to give birth vaginally.

Members of ICAN typically are women who have had a cesarean birth experience and are pregnant or planning another pregnancy, which they hope to complete by VBAC. They join ICAN for information, support, and referral to caregivers who agree with a generally non-interventionist approach to childbirth. Other participants include childbirth educators, nurses, other health care providers, and community members who are opposed to unnecessary cesarean births and supportive of organizations that empower women.

ICAN chapters hold monthly meetings that feature a variety of educational topics. The meetings also provide a forum for the exchange of ideas and a safe place in which to explore feelings and attitudes. Phone counseling is also available for women who are in need of information or emotional support. In addition, all members receive a quarterly newsletter, the *Clarion*.

It is difficult to evaluate the overall effect of an organization like ICAN. Historically, the impact of concerned citizens on the birth experience has been significant. Consumers have actively sought the opportunity for the family to participate more fully in the birth experience and changes such as the presence of a partner or other loved ones at birth, rooming-in, and early discharge have resulted. Moreover, the incidence of VBAC has risen markedly over the past 10 years as women actively challenged the old axiom, "Once a cesarean, always a cesarean." It is exciting, however, to see how a grassroots effort such as ICAN can take hold and flourish because it provides a valuable service to childbearing women and their families.

Source: Personal communication with April Kubachka, President of ICAN, and ICAN literature.

known. Until the twentieth century, cesareans were primarily equated with an attempt to save the fetus of a dying pregnant woman. Currently, cesarean birth is the method of birth for approximately 23 percent of all births in the United States (Woolbright 1996). This rate is the lowest since 1988 (Clarke and Taffel 1996).

Indications

Cesarean births are performed in cases of placenta previa, prolapsed cord, absolute CPD, active genital herpes, and transverse lie. These indications account for approximately 20 percent of the total number of cesarean births. The other 80 percent of cesareans are done in cases of failure to progress because of narrowed measurements of the maternal pelvis, breech presentation, fetal distress, and repeat cesarean births (Woolbright 1996).

Maternal Mortality and Morbidity

Maternal mortality for cesarean births is several-fold higher than for vaginal births, although it is still low (approximately 1 to 2 deaths per 1000 cesareans as opposed to 0.06 deaths per 1000 live vaginal births) (Depp 1996). Maternal morbidity is associated with a fairly wide variety of complications, such as unexplained fever, endometritis, wound infection, urinary tract infection, atelectasis, thrombophlebitis, and pulmonary embolism (Scott 1994).

Surgical Techniques

Skin Incisions

The skin incision for a cesarean birth is either transverse (Pfannenstiel) or vertical and is not indicative of the type of incision made into the uterus. The transverse incision is made across the lowest and narrowest part of the abdomen. Since the incision is made just below the pubic hair line, it is almost invisible after healing. The limitation of this type of skin incision is that it does not allow for extension of the incision if needed. Since it usually requires more time, this incision is used when time is not of the essence (eg, with CPD or failure to progress and no fetal or maternal distress). The vertical incision is made between the navel and the symphysis pubis. This type of incision is quicker and is therefore preferred in cases of fetal distress, when rapid birth is desired, with preterm or macrosomic infants, or when the woman is obese (Cunningham et al 1997). The type of skin incision is determined by time factor, client preference, or physician preference.

Uterine Incisions

The type of uterine incision depends on the need for the cesarean. The choice of incision affects the woman's opportunity for a subsequent vaginal birth and her risks of a ruptured uterine scar with a subsequent pregnancy.

The two major locations of uterine incisions are in the lower uterine segment or in the upper segment of the uterine corpus. The lower uterine segment incision most commonly used is a transverse incision, although a vertical incision may also be used (Figure 20–6). The *transverse incision* is preferred for the following reasons (Cunningham et al 1997):

- The lower segment is the thinnest portion of the uterus and involves less blood loss.
- It requires only moderate dissection of bladder from underlying myometrium.
- It is easier to repair.
- The site is less likely to rupture during subsequent pregnancies.
- There is a decreased chance of adherence of bowel or omentum to the incision line.

The disadvantages are the following:

- It takes longer to make and repair this incision.
- It is limited in size because of the presence of major blood vessels on either side of the uterus.
- It has a greater tendency to extend laterally into the uterine vessels.
- The incision may stretch and become a thin window, but it usually does not create problems clinically until a subsequent labor ensues.

The *lower uterine segment vertical incision* is preferred for multiple gestation, abnormal presentation, placenta previa, fetal distress, and preterm and macrosomic fetuses. Disadvantages of this incision include the following:

- The incision may extend downward into the cervix.
- More extensive dissection of the bladder is needed to keep the incision in the lower uterine segment.
- If it extends upward into the upper segment, hemostasis and closure are more difficult.
- It increases the chance of rupture with subsequent labor (Cunningham et al 1997; Martin et al 1993).

One other incision, the *classic incision,* was the method of choice for many years but is rarely used now. This vertical incision was made into the upper uterine segment. There was more blood loss, and it was difficult to repair. Most important, there was an increased risk of uterine rupture with subsequent pregnancy, labor, and birth, because the upper uterine segment is the most contractile portion of the uterus.

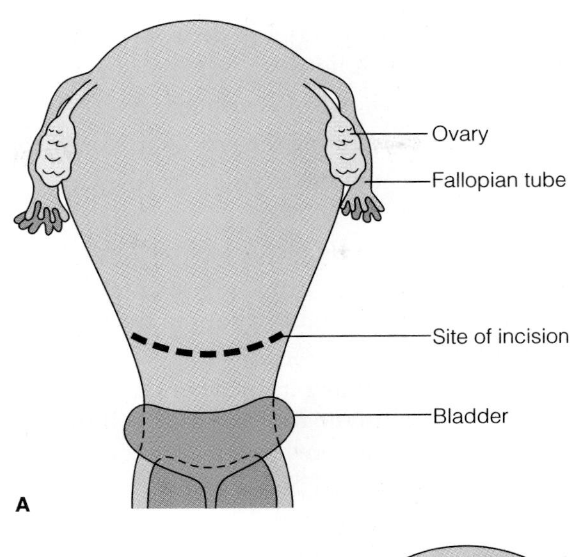

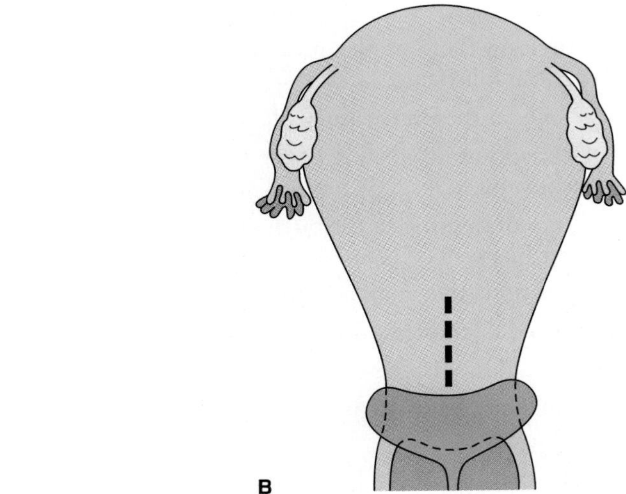

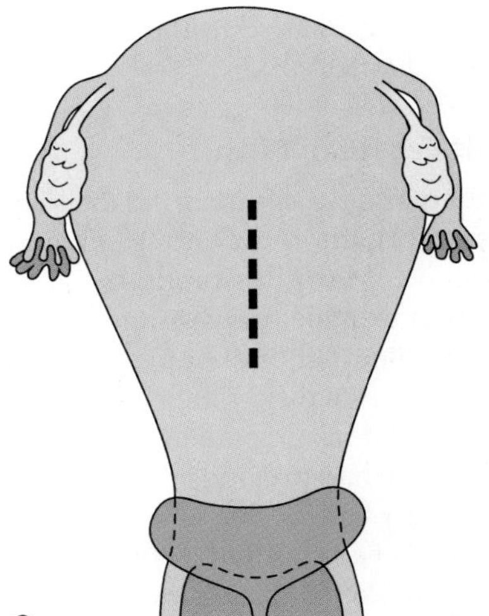

FIGURE 20–6 Uterine incisions for a cesarean birth. ***A*** This transverse incision in the lower uterine segment is called a Kerr incision. ***B*** The Sellheim incision is a vertical incision in the lower uterine segment. ***C*** This view illustrates the classic uterine incision that is done in the body (corpus) of the uterus. The classic incision was commonly done in the past but is associated with increased risk of uterine rupture in subsequent pregnancies and labor.

Nursing Care

Preparation for Cesarean Birth

Cesarean birth is an alternative method of childbirth. Given that 1 out of every 4 or 5 births is a cesarean, preparation for this possibility should be an integral part of every childbirth education curriculum. (See the discussion in Chapter 6.) Ideally all couples should be encouraged to discuss the possibility of a cesarean birth with their physician/certified nurse-midwife. They can also discuss their specific needs and desires. Their preferences may include the following:

- Participating in the choice of anesthetic
- Partner being present during the procedures or birth
- Partner being present in the recovery or postpartum room
- Audio recording or taking pictures of the birth
- Delayed instillation of eye drops to promote eye contact between parent and newborn in the first hours after birth
- Physical contact or holding the newborn while on the delivery table or in the recovery room. (If the mother cannot hold the newborn, her partner can hold the baby for her.)
- Breastfeeding at the time of birth or in the recovery room

Information that couples need about cesarean birth includes the following:

- Events in the preparatory phase
- Description or viewing of the birthing room or surgical suite
- Types of anesthesia for birth and analgesia available after birth
- Sensations that may be experienced
- Roles of significant others
- Interaction with newborn
- Immediate recovery phase
- Postpartal phase

The context in which this information is given should be birth oriented rather than surgery oriented.

Additional information is presented in the Cesarean Birth Critical Pathway in Chapter 29.

Preparation for Repeat Cesarean Birth

When the couple is anticipating a cesarean birth, they have time to take in the information they are given and prepare for the experience. Many hospitals or local groups (such as C-Sec, Inc.) provide preparation classes for cesarean birth. The instructor should impart factual information and a feeling of normality, which will allow the couple to make choices and participate in their birth experience. Couples who have had previous negative experiences need an opportunity to describe what they felt contributed to these events. They should be encouraged to identify what they would like to have altered and to list interventions that would make the experience more positive. Those who have had positive experiences need reassurance that their needs and desires will be met in the same manner. In addition, couples should have an opportunity to discuss any fears or anxieties.

A specific concern of the woman facing a repeat cesarean is anticipation of pain. She needs reassurance that subsequent cesareans are often less painful than the first. She may not experience the extreme fatigue that followed the primary cesarean if it was preceded by a long or strenuous labor. Giving this information will enable the woman to cope more effectively with stressful stimuli, including pain. The nurse can remind the woman that she has already had experience with how to prevent, cope with, and alleviate painful stimuli.

Preparation for Emergency Cesarean Birth

The period preceding surgery must be used to its greatest advantage. The couple needs some time for privacy to assimilate the information given to them and to ask for additional information. It is imperative that caregivers use their most effective communication skills. The nurse must address what the couple may anticipate during the next few hours. Asking the couple "What questions do you have about the decision?" gives the couple an opportunity for further clarification. The nurse can prepare the woman in stages, giving her information and the rationale for each procedure before beginning the procedure. Before carrying out a procedure it is essential to tell the woman (a) what is going to happen, (b) why it is being done, and (c) what sensations she may experience. This enables the woman to give informed consent to the procedure. The woman experiences a sense of control and therefore feels less helpless.

Preparation of the woman for surgery involves more than the procedures of establishing intravenous lines and a urinary catheter or doing an abdominal prep. As discussed previously, good communication skills are useful in helping the woman feel in control. For some women, the use of touch, empathetic listening, and eye contact do much to maintain their reality orientation and control. These measures reduce anxiety for the woman during the stressful preparatory period.

If the cesarean is scheduled and not an emergency, the nurse has ample time for preoperative teaching. The woman needs to practice her turning, coughing, and deep breathing. It is helpful if she is taught to splint her abdominal muscles when she coughs. Holding her muscles with her arms or a pillow decreases discomfort in the incisional area. She must sign an informed consent for surgery.

In preparation for surgery, the woman is given nothing by mouth. To reduce the likelihood of serious pulmonary damage, should aspiration of gastric contents occur, antacids may be administered within 30 minutes of surgery. If epidural anesthesia is used, the nurse may assist with the procedure, monitor the woman's blood pressure and response, and continue EFM. An abdominal and perineal prep is done and an indwelling catheter is inserted to prevent bladder distention. An intravenous line is started, with a needle of adequate size to permit blood administration, and preoperative medication is ordered. The pediatrician should be notified and adequate preparation made to receive the newborn. The nurse should make sure that the infant warmer is functional and that appropriate resuscitation equipment is available. The circulating nurse assists in positioning the woman on the operating table. Fetal heart rate should be ascertained before surgery, during preparation, and until immediately before the surgery. A wedge needs to be placed under the woman's right hip to tilt the uterus slightly and thus avoid vena caval syndrome.

Birth

Every effort should be made to include the father or partner in the birth experience. When the father attends the cesarean birth, he must scrub and wear a surgical gown and mask as do others in the operating suite. A stool can be placed beside the woman's head so that the father can sit nearby to provide physical touch, visual contact, and verbal reassurance to his partner.

Other measures can be taken to promote the participation of the father or partner who chooses not to be in the delivery room. These include:

- Allowing the father or partner to be near the delivery or operating room, where he can hear the newborn's first cry
- Encouraging the father or partner to carry or accompany the infant to the nursery for the initial assessment
- Involving the father or partner in postpartal care in the recovery room

After birth the nurse assesses the Apgar score and completes the initial assessment and identification procedures as after a vaginal birth. Every effort must be made to assist the parents in bonding with the infant. If the mother is awake, one of her arms should be freed to enable her to touch and stroke the infant. The baby can be given to the father to hold until she or he must be taken to the nursery. Facilitation of parent-infant interaction following birth is discussed in Chapter 16.

Immediate Postpartal Recovery Period

The physical care of the woman in the immediate recovery period assumes the highest priority, because her physiologic processes need to stabilize after surgery. The recovery room nurse checks the woman's vital signs every 5 minutes until they are stable, then every 15 minutes for an hour, then every 30 minutes until she is discharged to the postpartal floor. The nurse remains with the woman until she is stable.

The dressing and perineal pad must be checked every 15 minutes for at least an hour, and the fundus should be gently palpated to determine whether it is remaining firm. The fundus may be palpated from the side while the incision is supported with the other hand. Oxytocin is usually administered intravenously to promote the contractility of the uterine muscles. If the woman has been under general anesthesia, she should be positioned on her side to facilitate drainage of secretions, turned, and assisted with coughing and deep breathing every 2 hours for at least 24 hours. If she has received a spinal anesthetic, the level of anesthesia should be checked every 15 minutes until sensation has fully returned. The nurse monitors intake and output and observes the urine for bloody tinge, which could mean surgical trauma to the bladder. The physician prescribes medication, which should be administered as needed, to relieve the mother's pain and nausea.

Psychologic aspects of nursing care are also very important. The nurse provides support to the mother through the way that nursing care is organized and communicated. The nurse gives explanations for all assessments, maintains rapport with the couple, and helps with the difficult tasks that are part of this recovery period. If the woman's condition permits (vital signs are stable and the woman is awake), the mother, father (or support person) and infant may spend time together, and the mother may even wish to breastfeed. Women need to be supported in their decisions regarding interactions with support persons and the baby. Some women may wish to be alone and need to devote all their energy to this initial recovery time; others may want other people and the baby with them. These decisions are based on the woman's personal preferences and on the type of anesthesia used. Pertinent areas of nursing care are addressed in the Cesarean Birth Critical Pathway in Chapter 29.

Care of the Woman Undergoing Vaginal Birth After Cesarean Birth (VBAC)

There is an increasing trend to have a trial of labor and vaginal birth after a previous cesarean birth in cases of nonrecurring indications (such as prolapsed cord, placenta previa, or fetal distress). This trend has certainly been influenced by consumers and the goal of decreasing the rate of cesarean births in our country.

The ACOG guidelines (1988) state that the following aspects need to be considered for **vaginal birth after cesarean (VBAC):**

- A woman with one previous cesarean birth and a low transverse uterine incision should be counseled and encouraged to attempt VBAC.
- A woman with two or more previous cesareans may attempt VBAC.
- A classic uterine incision is a contraindication.
- It must be possible to do a cesarean in 30 minutes.
- A physician who is able to do a cesarean must be available.

Support of the laboring woman undergoing VBAC is the same as it would be for any laboring woman. Early ambulation, as well as adequate rest, is also encouraged. Warm baths, showers, and a variety of alternative positions are used to promote comfort.

CHAPTER HIGHLIGHTS

- An external (or cephalic) version may be done after 37 weeks' gestation to change a breech presentation to a cephalic presentation. The benefits of version are that a lower-risk vaginal birth may be anticipated. The version is accomplished with the use of tocolytics to relax the uterus. An internal (podalic) version is used only when needed during the vaginal birth of a second twin.
- Amniotomy (AROM) is performed to hasten labor. The risks are prolapse of the umbilical cord and infection.
- Prostaglandin E_2 may be inserted into the vagina before an induction of labor to soften the cervix (called cervical ripening).
- Indicated induction of labor is done for many reasons. The methods include amniotomy and intravenous oxytocin infusion. Nursing responsibilities are heightened during an induced labor.
- An episiotomy may be done just before birth of the fetus. Although in this country it is very prevalent, it is becoming somewhat controversial.
- Forceps-assisted birth can be accomplished with outlet, low, or midforceps. Outlet forceps are the most common and are associated with few maternal-fetal complications. Midforceps are associated with more complications but, when needed, are an important aid to birth.
- A vacuum extractor is a soft, pliable cup attached to suction that can be applied to the fetal head and used in much the same way as forceps.
- At least 1 in 3–4 births is now accomplished by cesarean. The nurse has a vital role in providing information, support, and encouragement to the couple participating in a cesarean birth.
- Vaginal birth after cesarean (VBAC) is becoming more popular. Overcoming the old fears of uterine rupture is a high priority for both the parents and the medical and nursing community.

REFERENCES

Albers LL et al: Factors related to perineal trauma in childbirth. *J Nurse-Midwifery* July/August 1996; 41:269.

American College of Obstetricians and Gynecologists: *Guidelines for Vaginal Delivery After a Previous Cesarean Birth.* ACOG Committee Opinion No. 64. Washington, DC: Author, October 1988.

American College of Obstetricians and Gynecologists: *Induction and Augmentation of Labor.* Technical Bulletin No. 157. Washington, DC: Author, 1991.

American College of Obstetricians and Gynecologists: *Prostaglandin E Gel for Cervical Ripening.* ACOG Committee Opinion No. 123. Washington, DC: Author, October 1993.

Arias F: *Practical Guide to High-Risk Pregnancy and Delivery.* St Louis: Mosby-Year Book, 1993.

Association of Women's Health, Obstetric, and Neonatal Nurses: *Cervical Ripening and Induction and Augmentation of Labor.* Washington, DC: Author, 1993.

Bachman J, Kendrick JM: Childbirth. In *AWHONN Perinatal Nursing.* Simpson KR, Creehan PA (editors). Philadelphia: Lippincott-Raven, 1996.

Bishop EH: Pelvic scoring for elective inductions. *Obstet Gynecol* 1964; 24:266.

Clarke SC, Taffel SM: Rates of cesarean and VBAC delivery: United States 1994. *Birth* 1996; 23:166.

Crawford LA et al: Incontinence following rupture of the anal sphincter during delivery. *Obstet Gynecol* 1993; 82:527.

Cunningham FG et al: *Williams Obstetrics,* 20th ed. Stamford, CT: Appleton & Lange, 1997.

Day ML, Snell BJ: Use of prostaglandins for induction of labor. *J Nurse-Midwifery* March/April 1993; 38:72S.

Depp R: Cesarean birth. In: *Obstetrics: Normal and Problem Pregnancies,* 3rd ed. Gabbe SG, Niebyl JR, Simpson JL (editors). New York: Churchill Livingstone, 1996.

Dunn LJ: Cesarean section and other obstetric operations. Chapter 31 in: *Danforth's Obstetrics and Gynecology,* 6th ed. Scott JR et al (editors). Philadelphia: Lippincott, 1990.

Forrest Pharmaceuticals Inc. UAD Laboratories St Louis: MO Drug Insert: Cervidil Dinoprostone 10 mg Vaginal Insert. 1995.

Fraser WD, Sokol R: Amniotomy and maternal position in labor. *Clin Obstet Gynecol* 1992; 35:535.

Henriksen TB et al: Episiotomy and perineal lesions in spontaneous vaginal deliveries. *Br J Obstet Gynecol* December 1992; 99:950.

Kochenour NK: Normal pregnancy and prenatal care. In: *Danforth's Obstetrics and Gynecology,* 7th ed. Scott JR et al (editors). Philadelphia: Lippincott, 1994.

Marshall C: The art of induction/augmentation of labor. *JOGNN* January/February 1985; 14:22.

Martin RW, Wiser WL, Morrison JC: Cesarean birth—Surgical techniques. Chapter 83 in: *Gynecology and Obstetrics, Vol. 2.* Dilts PV, Sciarra JJ (editors). Philadelphia: Lippincott, 1993.

Niswander KR, Evans AT: *Manual of Obstetrics.* Boston: Little, Brown, 1991.

O'Brien WF, Cefalo RC: Labor and delivery. In: *Obstetrics: Normal and Problem Pregnancies,* 3rd ed. Gabbe SG, Niebyl JR, Simpson JL (editors). New York: Churchill Livingstone, 1996

Owen J, Hauth JC: Oxytocin for the induction or augmentation of labor. *Clin Obstet Gynecol* 1992; 35:464.

Scott JR et al: *Danforth's Obstetrics and Gynecology,* 7th ed. Philadelphia: Lippincott, 1994.

Trofatter KF: Cervical ripening. *Clin Obstet Gynecol* 1992; 35:476.

Wenstrom K, Andrews WW, Maher JE: Amnioinfusion survey: Prevalence, protocols, and complications. *Obstet Gynecol* 1995; 86:572.

Woolbright LA: Why is the cesarean delivery rate so high in Alabama? An examination of risk factors, 1991–1993. *Birth* March 1996; 23:20.

Woolley RJ: Benefits and risks of episiotomy: A review of the English language literature since 1980. Part II. *Obstet Gynecol Surv* 1996; 50:821.

Zatuchni GI, Slupik RI: *Obstetrics and Gynecology Drug Handbook,* 2nd ed. St Louis: Mosby, 1996.

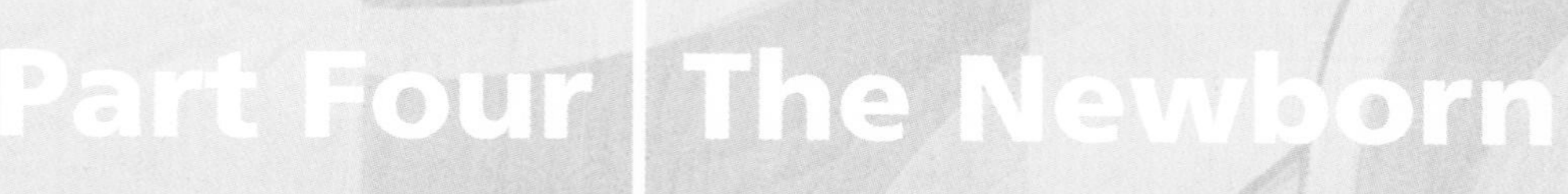

Part Four The Newborn

This moment of meeting seemed to be a birthtime for both of us; her first and my second life. Nothing, I knew, could ever be the same again.

—Laurie Lee, *Two Women*

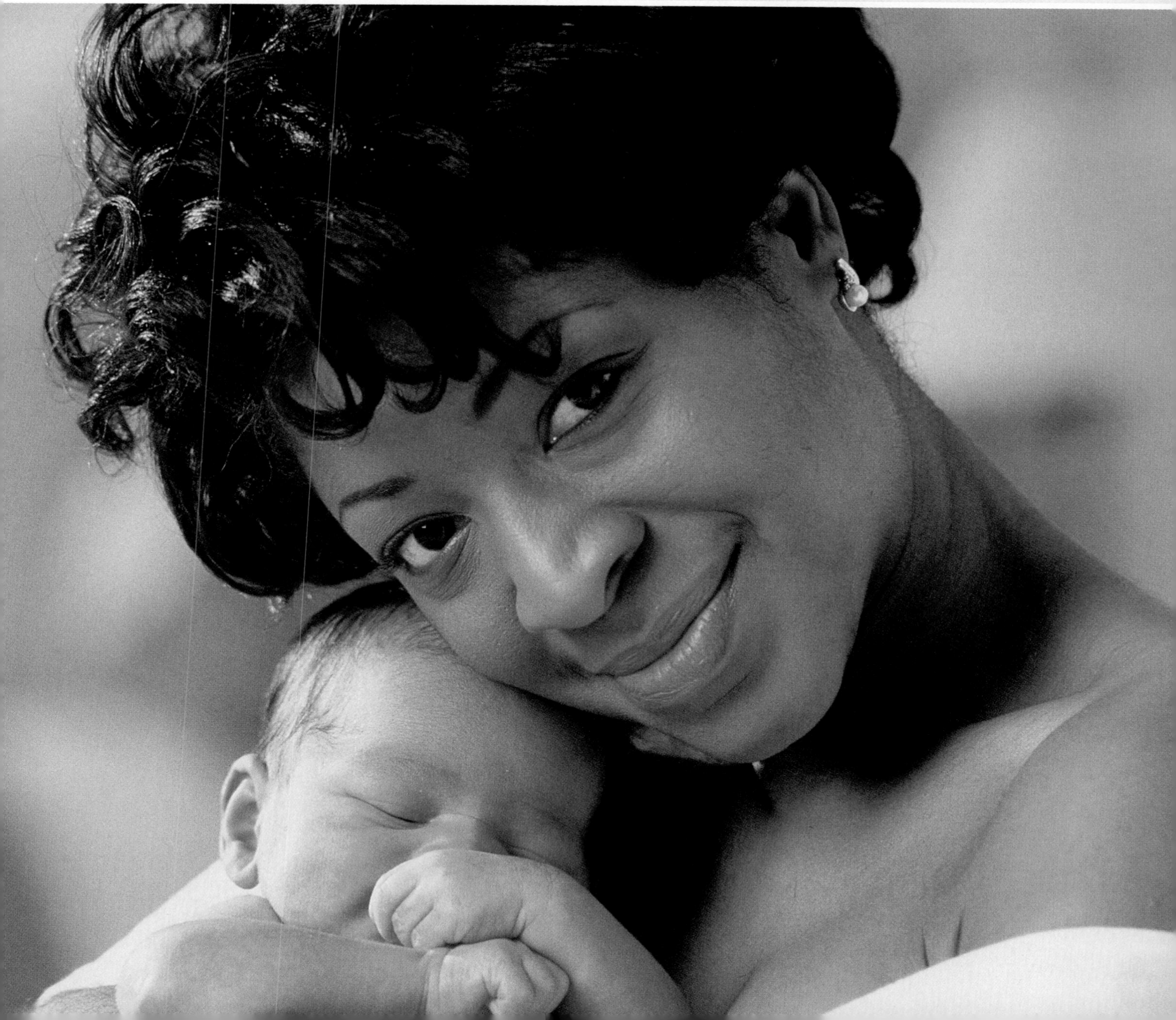

Chapter 21 The Physiologic Responses of the Newborn to Birth

OBJECTIVES

- Summarize the respiratory and cardiovascular changes that occur during the transition to extrauterine life.
- Describe how various factors affect the newborn's blood values.
- Correlate the major mechanisms of heat loss in the newborn to the process the newborn uses to produce heat.
- Explain the steps involved in conjugation and excretion of bilirubin in the newborn.
- Discuss the reasons why the newborn may develop jaundice.
- Describe the functional abilities of the newborn's gastrointestinal tract and liver.
- Identify three reasons why the newborn's kidneys have difficulty in maintaining fluid and electrolyte balance.
- List the immunologic responses available to the newborn.
- Explain the physiologic and behavioral responses of newborns during the periods of reactivity and identify possible interventions.
- Describe the normal sensory/perceptual abilities and behavioral states seen in the newborn period.

KEY TERMS

Active acquired immunity
Brown adipose tissue (BAT)
Cardiopulmonary adaptation
Conduction
Convection
Evaporation
Habituation
Meconium
Neonatal transition
Orientation
Passive acquired immunity
Periodic breathing
Periods of reactivity
Physiologic anemia of infancy
Physiologic jaundice
Radiation
Self-quieting ability
Surfactant
Thermal neutral zone (TNZ)

The newborn period includes the time from birth through the 28th day of life. During this period, the newborn adjusts from intrauterine to extrauterine life. The nurse needs to be knowledgeable about a newborn's normal physiologic and behavioral adaptations and to recognize alterations from normal.

To begin life as a separate being, the newborn must immediately establish respiratory gas exchange in conjunction with marked circulatory changes. These radical and rapid changes are crucial to the maintenance of extrauterine life. The first few hours of life, in which the newborn stabilizes respiratory and circulatory functions, are called **neonatal transition.** All other newborn body systems change their level of functioning and become established over a longer time period.

Respiratory Adaptations

Although significant respiratory events occur at birth, certain intrauterine factors also enhance the newborn's ability to breathe.

Intrauterine Factors Supporting Respiratory Function

Fetal Lung Development

The respiratory system is in a continuous state of development during fetal life, and lung development continues into the newborn period. During the first 20 weeks of gestation, development is limited to the differentiation of pulmonary, vascular, and lymphatic structures.

At 20–24 weeks, alveolar ducts begin to appear, followed by primitive alveoli at 24–28 weeks. During this time, the alveolar epithelial cells begin to differentiate into type I cells (structures necessary for gas exchange) and type II cells (structures that provide for the synthesis and storage of surfactant). **Surfactant** is composed of a group of surface-active phospholipids that are critical for alveolar stability.

At 28–32 weeks of gestation, the number of type II cells increases further, and surfactant is produced by a choline pathway within the type II cells. Surfactant production by this pathway peaks at about 35 weeks of gestation and remains high until term, paralleling late fetal lung development. At this time, the lungs are structurally developed enough to permit maintenance of good lung expansion and adequate exchange of gases.

Clinically, the peak production of lecithin corresponds closely with the marked decrease in incidence of respiratory distress syndrome for babies born after 35 weeks of gestation. Production of sphingomyelin (one component of surfactant) remains constant throughout gestation. The newborn born before the lecithin/sphingomyelin (L/S) ratio is 2:1 will have varying degrees of respiratory distress. (See discussion of L/S ratio in Chapter 26.)

Fetal Breathing Movements

The ability of the newborn to breathe air immediately when exposed to air in the extrauterine environment appears to be the consequence of weeks of intrauterine practice. In this respect, breathing can be perceived as a continuation of an intrauterine process as the lungs convert from a fluid-filled to a gas-filled organ. Fetal breathing movements (FBM) occur as early as 11 weeks' gestation (see Chapter 14 for discussion). These breathing movements are essential for developing the chest wall muscles and the diaphragm and, to a lesser extent, for regulating lung fluid volume and resultant lung growth.

Initiation of Breathing

To maintain life, the lungs must function immediately after birth. Two radical changes must take place for the lungs to function:

1. Pulmonary ventilation is established through lung expansion after birth.
2. Pulmonary circulation must increase markedly.

The first breath of life—the gasp in response to mechanical, chemical, thermal, and sensory changes associated with birth—initiates the serial opening of the alveoli. Thus begins the transition from a fluid-filled environment to an air-breathing, independent, extrauterine life. Figure 21–1 summarizes the initiation of respiration.

Mechanical Events

During the latter half of gestation, the fetal lungs produce fluid continuously. This fluid expands the lungs almost completely, filling the air spaces. Some of the lung fluid moves up into the trachea and into the amniotic fluid and is then swallowed by the fetus.

Production of lung fluid diminishes 2–4 days before onset of labor (Eden and Boehm 1990). However, approximately 80–110 mL of fluid remains in the respiratory passages of a normal full-term fetus at birth. This fluid must be removed from the lungs to permit adequate movement of air.

The primary mechanical events that initiate respiration involve the removal of fluid from the lungs as the fetus passes through the birth canal. During the birth process the fetal chest is compressed, increasing intrathoracic pressure, and approximately one-third of the

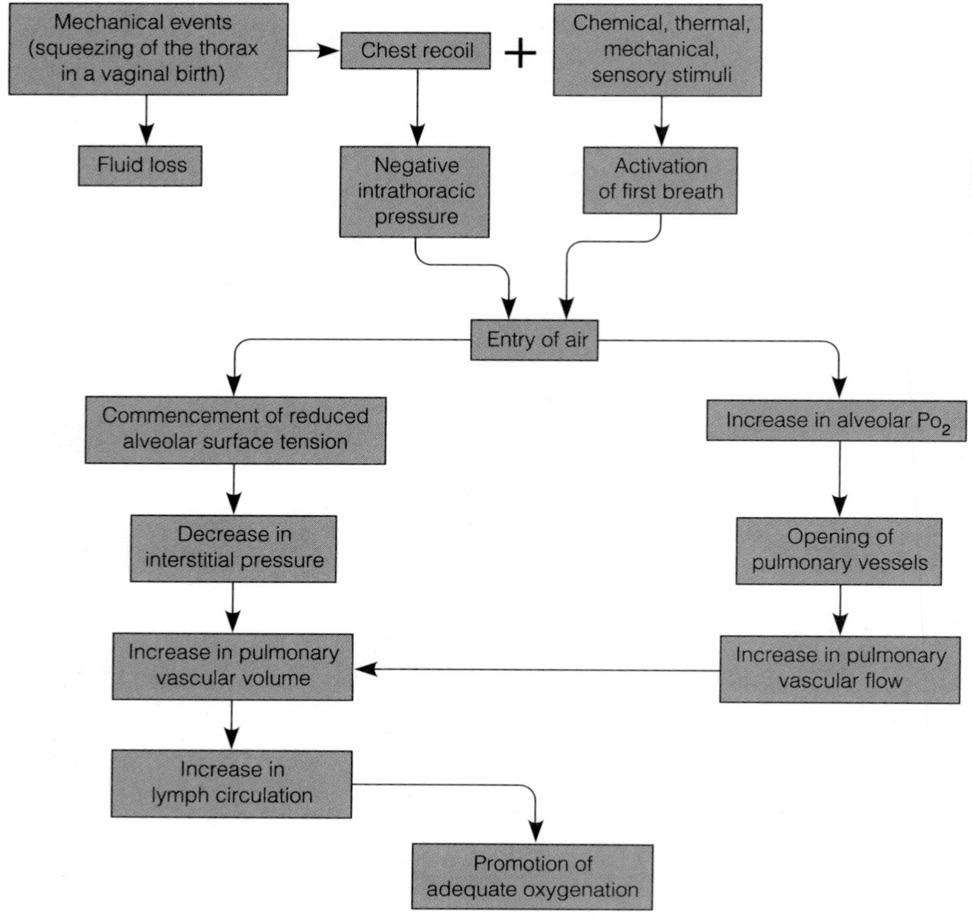

FIGURE 21–1 Initiation of respiration in the newborn.

fluid is squeezed out of the lungs. After the birth of the newborn's trunk, the chest wall recoils. This chest recoil creates a negative intrathoracic pressure which is thought to produce a small, passive inspiration of air that replaces the squeezed-out fluid. After this first inspiration, the newborn exhales, with crying, against a partially closed glottis, creating a positive intrathoracic pressure. The high positive intrathoracic pressure distributes the inspired air throughout the alveoli and begins the establishment of *functional residual capacity (FRC)*. The higher intrathoracic pressure also increases absorption of fluid via the capillaries and lymphatic system. The negative intrathoracic pressure resulting from downward movement of the diaphragm with inspiration causes lung fluid to flow from the alveoli across the alveolar membranes into the pulmonary interstitial tissue.

With each succeeding breath, the lungs expand. Since the protein concentration is higher in the pulmonary capillaries, oncotic pressure draws the interstitial fluid into the capillaries and lymphatic system. As pulmonary vascular resistance decreases, pulmonary blood flow increases, and more fluid is absorbed into the bloodstream. In the normal term newborn, movement of lung fluid to the interstitial tissue is rapid, but movement into lymph and blood vessels may take several hours. About 80 percent of the alveoli fluid is absorbed within 2 hours after birth, and it is completely absorbed within 12 to 24 hours of birth.

Although the initial chest compression and recoil should clear the airways of accumulated fluid and permit further inspiration, some clinicians feel it is wise to suction mucus and fluid from the newborn's mouth and oropharynx. They use a mucus trap attached to suction as soon as the newborn's head and shoulders are born and again as the newborn adapts to extrauterine life and stabilizes (see Procedure 17–1, and Chapter 17).

A variety of factors may cause problems associated with lung fluid clearance and initiation of respiratory activity. The lymphatic system may be underdeveloped, thus decreasing the rate at which the fluid is absorbed from the lungs. Complications that occur antenatally or during labor and birth can interfere with adequate lung expansion, causing failure to decrease pulmonary vascular resistance and thus decreasing blood flow. These complications include inadequate compression of the chest wall in a very small newborn, the absence of chest wall compression in the newborn delivered by cesarean birth, severe asphyxia at birth, respiratory depression due to maternal anesthesia, or aspiration of amniotic fluid or meconium.

Chemical Stimuli

An important chemical stimulator that contributes to the onset of breathing is transitory asphyxia of the fetus and newborn. The first breath is an inspiratory gasp triggered by elevation in PCO_2 and decrease in pH and PO_2, which are the natural outcomes of a normal vaginal birth with cessation of placental gas exchange when the cord is clamped. These changes, which are present in all newborns to some degree, stimulate the aortic and carotid chemoreceptors, initiating impulses that trigger the medulla's respiratory center. Although brief periods of asphyxia are a significant stimulator, prolonged asphyxia is abnormal and acts as a CNS respiratory depressant.

Thermal Stimuli

The significant decrease in environmental temperature after birth (from 98.6F to 70–75F, or 37C to 21–23.9C) is enough thermal stimulus to initiate breathing. The cold stimulates skin nerve endings, and the newborn responds with rhythmic respirations. Normal temperature changes that occur at birth are apparently within acceptable physiologic limits. Excessive cooling may result in profound depression and evidence of cold stress (see Chapter 26 for discussion of cold stress).

Sensory Stimuli

As the fetus moves from a familiar, comfortable, quiet environment to one of sensory abundance, a number of physical and sensory influences help respiration begin. They include the numerous tactile, auditory, and visual stimuli of birth. Historically, vigorous stimulation was provided by slapping the buttocks or heels of the newborn, but the emphasis today is on gentle physical contact. Thoroughly drying the newborn and placing it in skin-to-skin contact with the mother's chest and abdomen provides ample stimulation in a far more comforting way and also decreases heat loss.

Factors Opposing the First Breath

Three major factors may oppose the initiation of respiratory activity: (1) alveolar surface tension, (2) viscosity of lung fluid within the respiratory tract, and (3) degree of lung compliance.

The contracting force between the moist surfaces of the alveoli is called *alveolar surface tension.* This tension, which is necessary for healthy respiratory function, would nevertheless cause the small airways and alveoli to collapse between each inspiration were it not for the presence of surfactant. By reducing the attracting force between alveoli, surfactant prevents the alveoli from completely collapsing with each expiration and thus promotes lung expansion. Similarly, surfactant promotes lung *compliance,* the ability of the lung to fill with air easily. When surfactant decreases, compliance also decreases, and the pressure needed to expand the alveoli with air increases. Resistive forces of the fluid-filled lung, combined with the small radii of the airways, necessitate pressures of 20–25 cm of water to open the lung initially (James and Adamsons 1994). The first breath usually establishes an FRC that is 30 to 40 percent of the fully expanded lung volume. This FRC allows alveolar sacs to remain partially expanded on expiration. The remaining air in the lung after expiration or FRC decreases the need for continuous high pressures for each of the following breaths. Subsequent breaths require only 6–8 cm H_2O pressure to open alveoli during inspiration. Therefore, the first breath of life is usually the most difficult.

Cardiopulmonary Physiology

The onset of respiration stimulates changes in the cardiovascular system that are necessary for successful transition to extrauterine life, hence the term **cardiopulmonary adaptation.** As air enters the lungs, PO_2 rises in the alveoli, which stimulates the relaxation of the pulmonary arteries and triggers a decrease in the pulmonary vascular resistance. As pulmonary vascular resistance decreases, the vascular flow in the lung increases to 100 percent at 24 hours of life. This movement of greater blood volume to the lungs contributes to the conversion from fetal circulation to newborn circulation. After pulmonary circulation is established, blood is distributed throughout the lung, although the alveoli may or may not be fully open. For adequate oxygenation to occur, the heart must deliver sufficient blood to functional, open alveoli. Shunting of blood is common in the early newborn period. Bidirectional blood flow, or right-to-left shunting through the ductus arteriosus, may divert a significant amount of blood away from the lungs, depending on the pressure changes of respiration, crying, and the cardiac cycle. This shunting in the newborn period is also responsible for the unstable transitional period in cardiopulmonary function.

Oxygen Transport

The transportation of oxygen to the peripheral tissues depends on the type of hemoglobin in the red blood cells. In the fetus and newborn, a variety of hemoglobins exist, the most significant being fetal hemoglobin (Hb F) and adult hemoglobin (Hb A). Approximately 70 to 90 percent of the hemoglobin in the fetus and newborn is of the fetal variety. The greatest difference between Hb F and Hb A is related to the transport of oxygen.

Since Hb F has a greater affinity for oxygen than Hb A, the oxygen saturation in the newborn's blood is greater than in the adult's, but the amount of oxygen available to the tissues is less. This is beneficial prenatally, because the fetus must maintain adequate oxygen uptake in the presence of very low oxygen tension (umbilical venous PO_2 cannot exceed the uterine venous PO_2). Because of this high concentration of oxygen in the blood, hypoxia in the newborn is particularly difficult to recognize. Clinical manifestations of cyanosis do not appear until low blood levels of oxygen are present. In addition, alkalosis (increased pH) and hypothermia can result in less oxygen being available to the body tissues, whereas acidosis, hypercarbia, and hyperthermia can result in less oxygen being bound to hemoglobin and more oxygen being released to the body tissues.

Maintaining Respiratory Function

The ability of the lung to maintain oxygen (oxygenation) and carbon dioxide exchange (ventilation) is influenced by such factors as lung compliance and airway resistance. Lung compliance is influenced by the elastic recoil of the lung tissue and by anatomic differences in the newborn. The newborn has a relatively large heart, as well as mediastinal structures that reduce available lung space. Anatomically the newborn chest is equipped with weak intercostal muscles and a rigid rib cage with horizontal ribs and a high diaphragm that restricts the space available for lung expansion. The newborn's large abdomen further encroaches on the high diaphragm to decrease lung space. Ventilation is also limited by airway resistance, which depends on the radii, length, and number of airways.

Characteristics of Newborn Respiration

The normal newborn respiratory rate is 30–60 breaths per minute. Initial respirations may be largely diaphragmatic and shallow and irregular in depth and rhythm. The abdomen's movements are synchronous with the chest movements. When the breathing pattern is characterized by pauses lasting 5–15 seconds, **periodic breathing** is occurring. Periodic breathing is rarely associated with differences in skin color or heart rate changes, and it does not have prognostic significance. Tactile or other sensory stimulation increases the inspired oxygen and converts periodic breathing patterns to normal breathing patterns during neonatal transition. Newborn sleep states in particular influence respiratory patterns. With deep sleep, the pattern is reasonably regular. Periodic breathing occurs with rapid-eye-movement (REM) sleep, and grossly irregular breathing is evident with motor activity, sucking, and crying. Cessation of breathing lasting more than 20 seconds is defined as *apnea* and is abnormal in term newborns. Apnea may or may not be associated with changes in skin color or heart rate (drop below 100 beats per minute). Apnea always needs to be further evaluated.

The newborn is an obligatory nose breather, and any obstruction will cause respiratory distress, so it is important to keep the throat and nose clear. Immediately after birth, and for about 2 hours after birth, respiratory rates of 60–70 breaths per minute are normal. Some cyanosis and acrocyanosis are normal for several hours; thereafter the infant's color improves steadily. If respirations drop below 30 or exceed 60 per minute when the infant is at rest, or if retractions, cyanosis, or nasal flaring and expiratory grunting occur, the clinician should be notified. Any increased use of the intercostal muscles (retractions) may indicate respiratory distress. (See Chapter 26 and Table 26–1 for signs of respiratory distress.)

Cardiovascular Adaptations

As described earlier, blood flow to the lungs increases after the first respirations of the normal newborn. This greater blood volume contributes to the conversion from fetal circulation to neonatal circulation.

TABLE 21–1 Fetal and Neonatal Circulation

System	Fetal	Neonatal
Pulmonary blood vessels	Constricted with very little blood flow; lungs not expanded	Vasodilation and increased blood flow; lungs expanded; increased oxygen stimulates vasodilation.
Systemic blood vessels	Dilated with low resistance; blood mostly in placenta	Arterial pressure rises due to loss of placenta; increased systemic blood volume and resistance.
Ductus arteriosus	Large with no tone; blood flow from pulmonary artery to aorta	Reversal of blood flow. Now from aorta to pulmonary artery due to increased left atrial pressure. Ductus is sensitive to increased oxygen and body chemicals and begins to constrict.
Foramen ovale	Patent with large blood flow from right atrium to left atrium	Increased pressure in left atrium attempts to reverse blood flow and shuts one-way valve.

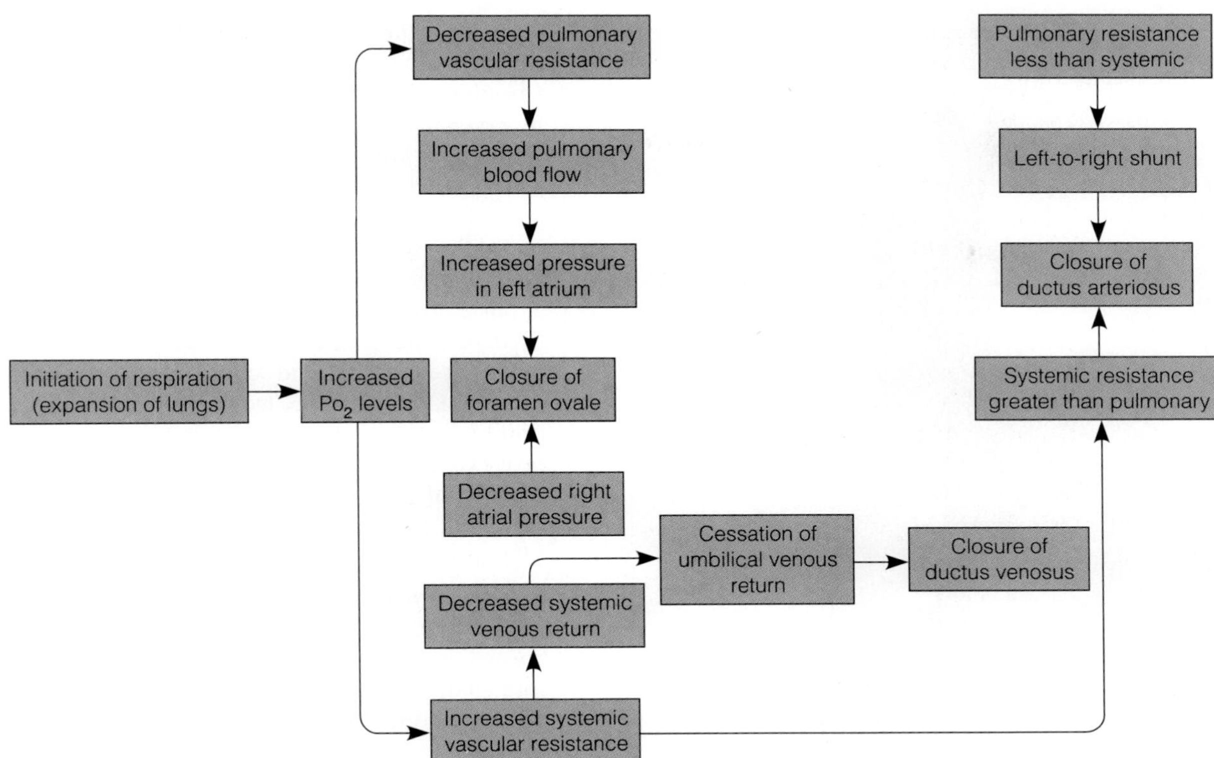

FIGURE 21–2 Transitional circulation: conversion from fetal to neonatal circulation.

Fetal-Neonatal Transitional Physiology

During fetal life, blood with higher oxygen content is diverted to the heart and brain. Blood in the descending aorta is less oxygenated and supplies the kidney and intestinal tract before it is returned to the placenta. Limited amounts of blood, pumped from the right ventricle toward the lungs, enter the pulmonary vessels. In the fetus, increased pulmonary resistance forces most of this blood through the ductus arteriosus into the descending aorta (see Table 21–1).

Marked changes occur in the cardiovascular system at birth. Expansion of the lungs with the first breath decreases pulmonary vascular resistance and increases pulmonary blood flow. Left atrial pressure increases as blood returns from the pulmonary veins. Right atrial pressure drops, and systematic vascular resistance increases as umbilical venous blood flow halts when the cord is clamped. These physiologic mechanisms mark the transition from fetal to neonatal circulation and show the interplay of cardiovascular and respiratory systems (Figure 21–2) (Sansoucie and Cavaliere 1995). Five major areas of change occur in cardiopulmonary adaptation (Figure 21–3):

1. *Increased aortic pressure and decreased venous pressure.* The cutting of the cord eliminates the placental vascular bed and reduces the intravascular space. Consequently, aortic (systemic) blood pressure increases. At the same time, blood return via the inferior vena cava decreases, resulting in a decreased right atrial pressure and a small decrease in pressure within the venous circulation.
2. *Increased systemic pressure and decreased pulmonary artery pressure.* With the loss of the low-resistance placenta, pressure increases in the systemic circulation, resulting in greater systemic resistance. At the same time, lung expansion promotes increased pulmonary blood flow, and the increased blood Po_2 associated with initiation of respirations produces vasodilation of pulmonary blood vessels. The combination of increased pulmonary blood flow and vasodilation decreases pulmonary artery resistance. As a result of opening the pulmonary vascular beds, the systemic vascular pressure increases, enhancing perfusion of the other body systems.
3. *Closure of the foramen ovale.* Closure of the foramen ovale is a function of atrial pressures. In utero, blood flow and pressure are greater in the right atrium, and the foramen ovale is open. After birth, decreased pulmonary resistance and increased pulmonary blood flow increase the pulmonary venous

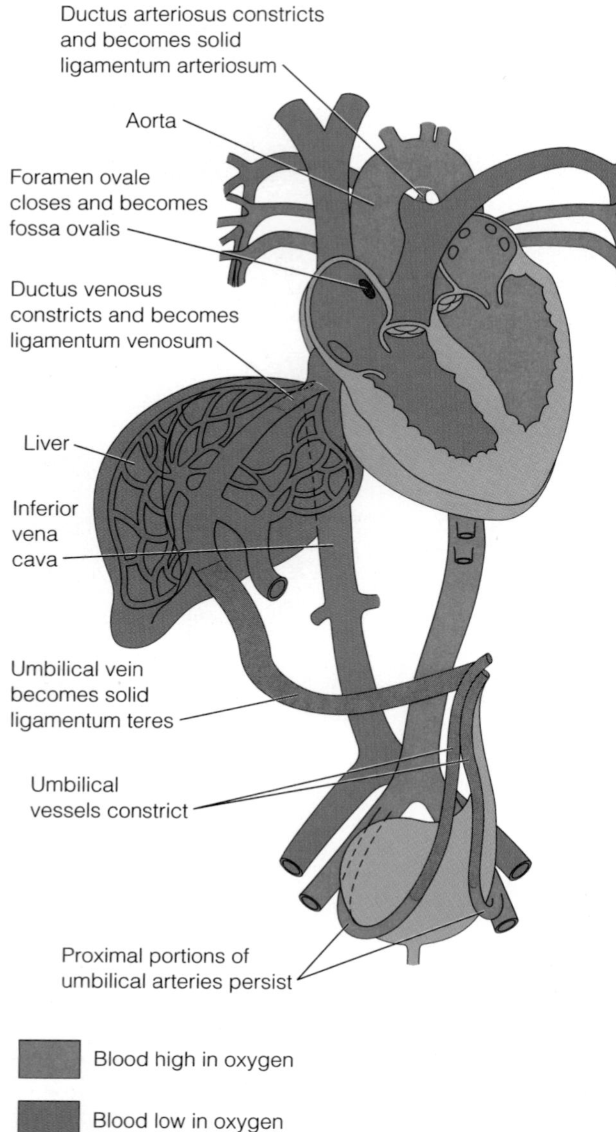

FIGURE 21–3 Major changes that occur in the newborn's circulatory system.

Source: Hole JW: *Human Anatomy and Physiology,* 6th ed. Dubuque, IA: WC Brown, 1993.

return into the left atrium, thereby increasing left atrial pressure slightly. The decreased pulmonary vascular resistance also decreases right atrial pressure. The pressure gradients are now reversed, left atrial pressure is greater, and the foramen ovale is functionally closed 1–2 hours after birth. However, a slight right-to-left shunting may occur in the early newborn period. Any increase in pulmonary resistance or right atrial pressure, such as occurs with crying, hypothermia, or acidosis, may result in reopening of the foramen ovale, causing a right-to-left shunt. Permanent closure occurs within 6 months.

4. *Closure of the ductus arteriosus.* Initial elevation of the systemic vascular pressure above the pulmonary vascular pressure increases pulmonary blood flow by reversing the flow through the ductus arteriosus. Blood now flows from the aorta into the pulmonary artery. Furthermore, although the presence of oxygen dilates the pulmonary arterioles, an increase in blood Po_2 triggers the opposite response in the ductus arteriosus—it constricts.

   In utero, the placenta provides prostaglandin E_2 (PGE_2), which causes ductus vasodilation. With the loss of the placenta and increased pulmonary blood flow, PGE_2 levels drop, leaving the active constriction by Po_2 unopposed. If the lungs fail to expand or if Po_2 levels drop, the ductus remains patent. Fibrosis of the ductus occurs within 3 weeks after birth, but functional closure is accomplished within 15 hours after birth (Nelson 1994, Long 1990).
5. *Closure of the ductus venosus.* Although the mechanism initiating closure of the ductus venosus is not known, it appears to be related to mechanical pressure changes after severing of the cord, redistribution of blood, and cardiac output. Closure of the bypass forces perfusion of the liver. Anatomic fibrosis occurs within 2 months (Long 1990).

Characteristics of Cardiac Function

Heart Rate

Shortly after the first cry and the beginning of changes in cardiopulmonary circulation, the newborn heart rate accelerates to 175–180 beats per minute. The average resting heart rate in the first week of life is 125–130 beats per minute in a quiet, full-term newborn (Fanaroff and Martin 1992). The range of the heart rate in the full-term newborn is 100 beats per minute while asleep and 120–160 while awake. Resting heart rates as low as 85–90 and rates above 180 while crying are sometimes seen (Taeusch et al 1991). Apical pulse rates should be obtained by auscultation for a full minute, preferably when the newborn is asleep. Peripheral pulses of all extremities should also be evaluated to detect any inequalities or unusual characteristics.

Blood Pressure

The blood pressure tends to be highest immediately after birth and descends to its lowest level at about 3 hours of age. By days 4 to 6 of life, the blood pressure rises and plateaus at a level approximately the same as the initial level. Blood pressure is particularly sensitive to the changes in blood volume that occur in the transition to newborn circulation (Figure 21–4). Capillary refill should be less than 2–3 seconds when the skin is blanched.

Blood pressure values during the first 12 hours of life vary with the birth weight. In the full-term, resting newborn, the average blood pressure is 72/47 mm Hg; in the preterm newborn, it averages 64/39 mm Hg (Fanaroff and Martin 1997). Crying may cause an elevation of 20 mm Hg in both the systolic and diastolic blood pressure, so accurate measurement is more likely in the quiet newborn. The best way to measure blood pressure is to use the Doppler technique or a 1- to 2-inch cuff and a stethoscope over the brachial artery.

Heart Murmurs

Murmurs are produced by turbulent blood flow. Murmurs may be heard when blood flows across an abnormal valve or across a stenosed valve, when there is an atrial or ventricular septal defect, or when there is increased flow across a normal valve. In newborns, 90 percent of all murmurs are transient and not associated with anomalies. With early discharge, murmurs associated with ventricular septal defect and patent ductus arteriosus are not being picked up until the first well-baby checkup at 4–6 weeks of age. Murmurs are sometimes absent even in seriously malformed hearts (Fletcher 1994).

Cardiac Workload

Before birth the right ventricle does approximately two-thirds of the cardiac work, resulting in increased size and thickness of the right ventricle at birth. After birth the left ventricle must assume a larger share of the cardiac workload, and it progressively increases in size and thickness (Blackburn and Loper 1992). This may explain why right sided heart defects are better tolerated than left sided ones and why left sided heart defects rapidly become symptomatic after birth.

Hematopoietic System

Fetal erythrocytes are large but few in number. After birth, the red blood cell (RBC) count gradually increases as cell size decreases. Neonatal RBCs have a life span of 80–100 days, approximately two-thirds the life span of an adult's RBC. About 5 percent of neonatal RBCs retain their nucleus. In the first days of life, hematocrit may rise 1–2 g/dL above fetal levels as a result of placental transfusion, low oral fluid intake, and diminished extracellular fluid volume. By 1 week postnatally, peripheral hemoglobin is comparable to fetal blood counts. The hemoglobin level declines progressively over the first 2 to 3 months of life (Polin and Fox 1992). This initial decline in hemoglobin creates a phenomenon known as **physiologic anemia of infancy.**

Leukocytosis is a normal finding, because the stress of birth stimulates increased production of neutrophils during the first few days of life. Neutrophils then decrease to 35 percent of the total leukocyte count by 2 weeks of age. Eventually, lymphocytes become the predominant type of leukocyte and the total white blood count falls.

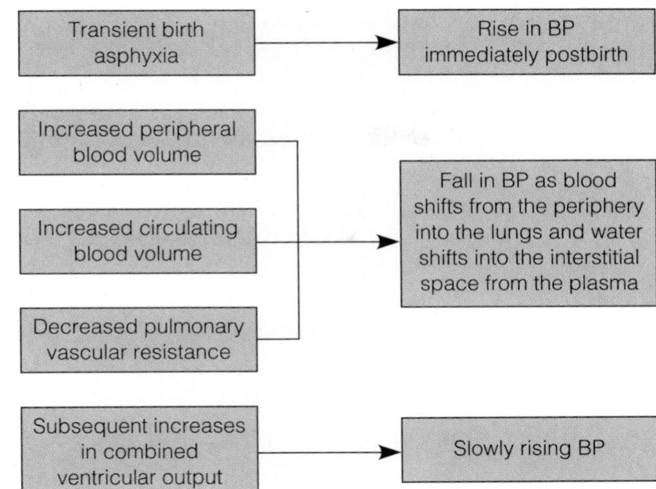

FIGURE 21–4 Response of blood pressure (BP) to neonatal changes in blood volume.

Blood volume of the term infant is estimated to be 80–85 mL/kg of body weight. For example, an 8 lb (3.6 kg) newborn has a blood volume of 290–309 mL. Blood volume varies, based on the amount of placental transfusion received during the delivery of the placenta, as well as other factors, including the following:

1. *Delayed cord clamping and the normal shift of plasma to the extravascular spaces.* Newborn hemoglobin and hematocrit values are higher when a placental transfusion occurs after birth. Placental vessels contain about 100 mL of blood at term, most of which can be transfused into the newborn by holding the newborn below the level of the placenta and delaying clamping of the cord. Blood volume increases by 50 percent with delayed cord clamping (Polin and Fox 1992). The increase is reflected by a rise in hemoglobin level and an increase in the hematocrit to about 65 percent after birth (compared with 48 percent when the cord is clamped immediately). For greatest accuracy, the initial hemoglobin and hematocrit levels should be measured in the cord blood, although this is not a routine practice.
2. *Gestational age.* There appears to be a positive association between gestational age, red blood cell numbers, and hemoglobin concentration.
3. *Prenatal and/or perinatal hemorrhage.* Significant prenatal or perinatal bleeding decreases the hematocrit level and causes hypovolemia.

TABLE 21–2 Normal Term Newborn Blood Values

Laboratory Data	Normal Range
Hemoglobin	15–20 g/dL
Hematocrit	43%–61%
WBC	10,000–30,000/mm^3
Neutrophils	40%–80%
Immature WBC	3%–10%
Platelets	100,000–280,000/mm^3
Reticulocytes	3%–6%
Blood volume	82.3 mL/kg (third day after early cord clamping)
	92.6 mL/kg (third day after delayed cord clamping)
Sodium	124–156 mmol/L
Potassium	5.3–7.3 mmol/L
Chloride	90–111 mmol/L
Calcium	7.3–9.2 mg/dL
Glucose	40–97 mg/dL

4. *The site of the blood sample.* Hemoglobin and hematocrit levels taken simultaneously are significantly higher in capillary blood than in venous blood. Sluggish peripheral blood flow creates red blood cell stasis, thereby increasing their concentration in the capillaries. Because of this, blood samples taken from venous blood sites are more accurate.

The concentration of serum electrolytes in the blood indicates the fluid and electrolyte status of the newborn. See Table 21–2 for normal term newborn electrolyte and blood values.

Temperature Regulation

Temperature regulation is the maintenance of thermal balance by the loss of heat to the environment at a rate equal to the production of heat. Newborns are *homeothermic;* they attempt to stabilize their internal body temperatures within a narrow range in spite of significant temperature variations in their environment.

Thermoregulation in the newborn is closely related to the rate of metabolism and oxygen consumption. Within a specific environmental temperature range, called the **thermal neutral zone (TNZ),** the rates of oxygen consumption and metabolism are minimal, and internal body temperature is maintained (Table 21–3). For an unclothed, full-term newborn, the TNZ is an ambient environmental temperature range of 32–34C (89.6–93.2F). The limits for an adult are 26–28C (78.8–82.4F) (Polin and Fox 1992). Thus the normal newborn requires higher environmental temperatures to maintain a thermal neutral environment.

Several newborn characteristics affect the establishment of a TNZ:

- The newborn has decreased subcutaneous fat and a thin epidermis.
- Blood vessels are closer to the skin than those of an adult. Therefore, the circulating blood is influenced by changes in environmental temperature, and in turn influences the hypothalamic temperature-regulating center.
- The flexed posture of the term newborn decreases the surface area exposed to the environment, thereby reducing heat loss.

Size and age may also affect the establishment of a TNZ. For example, preterm, small-for-gestational-age (SGA) newborns require higher environmental temperatures to achieve a thermal neutral environment, while larger, well-insulated newborns may be able to cope with lower environmental temperature. If the environmental temperature falls below the lower limits of the TNZ, the newborn responds with increased oxygen consumption and metabolism, which results in greater heat production. Prolonged exposure to the cold may result in depleted glycogen stores and acidosis. Oxygen consumption also increases if the environmental temperature is above the TNZ.

Heat Loss

A newborn is at a distinct disadvantage in maintaining a normal temperature. With a larger body surface in relation to mass, and a limited amount of insulating subcutaneous fat, the newborn loses about four times the heat of an adult (Cunningham et al 1997). The newborn's poor thermal stability is primarily due to excessive heat loss, rather than impaired heat production. Because of the risk of hypothermia and possible cold stress, minimizing heat loss in the newborn after birth is essential (see Chapter 17 and Chapter 23 for nursing measures).

Two major routes of heat loss are from the internal core of the body to the body surface and from the external surface to the environment. Usually the core temperature is higher than the skin temperature, resulting in continuous transfer of heat to the surface (Fanaroff and Martin 1997). The greater the difference in temperature between core and skin, the more rapid the transfer. Heat loss from the body surface to the environment takes place in four ways—convection, radiation, evaporation, and conduction (Figure 21–5, p 508).

- **Convection** is the loss of heat from the warm body surface to the cooler air currents. Air-conditioned rooms, air currents with a temperature below the infant's skin temperature, oxygen by mask, and

TABLE 21–3 Neutral Thermal Environmental Temperatures

Age and Weight	Range of Temperature (C)
0–6 Hours	
Under 1200 g	34.0–35.4
1200–1500 g	33.9–34.4
1501–2500 g	32.8–33.8
Over 2500 (and >36 weeks)	32.0–33.8
6–12 Hours	
Under 1200 g	34.0–35.4
1200–1500 g	33.5–34.4
1501–2500 g	32.2–33.8
Over 2500 (and >36 weeks)	31.4–33.8
12–24 Hours	
Under 1200 g	34.0–35.4
1200–1500 g	33.3–34.3
1501–2500 g	31.8–33.8
Over 2500 (and >36 weeks)	31.0–33.7
24–36 Hours	
Under 1200 g	34.0–35.0
1200–1500 g	33.1–34.2
1501–2500 g	31.6–33.6
Over 2500 (and >36 weeks)	30.7–33.5
36–48 Hours	
Under 1200 g	34.0–35.0
1200–1500 g	33.0–34.1
1501–2500 g	31.4–33.5
Over 2500 (and >36 weeks)	30.5–33.3
48–72 Hours	
Under 1200 g	34.0–35.0
1200–1500 g	33.0–34.0
1501–2500 g	31.2–33.4
Over 2500 (and >36 weeks)	30.1–33.2
72–96 Hours	
Under 1200 g	34.0–35.0
1200–1500 g	33.0–34.0
1501–2500 g	31.1–33.2
Over 2500 (and >36 weeks)	29.8–32.8
4–12 Days	
Under 1500 g	33.0–34.0
1501–2500 g	31.0–33.2
Over 2500 (and >36 weeks)	
4–5 days	29.5–32.6
5–6 days	29.4–32.3
6–8 days	29.0–32.2
8–10 days	29.0–31.8
10–12 days	29.0–31.4
12–14 Days	
Under 1500 g	32.6–34.0
1500–2500 g	31.0–33.2
Over 2500 (and >36 weeks)	29.0–30.8
2–3 Weeks	
Under 1500 g	32.2–34.0
1500–2500 g	30.5–33.0
3–4 Weeks	
Under 1500 g	31.6–33.6
1500–2500 g	30.0–32.7
4–5 Weeks	
Under 1500 g	31.2–33.0
1500–2500 g	29.5–32.2
5–6 Weeks	
Under 1500 g	30.6–32.3
1500–2500 g	29.0–31.8

*Generally speaking, the smaller infants in each weight group will require a temperature in the higher portion of the temperature range. Within each time range, the younger the infant, the higher the temperature required.

Source: Adapted from Scopes and Ahmed (1966). (For his table Scopes had the walls of the incubator 1–2 degrees warmer than the ambient air temperatures.) Reproduced, with permission, from Klaus MH, Fanaroff, AA: *Care of the High-Risk Neonate,* 3rd ed. Philadelphia: Saunders, 1986, p 103.

removal from an incubator for procedures increase convective heat loss in the newborn.

- **Radiation** losses occur when heat transfers from the heated body surface to cooler surfaces and objects not in direct contact with the body. The walls of a room or of an incubator are potential causes of heat loss by radiation, even if the ambient temperature of the incubator is within the thermal neutral range for that infant. Placing cold objects (such as ice for blood gases) onto the incubator or near the infant in the radiant warmer will increase radiant losses.
- **Evaporation** is the loss of heat incurred when water is converted to a vapor. The newborn is particularly prone to lose heat by evaporation immediately after birth when wet with amniotic fluid, and during baths; therefore, drying the newborn is critical.
- **Conduction** is the loss of heat to a cooler surface by direct skin contact. Chilled hands, cool scales, cold examination tables, and cold stethoscopes can cause loss of heat by conduction.

Once the infant has been dried after birth, the highest losses of heat generally result from radiation and convection because of the newborn's large body surface compared with weight, and from thermal conduction because of the marked difference between core temperature and skin temperature. The newborn can respond to the cooler environmental temperature with adequate peripheral vasoconstriction, but this mechanism is less effective because of the minimal amount of fat insulation present, the large body surface, and ongoing thermal conduction. Because of these factors, minimizing the baby's heat loss and preventing hypothermia are imperative. (See Chapter 26 for nursing measures to prevent hypothermia and cold stress.)

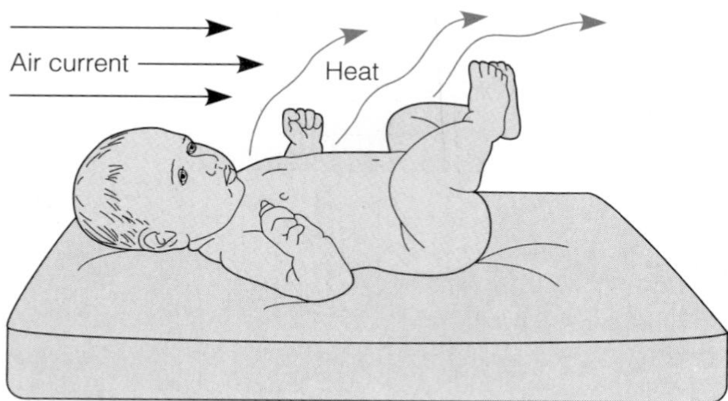

A Convection

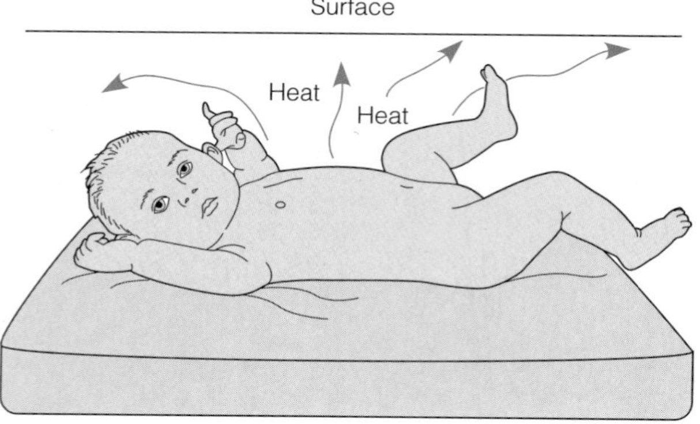

B Radiation

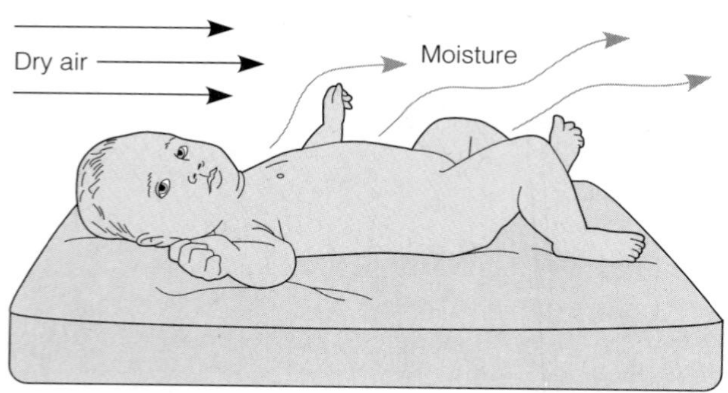

C Evaporation

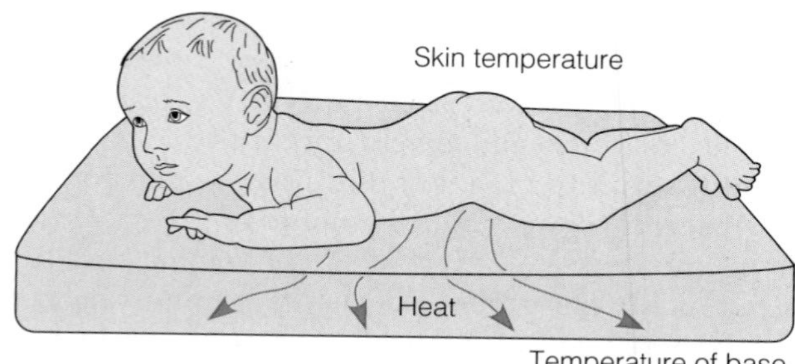

D Conduction

FIGURE 21–5 Methods of heat loss.

Heat Production (Thermogenesis)

When exposed to a cool environment, the newborn requires additional heat. The newborn has several physiologic mechanisms that increase heat production, or *thermogenesis*. These include increased basal metabolic rate, muscular activity, and chemical thermogenesis (also called *nonshivering thermogenesis*) (Hey 1994).

Nonshivering thermogenesis (NST), an important mechanism of heat production unique to the newborn, occurs when skin receptors perceive a drop in the environmental temperature and, in response, transmit sensations to the central nervous system, which in turn stimulates the sympathetic nervous system. NST uses the infant's stores of **brown adipose tissue (BAT)** (also called *brown fat*) as the primary source of heat in the cold-stressed newborn. It first appears in the fetus at about 26–30 weeks of gestation and continues to increase until 2–5 weeks after the birth of a term infant, unless the fat is depleted by cold stress. BAT is deposited in the midscapular area, around the neck, and in the axillas, with deeper placement around the trachea, esophagus, abdominal aorta, kidneys, and adrenal glands (Figure 21–6). BAT constitutes 2 to 6 percent of the newborn's total body weight.

Brown fat receives its name from the dark color caused by its enriched blood supply. It has a dense cellular content and abundant nerve endings. The large numbers of brown fat cells increase the speed with which triglycerides are metabolized to produce heat. In addition, brown fat's rich blood supply enhances distribution of heat throughout the body, and its nerve supply initiates metabolic activity.

Shivering is rarely seen in the newborn, although it has been observed at ambient temperatures of 15C (59F) or less (Polin and Fox 1992). If shivering does appear, it means the newborn's metabolic rate has already doubled, and the extra muscular activity does little to produce needed heat.

Thermographic studies of newborns exposed to cold show an increase in the skin heat over the newborn's brown fat deposits between 1 and 14 days of age. If the brown fat supply has been depleted, the metabolic response to cold will be limited or lacking. An increase in basal metabolism as a result of hypothermia results in an increase in oxygen consumption. A decrease in the environmental temperature of 2C, from 33C to 31C, is a drop sufficient to double the oxygen consumption of a term newborn. Keeping the normal newborn warm promotes normal oxygen requirements, while chilling can cause the newborn to show signs of respiratory distress.

Hypoxia, and the effect of certain drugs such as meperidine (Demerol), may prevent metabolism of brown fat. Meperidine given to the laboring woman leads to a greater fall in the newborn's body temperature during the neonatal period. Newborn hypothermia prolongs as well as potentiates the effects of many analgesic and anesthetic drugs in the newborn.

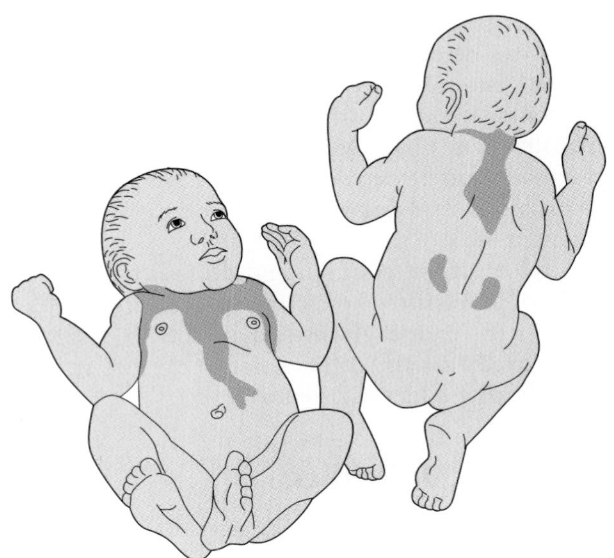

FIGURE 21–6 The distribution of brown adipose tissue (brown fat) in the newborn.

Source: Adapted from Davis V: Structure and function of brown adipose tissue in the neonate. *J Obstet Gynecol Neonat Nurs* November/December 1980; 9:364.

Hepatic Adaptation

In the newborn, the liver is frequently palpable 2–3 cm below the right costal margin. It is relatively large and occupies about 40 percent of the abdominal cavity. The newborn liver plays a significant role in iron storage, carbohydrate metabolism, conjugation of bilirubin, and coagulation.

Iron Storage and Red Blood Cell Production

As red blood cells are destroyed after birth, the iron is stored in the liver until needed for new red blood cell production. Newborn iron stores are determined by total body hemoglobin content and length of gestation. The term newborn has about 270 mg of iron at birth, and about 140–170 mg of this amount is in the hemoglobin. If the mother's iron intake has been adequate, enough iron will be stored to last until about 5 months of age. After about 6 months of age, foods containing iron or iron supplements must be given to prevent anemia.

Carbohydrate Metabolism

At term, the newborn's cord blood glucose is 70 to 80 percent of the maternal blood glucose level. Newborn carbohydrate reserves are relatively low. One-third of this reserve is in the form of liver glycogen. Newborn glycogen stores are twice that of the adult. The newborn enters an energy crunch at the time of birth, with the removal of the maternal glucose supply and the increased energy expenditure associated with the birth process and extrauterine life. Fuel sources are consumed at a faster rate because of the work of breathing, loss of heat when exposed to cold, activity, and activation of muscle tone.

Glucose is the main source of energy in the first 4–6 hours after birth. The blood glucose level falls rapidly, reaching a low point by 60–90 minutes of age, and then stabilizes at 50–60 mg/dL for several days; by the third day postnatally, the mean values increase to 60–70 mg/dL (Karp et al 1995). Glucose level is assessed by using a Chemstrip method upon admission and at 4 hours of age. If the fetus or newborn experiences hypoxia, the glycogen stores are used and may be depleted to meet metabolic requirements. As stores of liver and muscle glycogen and blood glucose decrease, the newborn compensates by changing from a predominantly carbohydrate metabolism to fat metabolism. Energy can be derived from fat and protein as well as from carbohydrates. The amount and availability of each of these "fuel substrates" depends on the ability of immature metabolic pathways (lack of specific enzymes or hormones) to function in the first few days of life.

Conjugation of Bilirubin

Conjugation of bilirubin is the conversion of yellow lipid-soluble pigment into water-soluble pigment. Unconjugated (indirect) bilirubin is a breakdown product derived from hemoglobin released primarily from destroyed red blood cells. Unconjugated bilirubin is not in excretable form and is a potential toxin. Total serum bilirubin is the sum of direct (conjugated) and indirect bilirubin.

Fetal unconjugated bilirubin crosses the placenta to be excreted, so the fetus doesn't need to conjugate bilirubin. Total bilirubin at birth is usually less than 3 mg/dL unless an abnormal hemolytic process has been present in utero. After birth the newborn's liver must begin to conjugate bilirubin. This produces a rise in serum bilirubin in the first few days of life. The newborn liver has relatively less glucuronyl transferase activity at birth and in the first few weeks of life than an adult liver. This reduction in hepatic activity along with a relatively large bilirubin load decreases the liver's ability to conjugate bilirubin and increases susceptibility to jaundice.

The bilirubin formed after red blood cells are destroyed is transported in the blood bound to albumin. The bilirubin is transferred into the hepatocytes and bound to two intracellular binding proteins. These two proteins determine the amount of bilirubin held in a

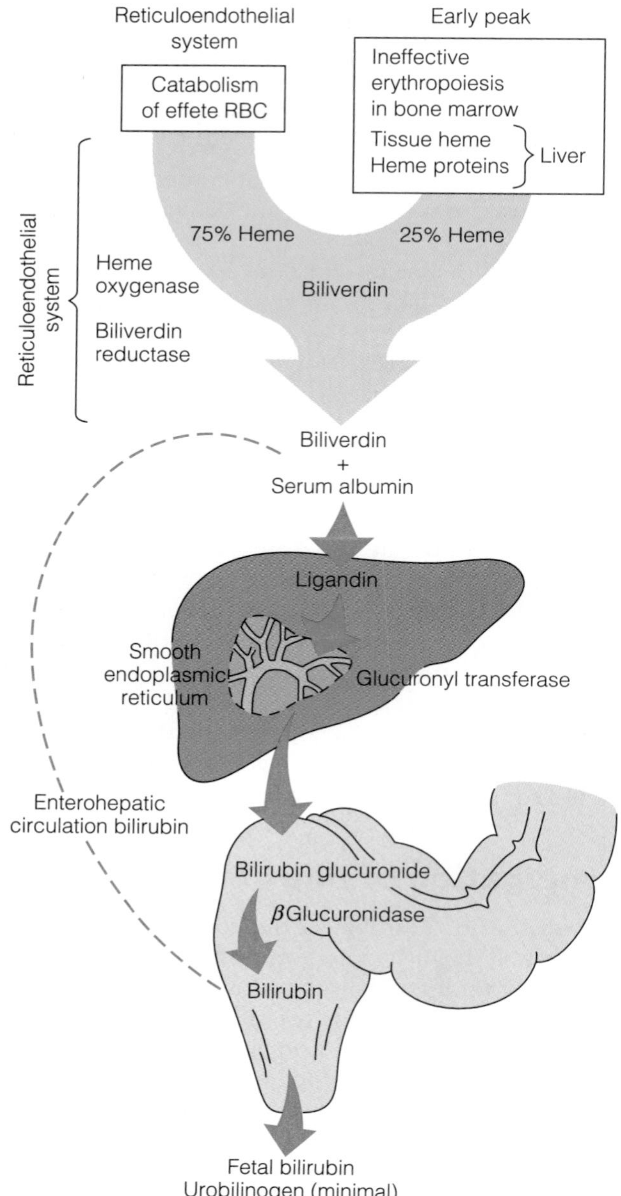

FIGURE 21–7 Conjugation of bilirubin in the newborn.

Source: Avery GB, Fletcher MA, MacDonald MG: *Neonatology: Pathophysiology and Management of the Newborn,* 4th ed. Philadelphia: Lippincott, 1994, p 635.

liver cell for processing and consequently determine the amount of bilirubin uptake into the liver. Activity of glucuronyl transferase results in the attachment of unconjugated bilirubin to glucuronic acid (product of liver glycogen), producing conjugated, direct bilirubin. Direct bilirubin is excreted into the common duct and duodenum. The (direct) conjugated bilirubin then progresses down the intestines, where bacteria transform it into urobilinogen. This product is not reabsorbed, but is excreted as a yellow-brown pigment in the stools.

Even after the bilirubin has been conjugated and bound, it can be changed back to unconjugated bilirubin via the enterohepatic circulation. In the intestines β-glucuronidase enzyme acts to split off (deconjugate) the bilirubin from glucuronic acid if it has not first been acted upon by gut bacteria to produce urobilinogen; the free bilirubin is reabsorbed through the intestinal wall and brought back to the liver via portal vein circulation. This recycling of the bilirubin and decreased ability to clear bilirubin from the system are prevalent in babies who have very high β-glucuronidase activity levels as well as delayed bacterial colonization of the gut (such as with the use of antibiotics) (Figure 21–7).

Physiologic Jaundice

Physiologic jaundice is caused by accelerated destruction of fetal RBCs, impaired conjugation of bilirubin, and increased bilirubin reabsorption from the intestinal tract. This condition does not have a pathologic basis but is a normal biologic response of the newborn.

Maisels (1994) describes six factors whose interactions may give rise to physiologic jaundice:

1. *Increased amounts of bilirubin delivered to the liver.* The increased blood volume due to delayed cord clamping combined with faster RBC destruction in the newborn leads to an increased bilirubin level in the blood. A proportionately larger amount of nonerythrocyte bilirubin forms in the newborn. Therefore, newborns have two to three times greater production or breakdown of bilirubin. The use of forceps, which sometimes causes facial bruising and/or cephalhematoma (entrapped hemorrhage), can increase the amount of bilirubin to be handled by the liver.
2. *Defective uptake of bilirubin from the plasma.* If the newborn does not ingest adequate calories, the formation of hepatic binding proteins diminishes, resulting in higher bilirubin levels.
3. *Defective conjugation of the bilirubin.* Decreased glucuronyl-transferase activity, as in hypothyroidism, and inadequate caloric intake results in greater unconjugated bilirubin levels in the blood. The fatty acids in breast milk are thought to compete with bilirubin for albumin binding sites and therefore impede bilirubin processing.
4. *Defect in bilirubin excretion.* A congenital infection may cause impaired excretion. Delay in introduction of bacterial flora and decreased intestinal motility can also delay excretion and increase enterohepatic circulation of bilirubin.
5. *Inadequate hepatic circulation.* Decreased oxygen supplies to the liver associated with neonatal hypoxia or congenital heart disease lead to a rise in the bilirubin level.

6. *Increased reabsorption of bilirubin from the intestine.* Reduced bowel motility, intestinal obstruction, or delayed passage of meconium increases the circulation of bilirubin in the enterohepatic pathway, thereby resulting in higher bilirubin values.

About 50 percent of term and 80 percent of preterm newborns exhibit physiologic jaundice on about the second or third day after birth. The characteristic yellow color results from increased levels of (indirect) unconjugated bilirubin, which are a normal product of RBC breakdown and reflect the body's temporary inability to eliminate bilirubin. Serum levels of bilirubin are about 4–6 mg/dL before the yellow coloration of the skin and sclera appears. The signs of physiologic jaundice appear *after* the first 24 hours postnatally. This differentiates physiologic jaundice from pathologic jaundice (Chapter 26), which is clinically seen at birth or within the first 24 hours of postnatal life.

In the past, the recommendation was that during the first week unconjugated bilirubin levels in physiologic jaundice should not exceed 13 mg/dL in the term or preterm newborn. Peak bilirubin levels are reached between days 3 and 5 in the term infant and between days 5 and 7 in the preterm infant. These values are established for European and American newborns. Chinese, Japanese, Korean, and Native American newborns have considerably higher bilirubin levels that are not as apparent and that persist for longer periods with no apparent ill effects (Maisels 1994). Some recent studies propose levels up to 22 mg/dL (300–375 μmol/L) in well babies (Newman and Maisels 1992).

Nursery or postpartum room environment, including lighting, hinders the early detection of the degree and type of jaundice. Pink walls and artificial lights mask the beginning of jaundice in newborns. Daylight assists the observer in early recognition by eliminating distortions caused by artificial light.

If jaundice is suspected, the nurse can quickly assess the newborn's coloring by pressing the skin, generally on the forehead or nose, with a finger. As blanching occurs, the nurse can observe the icterus (yellow coloring).

The following nursery or newborn care procedures are designed to decrease the probability of high bilirubin levels:

- Maintain the newborn's skin temperature at 36.5C (97.8F) or above, since chilling results in acidosis. Acidosis in turn decreases available serum albumin–binding sites, weakens albumin-binding powers, and causes elevated unconjugated bilirubin levels.
- Monitor stool for amount and characteristics. Bilirubin is eliminated in the feces; inadequate stooling may result in reabsorption and recycling of bilirubin. Encourage early breastfeeding because the laxative effect of colostrum increases excretion of stool.
- Encourage early feedings to promote intestinal elimination and bacterial colonization and provide caloric intake necessary for formation of hepatic binding proteins (Wilkerson 1988).

If jaundice becomes apparent, nursing care is directed toward keeping the newborn well hydrated and promoting intestinal elimination. For specific nursing management and therapies, see the Critical Pathway for the Newborn with Hyperbilirubinemia in Chapter 26.

Physiologic jaundice may be very upsetting to parents; they require emotional support and thorough explanation of the condition. If the baby is placed under phototherapy, a few additional days of hospitalization may be required. This may also be disturbing to parents. They should be encouraged to provide for the emotional needs of their newborn by continuing to feed, hold, and caress the infant. If the mother is discharged, the parents should be encouraged to return for feedings and feel free to telephone or visit whenever possible. In many instances, the mother, especially if she is breastfeeding, may elect to remain hospitalized with her newborn; this decision should be supported. As an alternative to continued hospitalization, some newborns are treated in home phototherapy programs.

Breastfeeding Jaundice

Breastfeeding is implicated in prolonged jaundice in some newborns. From 1 to 5 percent of newborns being breastfed will develop breastfeeding jaundice. The breastfed jaundiced newborn's bilirubin level begins to rise after the first week of life when physiologic jaundice is waning after the mother's milk has come in. The level peaks at 2–3 weeks of age and may reach 20–25 mg/dL without intervention (Maisels 1994).

Some women's breast milk may contain several times the normal concentration of certain free fatty acids. These free fatty acids may inhibit the conjugation of bilirubin or increase lipase activity, which disrupts the red blood cell membrane. Increased lipase activity enhances absorption of bile across the GI tract membrane, thereby increasing the enterohepatic circulation of bilirubin. In the past it was thought that the breast milk of women whose newborns have breastfeeding jaundice contained an enzyme that inhibited glucuronyl transferase (Blackburn 1995).

Newborns with breastfeeding jaundice appear well, and at present there is an absence of documented kernicterus with this type of jaundice. Temporary cessation of nursing may be advised if bilirubin reaches presumed toxic levels of approximately 20 mg/dL, or if the interruption is necessary to establish the cause of the hyperbilirubinemia (Maisels 1994). Within 24–36 hours after discontinuing breastfeeding, the newborn's serum bilirubin levels begin to fall dramatically and breastfeeding should be resumed.

KEY FACTS TO REMEMBER

Jaundice

Physiologic Jaundice

Physiologic jaundice occurs *after* the first 24 hours of life.

During the first week of life, bilirubin should not exceed 13 mg/dL. Some pediatricians allow levels up to 15 mg/dL.

Bilirubin levels peak at 3 to 5 days in term infants.

Breast Milk Jaundice

Bilirubin levels begin to rise about the fourth day after mature breast milk comes in.

Peak of 20–25 mg/dL is reached at 2 to 3 weeks of age.

It may be necessary to interrupt nursing for a short period when bilirubin reaches 20 mg/dL.

Pathologic Jaundice

- Occurs before 24 hours of life.
- Requires medical intervention.

Many physicians believe that breastfeeding may be resumed once other causes of jaundice have been ruled out and breastfeeding is determined to be the cause. The bilirubin concentration may rise 2–3 mg/dL with a subsequent decline (Maisels 1994). Nursing mothers need encouragement and support in their desire to breastfeed, assistance and instruction regarding pumping and expressing milk during the interrupted nursing period, and reassurance that nothing is wrong with their milk or mothering abilities. (See Key Facts to Remember: Jaundice.)

Coagulation

The liver plays an important part in blood coagulation during fetal life and continues this function to some degree during the first few months after birth. Coagulation factors II, VII, IX, and X (synthesized in the liver) are activated under the influence of vitamin K and therefore are considered vitamin K–dependent. The absence of normal flora needed to synthesize vitamin K in the newborn gut results in low levels of vitamin K and creates a transient blood coagulation alteration between the second and fifth day of life. From a low point at about 2 to 3 days after birth, these coagulation factors rise slowly, but they do not approach adult levels until 9 months of age or later. Other coagulation factors with low umbilical cord blood levels are XI, XII, and XIII. Fibrinogen and factors V and VII are near adult ranges (Eden and Boehm 1990).

Although newborn bleeding problems are rare, an injection of vitamin K (AquaMEPHYTON) is given prophylactically on the day of birth to combat potential clinical bleeding problems. (Chapter 26 discusses hemorrhagic disease of the newborn in more depth.)

Platelet counts at birth are in the same range as for older children, but newborns may manifest mild transient difficulty in platelet aggregation functioning. This platelet problem is accentuated by phototherapy (Eden and Boehm 1990).

Prenatal maternal therapy with phenytoin sodium (Dilantin) or phenobarbital also causes abnormal clotting studies and newborn bleeding in the first 24 hours after birth. Infants born to mothers receiving warfarin sodium (Coumadin) may bleed, because these agents cross the placenta and accentuate existing vitamin K–dependent factor deficiencies.

Gastrointestinal Adaptation

By 36–38 weeks of fetal life, the gastrointestinal system is adequately mature, with enzymatic activity and the ability to transport nutrients. The term newborn has adequate intestinal and pancreatic enzymes to digest most simple carbohydrates, proteins, and fats.

The carbohydrates requiring digestion in the newborn are usually disaccharides (lactose, maltose, and sucrose). Lactose is the primary carbohydrate in the breastfeeding newborn and is generally easily digested and well absorbed. The only enzyme lacking is pancreatic amylase, which remains relatively deficient during the first few months of life. Therefore, newborns have trouble digesting starches (changing more complex carbohydrates into maltose).

Although proteins require more digestion than carbohydrates, they are well digested and absorbed from the newborn intestine.

The newborn digests and absorbs fats less efficiently because of the minimal activity of the pancreatic enzyme lipase. The newborn excretes about 10–20 percent of the dietary fat intake, compared with 10 percent for the adult. The newborn absorbs the fat in breast milk more completely than the fat in cows' milk, because breast milk consists of more medium-chain triglycerides and contains lipase. (See Chapter 24 for further discussion of infant nutrition.) In utero, swallowing is accompanied by gastric emptying and peristalsis of the fetal intestinal tract. By the end of gestation, in preparation for extrauterine life, peristalsis becomes much more active.

Air enters the stomach immediately after birth. The small intestine is air-filled within 2–12 hours and the large bowel within 24 hours. The salivary glands are immature at birth, and the newborn produces little saliva until about age 3 months. The newborn's stomach has a

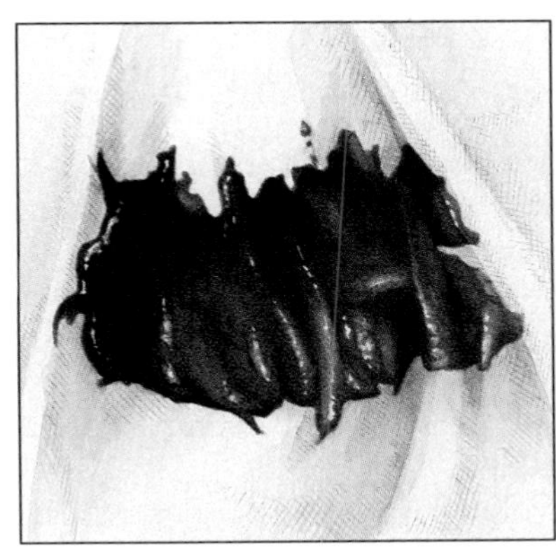

A

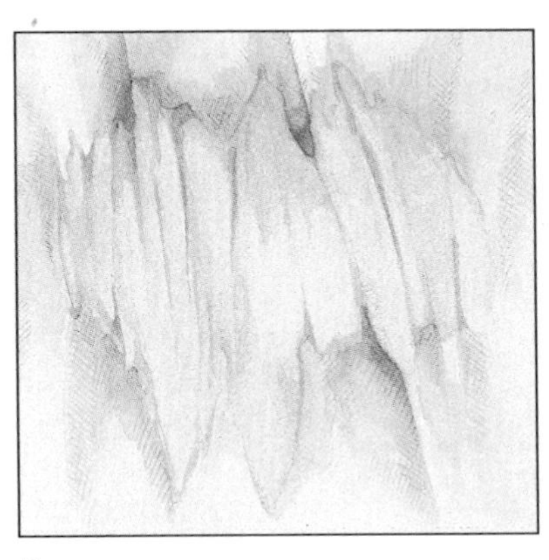

B

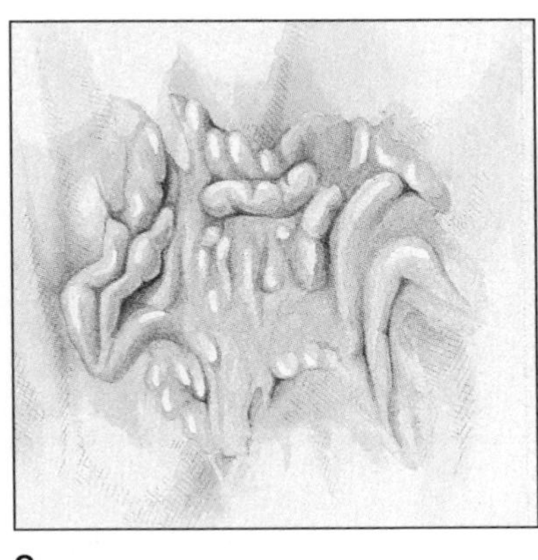

C

FIGURE 21–8 Newborn stool samples. ***A*** Meconium stool. ***B*** Breast milk stool. ***C*** Cow's milk stool.

capacity of about 50–60 mL. It empties intermittently, starting within a few minutes of the beginning of a feeding and ending 2–4 hours after feeding. The newborn's gastric pH becomes less acidic about a week after birth and remains less acidic than that of adults for the next 2–3 months.

The cardiac sphincter is immature, as is neural control of the stomach, so some regurgitation may be noted in the newborn period. Regurgitation of the first few feedings during the first day or two of life can usually be lessened by avoiding overfeeding and by burping the newborn well during and after the feeding.

When no other signs and symptoms are evident, vomiting is often self-limiting and ceases within the first few days of life. Continuous vomiting or regurgitation should be observed closely. If the newborn has swallowed bloody or purulent amniotic fluid, lavage of the stomach may be indicated in the term newborn to relieve the problem.

Adequate digestion and absorption are essential for newborn growth and development. If optimal nutritional support is available, postnatal growth should parallel intrauterine growth; that is, after 30 weeks of gestation, the fetus gains 30 g per day and adds 1.2 cm to body length daily. To gain weight at the intrauterine rate, the term newborn requires 120 cal/kg/day. After birth, caloric intake is often insufficient for weight gain until the newborn is 5–10 days old. During this time, there may be a weight loss of 5–10 percent in term newborns. A shift of intracellular water to extracellular space and insensible water loss account for the 5–10 percent weight loss; thus, failure to lose weight when caloric intake is inadequate may indicate fluid retention.

Term newborns usually pass meconium within 8–24 hours of life—and almost always within 48 hours. **Meconium** is formed in utero from the amniotic fluid and its constituents, intestinal secretions, and shed mucosal cells. It is recognized by its thick, tarry black or dark-green appearance. Transitional (thin brown to green) stools consisting of part meconium and part fecal material are passed for the next day or two, and then the stools become entirely fecal. Generally the stools of a breastfed newborn are pale yellow (but may be pasty green); they are more liquid and more frequent than those of formula-fed newborns, whose stools are paler (Figure 21-8) (Salariya and Robertson 1993). Frequency of bowel movement varies, but ranges from one every 2 to 3 days to as many as ten daily. Totally breastfed infants often progress to stools that occur every 5–7 days. Mothers should be counseled that the newborn is not constipated as long as the bowel movement remains soft. (See Key Facts to Remember: Physiologic Adaptations to Extrauterine Life.)

KEY FACTS TO REMEMBER

Physiologic Adaptations to Extrauterine Life

Periodic breathing may be present.

Desired skin temperature 36–36.5C (96.8–97.7F), stabilizes 4 to 6 hours after birth.

Desired blood glucose level reaches 60–70 mg/dL by third postnatal day.

Stools (progress from):

- Meconium (thick, tarry, black)
- Transitional stools (thin, brown to green)
- Breastfed infants (yellow-gold, soft, or mushy)
- Bottle-fed infants (pale yellow, formed, and pasty)

TABLE 21–4 Newborn Urinalysis Values
Protein < 5–10 mg/dL
WBC < 2–3
RBC 0
Casts 0
Bacteria 0
Specific gravity 1.001–1.025
Color pale yellow

Urinary Adaptations

Kidney Development and Function

Certain physiologic features of the newborn's kidneys are important to consider when looking at the newborn's ability to handle body fluids and excrete urine.

1. The term newborn's kidneys have a full complement of functioning nephrons by 34–36 weeks of gestation (Seaman 1995).
2. The glomerular filtration rate of the newborn's kidney is low compared to the adult rate. Because of this physiologic inefficiency, the newborn's kidney is unable to dispose of water rapidly when necessary because it favors reabsorption of sodium (Seaman 1995).
3. The juxtamedullary portion of the nephron has limited capacity to reabsorb HCO_3^- and H^+ and concentrate urine. The limitation of tubular reabsorption can lead to inappropriate loss of substances present in the glomerular filtrate, such as amino acids, bicarbonate, glucose, and sodium.

Term newborns are less able than adults to concentrate urine (reabsorb water back into the blood) because the tubules are short and narrow. There is a greater capacity for glomerular filtration than for tubular reabsorption-secretion. Although feeding practices may affect the osmolarity of the urine, the maximum concentrating ability of the newborn is a specific gravity of 1.025. The inability to concentrate urine is due to the limited excretion of solutes (principally sodium, potassium, chloride, bicarbonate, urea, and phosphate) in the growing newborn. The ability to concentrate urine fully is attained by 3 months of age.

Since the newborn has difficulty concentrating urine, the effect of excessive insensible water loss or restricted fluid intake is unpredictable. The newborn kidney is also limited in its dilutional capabilities. Maximal dilution ability is a specific gravity of 1.001. Concentrating and dilutional limitations of renal function are important considerations in monitoring fluid therapy to avoid dehydration or overhydration (Blackburn 1994).

Characteristics of Newborn Urinary Function

Many newborns void immediately after birth, and it goes unnoticed. Among normal newborns, 93 percent void by 24 hours after birth and 98 percent void by 48 hours (Blackburn 1994). A newborn who has not voided by 48 hours should be assessed for adequacy of fluid intake, bladder distention, restlessness, and symptoms of pain. The appropriate clinical personnel should be notified if indicated.

The initial bladder volume is 6–44 mL of urine. Unless edema is present, normal urinary output is often limited, and the voidings are scanty until fluid intake increases. The fluid of edema is eliminated by the kidneys, so newborns with edema have a much higher urinary output. The first 2 days postnatally, the newborn voids 2–6 times daily, with a urine output of 15 mL per day. The newborn subsequently voids 5–25 times every 24 hours, with a volume of 25 mL/kg per day.

Following the first voiding, the newborn's urine frequently appears cloudy (due to mucus content) and has a high specific gravity, which decreases as fluid intake increases. Occasionally pink stains ("brick dust spots") appear on the diaper. These are caused by urates and are innocuous. Blood may occasionally be observed on the diapers of female newborns. This *pseudomenstruation* is related to the withdrawal of maternal hormones. Males may have bloody spotting from a circumcision. In the absence of apparent causes for bleeding, the clinician should be notified. Normal urine during early infancy is straw-colored and almost odorless, although odor occurs when certain drugs are given, metabolic disorders exist, or infection is present. Table 21–4 contains urinalysis values for the normal newborn.

Immunologic Adaptations

The cells that constitute the immune system appear early in fetal life, but usually are not fully activated until sometime after birth. The most common class of immune cells are *immunoglobulins,* a type of antibody secreted by lymphocytes and plasma cells into body fluids. Of the three major types of immunoglobulins primarily involved in immunity—IgG, IgA, and IgM—only IgG crosses the placenta.

The pregnant woman forms antibodies in response to illness or immunization. This process is called **active acquired immunity.** When IgG antibodies are transferred to the fetus in utero, **passive acquired immunity** results, since the fetus does not produce the antibodies itself. IgG immunoglobulins are very active against bacterial toxins.

Because the maternal immunoglobin is transferred primarily during the third trimester, preterm newborns (especially those born before 34 weeks) may be more susceptible to infection. In general, newborns have immunity to tetanus, diphtheria, smallpox, measles, mumps, poliomyelitis, and a variety of other bacterial and viral diseases. The period of resistance varies: Immunity against common viral infections such as measles may last 4–8 months, whereas immunity to certain bacteria may disappear within 4–8 weeks.

The normal newborn produces antibodies in response to an antigen but not as effectively as an older child would. It is customary to begin immunization at 2 months of age, and then the infant can develop active acquired immunity.

IgM immunoglobulins are produced in response to blood group antigens, gram-negative enteric organisms, and some viruses in the expectant mother. Because IgM does not normally cross the placenta, most or all is produced by the fetus beginning at 10–15 weeks' gestation. Elevated levels of IgM at birth may indicate placental leaks or, more commonly, antigenic stimulation in utero. Consequently elevations suggest that the newborn was exposed to an intrauterine infection such as syphilis or a TORCH infection. (For further discussion, see Chapter 13.) The lack of available maternal IgM in the newborn also accounts for the susceptibility to gram-negative enteric organisms such as *E coli.*

The functions of IgA immunoglobulins are not fully understood. IgA appears to provide protection mainly on secreting surfaces such as the respiratory tract, gastrointestinal tract, and eyes. Serum IgA does not cross the placenta and is not normally produced by the fetus in utero. Unlike the other immunoglobulins, IgA is not affected by gastric action. Colostrum, the forerunner of breast milk, is very high in the secretory form of IgA. Consequently it may be of significance in providing some passive immunity to the infant of a breastfeeding mother. Newborns begin to produce secretory IgA in their intestinal mucosa at about 4 weeks after birth.

Neurologic and Sensory/Perceptual Functioning

The newborn's brain is about one-quarter the size of an adult's, and myelination of nerve fibers is incomplete. Unlike the cardiovascular or respiratory systems, which undergo tremendous changes at birth, the nervous system is minimally influenced by the actual birth process.

Because many biochemical and histologic changes have yet to occur in the newborn's brain, the postnatal period is considered a time of risk with regard to the development of the brain and nervous system. For neurologic development—including development of intellect—to proceed, the brain and other nervous system structures must mature in an orderly, unhampered fashion. For discussion of cranial nerves, see Chapter 22.

Intrauterine Factors Influencing Newborn Behavior

Newborns respond to and interact with the environment in a predictable pattern of behavior that is somewhat shaped by their intrauterine experience. This intrauterine experience is affected by intrinsic factors such as maternal nutrition and external factors such as the mother's physical environment. Depending on the newborn's intrauterine experience, neonatal behavioral responses to various stresses vary from dealing quietly with the stimulation, to becoming overreactive and tense, to a combination of the two.

Brazelton and colleagues (1977) found a positive association between newborn behavior and the nutritional status of the pregnant woman. Newborns with higher birth weight attended and responded to visual and auditory cues and exhibited more mature motor activity than newborns with lower birth weights.

Factors such as exposure to intense auditory stimuli in utero can eventually be manifested in the behavior of the newborn. For example, the fetal heart rate initially increases when the pregnant woman is exposed to auditory stimuli, but repetition of the stimuli leads to decreased FHR. Thus the newborn who was exposed to intense noise during fetal life is significantly less reactive to loud sounds postnatally.

Characteristics of Newborn Neurologic Function

Partially flexed extremities with the legs near the abdomen is the usual position of the normal newborn. When awake, the newborn may exhibit purposeless, uncoordinated bilateral movements of the extremities.

The organization and quality of the newborn's motor activity are influenced by a number of factors, including the following (Brazelton 1984):

- Sleep-alert states
- Presence of environmental stimuli, such as heat, light, cold, and noise
- Conditions causing a chemical imbalance, such as hypoglycemia
- Hydration status
- State of health
- Recovery from the stress of labor and birth

Eye movements are observable during the first few days of life. An alert newborn is able to fixate on faces and geometric objects or patterns such as black-and-white stripes. A bright light shining in the newborn's eyes elicits the blinking reflex.

The cry of the newborn should be lusty and vigorous. High-pitched cries, weak cries, or no cries are all causes for concern.

Growth of the newborn's body progresses in a cephalocaudal (head-to-toe), proximal-distal fashion. The newborn is somewhat hypertonic; that is, there is resistance to extending the elbow and knee joints. Muscle tone should be symmetrical. Diminished muscle tone and flaccidity may indicate neurologic dysfunction.

Specific symmetrical deep tendon reflexes can be elicited in the newborn. Plantar flexion is present. The knee jerk is brisk; a normal ankle clonus may involve 3 to 4 beats. Other reflexes, including the Moro, grasping, Babinski, rooting, and sucking reflexes are characteristic of neurologic integrity (see Chapter 22).

The performance of complex behavioral patterns reflects the newborn's neurologic maturation and integration. Newborns who can bring a hand to their mouth may be demonstrating motor coordination as well as a self-quieting technique, thus increasing the complexity of the behavioral response. Newborns also possess complex, organized defensive motor patterns as exhibited by the ability to remove an obstruction, such as a cloth across the face.

Periods of Reactivity

The baby usually shows a predictable pattern of behavior during the first several hours after birth, characterized by two **periods of reactivity** separated by a sleep phase.

First Period of Reactivity

The first period of reactivity lasts approximately 30 minutes after birth. During this phase the newborn is awake and active and may appear hungry and have a strong sucking reflex. This is a natural opportunity to initiate breastfeeding if the mother has chosen it. Bursts of random, diffuse movements alternating with relative immobility may occur. Respirations are rapid, as high as 80 breaths/min, and there may be retraction of the chest, transient flaring of the nares, and grunting. The heart rate is rapid, and the rhythm may be irregular. Bowel sounds are usually absent.

Period of Inactivity to Sleep Phase

After about half an hour the newborn's activity gradually diminishes, and the heart rate and respirations decrease as the newborn enters the sleep phase. The sleep phase may last from a few minutes to 2–4 hours. During this period, the newborn will be difficult to awaken and will show no interest in sucking. Bowel sounds become audible, and cardiac and respiratory rates return to baseline values.

Second Period of Reactivity

During the second period of reactivity, the newborn is again awake and alert. This phase lasts 4–6 hours in the normal newborn. Physiologic responses are variable during this stage. The heart and respiratory rates increase; however, the nurse must be alert for apneic periods, which may cause a drop in the heart rate. The newborn is stimulated to continue breathing during such times. The newborn may develop rapid color changes and become mildly cyanotic or mottled during these fluctuations. Production of respiratory and gastric mucus increases, and the newborn responds by gagging, choking, and regurgitating.

Continued close observation and intervention may be required to maintain a clear airway during this period of reactivity. The gastrointestinal tract becomes more active. The first meconium stool is frequently passed during this second active stage, and the initial voiding may also occur at this time. The newborn will indicate readiness for feeding by such behaviors as sucking, rooting, and swallowing. If feeding was not initiated in the first period of reactivity, it is done at this time. See Chapter 24 for further discussion of this first feeding.

Behavioral States of the Newborn

The behavior of the newborn can be divided into two categories, the sleep state and the alert state (Brazelton 1984). These postnatal behavioral states are similar to those that have been identified during pregnancy. Subcategories are identified under each major category.

Sleep States

The sleep states are as follows:

1. *Deep or quiet sleep.* Deep sleep is characterized by closed eyes with no eye movements; regular, even breathing; and jerky motions or startles at regular intervals. Behavioral responses to external stimuli are likely to be delayed. Startles are rapidly suppressed, and changes in state are not likely to occur. Heart rate may range from 100 to 120 beats per minute.
2. *Active rapid eye movement (REM) sleep.* Irregular respirations, eyes closed with REM, irregular sucking motions, minimal activity, and irregular but smooth movement of the extremities can be observed in active REM sleep. Environmental and internal stimuli initiate a startle reaction and a change of state.

Sleep cycles in the newborn have been recognized and defined according to duration. The length of the cycle depends on the age of the newborn. At term, REM active sleep and quiet sleep occur in intervals of 45–50 minutes. About 45–50 percent of the total sleep of the newborn is active sleep, 35–45 percent is quiet sleep, and 10 percent of sleep is transitional between these two states. It is hypothesized that REM sleep stimulates the growth of the neural system. Over a period of time, the

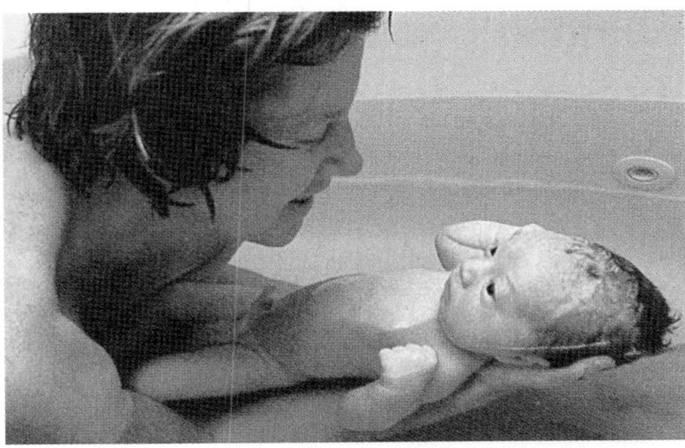

FIGURE 21–9 Mother and newborn gaze at each other. This quiet, alert state is the optimum state for interaction between baby and parents.

newborn's sleep-wake patterns become diurnal; that is, the newborn sleeps at night and stays awake during the day. (See Chapter 22 for a short discussion of Brazelton's assessment of newborn states.)

Alert States

In the first 30–60 minutes after birth, many newborns display a quiet alert state, characteristic of the first period of reactivity (Figure 21–9). Nurses should use these alert states to encourage bonding and breastfeeding. These periods of alertness tend to be short the first 2 days after birth to allow the baby to recover from the birth process. Subsequent alert states are of choice or of necessity (Brazelton 1984). Increasing choice of wakefulness by the newborn indicates a maturing capacity to achieve and maintain consciousness. Heat, cold, and hunger are but a few of the stimuli that can cause wakefulness by necessity. Once the disturbing stimuli are removed, sleep tends to recur.

The following are subcategories of the alert state (Brazelton 1984):

1. *Drowsy or semidozing.* The behaviors common to the drowsy state are open or closed eyes; fluttering eyelids; semidozing appearance; and slow, regular movements of the extremities. Mild startles may be noted from time to time. Although the reaction to a sensory stimulus is delayed, a change of state often results.
2. *Wide awake.* In the wide-awake state, the newborn is alert and follows and fixates on attractive objects, faces, or auditory stimuli. Motor activity is minimal, and the response to external stimuli is delayed.
3. *Active awake.* In the active-awake state, the newborn's eyes are open and motor activity is quite intense, with thrusting movements of the extremities. Environmental stimuli increase startles or motor activity, but individual reactions are difficult to distinguish because of the generally high activity level.
4. *Crying.* Intense crying is accompanied by jerky motor movements. Crying serves several purposes for the newborn. It may be a distraction from disturbing stimuli such as hunger and pain. Fussiness often allows the newborn to discharge energy and reorganize behavior. Most important, crying elicits an appropriate response of help from the parents.

Behavioral/Sensory Capacities of the Newborn

Habituation is the newborn's ability to process and respond to visual and auditory stimulation. For example, when a bright light is flashed into the newborn's eyes, the initial response is blinking, constriction of the pupil, and perhaps a slight startle reaction. However, with repeated stimulation, the newborn's response repertoire gradually diminishes and disappears. The capacity to ignore repetitious disturbing stimuli is a newborn defense mechanism readily apparent in the noisy, well-lighted nursery.

Orientation is the newborn's ability to be alert to, follow, and fixate on complex visual stimuli that are appealing and attractive. The newborn prefers the human face and eyes and bright shiny objects. As the face or object comes into the line of vision, the newborn responds with bright, wide eyes, still limbs, and fixed staring. This intense visual involvement may last several minutes, during which time the newborn is able to follow the stimulus from side to side. Figure 21–10 illustrates this response. The newborn uses this sensory capacity to become familiar with family, friends, and surroundings.

Self-quieting ability refers to newborns' ability to quiet and comfort themselves. Their repertoire includes hand-to-mouth movements, sucking on a fist or tongue,

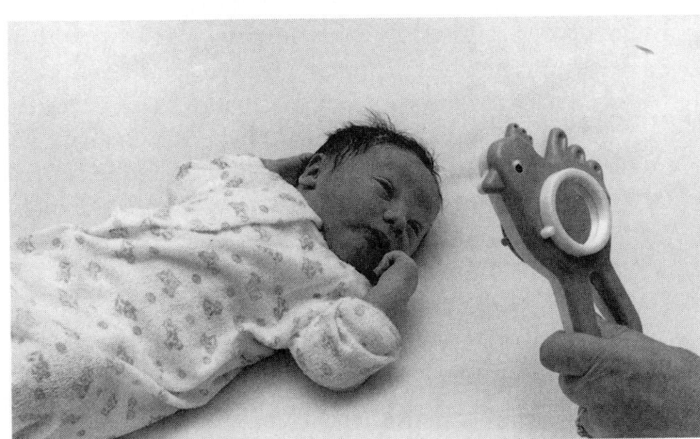

FIGURE 21–10 Head turning to follow movement.

and attending to external stimuli. Neurologically impaired newborns are unable to use self-quieting activities and require more frequent comforting from caregivers when stimulated. For example, drug-positive newborns often exhibit abnormal sleep and feeding patterns and irritability (Taeusch et al 1991).

Auditory Capacity

The newborn responds to auditory stimulation with a definite, organized behavior repertoire. The stimulus used to assess auditory response should be selected to match the state of the newborn. A rattle is appropriate for light sleep, a voice for an awake state, and a clap for deep sleep. As the newborn hears the sound, the cardiac rate rises, and a minimal startle reflex may be observed. If the sound is appealing, the newborn will become alert and search for the site of the auditory stimulus.

Olfactory Capacity

Newborns are apparently able to select people by smell. In one study, newborns were able to distinguish their mothers' breast pads from those of other mothers at just 1 week postnatally (Brazelton 1984).

Taste and Sucking

The newborn responds differently to varying tastes. Sugar, for example, increases sucking. Sucking pattern variations also exist in newborns fed with a rubber nipple versus the breast. When breastfeeding, the newborn sucks in bursts with frequent regular pauses. The bottle-fed newborn tends to suck at a regular rate with infrequent pauses.

When awake and hungry, the newborn displays rapid searching motions in response to the rooting reflex. Once feeding begins, the newborn establishes a sucking pattern according to the method of feeding. Finger sucking is present not only postnatally but also in utero. The newborn frequently uses nonnutritive sucking as a self-quieting activity, which assists in the development of self-regulation. Nonnutritive sucking with a pacifier should not be discouraged if the infant is bottle-fed. For breastfed infants pacifiers should be offered only after breastfeeding is well established. If the pacifier is offered too soon, a phenomenon called "nipple confusion" may occur in which the breastfed infant has difficulty learning to suck from the breast (see Chapter 24).

Tactile Capacity

The newborn is very sensitive to being touched, cuddled, and held. Often a mother's first response to an upset or crying newborn is touching or holding. Swaddling, placing a hand on the abdomen, or holding the arms to prevent a startle reflex are other methods of soothing the newborn. The settled newborn is then able to attend to and interact with the environment.

CHAPTER HIGHLIGHTS

- Newborn respiration is initiated primarily by chemical and mechanical events in association with thermal and sensory stimulation.
- The production of surfactant is crucial to keeping the lungs expanded during expiration by reducing alveolar surface tension.
- The newborn is an obligatory nose breather. Respirations move from being primarily shallow, irregular, and diaphragmatic to synchronous abdominal and chest breathing. Normal respiratory rate is 30–60 bpm.
- Periodic breathing is normal, and newborn sleep states affect breathing patterns.
- The status of the cardiopulmonary system may be measured by evaluating the heart rate, blood pressure, and presence or absence of murmurs. The normal heart rate is 120–160 bpm.
- Oxygen transport in the newborn is significantly affected by the presence of greater amounts of Hb F (fetal hemoglobin) than Hb A (adult hemoglobin); Hb F holds oxygen easier but releases it to the body tissues only at low PO_2 levels.
- Blood values in the newborn are modified by several factors such as site of the blood sample, gestational age, prenatal and/or perinatal hemorrhage, and the timing of the clamping of the umbilical cord.
- Blood glucose levels should reach 60–70 mg/dL by the third postnatal day.
- The newborn is considered to have established thermoregulation when oxygen consumption and metabolic activity are minimal.
- Evaporation is the primary heat-loss mechanism in newborns who are wet from amniotic fluid or a bath. In addition, excessive heat loss occurs from radiation and convection because of the newborn's larger surface area compared to weight, and from thermal conduction because of the marked difference between core temperature and skin temperature.
- The primary source of heat in the cold-stressed newborn is brown adipose tissue.
- The normal newborn possesses the ability to digest and absorb nutrients necessary for newborn growth and development.
- The newborn's liver plays a crucial role in iron storage, carbohydrate metabolism, conjugation of bilirubin, and coagulation.
- The newborn's stools change from meconium (thick, tarry, dark green) to transitional stools (thin, brown-to-green) and then to the distinct forms for

either breastfed newborns (yellow-gold, soft, or mushy) or bottle-fed newborns (pale yellow, formed, and pasty). Most newborns pass their first stool within 24 hours of birth.

- Controversy continues about the relationship of breastfeeding and the development of prolonged jaundice.
- The newborn's kidneys are characterized by a decreased rate of glomerular flow, limited tubular reabsorption, limited excretion of solutes, and limited ability to concentrate urine. Most newborns void within 24 hours of birth.
- The immune system in the newborn is not fully activated until sometime after birth, but the newborn does possess some immunologic abilities.
- Neurologic and sensory/perceptual functioning in the newborn is evident from the newborn's interaction with the environment, synchronized motor activity, and well-developed sensory capacities.
- The first period of reactivity lasts for 30 minutes after birth. The newborn is alert and hungry at this time, making this a natural opportunity to promote attachment.
- The second period of reactivity requires close monitoring by the nurse as apnea, decreased heart rate, gagging, choking, and regurgitation are likely to occur and require nursing intervention.
- The behavioral states in the newborn can be divided into sleep states and alert states.

REFERENCES

Blackburn S: Hyperbilirubinemia and neonatal jaundice. *Neonatal Network* 1995; 14(7):15.

Blackburn ST: Renal function in the neonate. *J Perinat Neonatal Nurs* 1994; 8(1):37.

Blackburn ST, Loper DL: *Maternal, Fetal, and Neonatal Physiology: A Clinical Perspective.* Philadelphia: Saunders, 1992.

Brazelton TB et al: The behavior of nutritionally deprived Guatemalan neonates. *Dev Med Child Neurol* 1977; 19:364.

Brazelton TB: *Neonatal Behavioral Assessment Scale,* 2nd ed. London: Heineman, 1984.

Cunningham FG, MacDonald PC, Gant NG: *Williams Obstetrics,* 20th ed. Stamford, CT: Appleton & Lange, 1997.

Eden RD, Boehm FH (editors): *Assessment and Care of the Fetus: Physiological, Clinical, and Medicolegal Principles.* Norwalk, CT: Appleton & Lange, 1990.

Fanaroff AA, Martin RJ: *Neonatal-Perinatal Medicine,* 6th ed. St Louis: Mosby, 1997.

Fletcher ME: Physical assessment and classification. In: *Neonatology: Pathophysiology and Management of the Newborn,* 4th ed. Avery GB, Fletcher M, MacDonald MG (editors). Philadelphia: Lippincott, 1994.

Hey E: Thermoregulation. In: *Neonatology: Pathophysiology and Management of the Newborn,* 4th ed. Avery GB, Fletcher M, MacDonald MG (editors). Philadelphia: Lippincott, 1994.

James LS, Adamsons K: The neonate and resuscitation. In: *Danforth's Obstetrics and Gynecology,* 7th ed. Scott JR et al (editors). Philadelphia: Lippincott, 1994.

Karp TB, Scardino C, Butler LA: Glucose metabolism in the neonate: The short and sweet of it. *Neonatal Network* 1995; 14(8):17.

Long WA: *Fetal and Neonatal Cardiology.* Philadelphia: Saunders, 1990.

Maisels MJ: Jaundice. In: *Neonatology: Pathophysiology and Management of the Newborn,* 4th ed. Avery GB, Fletcher M, MacDonald MG (editors). Philadelphia: Lippincott, 1994.

Nelson N: Physiology of transitions. In: *Neonatology: Pathophysiology and Management of the Newborn,* 4th ed. Avery GB, Fletcher M, MacDonald MG (editors). Philadelphia: Lippincott, 1994.

Newman TB, Maisels MJ: Evaluation and treatment of jaundice in the term newborn: A kinder, gentler approach. *Pediatrics* 1992; 89(5):809.

Polin RA, Fox WW: *Fetal and Neonatal Physiology.* Philadelphia: Saunders, 1992.

Salariya EM, Robertson CM: The development of a neonatal stool colour comparator. *Midwifery* 1993; 9:35.

Sansoucie DA, Cavaliere TA: Transition from fetal to extrauterine circulation. *Neonatal Network* 1995; 16(2):5.

Seaman SL: Renal physiology: II. Fluid and electrolyte regulation. *Neonatal Network* 1995; 14(5):5.

Taeusch HW, Ballard RA, Avery ME: *Schaffer and Avery's Diseases of the Newborn,* 6th ed. Philadelphia: Saunders, 1991.

Wilkerson NN: A comprehensive look at hyperbilirubinemia. *MCN* 1988; 13:360.

Chapter 22 Nursing Assessment of the Newborn

OBJECTIVES

- Describe the normal physical and behavioral characteristics of the newborn.
- Summarize the components of a complete newborn assessment and the significance of normal variations and abnormal findings.
- Explain the various components of the gestational age assessment.
- Discuss the neurologic or neuromuscular characteristics of the newborn and the reflexes that may be present at birth.
- Describe the categories of the newborn behavioral assessment.

KEY TERMS

Acrocyanosis
Babinski reflex
Barlow's maneuver
Brazelton's neonatal behavioral assessment
Caput succedaneum
Cephalhematoma
Chemical conjunctivitis
Epstein's pearls
Erb-Duchenne paralysis (Erb's palsy)
Erythema toxicum
Gestational age assessment tools
Grasping reflex
Harlequin sign
Jaundice
Milia
Molding
Mongolian spots
Moro reflex
Mottling
Nevus flammeus (port-wine stain)
Nevus vasculosus (strawberry mark)
Ortolani's maneuver
Pseudomenstruation
Rooting reflex
Skin turgor
Subconjunctival hemorrhage
Sucking reflex
Telangiectatic nevi (stork bites)
Thrush *(Candida albicans)*
Tonic neck reflex
Trunk incurvation (Galant reflex)
Vernix caseosa

Unlike the adult, the newborn communicates needs primarily by behavior. Because the nurse is the most consistent observer of the newborn, he or she can translate this behavior into information about the newborn's condition and respond with appropriate nursing interventions. This chapter focuses on the assessment of the newborn and the interpretation of the findings. Assessment of the newborn is a continuous process designed to evaluate development and adjustments to extrauterine life. In the birth setting, the Apgar scoring procedure (see Chapter 17 for discussion) and careful observation form the basis of assessment and are correlated with information such as

- Maternal prenatal care history
- Birthing history
- Maternal analgesia and anesthesia
- Complications of labor or birth
- Treatment instituted immediately after birth, in conjunction with determination of clinical gestational age
- Consideration of the classification of newborns by weight and gestational age and by neonatal mortality risk
- Physical examination of the newborn

The nurse incorporates data from these sources with the assessment findings during the first 1–4 hours after birth to formulate a plan for nursing intervention. The various newborn assessments and the data obtained from them are only as effective as the degree to which the findings are shared with the parents. The parents must be included in the assessment process from the moment of their child's birth. The Apgar score and its meaning should be explained immediately to the family. As soon as possible, the parents should take part in the physical and behavioral assessments.

The nurse encourages the parents to identify the unique behavioral characteristics of their newborn and to learn nurturing activities. Attachment progresses when parents can explore their newborn in private, identifying individual physical and behavioral characteristics. The nurse provides supportive responses to their questions and observations throughout the assessment process. The newborn physical examination therefore is the beginning of newborn health surveillance and health education for the newborn's family that continues into the community (Fowlie and Forsyth 1995).

Timing of Newborn Assessments

The first 24 hours of life are significant, because during this period the newborn makes the critical transition from intrauterine to extrauterine life. The risk of mortality and morbidity is statistically high during this period. Assessment of the newborn is essential to ensure that the transition is proceeding successfully.

There are three major time frames for assessments of newborns while they are in the birth facility:

- The first assessment is done in the birthing area immediately after birth to determine the need for resuscitation or other interventions. The newborn who is stable can stay with the family after birth to initiate early attachment. The newborn who has complications is usually taken to the nursery for further evaluation and intervention.
- A second assessment is done in the first 1–4 hours after birth as part of routine admission procedures. During this assessment, the nurse carries out a brief physical examination to estimate gestational age and evaluate the newborn's adaptation to extrauterine life. The nurse further assesses any problems that place the newborn at risk during this time.
- Prior to discharge, a certified nurse-midwife, physician, or nurse practitioner does a behavioral assessment and a complete physical examination to detect any emerging or potential problems.

This chapter presents the procedures for estimating gestational age and performing the complete physical examination and behavioral assessment. Chapter 17 discusses the immediate postbirth assessment. See Key Facts to Remember: Timing and Types of Newborn Assessments.

KEY FACTS TO REMEMBER

Timing and Types of Newborn Assessments

Assess immediately after birth: need for resuscitation or if newborn is stable and can be placed with parents to initiate early attachment/bonding

Assessments within 1 to 4 hours after birth:

- Progress of newborn's adaptation to extrauterine life
- Determination of gestational age
- Ongoing assessment for high-risk problems

Assessment procedures within first 24 hours or prior to discharge:

- Complete physical examination (Depending on agency protocol, the nurse may complete some components independently with the certified nurse-midwife/physician/nurse practitioner completing the exam prior to discharge.)
- Nutritional status and ability to bottle- or breastfeed satisfactorily.
- Behavioral state organization abilities

Estimation of Gestational Age

The nurse must establish the newborn's gestational age in the first 4 hours after birth so that careful attention can be given to age-related problems (Alexander and Allen 1996). Traditionally a newborn's gestational age was determined from the date of the pregnant woman's last menstrual period. This method was accurate only 75 to 85 percent of the time. Because of the problems that develop with the preterm newborn, or the newborn whose weight is inappropriate for gestational age, a postnatal system was developed to evaluate the newborn. Once learned, the nurse can do this procedure in a few minutes. *The nurse must wear gloves when assessing the newborn in these early hours after birth and before the first bath.*

Clinical **gestational age assessment tools** have two components: external physical characteristics and neurologic or neuromuscular development. Physical characteristics generally include sole creases, amount of breast tissue, amount of lanugo, cartilaginous development of the ear, testicular descent, and scrotal rugae or labial development. These objective clinical criteria are not influenced by labor and birth and do not change significantly within the first 24 hours after birth.

During the first 24 hours of life, the newborn's nervous system is unstable; thus neurologic findings based on reflexes or assessments that depend on the higher brain centers may not be reliable. If the neurologic findings drastically deviate from the gestational age derived by evaluation of external characteristics, caregivers do a second assessment within 24 hours.

The neurologic assessment components (excluding reflexes) can aid in assessing the gestational age of newborns of less than 34 weeks' gestation. Between 26 and 34 weeks, neurologic changes are significant, whereas significant physical changes are less evident. Important neurologic changes consist of replacement of extensor tone by flexor tone in a *caudocephalad* (tail-to-head) progression. Neurologic examination facilitates assessment of functional or physiologic maturation in addition to physical development.

Ballard's (1979) *estimation of gestational age by maturity* rating is a simplified version of the well researched Dubowitz tool (Dubowitz and Dubowitz 1977). The Ballard tool omits some of the neuromuscular tone assessments such as head lag, ventral suspension (which is difficult to assess in ill newborns or those on respirators), and leg recoil. In Ballard's tool each physical and neuromuscular finding is given a value, and the total score is matched to a gestational age (Figure 22–1). The maximum score on Ballard's tool is 50, which corresponds to a gestational age of 44 weeks.

For example, upon completing a gestational assessment of a 1-hour-old newborn, the nurse gives a score of 3 to all the physical characteristics, for a total of 18, and gives a score of 3 to all neuromuscular assessments, for a total of 18. The physical and neuromuscular scores are added together for a total score of 36, which correlates with 38+ weeks' gestation. Because all newborns vary slightly in the development of physical characteristics and maturation of neurologic function, scores usually vary instead of all being 3 as in this example.

Current postnatal gestational age assessment tools can overestimate preterm gestational age and underestimate postterm gestational age (Alexander and Allen 1996). The tools lose accuracy when used for newborns of fewer than 28 weeks' or more than 43 weeks' gestation. Ballard added criteria for more accurate assessment of the gestational age of newborns 20–28 weeks old (especially infants of fewer than 23 weeks' gestation) and less than 1500 g. Ballard (1991) suggests that the assessment be made within 12 hours of birth to optimize accuracy.

In carrying out gestational age assessments, the nurse keeps in mind that some maternal conditions, such as pregnancy-induced hypertension (PIH), diabetes, and maternal analgesia and anesthesia, may affect certain gestational assessment components and warrant further study. Maternal diabetes, although it appears to accelerate fetal physical growth, seems to retard maturation. Maternal hypertensive states, which retard fetal physical growth, seem to speed maturation.

Newborns of women with PIH have a poor correlation with the criteria involving active muscle tone and edema. Maternal analgesia and anesthesia may cause respiratory depression in the baby. Newborns with respiratory distress syndrome (RDS) tend to be flaccid and edematous and to assume a "froglike" posture. These characteristics affect the scoring of the neuromuscular components of the assessment tool used.

Assessment of Physical Characteristics

The nurse first evaluates observable characteristics without disturbing the newborn. Selected physical characteristics common to all gestational assessment tools appear here in the order in which they are evaluated most effectively:

1. *Resting posture,* although a neuromuscular component, should be assessed as the baby lies undisturbed on a flat surface (Figure 22–2).
2. *Skin* in the preterm newborn appears thin and transparent, with veins prominent over the abdomen early in gestation. As term approaches, the skin appears opaque because of increased subcutaneous tissue. Disappearance of the protective vernix caseosa promotes skin desquamation and is commonly seen in postmature infants (infants with

NEWBORN MATURITY RATING & CLASSIFICATION

ESTIMATION OF GESTATIONAL AGE BY MATURITY RATING

Symbols: X - 1st Exam O - 2nd Exam

NEUROMUSCULAR MATURITY

	−1	0	1	2	3	4	5
Posture							
Square Window (wrist)	>90°	90°	60°	45°	30°	0°	
Arm Recoil		180°	140°–180°	110°–140°	90°–110°	<90°	
Popliteal Angle	180°	160°	140°	120°	100°	90°	<90°
Scarf Sign							
Heel to Ear							

Gestation by Dates ________________ wks

Birth Date __________ Hour __________ am pm

APGAR __________ 1 min __________ 5 min

MATURITY RATING

score	weeks
−10	20
−5	22
0	24
5	26
10	28
15	30
20	32
25	34
30	36
35	38
40	40
45	42
50	44

PHYSICAL MATURITY

Skin	sticky friable transparent	gelatinous red, translucent	smooth pink, visible veins	superficial peeling &/or rash, few veins	cracking pale areas rare veins	parchment deep cracking no vessels	leathery cracked wrinkled
Lanugo	none	sparse	abundant	thinning	bald areas	mostly bald	
Plantar Surface	heel-toe 40–50mm:−1 <40mm:−2	>50mm no crease	faint red marks	anterior transverse crease only	creases ant. 2/3	creases over entire sole	
Breast	imperceptible	barely perceptible	flat areola no bud	stippled areola 1–2mm bud	raised areola 3–4mm bud	full areola 5–10mm bud	
Eye/Ear	lids fused loosely:−1 tightly:−2	lids open pinna flat stays folded	sl. curved pinna; soft; slow recoil	well curved pinna; soft but ready recoil	formed & firm instant recoil	thick cartilage ear stiff	
Genitals male	scrotum flat, smooth	scrotum empty faint rugae	testes in upper canal rare rugae	testes descending few rugae	testes down good rugae	testes pendulous deep rugae	
Genitals female	clitoris prominent labia flat	prominent clitoris small labia minora	prominent clitoris enlarging minora	majora & minora equally prominent	majora large minora small	majora cover clitoris & minora	

SCORING SECTION

	1st Exam = X	2nd Exam = 0
Estimating Gest Age by Maturity Rating	______Weeks	______Weeks
Time of Exam	Date ________ Hour______ am pm	Date ________ Hour______ am pm
Age at Exam	______ Hours	______ Hours
Signature of Examiner	____________ M.D.	____________ M.D.

FIGURE 22–1 Newborn maturity rating and classification. If a 1-hour-old newborn is given a score of 3 for each of the physical characteristics and neuromuscular assessments, the newborn's total score would be 36. A total score of 36 correlates with 38+ weeks' gestation.

Source: Ballard JL et al: New Ballard score, expanded to include extremely premature infants. *J Pediatr* 1991; 119:417.

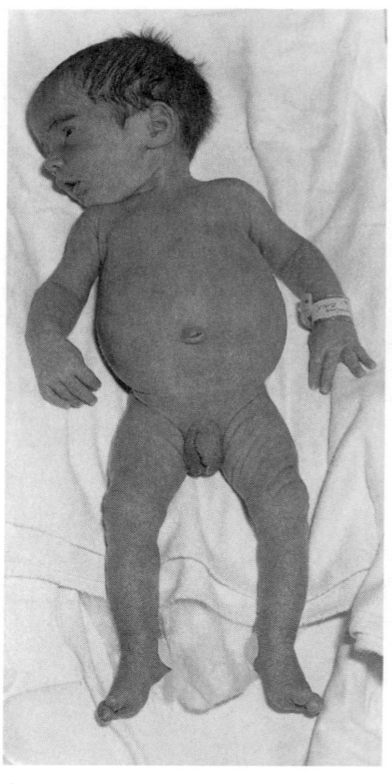

A

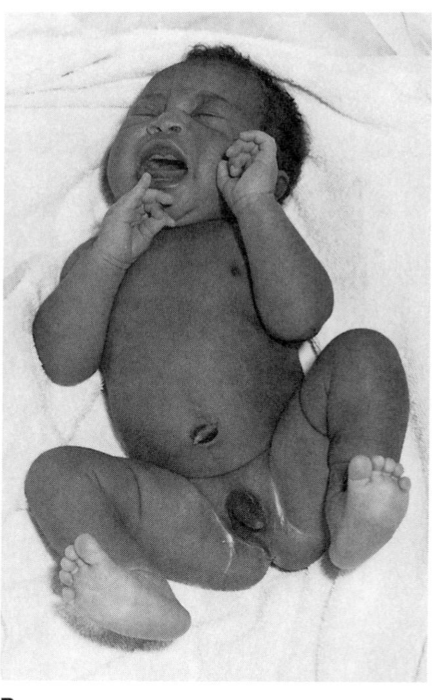

B

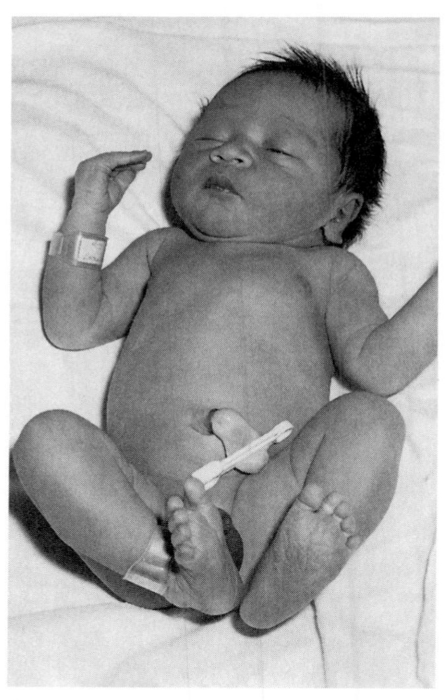

C

FIGURE 22–2 Resting posture. ***A*** Newborn exhibits beginning of flexion of the thigh. The gestational age is approximately 31 weeks. Note the extension of the upper extremities. ***B*** Newborn exhibits stronger flexion of the arms, hips, and thighs. The gestational age is approximately 35 weeks. ***C*** The full-term newborn exhibits hypertonic flexion of all extremities.

Source: Dubowitz L, Dubowitz V: *The Gestational Age of the Newborn.* Menlo Park, CA: Addison-Wesley, 1977. Reprinted by permission of V Dubowitz, MD, Hammersmith Hospital, London, England.

42+ weeks' gestational age and showing signs of placental insufficiency; see Chapter 25).

3. *Lanugo,* a fine hair covering, decreases as gestational age increases. The amount of lanugo is greatest at 28–30 weeks, and then it disappears, first from the face and then from the trunk and extremities.
4. *Sole (plantar) creases* are reliable indicators of gestational age in the first 12 hours of life. After this, the skin of the foot begins drying, and superficial creases appear. Development of sole creases begins at the top (anterior) portion of the sole and, as gestation progresses, proceeds to the heel (Figure 22–3). Peeling may also occur. Plantar creases vary with race. In newborns of African descent, sole creases may be less developed at term.
5. The nurse inspects the *areola* and gently palpates the *breast bud tissue* by applying the forefinger and middle finger to the breast area and measuring the tissue between them in centimeters or millimeters (Figure 22–4). At term gestation, the tissue measures between 0.5 and 1 cm (5–10 mm). During the assessment, the nipple should not be grasped, because skin and subcutaneous tissue will prevent accurate estimation of size. The nurse must do this procedure gently to avoid causing trauma to the breast tissue.

   As gestation progresses, the breast tissue mass and areola enlarge. However, a large breast tissue mass can occur as a result of specific conditions. The newborn of a diabetic mother tends to be large for gestational age (LGA) and the accelerated development of breast tissue is a reflection of subcutaneous fat deposits. Small-for-gestational-age (SGA) term or postterm newborns may have used subcutaneous fat (which would have been deposited as breast tissue) to survive in utero; as a result, their lack of breast tissue may indicate a gestational age of 34 to 35 weeks, even though other factors indicate a *term* or *postterm* newborn.
6. *Ear form and cartilage distribution* develop with gestational age. The cartilage gives the ear its shape and substance (Figure 22–5). In a newborn of less than 34 weeks' gestation, the ear is relatively shapeless and flat; it has little cartilage, so the ear folds over on itself and remains folded. By approximately 36 weeks' gestation, some cartilage and slight incurving of upper pinna are present, and the pinna springs back slowly when folded. (The nurse tests this response by holding the top and bottom of the

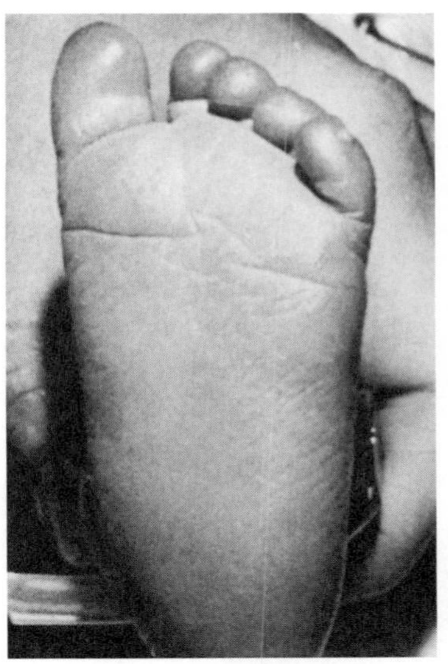

A

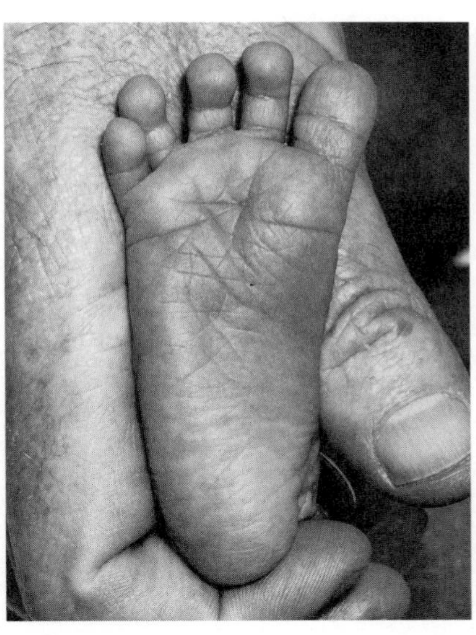

B

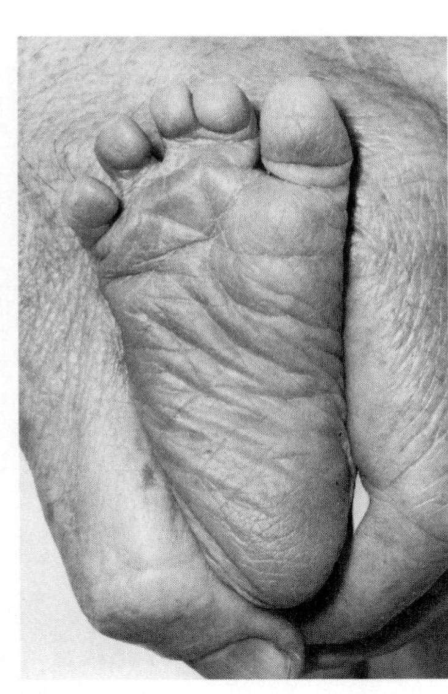

C

FIGURE 22–3 Sole creases. ***A*** Newborn has a few sole creases on the anterior portion of the foot. Note the slick heel. The gestational age is approximately 35 weeks. ***B*** Newborn has a deeper network of sole creases on the anterior two-thirds of the sole. Note the slick heel. The gestational age is approximately 37 weeks. ***C*** The term newborn has deep sole creases down to and including the heel as the skin loses fluid and dries after birth. Sole (plantar) creases can be seen even in preterm newborns.

Source: *B* and *C* from Dubowitz L, Dubowitz V: *The Gestational Age of the Newborn.* Menlo Park, CA: Addison-Wesley, 1977. Reprinted by permission of V Dubowitz, MD, Hammersmith Hospital, London, England.

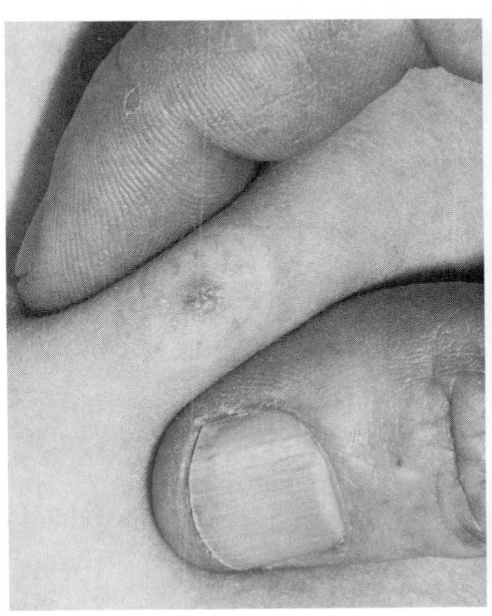

A

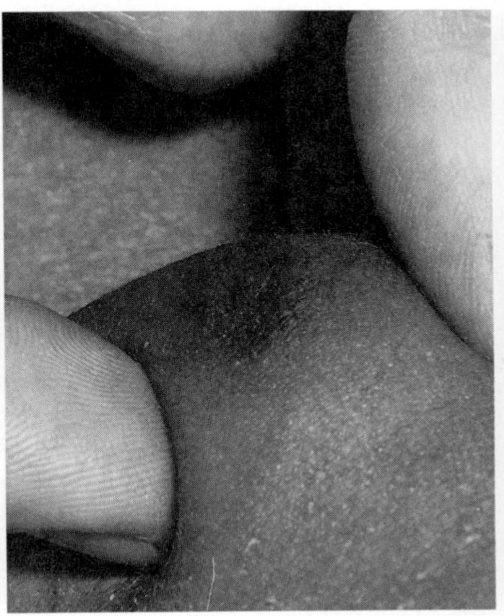

B

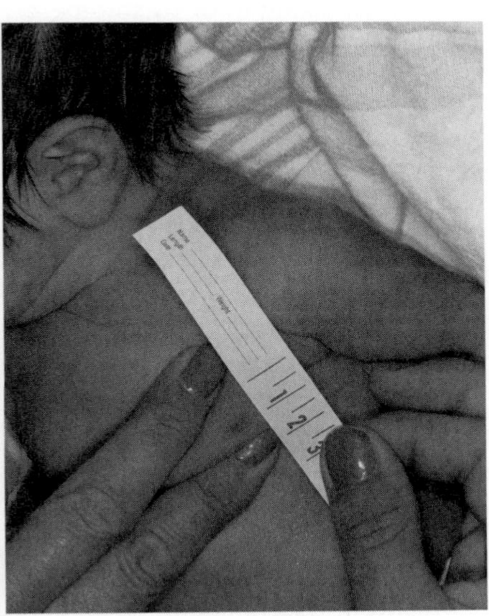

C

FIGURE 22–4 Breast tissue. ***A*** Newborn has a visible raised area. On palpation the area is 4 mm. The gestational age is 38 weeks. ***B*** Newborn has 10 mm breast tissue area. The gestational age is 49 to 44 weeks. ***C*** Gently compress the tissue between the middle and index fingers, and measure the tissue in centimeters or millimeters. Absence of or decreased breast tissue often indicates premature or SGA newborn.

Source: *A* and *B* from Dubowitz L, Dubowitz V: *The Gestational Age of the Newborn.* Menlo Park, CA: Addison-Wesley, 1977. Reprinted by permission of V Dubowitz, MD, Hammersmith Hospital, London, England.

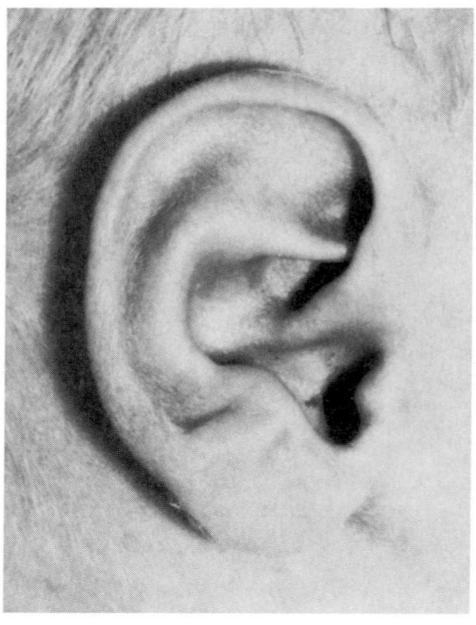
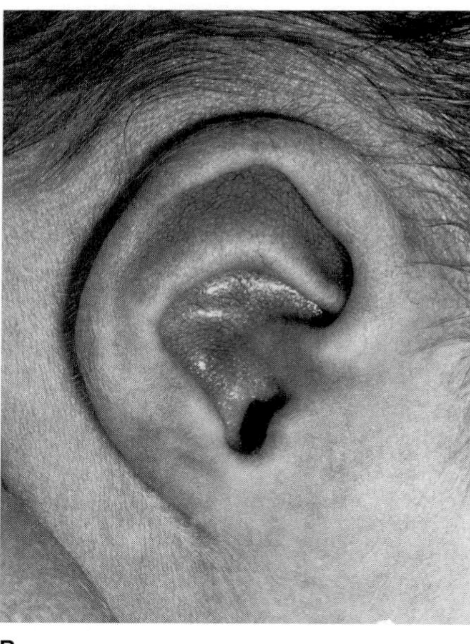
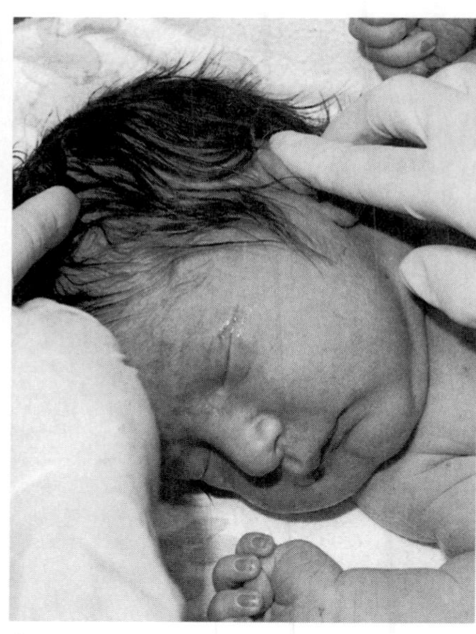

A B C

FIGURE 22–5 Ear form and cartilage. ***A*** The ear of the infant at approximately 36 weeks' gestation shows incurving of the upper two-thirds of the pinna. ***B*** Infant at term shows well-defined incurving of the entire pinna. ***C*** If the auricle stays in the position in which it is pressed or returns slowly to its original position, it usually means the gestational age is less than 38 weeks.

Source: *A* and *B* from Dubowitz L, Dubowitz V: *The Gestational Age of the Newborn.* Menlo Park, CA: Addison-Wesley, 1977. Reprinted by permission of V Dubowitz, MD, Hammersmith Hospital, London, England.

pinna together with the forefinger and thumb and then releasing it, or by folding the pinna of the ear forward against the side of the head, releasing it, and observing the response.) By term, the newborn's pinna is firm, stands away from the head, and springs back quickly from the folding.

7. *Male genitals* are evaluated for size of the scrotal sac, presence of rugae (wrinkles and ridges in the scrotum), and descent of the testes (Figure 22–6). Prior to 36 weeks, the scrotum has few rugae, and the testes are palpable in the inguinal canal. By 36 to 38 weeks, the testes are in the upper scrotum, and rugae have developed over the anterior portion of the scrotum. By term, the testes are generally in the lower scrotum, which is pendulous and covered with rugae.
8. The appearance of the *female genitals* depends in part on subcutaneous fat deposition and therefore relates to fetal nutritional status (Figure 22–7). The clitoris varies in size, and occasionally is so large that it is difficult to identify the sex of the newborn. This may be caused by adrenogenital syndrome, which causes the adrenals to secrete excessive amounts of androgen and other hormones. At 30 to 32 weeks' gestation, the clitoris is prominent, and the labia majora are small and widely separated. As gestational age increases, the labia majora increase in size. At 36 to 40 weeks, they nearly cover the clitoris. At 40 weeks and beyond, the labia majora cover the labia minora and clitoris.

Other physical characteristics assessed by some gestational age scoring tools include the following:

1. *Vernix* covers the preterm newborn. The postterm newborn has no vernix. After noting vernix distribution, the birthing area nurse (wearing gloves) dries the newborn to prevent evaporative heat loss, thus disturbing the vernix and potentially altering this gestational age criterion. The birthing area nurse must communicate to the newborn nurse the amount of vernix and the areas of vernix coverage.
2. *Hair* of the preterm newborn has the consistency of matted wool or fur and lies in bunches rather than in the silky, single strands of the term newborn's hair.
3. *Skull firmness* increases as the fetus matures. In a term newborn the bones are hard, and the sutures are not easily displaced. The nurse should not attempt to displace the sutures forcibly.
4. *Nails* appear and cover the nail bed at about 20 weeks' gestation. Nails extending beyond the fingertips may indicate a postterm newborn.

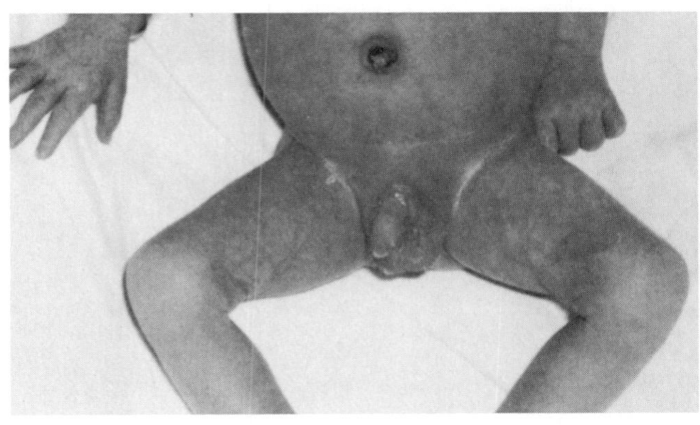

A

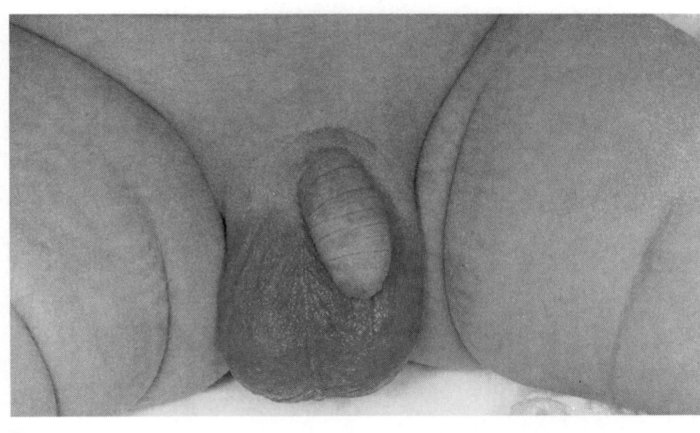

B

FIGURE 22–6 Male genitals. ***A*** Preterm newborn's testes are not within the scrotum. The scrotal surface has few rugae. ***B*** Term newborn's testes are generally fully descended. The entire surface of the scrotum is covered by rugae.

Source: *A* from Dubowitz L, Dubowitz V: *The Gestational Age of the Newborn.* Menlo Park, CA: Addison-Wesley, 1977. Reprinted by permission of V Dubowitz, MD, Hammersmith Hospital, London, England.

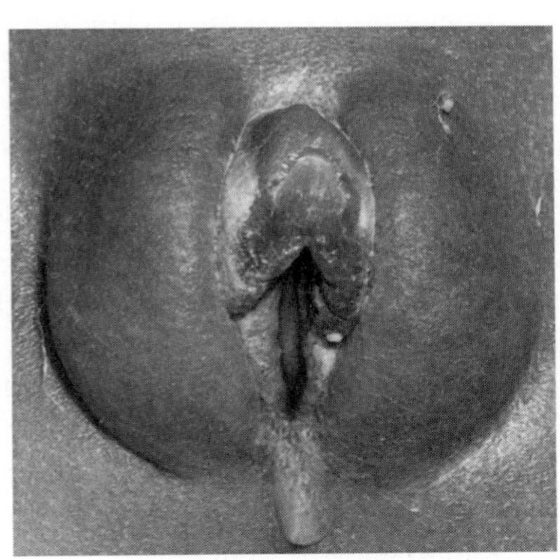

A

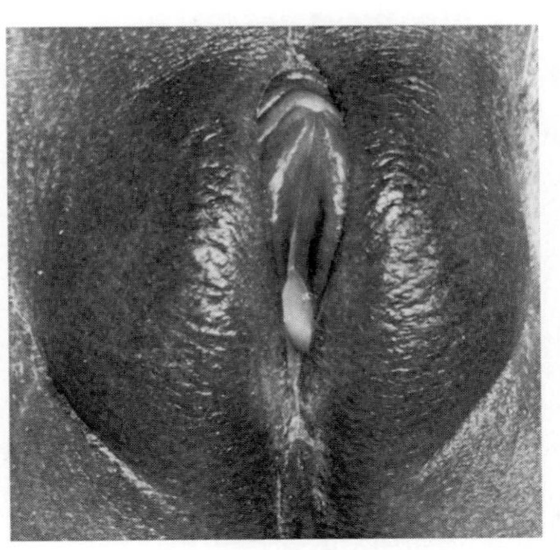

B

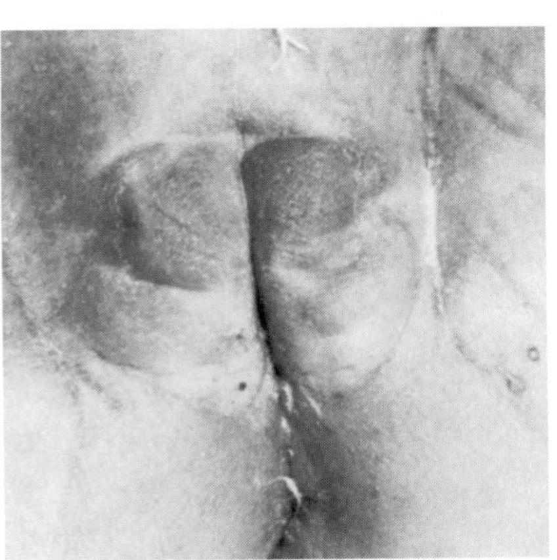

C

FIGURE 22–7 Female genitals. ***A*** Newborn has a prominent clitoris. The labia majora are widely separated, and the labia minora, viewed laterally, would protrude beyond the labia majora. The gestational age is 30–36 weeks. ***B*** The clitoris is still visible. The labia minora are now covered by the larger labia majora. The gestational age is 36–40 weeks. ***C*** The term newborn has well-developed, large labia majora that cover both clitoris and labia minora.

Source: Dubowitz L, Dubowitz V: *The Gestational Age of the Newborn.* Menlo Park, CA: Addison-Wesley, 1977. Reprinted by permission of V Dubowitz, MD, Hammersmith Hospital, London, England.

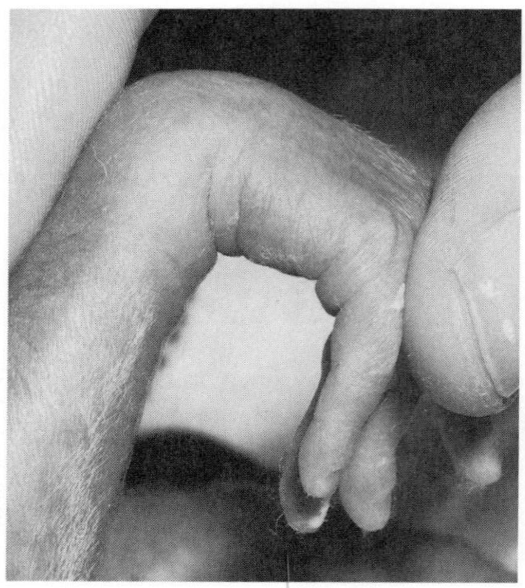
A

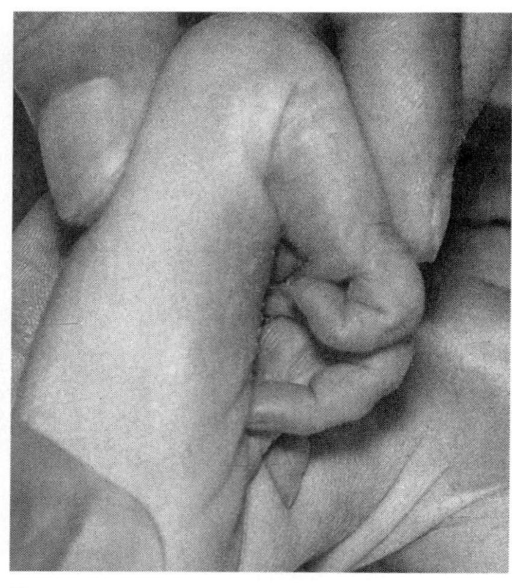
B

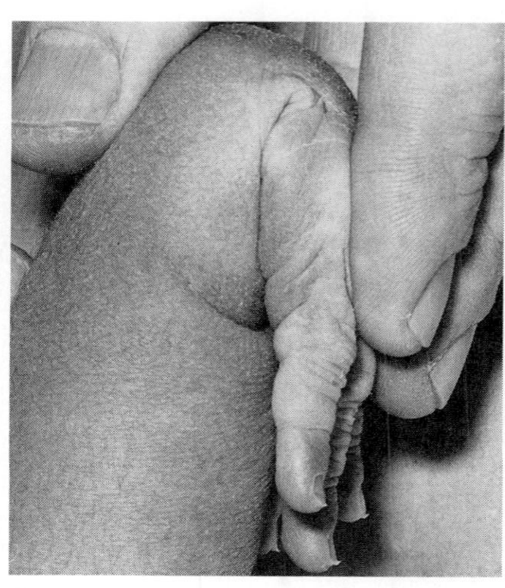
C

FIGURE 22–8 Square window sign. ***A*** This angle is 90 degrees and suggests an immature newborn of 28–32 weeks' gestation. ***B*** A 30-degree angle is commonly found from 39 to 49 weeks' gestation. ***C*** A 0-degree angle occurs from 40 to 42 weeks.

Source: Dubowitz L, Dubowitz V: *The Gestational Age of the Newborn.* Menlo Park, CA: Addison-Wesley, 1977. Reprinted by permission of V Dubowitz, MD, Hammersmith Hospital, London, England.

Assessment of Neuromuscular Maturity Characteristics

The central nervous system of the fetus matures at a fairly constant rate. Tests have been designed to evaluate neurologic status as manifested by neuromuscular tone development and correlated with gestational ages. In the fetus, neuromuscular tone develops from the lower to the upper extremities.

The neuromuscular evaluation (refer to Figure 22–1) is best performed when the newborn has stabilized. The nurse evaluates the following characteristics:

1. The *square window sign* is elicited by gently flexing the newborn's hand toward the ventral forearm until there is resistance and measuring the angle formed at the wrist (Figure 22–8).
2. *Recoil* is a test of flexion development. Because flexion first develops in the lower extremities, the nurse first tests recoil in the legs. Placing the newborn on its back on a flat surface, with a hand on the newborn's knees, the nurse places the newborn's legs in flexion and then extends them parallel to each other and flat on the surface. The response to this maneuver is recoil of the newborn's legs. According to gestational age, they may not move or they may return slowly or quickly to the flexed position. Preterm infants have less muscle tone than term infants, so preterm infants have less recoil.

   Arm recoil is tested by flexion at the elbow and extension of the arms at the newborn's side. While the baby is in the supine position, the nurse completely flexes both elbows, holds them in this position for 5 seconds, extends the arms at the baby's side, and releases them. Upon release, the elbows of a full-term newborn form an angle of less than 90 degrees and rapidly recoil back to flexed position. The elbows of preterm newborns have slower recoil time and form an angle of less than 90 degrees. Arm recoil is also slower in healthy but fatigued newborns after birth; therefore arm recoil is best elicited after the first hour of birth when the baby has had time to recover from the stress of the birth. Deep sleep state also decreases the arm recoil response. Assessment of arm recoil should be bilateral to rule out brachial palsy.
3. The *popliteal angle* (degree of knee flexion) is determined with the newborn flat on its back. The nurse flexes the newborn's thigh on the abdomen/chest and places the index finger of the other hand behind the newborn's ankle to extend the lower leg until resistance is met. The angle formed is then measured. Results vary from no resistance in the very immature newborn to an 80-degree angle in the term newborn.
4. The *scarf sign* is elicited by placing the newborn supine and drawing an arm across the chest toward the newborn's opposite shoulder until there is resistance. The nurse then notes the location of the elbow in relation to the midline of the chest (Figure 22–9).
5. The *heel-to-ear extension* is performed by placing the newborn in a supine position and then gently drawing the foot toward the ear on the same side until there is resistance. The nurse should allow the knee to bend during the test. It is important to hold the buttocks down to keep from rolling the baby.

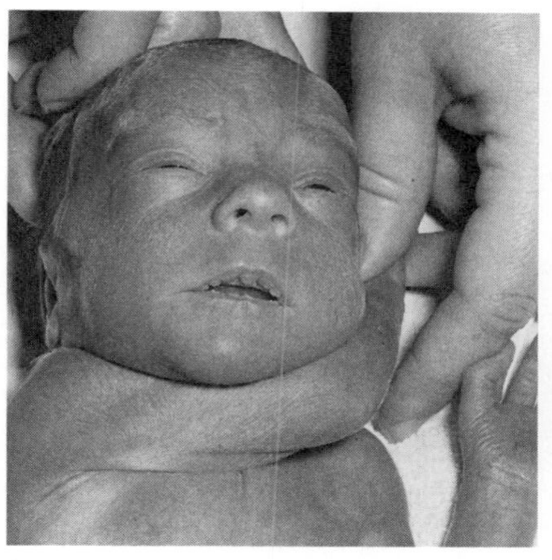

A

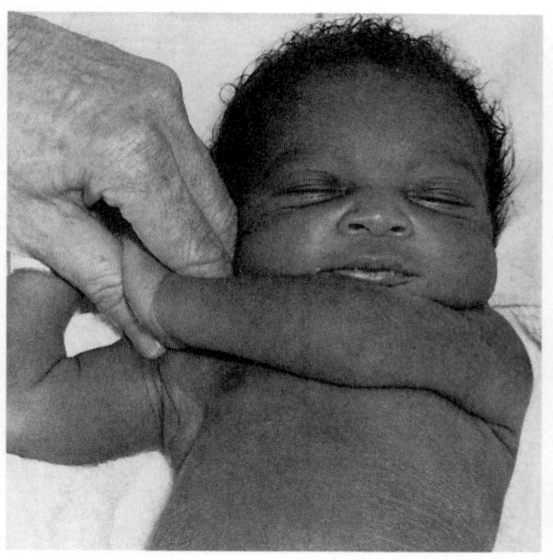

B

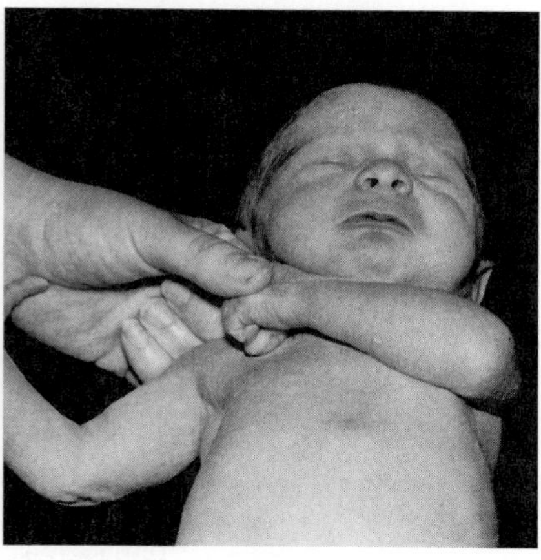

C

FIGURE 22–9 Scarf sign. ***A*** No resistance is noted until after 30 weeks' gestation. The elbow moves readily past the midline. ***B*** The elbow is at midline at 36 to 40 weeks' gestation. ***C*** Beyond 40 weeks' gestation the elbow will not reach the midline.

Source: Dubowitz L, Dubowitz V: *The Gestational Age of the Newborn.* Menlo Park, CA: Addison-Wesley, 1977. Reprinted by permission of V Dubowitz, MD, Hammersmith Hospital, London, England.

The nurse assesses both the proximity of foot to ear and the degree of knee extension. A preterm, immature newborn's leg will remain straight and the foot will go to the ear or beyond. With advancing gestational age the newborn demonstrates increasing resistance to this maneuver. Maneuvers involving the lower extremities of newborns who had frank breech presentation should be delayed to allow for resolution of leg positioning (Ballard et al 1979).

6. *Ankle dorsiflexion* is determined by flexing the ankle on the shin. The nurse uses a thumb to push on the sole of the newborn's foot while the fingers support the back of the leg and then measures the angle between the foot and the interior leg (Figure 22–10). This sign can be influenced by intrauterine position and congenital deformities.
7. *Head lag* (neck flexors) is measured by pulling the newborn to a sitting position and noting the degree of head lag. Total lag is common in newborns up to 34 weeks' gestation, whereas postterm newborns (42+ weeks) hold their heads in front of their body lines. Normal term newborns can support their heads momentarily.
8. *Ventral suspension* (horizontal position) is evaluated by holding the newborn prone on the examiner's hand. The nurse notes position of head and back and degree of flexion in the arms and legs. Some flexion of arms and legs indicates 36–38

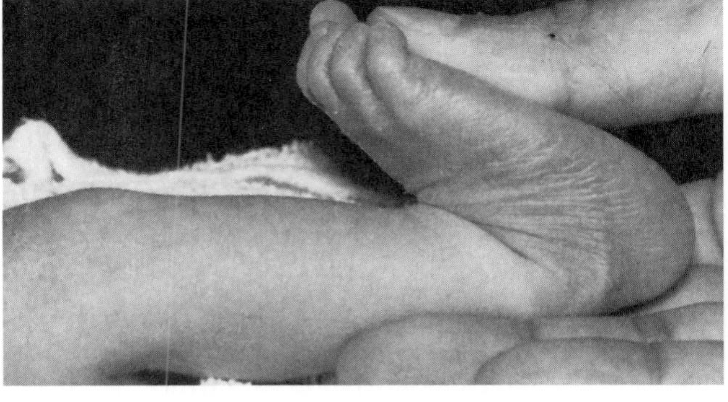

A

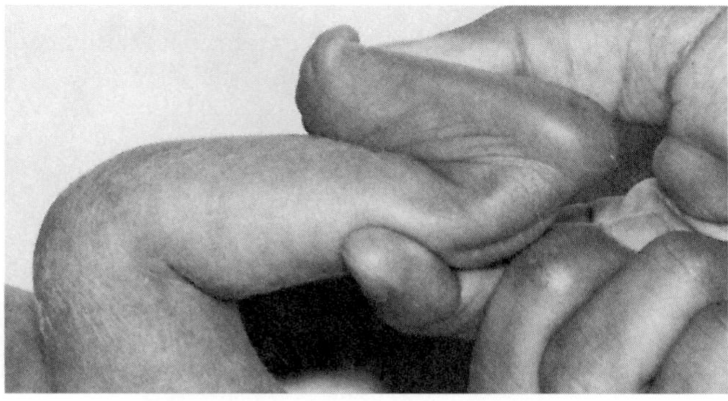

B

FIGURE 22–10 Ankle dorsiflexion. ***A*** A 45-degree angle indicates 32–36 weeks' gestation. A 20-degree angle indicates 36–40 weeks' gestation. ***B*** A 0-degree angle is common at 40 weeks' or more gestational age.

Source: Dubowitz L, Dubowitz V: *The Gestational Age of the Newborn.* Menlo Park, CA: Addison-Wesley, 1977. Reprinted by permission of V Dubowitz, MD, Hammersmith Hospital, London, England.

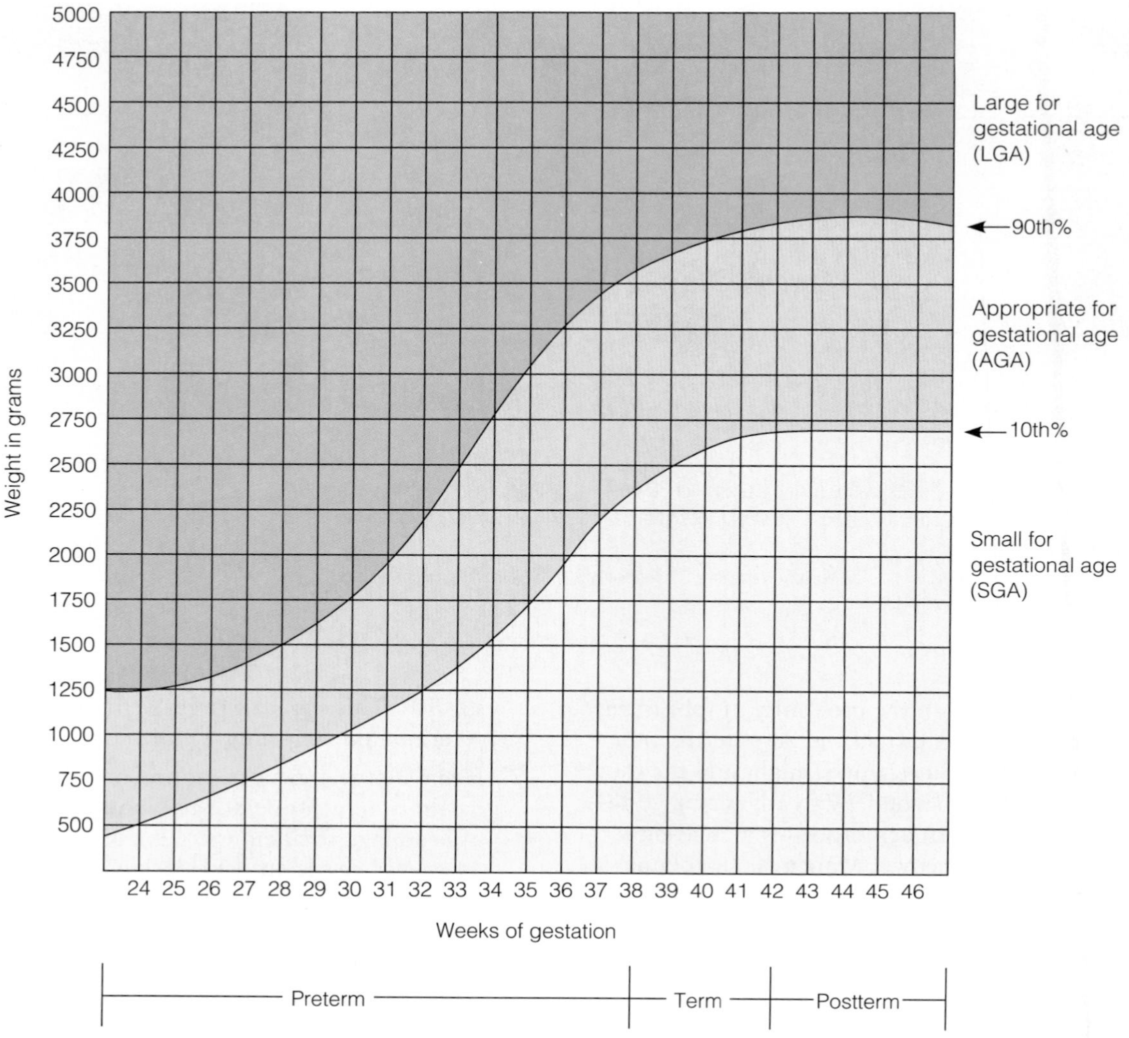

FIGURE 22–11 Classification of newborns by birth weight and gestational age. The nurse places the newborn's birth weight and gestational age on the graph and classifies the newborn as large for gestational age (LGA), appropriate for gestational age (AGA), or small for gestational age (SGA).

Source: Battaglia FC, Lubchenco LO: A practical classification of newborn infants by weight and gestational age. *J Pediatr* 1967; 71:161.

weeks' gestation; fully flexed extremities, with head and back even, are characteristic of a term newborn.

9. The nurse also evaluates major reflexes such as sucking, rooting, grasping, Moro, tonic neck, Babinski, and others during the newborn exam.

When the gestational age determination and birth weight are considered together, the newborn can be identified as one whose *growth is below the 10th percentile or small for gestational age (SGA); appropriate for gestational age (AGA); or above the 90th percentile or large for gestational age (LGA)* (Figure 22–11). This determination enables the nurse to anticipate possible physiologic problems and, in conjunction with a complete physical examination, to establish a plan of care appropriate for the individual newborn (Dodd 1995). For example, an SGA newborn often requires frequent glucose monitoring and early feedings. See Chapter 25 for more complete discussion of these categories and their potential problems.

The nurse also plots the gestational age against the newborn's length, head circumference, and weight on the appropriate growth chart to determine if these measurements fall within the average range—the 10th to 90th percentile for the corresponding gestational age (Figure 22–12). These correlations further document the level of maturity and appropriate category for the newborn. The comparison of the infant's weight-length ratio further facilitates identification of SGA infants as being symmetrically or asymmetrically growth retarded. See Chapter 25 for further discussion.

CLASSIFICATION OF NEWBORNS— BASED ON MATURITY AND INTRAUTERINE GROWTH

Symbols: X-1st Exam O-2nd Exam

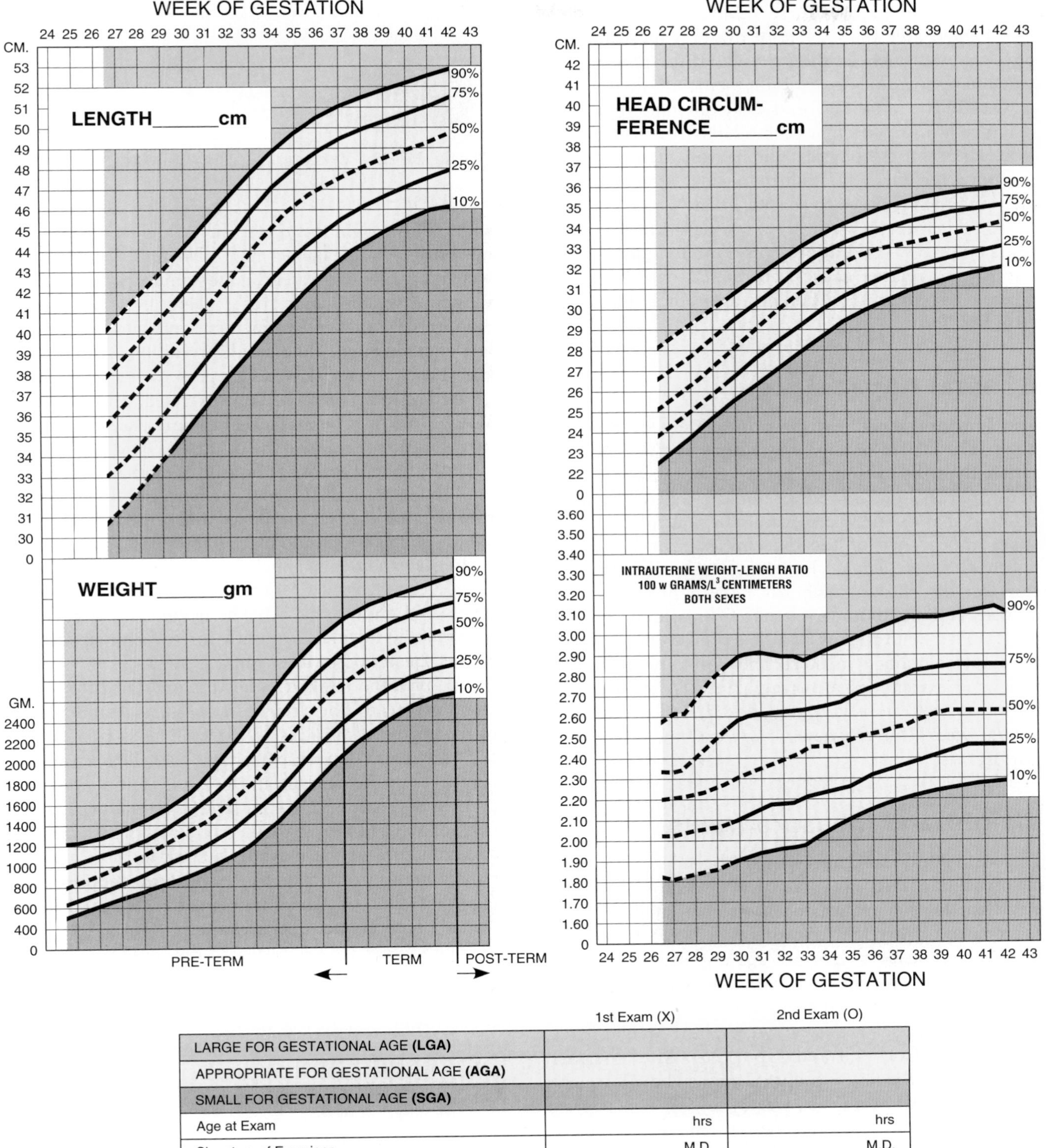

	1st Exam (X)	2nd Exam (O)
LARGE FOR GESTATIONAL AGE **(LGA)**		
APPROPRIATE FOR GESTATIONAL AGE **(AGA)**		
SMALL FOR GESTATIONAL AGE **(SGA)**		
Age at Exam	hrs	hrs
Signature of Examiner	M.D.	M.D.

FIGURE 22–12 Classification of newborns based on maturity and intrauterine growth.

Sources: Adapted from Lubchenco LO, Hansman C, Boyd E: *Pediatrics* 1966; 37:403; Battaglia FC, Lubchenco LO: A practical classification of newborn infants by weight and gestational age. *J Pediatr* 1967; 71:159.

Physical Assessment

After the initial determination of gestational age and related potential problems, a more extensive physical assessment is done. The nurse should choose a warm, well-lighted area that is free of drafts. Completing the physical assessment in the presence of the parents provides an opportunity to acquaint them with their unique newborn. The nurse performs the examination in a systematic, head-to-toe manner and records all findings. When assessing the physical and neurologic status of the newborn, the nurse should first consider general appearance and then proceed to specific areas.

A guide for systematically assessing the newborn appears on pp 550–564. It presents normal findings, alterations, and related causes, correlated with suggested nursing responses. The findings are typical for a full-term newborn.

General Appearance

The newborn's head is disproportionately large for the body. The center of the baby's body is the umbilicus rather than the symphysis pubis (as in the adult). The body appears long and the extremities short. The flexed position that the newborn maintains contributes to the short appearance of the extremities. The hands are tightly clenched. The neck looks short because the chin rests on the chest. Newborns have a prominent abdomen, sloping shoulders, narrow hips, and rounded chests. They tend to stay in a flexed position similar to the one maintained in utero and will offer resistance when the extremities are straightened. After a breech birth, the feet are usually dorsiflexed, and it may take several weeks for the newborn to assume the typical posture.

Weight and Measurements

The normal full-term caucasian newborn has an average birth weight of 3405 g (7 lb 8 oz). Newborns of African or Asian descent are usually somewhat smaller (Wen, Kramer, and Usher 1995; Brooks et al 1995). Other factors that influence weight are age and size of parents, health of mother (smoking and malnutrition decrease birth weight) and the interval between pregnancies (if too close together, such as every year, birth weight tends to decrease) (Cogswell and Yip 1995). After the first week, and for the first 6 months, the newborn's weight increases about 198 g (7 oz) weekly.

Approximately 70 to 75 percent of the newborn's body weight is water. During the initial newborn period (the first 3 or 4 days), there is a physiologic weight loss of about 5 to 10 percent for term newborns because of fluid shifts. This weight loss may reach 15 percent for preterm newborns. Large babies may also tend to lose more weight because of greater fluid loss in proportion to birth weight. If weight loss is greater than 10 percent, clinical reappraisal is indicated. Factors contributing to weight loss include small fluid intake resulting from delayed breastfeeding or a slow adjustment to the formula, increased volume of meconium excreted, and urination. Weight loss may be marked in the presence of temperature elevation (because of associated dehydration) or consistent chilling (because of nonshivering thermogenesis).

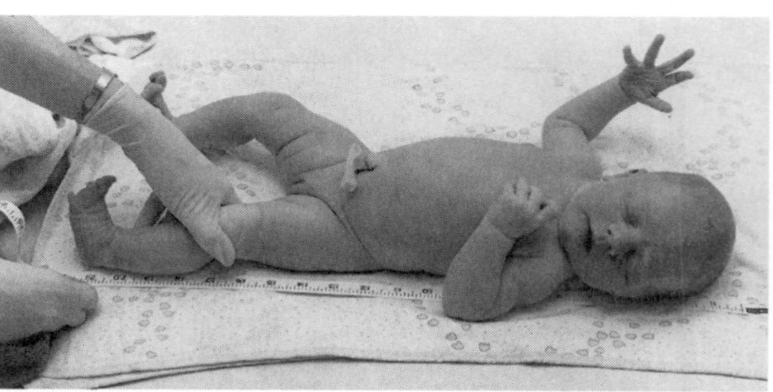

FIGURE 22–13 Measuring the length of the newborn.

The length of the normal newborn is difficult to measure because the legs are flexed and tensed. To measure length, the nurse should place babies flat on their backs with legs extended as much as possible (Figure 22–13). The average length is 50 cm (20 in), with the range being 45–55 cm (18–22 in). The newborn will grow approximately an inch a month for the next 6 months. This is the period of most rapid growth.

At birth the newborn's head is one-third the size of an adult's head. The circumference (biparietal diameter) of the newborn's head is 32–37 cm (12.5–14.5 in). For accurate measurement, place tape over the most prominent part of the occiput and bring it to just above the eyebrows (Figure 22–14*A*). The circumference of the newborn's head is approximately 2 cm greater than the circumference of the newborn's chest at birth and will remain in this proportion for the next few months. (Factors that alter this measurement are discussed in the "Head" section later in this chapter.)

The average circumference of the chest at birth is 32 cm (12.5 in) and ranges from 30 to 35 cm. The nurse should take chest measurements with the tape measure at the lower edge of the scapulas and directly over the nipple line (Figure 22–14*B*). Also measure the abdominal circumference, or girth, at this time by placing the tape around the newborn's abdomen at the level of the umbilicus, with the bottom edge of the tape at the top edge of the umbilicus. (See Key Facts to Remember: Newborn Measurements.)

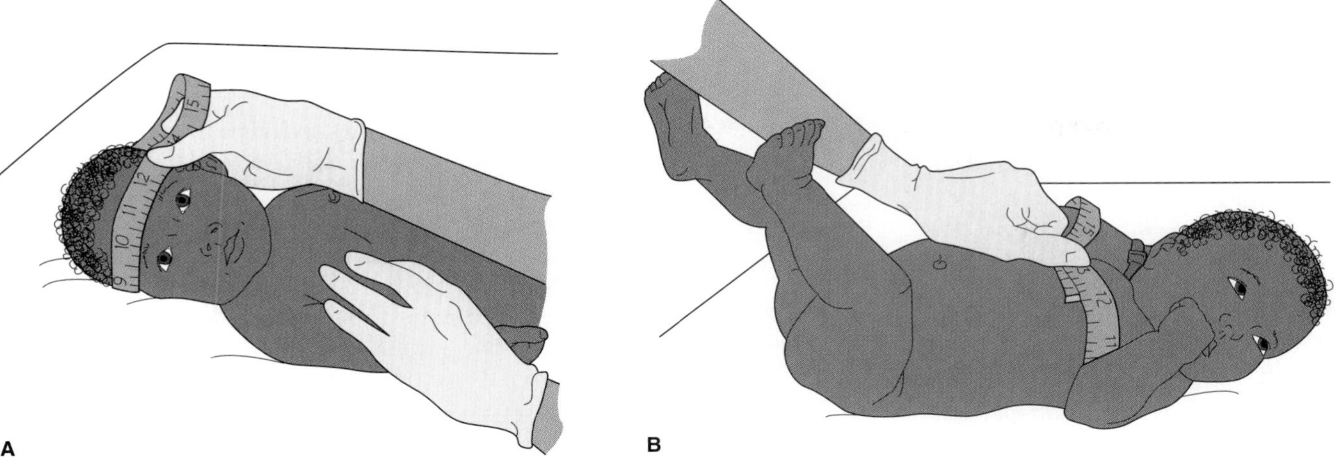

FIGURE 22–14 ***A*** Measuring the head circumference of the newborn. ***B*** Measuring the chest circumference of the newborn.

Temperature

Initial assessment of the newborn's temperature is critical. In utero, the temperature of the fetus is about the same as, or slightly higher than, the expectant mother's. When babies enter the outside world, their temperature can suddenly drop as a result of exposure to cold drafts and the skin's heat-loss mechanisms.

If no heat conservation measures are started, the normal term newborn's deep body temperature falls 0.1C (0.2F) per minute; skin temperature drops 0.3C (0.5F) per minute. Marked decrease in skin temperature occurs within 10 minutes after exposure to room air. The temperature should stabilize within 8 to 12 hours. Temperature is monitored when the newborn is admitted to the nursery and at least every 30 minutes until the newborn's status has remained stable for 2 hours. After that, the nurse should assess temperature at least once every 8 hours, or according to institutional policy (AAP 1992). (See Chapter 21 for a discussion of the physiology of temperature regulation.)

Body temperature can be assessed by the axillary skin method, a continuous skin probe, or the rectal route, or by using a tympanic thermometer. Axillary temperature reflects body temperature and the body's compensatory response to the thermal environment. Axillary temperatures are the preferred method, and are considered to be a close estimation of the rectal temperature. In preterm and term newborns, there is less than 0.10C (0.20F) difference between the two sites. With the axillary method, the thermometer must remain in place at least 3 minutes unless an electronic thermometer is used (Figure 22–15). Normal axillary temperature ranges from 36.4–37.2C (97.5–99F). Axillary temperatures can be misleading, because the friction caused by apposition of the inner arm skin and upper chest wall, and the nearness of brown fat to the probe, may elevate the temperature. Parents need to be aware that current research on forehead strip thermometers indicates that they do not reflect core temperature as accurately as the axillary method does (Shann and Mackenzie 1996).

The best measure of skin temperature is by means of continuous skin probe, especially for small newborns or newborns maintained in incubators or under radiant

KEY FACTS TO REMEMBER

Newborn Measurements

Weight

Average: 3405 g (7 lb, 8 oz)

Range: 2500–4000 g (5 lb, 8 oz–8 lb, 13 oz)

Weight is influenced by racial origin and maternal age and size.

Physiologic weight loss: 5%–10% for term newborns, up to 15% for preterm newborns

Growth: 198 g (7 oz) per week for first 6 months

Length

Average: 50 cm (20 in)

Range: 45–55 cm (18–22 in)

Growth: 2.5 cm (1 in) per month for first 6 months

Head Circumference

32–37 cm (12.5–14.5 in)

Approximately 2 cm larger than chest circumference

Chest Circumference

Average: 32 cm (12.5 in)

Range: 30–35 cm (12–14 in)

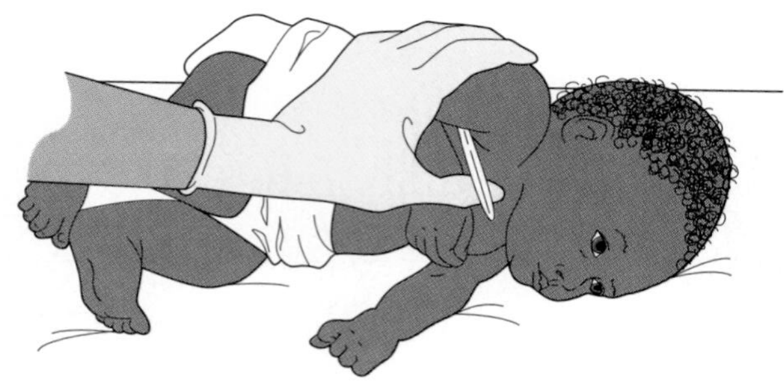

FIGURE 22–15 Axillary temperature measurement. The thermometer should remain in place for 3 minutes. The nurse presses the newborn's arm tightly but gently against the thermometer and the newborn's side as illustrated.

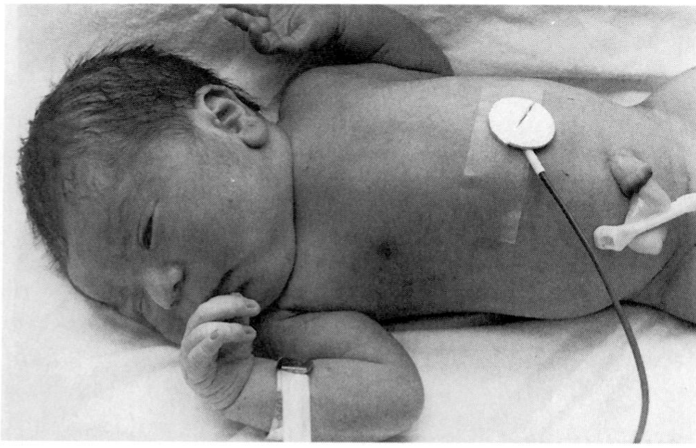

FIGURE 22–16 Temperature monitoring for the newborn. A skin thermal sensor is placed on the newborn's abdomen, upper thigh, or arm and secured with porous tape or a foil-covered foam pad.

warmers. Normal skin temperature is 36–36.5C (96.8–97.7F). Skin temperature assessment allows time for initiation of interventions before a more serious fall in core temperature occurs (Figure 22–16).

Rectal temperature is assumed to be the closest approximation to core temperature, but this depends on the depth of the thermometer insertion. Normal rectal temperature is 36.6–37.2C (97.8–99F). The rectal route is not recommended as a routine method, because it may irritate the rectal mucosa and increase chances of perforation. If the temperature must be taken rectally, the nurse inserts the lubricated thermometer to the depth of no greater than 1.27 cm (0.5 in) into the rectum and continuously holds it in the rectum while stabilizing the infant's lower extremities.

Some institutions may be using tympanic thermometers. These are portable sensor probes with disposable covers that are placed in the auditory canal. The probe uses infrared technology to measure the temperature of the internal carotid artery blood flow within several seconds. Early research findings indicate that tympanic temperatures are as accurate as axillary temperatures (Hicks 1996).

Temperature instability, a deviation of more than 1C (2F) from one reading to the next, or a subnormal temperature may indicate an infection. In contrast to an elevated temperature in older children, an increased temperature in a newborn may indicate reactions to too much covering, too hot a room, or dehydration. Dehydration, which tends to increase body temperature, occurs in newborns whose feedings have been delayed for any reason. Newborns may respond to overheating (a temperature greater than 37.5C, or 99.5F) by increased restlessness and eventually by perspiration. The perspiration appears initially on the head and face and then on the chest. Many newborns initially cannot perspire, so they increase their respiratory and heart rates, which increases oxygen consumption.

Skin Characteristics

Although the newborn's skin color varies with genetic background, all healthy newborns have a pink tinge to their skin. The ruddy hue results from increased red blood cell concentrations in the blood vessels and limited subcutaneous fat deposits.

Skin pigmentation is slight in the newborn period, so color changes may be seen even in darker-skinned babies. A newborn who is cyanotic at rest and pink only with crying may have choanal atresia (congenital blockage of the passageway between the nose and pharynx). If crying increases the cyanosis, heart or lung problems may be suspected. Very pale newborns may be anemic or have hypovolemia (low BP) and should be evaluated for these problems.

Acrocyanosis

Acrocyanosis (bluish discoloration of the hands and feet) may be present in the first 2 to 6 hours after birth (Figure 22–17). This condition is caused by poor peripheral circulation, which results in vasomotor instability and capillary stasis, especially when the newborn is exposed to cold. If the central circulation is adequate, the blood supply should return quickly when the skin is blanched with a finger. Blue hands and nails are a poor indicator of oxygenation in a newborn. The nurse should assess the face and mucous membranes for pinkness reflecting adequate oxygenation.

Mottling (lacy pattern of dilated blood vessels under the skin) is the result of general circulation fluctuations. It may last several hours to several weeks or may come and go periodically (Hockelman et al 1992). Mottling may be related to chilling or prolonged apnea.

Harlequin Sign

Harlequin sign (clown) color change is occasionally noted: A deep red color develops over one side of the newborn's body while the other side remains pale, so that the skin resembles a clown's suit. This color change results from a vasomotor disturbance in which blood vessels on one side dilate while the vessels on the other side constrict. It usually lasts from 1 to 20 minutes. Affected newborns may have single or multiple episodes, but they are transient and not of clinical significance.

Jaundice

Jaundice is first detectable on the face (where skin overlies cartilage) and the mucous membranes of the mouth. It is evaluated by blanching the tip of the nose, the forehead, the sternum, or the gum line. This procedure must be carried out in appropriate lighting. If jaundice is present, the area will appear yellowish immediately after blanching. Another area to assess for jaundice is the sclera. Evaluation and determination of the cause of jaundice must be initiated immediately to prevent possibly serious sequelae. The jaundice may be related to breastfeeding (small incidence), hematomas, immature liver function, or bruises from forceps, or it may be caused by blood incompatibility, oxytocin (pitocin) augmentation or induction, or severe hemolysis process. The nurse should report to the physician any jaundice noted before 24 hours of age. For detailed discussion of causes and assessment of jaundice, see Chapter 26.

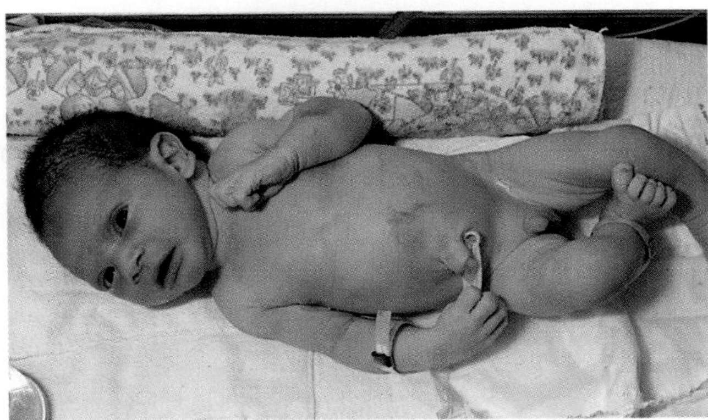

FIGURE 22–17 Acrocyanosis.

Erythema Toxicum

Erythema toxicum is a perifollicular eruption of lesions that are firm, vary in size from 1 to 3 mm, and consist of a white or pale yellow papule or pustule with an erythematous base. It is often called "newborn rash" or "flea bite" dermatitis. The rash may appear suddenly, usually over the trunk and diaper area, and is frequently widespread (Figure 22–18). The lesions do not appear on the palms of the hands or the soles of the feet. The peak incidence is at 24–48 hours of life. The condition rarely presents at birth or after 5 days of life (Hockelman et al 1992). The cause is unknown, and no treatment is necessary. Some clinicians feel it may be caused by irritation from clothing. The lesions disappear in a few hours or days. Should a maculopapular rash appear, a smear of the aspirated papule will show numerous eosinophils on staining; no bacteria will be cultured.

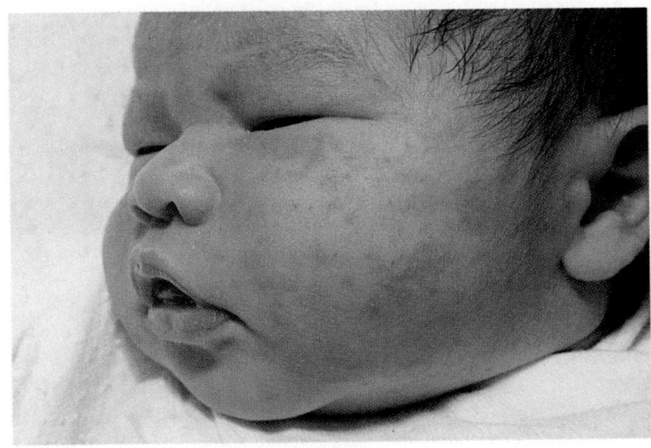

FIGURE 22–18 Erythema toxicum.

Milia

Milia, which are exposed sebaceous glands, appear as raised white spots on the face, especially across the nose (Figure 22–19). No treatment is necessary, as they will clear up spontaneously within the first month (Hockelman et al 1992). Infants of African heritage have a similar condition called transient neonatal pustular melanosis (Taeusch et al 1991).

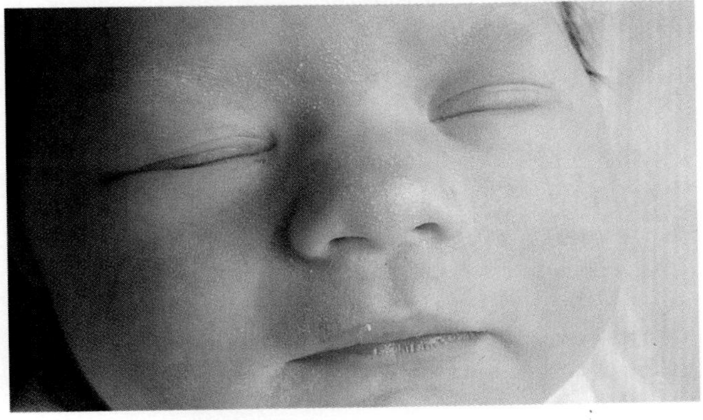

FIGURE 22–19 Facial milia.

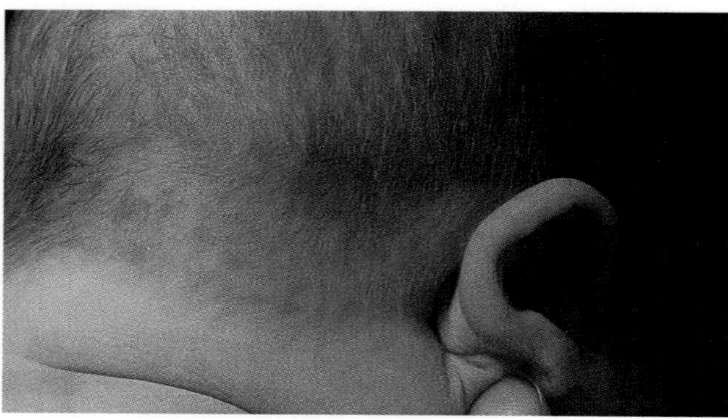

FIGURE 22–20 Stork bites.

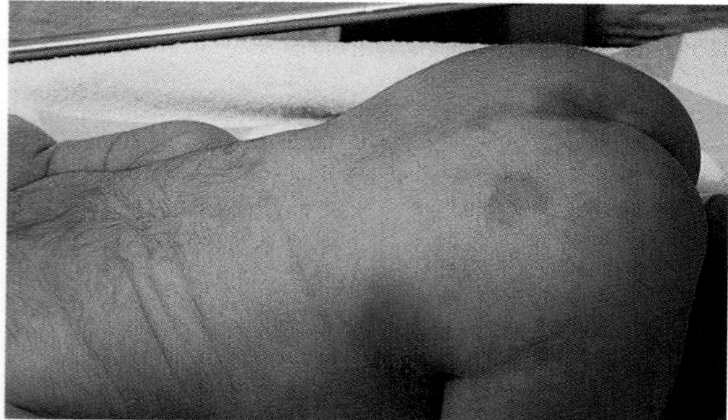

FIGURE 22–21 Mongolian spots.

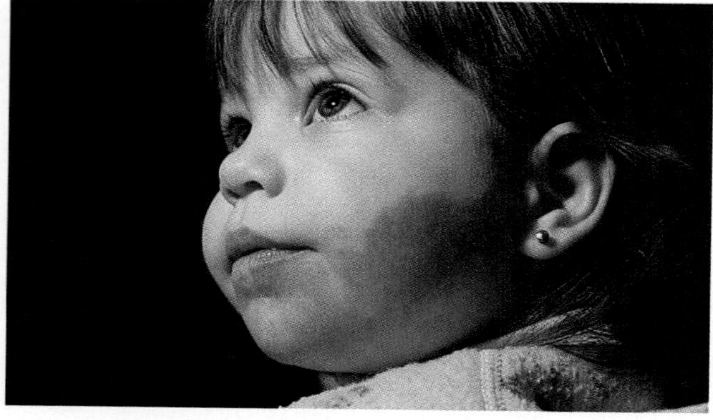

FIGURE 22–22 Port-wine stain.

Skin Turgor

Skin turgor is assessed to determine hydration status, the need to initiate early feedings, and the presence of any infectious processes. The usual place to assess skin turgor is over the abdomen or the thigh. Skin should be elastic and should return to its original shape.

Vernix Caseosa

Vernix caseosa, a whitish cheeselike substance, covers the fetus while in utero and lubricates the skin of the newborn. The skin of the term or postterm newborn has less vernix and is frequently dry; peeling is common, especially on the hands and feet.

Forceps Marks/Vacuum Extractor Marks

Forceps marks may be present after a difficult forceps birth. The newborn may have reddened areas over the cheeks and jaws. It is important to reassure the parents that these will disappear, usually within 1 or 2 days. Transient facial paralysis resulting from the forceps pressure is a rare complication. Suction marks on the vertex of the scalp are often seen when vacuum extractors are used to assist with the birth. These are benign and do not indicate any underlying brain lesions (Hockelman et al 1992).

Birthmarks

Telangiectatic Nevi

Telangiectatic nevi (stork bites) appear as pale pink or red spots and are frequently found on the eyelids, nose, lower occipital bone, and nape of the neck (Figure 22–20). These lesions are common in light-complexioned newborns and are more noticeable during periods of crying. These areas have no clinical significance, and usually fade by the second birthday.

Mongolian Spots

Mongolian spots are macular areas of bluish-black or gray-blue pigmentation on the dorsal area and the buttocks (Figure 22–21). They are common in newborns of Asian and African descent and other dark-skinned races. They gradually fade during the first or second year of life. They may be mistaken for bruises and should be documented in the newborn's chart.

Nevus Flammeus

Nevus flammeus (port-wine stain) is a capillary angioma directly below the epidermis. It is a nonelevated, sharply demarcated, red-to-purple area of dense capillaries (Figure 22–22). In infants of African descent, it may appear as a purple-black stain. The size and shape vary, but it commonly appears on the face. It does not grow in size, does not fade with time, and does not blanch as a rule. The birthmark may be concealed by using an opaque cosmetic cream. Convulsions and other neurologic problems accompanying the nevus flammeus are suggestive of Sturge-Weber syndrome with involvement of the fifth cranial nerve (the ophthalmic branch of the trigeminal nerve).

Nevus Vasculosus

Nevus vasculosus (strawberry mark) is a capillary hemangioma. It consists of newly formed and enlarged capillaries in the dermal and subdermal layers. It is a raised, clearly delineated, dark red, rough-surfaced birthmark commonly found in the head region. Such marks usually grow (often rapidly) for several months, becoming fixed in size by 8 months. They begin to shrink and start to resolve spontaneously several weeks to months after they reach peak growth. About 90 percent of cases resolve completely by the time the child is 9 years old (Hockelman et al 1992). Parents can be told that resolution is heralded by a pale purple or gray spot on the surface of the hemangioma. The best cosmetic effect is achieved when the lesions are allowed to resolve spontaneously.

Birthmarks are frequently a cause of concern for parents. The mother may be especially anxious, fearing that she is to blame ("Is my baby 'marked' because of something I did?"). Guilt feelings are common in the presence of misconceptions about the cause. The nurse should identify birthmarks and explain them to the parents. By providing appropriate information about the cause and course of birthmarks, the nurse frequently relieves the fears and anxieties of the family. The nurse should note any bruises, abrasions, or birthmarks seen upon admission to the nursery.

Head

General Appearance

The newborn's head is large (approximately one-fourth of the body size), with soft, pliable skull bones. The head may appear asymmetrical in the newborn of a vertex birth. This asymmetry, called **molding,** is caused by overriding of the cranial bones during labor and birth (Figure 22–23). The degree of molding varies with the amount and length of pressure exerted on the head. Within a few days after birth, the overriding usually diminishes and the suture lines become palpable. Because head measurements are affected by molding, a second measurement is indicated a few days after birth. The heads of breech-born newborns and those born by elective cesarean are characteristically round and well shaped because no pressure was exerted on them during birth. Any extreme differences in head size may indicate microcephaly or hydrocephalus. Variations in the shape, size, or appearance of the head measurements may be due to *craniostenosis* (premature closure of the cranial sutures), which will need to be corrected through surgery to allow brain growth, and *plagiocephaly* (asymmetry caused by pressure on the fetal head during gestation).

Two *fontanelles* ("soft spots") may be palpated on the newborn's head. Fontanelles, which are openings at the juncture of the cranial bones, can be measured with the fingers. Accurate measurement necessitates that the examiner's finger be measured in centimeters. The assessment should be carried out with the newborn in sitting position and not crying. The diamond-shaped *anterior fontanelle* is approximately 3–4 cm long by 2–3 cm wide. It is located at the juncture of the frontal and parietal bones. The *posterior fontanelle,* smaller and triangular, is formed by the parietal bones and the occipital bone and is 0.5 cm by 1 cm. Newborns of African descent have larger anterior and posterior fontanelles than caucasian newborns (Faix 1982). The fontanelles will be smaller immediately after birth than several days later because of molding. The anterior fontanelle closes within 18 months, whereas the posterior fontanelle closes within 8–12 weeks.

The fontanelles are a useful indicator of the newborn's condition. The anterior fontanelle may swell when the newborn cries or passes a stool, or may pulsate with the heartbeat, which is normal. A bulging fontanelle usually signifies increased intracranial pressure, and a depressed fontanelle indicates dehydration. The sutures between the cranial bones should be palpated for amount of overlapping. In growth-retarded newborns the sutures may be wider than normal, and the fontanelles may also be larger due to impaired growth of the cranial bones.

In addition to inspecting the newborn's head for degree of molding and size, the nurse should evaluate it for soft tissue edema and bruising.

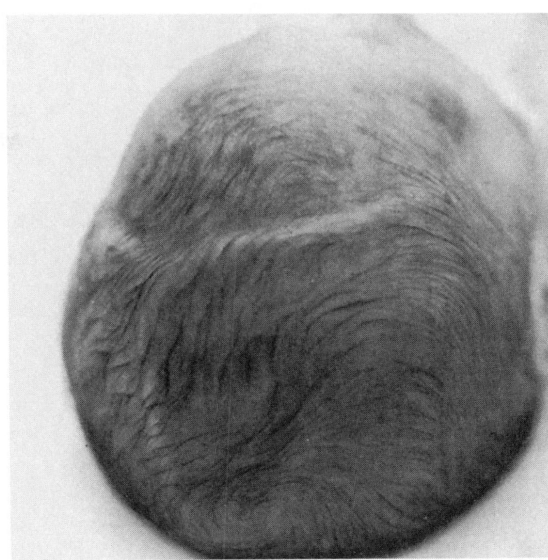

FIGURE 22–23 Overlapped cranial bones produce a visible ridge in a small, premature newborn. Easily visible overlapping does not occur often in term infants.

Source: Korones SB: *High-Risk Newborn Infants,* 4th ed. St Louis: Mosby, 1986.

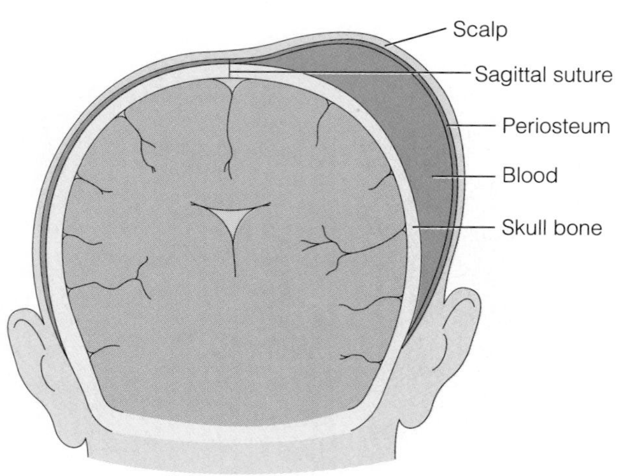

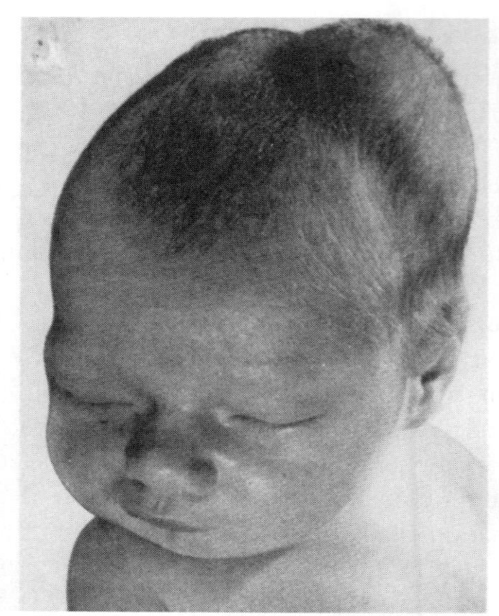

FIGURE 22–24 Cephalhematoma is a collection of blood between the surface of a cranial bone and the periosteal membrane. This is a cephalhematoma over the left parietal bone.

Source: Potter EL, Craig JM: *Pathology of the Fetus and Infant,* 3rd ed. Chicago: Year Book Medical Publishers, 1975. Reproduced with permisssion.

Cephalhematoma

Cephalhematoma is a collection of blood resulting from ruptured blood vessels between the surface of a cranial bone (usually parietal) and the periosteal membrane (Figure 22–24). The scalp in these areas feels loose and slightly edematous. These areas emerge as defined hematomas between the first and second day. Although external pressure may cause the mass to fluctuate, it does not increase in size when the newborn cries. Cephalhematomas may be unilateral or bilateral and do not cross suture lines. They are relatively common in vertex births and may disappear within 2 to 3 weeks, or very slowly over subsequent months. They may be associated with physiologic jaundice, because there are extra RBCs being destroyed within the cephalhematoma.

KEY FACTS TO REMEMBER

Comparison of Cephalhematoma and Caput Succedaneum

Cephalhematoma

Collection of blood between cranial (usually parietal) bone and periosteal membrane

Does not cross suture lines

Does not increase in size with crying

Appears on first and second day

Disappears after 2 to 3 weeks or may take months

Caput Succedaneum

Collection of fluid, edematous swelling of the scalp

Crosses suture lines

Present at birth or shortly thereafter

Reabsorbed within 12 hours or a few days after birth

Caput Succedaneum

Caput succedaneum is a localized, easily identifiable, soft area of the scalp, generally resulting from a long and difficult labor or vacuum extraction. The sustained pressure of the presenting part against the cervix compresses local blood vessels and slows venous return. This causes an increase in tissue fluids, an edematous swelling, and occasional bleeding under the periosteum. The caput may vary from a small area to a severely elongated head. The fluid in the caput is reabsorbed within 12 hours to a few days after birth. Caputs resulting from vacuum extractors are sharply outlined, circular areas up to 2 cm thick. They disappear more slowly than naturally occurring edema. It is possible to distinguish between a cephalhematoma and a caput because the caput overrides suture lines (Figure 22–25), whereas the cephalhematoma, because of its location, never crosses a suture line. Also, caput succedaneum is present at birth, whereas cephalhematoma is not. See Key Facts to Remember: Comparison of Cephalhematoma and Caput Succedaneum.

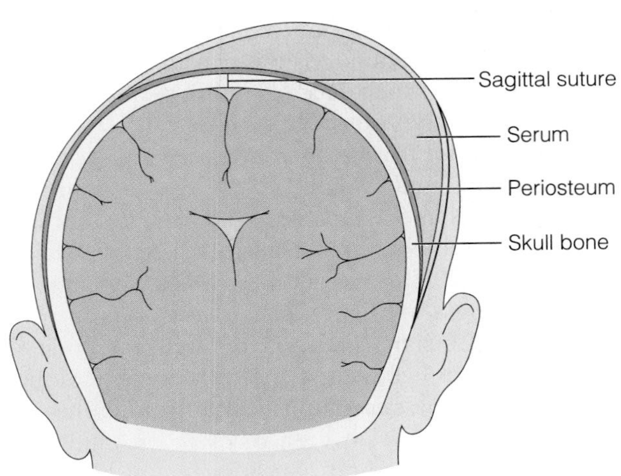

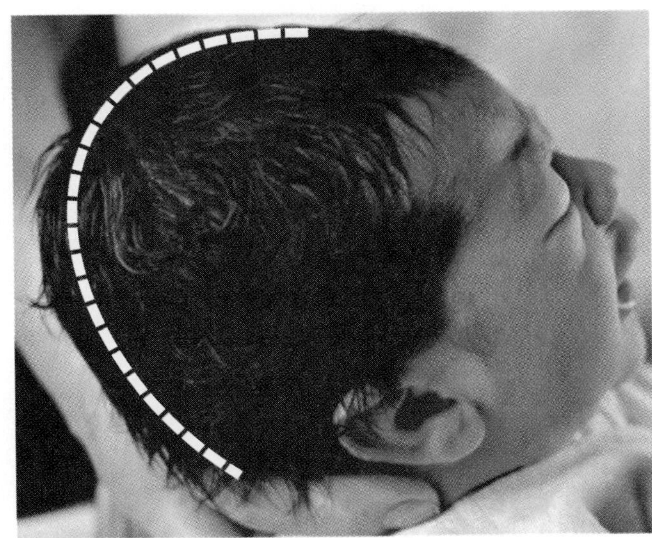

FIGURE 22–25 Caput succedaneum is a collection of fluid (serum) under the scalp.
Source: Photo courtesy of Mead Johnson Laboratories, Evansville, IN.

Face

The newborn's face is well designed to help the newborn suckle. Sucking (fat) pads are located in the cheeks, and a labial tubercle (sucking callus) is frequently found in the center of the upper lip. The chin is recessed, and the nose is flattened. The lips are sensitive to touch, and the sucking reflex is easily initiated. The nurse evaluates symmetry of the eyes, nose, and ears. See the Newborn Physical Assessment Guide on pp 553–557 for deviations in symmetry and variations in size, shape, and spacing of facial features.

The nurse should assess facial movement symmetry to determine the presence of facial palsy, which can be seen when the newborn cries; the affected side is immobile and the palpebral (eyelid) fissure widens (Figure 22–26). Paralysis may result from forceps-assisted birth or pressure on the facial nerve from the maternal pelvis during birth. Facial paralysis usually disappears within a few days to 3 weeks, although in some cases it may be permanent.

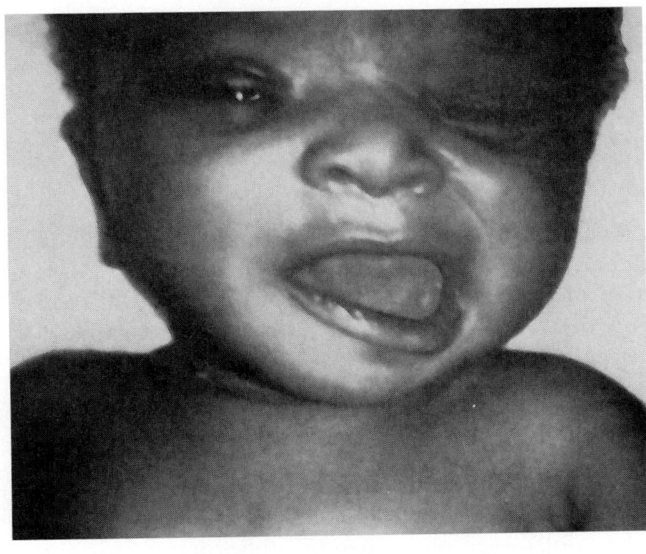

FIGURE 22–26 Facial paralysis. Paralysis of the right side of the face from injury to right facial nerve.
Source: Courtesy of Dr Ralph Platow. In: *Pathology of the Fetus and Infant,* 3rd ed. Potter EL, Craig JM. Chicago: Year Book Medical Publishers, 1975.

Eyes

The eyes of the newborn of Northern European descent are a blue- or slate-blue gray. Scleral color tends to be bluish-white because of its relative thinness. A blue sclera is associated with osteogenesis imperfecta (Tappero and Honeyfield 1996). The infant's eye color is usually established at approximately 3 months, although it may change any time up to 1 year. Dark-skinned newborns tend to have dark eyes at birth.

The eyes should be checked for size, equality of pupil size, reaction of pupils to light, blink reflex to light, and edema and inflammation of the eyelids. The eyelids are usually edematous during the first few days of life because of the trauma of birth.

Erythromycin and tetracycline are now frequently used prophylactically instead of silver nitrate and usually don't cause chemical irritation of the eye. The instillation of silver nitrate drops in the newborn's eyes may

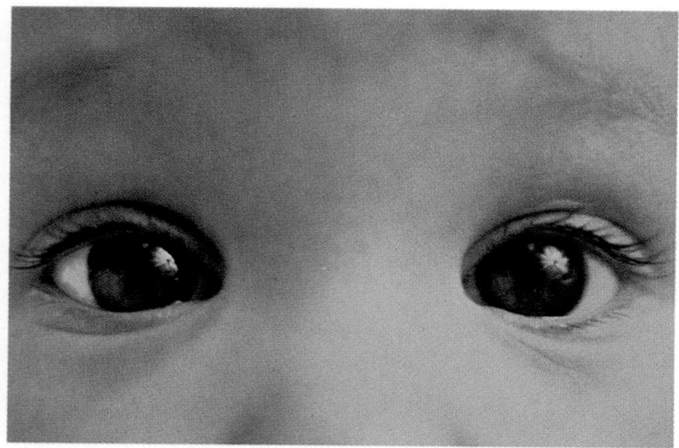

FIGURE 22–27 Transient strabismus may be present in the newborn due to poor neuromuscular control.

Source: Photo courtesy of Mead Johnson Laboratories, Evansville, IN.

cause edema, and **chemical conjunctivitis** may appear a few hours after instillation, but it disappears in 1–2 days. If infectious conjunctivitis exists, the newborn has the same purulent (greenish-yellow) discharge exudate as in chemical conjunctivitis, but it is caused by gonococcus, *Chlamydia,* staphylococci, or a variety of gram-negative bacteria and requires treatment with ophthalmic antibiotics. Onset is usually after the second day. Edema of the orbits or eyelids may persist for several days, until the newborn's kidneys can eliminate the fluid.

Small **subconjunctival hemorrhages** appear in about 10 percent of newborns and are commonly found on the sclera. These are caused by the changes in vascular tension or ocular pressure during birth. They will remain for a few weeks and are of no pathologic significance. Parents need reassurance that the newborn is not bleeding from within the eye and that vision will not be impaired.

The newborn may demonstrate transient strabismus caused by poor neuromuscular control of eye muscles (Figure 22–27). This gradually regresses in 3–4 months. The "doll's eye" phenomenon is also present for about 10 days after birth. As the newborn's head position is changed to the left and then to the right, the eyes move to the opposite direction. This results from underdeveloped integration of head-eye coordination.

The nurse should observe the newborn's pupils for opacities or whiteness. Congenital cataracts should be suspected in newborns of mothers with a history of rubella, cytomegalic inclusion disease, or syphilis. The nurse assesses both eyes for a symmetrical red reflex (Fowlie and Forsyth 1995).

The cry of the newborn is commonly tearless because the lacrimal structures are immature at birth and are not usually fully functional until the second month of life. However, some babies produce tears during the newborn period. Poor oculomotor coordination and absence of accommodation limit visual abilities, but newborns do have peripheral vision; can fixate on objects near (10 to 20 in) their face for short periods; can accommodate to large objects (3 inches tall by 3 inches wide); and can seek out high-contrast geometric shapes (Ludington-Hoe and Golani 1988). The newborn can perceive faces, shapes, and colors and begins to show visual preferences early. Visual acuity has been reported to be 20/100 and 20/400 (Steinkuller 1988). The newborn blinks in response to bright lights, to a tap on the bridge of the nose (glabellar reflex), or to a light touch on the eyelids. Pupillary light reflex is also present. Examination of the eye is best accomplished by rocking the newborn from an upright position to the horizontal a few times or by other methods, such as diminishing overhead lights, that elicit an opened-eye response.

Nose

The newborn's nose is small and narrow. Newborns are characteristically nose breathers for the first few months of life. The newborn generally removes obstructions by sneezing. Nasal patency is assured if the newborn breathes easily with the mouth closed. If respiratory difficulty occurs, the nurse checks for *choanal atresia* (congenital blockage of the passageway between nose and pharynx).

The newborn has the ability to smell after the nasal passages are cleared of amniotic fluid and mucus. This ability is demonstrated by the search for milk. Newborns turn their heads toward a milk source, whether bottle or breast.

Mouth

The lips of the newborn should be pink, and a touch on the lips should produce sucking motions. Saliva is normally scant. The taste buds develop before birth, and the newborn can easily discriminate between sweet and bitter flavors.

The easiest way to examine the mouth completely is to gently depress the tongue, which stimulates crying and causes the newborn to open the mouth fully. It is extremely important to observe the entire mouth to check for a cleft palate, which can be present even in the absence of a cleft lip (Fowlie and Forsyth 1995). The examiner also moves a gloved index finger along the hard and soft palates to feel for any openings (Figure 22–28). The nurse should remove any glove powder before examining the newborn's mouth.

An examination of the gums occasionally reveals *precocious teeth* on the lower central incisor. If they appear loose, they should be removed to prevent aspiration. Gray-white lesions *(inclusion cysts)* on the gums may be confused with teeth. On the hard palate and gum margins, **Epstein's pearls,** small glistening white

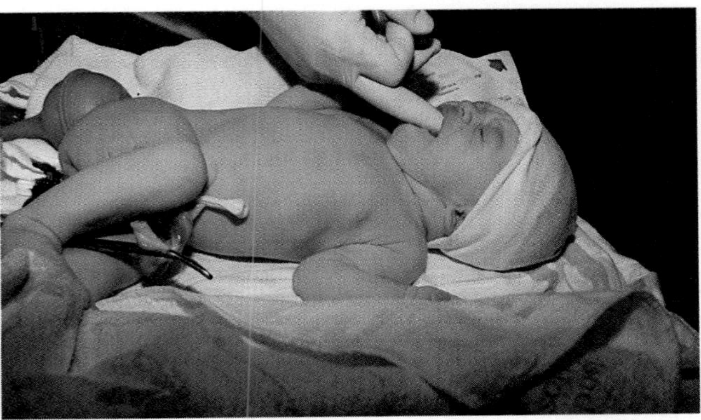

FIGURE 22–28 The nurse inserts a gloved index finger into the newborn's mouth and feels for any openings along the hard and soft palates. Note: Gloves or a finger cot are always worn to examine the palate.

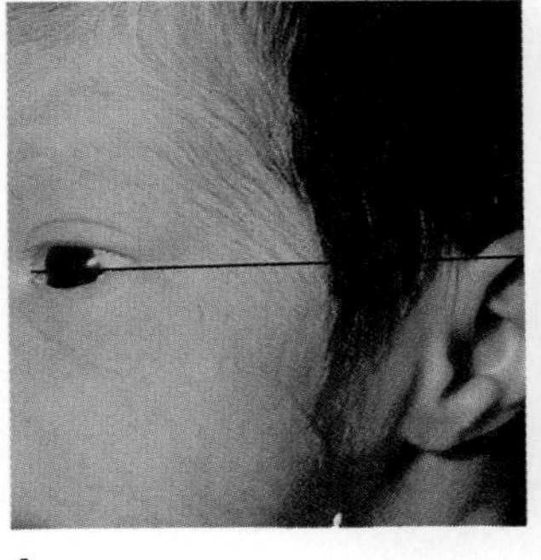

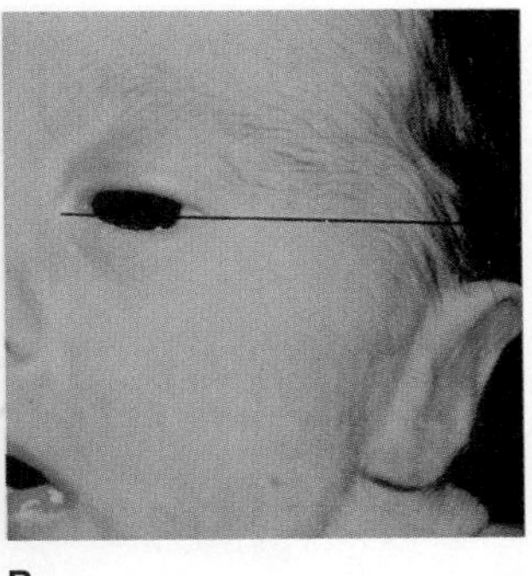

A B

FIGURE 22–29 The position of the external ear may be assessed by drawing a line across the inner and outer canthus of the eye to the insertion of the ear. ***A*** Normal position. ***B*** True low-set position.

Source: Photo courtesy of Mead Johnson Laboratories, Evansville, IN.

specks (keratin-containing cysts) that feel hard to the touch, are often present. These usually disappear in a few weeks and are of no significance. **Thrush** may appear as white patches that look like milk curds adhering to the mucous membranes and cause bleeding when removed. Thrush is caused by *Candida albicans,* often acquired from an infected vaginal tract during birth or if the mother uses poor hand washing when handling her newborn. Thrush is treated with a preparation of nystatin (Mycostatin).

A newborn who is *tongue-tied* has a ridge of frenulum tissue attached to the underside of the tongue at varying lengths from its base, causing a heart shape at the tip of the tongue. "Clipping the tongue," or cutting the ridge of tissue, is not recommended. This ridge does not affect speech or eating, but cutting does create an entry for infection.

Transient nerve paralysis resulting from birth trauma may be manifested by asymmetrical mouth movements when the newborn cries or by difficulty with sucking and feeding.

Ears

The ears of the newborn should be soft and pliable and should recoil readily when folded and released. In the normal newborn, the top of the ear (pinna) should be parallel to the outer and inner canthus of the eye. The ears should be inspected for shape, size, position, and firmness of cartilage. *Low-set ears* are characteristic of many syndromes and may indicate chromosomal abnormalities (especially trisomies 13 and 18), mental retardation, and internal organ abnormalities, especially bilateral renal agenesis as a result of embryologic developmental deviations (Figure 22–29). *Preauricular skin tags* may be present just in front of the ear. They are ligated at the base and allowed to slough off.

Following the first cry, the newborn's hearing becomes acute as mucus from the middle ear is absorbed, the eustachian tube becomes aerated, and the tympanic membrane becomes visible. The nurse evaluates the newborn's hearing by noting the baby's response to loud or moderately loud noises unaccompanied by vibrations. The sleeping newborn should stir or awaken in response to nearby sounds. (This is not a very accurate test but it may alert the examiner to a possible problem.) The newborn can discriminate the individual characteristics of the human voice and is especially sensitive to sound levels within the normal conversational range (Peck 1995). The newborn in a noisy nursery may habituate to the sounds and not stir unless the sound is sudden or much louder.

Neck

The normal newborn's neck is short and creased with skin folds. Because muscle tone is not well developed, the neck cannot support the full weight of the head, which rotates freely. The head lags considerably when the newborn is pulled from a supine to a sitting position, but the prone newborn is able to raise the head slightly. The nurse palpates the neck for masses and the presence of lymph nodes and inspects it for webbing. Adequacy of range of motion and neck muscle function is determined by fully extending the head in all directions. Injury to the sternocleidomastoid muscle (congenital torticollis) must be considered in the presence of neck rigidity.

The clavicles are evaluated for evidence of fractures, which occasionally occur during difficult births or in newborns with broad shoulders. The normal clavicle is straight. If fractured, a lump and a grating sensation (crepitus) during movements may be palpated along the course of the side of the break. The Moro reflex (p 547) is also elicited to evaluate bilateral equal movement of the arms. If the clavicle is fractured, the response will be demonstrated only on the unaffected side.

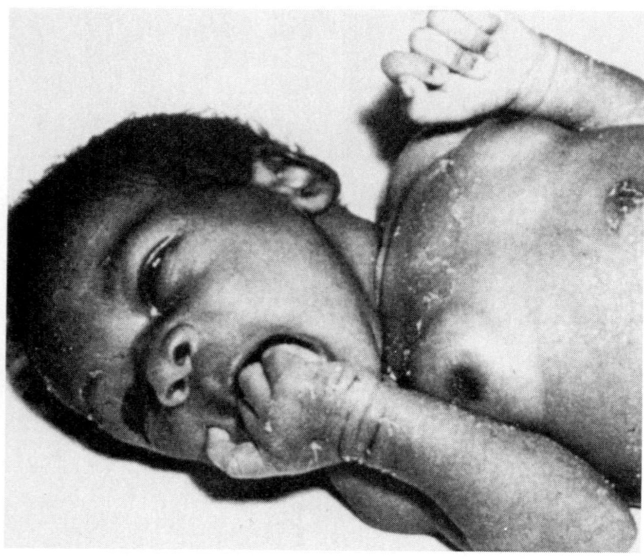

FIGURE 22–30 Breast hypertrophy.

Source: Korones SB: *High-Risk Newborn Infants,* 4th ed. St Louis: Mosby, 1986.

Chest

The thorax is cylindrical at birth, and the ribs are flexible. The nurse should assess the general appearance of the chest. A protrusion at the lower end of the sternum, called the *xiphoid cartilage,* is frequently seen. It is under the skin, and will become less apparent after several weeks as the newborn accumulates adipose tissue.

Engorged breasts occur frequently in both male and female newborns. This condition, which occurs by the third day, is a result of maternal hormonal influences and may last up to 2 weeks (Figure 22–30). A whitish secretion from the nipples may also be noted. The newborn's breast should not be massaged or squeezed, because this may cause a breast abscess. Extra nipples, or *supernumerary nipples* are occasionally noted below and medial to the true nipples. These harmless pink or brown (in darker-skinned newborns) spots vary in size and do not contain glandular tissue. Accessory nipples can be differentiated from a pigmented nevi (mole) by placing the fingertips alongside the accessory nipple and pulling the adjacent tissue laterally. The accessory nipple will appear dimpled. At puberty the accessory nipple may darken.

Cry

The newborn's cry should be strong, lusty, and of medium pitch. A high-pitched, shrill cry is abnormal and may indicate neurologic disorders or hypoglycemia. Periods of crying usually vary in length after consoling measures are used. Crying is an important method of communication and alerts caregivers to changes in the baby's condition and needs.

Respiration

Normal breathing for a term newborn is 30–60 respirations per minute, and predominantly diaphragmatic, with associated rising and falling of the abdomen during inspiration and expiration. The nurse should note any signs of respiratory distress, nasal flaring, intercostal or xiphoid retraction, expiratory grunt or sigh, seesaw respirations, or tachypnea (greater than 60/min or sustained). Hyperextension (chest appears high) or hypoextension (chest appears low) of the anteroposterior diameter of the chest should also be noted. The examiner auscultates both the anterior and posterior chest. Some breath sounds are more audible when the newborn is crying, but localization and identification of breath sounds are difficult in the newborn. Upper airway noises and bowel sounds may also be heard over the chest wall and make auscultation difficult. Because sounds may be transmitted from the unaffected lung to the affected lung, the absence of breath sounds may not be diagnosed. Air entry may be noisy in the first couple of hours until lung fluid resolves, especially after cesarean births. Brief periods of apnea (episodic breathing) occur, but no color or heart-rate changes occur in healthy term newborns.

Heart

Heart rates can be as rapid as 180 beats per minute in newborns, and they fluctuate a great deal, especially if the baby moves or is startled. Normal range is 120–160 beats per minute. The heart is examined for rate and rhythm, position of the apical impulse, and heart sound intensity. The physician should reassess dysrhythmias.

The pulse rate is variable and is influenced by physical activity, crying, state of wakefulness, and body temperature. The examiner auscultates over the entire heart region (precordium), below the left axilla, and below the scapula. Apical pulse rates are obtained by auscultation for a full minute, preferably when the newborn is asleep.

The placement of the heart in the chest should be determined when the newborn is in a quiet state. The heart is relatively large at birth and is located high in the chest, with its apex somewhere between the fourth and fifth intercostal space. A shift of heart tones in the mediastinal area to either side may indicate pneumothorax, dextrocardia (heart placement on the right side of the chest), or a diaphragmatic hernia. The experienced nurse can diagnose these and many other problems early with a stethoscope.

Normally, the heart beat has a "toc tic" sound. A slur or slushing sound (usually after the first sound) may

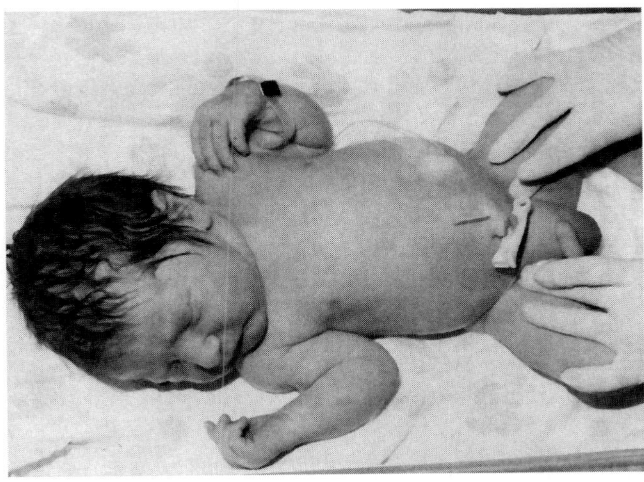

A

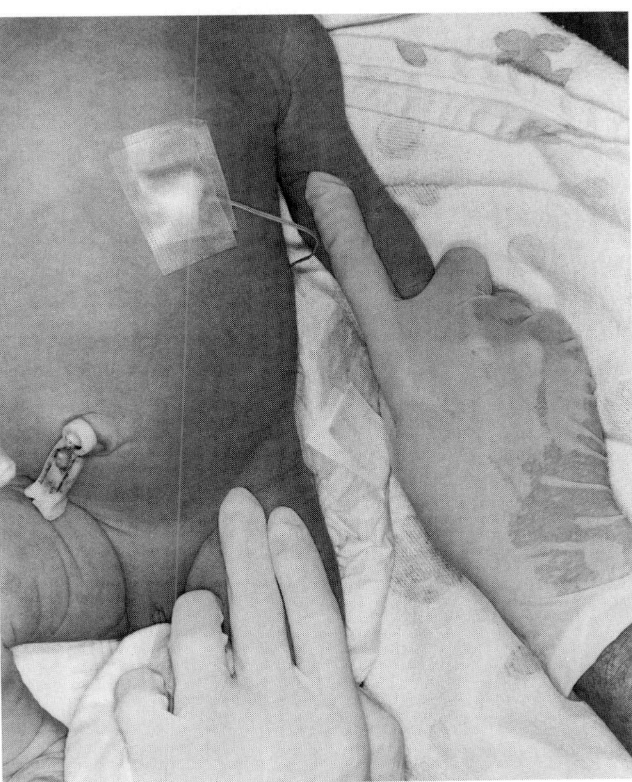

B

FIGURE 22–31 ***A*** Bilaterally palpate the femoral arteries for rate and intensity of the pulses. Press fingertip gently at the groin as shown.
B Compare the femoral pulses to the brachial pulses by palpating the pulses simultaneously for comparison of rate and intensity.

indicate a *murmur.* Although 90 percent of all murmurs are transient and are considered normal, a physician should observe them closely. Many murmurs are related to a patent ductus arteriosus, which closes in about 1 to 2 days. In newborns, a low-pitched, musical murmur heard just to the right of the apex of the heart is fairly

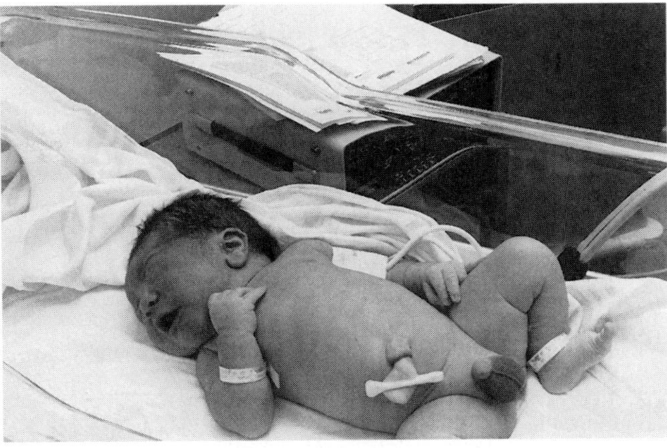

FIGURE 22–32 Blood pressure measurement using a Doppler device. The cuff can be applied to the upper arm or thigh.

common. Occasionally, significant murmurs will be heard, including the murmur of a patent ductus arteriosus, aortic or pulmonary stenosis, or small ventricular septal defect. See Chapter 25 for a discussion of congenital heart defects.

Also evaluate peripheral pulses (brachial, femoral, pedal) to detect any lags or unusual characteristics. Brachial pulses are palpated bilaterally for equality and compared with the femoral pulses. Femoral pulses are palpated by applying gentle pressure with the middle finger over the femoral canal (Figure 22–31). Decreased or absent femoral pulses indicate coarctation of the aorta and require additional investigation. A wide difference in blood pressure between the upper and lower extremities also indicates coarctation.

The measurement of blood pressure is best accomplished by using the Doppler technique or a 1- to 2-inch cuff and a stethoscope over the brachial artery (Figure 22–32). If a Doppler device is used, the newborn's extremities must be immobilized during the assessment, and the cuff should cover two-thirds of the upper arm or upper leg. Movement, crying, and inappropriate cuff size can give inaccurate measurements of the blood pressure.

Blood pressure may not be measured routinely on healthy newborns, but it is a routine measurement on newborns who are having distress, are premature, or are suspected of cardiac anomaly (Taeusch et al 1991). Infants with birth asphyxia and on ventilators have significantly lower systolic and diastolic blood pressures than healthy infants (Hegyi et al 1996). If cardiac anomaly is suspected, blood pressure is palpated in all four extremities (Key Facts to Remember: Newborn Vital Signs).

Abdomen

The newborn's abdomen should be cylindrical and protrude slightly. A certain amount of laxness of the

KEY FACTS TO REMEMBER

Newborn Vital Signs

Pulse

120–160 bpm

During sleep as low as 100 bpm; if crying, up to 180 bpm

Apical pulse counted for 1 full minute

Respirations

30–60 respirations/minute

Predominantly diaphragmatic but synchronous with abdominal movements

Respirations are counted for 1 full minute

Blood Pressure

80–60/45–40 mm Hg at birth

100/50 mm Hg at day 10

Temperature

Normal range: 36.5–37.5C (97.7–99.4F)

Axillary: 36.4–37.2C (97.5–99F)

Skin: 36–36.5C (96.8–97.7F)

Rectal: 36.6–37.2C (97.8–99F)

abdominal muscles is normal. A scaphoid (hollow-shaped) appearance suggests the absence of abdominal contents. No cyanosis should be present, and few if any blood vessels should be apparent to the eye. There should be no gross distention or bulging. The more distended the abdomen, the tighter the skin becomes, with engorged vessels appearing. Distention is the first sign of many of the abnormalities found in the gastrointestinal tract.

Before palpation of the abdomen, the nurse should auscultate for the presence or absence of bowel sounds in all four quadrants. Bowel sounds may be present by one hour after birth. Palpation can cause a transient decrease in intensity of the bowel sounds.

Abdominal palpation should be done systematically. The nurse palpates each of the four abdominal quadrants and moves in a clockwise direction until all four quadrants have been palpated for softness, tenderness, and the presence of masses.

Umbilical Cord

Initially the umbilical cord is white and gelatinous in appearance, with the two umbilical arteries and one umbilical vein readily apparent. Because a single umbilical artery is frequently associated with congenital anomalies, the nurse should count the vessels during the newborn assessment. The cord begins drying within 1 or 2 hours of birth and is shriveled and blackened by the second or third day. Within 7 to 10 days, it sloughs off, although a granulating area may remain for a few more days.

Cord bleeding is abnormal and may result when the cord was inadvertently pulled or the cord clamp loosened. Foul-smelling drainage is also abnormal and is generally caused by infection. Such infection requires immediate treatment to prevent the development of septicemia. If the newborn has a patent urachus (abnormal connection between the umbilicus and bladder), moistness or draining urine may be apparent at the base of the cord.

Serous or serosanguineous drainage that continues after the cord falls off may indicate a granuloma. It appears as a small, red button deep in the umbilicus. Treatment involves cauterization by a physician with a silver nitrate stick. Another umbilical cord anomaly that must be assessed before cord clamping is umbilical cord hernia and associated patent omphalomesenteric duct (Jona 1996).

Genitals

Female Infants

The nurse examines the labia majora, labia minora, and clitoris and notes the size of each as appropriate for gestational age. A vaginal tag or hymenal tag is often evident and will usually disappear in a few weeks. During the first week of life, the newborn may have a vaginal discharge composed of thick whitish mucus. This discharge, which can become tinged with blood, is called **pseudomenstruation** and is caused by the withdrawal of maternal hormones. Smegma, a white cheeselike substance, is often present between the labia. Removing it may traumatize tender tissue.

Male Infants

The penis is inspected to determine whether the urinary orifice is correctly positioned. *Hypospadias* occurs when the urinary meatus is located on the ventral surface of the penis. It occurs most commonly among caucasians in the United States. *Phimosis* is a condition occurring in newborn males in which the opening of the foreskin (prepuce) is small and the foreskin cannot be pulled back over the glans at all. This condition may interfere with urination, so the adequacy of the urinary stream should be evaluated.

The nurse inspects the scrotum for size and symmetry, palpating to verify the presence of both testes and to rule out cryptorchidism (failure of testes to descend). The testes are palpated separately between the thumb and forefinger, with the thumb and forefinger of the other hand placed together over the inguinal canal.

Scrotal edema and discoloration are common in breech births. *Hydrocele* (a collection of fluid surrounding the testes in the scrotum) is common in newborns and should be identified. It usually resolves without intervention. The presence of a hard testis should raise the suspicion of perinatal torsion (Baptist and Amin 1996).

Anus

The anal area is inspected to verify that it is patent and has no fissure. The nurse rules out imperforate anus and rectal atresia by digital examination and notes the passage of the first meconium stool. Atresia of the gastrointestinal tract or meconium ileus with resultant obstruction must be considered if the newborn does not pass meconium in the first 24 hours of life.

Extremities

Extremities are examined for gross deformities, extra digits or webbing, clubfoot, and range of motion. Normal newborn extremities appear short, are generally flexible, and move symmetrically.

Arms and Hands

Nails extend beyond the fingertips in term newborns. The nurse should count fingers and toes. *Polydactyly* is the presence of extra digits on either the hands or the feet. *Syndactyly* refers to fusion (webbing) of fingers or toes. The nurse should inspect the hands for normal palmar creases. A single palmar crease, called *simian line* (see Figure 4–17), is frequently present in children with Down syndrome.

Brachial palsy, which is partial or complete paralysis of portions of the arm, results from trauma to the brachial plexus during a difficult birth. It occurs most commonly when strong traction is exerted on the head of the newborn in an attempt to deliver a shoulder lodged behind the symphysis pubis in the presence of shoulder dystocia. Brachial palsy may also occur during a breech birth if an arm becomes trapped over the head and traction is exerted.

The affected portion of the arm is determined by the nerves damaged. **Erb-Duchenne paralysis (Erb's palsy)** involves damage to the upper arm (fifth and sixth cervical nerves) and is the most common type. Injury to the eighth cervical and first thoracic nerve roots and the lower portion of the plexus produces the relatively rare *lower arm injury.* The *whole arm type* results from damage to the entire plexus.

With Erb-Duchenne paralysis the newborn's arm lies limply at the side. The elbow is held in extension, with the forearm pronated. The newborn is unable to elevate the arm, and the Moro reflex cannot be elicited on the affected side (Figure 22–33). Lower arm injury causes paralysis of the hand and wrist; complete paralysis of the limb occurs with the whole-arm type.

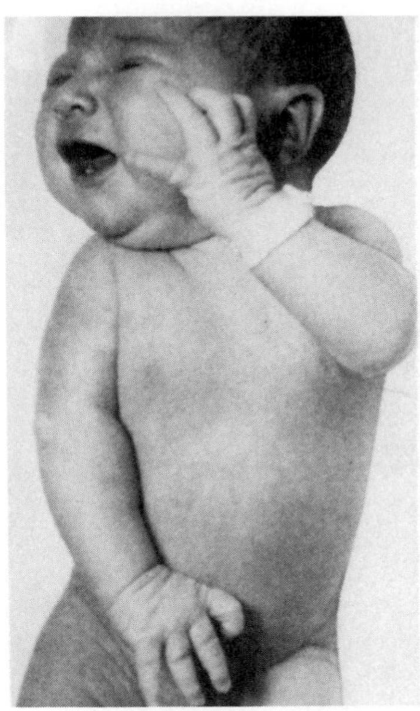

FIGURE 22–33 Right Erb palsy resulting from injury to the fifth and sixth cervical roots of the brachial plexus.

Source: Potter EL, Craig JM: *Pathology of the Fetus and Infant,* 3rd ed. Chicago: Year Book Medical Publishers, 1975. Reproduced with permisssion.

The nurse carefully instructs the parents in the correct method of performing passive range of motion exercises (to prevent muscle contractures and restore function) and arranges supervised practice sessions. In more severe cases, splinting of the arm is indicated until the edema decreases. The arm is held in a position of abduction and external rotation with the elbow flexed 90 degrees. The "Statue of Liberty" splint is commonly used, although similar results are obtained by attaching a strip of muslin to the head of the crib and tying the other end around the wrist, thereby holding the arm up.

Prognosis is related to the degree of nerve damage resulting from trauma and hemorrhage within the nerve sheath. Complete recovery occurs within a few months with minimal trauma. Routine orthopedic follow-up should occur in all cases, as growth plate problems can occur years later. Moderate trauma may result in some partial paralysis. Recovery is unlikely with severe trauma, and muscle wasting may develop.

Legs and Feet

The legs of the newborn should be of equal length, with symmetrical skin folds. However, they may assume a "fetal posture" secondary to position in utero, and it may take several days for the legs to relax into normal position. The nurse performs **Ortolani's maneuver** to

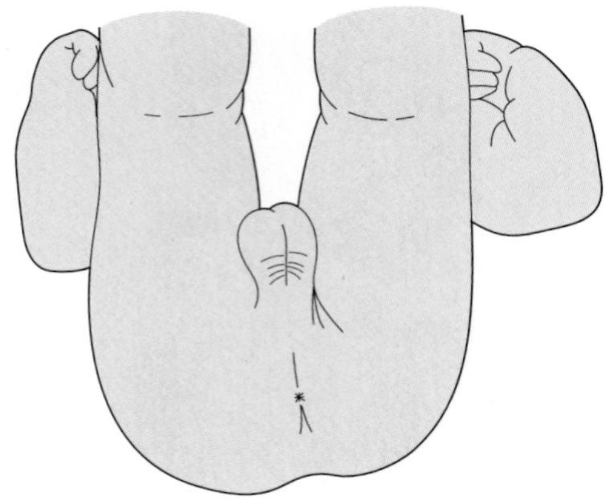
A

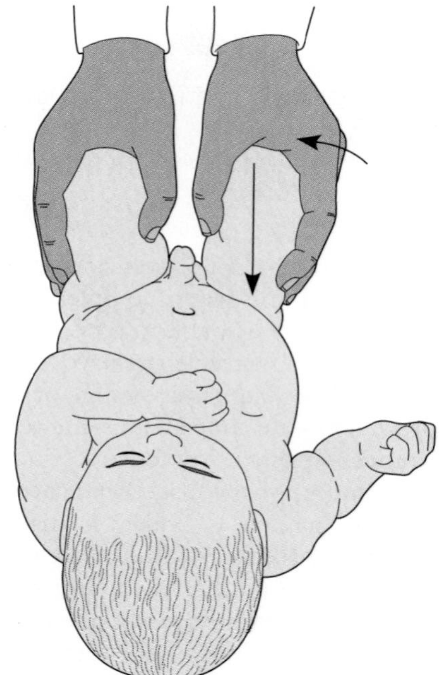

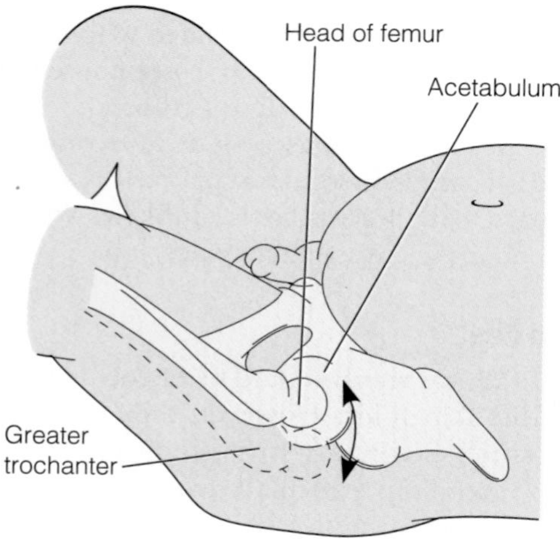

B

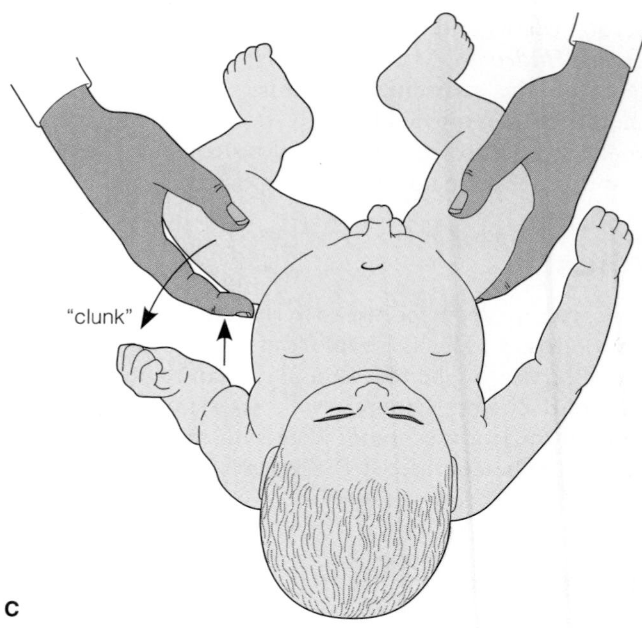

C

FIGURE 22–34 ***A*** Congenitally dislocated right hip in a young infant as seen on gross inspection. ***B*** Barlow's (dislocation) maneuver. Baby's thigh is grasped and adducted with gently downward pressure. Dislocation is palpable as femoral head slips out of acetabulum. ***C*** Ortolani's maneuver puts downward presure on the hip and then inward rotation. If the hip is dislocated, this forces the femoral head over the acetabular rim with a noticeable "clunk."

rule out the possibility of congenital hip dysplasia (hip dislocation). With the newborn relaxed and quiet on a firm surface, with hips and knees flexed at a 90-degree angle, the nurse grasps the infant's thigh with the middle finger over the greater trochanter and lifts the thigh to bring the femoral head from its posterior position toward the acetabulum. With gentle abduction of the thigh the femoral head is returned to the acetabulum. Simultaneously, the examiner feels a sense of reduction or a "clunk" as the femoral head returns. This reduction is audible. With **Barlow's maneuver,** the nurse grasps and adducts the infant's thigh and applies gentle downward pressure. Dislocation is felt as the femoral head is then returned to the acetabulum using Ortolani's maneuver, confirming the diagnosis of an unstable or dislocated hip (Figure 22–34).

The nurse examines the feet for evidence of clubfoot. Intrauterine position frequently causes the feet to appear to turn inward (Figure 22–35). This is termed a "positional" clubfoot. If the feet can easily be returned to the midline by manipulation, no treatment is indicated and the nurse teaches range of motion exercises to the family. Further investigation is indicated when the foot will not turn to a midline position or align readily. This is a severe "true clubfoot," or talipes equinovarus.

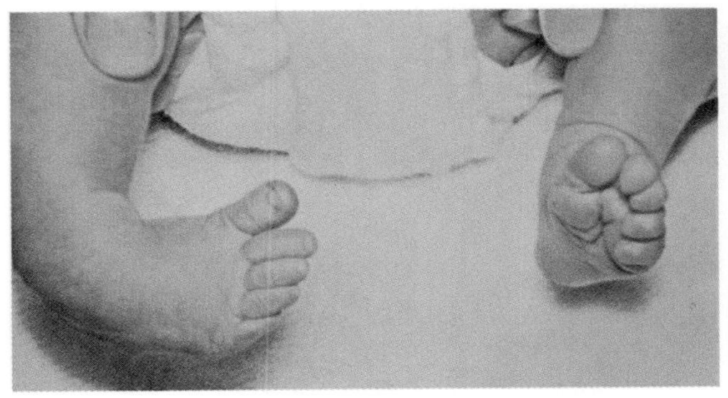

A

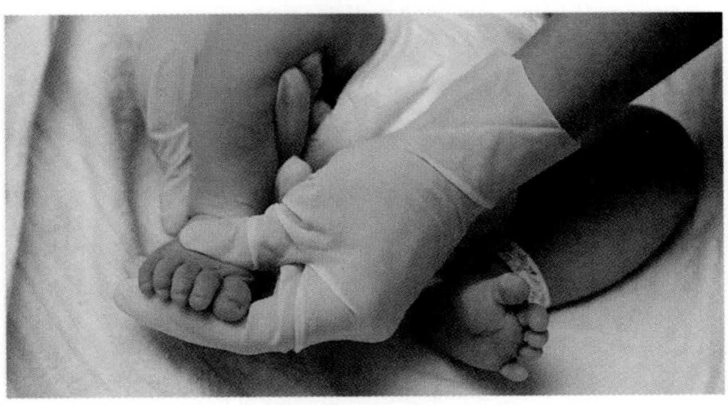

B

FIGURE 22–35 ***A*** Unilateral talipes equinovarus (clubfoot). ***B*** To determine the presence of clubfoot, the nurse moves the foot to the midline. Resistance indicates true clubfoot.

Back

With the newborn prone, the nurse examines the back. The spine should appear straight and flat, since the lumbar and sacral curves do not develop until the newborn begins to sit. The nurse then examines the base of the spine for a dermal sinus. The nevus philosus ("hairy nerve") is only occasionally found at the base of the spine in newborns, but it is significant because it is frequently associated with spina bifida. A pilonidal dimple should be examined to ascertain that there is no connection to the spinal canal.

Assessment of Neurologic Status

The neurologic examination should begin with a period of observation, noting the general physical characteristics and behaviors of the newborn. Important behaviors to assess are the *state of alertness, resting posture, cry, and quality of muscle tone and motor activity.*

The usual position of the newborn is with partially flexed extremities with the legs abducted to the abdomen. When awake, the newborn may exhibit purposeless, uncoordinated bilateral movements of the extremities. If these movements are absent, minimal, or obviously asymmetrical, neurologic dysfunction should be suspected. Eye movements are observable during the first few days of life. An alert newborn is able to fixate on faces and brightly colored objects. A bright light shining in the newborn's eyes elicits the blinking response.

The nurse evaluates muscle tone by moving various parts of the body while the head of the newborn is in a neutral position. The newborn is somewhat hypertonic; that is, there should be resistance to extending the elbow and knee joints. Muscle tone should be symmetrical. Diminished muscle tone and flaccidity require further evaluation.

Tremors are common in the full-term newborn and must be evaluated to differentiate them from convulsions. A fine jumping of the muscle is likely to be a CNS disorder and requires further evaluation. Tremors may also be related to hypoglycemia or hypocalcemia. Newborn seizures may consist of no more than chewing or swallowing movements, deviations of the eyes, rigidity, or flaccidity because of CNS immaturity.

The nurse can elicit specific deep tendon reflexes, but they have limited value unless they are obviously asymmetrical. The knee jerk is brisk; a normal ankle clonus may involve three or four beats. Plantar flexion is present.

The immature central nervous system of the newborn is characterized by a variety of reflexes. Because the newborn's movements are uncoordinated, methods of communication are limited, and control of bodily functions is drastically limited, the reflexes serve a variety of purposes. Some are protective (blink, gag, sneeze), some aid in feeding (rooting, sucking) and may not be very active if the infant has eaten recently, and some stimulate human interaction (grasping). Newborn reflex and general neurologic activity should be carefully assessed.

The most common reflexes found in the normal newborn are the following:

- The **tonic neck reflex** (fencer position) is elicited when the newborn is supine and the head is turned to one side. In response, the extremities on the same side straighten, whereas on the opposite side they flex (Figure 22–36). This reflex may not be seen during the early newborn period, but once it appears it persists until about the third month.
- The **Moro reflex** is elicited when the newborn is startled by a loud noise or lifted slightly above the crib and then suddenly lowered. In response, the

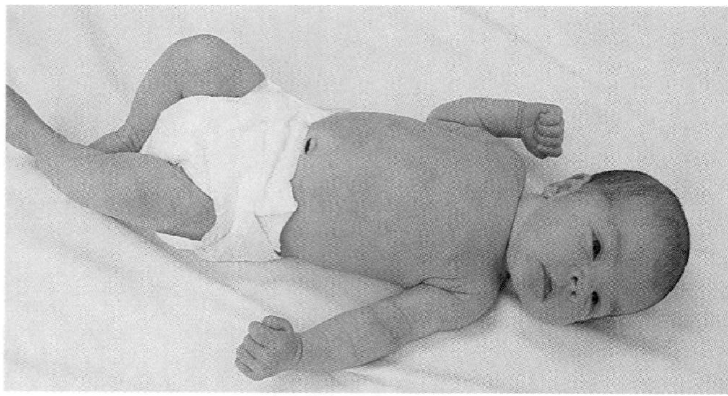

FIGURE 22–36 Tonic neck reflex.

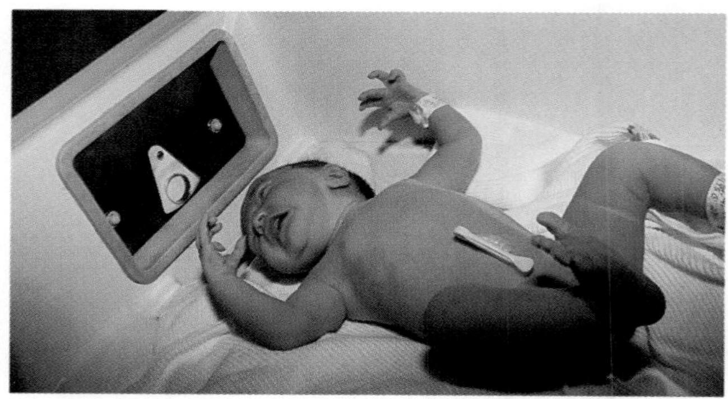

FIGURE 22–37 Moro reflex.

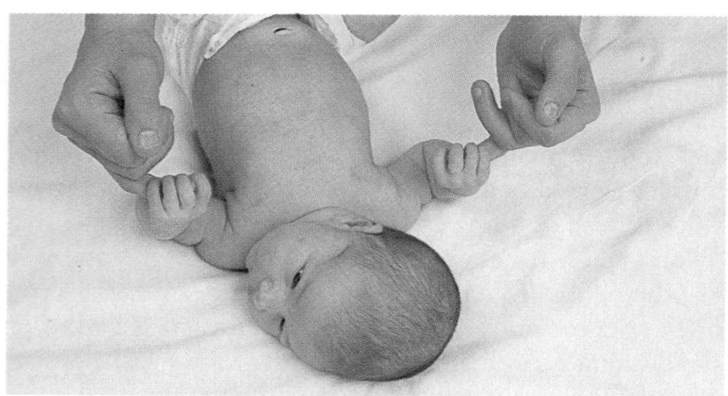

FIGURE 22–38 Grasping reflex.

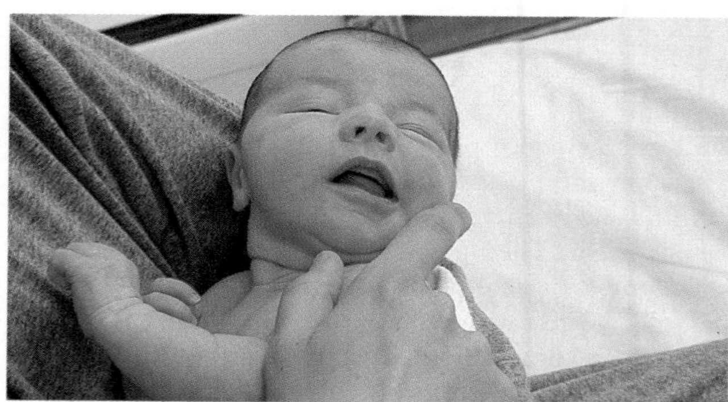

FIGURE 22–39 Rooting reflex.

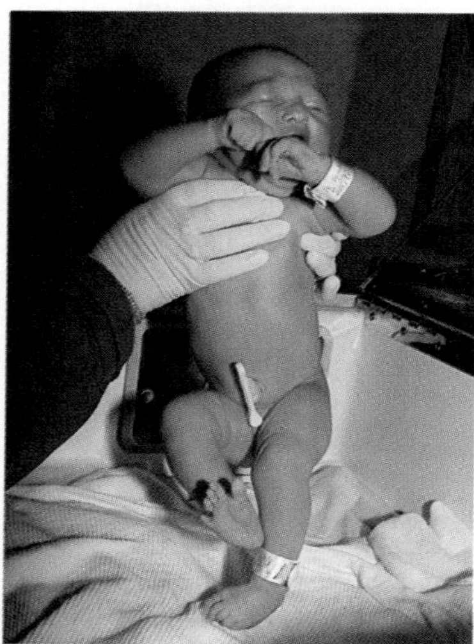

FIGURE 22–40 The stepping reflex disappears after about 4–5 months.

newborn straightens arms and hands outward while the knees flex. Slowly the arms return to the chest, as in an embrace. The fingers spread, forming a C, and the newborn may cry (Figure 22–37). This reflex may persist until about 6 months of age.

- The **grasping reflex** is elicited by stimulating the newborn's palm with a finger or object; the newborn grasps and holds the object or finger firmly enough to be lifted momentarily from the crib (Figure 22–38).
- The **rooting reflex** is elicited when the side of the newborn's mouth or cheek is touched. In response, the newborn turns toward that side and opens the lips to suck (if not fed recently) (Figure 22–39).
- The **sucking reflex** is elicited when an object is placed in the newborn's mouth or anything touches the lips. Newborns suck even while sleeping; this is called nonnutritive sucking, and it can have a quieting effect on the baby.
- The **Babinski reflex,** or fanning and hyperextension of all toes, occurs when the lateral aspect of the sole is stroked from the heel upward across the ball of the foot. In adults, the toes flex.
- **Trunk incurvation** (Galant reflex) is seen when the newborn is prone. Stroking the spine causes the pelvis to turn to the stimulated side.

In addition to these reflexes, newborns can *blink, yawn, cough, sneeze,* and *draw back from pain* (protective reflexes). They can even move a little on their own.

When placed on their stomachs, they push up and try to crawl *(prone crawl)*. When held upright with one foot touching a flat surface, the newborn puts one foot in front of the other and "walks" *(stepping reflex)* (Figure 22–40). This reflex is more pronounced at birth and is lost in 4 to 5 months.

The Newborn Physical Assessment Guide summarizes the stimulus for, and response of, the common newborn reflexes.

Brazelton (1984) recommends the following steps as a means of assessing CNS integration:

1. Insert a gloved finger into the newborn's mouth to elicit a sucking reflex.
2. As soon as the newborn is sucking vigorously, assess hearing and vision responses by noting changes in sucking in the presence of a light, a rattle, and a voice.
3. The newborn should respond to such stimuli with a brief cessation of sucking followed by continuous sucking with repetitious stimulation.

This examination demonstrates auditory and visual integrity as well as the ability for complex behavioral interactions.

Newborn Physical Assessment Guide

Following is a guide for systematically assessing the newborn (pages 550–564). Normal findings, alterations, and related causes are presented, correlated with suggested nursing responses. The findings are typical for a full-term newborn.

Newborn Behavioral Assessment

Two conflicting forces influence parents' perceptions of their newborn. One is their preconceptions, based on hopes and fears, of what their newborn will be like. The other is their initial reaction to the baby's temperament, behaviors, and physical appearance. Nurses can assist parents in identifying their baby's specific behaviors.

Brazelton's neonatal behavioral assessment scale provides valuable guidelines for assessing the newborn's state changes, temperament, and individual behavior patterns. It provides a means by which the health care provider, in conjunction with the parents (primary caregivers), can identify and understand the individual newborn's states and capabilities. Families learn which responses, interventions, or activities best meet the special needs of their newborn, and this understanding fosters positive attachment experiences.

The assessment tool attempts to identify the newborn's repertoire of behavioral responses to the environment and also documents the newborn's neurologic adequacy and capabilities. The examination usually takes 20 to 30 minutes and involves about 30 tests.

Some items are scored according to the newborn's response to specific stimuli. Others, such as consolability and alertness, are scored as a result of continuous behavioral observations throughout the assessment. (For a complete discussion of all test items and maneuvers, see Brazelton 1973.)

Assessment of the newborn should be carried out initially in a quiet, softly lit room, if possible. First the nurse determines the newborn's state of consciousness, because scoring and introduction of the test items are correlated with the sleep or waking state. The newborn's state depends on physiologic variables, such as the amount of time from the last feeding, positioning, environmental temperature, and health status; presence of such external stimuli as noises and bright lights; and the wake-sleep cycle of the newborn. An important characteristic of the newborn period is the *pattern of states,* as well as the transitions from one state to another. The pattern of states is a predictor of the newborn's receptivity and ability to respond to stimuli in a cognitive manner. Babies learn best in a quiet, alert state and in an environment that is supportive and protective and that provides appropriate stimuli.

The nurse should observe the newborn's sleep-wake patterns (as discussed in Chapter 23), including the rapidity with which the newborn moves from one state to another; ability to be consoled; and ability to diminish the impact of disturbing stimuli. The following questions may provide the nurse with a framework for assessment:

- Does the newborn's response style and ability to adapt to stimuli indicate a need for parental interventions that will alert the newborn to the environment so that he or she can grow socially and cognitively?
- Are parental interventions necessary to lessen the outside stimuli, as in the case of the baby who responds to sensory input with intensity?
- Can the baby control the amount of sensory input that he or she must deal with?

The behaviors, and the sleep-wake states in which they are assessed, are categorized as follows:

1. *Habituation.* The newborn's ability to diminish or shut down innate responses to specific repeated stimuli, such as a rattle, bell, light, or pinprick to heel.
2. *Orientation to inanimate and animate visual and auditory assessment stimuli.* The nurse observes

Text continues on page 564

NEWBORN PHYSICAL ASSESSMENT GUIDE

Assessment and Normal Findings	Alterations and Possible Causes*	Nursing Responses to Data[†]
Vital Signs		
Blood pressure (BP) At birth: 80–60/45–40 mm Hg Day 10: 100/50 mm Hg (may be unable to measure diastolic pressure with standard sphygmomanometer)	Low BP (hypovolemia, shock)	Monitor BP in all cases of distress, prematurity, or suspected anomaly. Low BP: Refer to physician immediately so measures to improve circulation are begun.
Pulse 120–160 bpm (if asleep 100 bpm; if crying, up to 180 bpm)	Weak pulse (decreased cardiac output) Bradycardia (severe asphyxia, arrhythmia) Tachycardia (over 160 bpm at rest) (infection, central nervous system problems, arrhythmia)	Assess skin perfusion by blanching (capillary refill test). Correlate finding with BP assessments; refer to physician. Carry out neurologic and thermoregulation assessments.
Respirations 30–60 breaths/minute Synchronization of chest and abdominal movements Diaphragmatic and abdominal breathing	Tachypnea (pneumonia, respiratory distress syndrome [RDS]) Rapid, shallow breathing (hypermagnesemia due to large doses given to mothers with PIH) Respirations below 30 breaths/minute (maternal anesthesia or analgesia)	Identify sleep-wake state; correlate with respiratory pattern. Evaluate for all signs of respiratory distress; report findings to physician.
Transient tachypnea	Expiratory grunting, subcostal and substernal retractions; flaring of nares (respiratory distress); apnea (cold stress, respiratory disorder)	Evaluate for cold stress. Report findings to physician/nurse practitioner.
Crying Strong and lusty Moderate tone and pitch Cries vary in length from 3 to 7 minutes after consoling measures are used	High pitched, shrill (neurologic disorder, hypoglycemia) Weak or absent (CNS disorder, laryngeal problem)	Discuss newborn's use of cry for communication. Assess and record abnormal cries. Reduce environmental noises.
Temperature Axilla 36.4–37.2C (97.5–99F) Rectal 36.6–37.2C (97.8–99F); 36.8C (98.8F) desired Heavier neonates tend to have higher body temperatures	Elevated temperature (room too warm, too much clothing or covers, dehydration, sepsis, brain damage) Subnormal temperature (brain stem involvement, cold, sepsis) Swings of more than 2F from one reading to next or subnormal temperature (infection)	Notify physician of elevation or drop. Counsel parents on possible causes of elevated or low temperatures, appropriate home-care measures, when to call physician. Teach parents how to take rectal and/or axillary temperature; assess parents' information regarding use of thermometer; provide teaching as needed.
Weight 2500–4000 g (5–8.75 lb)	$<$ 2748 g ($<$ 6 lb) = SGA or preterm infant $>$ 4050 g ($>$ 9 lb) = LGA or infants of diabetic mothers	Plot weight and gestational age on growth chart to identify high-risk infants. Ascertain body build of parents. Counsel parents regarding appropriate caloric intake.

*Possible causes of alterations are placed in parentheses.

[†]This column provides guidelines for further assessment and initial nursing interventions.

NEWBORN PHYSICAL ASSESSMENT GUIDE continued

Assessment and Normal Findings	Alterations and Possible Causes*	Nursing Responses to Data†
Within first 3 to 4 days, normal weight loss of 5%–10% Large babies tend to lose more due to greater fluid loss in proportion to birth weight except infants of diabetic mother	Loss greater than 15% (small fluid intake, loss of meconium and urine, feeding difficulties)	Notify physician of net losses or gains. Calculate fluid intake and losses from all sources (insensible water loss, radiant warmers, and phototherapy lights).
Length		
45–55 cm (18–22 in) Grows 10 cm (3 in) during first 3 months	Less than 45 cm (congenital dwarf) Short/long bones proximally (achondroplasia) Short/long bones distally (Ellis-Van Creveld syndrome)	Assess for other signs of dwarfism. Determine other signs of skeletal system adequacy. Plot progress at subsequent well-baby visits.
Posture Body usually flexed, hands may be tightly clenched, neck appears short as chin rests on chest In breech births feet are usually dorsiflexed	Only extension noted, inability to move from midline (trauma, hypoxia, immaturity) Constant motion (maternal caffeine intake)	Record spontaneity of motor activity and symmetry of movements. If parents express concern about newborn's movement patterns, reassure and evaluate further if appropriate.
Skin		
Color		
Color consistent with genetic background Newborns of European descent: pink-tinged or ruddy color over face, trunk, extremities Newborns of African or Native American descent: pale pink with yellow or red tinge Newborns of Asian descent: pink or rosy red to yellow tinge	Pallor of face, conjunctiva (anemia, hypothermia, anoxia) Beefy red (hypoglycemia, immature vasomotor reflexes, polycythemia)	Discuss with parents common skin color variations to allay fears. Document extent and time of occurrence of color change.
Common variations: acrocyanosis, circumoral cyanosis, or harlequin color change	Meconium staining (fetal distress) Jaundice (hemolytic reaction from blood incompatibility within first 24 hours, sepsis)	Obtain Hb and hematocrit values; obtain bilirubin levels. Assess for respiratory difficulty. Differentiate between physiologic and pathologic jaundice.
Mottled when undressed	Cyanosis (choanal atresia, CNS damage or trauma, respiratory or cardiac problem, cold stress)	Assess degree of (central or peripheral) cyanosis and possible causes; refer to physician.
Minor bruising over buttocks in breech presentation and over eyes and forehead in facial presentations		Discuss with parents cause and course of minor bruising related to labor and birth.
Texture		
Smooth, soft, flexible; may have dry, peeling hands and feet	Generalized cracked or peeling skin (SGA or postterm; blood incompatibility; metabolic, kidney dysfunction)	Report to physician.
	Seborrheic-dermatitis (cradle cap) Absence of vernix (postmature) Yellow vernix (bilirubin staining)	Instruct parents to shampoo the scalp and anterior fontanelle areas daily with soap; rinse well; avoid use of oil.

*Possible causes of alterations are placed in parentheses.

†This column provides guidelines for further assessment and initial nursing interventions.

NEWBORN PHYSICAL ASSESSMENT GUIDE continued

Assessment and Normal Findings	Alterations and Possible Causes*	Nursing Responses to Data[†]
Turgor		
Elastic, returns to normal shape after pinching	Maintains tent shape (dehydration)	Assess for other signs and symptoms of dehydration.
Pigmentation		
Clear; milia across bridge of nose, forehead, or chin will disappear within a few weeks		Advise parents not to pinch or prick these pimplelike areas.
Café-au-lait spots (one or two)	Six or more (neurologic disorder such as Von Recklinghausen disease, cutaneous neurofibromatosis)	If there are six or more café-au-lait spots, refer for genetic and neurologic consult.
Mongolian spots common over dorsal area and buttocks in dark-skinned infants		Assure parents of normalcy of this pigmentation; it will fade in first year or two.
Erythema toxicum	Impetigo (group A β-hemolytic streptococcus or *Staphylococcus aureus* infection)	If impetigo occurs, instruct parents about hand washing and linen precautions during home care.
Telangiectatic nevi	Hemangiomas: Nevus flammeus (port wine stain) Nevus vascularis (strawberry hemangioma) Cavernous hemangiomas	Collaborate with physician. Counsel parents about birthmark's progression to allay misconceptions. Record size and shape of hemangiomas. Refer for follow-up at well-baby clinic.
Rashes	Rashes (infection)	Assess location and type of rash (macular, papular, vesicular). Obtain history of onset, prenatal history, and related signs and symptoms.
Petechiae of head or neck (breech presentation, cord around neck)	Generalized petechiae (clotting abnormalities)	Determine cause; advise parents if further health care is needed.
Head		
General appearance, size, movement Round, symmetric, and moves easily from left to right and up and down; soft and pliable	Asymmetric, flattened occiput on either side of the head (plagiocephaly) Head held at angle (torticollis)	Instruct parents to change infant's sleeping positions frequently.
	Unable to move head side to side (neurologic trauma)	Determine adequacy of all neurologic signs.
Circumference: 32–37 cm (12.5–14.5 in); 2 cm greater than chest circumference Head one-fourth of body size	Extreme differences in size may be microencephaly (Cornelia de Lange syndrome, cytomegalic inclusion disease [CID]), rubella, toxoplasmosis, chromosome abnormalities), hydrocephalus (meningomyelocele, achondroplasia), anencephaly (neural tube defect) Head is 3 cm or more larger than chest circumference (preterm, hydrocephalus)	Measure circumference from occiput to frontal area using metal or paper tape. Measure chest circumference using metal or paper tape and compare to head circumference. Record measurements on growth chart. Reevaluate at well-baby visits.
Common variations		
Molding Breech and cesarean newborns' heads are round and well shaped	Cephalhematoma (trauma during birth persists up to 3 weeks) Caput succedaneum (long labor and birth; disappears in 1 week)	Evaluate neurologic response. Observe for hyperbilirubinemia. Reassure parents regarding common manifestations due to birth process and when they should disappear.

*Possible causes of alterations are placed in parentheses.

[†]This column provides guidelines for further assessment and initial nursing interventions.

NEWBORN PHYSICAL ASSESSMENT GUIDE continued

Assessment and Normal Findings	Alterations and Possible Causes*	Nursing Responses to Data†
Fontanelles		
Palpation of juncture of cranial bones Anterior fontanelle: 3–4 cm long by 2–3 cm wide, diamond shaped Posterior fontanelle: 1–2 cm at birth, triangle shaped	Overlapping of anterior fontanelle (malnourished or preterm newborn) Premature closure of sutures (craniostenosis) Late closure (hydrocephalus)	Discuss normal closure times with parents and care of "soft spots" to allay misconceptions. Refer to physician. Observe for signs and symptoms of hydrocephalus.
Slight pulsation	Moderate to severe pulsation (vascular problems)	Refer to physician.
Moderate bulging noted with crying, stooling, or pulsations with heartbeat	Bulging (increased intracranial pressure, meningitis) Sunken (dehydration)	Evaluate hydration status. Evaluate neurologic status. Report to physician.
Hair		
Texture		
Smooth with fine texture variations (Note: Variations depend on ethnic background.)	Coarse, brittle, dry hair (hypothyroidism) White forelock (Waardenburg syndrome)	Instruct parents regarding routine care of hair and scalp.
Distribution		
Scalp hair high over eyebrows (Spanish-Mexican hairline begins mid-forehead and extends down back of neck.)	Low forehead and posterior hairlines may indicate chromosomal disorders.	Assess for other signs of chromosomal aberrations. Refer to physician.
Face		
Symmetric movement of all facial features, normal hairline, eyebrows and eyelashes present		Assess and record symmetry of all parts, shape, regularity of features, sameness or differences in features.
Spacing of features		
Eyes at same level, nostrils equal size, cheeks full, and sucking pads present	Eyes wide apart—ocular hypertelorism (Apert syndrome, cri-du-chat, Turner syndrome)	Observe for other signs and symptoms indicative of disease states or chromosomal aberrations.
Lips equal on both sides of midline	Abnormal face (Down syndrome, cretinism, gargoylism)	
Chin recedes when compared to other bones of face	Abnormally small jaw—micrognathia (Pierre Robin syndrome, Treacher Collins syndrome)	Maintain airway; do not position supine. Initiate surgical consultation and referral.
Movement		
Makes facial grimaces	Inability to suck, grimace, and close eyelids (cranial nerve injury)	Initiate neurologic assessment and consultation.
Symmetric when resting and crying	Asymmetry (paralysis of facial cranial nerve)	Assess and record symmetry of all parts, shape, regularity of features, and sameness or differences in features.

*Possible causes of alterations are placed in parentheses.

†This column provides guidelines for further assessment and initial nursing interventions.

NEWBORN PHYSICAL ASSESSMENT GUIDE continued

Assessment and Normal Findings	Alterations and Possible Causes*	Nursing Responses to Data†
Eyes		
General placement and appearance		
Bright and clear; even placement; slight nystagmus (involuntary cyclical eye movements)	Gross nystagmus (damage to third, fourth, and sixth cranial nerves)	
Concomitant strabismus	Constant and fixed strabismus	Reassure parents that strabismus is considered normal up to 6 months.
Move in all directions		
Blue- or slate-blue gray	Lack of pigmentation (albinism) Brushfield spots may indicate Down syndrome (a light or white speckling of the outer two-thirds of the iris)	Discuss with parents any necessary eye precautions. Assess for other signs of Down syndrome.
Brown color at birth in dark-skinned infants		Discuss with parents that permanent eye color is usually established by 3 months of age.
Eyelids		
Position: above pupils but within iris, no drooping	Elevation or retraction of upper lid (hyperthyroidism)	Assess for signs of hydrocephalus and hyperthyroidism.
	"Sunset sign" lid retraction and downward gaze (hydrocephalus), ptosis (congenital or paralysis of oculomotor muscle)	Evaluate interference with vision in subsequent well-baby visits.
Eyes on parallel plane Epicanthal folds in Asian and 20% of newborns of Northern European descent	Upward slant in non-Asians (Down syndrome) Epicanthal folds (Down syndrome, cri-du-chat syndrome)	Assess for other signs of Down syndrome.
Movement		
Blink reflex in response to light stimulus Eyes open wide in dimly lit room	Blink absent (CNS injury)	Evaluate neurologic status. Refer to physician.
Inspection		
Edematous for first few days of life, resulting from birth and instillation of silver nitrate (chemical conjunctivitis); no lumps or redness	Purulent drainage (infection); infectious conjunctivitis (gonococcus, chlamydia, staphylococcus, or gram-negative organisms) Marginal blepharitis (lid edges red, crusted, scaly)	Initiate good hand washing. Refer to physician. Evaluate infant for seborrheic dermatitis; scales can be removed easily.
Cornea		
Clear Corneal reflex present	Ulceration (herpes infection); large cornea or corneas of unequal size (congenital glaucoma) Clouding, opacity of lens (cataract)	Refer to ophthalmologist. Assess for other manifestations of congenital herpes; institute nursing care measures.
Sclera		
May appear bluish in newborn, then white; slightly brownish color frequent in newborns of African descent	True blue sclera (osteogenesis imperfecta)	Refer to physician.

*Possible causes of alterations are placed in parentheses.

†This column provides guidelines for further assessment and initial nursing interventions.

NEWBORN PHYSICAL ASSESSMENT GUIDE continued

Assessment and Normal Findings	Alterations and Possible Causes*	Nursing Responses to Data†
Pupils		
Pupils equal in size, round, and react to light by accommodation	Anisocoria—unequal pupils (CNS damage) Dilation or constriction (intracranial damage, retinoblastoma, glaucoma) Pupils nonreactive to light or accommodation (brain injury)	Refer for neurologic examination.
Slight nystagmus in newborn who has not learned to focus Pupil light reflex demonstrated at birth or by 3 weeks of age	Nystagmus (labyrinthine disturbance, CNS disorder)	
Conjunctiva		
Chemical conjunctivitis Subconjunctival hemorrhage	Pale color (anemia)	Obtain hematocrit and hemoglobin. Reassure parents that chemical conjunctivitis will subside in 1 to 2 days and subconjunctival hemorrhage disappears in a few weeks.
Palpebral conjunctiva (red but not hyperemic)	Inflammation or edema (infection, blocked tear duct)	
Vision		
20/150 Tracks moving object to midline Fixed focus on objects at a distance of about 10–20 in; may be difficult to evaluate in newborn Prefers faces, geometric designs, and black and white to colors	Cataracts (congenital infection)	Record any questions about visual acuity, and initiate follow-up evaluation at first well-baby checkup.
Lashes and lacrimal glands		
Presence of lashes (lashes may be absent in preterm newborns)	No lashes on inner two-thirds of lid (Treacher Collins syndrome); bushy lashes (Hurler syndrome); long lashes (Cornelia de Lange syndrome)	
Cry commonly tearless	Excessive tearing (plugged lacrimal duct, natal narcotic withdrawal), glaucoma	Demonstrate to parents how to milk blocked tear duct. Refer to ophthalmologist if tearing is excessive before third month of life.
Nose		
Appearance of external nasal aspects		
May appear flattened as a result of birth process	Continued flat or broad bridge of nose (Down syndrome)	Arrange consultation with specialist.
Small and narrow in midline, even placement in relationship to eyes and mouth	Low bridge of nose, beaklike nose (Apert syndrome, Treacher Collins syndrome) Upturned (Cornelia de Lange syndrome)	Initiate evaluation of chromosomal abnormalities.

*Possible causes of alterations are placed in parentheses.

†This column provides guidelines for further assessment and initial nursing interventions.

NEWBORN PHYSICAL ASSESSMENT GUIDE continued

Assessment and Normal Findings	Alterations and Possible Causes*	Nursing Responses to Data[†]
Patent nares bilaterally (nose breathers)	Blockage of nares (mucus and/or secretions), choanal atresia	Inspect for obstruction of nares.
Sneezing common to clear nasal passages	Flaring nares (respiratory distress)	Maintain oral airway until surgical correction is made.
Responds to odors, may smell breast milk	No response to stimulating odors	Inspect for obstruction of nares.
Mouth		
Function of facial, hypoglossal, glossopharyngeal, and vagus nerves		
Symmetry of movement and strength	Mouth draws to one side (transient seventh cranial nerve paralysis due to pressure in utero or trauma during birth, congenital paralysis)	Initiate neurologic consultation. Administer eye care if eye on affected side of face is unable to close.
	Fishlike shape (Treacher Collins syndrome)	
Presence of gag, swallowing, coordinated with sucking reflexes Adequate salivation	Suppressed or absent reflexes	Evaluate other neurologic functions of these nerves.
Palate (soft and hard)		
Hard palate dome-shaped Uvula midline with symmetrical movement of soft palate	High-steepled palate (Treacher Collins syndrome), bivid uvula (congenital anomaly)	Assess for other congenital anomalies.
Palate intact, sucks well when stimulated	Clefts in either hard or soft palate (polygenic disorder)	Initiate a surgical consultation referral.
Epithelial (Epstein's) pearls appear on mucosa		Assure parents that these are normal and will disappear at 2 or 3 months of age.
Esophagus patent, some drooling common in newborn	Excessive drooling or bubbling (esophageal atresia)	Test for patency of esophagus.
Tongue		
Free moving in all directions, midline	Lack of movement or asymmetric movement (neurologic damage) Tongue-tied	Further assess neurologic functions. Test reflex elevation of tongue when depressed with tongue blade.
	Deviations from midline (cranial nerve damage)	Check for signs or weakness or deviation.
Pink color, smooth to rough texture, noncoated	White cheesy coating (thrush) Tongue has deep ridges	Differentiate between thrush and milk curds. Reassure parents that tongue pattern may change from day to day.
Tongue proportional to mouth	Large tongue with short frenulum (cretinism, Down syndrome, other syndromes)	Evaluate in well-baby clinic to assess development delays. Initiate referrals.

*Possible causes of alterations are placed in parentheses.

[†]This column provides guidelines for further assessment and initial nursing interventions.

NEWBORN PHYSICAL ASSESSMENT GUIDE continued

Assessment and Normal Findings	Alterations and Possible Causes*	Nursing Responses to Data[†]
Ears		
External ear		
Without lesions, cysts, or nodules	Nodules, cysts, or sinus tracts in front of ear Adherent earlobes Low set	Evaluate characteristics of lesions. Counsel parents to clean external ear with washcloth only; discourage use of cotton-tip applicators.
	Preauricular skin tags	Refer to physician for ligation.
Hearing		
Eustachian tubes are cleared with first cry Absence of all risk factors	Presence of one or more risk factors	Assess history of risk factors for hearing loss.
Attends to sounds; sudden or loud noise elicits Moro reflex	No response to sound stimuli (deafness)	Test for Moro reflex.
Neck		
Appearance		
Short, straight, creased with skin folds	Abnormally short neck (Turner syndrome) Arching or inability to flex neck (meningitis, congenital anomaly)	Report findings to physician.
Posterior neck lacks loose extra folds of skin	Webbing of neck (Turner syndrome, Down syndrome, trisomy 18)	Assess for other signs of the syndromes.
Clavicles		
Straight and intact	Knot or lump on clavicle (fracture during difficult birth)	Obtain detailed labor and birth history; apply figure-8 bandage.
Moro reflex elicitable	Unilateral Moro reflex response on unaffected side (fracture of clavicle, brachial palsy, Erb-Duchenne paralysis)	Collaborate with physician.
Symmetric shoulders	Hypoplasia	
Chest		
Appearance and size		
Circumference: 32.5 cm, 1–2 cm less than head Wider than it is long		Measure at level of nipples after exhalation.
Normal shape without depressed or prominent sternum Lower end of sternum (xiphoid cartilage) may be protruding; is less apparent after several weeks Sternum 8 cm long	Funnel chest (congenital or associated with Marfan syndrome) Continued protrusion of xiphoid cartilage (Marfan syndrome, "pigeon chest") Barrel chest	Determine adequacy of other respiratory and circulatory signs. Assess for other signs and symptoms of various syndromes.

*Possible causes of alterations are placed in parentheses.

[†]This column provides guidelines for further assessment and initial nursing interventions.

NEWBORN PHYSICAL ASSESSMENT GUIDE continued

Assessment and Normal Findings	Alterations and Possible Causes*	Nursing Responses to Data[†]
Expansion and retraction		
Bilateral expansion	Unequal chest expansion (pneumonia, pneumothorax, respiratory distress)	Assess respiratory effort regularity, flaring of nares, difficulty on both inspiration and expiration.
No intercostal, subcostal, or supracostal retractions	Retractions (respiratory distress) See-saw respirations (respiratory distress)	Record and consult physician.
Auscultation		
Breath sounds are louder in infants	Decreased breath sounds (decreased respiratory activity, atelectasis, pneumothorax)	Perform assessment and report to physician any positive findings.
Chest and axilla clear on crying	Increased breath sounds (resolving pneumonia or in cesarean births)	
Bronchial breath sounds (heard where trachea and bronchi closest to chest wall, above sternum and between scapulae): Bronchial sounds bilaterally Air entry clear Rales may indicate normal newborn atelectasis Cough reflex absent at birth, appears in 2 or more days	Adventitious or abnormal sounds (respiratory disease or distress)	Evaluate color for pallor or cyanosis. Report to physician.
Breasts		
Flat with symmetric nipples Breast tissue diameter 5 cm or more at term Distance between nipples 8 cm	Lack of breast tissue (preterm or SGA) Discharge Enlargement	Evaluate for infection.
Breast engorgement occurs on third day of life; liquid discharge may be expressed in term newborns	Breast abscesses	Reassure parents of normality of breast engorgement.
Nipples	Supernumerary nipples Dark-colored nipples	No intervention is necessary.
Heart		
Auscultation		
Location: lies horizontally, with left border extending to left of midclavicle		
Regular rhythm and rate	Arrhythmia (anoxia), tachycardia, bradycardia	Refer all arrhythmia and gallop rhythms.
Determination of point of maximal impulse (PMI) Usually lateral to midclavicular line at third or fourth intercostal space	Malpositioning (enlargement, abnormal placement, pneumothorax, dextrocardia, diaphragmatic hernia)	Initiate cardiac evaluation.
Functional murmurs No thrills	Location of murmurs (possible congenital cardiac anomaly)	Evaluate murmur: location, timing, and duration; observe for accompanying cardiac pathology symptoms; ascertain family history.
Horizontal groove at diaphragm shows flaring of rib cage to mild degree	Marked rib flaring (vitamin D deficiency) Inadequacy of respiratory movement	Initiate cardiopulmonary evaluation; assess pulses and blood pressures in all four extremities for equality and quality.

*Possible causes of alterations are placed in parentheses.

[†]This column provides guidelines for further assessment and initial nursing interventions.

NEWBORN PHYSICAL ASSESSMENT GUIDE continued

Assessment and Normal Findings	Alterations and Possible Causes*	Nursing Responses to Data†
Abdomen		
Appearance		
Cylindrical with some protrusion, appears large in relation to pelvis, some laxness of abdominal muscles No cyanosis, few vessels seen Diastasis recti—common in infants of African descent	Distention, shiny abdomen with engorged vessels (gastrointestinal abnormalities, infection, congenital megacolon) Scaphoid abdominal appearance (diaphragmatic hernia) Increased or decreased peristalsis (duodenal stenosis, small bowel obstruction) Localized flank bulging (enlarged kidneys, ascites, or absent abdominal muscles)	Examine abdomen thoroughly for mass or organomegaly. Measure abdominal girth. Report deviations of abdominal size. Assess other signs and symptoms of obstruction. Refer to physician.
Umbilicus		
No protrusion of umbilicus (protrusion of umbilicus common in infants of African descent) Bluish-white color Cutis navel (umbilical cord projects), granulation tissue present in navel	Umbilical hernia Patent urachus (congenital malformation) Omphalocele Gastroschisis Redness or exudate around cord (infection) Yellow discoloration (hemolytic disease, meconium staining)	Measure umbilical hernia by palpating the opening and record; it should close by 1 year of age; if not, refer to physician. Cover omphalocele with sterile, moist dressing. Instruct parents on cord care and hygiene.
Two arteries and one vein apparent Begins drying 1 to 2 hours after birth No bleeding	Single umbilical artery (congenital anomalies) Discharge or oozing of blood from the cord	Refer anomalies to physician.
Auscultation and percussion Soft bowel sounds heard shortly after birth every 10–30 seconds	Bowel sounds in chest (diaphragmatic hernia) Absence of bowel sounds Hyperperistalsis (intestinal obstruction)	Collaborate with physician. Assess for other signs of dehydration and/or infection.
Femoral pulses		
Palpable, equal, bilateral	Absent or diminished femoral pulses (coarctation of aorta)	Monitor blood pressure in upper and lower extremities.
Inguinal area		
No bulges along inguinal area No inguinal lymph nodes felt	Inguinal hernia	Initiate referral. Continue follow-up in well-baby clinic.
Bladder		
Percusses 1–4 cm above symphysis Emptied about 3 hours after birth; if not, at time of birth Urine—inoffensive, mild odor	Failure to void within 24–48 hours after birth Exposure of bladder mucosa (exstrophy of bladder) Foul odor (infection)	Check whether baby voided at birth. Obtain urine specimen if infection is suspected. Consult with clinician.

*Possible causes of alterations are placed in parentheses.

†This column provides guidelines for further assessment and initial nursing interventions.

NEWBORN PHYSICAL ASSESSMENT GUIDE continued

Assessment and Normal Findings	Alterations and Possible Causes*	Nursing Responses to Data[†]
Genitals		
Gender clearly delineated	Ambiguous genitals	Refer for genetic consultation.
MALE		
Penis		
Slender in appearance, about 2.5 cm long, 1 cm wide at birth	Micropenis (congenital anomaly) Meatal atresia	Observe and record first voiding.
Normal urinary orifice, urethral meatus at tip of penis	Hypospadias, epispadias	Collaborate with physician in presence of abnormality. Delay circumcision.
Noninflamed urethral opening	Urethritis (infection)	Palpate for enlarged inguinal lymph nodes and record painful urination.
Foreskin adheres to glans	Ulceration of meatal opening (infection, inflammation)	Evaluate whether ulcer is due to diaper rash; counsel regarding care.
Uncircumcised foreskin tight for 2 to 3 months	Phimosis—if still tight after 3 months	Instruct parents on how to care for uncircumcised penis.
Circumcised Erectile tissue present		Teach parents how to care for circumcision.
Scrotum		
Skin loose and hanging or tight and small; extensive rugae and normal size Normal skin color Scrotal discoloration common in breech	Large scrotum containing fluid (hydrocele) Red, shiny scrotal skin (orchitis) Minimal rugae, small scrotum	Shine a light through scrotum (transilluminate) to verify diagnosis. Assess for prematurity.
Testes		
Descended by birth; not consistently found in scrotum	Undescended testes (cryptorchidism)	If testes cannot be felt in scrotum, gently palpate femoral, inguinal, perineal, and abdominal areas for presence.
Testes size 1.5–2 cm at birth	Enlarged testes (tumor) Small testes (Klinefelter syndrome or adrenal hyperplasia)	Refer and collaborate with physician for further diagnostic studies.
FEMALE		
Mons		
Normal skin color, area pigmented in dark-skinned infants Labia majora cover labia minora in term and postterm newborns; symmetric size appropriate for gestational age	Hematoma, lesions (trauma) Labia minora prominent	Evaluate for recent trauma. Assess for prematurity.
Clitoris		
Normally large in newborn Edema and bruising in breech birth	Hypertrophy (hermaphroditism)	Refer for genetic workup.

*Possible causes of alterations are placed in parentheses.

[†]This column provides guidelines for further assessment and initial nursing interventions.

NEWBORN PHYSICAL ASSESSMENT GUIDE continued

Assessment and Normal Findings	Alterations and Possible Causes*	Nursing Responses to Data[†]
Vagina		
Urinary meatus and vaginal orifice visible (0.5 cm circumference) Vaginal tag or hymenal tag disappears in a few weeks	Inflammation; erythema and discharge (urethritis) Congenital absence of vagina	Collect urine specimen for laboratory examination. Refer to physician.
Discharge; smegma under labia	Foul-smelling discharge (infection)	Collect data and further evaluate reason for discharge.
Bloody or mucoid discharge	Excessive vaginal bleeding (blood coagulation defect)	
Buttocks and Anus		
Buttocks symmetric	Pilonidal dimple	Examine for possible sinus. Instruct parents about cleansing this area.
Anus patent and passage of meconium within 24–48 hours after birth	Imperforate anus, rectal atresia (congenital gastrointestinal defect)	Evaluate extent of problems. Initiate surgical consultation. Perform digital examination to ascertain patency if patency uncertain.
No fissures, tears, or skin tags	Fissures	
Extremities and Trunk		
Short and generally flexed, extremities move symmetrically through range of motion but lack full extension	Unilateral or absence of movement (spinal cord involvement) Fetal position continued or limp (anoxia, CNS problems, hypoglycemia)	Review birth record to assess possible cause.
All joints move spontaneously; good muscle tone, of flexor type, birth to 2 months	Spasticity when infant begins using extensors (cerebral palsy, lack of muscle tone, "floppy baby" syndrome) Hypotonia (Down syndrome)	Collaborate with physician.
Arms		
Equal in length Bilateral movement Flexed when quiet	Brachial palsy (difficult birth) Erb-Duchenne paralysis Muscle weakness, fractured clavicle Absence of limb or change of size (phocomelia, amelia)	Report to clinician.
Hands		
Normal number of fingers	Polydactyly (Ellis-Van Creveld syndrome) Syndactyly—one limb (developmental anomaly) Syndactyly—both limbs (genetic component)	Report to clinician.
Normal palmar crease	Simian line on palm (Down syndrome)	Refer for genetic workup.
Normal size hands	Short fingers and broad hand (Hurler syndrome)	
Nails present and extend beyond fingertips in term newborn	Cyanosis and clubbing (cardiac anomalies) Nails long or yellow stained (postterm)	Evaluate for history of distress in utero.

*Possible causes of alterations are placed in parentheses.

[†]This column provides guidelines for further assessment and initial nursing interventions.

NEWBORN PHYSICAL ASSESSMENT GUIDE continued

Assessment and Normal Findings	Alterations and Possible Causes*	Nursing Responses to Data†
Spine		
C-shaped spine Flat and straight when prone Slight lumbar lordosis Easily flexed and intact when palpated At least half of back devoid of lanugo Full-term infant in ventral suspension should hold head at 45-degree angle, back straight	Spina bifida occulta (nevus pilosus) Dermal sinus Myelomeningocele Head lag, limp, floppy trunk (neurologic problems)	Evaluate extent of neurologic damage; initiate care of spinal opening.
Hips		
No sign of instability	Sensation of abnormal movement, jerk, or snap of hip dislocation	Examine all newborn infants for dislocated hip prior to discharge from birthing center.
Hips abduct to more than 60 degrees		If this is suspected, refer to orthopedist for further evaluation. Reassess at well-baby visits.
Inguinal and buttock skin creases		
Symmetric inguinal and buttock creases	Asymmetry (dislocated hips)	Refer to orthopedist for evaluation. Counsel parents regarding symptoms of concern, and discuss therapy.
Legs		
Legs equal in length Legs shorter than arms at birth	Shortened leg (dislocated hips) Lack of leg movement (fractures, spinal defects)	Refer to orthopedist for evaluation. Counsel parents regarding symptoms of concern, and discuss therapy.
Feet		
Foot is in straight line Positional clubfoot—based on position in utero	Talipes equinovarus (true clubfoot)	Discuss differences between positional and true clubfoot with parents. Teach parents passive manipulation of foot.
Fat pads and creases on soles of feet	Incomplete sole creases in first 24 hours of life (premature)	Refer to orthopedist if not corrected by 3 months of age.
Talipes planus (flat feet) normal under 3 years of age		Reassure parents that flat feet are normal in infants.
Neuromuscular		
Motor function		
Symmetric movement and strength in all extremities	Limp, flaccid, or hypertonic (CNS disorders, infection, dehydration, fracture)	Appraise newborn's posture and motor functions by observing activities and motor characteristics.
May be jerky or have brief twitchings	Tremors (hypoglycemia, hypocalcemia, infection, neurologic damage)	Evaluate electrolyte imbalance, hypoglycemia, and neurologic functioning.
Head lag not over 45 degrees	Delayed or abnormal development (preterm, neurologic involvement)	

*Possible causes of alterations are placed in parentheses.

†This column provides guidelines for further assessment and initial nursing interventions.

NEWBORN PHYSICAL ASSESSMENT GUIDE continued

Assessment and Normal Findings	Alterations and Possible Causes*	Nursing Responses to Data†
Neck control adequate to maintain head erect briefly	Asymmetry of tone or strength (neurologic damage)	Refer for genetic evaluation.
Reflexes		
Blink		
Stimulated by flash of light; response is closure of eyelids	Lack of blink response (damage to cranial nerve, CNS injury)	Assess neurologic status.
Pupillary reflex		
Stimulated by flash of light; response is constriction of pupil	Lack of reflex (damage to cranial nerve, CNS injury)	
Moro		
Response to sudden movement or loud noise should be one of symmetric extension and abduction of arms with fingers extended; then return to normal relaxed flexion Infant lying on back: slightly raised head suddenly released; infant held horizontally, lowered quickly about 6 in, and stopped abruptly Fingers form a C Present at birth; disappears by 6 months of age	Asymmetry of body response (fractured clavicle, injury to brachial plexus) Consistent absence (brain damage)	Discuss normality of this reflex in response to loud noises and/or sudden movements. Absence of reflex requires neurologic evaluation.
Rooting and sucking		
Turns in direction of stimulus to cheek or mouth; opens mouth and begins to suck rhythmically when finger or nipple is inserted into mouth; difficult to elicit after feeding; disappears by 4 to 7 months of age Sucking is adequate for nutritional intake and meeting oral stimulation needs; disappears by 12 months	Poor sucking or easily fatigable (preterm, breastfed infants of barbiturate-addicted mothers, possible cardiac problem) Absence of response (preterm, neurologic involvement, depressed newborns)	Evaluate strength and coordination of sucking. Observe newborn during feeding, and counsel parents about mutuality of feeding experience and newborn's responses.
Palmar grasp		
Fingers grasp adult finger when palm is stimulated and hold momentarily; lessens at 3 to 4 months of age	Asymmetry of response (neurologic problems)	Evaluate other reflexes and general neurologic functioning.
Plantar grasp		
Toes curl downward when sole of foot is stimulated; lessens by 8 months	Absent (defects of lower spinal column)	Assess for other lower extremity neurologic problems.

*Possible causes of alterations are placed in parentheses.

†This column provides guidelines for further assessment and initial nursing interventions.

NEWBORN PHYSICAL ASSESSMENT GUIDE continued

Assessment and Normal Findings	Alterations and Possible Causes*	Nursing Responses to Data†
Stepping		
When held upright and one foot touching a flat surface, will step alternately; disappears at 4 to 5 months of age	Asymmetry of stepping (neurologic abnormality)	Evaluate muscle tone and function on each side of body. Refer to specialist.
Babinski		
Fanning and extension of all toes when one side of sole is stroked from heel upward across ball of foot; disappears at about 12 months	Absence of response (low spinal cord defects)	Refer for further neurologic evaluation.
Tonic neck		
Fencer position—when head is turned to one side, extremities on same side extend and on opposite side flex; this reflex may not be evident during early neonatal period; disappears at 3 to 4 months of age Response often more dominant in leg than in arm	Absent after 1 month of age or persistent asymmetry (cerebral lesion)	Assess neurologic functioning.
Prone crawl		
While on abdomen, neonate pushes up and tries to crawl	Absence or variance of response (preterm, weak, or depressed newborns)	Evaluate motor functioning. Refer to specialist.
Trunk incurvation (Galant)		
In prone position stroking of spine causes pelvis to turn to stimulated side	Failure to rotate to stimulated side (neurologic damage)	

*Possible causes of alterations are placed in parentheses.

†This column provides guidelines for further assessment and initial nursing interventions.

how often and where the newborn attends to auditory and visual stimuli. Orientation to the environment is determined by an ability to respond to clues given by others and by a natural ability to fix on and follow a visual object horizontally and vertically. This capacity, and parental appreciation of it, are important for positive communication between infant and parents; the parents' visual *(en face)* and auditory (soft, continuous voice) presence stimulates their newborn to orient to them. Inability or lack of response may indicate visual or auditory problems. It is important for parents to know that their newborn can turn to voices soon after birth or by 3 days of age and can become alert at different times with a varying degree of intensity in response to sounds.

3. *Motor activity.* Several components are evaluated. Motor tone of the newborn is assessed in the most characteristic state of responsiveness. This summary assessment includes overall use of tone as the newborn responds to being handled—whether during spontaneous activity, prone placement, or horizontal holding—and overall assessment of body tone as the newborn reacts to all stimuli.
4. *Variations.* Frequency of alert states, state changes, color changes (throughout all states as examination progresses), activity, and peaks of excitement are assessed.
5. *Self-quieting activity.* This assessment is based on how often, how quickly, and how effectively newborns can use their resources to quiet and console themselves when upset or distressed. Considered in this assessment are such self-consolatory activities as putting hand to mouth, sucking on a fist or the tongue, and attuning to an object or sound. The

CRITICAL THINKING IN ACTION

Maria Reyes, a 19-year-old G2 now P2 mother, delivered a 40-week-old female neonate 24 hours ago. The newborn exam was normal. Mrs Reyes asks about the newborn's exam. She says she has noticed that the baby cries more than her first child and seems to require holding for longer periods of time after feeding before "quieting down." She is concerned that there is something she is doing wrong and wants to know when her newborn will start to act like her first baby. What should you discuss with her about newborn behavior?

Answers can be found in Appendix H.

newborn's need for outside consolation must also be considered (for example, seeing a face; being rocked, held, or dressed; using a pacifier; and being swaddled).

6. *Cuddliness or social behaviors.* This area encompasses the newborn's need for, and response to, being held. Also considered is how often the newborn smiles. These behaviors influence the couple's self-esteem and feelings of acceptance or rejection. Cuddling also appears to be an indicator of personality. Cuddlers appear to enjoy, accept, and seek physical contact; are easier to placate; sleep more; and form earlier and more intense attachments. Noncuddlers are active, restless, have accelerated motor development, and are intolerant of physical restraint. Smiling, even as a grimace reflex, greatly influences parent-newborn feedback. Parents identify this response as positive.

CHAPTER HIGHLIGHTS

- A perinatal history, determination of gestational age, physical examination, and behavior assessment form the basis for a complete newborn assessment.
- The common physical characteristics included in the gestational age assessment are skin, lanugo, sole (plantar) creases, breast tissue and size, ear form and cartilage, and genitalia.
- The neuromuscular components of gestational age scoring tools are usually posture, square window sign, popliteal angle, arm recoil, heel-to-ear, and scarf sign.
- By assessing the physical and neuromuscular components of a gestational age tool, the nurse can determine the gestational age of the newborn.
- After determining the gestational age of the baby, the nurse can assess how the newborn will make the transition to extrauterine life and anticipate potential physiologic problems.
- The nurse identifies the newborn as SGA, AGA, or LGA and prioritizes individual needs.
- Normal ranges for vital signs assessed in the newborn are: heart rate, 120–160 beats/min; respirations, 30–60 respirations/min; axillary temperature, 36.4–37.2C (97.5–99F); skin temperature, 36–36.5C (96.8–97.7F); rectal temperature, 36.6–37.2C (97.8–99F); and blood pressure at birth of 80–60/45–40 mm Hg.
- Normal newborn measurements include: weight range, 2500–4000 g (5 lb 8 oz–8 lb 13 oz), with weight dependent on maternal size and age; length range, 45–55 cm (18–22 in); and head circumference range of 32–37 cm (12.5–14.5 in)—approximately 2 cm larger than the chest circumference.
- Commonly elicited newborn reflexes are tonic neck, Moro, grasp, rooting, sucking, and blink.
- Newborn behavioral abilities include habituation, orientation to visual and auditory stimuli, motor activity, cuddliness, and self-quieting activity.
- An important role of the nurse during the physical and behavioral assessments of the newborn is to teach parents about their newborn and involve them in their baby's care. This facilitates the parents' identification of their newborn's uniqueness and allays their concerns.

REFERENCES

AAP Committee on Fetus and Newborn and ACOG Committee on Obstetrics: *Guidelines for Perinatal Care.* Evanston, IL: American Academy of Pediatrics, 1992.

Alexander GR, Allen MC: Conceptualization, measurement, and use of gestational age: I. Clinical and public health practice. *J Perinatol* 1996; 16(1):53.

Ballard JL et al: New Ballard score, expanded to include extremely premature infants. *J Pediatr* 1991; 119:417.

Ballard JL et al: A simplified score for assessment of fetal maturation of newly born infants. *J Pediatr* November 1979; 95:769.

Baptist EC, Amin PV: Perinatal testicular torsion and the hard testicle. *J Perinatol* 1996; 16(1):67.

Brazelton TB: Neonatal behavior and its significance. In: *Schaeffer's Diseases of the Newborn.* Avery ME, Taeusch HW (editors). Philadelphia: Saunders, 1984.

Brazelton TB: *The Neonatal Behavioral Assessment Scale.* Philadelphia: Lippincott, 1973.

Brooks AA et al: Birth weight: Nature or nuture? *Early Human Development* 1995; 42:29.

Cogswell ME, Yip R: The influence of fetal and maternal factors on the distribution of birthweight. *Semin Perinatol* 1995; 19(3):222.

Dodd V: Gestational age assessment. *Neonatal Network* 1995; 15(1):27.

Dubowitz L, Dubowitz V: *Gestational Age of the Newborn.* Menlo Park, CA: Addison-Wesley, 1977.

Faix RG: Fontanelle size in Black and White term infants. *J Pediatr* 1982; 100:304.

Fowlie P, Forsyth S: Examination of the newborn infant. *Modern Midwife* 1995: 1:15.

Hegyi T et al: Blood pressure ranges in premature infants: II. The first week of life. *Pediatrics* 1996; 97(3):336.

Hicks MA: A comparison of the tympanic and axillary temperatures of the preterm and term infant. *J Perinatol* 1996; 16(4):261.

Hockelman RA et al: *Primary Pediatric Care,* 2nd ed. St Louis: Mosby, 1992.

Jona JZ: Congenital hernia of the cord and associated patent omphalomesenteric duct: A frequent neonatal problem? *Am J Perinatol* 1996; 13(4):223.

Ludington-Hoe SM, Golani S: *How to Have a Smarter Baby.* New York: Bantam, 1988.

Peck JE: Development of hearing: Part III. Postnatal development. *J Am Acad Audiol* 1995; 6(2):113.

Shann F, Mackenzie A: Comparison of rectal, axillary, and forehead temperatures. *Arch Pediatr Adolesc Med* 1996; 150:74.

Steinkuller PG: *Best Methods for Visual Assessment in Children.* Paper presented at the Cullen Course, Baylor College of Medicine, Dallas, March 1988.

Taeusch HW, Ballard RA, Avery ME: *Schaffer and Avery's Diseases of the Newborn,* 6th ed. Philadelphia: Saunders, 1991.

Tappero EP, Honeyfield ME: *Physical Assessment of the Newborn,* 2nd ed. Petaluma, CA: NICU Ink, 1996.

Wen SW, Kramer MS, Usher RH: Comparison of birth weight distribution between Chinese and Caucasian infants. *Am J Epidemiol* 1995; 141(12):1177.

Chapter 23 The Normal Newborn: Needs and Care

OBJECTIVES

- Summarize the essential areas of information to be obtained about a newborn's birth experience and immediate postnatal period.
- Explain the physiologic and behavioral responses of newborns and possible interventions needed.
- Discuss the major nursing considerations and activities to be carried out during the first 4 hours after birth (admission and transitional period) and subsequent daily care.
- Identify the activities that should be included in a daily care plan for a normal newborn.
- Determine common family concerns about their newborns.
- Describe the topics and related content to be included in parent education classes on newborn/infant care.
- Identify opportunities to individualize parent teaching and enhance each parent's abilities and confidence while providing infant care in the birthing unit.
- Identify the information to be included in discharge planning with the newborn's family.

KEY TERMS

Circumcision
Newborn screening tests
Parent-infant attachment

At the moment of birth, numerous physiologic adaptations begin to take place in the newborn's body. Because of these dramatic changes, newborns require close observation to determine how smoothly they are making the transition to extrauterine life. Newborns also require care that enhances their chances of making the transition successfully.

The two broad goals of nursing care during this period are to promote the physical well-being of the newborn and to promote the establishment of a functioning family unit. The nurse meets the first goal by providing comprehensive care to the newborn in the mother-baby unit. The nurse meets the second goal by teaching family members how to care for their new baby and by supporting their efforts so that they feel confident and competent. Thus the nurse must be knowledgeable about family adjustments that need to be made as well as the health care needs of the newborn. It is important that the family return home with the positive feeling that they have the support, information, and skills to care for their newborn. Equally important is the need for each member of the family to begin a unique relationship with the newborn. The cultural and social expectations of individual families and communities affect the way in which normal newborn care is carried out.

The previous two chapters presented an informational database of the physiologic and behavioral changes occurring in the newborn and the pertinent nursing assessments that are needed. This chapter discusses the nursing care required during the newborn period. The Newborn Critical Pathway starts on p 570.

Nursing Diagnosis During Admission and the First 4 Hours

Nursing diagnoses are based on an analysis of the assessment findings. Physiologic alterations of the newborn form the basis of many nursing diagnoses, as does the family's incorporation of them in caring for their new baby. Nursing diagnoses that may apply to newborn and family include

- Ineffective airway clearance related to presence of mucus and retained lung fluid
- High risk for altered body temperature related to evaporative, radiant, conductive, and convective heat losses
- Altered nutrition: less than body requirements related to limited fluid intake
- Pain related to heelsticks for glucose, hematocrit, or vitamin K administration
- Altered peripheral tissue perfusion related to decreased thermoregulation

Many of these nursing diagnoses and associated interventions must be identified and implemented very quickly during this period.

Nursing Plan and Implementation During Admission and First 4 Hours

The nurse initiates newborn admission procedures and evaluates the newborn's need to remain under observation. The nurse monitors the newborn's ability to maintain a clear airway and stable vital signs, maintain body temperature, demonstrate normal neurologic status and no observable complications, and tolerate the first feeding. If these criteria are met, it indicates a successful beginning adaptation to extrauterine life, and the baby is moved to a regular nursery or back to the mother's room. This transfer usually takes place between 2 and 6 hours after birth.

Initiation of Admission Procedures

After birth, the baby is formally admitted to the health care facility. The admission procedures include an assessment to ensure that the newborn's adaptation to extrauterine life is proceeding normally and several interventions to promote successful adaptation. (See Essential Precautions for Practice: During Newborn Care.)

If the initial assessment indicates that the newborn is not at risk physiologically, the nurse performs many of the routine admission procedures in the presence of the parents in the birthing area. The nurse may perform the care measures indicated by the assessment findings or may have the parents perform them with the nurse's guidance in an effort to educate and support the family. Other interventions may be delayed until the newborn has been transferred to an observational nursery.

The nurse responsible for the newborn first checks and confirms the newborn's identification and then obtains and records all significant information. The essential data to be recorded on the newborn's chart include the following:

1. *Condition of the newborn.* Pertinent information includes the newborn's Apgar scores at 1 and 5 minutes, resuscitative measures required in the birthing area, vital signs, voidings, and passing of meconium. Complications to be noted are excessive mucus, delayed spontaneous respirations or responsiveness, abnormal number of cord vessels, and obvious physical abnormalities.
2. *Labor and birth record.* The nurse should place a copy of the labor and birth record in the newborn's

ESSENTIAL PRECAUTIONS FOR PRACTICE

During Newborn Care

Examples of procedures for which disposable gloves are recommended include

- Handling baby before first bath and removal of all blood and amniotic fluid
- Oral or nasal suctioning after birth when blood or amniotic fluid is present in secretions
- Carrying out blood work (ie, glucose, hematocrit, newborn screen)
- Administer vitamin K and eye prophylaxis
- Changing linen soiled with blood or amniotic fluid

REMEMBER to wash your hands before putting on the disposable gloves and AGAIN immediately after you remove the gloves.

Examples of body fluids and procedures for which only hand washing is recommended include

- Breast milk
- Urine
- Stool
- Vomitus
- Tears
- Nasal secretions
- Oral secretions
- Diaper change

If the body fluids and excretions contain visible blood, gloves are warranted.

For further information, consult OSHA and CDC guidelines.

chart. The record contains all the significant data about the birth—for example, duration, course, and status of mother and fetus throughout labor and birth and any analgesia or anesthesia administered to the mother. Particular care is taken to note any variation or difficulties, such as prolonged rupture of membranes, abnormal fetal position, meconium-stained amniotic fluid, signs of fetal distress during labor, nuchal cord (cord around the newborn's neck at birth), precipitous birth, use of forceps, and maternal analgesics and anesthesia received within 1 hour before birth.

3. *Antepartal history.* Any maternal problems that may have compromised the fetus in utero, such as PIH, spotting, illness, recent infections, rubella status, serology results, hepatitis B screen results, exposure to group β streptococci (AAP 1992), or a history of maternal substance abuse, are of immediate concern in the assessment of the newborn. The chart should also include information about maternal age, estimated date of birth (EDB), previous pregnancies, and presence of any congenital anomalies.
4. *Parent-newborn interaction information.* The nurse notes parents' interactions with their newborn, and their desires regarding care, such as rooming-in, circumcision, and the type of feeding, are noted. Information about other children in the home, available support systems, and interactional patterns within each family unit assists in providing comprehensive care.

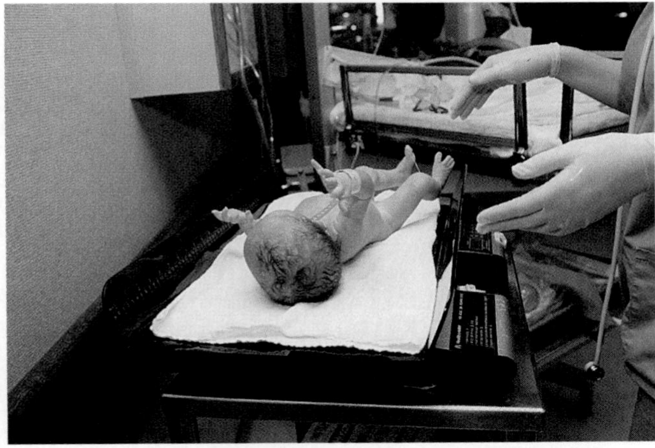

FIGURE 23–1 Weighing of newborns. The scale is balanced before each weighing, with the protective pad in place. The caregiver's hand is poised above the newborn as a safety measure.

As discussed in Chapter 21, the newborn's physiologic adaptations to extrauterine life occur rapidly. All the body systems are affected. The nurse must be able to monitor the newborn's physiologic adaptation and behavior during the transitional periods of the first few hours of life to identify any deviation from normal immediately. (See Key Facts to Remember: Signs of Newborn Transition on p 572.)

As part of the admission procedure, the nurse weighs the newborn in both grams and pounds; parents understand weights best when stated in pounds and ounces (Figure 23–1). The scales are cleaned and covered each time a newborn is weighed to prevent cross-infection and heat loss from conduction.

The nurse then measures the newborn and records the measurements in both centimeters and inches. Three routine measurements are (a) length, (b) circumference of the head, and (c) circumference of the chest. Some facilities also measure the abdominal girth. The nurse rapidly assesses the baby's color, muscle tone, alertness, and general state. Remember that the first period of reactivity may have concluded, and the baby may be in the sleep-inactive phase, which makes the infant hard to arouse. The nurse does basic assessments for estimating

Text continues on page 572

NEWBORN CRITICAL PATHWAY

Category	First 4 Hours	4–8 Hours Past Birth	8–12 Hours Past Birth
Referral	Review labor/birth record Review transitional nursing record Check ID bands	Check ID bands Transfer to mother/baby care at 4 hours of age Circumcision permit signed	Check ID bands q shift
Assessments	Continue assessments begun first hour after birth Vital signs: T, P, R, B/P, q1h × 4 (skin temp 97.8–98.6F, resp may be irregular but within 30–60 per min) Newborn assessments include: • Respiratory status with resp distress scale × 1 then prn If resp distress, assess q5–15min • Cord—bluish white color, clamp in place • Skin, mucous membranes, extremities—color (trunk pinkish with slight acrocyanosis of hands and feet) • Wt (5 lb 8 oz–8 lb 13 oz), Length (18–22 in), HC (12.5–14.5 in), CC (32.5 cm, 1–2 cm less than head) • Extremity movement—may be jerky or brief twitches • GA classification—Term AGA • Anomalies (cong. anomalies can interfere with normal extrauterine adaptation)	Assess newborn's progress thru periods of reactivity Vital signs: T, P, R, B/P q4h Newborn assessments include: • Skin color q4h (circulatory system stabilizing, acrocyanosis decreased) • Eyes for drainage, redness, hemorrhage • Ausculate lungs q4h (noisy wet resp normal) • Increased mucus production (normal in 2nd period of reactivity) • Check apical pulse q4h • Umbilical cord base for redness, drainage, foul odor, drying. Clamp remains in place. • Extremity movement q4h • Check for expected reflexes (suck, rooting, Moro, grasp, blink, yawn, sneeze, tonic neck, Babinski) • Note common normal variations • Assess suck and swallow during feeding • Note behavioral characteristics • Temp before and after admission bath	VS q4h–range: T, 97.5–99F; P, 120–160; R, 30–60; B/P, 60–80/45–40 mm Hg Continue newborn assessments: • Skin color q4h • Signs of drying or infection in cord area • Check cord clamp in place until removed before discharge • Check circ for bleeding after procedure, then q30min × 2, then at least q4h
Teaching/ psychosocial	Admission activities performed at mother's bedside if possible Teach parents use of bulb syringe, signs of choking, positioning, and when to call for assistance Teach reasons for radiant warmer use and the need to wrap baby in warmed blankets when out of warmer	Reinforce teaching about choking, bulb syringe, positioning, maintaining warmth by use of blankets and clothing Teach infant positioning to facilitate breathing and digestion Teach new parents holding and feeding skills Teach parents soothing/calming techniques	Teach parents re: diapering, normal void and stool patterns, bathing, nail and cord care, circumcision/uncircumcised penis care, rashes, jaundice, sleep/wake cycles and soothing activities, taking temperatures and reading thermometer Explain S&S of illness and when to call health care provider No tub bath until cord falls off
Therapeutic nursing interventions and reports	Place under radiant warmer Put hat on newborn (decreases convection heat loss) Suction nares/mouth with bulb syringe prn Keep bulb syringe in crib Obtain lab tests: blood type, Rh, Coombs on cord blood as needed; glucose, HSV culture if hx of maternal or paternal HSV	Keep under radiant warmer as needed Bathe infant if temp > 97.8F Position on side Suction nares (esp during 2nd period of reactivity) Obtain peripheral Hct per protocol Cord care per protocol (alcohol or triple dye prn) Fold diaper below cord (for plastic diapers, turn plastic layer away from skin)	Check for hearing test results Weigh before discharge Cord care q shift DC cord clamp before discharge Perform newborn screening blood tests before discharge Circumcision care: position on side, change dressing when soiled

NEWBORN CRITICAL PATHWAY continued

Category	First 4 Hours	4–8 Hours Past Birth	8–24 Hours Past Birth
Activity and comfort	Place under radiant warmer or wrap in prewarmed blankets until stable Soothe baby as needed with voice and/or touch	Leave in warmer until stable, then swaddle Position on side or abd after each feeding	Place in open crib Swaddle and allow movement of extremities in blanket
Nutrition	Assist newborn to breastfeed as soon as mother/baby condition allows Initiate bottle-feeding within first hour Gavage feed if necessary to prevent hypo-glycemia Supplement breast only when medically indicated or per agency policy	Breastfeed at least q3–4h or on demand Bottle-feed q3–6h or on demand Determine readiness to feed and feeding tolerance	Continue breast/bottle-feeding pattern Assess feeding tolerance q4h Discuss normal feeding requirements, signs of hunger and satiation, handling feeding problems, and when to seek help
Elimination	Note first void and stool if not done at birth	Note all voids and color of stools q4h	Evaluate all voids and color of stools q8h
Medication	Prophylactic ophthalmic ointment OU after baby makes eye contact with parents within 1 h after birth Administer vitamin K injection, 1 mg IM per agency protocol	Hepatitis B if ordered by Dr or consent signed by parent	Hepatitis B vaccine before dishcarge
Discharge planning/ home care	Hepatitis B form signed Hearing and screen consent signed Plan discharge call with parent/guardian in 24 hours to 2 days Assess parents' discharge plans and support systems	Review/reinforce teaching with mother and significant other	Initial newborn screening tests (hearing, blood tests, ie, PKU) before discharge Bath and feeding classes, videos, or written information given Give written copy of discharge instructions Set up appointment for follow-up PKU test Discuss infant safety needs Have car seat available before discharge All discharge referrals made Give hepatitis B vaccine as ordered
Family involvement	Facilitate early investigation of baby's physical characteristics (maintain temp during unwrapping), hold infant en face Dim lights to help infant keep eyes open Provide uninterrupted time with family	Assess parents' knowledge of newborn behaviors, such as alertness, suck and rooting behavior, and attention to human voice and soothing techniques	Assess mother-baby bonding/interaction Incorporate father and sibs into care Enhance parent-infant interaction by sharing characteristics & behavioral assessment Support positive parenting behaviors Identify community referral needs and refer to community agencies
Date			

KEY FACTS TO REMEMBER

Signs of Newborn Transition

Normal findings for the newborn during the first few days of life include the following:

Pulse: 120–160 beats/minute
- During sleep as low as 100 beats/minute
- If crying, up to 180 beats/minute
- Apical pulse is counted for 1 full minute because rate may fluctuate.

Respirations: 30–60 respirations/minute
- Predominantly diaphragmatic but synchronous with abdominal movements
- Brief periods of apnea (5–10 seconds) with no color or heart rate changes

Temperature:
- Axillary: 36.4–37C (97.5–99F)
- Skin: 36–36.5C (96.8–97.7F)

Blood pressure:
- 80–60/45–40 mm Hg at birth
- 100/50 mm Hg at day 10

Chemstrip: greater than 40 mg%

Hematocrit: less than 65%–70% central venous sample

gestational age and completes the physical assessment (see Chapter 22).

In addition to obtaining vital signs, the nurse may perform a hematocrit and blood glucose evaluation on all newborns or as clinically indicated (such as for small-for-gestational-age [SGA] or large-for-gestational-age [LGA] infants, or if the newborn is jittery). These procedures may be done on admission or within the first 4 hours after birth (AAP 1992). (See Procedure 26–1, p 690.)

Maintenance of a Clear Airway and Stable Vital Signs

The nurse positions the newborn on his or her side. If necessary, the nurse uses a bulb syringe or DeLee wall suction (Procedure 17–1, p 416) to remove mucus from the newborn's nasal passages and oral cavity. A DeLee catheter attached to suction may be used to remove mucus from the stomach to help prevent possible aspiration. This procedure also ensures that the esophagus is patent prior to the newborn's first feeding. Gastric suctioning can cause vagal nerve stimulation, which may result in bradycardia and apnea in the unstabilized newborn.

In the absence of any newborn distress, the nurse continues with the admission by taking the newborn's vital signs. The initial temperature is taken by the axillary method. A wider range of normal for axillary temperature is recommended (Merestein and Gardner 1992). This range is 36.5–37C (97.7–98.6F).

Once the initial temperature is taken, the core temperature is monitored either by obtaining axillary temperatures at intervals or by placing a skin sensor on the newborn for continuous reading. The usual skin sensor placement site is the newborn's abdomen, but placement on the upper thigh or arm can give a reading closely correlated with the mean body temperature. Nurses should monitor the vital signs for a healthy term newborn at least every 30 minutes until the newborn's condition has remained stable for 2 hours (AAP 1992). The newborn's respirations may be irregular and still be normal. Brief periods of apnea, lasting only 5–10 seconds with no color or heart rate changes, are considered normal. The normal pulse range is 120–160 beats per minute, and the normal respiratory range is 30–60 respirations per minute.

Maintenance of a Neutral Thermal Environment

A neutral thermal environment is essential to minimize the newborn's need for increased oxygen consumption and use of calories to maintain body heat in the optimal range of 36.4–37.2C (97.5–99F). If the newborn becomes hypothermic, the body's response can lead to metabolic acidosis, hypoxia, and shock.

A neutral thermal environment is best achieved by performing the newborn assessment and interventions with the newborn unclothed and under a radiant warmer. The thermostat of the radiant warmer is controlled by the thermal skin sensor taped to the newborn's abdomen, upper thigh, or arm. The sensor indicates when the newborn's temperature exceeds or falls below the acceptable temperature range. The nurse should be aware that leaning over the newborn may block the radiant heat waves from reaching the newborn.

It is common practice in some institutions to cover the newborn's head with a stockinette or knit cap to prevent further heat loss, in addition to placing the baby under a radiant warmer. Ruchala (1985) compared axillary temperatures of newborns whose heads were covered and those remaining uncovered and found no significant difference 2 hours after birth. More definitive studies are necessary. However, these limited results raise the question whether heat can more effectively be retained by using a head covering while the newborn is outside the radiant warmer but not when the newborn is under the radiant warmer (to avoid a barrier effect).

DRUG GUIDE Vitamin K_1 Phytonadione (AquaMEPHYTON)

Overview of Neonatal Action

Phytonadione is used in prophylaxis and treatment of hemorrhagic disease of the newborn. It promotes liver formation of the clotting factors II, VII, IX, and X. At birth the neonate does not have the bacteria in the colon that are necessary for synthesizing fat-soluble vitamin K_1. Therefore the newborn may have decreased levels of prothrombin during the first 5–8 days of life reflected by a prolongation of prothrombin time.

Route, Dosage, Frequency

Intramuscular injection is given in the vastus lateralis thigh muscle. A one-time-only prophylactic dose of 0.5–1 mg IM is given in the birthing area or upon admission to the newborn nursery. A one-time dose of 2 mg is given if the route of administration is by mouth. If the mother received anticoagulants during pregnancy, an additional dose may be ordered by the physician and is given at 6–8 hours post first injection.

Neonatal Side Effects

Pain and edema may occur at injection site. Possible allergic reactions such as rash and urticaria.

Nursing Considerations

Observe for bleeding (usually occurs on second or third day). Bleeding may be seen as generalized ecchymoses or bleeding from umbilical cord, circumcision site, nose, or gastrointestinal tract. Results of serial PT and PTT should be assessed.

Observe for jaundice and kernicterus, especially in preterm infants.

Observe for signs of local inflammation.

Protect drug from light.

Give vitamin K_1 before circumcision procedure.

When the newborn's temperature is normal and vital signs are stable (about 2 to 4 hours after birth), the nurse may give the baby a sponge bath. However, this admission bath may be postponed for some hours if the newborn's condition dictates or the parents wish to give the first bath. A recent study provides some reassurances, in light of early discharge practices (12–48 hrs), that healthy term infants can safely be bathed immediately after the admission assessment is completed (Penny-MacGillivray 1996). The baby is bathed while still under the radiant warmer. This can be done in the parents' room. Bathing the newborn offers an excellent opportunity for teaching and welcoming parent involvement in the care of their baby.

The nurse rechecks the baby's temperature after the bath and, if it is stable, dresses, wraps, and places the newborn in an open crib at room temperature. If the baby's axillary temperature is below 36.4C (97.5F), the baby returns to the radiant warmer. The rewarming process should be gradual to prevent hyperthermia. Slow rewarming is accomplished by maintaining the ambient temperature 1.5C (3F) higher than the newborn's current skin temperature (Neonatal Thermoregulation 1990). When this new skin temperature is reached, the control point of the heater can be set another 1.5C higher until the desired skin temperature is reached. Once the newborn is rewarmed, the nurse implements measures to prevent further heat loss, such as keeping the newborn dry, double-wrapped with hat on, and away from cool surfaces or instruments. The nurse also protects the newborn from drafts, open windows or doors, and air conditioners and stores blankets and clothing in a warm place. See Temperature Regulation in Chapter 21 and Procedure 23–1: Thermoregulation of the Newborn on pp 575–576.

Prevention of Complications of Hemorrhagic Disease of Newborn

A prophylactic injection of vitamin K_1 (AquaMEPHYTON) is given to prevent hemorrhage, which can occur due to low prothrombin levels in the first few days of life (see the accompanying Drug Guide: Vitamin K_1 Phytonadione [AquaMEPHYTON]). The potential for hemorrhage is considered to result from the absence of gut bacterial flora, which influences the production of vitamin K_1 in the newborn (see Chapter 26 for further discussion). Controversy exists over whether the administration of vitamin K_1 may predispose the newborn to significant hyperbilirubinemia. However, Cunningham, MacDonald, and Grant (1997) indicate there is no evidence to support this concern as long as a standard dose of 1 mg is given. Some people have questioned whether research supports giving vitamin K_1 to newborns who have had a nontraumatic birth.

The vitamin K_1 injection is given intramuscularly in the middle one-third of the vastus lateralis muscle located in the lateral aspect of the thigh (Figure 23–2). Before injecting, the nurse cleans the area thoroughly with a small alcohol swab. The nurse uses a 25-gauge, ⅝-in needle for the injection. An alternate site is the rectus femoris muscle in the anterior aspect of the thigh. However, this site is near the sciatic nerve and femoral artery and should be used with caution (Figure 23–3). Remember that vitamin K_1 needs to be protected from the light.

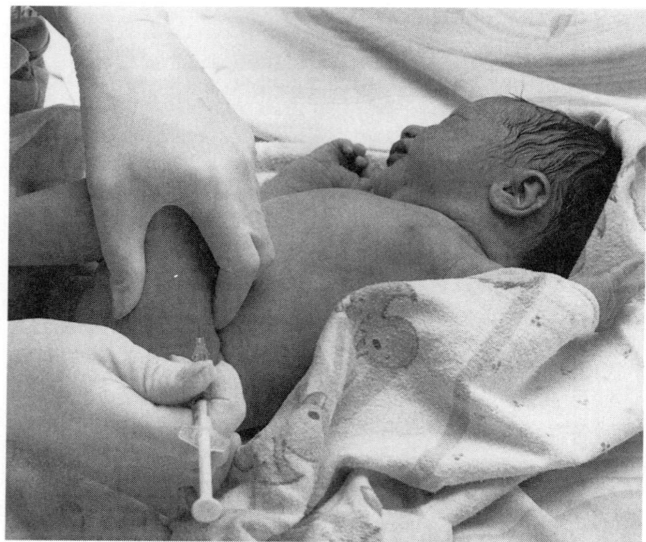

FIGURE 23–2 Procedure for vitamin K injection. Cleanse area thoroughly with alcohol swab and allow skin to dry. Bunch the tissue of the upper thigh (vastus lateralis muscle) and quickly insert a 25-gauge 5/8 inch needle at a 90-degree angle to the thigh. Aspirate, then slowly inject the solution to distribute the medication evenly and minimize the baby's discomfort. Remove the needle and massage the site with an alcohol swab.

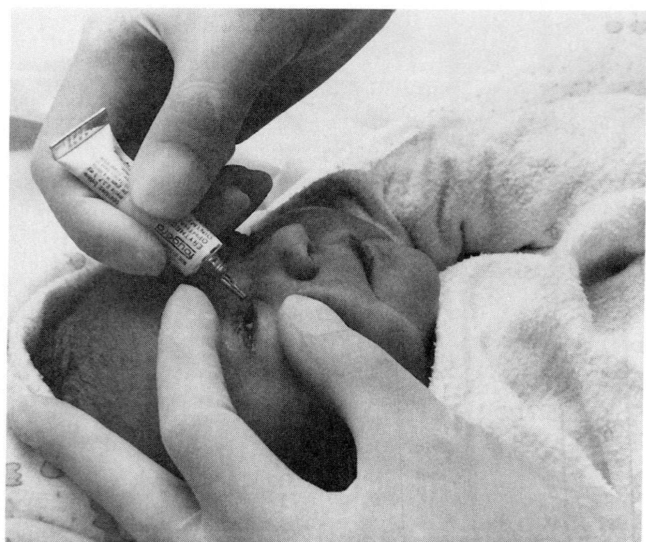

FIGURE 23–4 Ophthalmic ointment. Retract lower eyelid outward to instill 1/4 inch long strand of ointment from a single-dose ampule along the lower conjunctival surface.

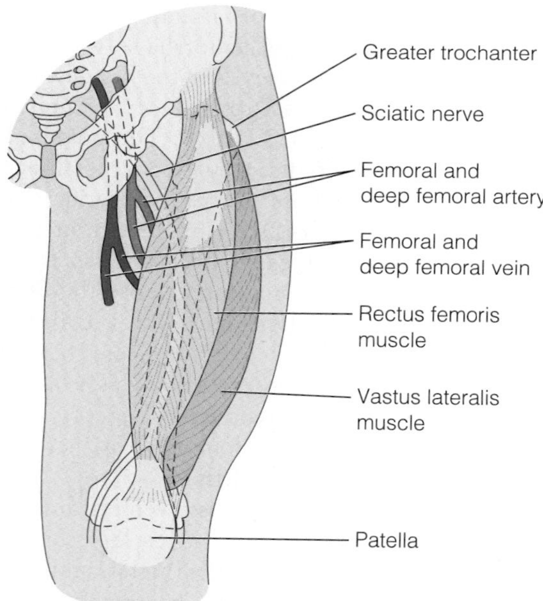

FIGURE 23–3 Injection sites: The middle third of the vastus lateralis muscle is the preferred site for intramuscular injection in the newborn. The middle third of the rectus femoris is an alternate site, but its proximity to major vessels and the sciatic nerve requires caution in using this site for injection.

Prevention of Eye Infection

The nurse is also responsible for giving the legally required prophylactic eye treatment for *Neisseria gonorrhoeae,* which may have infected the newborn of an infected mother during the birth process. In the past, the drug of choice was 1 percent silver nitrate solution. Other ophthalmic ointments used instead of silver nitrate are erythromycin (Ilotycin) (see the Drug Guide: Erythromycin, p 577), tetracycline, or penicillin; all are also effective against chlamydia, which has a higher incidence rate than gonorrhea. Zanoni and Isenberg (1992) showed that erythromycin and tetracycline weren't any more effective against *Chylamydia trachomatis* than silver nitrate.

The eyes should be treated within the first few hours after birth. Successful eye prophylaxis requires that the medication be instilled into the lower conjunctival sac (Figure 23–4). It may be delayed up to 1 hour after birth to allow eye contact during parent-newborn bonding (AAP 1992). (See Procedure 23–2 on p 576.)

Eye prophylaxis medications can cause chemical conjunctivitis, which gives the newborn some discomfort and may interfere with the ability to focus on the parents' faces. The resulting edema, inflammation, and discharge may cause concern if the parents have not been given information that the side effects will clear in 24–48 hours and that this prophylactic eye treatment is necessary for the newborn's well-being.

PROCEDURE 23–1 Thermoregulation of the Newborn

Nursing Action	Rationale
Objective: Prepare the warming equipment.	
• Prewarm the incubator or radiant warmer. Make sure warmed towels and/or lightweight blankets are available.	The change from a warm, moist intrauterine environment to a cool, dry, drafty environment stresses the newborn's immature thermoregulation mechanisms.
• Maintain the birthing room at 22C (71F), with a relative humidity of 60%–65%.	
Objective: Establish a stable temperature after birth.	
• Wipe the newborn free of blood and excessive vernix, especially from the head, with prewarmed towels.	This prevents loss of body heat from a large surface area through evaporation.
• Place the newborn under the radiant warmer.	The radiant warmer creates a heat-gaining environment.
• Wrap the newborn in a prewarmed blanket and transfer the newborn to the mother.	Use of the prewarmed blanket reduces convective heat loss and facilitates maternal-infant contact without compromising the newborn's thermo-regulation.
• Place the infant skin-to-skin with the mother under a warmed blanket.	Skin-to-skin contact with the mother or father helps maintain the newborn's temperature.
Objective: Maintain a stable infant temperature.	
• Diaper the newborn and place a stocking hat on its head. Place the newborn uncovered (except for diaper and hat) under the radiant warmer.	Radiant heat warms the outer surface skin, so the skin needs to be exposed.
• Tape a servocontrol probe on the newborn's anterior abdominal wall, with the metal side next to the skin, and cover the probe with an aluminum heat deflector patch.	The aluminum cover prevents heating of the probe directly and overheating the infant.
• Turn the heater to servocontrol mode so that the abdominal skin is maintained at 36.5–37C.	
• Monitor the newborn's axillary and skin probe temperature per institution's protocol.	The temperature indicator on the radiant warmer continually displays the newborn's probe temperature, so the axillary temperature is checked to ensure that the machine accurately reports the newborn's temperature.
• When the newborn's temperature reaches 37C (98.6F), remove the infant from the radiant warmer, and place a T-shirt, diaper and stocking hat on the newborn.	
• Double wrap (2 blankets) the newborn and place the newborn in an open crib.	
• Recheck the newborn's axillary temperature in 1 h.	It is important to monitor the infant's ability to maintain its own thermoregulation.
Objective: Rewarm the newborn gradually if temperature drops below 36.1C (97F).	
• Assess axillary temperature frequently, per agency routine; usually every 2–4 h.	Frequent assessment may detect hypothermia, which predisposes the newborn to cold stress.
• If the newborn needs rewarming, place the newborn (unclothed except for diaper) under the radiant warmer with a servocontrol probe on the abdomen.	
• Gradually rewarm back to normal temperature.	Rapid heating can lead to hyperthermia, which is associated with apnea, increased insensible water loss, and increased metabolic rate.

PROCEDURE 23–1 Thermoregulation of the Newborn continued

Nursing Action	Rationale
• Recheck the newborn's temperature in 30 min, then hourly. When the temperature reaches 37C (98.6F), remove the newborn from the radiant heater, dress the newborn, double wrap, and place in the open crib. Recheck the temperature in 1 h.	
Objective: Prevent drops in the newborn's temperature.	
The nurse carries out the following activities:	
• Keep the newborn's clothing and bedding dry.	
• Double wrap the newborn and put a stocking hat on.	
• Use the radiant warmer during procedures.	
• Reduce the newborn's exposure to drafts.	
• Warm objects that will come in contact with the newborn (eg, stethoscopes).	
• Encourage the mother to snuggle with the newborn under blankets or breastfeed the newborn with hat and light cover on.	

PROCEDURE 23–2 Instilling Ophthalmic Ilotycin Ointment

Nursing Action	Rationale
Objective: Provide newborn prophylactic eye care.	
• Wash your hands and put on gloves.	This prevents introduction of bacteria.
• Clean the infant's eyes to remove any drainage.	Removal of exudate will facilitate instillation and absorption of the ointment.
• Retract the lower eyelid outward with your forefinger.	
• Instill 1/4-inch strand of ointment along the lower conjunctival surface, beginning at the inner canthus.	This maximizes the absorption.
• Repeat the above process on the other eye. Instill only a single dose per eye.	Prophylaxis requires only a single dose.
• Wipe excess ointment away after 1 min (American Academy of Pediatrics 1992). Do not irrigate eyes.	Irrigation will remove the ointment.
• Assess for any sensitivity reaction such as edema, inflammation, or drainage.	Sensitivity reactions may interfere with the infant's ability to focus and with the bonding process.
Objective: Explain the procedure to the parents.	
• Explain the rationale for eye prophylaxis and that it may interfere with the newborn's ability to focus on the parents' faces and that there may be temporary side effects that usually disappear in 24–48 h.	The parents should understand that the instillation of ointment is required by law and is preventive treatment of gonorrhea and chlamydia infection, both of which can cause blindness.
Objective: Record the completion of the procedure on the newborn's chart.	This provides a permanent record to meet the legal requirements.

DRUG GUIDE | Erythromycin Ophthalmic Ointment (Ilotycin Ophthalmic)

Overview of Neonatal Action
Erythromycin (Ilotycin Ophthalmic) is used as prophylactic treatment of ophthalmia neonatorum, which is caused by the bacteria *Neisseria gonorrhoeae.* Preventive treatment of gonorrhea in the newborn is required by law. Erythromycin is also effective against ophthalmic chlamydial infections. It is either bacteriostatic or bactericidal, depending on the organisms involved and the concentration of drug.

Route, Dosage, Frequency
Ophthalmic ointment (0.5%) is instilled as a narrow ribbon or strand, 1/4 inch long, along the lower conjunctival surface of each eye, starting at the inner canthus. It is instilled only once in each eye. Administration may be done in the birthing area or later in the nursery so that eye contact is facilitated and the bonding process immediately after birth is not interrupted. After administration gently close eye and manipulate to ensure spread of ointment.

Neonatal Side Effects
Sensitivity reaction; may interfere with ability to focus and may cause edema and inflammation. Side effects usually disappear in 24–48 hours.

Nursing Considerations
Wash hands immediately prior to instillation to prevent introduction of bacteria.

Do not irrigate the eyes after instillation. Use new tube or single-use container for ophthalmic ointment administration shortly after birth. May wipe away excess after 1 minute.

Observe for hypersensitivity.

Teach parents about need for eye prophylaxis. Educate them regarding side effects and signs that need to be reported to the health care provider.

Early Assessment of Neonatal Distress

During the first 24 hours of life, the nurse is constantly alert for signs of distress. If the newborn is with his or her parents during this period, the nurse must take extra care to teach them how to maintain their newborn's temperature, recognize the hallmarks of newborn distress, and respond immediately to signs of respiratory problems. The parents should learn to observe the newborn for changes in color or activity, rapid breathing with chest retractions, or facial grimacing. Their interventions should include nasal and oral suctioning with bulb syringe, positioning, and vigorous fingertip stroking of the newborn's spine to stimulate respiratory activity if necessary. The nurse also must be available immediately should the newborn develop distress. (See Key Facts to Remember: Signs of Newborn Distress.)

Initiation of First Feeding

The timing of the first feeding varies depending on whether the newborn is to be breastfed or bottle-fed and whether there were any complications during pregnancy or birth (IDM, IUGR, and so forth). Mothers who choose to breastfeed their newborns may seek to put their baby to the breast while in the birthing area. This practice should be encouraged, since successful, long-term breastfeeding during infancy appears to be related to beginning breastfeedings in the first few hours of life. Bottle-fed newborns usually begin the first feedings by 5 hours of age, during the second period of reactivity when they awaken and appear hungry. Signs indicating newborn readiness for the first feeding are active bowel sounds, absence of abdominal distention, and a lusty cry that quiets with rooting and sucking behaviors when a stimulus is placed near the lips.

Facilitation of Parent-Newborn Attachment

Eye-to-eye contact between the parents and their newborn is extremely important during the early hours after

KEY FACTS TO REMEMBER

Signs of Newborn Distress

Increased rate (more than 60/minute) or difficult respirations
Sternal retractions
Nasal flaring
Grunting
Excessive mucus
Facial grimacing
Cyanosis (central: skin, lips, tongue)
Abdominal distention or mass
Vomiting of bile-stained material
Absence of meconium elimination within 24 hours of birth
Absence of urine elimination within 24 hours of birth
Jaundice of the skin within 24 hours of birth or due to hemolytic process
Temperature instability (hypothermia or hyperthermia)
Jitteriness or glucose less than 40 mg%

Source: Adapted from Tappero EP, Honeyfield ME: *Physical Assessment of the Newborn.* 2nd ed. Petaluma, CA: NICU Ink, 1996.

birth, when the newborn is in the first period of reactivity. The newborn is alert during this time, the eyes are wide open, and the baby often makes direct eye contact with human faces within optimal range for visual acuity (7 to 8 inches). It is theorized that this eye contact is an important foundation in establishing attachment in human relationships (Klaus and Klaus 1985). Consequently, the prophylactic eye medication is often delayed (but no more than 1 hour) to provide an opportunity for this period of eye contact between parents and their newborn, thus facilitating the attachment process (AAP 1992).

Nursing Diagnosis for Newborn Care During Stay in Birthing Unit

Possible nursing diagnoses for care of newborns during their stay in the birthing unit include

- Altered peripheral tissue perfusion related to transition to extrauterine environment
- Risk for ineffective breathing pattern related to periodic breathing
- Alteration in nutrition: less than body requirements related to limited nutritional/fluid intake and increased caloric expenditure
- Altered urinary elimination patterns related to meatal edema secondary to circumcision
- Altered bowel elimination related to immature gastrointestinal system or delayed passage of meconium
- Risk for infection related to umbilical cord healing, circumcision site, or immature immune system
- Knowledge deficit related lack of information about male circumcision or pros and cons of breastfeeding and bottle-feeding
- Risk for altered parenting related to lack of experience with infant care or transition to parental role
- Altered family processes related to integration of newborn into family unit or demands of newborn feeding schedule

Nursing Plan and Implementation of Newborn Care During Stay in Birthing Unit

Maintenance of Cardiopulmonary Function

The nurse takes *vital signs* every 6–8 hours or more, depending on the newborn's status.

The newborn should always be in a propped, side-lying position when left unattended to prevent aspiration and facilitate drainage of mucus (Infant Sleep Positioning and SIDS Position Statement 1992). A bulb syringe is within easy reach should the baby need oral-nasal suctioning. If the newborn has respiratory difficulty, clear the airway. Vigorous fingertip stroking of the baby's spine will frequently stimulate respiratory activity. A cardiorespiratory monitor can be used on newborns who are not being observed at all times and are at risk for decreased respiratory or cardiac function. Indicators of risk are pallor, cyanosis, ruddy color, apnea, or other signs of instability. Changes in skin color may indicate the need for closer assessment of temperature, cardiopulmonary status, hematocrit, and bilirubin levels.

Maintenance of Neutral Thermal Environment

The nurse makes every effort to maintain the newborn's temperature within the normal range. The nurse must make certain the newborn is undressed and exposed to the air as little as possible. A stockinette or knit head covering should be used for the small newborn who has less subcutaneous fat to act as insulation in maintaining body heat. The ambient temperature of the room where the newborn is kept should be monitored routinely and kept at approximately 32.5–33.9C (90.5–93.1F) for large babies and 35.4±0.5C for smaller babies (Merestein and Gardner 1992). Parents may be advised to dress the newborn in one more layer of clothing than is necessary for an adult to maintain thermal comfort. A newborn whose temperature falls below optimal levels will use calories to maintain body heat rather than for growth. Chilling also decreases the affinity of serum albumin for bilirubin, thereby increasing the likelihood of newborn jaundice. It also increases oxygen use and may cause respiratory distress.

An overheated newborn will increase activity and respiratory rate in an attempt to cool the body. Both measures deplete caloric reserves. In addition, the increased respiratory rate leads to increased insensible fluid loss.

Promotion of Adequate Hydration and Nutrition

Newborn nutrition is addressed in depth in Chapter 24. The nurse records caloric and fluid intake and enhances adequate hydration by maintaining a neutral thermal environment and offering early and frequent feedings. Early feedings promote gastric emptying and increase peristalsis, thereby decreasing the potential for hyperbilirubinemia by decreasing the amount of time fecal material is in contact with beta glucuronidase in the small intestine. This enzyme frees the bilirubin from the feces, allowing it to be reabsorbed into the vascular system. Voiding and stooling patterns are recorded. If 24 hours have passed and the first voiding and passage of stool has not occurred, the nurse continues the normal observation routine while also assessing for abdominal distention, status of bowel sounds, hydration, fluid intake, and temperature stability.

The nurse should weigh the newborn at the same time each day for accurate comparisons. A weight loss of up to 10 percent for term newborns is considered within normal limits during the first week of life. This is the result of limited intake, loss of excess extracellular fluid, and passage of meconium. Parents should be told about the expected weight loss, the reason for it, and the expectations for regaining the birth weight. Birth weight should be regained by 2 weeks if feedings are adequate.

Excessive handling can cause an increase in the newborn's metabolic rate and caloric use. The nurse should be alert to the newborn's subtle cues of fatigue. These include turning the head away from eye contact, decrease in muscle tension and activity in the extremities and neck, and loss of eye contact, which may be manifested by fluttering or closure of the eyelids. The nurse quickly ceases stimulation when signs of fatigue emerge. The nurse's care should demonstrate to the parents the need for awareness of newborn cues and the use of periods of alertness for contact and stimulation. The nurse is also responsible for assessing the woman's comfort and latching-on techniques if breastfeeding or bottle-feeding.

Prevention of Complications and Promotion of Safety

Newborns are at continued risk for the complications of hemorrhage, late-onset cardiac symptoms, and infection. Pallor may be an early sign of hemorrhage and must be reported to the physician. The newborn is placed on a cardiorespiratory monitor to permit continuous assessment. Several newborn conditions put newborns at risk for hemorrhage, but this is especially true following a circumcision procedure (see p 587). The circumcision is assessed for signs of hemorrhage and infection. The first voiding after a circumcision is also a significant assessment in evaluating for possible urinary obstruction due to trauma and edema. Vaseline gauze is applied to the circumcision site to prevent bleeding and allow the gauze to be removed and replaced if it gets soiled.

The nurse assesses the umbilical cord for signs of bleeding or infection, such as oozing and foul smell. Triple dye is usually applied to the newborn's cord. Then the nurse is responsible for giving cord care with alcohol each time the diaper is changed.

Cyanosis that is not relieved by oxygen administration requires emergency intervention, may indicate a congenital cardiac condition or shock, and requires ongoing assessment.

Infection in the nursery is best prevented by requiring that all personnel having direct contact with newborns scrub for 2–3 minutes from fingertips to and including elbows at the beginning of each shift. The hands must also be washed with soap and rubbed vigorously for 15 seconds (Neonatal Skin Care 1992) before and after contact with every newborn or after touching any soiled surface such as the floor or one's hair or face. Parents are often instructed to use an antiseptic hand cleaner before touching the baby. Anyone with an infection should refrain from working with newborns until the infection has cleared. Some agencies ask family members to wear gowns (preferably disposable) over their street clothes. Parents need to be taught that everyone handling the baby should *always* wash their hands before doing so, even after the baby is home.

Safety of the newborn is provided through a variety of nursing interventions and institutional security measures. It is essential to verify the identity of the newborn by comparing the numbers and names on the identification bracelets of mother and newborn before giving a baby to a parent and to follow institutional policies for identification of all nursery personnel.

Enhancement of Parent-Infant Attachment and Parental Knowledge of Newborn Care

Parent-infant attachment is promoted by encouraging all family members to be involved with the new member of the family. For specific interventions see Chapters 17 and 28, and the Teaching Guide: Enhancing Attachment.

To meet parent needs for information, the nurse who is responsible for the care of the mother and newborn should assume the primary responsibility for education. Nearly every contact with the parents presents an opportunity for sharing information that can facilitate their sense of competence in newborn care. The nurse also needs to recognize and respect the fact that there are many good ways to provide safe care. Unless their care methods are harmful to the newborn, the parents' methods of giving care should be reinforced rather than contradicted. The nurse also needs to be sensitive to the cultural beliefs and values of the family (Table 23–1). The information that follows is provided to increase the nurse's knowledge of newborn care and can also be used to meet parents' needs for information.

Parents may be familiar with handling and caring for newborns, or this may be their first time to interact with a newborn. If the couple are new parents, the sensitive

TEACHING GUIDE Enhancing Attachment

Assessment

The nurse provides maximum opportunity for parents to interact with their infant immediately after birth and while in the birthing unit. Observation and documentation of these interactions will assist the nurse in determining family's needs for teaching, support, or interventions.

Nursing Diagnosis

The nursing diagnoses will probably be: Altered family processes related to addition of a new baby to the family or Knowledge deficit related to lack of information about emotional needs of newborn.

Nursing Plan and Implementation

The teaching plan includes information about the infant's physical status and normal characteristics, comforting techniques, and the baby's emotional needs immediately after birth and during the newborn period. Parents are encouraged to maintain continuous contact through rooming-in.

Parent Goals

At the completion of the teaching the parents will be able to

1. Demonstrate appropriate nurturing behaviors such as touching, bonding, talking to, kissing, and holding their baby
2. Discuss normal characteristics and emotional needs of the newborn
3. List at least three comforting techniques

Teaching Plan

Content	Teaching Method
Present information on periods of reactivity and expected newborn responses.	Discussion
Describe normal physical characteristics of newborn.	Discussion and presentation of slides showing newborn characteristics
Explain the bonding process, its gradual development, and the reciprocal interactive nature of the process.	
Discuss infant's capabilities for interaction, such as nonverbal communication abilities. The nonverbal communications include movement, gaze, touch, facial expressions, and vocalizations—including crying. Emphasize that eye contact is considered one of the cardinal factors in developing infant-parent attachment and will be integrated with touching and vocal behaviors.	Show video on interactive capabilities of newborns
Discuss that touching, including stroking, patting, massaging, and kissing, will progress to interactive touch between parent and infant; discuss need to assimilate these behaviors into daily routine with baby.	Discussion, demonstration, and handouts
Describe and demonstrate comforting techniques, including use of sound, swaddling, rocking, and stroking.	Demonstration and return demonstration
Discuss progression of the infant's behaviors as infant matures and importance of parents' consistent response to infant's cues and needs.	Discussion, time for questions
Provide information about available pamphlets, videos, and support groups in the community.	

Evaluation

The nurse may evaluate the learning by providing time for discussion, questions, and return demonstrations in the birthing unit, during postpartal return visit or home visit. Continued observation of parents' positive interaction with their baby during remainder of stay in birthing unit provides a beginning means of evaluating learning.

TABLE 23–1 Examples of Some Cultural Beliefs and Practices Regarding Baby Care

Umbilical Cord

People of Hispanic or Filipino cultural background may use an abdominal binder or bellyband to protect against dirt, injury, and umbilical hernia. They may also apply oils to the stump of the cord or tape metal to the umbilicus to ward off evil spirits.

People of northern European ancestry may expect a sterile cutting of the cord at birth. They may allow the stump to air dry and discard the cord once it falls off.

Mother-Infant Contact

People of Asian ancestry may pick up the baby as soon as it cries, or they may carry the baby at all times.

Some Native Americans, notably the Navajos, may use cradle boards.

Korean mothers may be slow to pick up, touch, or respond to their baby's cues because of focus on care of mother (Schneiderman 1996).

Feeding

Some people of Asian heritage may breastfeed their babies for the first 1 to 2 years of life.

Many Cambodian refugees practice breastfeeding on demand without restriction, or if bottle-feeding provide a "comfort bottle" in between feedings (Rasbridge and Kulig 1995).

People of Iranian heritage may breastfeed female babies longer than males.

Some people of African ancestry may wean their babies after they begin to walk.

Circumcision

People of Muslim and Jewish ancestry practice circumcision as a religious ritual (Hutchinson & Baqi-Aziz 1994).

Many natives of Africa and Australia practice circumcision as a puberty rite.

Most Native Americans and people of Asian and Hispanic cultures rarely perform circumcision.

Only 15% of the world's male population is circumcised.

Health/Illness

Some people from Hispanic cultural backgrounds may believe that touching the face or head of an infant when admiring it will ward off the "evil eye." They may also neglect to cut the baby's nails to avoid nearsightedness and instead put mittens on the baby's hands to prevent scratching. They also may believe that fat babies are healthy.

Some people of Asian heritage may not allow anyone to touch the baby's head without asking permission.

Some Orthodox Jews believe that saying the baby's name before the formal naming ceremony will harm the baby.

Some people of Vietnamese ancestry believe that cutting a baby's hair or nails will cause illness.

Note: The above are meant only as examples of some of the behaviors that may be found within certain cultures. Not all members of a culture will practice the behaviors described.

Source: Adapted from Andrews MM: Transcultural perspectives in the nursing care of children and adolescents. In: *Transcultural Concepts in Nursing Care,* 2nd ed, Andrews MM, Boyle JS (editors). Philadelphia: Lippincott, 1995; Riordan J, Auerbach KG: *Breastfeeding and Human Lactation.* Boston: Jones & Bartlett, 1993.

nurse gently teaches them by example and instructions geared to their needs and previous knowledge about the various aspects of newborn care.

The length of stay in the birthing unit for mother and baby after birth is often 48 hours or less. One proposal to deal with early discharge is for the labor and birthing nurse to start the newborn care by assessing vital signs and administering vitamin K and eye prophylaxis. Then admission nursery care is viewed as a continuation of newborn care and the time during this period is cut in half. This approach to newborn care also provides for earlier identification of those newborns in need of more aggressive intervention (McGregor 1994). The challenge for the nurse is to use every opportunity to teach, guide, and support individual parents, fostering their own capabilities and confidence in caring for their newborn. Including mother-baby care and home care instruction on the night shift assists with education needs for early discharge parents.

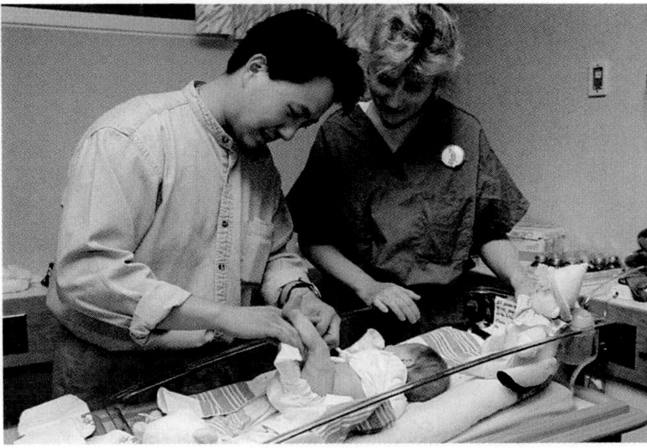

FIGURE 23–5 Individualizing family education. Father returns demonstration of diapering his son.

The nurse observes how parents interact with their newborn during feeding and caregiving activities. Even in a short time, there will be opportunities for the nurse to provide information and evaluate whether the parents are comfortable with changing diapers, wrapping, handling, and feeding their newborn. Do both parents get involved in the newborn's care? Is the mother depending on someone else to help her at home? Does she give excuses for not wanting to be involved in her newborn's care? ("I'm too tired," "My stitches hurt," or "I'll learn later.") All these considerations need to be taken into account when evaluating the educational needs of the parents.

Several methods may be used to teach families about newborn care. Group newborn care classes are a nonthreatening way to convey general information. Individual instruction is helpful to answer specific questions or to clarify something that may have been confusing in class (Figure 23–5). See Teaching Guide: What to Tell Parents About Infant Care. Bordman and Holzman (1996) found that many women pose questions about their baby's care to confirm that they are doing the right

TEACHING GUIDE What to Tell Parents About Infant Care

Assessment

The nurse determines parents' prior knowledge and experience with newborns and any concerns they may have about caring for their baby.

Nursing Diagnosis

The key nursing diagnoses would be: Knowledge deficit related to lack of information about ongoing newborn daily care needs and Altered parenting related to integration of new family member.

Nursing Plan and Implementation

The teaching plan will include information about sponge and tub baths, umbilical cord care, care of circumcised and uncircumcised infant, feeding techniques, positioning, elimination patterns, use of bulb syringe, signs and symptoms of illness, expected sleep patterns, comfort measures, and attachment behaviors.

Demonstration of bath, cord care, use of bulb syringe, thermometer, and comfort measures.

Parent Goals

At the completion of the class the parents will be able to

1. Demonstrate safe techniques of caring for their newborn, especially in use of bulb syringe, thermometer, cord cleaning, and comforting measures
2. List signs and symptoms of illness
3. Describe infant's sleep patterns and attachment behaviors
4. Demonstrate an emerging comfort level and confidence in their ability to care for their infant

Teaching Plan

Content	Teaching Method
Demonstrate sponge and tub bathing techniques, emphasizing safety and timing of cord separation. Demonstrate cord care to be carried out at home—see Teaching Guide: What to Tell Families About Home Cord Care on p 585 for specific techniques.	Discussion and demonstration. Stress basic useful information that new parents need. Avoid patronizing tone. Provide opportunities for parents to practice.
Discuss care required for circumcised and uncircumcised infants.	Demonstration, discussion.
Discuss the signs of illness (see Key Facts to Remember: Signs of Newborn Distress on p 577) and demonstrate use of thermometer and bulb syringe.	Discussion, handouts, pamphlets, and posters are helpful, as are videos.
Discuss normal newborn eating, sleep, and elimination patterns and behavioral characteristics.	
Demonstrate comfort measures for newborns.	Discussion, demonstration, and return demonstration.

Evaluation

Parents are able to describe general newborn care. Parents demonstrate use of bulb syringe, taking temperature, umbilical cord care, and care of circumcision (if appropriate) to primary nurse prior to discharge from birthing center.

Provide positive feedback to build confidence.

thing, not to receive absolute answers. With shorter stays most teaching unfortunately tends to focus on infant feeding and immediate physical care needs of the mothers, with limited anticipatory guidance provided in other areas (Brown et al 1996).

Discharge planning is essential to verify the family's knowledge when leaving the birthing unit. Follow-up calls and home visits after discharge lend added support by providing another opportunity for questions to be answered. Several programs link the birthing center and community-based nursing care to better meet the new family's educational and support needs. The Art Future Image (AFI) project assists teenage mothers to visualize incorporating their new parent roles and future goals (Walsh and Corbett 1995). Programs such as Birth Care Home Advantage provide a model where experienced birthing/mother-baby nurses are able to meet the family's ongoing education and support needs in the home setting (Mendler et al 1996). Methods of positioning, handling, nasal and oral suctioning, and wrapping the newborn are demonstrated as needed. As the family provides care, the nurse can instill confidence by giving them positive feedback. If the family encounters problems, the nurse can suggest alternatives and serve as a role model.

How to pick up a newborn is one of the first concerns of nurses as well as parents who have not had the

COMMUNITY IN FOCUS Center on Fathering

Fathers are often overlooked when resources and programs are designed for childbearing families, and only a few comprehensive programs designed for fathers are available nationwide. However, fathers play a vital role in the family as partner and parent, and research indicates that children with two involved, loving parents generally fare better throughout life. To address this need, Colorado Springs, Colorado, has established the Center on Fathering. This innovative organization, funded primarily by El Paso County Human Services, grants, and donations, is housed in a restored victorian home that provides an accessible, inviting location for fathers seeking information or support.

The mission of the Center is to provide programs and services to help fathers be actively and positively involved in the care and parenting of their children. The Center is open weekdays from 8–5 for drop-ins or appointments. Most classes and groups are held in the evening, however, to better accommodate the needs of working parents. The Center achieves its mission in a variety of ways, including the following:

- *A 12-week course on Fathering.* This course is designed to help fathers deal with parenting issues, child development, reading children's cues, discipline, and so forth.
- *A 2-hour class, "Now You're a Father."* Offered in cooperation with Bright Beginnings, this class is geared to expectant fathers and new fathers. It addresses issues such as what to expect of a newborn, how to maximize involvement with the infant in the early months, and available community resources.
- *A 4-week course on conflict resolution.* This course, part of a newly funded pilot program, is designed to help reduce youth violence by teaching conflict resolution skills to fathers, so they can, in turn, teach these approaches to their children.
- *Fathers' Support Group.* This group meets weekly to help dads who have issues related to any aspect of fathering from concerns about a child's behavior to disagreements with the partner about child discipline, to general family conflicts, to concerns of noncustodial fathers about relating to their children. The group is action oriented with specific topics of discussion, occasional guest speakers, and periodic group needs assessments. Typically 8–10 fathers participate at a given time; most fathers stay involved with the group for 6–10 months.
- *Resources library.* The Center on Fathering has a resource library of over 300 books available for check-out on a variety of topics ranging from the needs of new fathers to helping children cope with divorce.
- *Computer database.* The Center has an excellent database with articles on a wide range of topics. Interested individuals can stop by for information, copies of articles and handouts, and referral to other agencies as needed.
- *Mentoring program.* This program uses community volunteers to help other men improve their fathering skills through one-on-one interaction.

All too often, society devalues the importance of the father's role in child rearing and provides little support for fathers. The Colorado Springs community has acted to address this issue. The Center on Fathering is a creative, exciting model that communities everywhere would do well to emulate.

Source: Personal communication with Ken Sanders, Coordinator, Center on Fathering, Colorado Springs, Colorado.

experience. The newborn is easily picked up by sliding one hand under the neck and shoulders and the other hand under the buttocks or between the legs and then gently lifting the newborn. This technique provides security and support for the head (which the newborn is unable to support until 3 or 4 months of age). Remember that left-handed people tend to hold the baby over their right shoulder, and right-handed people do the opposite. This keeps the dominant hand free. However, most health personnel wear their name tags on the left side. To avoid scratching the baby's face, wear your name tag on the same side as your dominant hand.

CRITICAL THINKING IN ACTION

You are caring for a new mother who had her first child, a daughter, about 4 hours ago. She appears visibly upset when changing her infant's diaper and says she thinks something is wrong because her daughter has tissue protruding from her vagina and some blood in her diaper. What would you do?

Answers can be found in Appendix H.

Nasal and Oral Suctioning

Most newborns are obligatory nose breathers for the first months of life. They generally maintain air passage patency by coughing or sneezing. During the first few days of life, however, the newborn has increased mucus, and gentle suctioning with a bulb syringe may be indicated. The nurse can demonstrate the use of the bulb syringe in the mouth and nose and have the parents do a return demonstration. The parents should repeat this demonstration before discharge so they feel more confident about the procedure. Care should be taken to apply only gentle suction to avoid causing nasal bleeding.

To suction the newborn, compress the bulb syringe; place the tip in the nostril, taking care not to occlude the passageway; and permit the bulb to reexpand slowly by releasing the compression on the bulb (Figure 23–6). Remove the bulb syringe from the nostril and compress

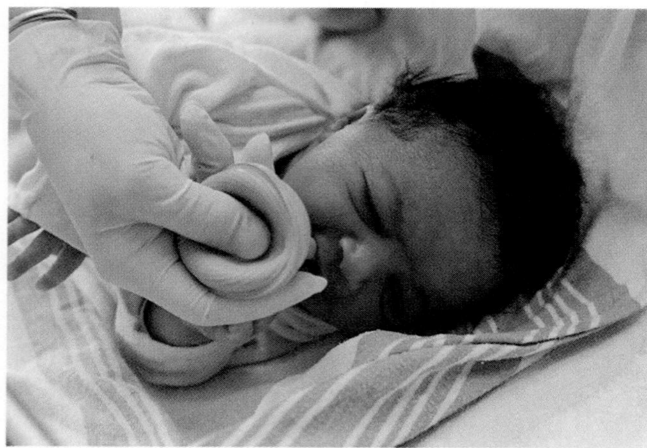

FIGURE 23–6 Nasal and oral suctioning. The bulb is compressed, the tip is placed in either the mouth or the nose, and the bulb is released.

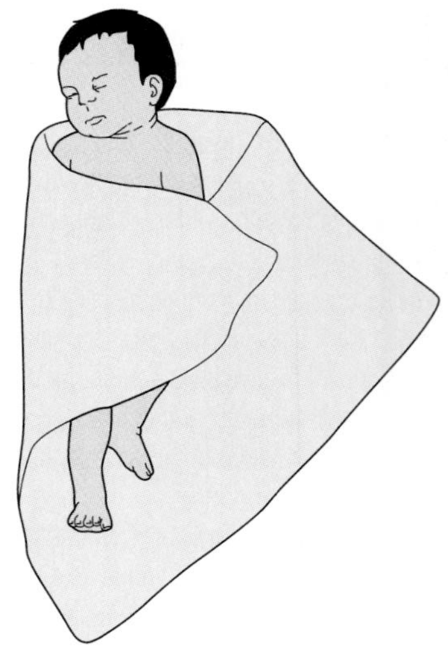

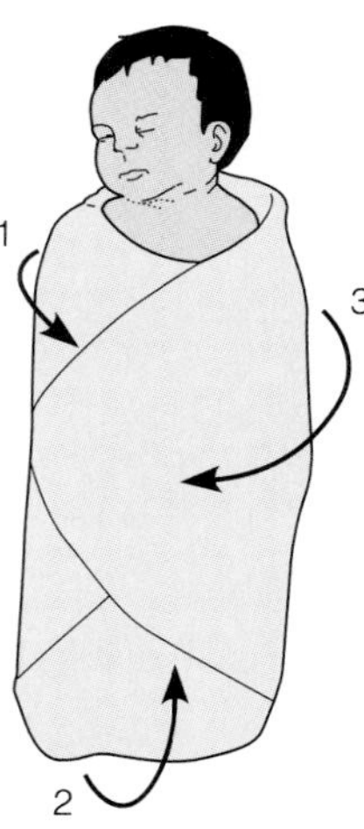

FIGURE 23–7 Steps used for wrapping a baby.

drainage out of the bulb onto a tissue. The bulb syringe may also be used in the mouth if the newborn is spitting up and unable to handle the excess secretions. The caregiver compresses the bulb, inserts the tip about 1 inch into one side of the newborn's mouth, and releases compression. This draws up the excess secretions. The procedure is repeated on the other side of the mouth. Avoid the roof of the mouth and back of the throat because suction in these areas might stimulate the gag reflex. The bulb syringe should be washed in warm, soapy water and rinsed in warm water daily. A bulb syringe should always be kept near the newborn. New parents and nurses who are inexperienced with newborns may fear that the baby will choke and will be relieved if they know what to do in such an event. They should be advised to turn the newborn's head to the side or down as soon as there is any indication of gagging or vomiting and to use the bulb syringe as needed.

Wrapping the Newborn

Wrapping (swaddling) helps the newborn maintain body temperature, provides a feeling of closeness and security, and may be effective in quieting a crying baby. When wrapping, a blanket is placed on the crib (or secure surface) in the shape of a diamond. The top corner of the blanket is folded down slightly, and the newborn's body is placed with the head at the upper edge of the blanket. The right corner of the blanket is wrapped around the newborn and tucked under the left side (not too tightly—allow a little room to move). The bottom corner is then pulled up to the chest, and the left corner wrapped around the newborn's right side (Figure 23–7). The nurse can show this wrapping technique to a new mother so she will feel more skilled in handling her baby.

An actual bath, cord care, and temperature assessment demonstration is the best way for the nurse to provide information on these topics to parents. Parents should be told to call their health care provider if bright red bleeding or puslike drainage occurs or if the area remains unhealed 2 to 3 days after the cord stump has sloughed off. See Teaching Guide: What to Tell Families About Cord Care.

The nurse demonstrates for the family how to take axillary and rectal temperatures and discusses the differ-

CRITICAL THINKING IN ACTION

A mother calls you to her room. She sounds frightened and says her baby can't breathe. You find the mother cradling her infant in her arms. The infant is mildly cyanotic, waving her arms, and has mucus coming from her nose and mouth. What would you do?

Answers can be found in Appendix H.

TEACHING GUIDE What to Tell Parents About Cord Care

Assessment

The nurse focuses on the family's previous experience with newborns and their understanding of what the umbilical cord is and what naturally happens during the first few weeks after birth.

Nursing Diagnosis

The essential nursing diagnoses would probably be: Knowledge deficit related to lack of information about home care of the umbilical cord and Risk for infection related to contamination of umbilical cord.

Nursing Plan and Implementation

The teaching plan will include information about the need for daily cleansing, expected changes in the umbilical cord, and demonstration of actual procedure for care of the umbilical cord.

Parent Goals

At the completion of the teaching session the parents will be able to

1. State the normal changes in the umbilical cord
2. List the signs of infection of the cord
3. Demonstrate proper cord care

Teaching Plan

Content

Clean the cord and skin around base of cord with a cotton ball or cotton-tipped swab using a cotton ball wet with 70% isopropyl alcohol. Lift the cord stump and wipe around the cord. Start at the top and wipe around halfway; then rotate cotton ball and start at the top again and wipe around the other half of the cord. Swabbing around the base of the cord cleans away drainage, and bacteria grows on dried drainage. Cord care should be done at least two to three times a day, or it could be done with each diaper change. The newborn may cry when the cold alcohol touches the abdomen; however, cord care is not painful because there are no nerve ends in the cord. No tub baths are given until the cord falls off in 7–14 days.

Fold diapers below umbilical cord to air-dry the cord. Contact with wet or soiled diapers slows the drying process and increases the possibility of infection.

Check cord each day for any odor, oozing of yellow puslike material, or reddened areas around the cord. Area around cord may also be tender. Report to health care provider any signs of infection.

Normal changes in cord: Cord should look dark and dry up before falling off. A little drop of blood may appear on the diaper as the cord is about to fall off. Never pull the cord or attempt to loosen it.

Teaching Method

Discussion: Use of poster showing cleaning techniques, position of diapers, and colored pictures of signs of infection. Demonstration of cord cleaning.

Evaluation

The nurse presented the information and demonstrated the proper procedure for cord care. Parents were able to identify the signs of infection and normal changes seen in the cord prior to its falling off and carried out proper cord care procedure before their newborn's discharge.

ent types of thermometers. It is important that families understand the differences and know how to select the appropriate one. The newborn's temperature needs to be taken only when signs of illness are present. Parents are advised to call their physician or pediatric nurse practitioner immediately if any signs of illness become apparent.

Sleep and Activity

Perhaps nothing is more individual to each newborn than the sleep-activity cycle. It is important for the nurse to recognize the individual variations of each newborn and to assist parents as they develop sensitivity to their newborn's communication signals and rhythms of activity and sleep.

Circumcision

Circumcision is a surgical procedure in which the prepuce, an epithelial layer covering the penis, is separated from the glans penis and excised. This permits exposure of the glans for easier cleaning.

The family makes the decision about circumcision for their newborn male child. In most cases the choice is based on cultural, social, and family tradition. To ensure informed consent, parents should be informed about possible long-term medical effects of circumcision and noncircumcision during the prenatal period.

Current Recommendations Recommendations about circumcision have varied in the past. Before about 1980, circumcision was recommended by the American Academy of Pediatrics; then, from 1980 to 1988, it was no longer recommended. However, cultural practices, social customs, parental wishes, and (sometimes) lack of knowledge about the procedure led many families to choose to have the male newborn circumcised. In 1989 the American Academy of Pediatrics wrote a position paper again recommending circumcision and citing the following medical reasons:

- It helps prevent phimosis (stenosis of the preputial space) and inflammation of the glans penis and foreskin.
- The incidence of penile cancer is lower in circumcised men in the United States.
- There is a decreased incidence of urinary tract infection in children under 1 year of age.

Circumcision should still be considered an elective procedure, but the procedure should not be performed if the newborn is premature or compromised, has a known bleeding problem, or is born with a genitourinary defect such as hypospadias or epispadias, which may necessitate the use of the foreskin in future surgical repairs (Reynolds 1996).

Circumcision was originally a religious rite practiced by Jews and Moslems. The practice gained widespread cultural acceptance in the United States but is done infrequently in many European countries. Many parents choose circumcision because they want the male child to have a similar physical appearance to the father or the majority of other children or because they feel that it is expected by society (O'Grady 1996). Another frequently cited reason for circumcising newborn males is to prevent the need for anesthesia, hospitalization, pain, and trauma should the procedure be needed later in life. O'Grady (1996) noted that only 2 to 10 percent of males are estimated to be in this category.

Nurse's Role The nurse plays an essential role in providing families with current information about circumcision. Nurses can facilitate parental informed consent because of their knowledge of the medical, social, and psychologic aspects of newborn circumcision (L'Archevesque and Goldstein-Lohman 1996). A well-informed nurse can allay parents' anxiety by sharing information and allowing them to express their concerns. Parents must be informed about potential risks and outcomes of circumcision. Hemorrhage, infection, difficulty in voiding, separation of the edges of the circumcision, discomfort, and restlessness are early potential problems. Later there is a risk that the glans and urethral meatus may become irritated and inflamed from contact with the ammonia in urine. Ulcerations and progressive stenosis may develop. Adhesions, entrapment of the penis, and damage to the urethra are all potential complications that could require surgical correction (O'Grady 1996).

Parents who are doubtful about their ability to use good hygienic practices in caring for their uncircumcised male child require information from the nurse. They should be told that the foreskin and glans are two similar layers of cells that separate from each other. The separation process begins prenatally and is normally completed between 3 and 5 years of age. In the process of separation, sterile sloughed cells build up between the layers. This buildup looks similar to the smegma secreted after puberty, and it is harmless. Occasionally during the daily bath, the parent can gently test for retraction. If retraction has occurred, daily gentle washing of the glans with soap and water is sufficient to maintain adequate cleanliness. The parents should teach the child to incorporate this practice into his daily self-care activities.

If circumcision is to be done, the procedure should be performed after the newborn is well established and has received his initial physical examination by a health care provider. The parents may also choose to have the circumcision done after discharge. However, they need to be advised that if the baby is older than 1 month, the current practice is to hospitalize him.

The nurse's responsibilities during a circumcision are to determine if the parents have any questions about the procedure and to ensure that the circumcision permit is signed. The nurse gathers the equipment and prepares the newborn by removing the diaper and placing him on a circumcision board or some other type of restraint but restraining only the legs (O'Grady 1996). In Jewish ceremonies, the infant is held by the father or godfather and given wine before the procedure (Reynolds 1996).

There are a variety of techniques for circumcision (Figures 23–8 and 23–9), and all produce minimal bleeding. During the procedure, the nurse assesses the newborn's response. One consideration is pain being experienced by the newborn. Some physicians use local anesthesia for this procedure. The American Academy of Pediatrics Committee on the Fetus and Newborn and Committee on Drugs (1987) have published a policy

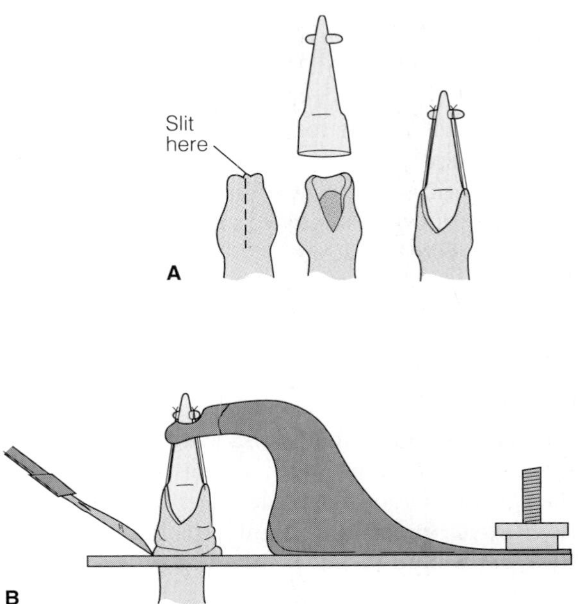

FIGURE 23–8 Circumcision using the Yellen or Gumco clamp: ***A*** The prepuce is drawn over the cone and ***B*** the clamp is applied. Pressure is maintained for 3–4 minutes, and then excess prepuce is cut away.

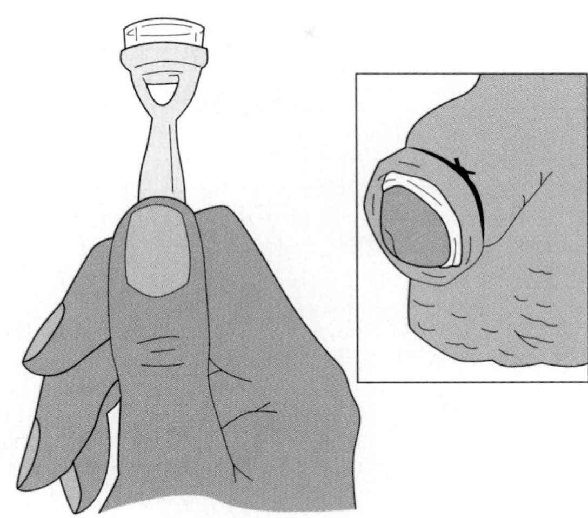

FIGURE 23–9 Circumcision using the Plastibell: The bell is fitted over the glans. A suture is tied around the bell's rim and the excess prepuce is cut away. The plastic rim remains in place for 3–4 days until healing occurs. The bell may be allowed to fall off; it is removed if still in place after 8 days.

statement endorsing the administration of local or systemic anesthesia to newborns undergoing surgical procedures. A dorsal penile nerve block (DPNB) using 1 percent Lidocaine without epinephrine significantly minimizes the pain and the shifts in behavioral patterns such as crying, irritability, and erratic sleep cycles (O'Grady 1996). Other studies are investigating the use of topical anesthetic (30 percent lidocaine cream) applied 20 minutes before prepuce removal, acetaminophen, and cryoanalgesia (O'Grady 1996; Weatherstone et al 1993). Wellington and Reider (1993) and O'Grady (1996) found that many physicians continue not to employ analgesics or use analgesics of questionable efficacy when performing newborn circumcisions.

The nurse can provide comfort measures such as lightly stroking the newborn's head, providing a plain or sucrose-flavored pacifier, and talking to him. Following the circumcision, he should be held and comforted by a family member or the nurse. The nurse must be alert to any cues that these measures are overstimulating the newborn instead of comforting him. Such cues include turning away of the head, increased generalized body movement, skin color changes, hyperalertness, and hiccoughing.

After the circumcision, A and D ointment is placed on the penis to keep the diaper from adhering to the site in all procedures except those using the Plastibell. New ointment is applied with each diaper change, or at least 4 to 5 times a day for at least 24–48 hours. Petroleum jelly or an antibiotic ointment may be used instead of A and D ointment.

Parents should assess the newborn's voiding for amount, adequacy of stream, and presence of blood. If bleeding does occur, they should apply light pressure intermittently to the site with a sterile gauze pad and notify their physician (Perlmutter et al 1995). The newborn may cry when he voids after circumcision. He should be positioned on his side with the diaper fastened loosely to prevent undue pressure. He may remain fussy for several hours and be less interested in feedings.

The parents should be instructed to squeeze water gently over the penis and pat it dry after each diaper change. The diaper is loosely fastened for 2 to 3 days, because the glans remains tender for this length of time. Before discharge, the parents should be instructed to observe the penis for bleeding or possible signs of infection. A whitish-yellow exudate around the glans is granulation tissue. It is normal and not indicative of an infection. The exudate may be noted for about 2 or 3 days and should not be removed.

If the Plastibell is used, families are informed that it may remain in place for up to 8 days and then fall off. If it is still in place after 8 days, it may require manual removal by the clinician.

A Letter From Your Baby

Dear Parents:

I come to you a small, immature being with my own style and personality. I am yours for only a short time; enjoy me.

1. Please take time to find out who I am, how I differ from you and how much I can bring you joy.
2. Please feed me when I am hungry. I never knew hunger in the womb, and clocks and time mean little to me.
3. Please hold, cuddle, kiss, touch, stroke, and croon to me. I was always held closely in the womb and was never alone before.
4. Please don't be disappointed when I am not the perfect baby that you expected, nor disappointed with yourselves that you are not the perfect parents.
5. Please don't expect too much from me as your newborn baby, or too much from yourself as a parent. Give us both six weeks as a birthday present—six weeks for me to grow, develop, mature and become more stable and predictable, and six weeks for you to rest and relax and allow your body to get back to normal.
6. Please forgive me if I cry a lot. Bear with me and in a short time, as I mature, I will spend less and less time crying and more time socializing.
7. Please watch me carefully and I can tell you the things that soothe, console and please me. I am not a tyrant who was sent to make your life miserable, but the only way I can tell you that I am not happy is with my cry.
8. Please remember that I am resilient and can withstand the many natural mistakes you will make with me. As long as you make them with love, you cannot ruin me.
9. Please take care of yourself and eat a balanced diet, rest and exercise so that when we are together, you have the health and strength to take care of me.
10. Please take care of your relationship with others. Relationships that are good for you, support both you and me.

Although I may have turned your life upside down, please realize that things will be back to normal before long.

Thank you,

Your Loving Child

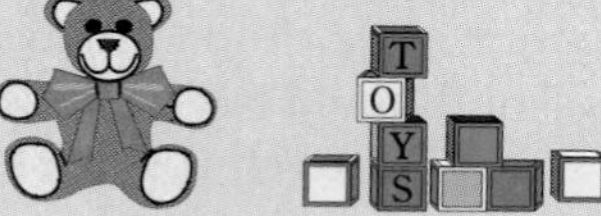

FIGURE 23–10 A letter from your baby.

Community-Based Nursing Care

The nurse can do much to help families feel comfortable with newborn care before they go home with their new baby and in preparation for ongoing care in the community. In addition to the information the nurse provides to parents during their stay in the birthing site, the nurse should provide information about safety, the newborn screening program, and community-based follow-up care before the mother and newborn are discharged. By discussing with parents how to meet their newborn's needs, ensure his or her safety, and appreciate their newborn's unique characteristics and behaviors and by assisting parents in establishing links with their community-based health care provider, the nurse can get the new family off to a good start. The nurse also plays a vital role in fostering parent-infant attachment (Figure 23–10). Parents need to know the signs of illness, how to reach the pediatrician or after-hours clinic, and the importance of follow-up after discharge. See Key Facts to Remember: When Parents Should Call Their Health Care Provider. Parents should also check with their clinician for advice about over-the-counter medications to be kept in the medicine cabinet.

Safety Considerations

The nurse can be an excellent role model for families in the area of safety. Gibson (1995) has reiterated the AAP's infant sleep position that healthy term infants be placed on their back or side to decrease the risk of sudden infant death syndrome. The nurse should demonstrate the proper positioning of the newborn and correct use of the bulb syringe. The newborn should never be left alone anywhere but in the crib. The nurse should remind the mother that while she and the newborn are together in the birthing unit, she should never leave the baby alone, because newborns spit up frequently the first day or two after birth.

Individual birthing units should practice safety measures to prevent infant abduction and provide teaching and information to parents regarding their role in this area.

Half of the children killed or injured in automobile accidents could have been protected by the use of federally approved car seats. Newborns should go home from the birthing unit in a car seat adapted to fit newborns (Figure 23–11). The seat should be positioned to face the rear of the car until the baby is a year old or weighs 20 pounds (9.09 kg). At this time the child's bone structure is adequately mineralized and better able to withstand a forward impact in a five-point harness restraint belt. In many states, the use of car seats for children up to the age of 4 is mandatory.

KEY FACTS TO REMEMBER

When Parents Should Call Their Health Care Provider

Temperature above 38.4C (101F) rectally or 38C (100.4F) axillary or below 36.1C (97F) rectally or 36.6C (97.8F) axillary

Continual rise in temperature

More than one episode of forceful vomiting or frequent vomiting over a 6-hour period

Refusal of two feedings in a row

Lethargy (listlessness), difficulty in awakening baby

Cyanosis with or without a feeding

Absence of breathing longer than 15 seconds

Inconsolable infant (quieting techniques are not effective) or continuous high-pitched cry

Discharge or bleeding from umbilical cord, circumcision, or any opening (except vaginal mucus or pseudomenstruation)

Two consecutive green, watery stools

No wet diapers for 18–24 hours or fewer than six to eight wet diapers per day

Development of eye drainage

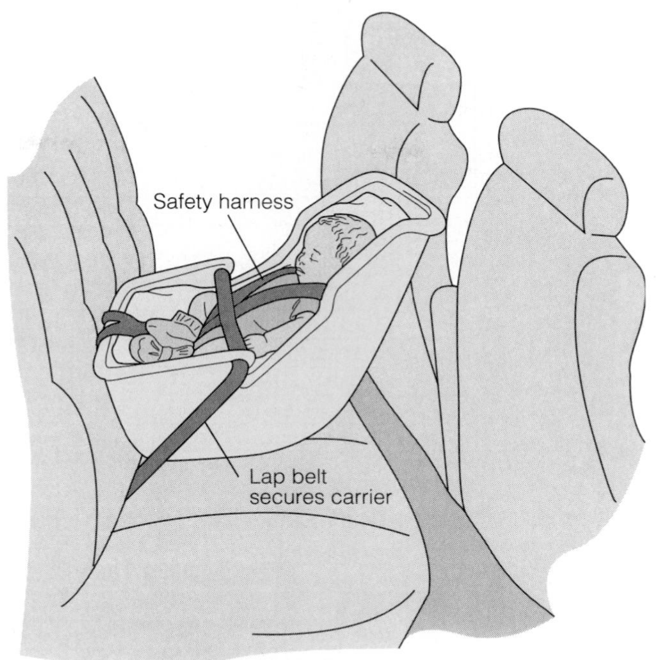

FIGURE 23–11 Infant car restraint for use from birth to about 12 months of age.

Source: Mott SR, James SD, Sperhac AM: *Nursing Care of Children and Families,* 2nd ed. Redwood City: Addison-Wesley, 1990, p 530.

Newborn Screening Program

Before the newborn and mother are discharged from the hospital, the nurse informs the parents about the normal **newborn screening tests** and tells them when to return to the birthing center or clinic if further tests are needed. The disorders that can be identified from a drop of blood obtained by a heel stick are galactosemia, homocystinuria, hypothyroidism, maple syrup urine disease, phenylketonuria (PKU), and sickle cell anemia. Early newborn discharge puts infants at risk for delayed or even missed diagnosis of PKU and congenital hypothyroidism because of decreased sensitivity of screening (Sinai et al 1995; Saslow et al 1996).

Immunization programs against the hepatitis B virus during the newborn period and infancy are in place in many states, at least 20 countries, and high-incidence areas such as Alaska and American Samoa (Freij and Sever 1994). Universal hepatitis B vaccination for all infants, regardless of maternal HBsAg status, is currently recommended by the CDC and American Academy of Pediatrics (Woodruff et al 1996). The current recommendation is that newborns receive the first dose within 12 hours of birth (0.5 mL of either vaccine preparation), a second dose at 1 month of age, and the last dose at 6 months of age (Freij and Sever 1994). See the Drug Guide: Recombinant Hepatitis B Vaccines on page 591. Parents need to be advised if their birthing center is doing newborn hepatitis vaccinations so that an adequate follow-up program can be set in motion (Woodruff et al 1996).

Early discharge has affected both the timing of newborn metabolic screening tests and the acquisition of subsequent immunization. For example, the accuracy of the test for PKU is directly related to the newborn's age. The likelihood of detecting PKU increases as the infant grows older; the infant needs to be at least 24 hours old for a valid test (Coody et al 1993).

The nurse should teach the family all necessary caregiving methods before discharge. A checklist may be helpful to make sure the teaching has been completed (Figure 23–12). The nurse needs to review with the couple all areas for understanding and any outstanding questions, without rushing, taking time to answer all queries. The mother should have the certified nurse-midwife/nurse practitioner/physician's phone number, address, and any specific instructions. Having the nursery phone number is also reassuring to a new family. The nurse encourages them to call with questions.

DATE AND TIME OF BIRTH ____________________

TOPICS:	TIME & DATE	INT.	COMMENTS:
I. PHYSICIAN INSTRUCTION BOOKLET			
II. INITIAL M/B CONTACT ON MATERNITY			
A. Orient to Mother/Baby			
B. Permits (PKU, Circ)			
C. Diapering & wrapping			
D. Crying			
E. Positioning in crib			
F. Bulb syringe			
G. Regurgitation			
III. BREASTFEEDING			
A. Mechanics & position			
B. Length of feeding			
C. Rooting reflex			
D. New bottle pc			
E. Expression/pump			
F. Burping			
G. Formula & preparation			
IV. BOTTLE FEEDING			
A. Mechanics			
B. Rooting reflex			
C. New bottle each feeding			
D. Propping			
E. Amount & time			
F. Burping			
G. Formula & preparation			
V. NEWBORN CHARACTERISTICS			
A. Rash, milia			
B. Vag. discharge			
C. Jaundice (Handout)			
D. Molding			
E. Coloring			
F. Vision & hearing			
VI. BATH DEMONSTRATION			
A. Cord care			
B. Genital care			
C. Circumcision care			
D. Support & safety			
VII. DISCHARGE INSTRUCTIONS			
A. Normal void & stool			
B. Constipation			
C. Car seats			
D. When to call Doctor			
E. Choking baby			
F. Use of thermometer			
G. Safety			
H. PKU			

I. Referral YES ___ NO ___

Parent's Signature ____________________ Comments: ____________________

Witness to Signature ____________________

FIGURE 23–12 Infant teaching checklist. Sections I and II are completed upon initial contact. Sections III and IV are completed by 4 hours from initial contact. Section V is completed by 12 hours from initial contact. Sections VI and VII are completed by the time of discharge.

Source: Adapted from Memorial Hospital, Colorado Springs.

DRUG GUIDE | Recombinant Hepatitis B Vaccine

Overview of Neonatal Action

Recombinant hepatitis B vaccine is used as a prophylactic treatment against all subtypes of hepatitis B virus. It provides passive immunization for newborns of HBsAg-negative and HBsAg-positive mothers. Hepatitis B can be transmitted across the placenta, but most newborns are infected during birth. It is produced from baker's yeast and plasmid containing the HBsAg gene.

Hepatitis B vaccine contains more than 95% HBsAg protein and is an inactivated (noninfective) product. Universal immunization is recommended.

Infants of HBsAg-positive mothers should concurrently receive 0.5 mL of hepatitis B immunoglobulin (HBIG) prophylaxis.

Route, Dosage, Frequency

The first dose of 0.5 mL (10 μg) is given intramuscularly into the anterolateral thigh within 12 hours of birth for infants born to HBsAg-positive mothers. The second dose of vaccine is given at 1 month of age and followed by a final dose at 6 months of age.

Infants born to HBsAg-negative mothers receive their first dose of vaccine at birth, the second dose at 1–2 months, and the third dose at 6–18 months (American Academy of Pediatrics 1992).

Infants whose mother's HBsAg status is unknown receive the same doses of vaccine as infants born to HBsAg-positive mothers.

Neonatal Side Effects

The only common side effect is soreness at the injection site. Occasionally, there is erythema, swelling, warmth, and induration at the injection site or a low-grade fever.

Nursing Considerations

Delay administration during active infection; the vaccine will not prevent infection during its incubation period.

The vaccine should be used as supplied. Do not dilute.

Do not inject intravenously or interdermally.

Monitor for adverse reactions. Monitor temperature closely.

Have epinephrine available to treat possible allergic reactions.

Responsiveness to the vaccine is age dependent. Preterm infants weighing less than 1000 g have lower seroconversion rates. Consider delaying the first dose until the infant is term PCA (postconceptual age) or use a four-dose schedule.

Documentation

The final step of discharge planning is documentation. Note any concerns of the parents or nurse and record which demonstrations or classes the parent(s) attended and their expressed understanding of the instructions given to them.

Education is a wonderful aspect of family-centered maternity care. The nurse who takes the time to get the family off to a good start can feel the satisfaction of providing optimal care.

Evaluation

When evaluating the nursing care provided during the newborn period, the following outcomes may be anticipated:

- The newborn's adaptation to extrauterine life is supported and complete.
- The newborn's physiologic and psychologic integrity is supported.
- The newborn feeding pattern is satisfactorily established.
- Parents demonstrate safe techniques for caring for their newborn.
- Parents express understanding of the bonding process and display attachment behaviors.
- Parents verbalize developmentally appropriate behavioral expectations of, and community-based follow-up care for, their newborn.

CHAPTER HIGHLIGHTS

- The overall goal of newborn nursing care is to provide comprehensive care while promoting the establishment of a functioning family unit.
- In the period immediately after birth, during which adaptation to extrauterine life occurs, the newborn requires close monitoring to identify any deviations from normal.
- Nursing goals during the first 4 hours after birth (admission period) are to maintain a clear airway, maintain a neutral thermal environment, prevent hemorrhage and infection, initiate oral feedings, and facilitate attachment.
- The newborn is routinely given prophylactic vitamin K to prevent possible hemorrhagic disease of the newborn.
- Prophylactic eye treatment for *Neisseria gonorrhoeae* is legally required on all newborns.

- Nursing goals in ongoing newborn care include maintenance of cardiopulmonary function, maintenance of neutral thermal environment, promotion of adequate hydration and nutrition, prevention of complications, promotion of safety, and enhancement of attachment and family knowledge of child care.

REFERENCES

American Academy of Pediatrics: *Guidelines for Perinatal Care,* 3rd ed. Chicago: American Academy, 1992.

American Academy of Pediatrics, Committee on Fetus and Newborn: Report of the Ad Hoc Task Force on Circumcision. *Pediatrics* 1989; 84:388.

American Academy of Pediatrics, Committee on Fetus and Newborn and Committee on Drugs: Neonatal anesthesia. *Pediatrics* 1987; 80:446.

Andrews MM: Transcultural perspectives in the nursing care of children and adolescents. In: *Transcultural Concepts in Nursing Care,* 2nd ed. Andrews MM, Boyle JS (editors). Philadelphia: Lippincott, 1995.

Bordman HB, Holzman UR: Infant care knowledge of primiparous urban mothers. *J Perinatol* 1996; 16(2):107.

Brown LP et al: Controversial issues surrounding early postpartum discharge. *Nurs Clin North Am* 1996; 31(2):333.

Coody D et al: Early hospital discharge and the timing of newborn metabolic screening. *Clin Pediatr* August 1993; 463.

Cunningham FG, MacDonald PC, Gant NG: *Williams' Obstetrics,* 20th ed. Stamford, CT: Appleton & Lange, 1997.

Freij BJ, Sever JL: Chronic infections. In: *Neonatalogy: Pathophysiology and Management of the Newborn,* 14th ed. Avery GB, Fletcher MA, MacDonald MG (editors). Philadelphia: Lippincott, 1994.

Gibson E et al: Infant sleep position following new AAP guidelines. *Pediatrics* 1995; 96(1):69.

Infant Sleep Positioning and SIDS Position Statement. Evanston, IL: American Academy of Pediatrics, 1992.

Hutchinson MK, Baqi-Aziz M: Nursing care of the childbearing Muslim family. *JOGNN* 1994; 23(9):767.

Klaus M, Klaus P: *The Amazing Newborn.* Menlo Park, CA: Addison-Wesley, 1985.

L'Archevesque CI, Goldstein-Lohman H: Ritual circumcision: Educating parents. *Pediatr Nurs* 1996; 22(3):228.

McGregor LA: Short, shorter, shortest: Improving the hospital stay for mothers and newborns. *MCN* 1994; 19(2):91.

Mendler VM et al: The conception, birth, and infancy of an early discharge program. *MCN* 1996; 21(5):241.

Merestein GB, Gardner SL: *Handbook of Neonatal Intensive Care,* 3rd ed. St Louis: Mosby, 1992.

Neonatal Skin Care. *NAACOG-OGN Nursing Practice Resource.* January 1992.

Neonatal Thermoregulation. *NAACOG-OGN Nursing Practice Resource.* February 1990.

O'Grady JP: Circumcision: Ritual and surgery. In: *Gynecology and Obstetrics Vol. 2.* Sciarra JJ (editors). Philadelphia: Harper & Row, 1996.

Penny-MacGillivray T: A newborn's first bath: When? *JOGNN* 1996; 25(6):481.

Perlmutter DF et al: Voiding after neonatal circumcision. *Pediatrics* 1995; 96(6):1111.

Rasbridge LA, Kulig JC: Infant feeding among Cambodian refugees. *MCN* 1995; 20(4):213.

Reynolds RD: Use of the Mogen Clamp for neonatal circumcision. *AFP* 1996; 54(1):177.

Riordan J, Auerbach KG: *Breastfeeding and Human Lactation.* Boston: Jones & Bartlett, 1993.

Ruchala P: The effect of wearing head covering on the axillary temperature of infants. *MCN* July/August 1985; 10:240.

Saslow JG, Post EM, Southard CA: Thyroid screening for early discharged infants. *Pediatrics* 1996; 98(1):41.

Schneiderman JU: Postpartum nursing for Korean mothers. *MCN* 1996; 21(3):155.

Sinai LN et al: Phenylketonuria screening: Effect of early newborn discharge. *Pediatrics* 1995; 96(4):605.

Walsh SM, Corbett RW: Helping postpartum rural adolescents visualize future goals. *MCN* 1995; 20(5):276.

Weatherstone KB et al: Safety and efficacy of a topical anesthetic for neonatal circumcision. *Pediatrics* 1993; 92(5):710.

Wellington N, Rieder MJ: Attitudes and practice regarding analgesia for newborn circumcision. *Pediatrics* 1993; 92:541.

Woodruff BA et al: Progress toward integrating hepatitis B vaccine into routine infant immunization schedules in the United States, 1991 through 1994. *Pediatrics* 1996; 97(6):798.

Zanoni D, Isenberg SJ, Apt L: A comparison of silver nitrate with erythromycin for prophylaxis against ophthalmia neonatorium. *Clin Pediatr* May 1992; 295.

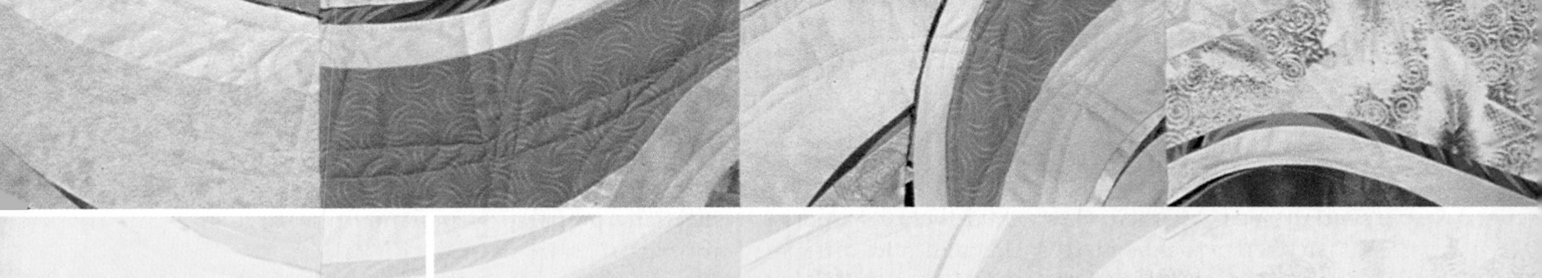

Chapter 24 | Newborn Nutrition

OBJECTIVES

- Compare the nutritional value and composition of breast milk and formula preparations.
- Discuss the advantages/disadvantages of breastfeeding and formula-feeding for both mother and newborn.
- Develop guidelines for helping both breastfeeding and bottle-feeding mothers to feed their newborns successfully.
- Delineate nursing responsibilities for client education about problems the breastfeeding mother may encounter at home.
- Describe an appropriate process for weaning an infant from breastfeeding.
- Incorporate knowledge of newborn nutrition and normal growth patterns into parent education and infant assessment.
- Recognize the influence of cultural values on infant care, especially feeding practices.

KEY TERMS

Colostrum
Foremilk
Hindmilk
La Leche League
Letdown reflex
Mature milk
Oxytocin
Prolactin
Transitional milk
Weaning

Feeding their newborn is an exciting, satisfying, but often worrisome task for parents. Meeting this essential need of their new child helps parents strengthen their attachment to their child and fosters their self-images as nurturers and providers. Whether a woman chooses to breast- or bottle-feed, she can be reassured that she can adequately meet her infant's needs. As questions about feeding arise, the nurse works with the woman to help her develop skill in her chosen method. In every interaction, it is the nurse's responsibility to support the parents and promote the family's sense of confidence.

Nutritional Needs of the Newborn

The newborn's diet must supply nutrients to meet the rapid rate of physical growth and development. A neonatal diet should include protein, carbohydrate, fat, water, vitamins, and minerals. The recommended dietary allowances (RDAs) for birth through the first 6 months are listed in Table 24–1.

The calories (50–55 kcal/lb/day or 105–110 kcal/kg/day) in the newborn's diet are divided among protein, carbohydrate, and fat and should be adjusted according to the newborn's weight. Protein is needed for rapid cellular growth and maintenance. Carbohydrates provide energy. The fat portion of the diet provides calories, regulates fluid and electrolyte balance, and develops the newborn brain and neurologic system. Water requirements are high (64–73 mL/lb/day or 140–160 mL/kg/day) because of the newborn's inability to concentrate urine. Fluid needs increase further during illness or hot weather. The infant's iron needs are affected by accumulation of iron stores during fetal life and the mother's iron and other food intake if she is breastfeeding. Ascorbic acid (usually in the form of fruit juices) and meat, poultry, and fish enhance absorption of iron in the mother just as they do later in the infant. See Key Facts to Remember: Newborn Caloric and Fluid Needs.

KEY FACTS TO REMEMBER

Newborn Caloric and Fluid Needs

- Caloric intake: 50–55 kcal/lb/day or 105–110 kcal/kg/day
- Fluid requirements: 64–73 mL/lb/day or 140–160 mL/kg/day
- Weight gain: First 6 months—1 oz/day
  Second 6 months—0.5 oz/day

Formula-fed babies do gain weight faster than breastfed babies because of the higher protein in commercially prepared formula and the larger volumes of formula that are needed to obtain the necessary nutrients. Bottle-fed infants up to 6 months of age can gain as much as 30 g (1 oz) per day and tend to regain their birth weight by 10 days after birth (Pipes 1989). Healthy breastfed babies gain approximately 15 g (0.5 oz) per day in the first 6 months of life (Sawley 1989) and tend to regain their birth weight by about 14 days after birth. Formula-fed infants generally double their weight within 3.5–4 months, whereas nursing infants double their weight at about 5 months of age.

Breast Milk

The composition of human milk varies with the stage of lactation, the time of the day, the time during the feeding, maternal nutrition, and gestational age of the newborn at birth. During the establishment of lactation there are three stages of human milk: (a) colostrum, (b) transitional milk, and (c) mature milk. **Colostrum** is a yellowish or creamy-appearing fluid that is thicker than the later milk and contains more protein, fat-soluble vitamins, and minerals (Wagner et al 1996). It also contains high levels of immunoglobulins (antibodies such as IgA), which are a source of passive immunity for the newborn. Colostrum production begins early in pregnancy and may last for several days after birth. However, in most cases colostrum is replaced by transitional milk within 2–4 days after birth. Even small amounts of colostrum are invaluable for the newborn. **Transitional milk** is produced from the end of colostrum production until approximately 2 weeks postpartum. This milk contains lactose, water-soluble vitamins, elevated levels of fat, and more calories than colostrum.

The final milk produced, **mature milk,** contains about 10 percent solids (carbohydrates, proteins, fats) for energy and growth; the rest is water, which is vital for maintaining hydration. The composition of mature milk varies according to the time during the feeding. **Foremilk** is the milk obtained at the beginning of the feeding. It is high in water content and contains vitamins and protein. **Hindmilk** is released after the initial letdown, or release of milk, and has a higher fat concentration. Although it appears similar to skim milk and may cause mothers to question whether their milk is "rich enough," mature breast milk provides 20 kcal/ounce, as do most prepared formulas. However, the percentage of calories derived from protein is lower in breast milk than in formulas, with a greater proportion of calories being derived from fat (Lawrence 1994a). In breastfed babies, protein metabolism produces less nitrogen waste, which has a positive effect on the infant's immature renal system.

The American Academy of Pediatrics Committee on Nutrition (1992) recommends breast milk as the optimal food for the first 6 to 12 months of life. Breastfeeding provides newborns and infants with immunologic, nutritional, and psychosocial advantages.

Immunologic Advantages

Immunologic advantages include varying degrees of protection from respiratory and gastrointestinal infections, otitis media, meningitis, sepsis, and allergies (Beaudry et al 1995; Wagner et al 1996). This protection has a positive effect on the breastfed baby's health in the newborn period. Secretory IgA, an immunoglobulin present in colostrum and breast milk, has antiviral, antibacterial, and antigenic-inhibiting properties. It is theorized that the infant's immature intestine allows antigenic macromolecules, such as those found in cow's milk, to cross the mucosa of the small intestine (Spencer 1996). Secretory IgA plays a role in decreasing the permeability of the intestine to these macromolecules. Other properties in colostrum and breast milk that act to inhibit the growth of bacteria and viruses are *Lactobacillus bifidus,* lysozymes, lactoperoxidase, lactoferrin, transferrin, and various immunoglobulins. Immunoglobulins to the poliomyelitis virus are also present in the breast milk of mothers who have immunity to this virus. Because the presence of these immunoglobulins may inhibit the desired intestinal infection and immune response of the infant, some clinics suggest that breastfeedings be withheld for 30 to 60 minutes following the administration of the Sabin oral polio vaccine. In addition to its immunologic properties, breast milk is known to be nonallergenic and is not affected by unsafe water or insect-carried disease (Lawrence 1994b).

Nutritional Advantages

Breast milk is composed of lactose, lipids, polyunsaturated fatty acids, and amino acids, especially taurine, and has a whey-to-casein protein ratio that facilitates its digestion, absorption, and full use compared to formulas (Spencer 1996). Some researchers feel the high concentration of cholesterol and the balance of amino acids in breast milk make it the best food for myelination and neurologic development. High cholesterol levels in breast milk may stimulate the production of enzymes that lead to more efficient metabolism of cholesterol, thereby reducing its harmful effects on the cardiovascular system (Lawrence 1994a).

Breast milk provides newborns with minerals in more acceptable doses than formulas do (Lawrence 1994a). The iron found in breast milk, even though much lower in concentration than that in prepared formulas, is much more readily and fully absorbed and appears sufficient to meet the infant's iron needs for the first 4 to 6 months. The American Academy of Pediatrics Committee on Nutrition (1992) states that there is generally no need to give supplemental iron to breastfed newborns before the age of 4–6 months. Supplemental iron may decrease the ability of breast milk to protect the newborn by interfering with lactoferrin, an iron-binding protein that enhances the absorption of iron and has anti-infective properties.

TABLE 24–1 Recommended Dietary Allowances for the Normal Newborn

Daily Requirements, Birth–6 Months	
Calories	108 kcal/kg
Protein	2.2 g/kg
Fat	30–35% total kcal
Carbohydrate	50–55% total kcal
Water	1.5 mL/kcal
Calcium	400 mg
Phosphorus	300 mg
Magnesium	40 mg
Iron	6 mg
Zinc	5 mg
Iodine	40 μg
Selenium	10 μg
Vitamins	
A	420 μg
B_6	0.3 mg
B_{12}	0.3 μg
D	400 IU
E	3 mg
K	5 μg
C	30 mg
Thiamine	0.3 mg
Riboflavin	0.4 mg
Niacin	5 mg
Folate	25 μg

Note: The allowances, expressed as average daily intakes, are intended to provide for individual variations among normal persons in the United States under usual environmental stresses.

Source: Food and Nutrition Board, National Academy of Sciences—National Research Council: *Recommended Dietary Allowances,* 10th ed. Washington, DC, 1989.

Another advantage of breast milk is that all its components are delivered to the infant in an unchanged form, and vitamins are not lost through processing and heating. If the breastfeeding mother is taking daily multivitamins and her diet is adequate, the only supplement the infant will need until the age of 6 months is fluoride (American Academy of Pediatrics Committee on Nutrition 1995, Spencer 1996). If the mother's diet or vitamin intake is inadequate or questionable, caregivers may choose to prescribe additional vitamins for the infant.

Psychosocial Advantages

The psychosocial advantages of breastfeeding are primarily those associated with maternal-infant attachment. The mother's level of oxytocin generally increases with breastfeeding, and studies indicate that this hormonal change coincides with more even mood responses and increased feelings of maternal well-being (Lawrence 1994b). Breastfeeding enhances attachment by providing the opportunity for frequent, direct skin contact between the newborn and the mother. The newborn's

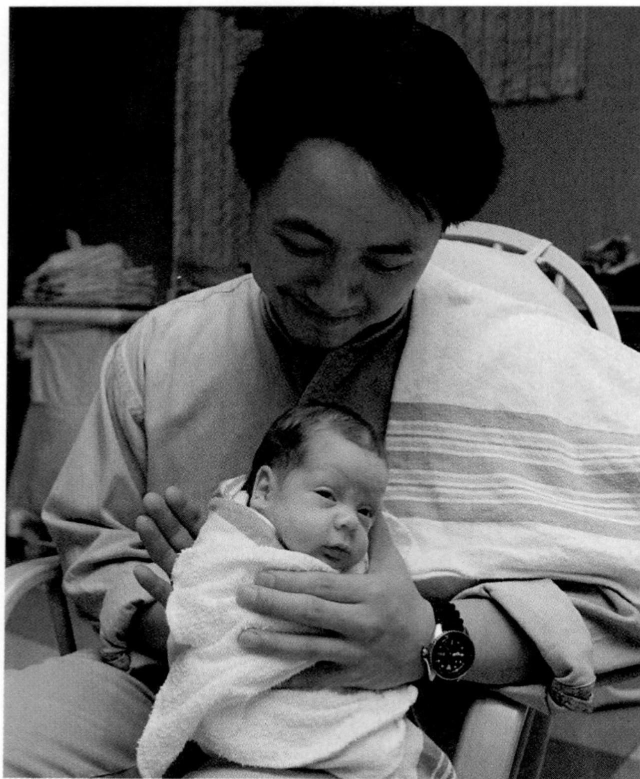

FIGURE 24–1 A father can nurture his baby in many ways.

sense of touch is highly developed at birth and is a primary means of communication. The tactile stimulation associated with breastfeeding can communicate warmth, closeness, and comfort. The increased closeness provides both newborn and mother with the opportunity to learn each other's behavioral cues and needs. The mother's sense of accomplishment in being able to satisfy her baby's needs for nourishment and comfort is enhanced when the newborn sucks vigorously and is satiated and calmed by the breastfeeding. Some mothers prefer breastfeeding as a means of extending the close, unique, nourishing relationship between mother and baby that existed before birth. In the event of a twin birth, breastfeeding not only is possible but also enhances the mother's individualization and attachment to each newborn. The fantasized single baby is replaced more readily with the reality of two individual babies when the mother has close and frequent contact with each (Sollid et al 1989). Fathers are encouraged to be a part of the feeding experience by offering fresh pumped or thawed (frozen) breast milk to the baby at one or more feedings daily.

Contraindications and Disadvantages

There are some medical contraindications to breastfeeding. A mother with a diagnosis of breast cancer should not breastfeed so that she may begin treatment immediately. The CDC recommends counseling the mother with AIDS against breastfeeding except in a country where the risk of neonatal death from diarrhea and other disease is 50 percent or greater (Lawrence 1994b). Breastfeeding is also contraindicated for the infant suffering from galactosemia (Eggert and Rayburn 1994; Lawrence 1994a). Maternal medications may preclude breastfeeding as discussed in Chapters 12 and 25. Cocaine in particular, because of its high lipid solubility, passes easily into breast milk and is harmful to the breastfeeding infant. At times management of newborn jaundice may include suspension of breastfeeding (see Chapter 26).

In the dominant Western culture, where women may need to pursue activities outside the home, being "tied down" to an infant for 9 to 12 feedings every day may be considered inconvenient and stressful. Another cited disadvantage of breastfeeding is exclusion of the father from the nurturing involved in feeding the infant. But, since nurturing encompasses more than just feeding, the father can comfort and attend to the baby in many other ways (Figure 24–1).

Opinion varies on the advisability of continuing breastfeeding during a pregnancy. Some feel the nutritional demands on the pregnant mother are too great and advocate gradual weaning. Others suggest that with adequate rest, a proper diet, and strong emotional support, continued breastfeeding during pregnancy is a valid choice. The practice of nursing one infant throughout pregnancy and then breastfeeding both infants after birth is called *tandem nursing* (Lawrence 1994b). When pregnancy occurs, the decision is best made on an individual basis after considering maternal health and motivation and the age of the first child.

Even though many mothers obtain information about breastfeeding from written sources, family and friends, and La Leche League (an international lay support and information group), the nurse needs to be a ready source of information, encouragement, and support as well. The nurse can be helpful when parents are deciding whether to breastfeed, after the birth process when breastfeedings are just being established, and after the family returns home.

Formula-Feeding

Although breastfeeding is increasing in popularity, formula-feeding is a viable and nurturing choice, particularly in developed countries. Formula-feeding can also meet the goal of successful growth of the baby. The closeness and warmth that can occur during breastfeeding is also an integral part of bottle-feeding. An advantage of bottle-feeding is that parents can share equally in this nurturing, caring experience with their baby. Numerous types of commercially prepared lactose formulas meet the nutritional needs of the infant. Some of the most common formulas are Similac, Enfamil, and SMA. These formulas contain more tyrosine and phenylalanine and less taurine than breast milk does.

KEY FACTS TO REMEMBER Comparison of Breast- and Bottle-Feeding continued

Breast	Bottle (Feeding Iron-Enriched Formula)
Nutrition	
Breast milk is species specific (ie, perfect balance of proteins, carbohydrates, fats, vitamins, and minerals for human infants).	Formula is as close to human milk as possible, but nutrients are not as efficiently utilized.
Breast milk contains higher levels of lactose, cystine, and cholesterol, which are necessary for brain and nerve growth.	Nutritional adequacy depends on proper preparation (overdilution results in decreased nutrients delivered to infant).
Proteins are easily digested and fats are well absorbed.	Some babies cannot tolerate the fats or carbohydrates found in regular formula. Companies are offering alternative formulas.
Composition varies according to gestational age and stage of lactation, thereby meeting the changing nutritional requirements of individual infants as they grow.	
Infants determine the volume of milk consumed.	Pediatrician or caregiver determines the volume consumed. Overfeeding may occur if caregiver is determined that baby will empty bottle.
Frequency of feeding is determined by infant cues rather than by time schedule.	Feeding commonly occurs according to a preset schedule.
Anti-Infective and Antiallergic Properties	
Breast milk contains immunoglobulins, enzymes, and leukocytes that protect against pathogens.	Formula is linked to an increased number of GI and respiratory infections.
Bacteriostatic properties permit storage at room temperature up to 6 hours, in refrigerator for 24 hours, and freezing for 6 months.	Potential for bacterial contamination exists during preparation and storage.
Breast milk decreases the incidence of allergy by eliminating exposure to potential antigens (cow and soy protein).	Some babies are allergic to cow or soy protein. Formula companies are offering alternative formulas suitable for babies who develop allergies.

Formulas contain mostly saturated fatty acids, whereas breast milk is higher in unsaturated fatty acids, long chain fats, and cholesterol. Calcium, sodium, and chloride occur in higher concentrations in some commercially made formulas, which may be detrimental to the newborn's kidneys. They may not be ready to handle such high loads of solutes. This high solute load may also lead to thirst in the formula-fed infant, causing overfeeding and possible obesity.

Another potential problem with formulas is an allergic reaction in the newborn. The small intestine of the infant is permeable to macromolecules such as those found in cow's milk and milk-based formulas. The introduction of formula's foreign protein can cause an allergic reaction, with such signs as vomiting, colic, diarrhea, colitis, reluctance to feed, and eczema (See Key Facts to Remember: Comparison of Breast- and Bottle-Feeding on pp 597 and 598.)

Clinicians recommend iron-fortified formulas or supplements when bottle-feeding with non-iron-fortified formulas, because iron deficiency anemia is still very prevalent. The RDA for iron is 6 mg per day from birth to 6 months and 10 mg per day from 6 to 12 months. However, the nurse must be aware that excess iron in the diet may interfere with the baby's natural ability to defend against disease. Parents also need to be informed about the constipation that sometimes results from iron-enriched formula and about various methods of alleviating it. Opinion varies about the use of vitamin supplements for newborns, but it is generally agreed that commercially prepared formulas adequately meet the needs of the healthy newborn and infant.

Many companies make an enriched formula that is similar to breast milk. These formulas all have sufficient levels of carbohydrate, protein, fat, vitamins, and minerals to meet the newborn's nutritional needs.

The American Academy of Pediatrics (1992a) recommends that infants be given breast milk or iron-fortified formula rather than whole milk until 1 year of age. Neither unmodified cow's milk, low iron formula, nor skim milk is an acceptable alternative for newborn feeding (Spencer 1996). The protein content in cow's milk is too high (50 to 75 percent more than human milk), is poorly digested, and may cause bleeding of the gastrointestinal tract. Cow's milk is also inadequate in vitamins. Skim milk lacks adequate calories, fat content, and

KEY FACTS TO REMEMBER Comparison of Breast- and Bottle-Feeding continued

Breast	Bottle (Feeding Iron-Enriched Formula)
Psychosocial Aspects	
Skin-to-skin contact enhances closeness.	Bottle-feeding can provide an opportunity for positive parent-infant interaction.
Hormones of lactation promote maternal feelings and sense of well-being.	
The value system of an industrial society can create barriers to successful breastfeeding: Mother may feel ashamed or embarrassed. Breastfeeding after return to work may be difficult.	
Father is not able to breastfeed, but he can feed expressed breast milk from a bottle and nurture the infant in ways other than feeding.	Father can feed the baby.
Cost	
Healthy diet for mother.	Formula is a major expense.
Optional, but recommended, items include nursing pads, nursing bras.	Bottles or disposable nursers with plastic liners, nipples, and nipple caps must be purchased.
A breast pump may be needed.	A refrigeration system is necessary if mixing formula for more than one feeding at a time or using large containers of ready-to-feed formula.
Convenience	
The milk is always the perfect temperature.	Varying amounts of time are involved in formula preparation.
No preparation time is needed.	Anyone can feed the baby.
The mother must be available to feed or provide expressed milk to be given in her absence.	
If she misses a feeding, the mother must express milk to maintain lactation.	
The mother may experience slight discomfort in the early days of lactation.	
Maternal medication may interrupt breastfeeding.	

essential fatty acids necessary for proper development of the newborn's neurologic system. Nutritionists advise against giving cow's milk with decreased fat content, or skim milk, to children under 2 years of age.

Newborn Feeding

Initial Feeding

The time when the first feeding is given is determined by the physiologic and behavioral cues of the newborn. The nurse should assess for active bowel sounds, absence of abdominal distention, and a lusty cry, which quiets and is replaced with rooting and sucking behaviors when a stimulus is placed near the lips. These signs are indicators that the newborn is hungry and physically ready to tolerate the feeding.

Bottle-feeding newborns are offered formula as soon as they show an interest and ability to suck and swallow. Many institutions offer the newborn who is to be formula-fed a few milliliters of sterile water or 5 percent dextrose 1 to 4 hours after birth. There is no current evidence to support this practice because it is the aspirated gastric contents with acid that are harmful and not the type of feeding (Fletcher 1994). The first feeding provides an opportunity for the nurse to assess the effectiveness of the newborn's suck, swallow, and gag reflexes.

The mother who plans to breastfeed is encouraged to nurse her newborn immediately after birth, allowing the baby to nurse to satiety.

Early feedings are of great benefit to the breastfeeding pair because oxytocin helps expel the placenta and prevent excessive maternal blood loss; the infant receives the immunologic protection of colostrum; the infant's peristalsis is stimulated, facilitating elimination of the byproducts of bilirubin conjugation, which decreases the risk of jaundice; lactation is accelerated; and maternal-infant attachment is enhanced (Riordan and Auerbach 1993).

TABLE 24–2 Infant Feeding Behaviors

Age	Hunger Behavior	Feeding Behavior	Satiety Behavior
Birth to 13 weeks (0–3 months)	Cries; hands fisted; body tense	Rooting reflex; medial lip closure; strong suck reflex; suck-swallow pattern; tongue thrust and retraction; palmomental reflex, gags easily, needs burping	Withdraws head from nipple; falls asleep; hands relaxed; relief of body tension
14–24 weeks (4–6 months)	Eagerly anticipates; grasps and draws bottle or breast to mouth; reaches with open mouth	Aware of hands; generalized reaching; intentional hand to mouth; tongue elevation; lips purse at corners—pucker; shifts food in mouth—prechewing; tongue protrudes in anticipation of nipple; tongue holds nipple firm; tongue projection strong; suck strength increases; coughs and chokes easily; preference for tastes	Tosses head back; fusses or cries; covers mouth with hands; ejects food; distracted by surroundings

Source: Mott S et al: *Nursing Care of Children and Families,* 2nd ed. Redwood City, CA: Addison-Wesley, 1990, p 155.

Throughout the first 2 hours after birth, especially during the first 20–30 minutes, the infant is usually alert and ready to nurse. However, newborn suckling patterns vary, and although many babies are eager to suckle at this time, many will simply lick or nuzzle the nipple. This behavior is beneficial because the licking stimulates the release of oxytocin, which aids uterine involution and lactation (letdown). The mother should be encouraged to interpret this as a positive breastfeeding interaction (Riordan and Auerbach 1993).

Assessment of the newborn's physiologic status is of primary and ongoing concern to the nurse throughout the first feeding. Extreme fatigue coupled with rapid respiration, circumoral cyanosis, and diaphoresis of the head and face may indicate cardiovascular complications and requires further assessment. The initial feeding also requires assessment of the infant for the congenital anomaly of tracheoesophageal fistula or esophageal atresia (see Chapter 25). Findings associated with esophageal anomalies include maternal polyhydramnios and increased oral mucus in the infant. In cases of esophageal atresia, the feeding is taken well initially, but as the esophageal pouch fills, the feeding is quickly regurgitated unchanged by stomach contents. If a fistula is present, the infant gags, chokes, regurgitates mucus, and may become cyanotic as fluid passes through the fistula into the lungs.

Because colostrum is not irritating if aspirated and is readily absorbed by the respiratory system, breastfeeding can usually begin immediately after birth. Contraindications to immediate nursing include heavy sedation of the mother and physical compromise of either mother or baby.

It is not unusual for the newborn to regurgitate some mucus and water following a feeding, even if it was taken without difficulty. Consequently, the nurse observes the newborn closely and positions the infant on the right side after a feeding to aid drainage and facilitate gastric emptying.

Establishing a Feeding Pattern

An "on demand" feeding program facilitates each baby's own rhythm and assists a new mother in establishing lactation. The newborn rapidly digests breast milk and may desire to nurse 8 to 10 times in a 24-hour period. After the initial period of alertness and eagerness to suckle, the infant progresses to light sleep, then deep sleep, followed by increased wakefulness and interest in nursing. As wakefulness and interest in nursing increase, the infant will often cluster 5 to 10 feeding episodes over 2 to 3 hours, followed by a 4- to 5-hour deep sleep. After this cluster of minifeeds and deep sleep, the infant will feed frequently, but at more regular intervals. Maternal medications received during labor may affect newborn feeding behavior by delaying early cluster feedings that usually occur in the initial 1 to 2 days after birth. Newborns whose mothers received epidural analgesia have been noted to be irritable and demonstrate reduced motor organization, poor self-quieting skills, and decreased visual skills and alertness (Riordan and Auerbach 1993).

Rooming-in permits the mother to learn about and respond to her infant's early feeding cues. Early cues that indicate a newborn is interested in feeding include hand-to-mouth motion, whimpering, sucking, and rooting (Mulford 1992). Crying is a late sign of hunger. When rooming-in is not available, a supportive nursing staff and flexible nursery policies will allow the mother to feed her infant on cue. It is very frustrating to a new mother to attempt to feed a newborn who is sound asleep because he or she is either not hungry or exhausted from crying. The nurse can use Table 24–2 to help parents identify their baby's cues for hunger and satiation.

Keefe's (1988) research study also showed that rooming-in mothers reported sleeping better than those whose babies were in a central nursery. Research also indicates that rooming-in babies experience more REM sleep and cry less. Although our society accepts crying as normal and healthy behavior for newborns, it may actually delay the transition to extrauterine life. Crying involves a Valsalva maneuver that increases pulmonary vascular pressure, which may cause unoxygenated blood to be shunted into systemic circulation through the foramen ovale and ductus arteriosus. Therefore, rooming-in may be advantageous for the baby because the mother will respond to the baby's needs quickly and thus minimize crying.

Formula-fed newborns may awaken for feedings every 2–5 hours but are frequently satisfied with feedings every 3–4 hours. Because infants digest formula more slowly, the bottle-fed infant may go longer between feedings but should not go longer than 4 hours. Babies may begin skipping the night feeding within about 8–12 weeks of age (Riordan and Auerbach 1993). This is very individual, depending on the size and development of the infant.

Both breastfed and bottle-fed infants experience growth spurts at certain times and require increased feeding. The mother of a breastfed infant may meet these increased demands by nursing more frequently to increase her milk supply; however, it will take about 24 hours for the milk supply to increase adequately to meet the new demand (Lawrence 1994b). A slight increase in feedings will meet the needs of the formula-fed infant.

Providing nourishment for her newborn is a major concern of the new mother. Her feelings of success or failure may influence her self-concept as she assumes her maternal role. With proper instruction, support, and encouragement from professionals, feeding becomes a source of pleasure and satisfaction to both parents and infant.

Community-Based Nursing Care

Promotion of Successful Infant Feeding

Parents may see feeding their baby as the center of the relationship between themselves and this new family member. Whether the mother has chosen to bottle- or breastfeed, the nurse can be instrumental in assisting the mother to have a successful experience while in the birthing unit and during the early days at home. Feeding and caring for newborns may be routine tasks for the nurse, but the mother's success or failure during the first few times may determine her feelings about herself as an adequate mother.

The newborn's response to caring is important. A parent may interpret the newborn's behavior as rejection, which may alter the progress of parent-child relationships. A parent may also interpret the sleepy infant's refusal to suck or inability to retain formula as evidence of parental incompetence. The breastfeeding mother may deduce that the newborn does not like her if he or she fails to take her nipple readily. Conversely, infants pick up messages from the muscular tension of those holding them.

A nurse who is sensitive to the needs of the mother can form a relationship with her that permits sharing of knowledge about techniques and emotions connected with the feeding experience. Breastfeeding women frequently express disappointment in the help given to them by birthing unit nurses, saying they would like more encouragement, support, and practical information about feeding their newborn, especially with very early discharges (Renfrew et al 1990). This desire and need also applies to nonnursing mothers. Consistency in teaching by nurses is essential. A new mother becomes very frustrated if she is shown a number of different methods of feeding her newborn. With the technologic advances in formula production and the availability of knowledge about breastfeeding techniques, the mother should be confident that the choice she makes will promote normal growth and development of her newborn.

The mother's decision to breast- or bottle-feed is usually made by the sixth month of pregnancy and often even before conception. The final decision, however, may not be made until the mother's admission to the birth center. The decision is frequently influenced by relatives, especially the baby's father and maternal grandmother (Littman et al 1994), friends, and social customs, rather than being based on knowledge about the nutritional and psychologic needs of herself and her newborn.

The goals of Healthy People 2000 are to have 75 percent of infants breastfeeding at birth and 50 percent feeding at least some human milk until age 6 months (Losch et al 1995). It is the health care provider's responsibility to provide the parents with accurate information about the distinct advantages of breastfeeding to the mother and infant. In times of short stays, the Baby Friendly Hospital Initiative program promotes breastfeeding by designating hospitals as centers for breastfeeding education (Pascale et al 1996). Many mothers who chose to bottle-feed say they could have been persuaded to breastfeed if someone had cared enough to tell them how important it is.

Once an *informed* choice of feeding method has been made, the nurse's primary responsibilities are to support the mother's decision and to help the family achieve a positive result. No woman should be made to feel either inadequate or superior because of her choice in feeding (Gigliotti 1995). There are advantages and disadvantages to breast- and bottle-feeding, but positive bonds in parent-child relationships can be developed with either method.

Before feeding, the mother should be as comfortable as possible. Preparations may include voiding, washing

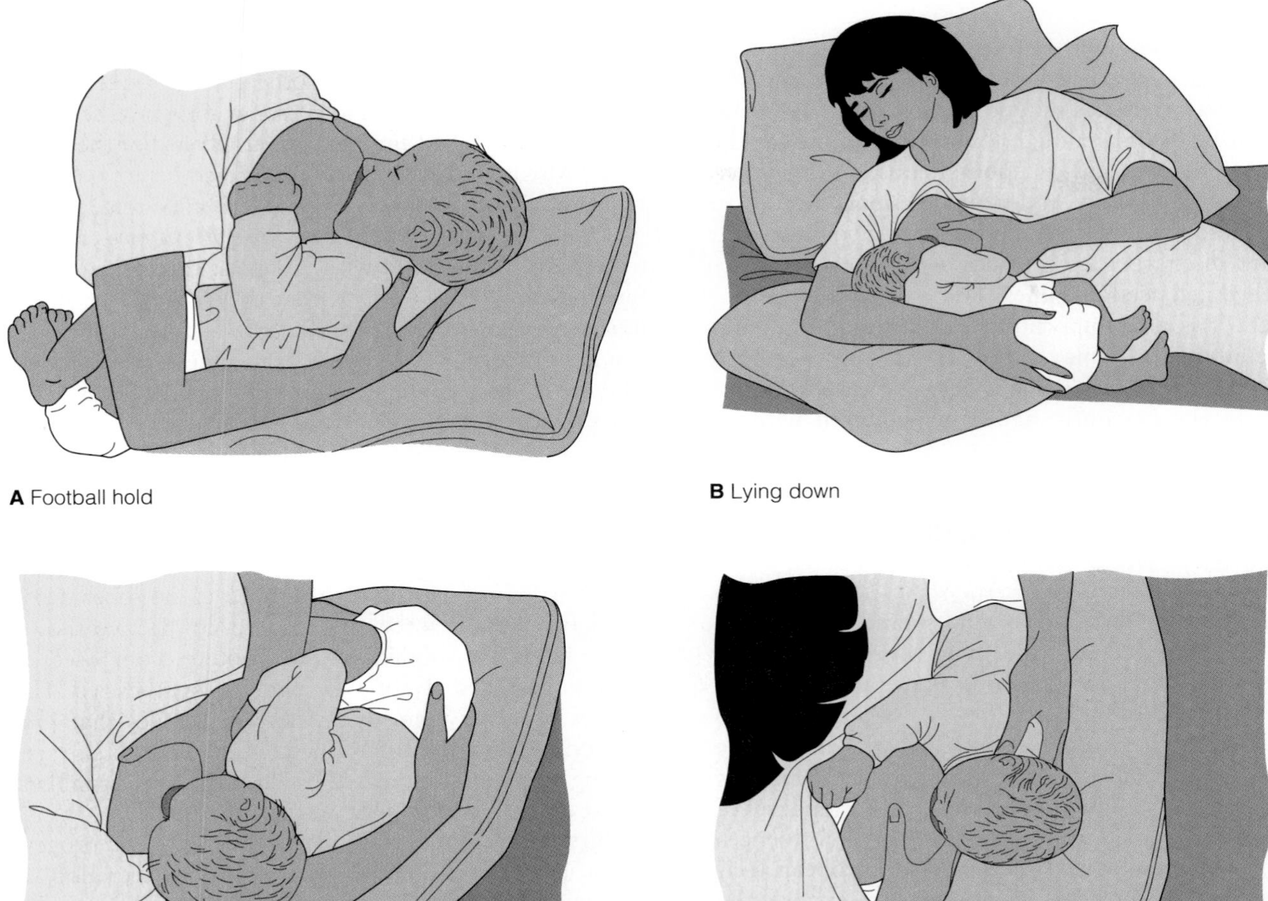

A Football hold

B Lying down

C Cradling

D Across the lap

FIGURE 24–2 Four common breastfeeding positions.

Source: *Breastfeeding: A Special Relationship.* Eagle Video Productions, Raleigh, NC. Copyright Lactation Consultants of NC.

her hands, and assuming a position of comfort. The woman who has had a cesarean birth needs support so that the infant does not rest on her abdomen for long periods of time. If she is breastfeeding, she may be more comfortable lying on her side with a pillow behind her back and one between her legs. The nurse can position the newborn next to the woman's breast and place a rolled towel or small pillow behind the infant for support. At first the mother will need assistance turning from side to side and burping the newborn. She may prefer to breastfeed sitting up with a pillow on her lap and the infant resting on the pillow rather than directly on her abdomen. It may be helpful to place a rolled pillow under the arm supporting the infant's head. An alternative position that avoids pressure on the incision while allowing for maximum visualization of the infant's face is the football hold. See Figure 24–2 for a variety of breastfeeding positions.

Bottle-feeding mothers who have undergone cesarean birth frequently use the sitting position also. If incisional pain makes this position difficult, the bottle-feeding mother may also find it helpful to assume the side-lying position. The infant can be positioned in a semisitting position against a pillow close to the mother.

Depending on the newborn's level of hunger, the parents may want to use the time before feeding to get acquainted with their infant. The presence of the nurse during part of this time to answer questions and provide reinforcement of parenting skills will be helpful for the family. For the sleepy baby, a period of playful activity—such as gently rubbing the feet and hands or adjusting clothing and loosening coverings to expose the infant to room air—may increase alertness so that, when the feeding is initiated, the infant is ready and sucks eagerly. If an infant is overly hungry and upset, talking quietly and rocking gently may provide the baby with an opportunity to calm down so that he or she can find and grasp the nipple effectively. After the feeding, when the infant is satisfied and asleep, parents may explore the characteristics unique to their newborn. Routines must be flexible enough to allow this time for the family. Rooming-in offers spontaneous, frequent encounters for the family and provides opportunities to practice handling skills, thereby increasing confidence in care after discharge. It also allows for demand rather than scheduled feeding times, and this should be encouraged. It is also important to understand and support the mother who may choose to have her newborn cared for in the nursery if she is being dismissed to care for herself, the newborn, and other children without adult help.

Cultural Considerations in Infant Feeding

It is important for the nurse to understand how culture and society influence infant feeding. Motherhood itself changes the woman's lifestyle. Perceptions of the mother's role and of breastfeeding as a biologic act also influence the mother's comfort with breastfeeding. Some mothers identify shame, modesty, and embarrassment as reasons they chose not to breastfeed. The amount of body contact considered acceptable also influences parental behaviors. North American and European societies sometimes consider it indecent to expose the breast, believe that too much handling spoils children, and regard weaning as a sign of infant development (Lawrence 1994b).

The nurse also needs to understand the impact of culture on the idiosyncrasies of specific feeding practices. For example, in many cultures (Mexican-American, Navajo, Filipino, and Vietnamese) and in some countries (Guinea, Pakistan) colostrum is not offered to the newborn (Gunnlaugsson et al 1994). Breastfeeding begins only after the milk flow is established. In many Asian cultures the newborn is given boiled water until the mother's milk flows. The newborn is fed on demand and cries are responded to immediately. If the crying continues, evil spirits may be blamed and a priest's blessing may be sought. Although many of the Hmong women of Laos combine breastfeeding with some bottle-feeding, they usually find it unacceptable to express their milk or pump their breasts. Thus other methods of providing relief should be suggested if breast engorgement develops (LaDu 1985). Most Muslim mothers breastfeed because the Qur'an encourages it until the child is 2 years old (Hutchinson and Baqi-Aziz 1994). Japanese women are returning to breastfeeding as the method of feeding for the baby's first year (Riordan 1991).

In the African-American culture, there tends to be an increased emphasis on plentiful feeding. Solid foods are introduced early and may even be added to the infant's formula. African-American mothers view frequent feeding as an expression of hardiness and a positive behavior characteristic for the future (Vezeau 1991). For the traditional Mexican, a fat baby is considered healthy and infants are fed on demand. "Spoiling" is encouraged.

These are but a few of the cultural practices related to feeding. When faced with an infant care practice different from the ones to which they are accustomed, nurses need to evaluate the effect of the practice. Just because a practice is different does not mean it is inferior. The nurse should intervene only if the practice is actually harmful to the mother and baby.

Physiology of the Breasts and Lactation

The female breast is divided into 15 to 24 lobes separated from one another by fat and connective tissue. These lobes are subdivided into lobules, composed of small units called alveoli where milk is synthesized. The lobules have a system of lactiferous ductiles that join larger ducts and eventually open onto the nipple surface. During pregnancy, increased levels of estrogen stimulate breast development in preparation for lactation.

Birth results in a rapid drop in estrogen and progesterone and a concomitant increase in the secretion of **prolactin.** This hormone promotes milk production by stimulating the alveolar cells of the breast. Prolactin levels rise in response to the infant suckling. **Oxytocin,** secreted by the posterior pituitary when the infant sucks on the mother's nipple, triggers the **letdown reflex,** or milk ejection reflex, and a flow of milk results. Mothers have described the letdown reflex as a prickling or tingling sensation during which they feel the milk coming down. Other signs of letdown include increased uterine cramps and increased lochia (during the early postpartum period), milk leaking from the other breast, and a feeling of relaxation. It is not unusual for the breasts to leak some milk before feeding.

The letdown reflex can be stimulated by the newborn's sucking, presence, or cry, or even by maternal thoughts about her baby. It may also occur during sexual orgasm because oxytocin is released. Conversely, the mother's lack of self-confidence or fear of embarrassment about, or pain connected with breastfeeding may prevent the milk from being ejected into the duct system.

Milk production decreases with repeated inhibition of the milk ejection reflex. Failure to empty the breasts frequently and completely also decreases production. As milk accumulates and is not withdrawn, the buildup of pressure in the alveoli suppresses secretion. Once lactation is well established, prolactin production decreases. Oxytocin and sucking continue to be the facilitators of milk production.

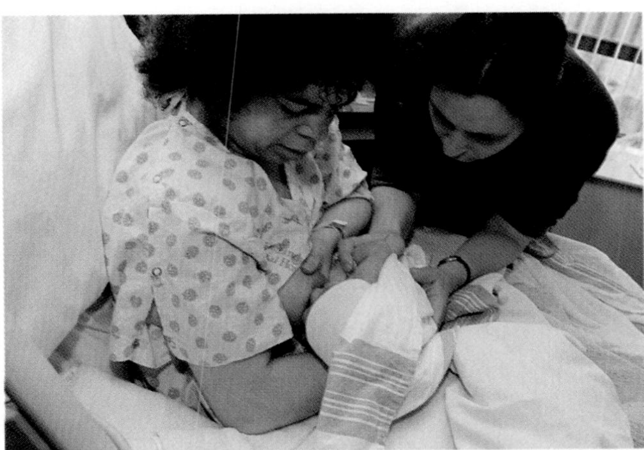

FIGURE 24–3 For many mothers, the nurse's support and knowledge are instrumental in establishing successful breastfeeding.

ESSENTIAL PRECAUTIONS FOR PRACTICE

During Breastfeeding

Examples of times when disposable gloves should be worn include the following:

- Assisting the mother to breastfeed the newborn immediately after birth
- Handling breast milk for breast milk banking
- Assisting with manual expression of breast milk
- Handling used breastfeeding pads

Excellent handwashing is essential when assisting a breastfeeding mother.

REMEMBER to wash your hands before putting on the disposable gloves and AGAIN immediately after you remove the gloves.

For further information consult OSHA and CDC guidelines.

Client Education for Breastfeeding Self-Care

Breastfeeding Process

The nurse caring for the breastfeeding mother should help the woman achieve independence and success in her feeding efforts (Figure 24–3). Prepared with a knowledge of the anatomy and physiology of the breast and lactation, the components and positive effects of breast milk, and techniques of breastfeeding, the nurse can help the woman and her family use their own resources to achieve a successful experience. The objectives involved in breastfeeding are to (a) provide adequate nutrition, (b) establish an adequate milk supply, and (c) prevent trauma to the nipples. All education is aimed toward these goals. When assisting the mother with breastfeeding, the nurse should use disposable gloves (see Essential Precautions for Practice: During Breastfeeding).

To facilitate successful breastfeeding, the nurse should arrange for privacy, help the mother find a comfortable position, and position the baby comfortably close to her. The mother should support her breast with her hand, using the C-hold or the scissors hold. In the C-hold the mother places her thumb well above the areola and the rest of her fingers below the areola and under the breast. For the scissors hold, the mother places her index finger above the areola and her other three fingers below the areola and under the breast. Either method of presenting the breast to the infant is acceptable as long as the mother's hand is well away from the nipple so the baby can "latch on" to the breast (Figure 24–4).

The mother should position the baby so that the nose is at the level of the nipple. She then lightly tickles the baby's lower lip with her nipple until the baby opens her or his mouth wide, and then brings the baby to the breast. The baby needs to take the whole nipple into the mouth so that the gums are on the areola. This allows the jaws to compress the milk ducts directly beneath the areola when the baby suckles. The baby's nose and chin should touch the breast. If the breast occludes the baby's airway, simply lifting up on the breast will usually clear the nares. The baby's lips should be relaxed and flanged outward with the tongue over the lower gum. At this point the baby should be facing the mother (tummy to tummy or chest to chest) with the ear, shoulder, and hip aligned (Figure 24–5).

During early feedings the infant should be offered both breasts at each feeding to stimulate the supply-demand response. In some cases the newborn will suckle only one breast well before falling asleep. As long as each breast is offered frequently (at least every 2 hours), single-breast feeds of whatever duration the baby wishes are appropriate until the baby shows a desire for both breasts (Woolridge and Baum 1993). The mother should breastfeed until she becomes relaxed to the point of sleepiness—a delightful side effect of oxytocin secretion (Mulford 1990)—or until she notes cues from the infant suggesting satiety (suckling activity ceases or the baby falls asleep). Recent literature suggests that imposing time limits for breastfeeding does not prevent nipple soreness and in fact interferes with successful feeding. For example, the length of nursing time necessary to stimulate the milk ejection reflex varies with the individual. If the mother feeds according to the clock and disengages the baby before letdown, the baby will not get the hindmilk. Because the hindmilk is higher in fat and

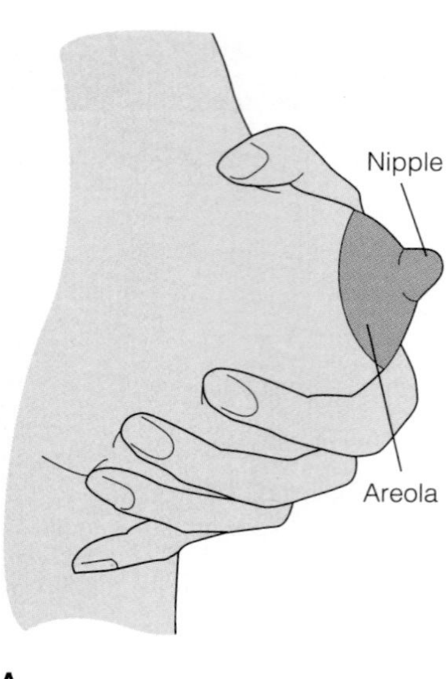

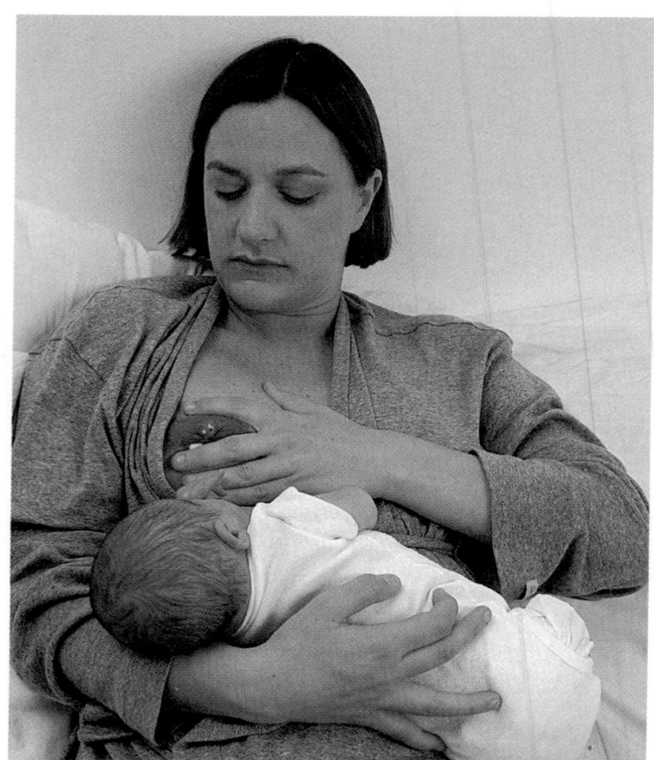

FIGURE 24–4 ***A*** C-hold. ***B*** Scissors hold.

Source: Courtesy Childbirth Graphics Ltd., Rochester, NY.

calories than the foremilk, the baby will be less satisfied, will need to nurse again sooner, and will gain less weight. The mother should learn to feed in response to her baby's cues and her body. If the mother wishes to end the feeding before the infant falls asleep or voluntarily detaches, she should break the suction by gently inserting her fingers between the baby's gums. Burping between feedings on each breast and at the end of the feeding continues to be necessary. If the infant has been crying, it is also advisable to burp before beginning feeding.

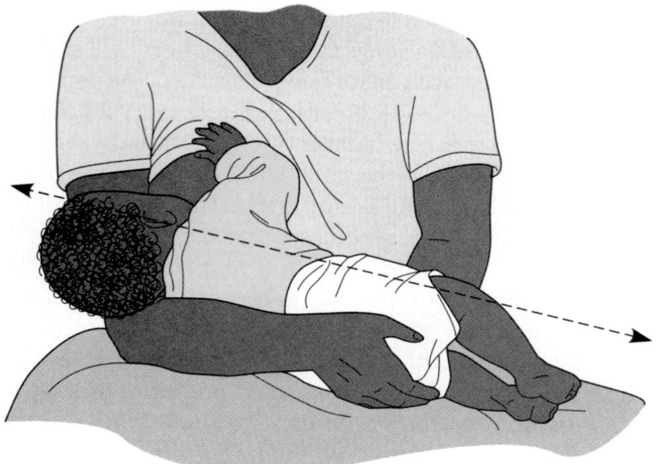

FIGURE 24–5 Infant in good breastfeeding position tummy-to-tummy, with ear, shoulder, and hip aligned.

Source: Adapted from Riodan J, Auerbach K: *Breastfeeding and Lactation.* Boston: Jones & Bartlett, 1993, p. 248.

Leaking

Initially more milk is produced than the infant requires. During the first few weeks, infant needs and maternal responses are not yet well attuned, daily variabilities of feeding frequency and duration are greatest, and most women experience breast leaking. The mother should expect this and use breast pads in her bra to absorb the secretions. She should be cautioned to remove wet pads frequently to avoid irritation to the nipples or infection. (Breast pads with plastic liners interfere with air circulation; the plastic should be removed before using them.) After breastfeeding is well established—usually after the first month—the mother may also be taught to apply direct pressure to the breast with her hand or forearm when leaking occurs.

Supplementary Feeding

The use of supplementary feedings for the breastfeeding infant may weaken or confuse the sucking reflex or decrease the infant's interest in nursing. The shape of the mouth and lips and the sucking mechanism needed for breastfeeding are different from those needed to suck on a bottle nipple. To suck on the breast, the infant's tongue moves front to back, squeezing the milk from the nipple. To suck on a rubber nipple, the tongue pushes forward against the nipple to control the milk flow. Some breastfeeding babies who are given supplementary bottles cannot adjust to these different techniques and push the mother's nipple out of their mouth in subsequent breastfeeding attempts. Breastfeeding mothers should avoid introducing bottles until breastfeeding is well established.

Often parents are concerned because they have no visual assurance about the amount consumed. The nurse should teach the mother the signs of milk transfer to the infant (audible swallowing, milk appearing in the baby's mouth, her breast feeling soft after feeding, milk leaking from the opposite breast) (Mulford 1992). In addition, if the infant gains weight and has six or more wet diapers without supplementary feedings of water or formula, he or she is receiving adequate amounts of milk. Activity levels and intervals between feedings may also indicate how satisfied the infant is. Parents should know that, because breast milk is more easily digested than formulas, the breastfed infant becomes hungry sooner. Thus the frequency of breastfeedings may be greater. The parents can also expect the infant to demand more frequent nursing during periods of growth spurts, such as 10 days to 2 weeks, 5 to 6 weeks, and 2.5 to 3 months (Bear and Tigges 1993).

Expression of Milk

If the mother who desires to breastfeed is unable to nurse for medical or workplace reasons, she must learn how to stimulate milk production and store the breast milk. The choice of method (manual or with breast pump) depends on the mother's physiologic capabilities to produce the desired amount of milk and her personal preference. During the early postpartum period, if the baby can't nurse at the breast (as in the case of some premature or sick infants), the mother needs frequent breast stimulation to establish and increase her milk supply to prepare for later breastfeeding (Lawrence 1994). She should use an electric breast pump at least eight times in each 24-hour period (Riordan and Auerbach 1993). Research has shown that a pulsatile electric pump and double setup (allowing both breasts to be stimulated simultaneously) results in higher prolactin levels and a greater volume of milk than does manual expression (Zinaman et al 1992). After lactation is established, milk expression may be accomplished by the method that the mother finds most effective and convenient.

To express her milk manually, the woman first washes her hands and then massages her breast to stimulate letdown. To massage her breast, the woman grasps the breast with both hands at the base of the breast near the chest wall. Using the palms of her hands she then firmly slides her hands toward her nipple. She repeats this process several times. She is then ready to begin hand expression. The woman generally uses her left hand for her right breast and right hand for her left breast. However, some women find it preferable to use the hand on the same side as the breast. The nurse should encourage the woman to use the method she finds most effective. She grasps the areola with her thumb on the top and her first two fingers on the lower portion (Figure 24–6). Without allowing her fingers to slide on her skin, she pushes inward toward the chest and then squeezes her fingers together while pulling forward on the areola. She can use a container to catch any fluid that is squeezed out. She then repositions her hand by rotating it slightly so that she can repeat the process. She continues to reposition her hand and repeat the process to empty all the milk sinuses.

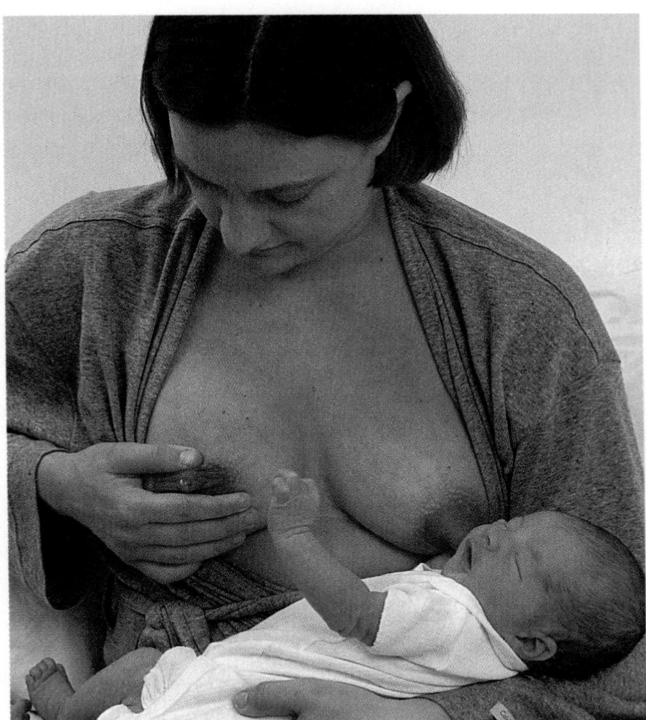

FIGURE 24–6 Hand position for manual expression of milk.

Breast pumps use suction to express milk. Some have collection systems to conveniently store the milk. Hand pumps are portable and inexpensive. Battery-operated pumps are more efficient than hand pumps but are also more expensive. Electric pumps (Figure 24–7) are more efficient but are bulky and expensive. They can be rented in many areas. Many agencies have a variety of pumps available and provide instruction on correct use (Table 24–3). Videotapes or photographs are also useful in demonstrating the process to new mothers.

TABLE 24–3 Recommendations for the Nursing Mother Who Uses a Pump

General Pumping Recommendations	Recommendations for Specific Types of Pumps
1. Read the instructions on the use and cleaning of a pump before expressing milk with any product. 2. Wash hands before each pumping session. 3. Frequency: For occasional pumping, pump during, after, or between feedings, whichever gives the best results. Most mothers tend to express more milk in the morning. For working mothers pumping should occur on a regular basis for the number of nursings that are missed. For premature or ill babies who are not at breast the number of pumpings should total eight or more in 24 hours. Initiation of pumping should be delayed no longer than 6 hours following birth unless medically indicated. This assures appropriate development and sensitivity of prolactin receptors. More frequent pumping will avoid the buildup of excessive back pressure of milk during engorgement. 4. Duration: With single-sided pumping optimal duration is 10 to 15 minutes with an electric pump and 10 to 20 minutes with a manual pump. If double pumping with an electric or two battery-operated pumps, 7 to 15 minutes is optimal. Encourage mothers to tailor these times to their own situation. 5. Technique: • Elicit the milk ejection reflex before using any pump. • Use only as much suction as is needed to maintain milk flow. • Massage the breast in quadrants during pumping to increase intramammary pressure. • Allow enough time for pumping to avoid anxiety. • Use inserts or different flanges if needed to obtain the best fit between pump and breast. • Avoid long periods of uninterrupted vacuum. • Stop pumping when the milk flow is minimal or has ceased.	1. Avoid pumps that use rubber bulbs to generate vacuum. 2. Cylinder pumps: • When "O" rings are used, they must be in place for proper suction. • Gaskets must be removed *after each use* for cleaning to avoid harboring bacteria in the pump. • The gasket on the inner cylinder may be rolled back and forth to restore it to its original shape. • The pump stroke may need to be shortened as the outer cylinder fills with milk. • The user may need to empty the outer cylinder once or twice during pumping. • Hand position should be palm up with the elbow held close to the body. 3. Battery-operated pumps: • Use alkaline batteries. • Replace batteries when cycles per minute decrease. • Interrupt vacuum frequently to avoid nipple pain and damage. • Use an AC adapter when possible, especially if the pump generates fewer than six cycles per minute. • Consider renting an electric pump for pumping that will continue for longer than 1 or 2 months. • Use two pumps simultaneously if pumping time is limited or to increase the quantity of milk obtained. • Choose a pump in which the vacuum can be regulated. • Massage the breast by quadrants during pumping. 4. Semiautomatic pumps: • Vacuum may be easier to control if the mother does not lift her finger completely off the hole but rolls it back and forth rhythmically so that the vacuum is efficient but not painful. 5. Automatic electric pumps: • Use the lowest pressure setting that is efficient. • Use a double setup (simultaneous pumping) when time is limited to increase the milk supply and for prematurity, maternal or infant illness, or other special situations.

Source: Riordan J, Auerbach K: *Breastfeeding and Human Lactation.* Boston: Jones & Bartlett, 1993, p 283.

Storing Breast Milk

Breast milk can be stored for up to 6 hours at room temperature or up to 5 days in a refrigerator. If breast milk is to be refrigerated and then fed to the infant, it should be stored in clean plastic containers because the white blood cells will adhere to glass, and their protective effect will be lost. Breast milk can be frozen in either glass or plastic because freezing destroys the white blood cells anyway. Breast milk can be stored in a freezer compartment inside the refrigerator for up to 2 weeks, in a self-contained freezer unit of a refrigerator for up to 1 month, and in a separate deep freeze unit at 0 degrees for up to 6 months. Frozen breast milk can be thawed by running warm water over the container. The container should then be shaken well to return the fat molecules, which separate during freezing, to suspension.

External Supports

Breastfeeding mothers who work outside the home and who receive support for their decision tend to breastfeed their infants for longer periods of time (Fendrick et al 1994).

La Leche League is an organized group of volunteers who work to provide education about breastfeeding and assistance to women who are breastfeeding infants. Organized as small, neighborhood-based groups, it sponsors activities, has printed material available, has electric breast pumps available for rental, offers one-to-one counseling to mothers with questions or problems, and provides group support to breastfeeding mothers. Lactation consultants offer a variety of services through private practice and health care facilities.

Numerous books and pamphlets are also available to help the breastfeeding mother. The mother needs the

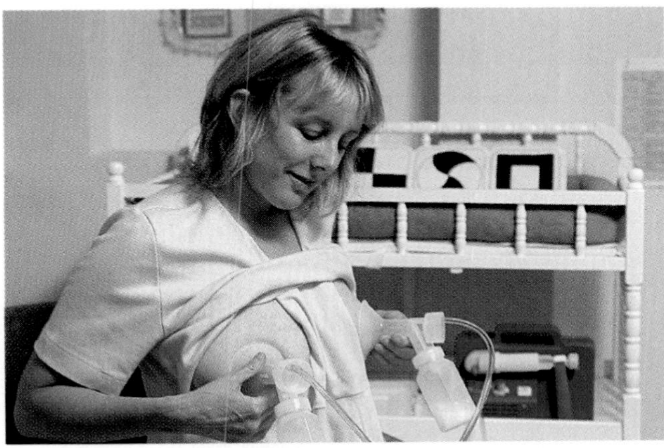

FIGURE 24–7 Mother using electric breast pump and double setup.

support of all family members, her physician/certified nurse-midwife, pediatrician or pediatric nurse practitioner, and all nursing personnel, because it is often the attitudes of these people that ultimately lead the woman to success or failure.

Drugs and Breastfeeding

It has long been recognized that certain medications taken by the mother may have an effect on her infant. It should be noted that: (1) most drugs pass into breast milk, (2) almost all medications appear in only small amounts in human milk (usually less than 1 percent of the maternal dosage), and (3) very few drugs are contraindicated for breastfeeding women. Concerns about the consequences of the presence of drugs in breast milk focus on the infant and on the milk volume.

Other variables that affect the passage of drugs into breast milk include the amount of the drug taken, the frequency and route of administration, and the timing of the dose in relationship to infant feeding. The drug's effects are influenced by the infant's age, the feeding frequency, the volume of milk taken, and the degree of absorption through the gastrointestinal tract.

Four adjustments should be made to decrease the effects on the infant when administering drugs to a nursing mother (Lawrence 1994):

1. Avoid long-acting forms of drugs. The infant may have difficulty excreting them and accumulation may be a problem.
2. Consider absorption rates and peak blood levels in scheduling the administration of the drugs. Less of the drug crosses into the milk if the medication is given immediately after the woman has nursed her baby.
3. Closely observe the infant for any signs of drug reaction, including rash, fussiness, lethargy, or changes in sleeping or feeding patterns.
4. Whenever alternatives are available, select the drug that shows the least tendency to pass into breast milk.

The mother should be given information about the potential of most drugs to cross into breast milk (American Academy of Pediatrics Committee on Drugs 1994). She must also be advised to tell any physician who may prescribe medications for her that she is breastfeeding.

In counseling the nursing mother, the health care provider should weigh the benefits of the medication against the possible risk to the infant and its possible effect on the breastfeeding process. The potential risk to the infant must also be weighed against the effect of interrupting breastfeeding.

Selected Potential Problems in Breastfeeding

Because mothers are discharged from the birthing unit before breastfeeding is well established, they are frequently alone when they encounter changes in the breastfeeding process. Many women stop nursing if the situations they encounter seem problematic. The nurse can offer anticipatory guidance regarding common breastfeeding phenomena and provide resources for the woman's use after discharge. Table 24–4 summarizes self-care measures the nurse can suggest to a woman with a breastfeeding problem.

Nipple Soreness The mother should be told that some discomfort often occurs initially with breastfeeding, peaking between the third and sixth days, and then receding (Riordan and Auerbach 1993). The infant should not be switched to bottle-feeding or have feedings delayed because these measures will cause engorgement and more soreness. Discomfort that lasts throughout the feeding or past the first week demands attention. The baby's position at the breast is one of the most critical factors in nipple soreness. The mother's hand should be off the areola, and the baby should be facing the mother's chest with ear, shoulder, and hip aligned (see Figure 24–5). Because the area of greatest stress to the nipple is in line with the newborn's chin and nose, nipple soreness may be decreased by encouraging the mother to rotate positions when feeding the infant. Changing positions alters the focus of greatest stress and promotes more complete breast emptying.

Nipple soreness may also develop if the infant has faulty sucking habits. Nipples may have injured tips that are bruised, scabbed, or blistered from the nipple entering the baby's mouth at an upward angle and rubbing against the roof of the mouth (Lawrence 1994b). Soreness may also be due to continuous negative pressure if the infant falls asleep with the breast in his or her mouth (Ziemer et al 1990).

Chewed nipples, which result from improper positioning, are cracked or tender at or near the base. In

TABLE 24–4 Breastfeeding Problems and Remedies

Nipples Not Graspable

Flat or inverted nipples

- Use Hoffman technique to break adhesions.
- Wear milk cups to encourage nipples to protrude.
- Use nipple tug and roll to increase protractility.
- Form the nipple prior to nursing by hand shaping, ice, wearing milk cups a half-hour before feeding.
- As a last resort, use nipple shield for first few minutes of feeding to draw out nipple; then place baby on breast.

Engorged breasts

- Treat engorgement by relieving fullness with hand expression of milk prior to nursing and instituting frequent feeding so nipple is more prominent.

Large breasts

- Support breast with opposite hand, or use rolled towel under breast to bring nipple to the level of baby's mouth.
- Use C-hold to make nipple accessible to baby.

Engorgement

Missed or infrequent feedings

- Nurse frequently (every $1\frac{1}{2}$ hours).
- Massage and hand express or pump to empty breasts completely when feedings are missed or when a full feeling develops in breasts and baby is not available or willing to nurse.

Breasts not emptied at feedings

- Nurse long enough to empty breasts (10–15 minutes on each side at each feeding).
- If baby will not nurse long enough to empty breasts, hand express or pump after feeding.

Inadequate letdown

- Use relaxation techniques, massage, and warm or cool compresses before nursing.
- Relax in warm shower with water running from back over shoulders and breasts, hand expressing to relieve fullness.
- If due to anxiety, try to eliminate the source of tension.

Baby sleepy or not eager to nurse

- Use rousing techniques (eg, hold baby upright, unwrap blanket, change diaper).
- Pre-express milk onto nipple or baby's lips to entice baby.
- Avoid use of bottles of water or formula; these will decrease baby's willingness to suckle.

Inadequate Letdown

Letdown not well established

- Give the baby ample time at the breast (at least 15 minutes per side) to allow for letdown and complete emptying.
- Nurse in a quiet spot away from distractions.
- Massage breasts before nursing.
- Drink juice, water, tea (no caffeine) before and during nursing.
- Condition letdown by setting up a routine for beginning feedings.
- Use relaxation and breathing techniques.
- Stimulate the nipple manually before nursing.
- Concentrate thought on the baby and milk flow; turn on a faucet so that the sound of running water helps stimulate letdown.
- Use synthetic oxytocin nasal spray several times during a feeding. (This should condition letdown within 24 hours. Then it is no longer needed. Spray must be prescribed by a doctor.)

Mother overtired or overextended

- Nap or rest when the baby rests.
- Lie down to nurse.
- Nurse the baby in bed at night.
- Simplify daily chores; set priorities.

Mother tense, pressured

- Identify the causes of tensions and eliminate or minimize them.
- Decrease fatigue.

Mother caught in cycle of little milk, worry, less milk

- Try all the actions above.
- Develop confidence in mothering skills. (A home visit by a counselor may help.)

Source: Adapted from Lauwers J, Woessner C: *Counseling the Nursing Mother: A Reference Handbook for Health Care Providers and Lay Counselors,* 2nd ed. Garden City Park, NY: Avery, 1990, pp 385–397.

these cases, the baby's jaws close only on the nipple instead of the areola, or the baby's mouth is not opened wide enough, or the infant's mouth has slipped down to the nipple from the areola as a result of engorgement. Soreness on the underside of the nipple is caused by the infant nursing with her or his bottom lip tucked in rather than out, causing a friction burn. Vigorous sucking produces little milk because the milk sinuses under the areola are not compressed. This results in a frustrated infant and marked soreness for the mother. The problem is overcome by positioning the infant with as much areola as possible in his or her mouth and rotating the baby's positions at the breast.

Nipple soreness is especially pronounced during the first few minutes of the feeding. If the mother is not expecting this, she may become discouraged and quickly stop. The letdown reflex may take a few minutes to activate, and it may not occur if the mother stops nursing too quickly. The problem is compounded if the infant is unsatisfied, and the possibility of breast engorgement increases.

Because nipple soreness can also result from an overeager infant, the mother may find it helpful to nurse more frequently. This helps ease the vigorous sucking of a ravenous infant. The woman can also apply ice to her nipples and areola for a few minutes before feeding. This promotes nipple erectness and numbs the tissue to ease the initial discomfort. To prevent excoriation and skin breakdown, the nipples and areola should be washed with water and then allowed to dry thoroughly. Drying may be accomplished by leaving the bra flaps down for a few minutes after feeding or by exposing the

TABLE 24–4 continued

Cracked Nipples

All causes of sore nipples carried to extreme

- Refer to all actions for sore nipples.
- Consult doctor about using aspirin, Tylenol, or other painkiller.
- Improve nutritional status, increasing protein, vitamin C, zinc.

Local infection (baby with staph or other organism may have infected mother's nipples)

- Refer to physician.

Plugged Ducts

Poor positioning

- Try a variety of positions for complete emptying.

Incomplete emptying of breast

- Nurse at least 10 minutes per side after letdown.
- Alternate nursing positions.
- If baby does not empty breasts, pump or express milk after feedings.

External pressure on breast

- Use larger size bras, insert bra extender, or go braless.
- Use nursing bra instead of pulling up conventional bra to nurse to avoid pressure on ducts.
- Avoid bunching up sweater or nightgown under arm during nursing.

Sore Nipples

Poor positioning

- Alternate nursing positions throughout the day.
- Bring the baby close to nurse so the baby does not pull on the breast.
- Place the nipple and some of the areola in the baby's mouth.
- Check to ensure the baby is put on and off the breast properly.
- Check to ensure the nipple is back far enough in the baby's mouth.
- Hold the baby closely during nursing so the nipple is not constantly being pulled.

Baby chewing or nuzzling onto nipple

- Form the nipple for the baby.
- Set up a pattern of getting the baby onto the breast using the rooting reflex.

Baby nursing on end of nipple

- Ensure the nipple is way back in the baby's mouth by getting the baby properly onto the breast.
- Check for an inverted nipple.
- Check for engorgement.

Baby chewing his or her way off the nipple (nipple being pulled out of baby's mouth at end of feeding)

- Remove the baby from the breast by placing a finger between the baby's gums to ensure suction is broken.
- End feeding when the baby's suckling slows, before he or she has a chance to chew on the nipple.

Baby overly eager to nurse

- Nurse more often.
- Pre-express milk to hasten letdown, avoiding vigorous suckling.

Dried colostrum or milk causing nipple to stick to bra or breast pads

- Moisten bra or pads before taking off so as not to remove keratin.

Nipples not allowed to dry

- Remove plastic liners from milk pads.
- Air dry breast completely after nursing.
- Change milk pads frequently.

Improper use of breast shield

- Use shield only to draw out nipple; then have the baby nurse on the breast.
- Cut tip of shield back bit by bit and eventually discard.

Nipple skin not resistant to stress

- Improve diet, especially adding fresh fruits and vegetables and vitamin supplements.
- Eliminate or decrease use of sugary foods, alcohol, caffeine, cigarettes.
- Check use of cleansing or drying agents.

Natural oils removed or keratin layers broken down by drying agents (soap, alcohol, shampoo, deodorant)

- Eliminate irritants.
- Wash breasts with water only.

nipples to sunlight or ultraviolet light, for 30 seconds at first and gradually increasing to 3 minutes. Drying the nipples with a hair dryer on low heat setting has been suggested as it also facilitates drying and promotes healing, especially if breast milk is allowed to dry on the nipples (Lawrence 1994b).

The use of substances such as lanolin, Massé Breast Cream, Eucerin cream, or A and D ointment on the nipples between feedings should be discouraged. These preparations may cause allergic reactions, and irritation may increase if the substance needs to be washed off before nursing. The substance may also be contaminated.

In very dry environments, however, creams may be appropriate. Lanolin is most hazardous to women with wool allergy (Lawrence 1994b). Lansinoh is a purified, alcohol-free, and "allergen-free" ointment that is considered safe if an ointment is indicated. Alternatively, applying breast milk and allowing it to dry on the nipples has been shown to heal sore nipples rapidly (Huml 1995). Breast milk is high in fat, fights infection, and will not irritate the nipples. An obvious advantage is that it is readily available at no cost to the mother.

If the woman finds that her bra or clothing rubs against her nipples and adds to her discomfort, she may insert shields into her bra. Both Medela Shells and Woolrich Shields, for example, relieve friction and promote air circulation. If a woman uses breast pads inside her bra to keep milk from leaking onto her clothes, she should change the pads frequently so the nipples remain dry.

CRITICAL THINKING IN ACTION

Ann calls you from home in tears on her third postpartum day. She states that, although breastfeeding was going well in the hospital, her breasts are now swollen, hard, and very painful, and her baby is refusing to suckle. Ann expresses extreme disappointment that "the breastfeeding didn't work" because she truly believes that breast milk is best for babies and she had enjoyed her breastfeeding experience in the hospital, especially nursing the baby immediately after delivery. But she also states she has not been able to stop crying all day and can no longer tolerate her painful breasts. In addition she says that the baby "seems happier" with the bottle. What would you do?

Answers can be found in Appendix H.

Older remedies for nipple soreness are receiving renewed acceptance. For instance, tea bags may be moistened in warm water and applied to the nipples. The tannic acid seems to help toughen the nipples, and the warmth is soothing and promotes healing. However, tannic acid can cause drying and cracking and is not appropriate in all situations (Lawrence 1994b).

Nipple dermatitis, which causes swollen, erythematous, burning nipples, is most commonly caused by thrush or by allergic response to breast cream preparations. If the nipple soreness has a sudden onset and is accompanied by burning or itching, shooting pains through the breast, and a deep pink coloration of the nipple, it may be caused by a thrush infection transmitted from the infant to the mother. White patches or streaks in the infant's mouth indicate a need for treatment of the mouth and nipple infection. The disease can be treated with a variety of antifungal preparations and does not preclude breastfeeding.

Cracked Nipples Nipple soreness is frequently coupled with cracked nipples. Whenever a breastfeeding mother complains of soreness, the nipples must be carefully examined for fissures or cracks, and the mother should be observed during breastfeeding to see whether the infant is correctly positioned at the breast. If the positioning is correct and cracks exist, interventions are necessary. The mother's first reaction may be to cease nursing on the sore breast, but this may aggravate the problem if engorgement and plugged ducts result. All the interventions described for sore nipples may be used. It may also help the mother to begin nursing on the breast that is less sore. This allows the letdown reflex to occur in the affected breast, and the infant does more vigorous sucking on the less tender breast, which decreases trauma to the cracked nipple.

With severe cases, the temporary use of a nipple shield for nursing may be necessary, although it is a last resort. For the mother's comfort, analgesics may be taken after nursing.

Breast Engorgement A distinction should be made between breast fullness and engorgement. All lactating women experience a transition fullness at first. This is caused by venous congestion and later by accumulating milk. However, this generally lasts only 24 hours, the breasts remain soft enough for the newborn to suckle, and there is no pain. Engorged breasts are hard, painful, and warm, and appear taut and shiny.

The infant should suckle for an average of 15 minutes per feeding and should feed at least eight times in 24 hours (Riordan and Auerbach 1993). If the baby is unable to nurse more frequently, the mother may express some milk manually or with a pump, being careful not to traumatize the breast tissue. Warm or cool compresses before nursing stimulate letdown and soften the breast so that the infant can more easily grasp the areola. The mother should wear a well-fitting nursing bra 24 hours a day. The bra supports the breasts and prevents further discomfort from tension and pulling on the Cooper's ligament. Analgesics such as acetaminophen or aspirin, alone or in combination with codeine, are appropriate, especially if taken just before nursing. The pain will be relieved, but the medication will not reach the milk for at least 30 minutes (Lawrence 1994b).

Plugged Ducts Some mothers experience plugging of one or more ducts, especially in conjunction with or following engorgement. This is often referred to as "caked breasts." Manifested as an area of tenderness or "lumpiness" in an otherwise well woman, plugging may be relieved by the use of heat and massage. The nurse can encourage the mother to massage her breasts from her chest wall forward to the nipple while standing in a warm shower or following the application of moist heat to the breast (Riordan and Auerbach 1993). She should then nurse her infant, starting on the unaffected breast if the plugged breast is tender. Frequent nursing and trying a variety of positions to ensure complete emptying will help prevent the problem. In cases of repeatedly plugged ducts or caked breasts, it may be necessary for the mother to limit her fat intake to polyunsaturated fats and to add lecithin to her diet (Lawrence 1994b).

Breastfeeding and the Working Mother

The best preparation for maintaining lactation after return to work is frequent, unlimited breastfeeding and enjoying the baby. Even when planned, the first day back to work may be fraught with emotional and physical distresses. Anticipatory guidance from the nurse may facilitate the transition from maternity leave to work. The earlier the breastfeeding mother returns to work, the more often she will need to pump her breasts to express the breast milk (Riordan and Auerbach 1993). Because milk production follows the principle of supply and demand, if breasts are not pumped, the milk supply will decrease. An electric breast pump and double collection system are considered the optimal means of milk expression. But this is not the only method; mechanical means may not suit some women (Neifert 1994). Sometimes a mother has a flexible schedule and can return home or have the baby brought to her to nurse at lunch time. If this is not possible, the infant may be fed expressed milk. For proper storage of breast milk, see Storing Breast Milk earlier in this chapter. When the mother is absent, the infant can be bottle-fed or spoon-fed. If the baby is 3 months or older, cup-feeding is an option. The mother should wait until lactation is well established before introducing the bottle. Most babies will adjust to the bottle within 7–10 days.

To maintain an adequate milk supply, the working mother must pay special attention to her fluid intake. She can ensure adequate intake by drinking extra fluid at each break and whenever possible during the day. It is also helpful to nurse more on weekends, nurse during the night, eat a nutritionally sound diet, and continue manual expression or pumping when not nursing (Neifert 1994).

Night nursing presents a dilemma: it may help a working mother maintain her milk supply, but it may also contribute to fatigue. Some women choose to have the infant sleep with them so that breastfeeding is more easily accomplished. Other women find it difficult to sleep soundly when the infant is in the same bed. For the mother who works long hours or has a rigid work schedule, the best alternative may be to limit breastfeeding to morning and evening feedings with supplemental feedings at other times. This choice allows her to maintain a close relationship with the infant and provides some of the unique benefits of breast milk. Pinella and Birch (1993) found that the use of focal feeds (feeding between 10 and midnight) and teaching parents how to help their babies develop self-soothing activities can help the infant and mother sleep for longer intervals at night.

Weaning

The decision to wean the baby from the breast may be made for a variety of reasons including family or cultural pressures, changes in the home situation, pressure from the woman's partner, or a personal opinion about when **weaning** should occur. For the woman who is comfortable with breastfeeding and well informed about the process, the appropriate time to wean her infant will become evident if she is sensitive to the child's cues. Often weaning falls between periods of great developmental activity for the child. Thus weaning commonly occurs at 8 to 9 months, 12 to 14 months, 18 months, 2 years, and 3 years of age. Within our society, however, weaning commonly occurs before the child is 9 months old, although it may occur any time from soon after birth to 4 years of age (Barness 1990). The infant may give weaning signals as early as 5 or 6 months of age (Furman 1995).

If weaning is timed to respond to the child's cues, and if the mother is comfortable with the timing, it can be accomplished with less difficulty than if the process begins before mother and child are ready emotionally. Nevertheless, weaning is a time of emotional separation for mother and baby; it may be difficult for them to give up the closeness of their nursing sessions. The nurse who is understanding about this possibility can help the mother see that her infant is growing up and plan other comforting, consoling, and play activities to replace breastfeeding. A gradual approach is the easiest and most comforting way to wean the child from breastfeedings. Other activities can enhance the parent-infant attachment process.

During weaning, the mother should substitute one cup-feeding or bottle-feeding for one breastfeeding session over a couple of days to a week so that her breasts gradually produce less milk. Eliminating the breastfeedings associated with meals first facilitates the mother's ability to wean the infant, as satiation with food lessens the desire for milk. Over a period of several weeks she needs to substitute more cup-feedings or bottle-feedings for breastfeedings. Many mothers continue to nurse once a day in the early morning or late evening for several months until the milk supply is gone. The slow method of weaning prevents breast engorgement, allows infants to alter their eating methods at their own rates, and provides time for psychologic adjustment.

Client Education for Bottle-Feeding

The mother who has chosen to bottle-feed her infant should be encouraged to assume a comfortable position with adequate arm support so she can easily hold her infant. Most women cradle their infants in the crook of the arm close to the body, which provides the intimacy and cuddling so essential to an infant and provides the same benefits of closeness as breastfeeding. With the great emphasis placed on successful breastfeeding, the teaching needs of the bottle-feeding new mother may be overlooked. If she has had only limited experience in feeding infants, she may need some guidelines to feed her newborn successfully. The nurse can provide teaching including the following important principles:

1. Always hold bottles; never prop them. Positional otitis media may develop if the infant is fed horizontally, because milk and nasal mucus may block the eustachian tube. Holding the infant provides social and close physical contact for the baby and an opportunity for parent-child interaction and bonding (Figure 24–8).

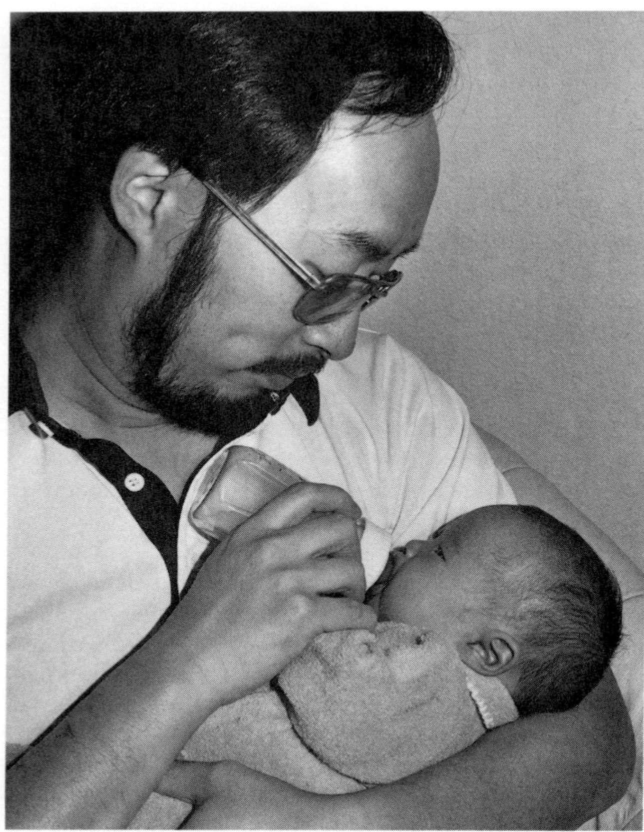

FIGURE 24–8 An infant is supported comfortably during bottle-feeding.

2. The nipple should have a hole big enough to allow milk to flow in drops when the bottle is inverted. Too large an opening may cause overfeeding or regurgitation because of rapid feeding. If feeding is too fast, change the nipple and help the infant to eat more slowly by stopping the feeding frequently for burping and cuddling.
3. Point the nipple directly into the mouth, not toward the palate or tongue, and place it on top of the tongue. The nipple should be full of liquid at all times to avoid ingestion of extra air, which decreases the amount of feeding and increases discomfort.
4. Burp the infant at intervals, preferably at the middle and end of the feeding. The infant who seems to swallow a great deal of air while sucking may need more frequent burping. In addition, if the infant has cried before being fed, air may have been swallowed, and the infant should be burped before beginning to feed or after taking enough to calm down. To burp, hold the infant upright on the shoulder or in a sitting position on the feeder's lap with chin and chest supported on one hand. Then gently pat or stroke the infant's back with the other hand. Too-frequent burping may confuse a newborn who is attempting to coordinate sucking, swallowing, and breathing.
5. Newborns frequently regurgitate small amounts of feedings. This may look like a large amount to the inexperienced parent, but it is normal. Initially it may be due to excessive mucus and gastric irritation from foreign substances in the stomach from birth. Later, regurgitation may result when the infant feeds too rapidly and swallows air. It may also occur when the infant is overfed and the cardiac sphincter allows the excess to be regurgitated. Because this is a common occurrence, experienced mothers and nurses generally keep a "burp cloth" available. Although regurgitation is normal, vomiting or a forceful expulsion of fluid is not. When forceful expulsion occurs, further evaluation may be indicated, especially if other symptoms are present.
6. A fat baby is not necessarily a healthy one. Avoid overfeeding or feeding infants every time they cry. Encourage but do not force the infant to feed and allow the infant to set the pace once feedings are established. Parents sometimes set artificial goals—"the baby must take all 5 ounces"—and keep feeding the child until those goals are met, even though the infant may not be hungry. Overfeeding results in infant obesity. During early feedings, however, the infant may need simple tactile stimulation—such as gently rubbing feet and hands, adjusting clothing, and loosening coverings—to maintain adequate sucking for a sufficient time to complete a full feeding.

It is important to discuss formula preparation and sterilization techniques with families. Cleanliness remains an essential component but sterilization is necessary only if the water source is questionable. Parents can prepare bottles in the dishwasher or thoroughly hand wash in warm soapy water and rinse well. Nipples may be weakened by the temperature of dishwashers and therefore should be washed thoroughly by hand and rinsed well. Tap water from an uncontaminated source may be used for mixing powdered formulas, which are less expensive than the concentrated or ready-to-use formulas. Honey should not be used as a sugar source because of the danger of infant botulism (Mott et al 1990).

Bottles may be prepared individually or a day's supply of formula may be prepared at one time. Extra bottles can be stored in the refrigerator and warmed slightly before feeding. Ready-to-use disposable bottles of formula are very convenient, but they are expensive. See Key Facts to Remember: Formula Preparation.

Nutritional Assessment of the Infant

During the early months of life, the food offered to and consumed by infants will be instrumental in their proper growth and development. At each well-baby visit the nurse assesses the nutritional status of the newborn. Assessment should include four components:

- Nutritional history from the parent
- Weight gain since the last visit
- Growth chart percentiles
- Physical examination

The nutritional history reports the type, amount, and frequency of milk, supplemental foods, vitamins, and minerals being given to the infant on a daily basis. If the baby is taking formula, the history also includes how the formula is mixed (checking for under- or over-dilution) and stored. The healthy formula-fed infant should generally gain 1 ounce per day for the first 6 months of life and 0.5 ounce per day for the second 6 months. Healthy breastfed babies may fall within these weight-gain parameters but may also be normal while gaining 0.5 ounce per day for the first 6 months.

Individual charts show the infant's growth with respect to height, weight, and head circumference. The important consideration is that infants continue to grow at their own individual rates.

If a breastfeeding mother is concerned about whether her infant is getting adequate nutrition, the nurse can recommend looking for an appearance of weight gain and counting the number of wet diapers in a 24-hour period. Six wet diapers or more in a day indicates adequate nutrition is being attained in the totally breastfed infant. If additional water is ingested, the diaper count should be higher. The presence of urine can most accurately be assessed when the diaper is free of feces, generally just before feedings. The gastrocolic reflex often stimulates stooling after a feeding. Another way for the anxious parents to reassure themselves of adequate intake and output is to keep a record of the frequency and duration of feedings and the exact number of wet or soiled diapers. Keeping a record tends to give the worried parent a sense of control and a tangible indication on which to rule out or base concern. See Key Facts to Remember: Successful Breastfeeding Evaluation.

The physical examination will assist in identifying any nutritional disorders. Iron deficiency should be suspected in an obese infant who is pale, diaphoretic, and irritable.

By calculating the nutritional needs of infants, the nurse can recommend a diet that supplies appropriate nutrition for infant growth and development. The assessment is especially helpful in counseling mothers of infants under 6 months of age, since there is a tendency

KEY FACTS TO REMEMBER

Formula Preparation

Ready to Feed (20 kcal/oz) (available in 32 oz cans or 4 oz bottles):

Use within 30 minutes to 1 hour once opened.

Do not dilute. Use directly from can, no mixing required.

Just add clean nipple to bottle.

Most expensive type of formula preparation.

Formula Concentrate (available in 13 oz cans):

Mix equal amounts of concentrate and water from uncontaminated source. This provides a 20 kcal/30 mL (1 oz) dilution. For example, for a 4 oz feeding mix 2 oz of formula concentrate with 2 oz water.

Wash punch-type can opener and top of formula can before opening.

Prepare a single feeding by measuring water and liquid directly into nursing bottle.

Cover opened concentrate formula cans with foil or plastic wrap and refrigerate until next bottle is made up.

Powdered Formula (52 scoops per can):

Mix one unpacked level scoop of powdered formula with each 60 mL (2 oz) of warm water.

Always pour water into bottle first; then add powder and stir well.

Make sure the powder and water are well mixed to ensure the formula composition is 20 kcal/30 mL (1 oz).

After opening, keep can tightly covered and use contents within 1 month to assure freshness.

Least expensive type.

KEY FACTS TO REMEMBER

Successful Breastfeeding Evaluation

Babies are probably getting enough milk if:

They are nursing at least eight times in 24 hours.

In a quiet room, their mothers can hear them swallow while nursing.

Their mothers' breasts appear to soften after nursing.

The number of wet diapers increases by the fourth or fifth day after birth, or there are at least six to eight wet diapers every 24 hours after day 5.

The baby's stools are yellow (mustard) in color and cottage cheese by the fourth or fifth day after birth.

Offering a supplemental bottle is not a reliable indicator because most babies will take a few ounces even if they are getting enough breast milk (Neifert 1994).

to add too many supplemental foods or offer too much formula to infants of this age. Clinicians generally advise that an infant not be given more than 32 ounces of formula in a day. If additional calories are needed, supplemental foods can be added to the diet. Conversely, if the caloric intake is adequate or excessive, formula alone gives the infant enough calories and introduction of solid foods can be delayed until later.

When an infant's caloric intake and weight gain is found to be excessive, clinicians do not advise putting the infant on a weight reduction diet, because tissue growth is rapid during this period and must be supported. The appropriate advice is to provide a maintenance caloric intake as a means of allowing the infant to maintain weight while maturing and growing in length.

Identification of appropriate nutritional intake can be done by comparing the infant's dietary intake with the desired caloric intake for the infant's weight and age. Most commercial formulas prescribed for the normal healthy newborn contain 20 calories per ounce. If the infant is eating solids, the caloric value of those foods must be determined and included in the calculation of nutritional intake. With knowledge of the amount of calories needed by the infant according to weight (108 kcal/kg/day [55 kcal/lb]), the nurse can counsel the parents about how many ounces per day the infant needs to meet caloric requirements.

CHAPTER HIGHLIGHTS

- The RDA for calories for the newborn is 105–110 kcal/kg/day (50–55 kcal/lb/day).
- Breast milk has immunologic and nutritional properties that make it the optimal food for the first year of life.
- Signs indicating newborn readiness for the first feeding are active bowel sounds, absence of abdominal distention, and a lusty cry that quiets with rooting and sucking behaviors when a stimulus is placed near the lips.
- Mature breast milk and commercially prepared formulas (unless otherwise noted) provide 20 kcal/oz.
- Breastfed infants need supplements of vitamin D and fluoride. However, there is no need to give supplemental iron to breastfed infants before 6 months of age.
- Nurses must recognize that cultural values influence infant feeding practices, be sensitive to ethnic backgrounds of minority populations, and understand that the dominant culture in any society defines "normal" maternal-infant feeding interactions.
- Breastfed infants are getting adequate nutrition if they are gaining weight and have at least six wet diapers a day when not receiving additional water supplements.
- Breastfeeding mothers should be encouraged to ensure that the infant is correctly positioned at the breast, with a large portion of the areola in his or her mouth. The mother is advised to rotate positions to ensure that all ducts are emptied.
- Most maternal medications are transmitted through breast milk. The effects on the infant and lactation depend on a variety of factors, including route of administration, timing of the dose with respect to feeding time, and multiple properties of the medication.
- To prevent sore nipples the nurse can encourage the breastfeeding mother to allow her breasts to air dry after feeding.
- Formula-fed infants regain their birth weight by 10 days of age and gain 1 oz/day for the first 6 months and 0.5 oz/day for the second 6 months; birth weight is doubled at 3.5–4 months of age. Healthy breastfed babies gain approximately 0.5 oz/day in the first 6 months of life, regain their birth weight by about 14 days of age, and double their birth weight at approximately 5 months of age.
- Formula-fed infants need no vitamin or mineral supplements other than iron, if it is not already in the formula, and fluoride, if it is not obtained in the water system.
- The bottle-feeding mother may require assistance with feeding and burping her infant. She will also benefit from information about feeding schedules and types of formula.
- The use of skim milk, cow's milk with lowered fat content, or unmodified cow's milk is not recommended for children under 2 years old.
- Nutritional assessment of the infant includes nutritional history from the parents, weight gain, growth chart percentiles, and physical examination.

REFERENCES

American Academy of Pediatrics, *Committee on Fetus and Newborn: Guidelines for Perinatal Care,* 3rd ed. Elk Grove Village, IL: AAP, 1992a.

American Academy of Pediatrics, Committee on Drugs: The transfer of drugs and other chemicals into human milk. *Pediatrics* 1994; 93(1):137.

American Academy of Pediatrics, Committee on Nutrition: Follow-up of weaning formulas. *Pediatrics* 1992b; 89:1105.

American Academy of Pediatrics, Committee on Nutrition. Fluoride supplementation for children: Interim policy recommendations. *Pediatrics* 1995; 95:777.

Barness LA: Bases of weaning recommendations. *J Pediatr* 1990; 117:S84.

Bear K, Tigges BB: Management strategies for promoting successful breastfeeding. *Nurse Pract* 1993; 18(6):50.

Beaudry M, DuFour R, Marcoux S: Relation between infant feeding and infections during the first six months of life. *J Pediatr* 1995; 126:191.

Eggert JV, Rayburn WF: Nutrition and lactation. In: *Gynecology and Obstetrics, Vol 2.* Sciarra JJ (editor). Philadelphia: HarperCollins, 1994.

Fendrick SM, Major AL, Brown FR: Nursing mothers service: A community breast-feeding program. *Pediatr Nurs* 1994; 20(3):241.

Fletcher AB: Nutrition. In: *Neonatology: Pathophysiology and Management of the Newborn,* 4th ed. Avery GB et al (editors). Philadelphia: Lippincott, 1994.

Food and Nutrition Board, National Academy of Sciences—National Research Council: *Recommended Dietary Allowances,* 10th ed. Washington, DC, 1989.

Furman L: A developmental approach to weaning. *MCN* 1995; 20(6):322.

Gigliotti E: When women decide not to breastfeed. *MCN* 1995; 20(6):315.

Gunnlaugsson G, da Silva MC, Smedman L: Age at breast feeding start and postnatal growth and survival. *Arch Dis Child* 1994; 69:134.

Huml SC: Cracked nipples in the breastfeeding mother: Looking at an old problem in a new way. *Advance for Nurse Practitioners.* April 1995.

Huggins K: *The Nursing Mother's Companion.* Boston: The Harvard Common Press, 1990.

Hutchinson MK, Baqi-Aziz M: Nursing care of the childbearing Muslim family. *JOGNN* 1994; 23(9):767.

Keefe M: The impact of rooming-in on maternal sleep at night *JOGNN* 1988; 17(2):122.

LaDu EB: Childbirth care for Hmong families. *MCN* November/December 1985; 10:382.

Lawrence PB: Breast milk. *Ped Clin North Am.* 1994a; 41(5):925.

Lawrence RA: *Breastfeeding: A Guide for the Medical Profession,* 4th ed. St Louis: Mosby, 1994b.

Littman H, VanderBrug Medenforp S, Goldfarb J: The decision to breastfeed. *Clin Pediatr* 1994; 214.

Losch M et al: Impact of attitudes on maternal decisions regarding infant feeding. *J Pediatr* 1995; 126(4):507.

Mott SR et al: *Nursing Care of Children and Families,* 2nd ed. Redwood City, CA: Addison-Wesley, 1990.

Mulford C: Subtle signs and symptoms of the milk ejection reflex. *J Hum Lact* 1990; 6:177.

Mulford C: The mother-baby assessment (MBA): An "Apgar score" for breastfeeding. *J Hum Lact* 1992; 8:79.

Neifert M: *Criteria for Assessing Early Breastfeeding.* Denver, CO: The Lactation Program, 1994.

Pascale JA et al: Breastfeeding, dehydration, and shorter maternity stays. *Neonatal Network* 1996; 15(7):37.

Pinella T, Birch LL: Help me make it through the night: Behavioral entrainment of breast-fed infants' sleep patterns. *Pediatrics* 1993; 91(2):436.

Pipes P: *Nutrition in Infancy and Childhood,* 4th ed. St Louis: Mosby, 1989.

Renfrew M, Fisher C, Arms S: *Breastfeeding: Getting Breastfeeding Right for You.* Berkeley: Celestial Arts, 1990.

Riordan J: *A Practical Guide to Breastfeeding.* St Louis: Mosby, 1991.

Riordan J, Auerbach K: *Breastfeeding and Human Lactation.* Boston: Jones & Bartlett, 1993.

Sawley L: Infant feeding. *Nursing* 1989; 39(3):18.

Sollid DT et al: Breastfeeding multiples. *J Perinatal Neonatal Nurs* 1989; 3(1):46.

Spencer JP: Practical nutrition for the healthy term infant. AFP 1996; 54(1):138.

Vezeau TM: Investigating "Greedy." *MCN* 1991; 16:337.

Wagner CL, Anderson DM, Pittard WB: Special properties of human milk. *Clin Pediatr* 1996; June:283.

Woolridge MW, Baum JD: Recent advances in breast feeding. *Acta Paediatr Japonica* 1993; 35:12.

Ziemer MM et al: Methods to prevent and manage nipple pain in breastfeeding women. *West J Nurs Res* 1990; 12(6):732.

Zinaman MJ et al: Acute prolactin, oxytocin responses and milk yield to infant sucking and artificial methods of expression in lactating women. *Pediatrics* 1992; 89:437.

Chapter 25 The Newborn at Risk: Conditions Present at Birth

OBJECTIVES

- Identify factors that may put a newborn at risk.
- Compare the underlying etiologies of the similar physiologic complications of small-for-gestational-age (SGA) newborns and preterm appropriate-for-gestational-age (Pr AGA) newborns.
- Describe the impact maternal diabetes mellitus has on the newborn.
- Compare the characteristics and potential complications of the postterm newborn and the newborn with postmaturity syndrome.
- Discuss the physiologic characteristics of the preterm newborn that predispose each body system to various complications of prematurity.
- Identify the data used in developing the nursing diagnoses required to plan interventions for the care of the preterm AGA newborn.
- Explain the special care needed by alcohol- or drug-exposed newborns.
- Relate the consequences of maternal AIDS to the management of the infant in the newborn period.
- Identify the nursing assessments that would make the nurse suspect a congenital cardiac defect during the early newborn period.
- Discuss the nursing assessments of, and initial interventions in, selected congenital anomalies.
- Explain the special care needed by newborns with inborn errors of metabolism.
- Delineate interventions to facilitate parental attachment with the at-risk newborn.
- Identify the nursing actions necessary to support family members dealing with the birth of an at-risk infant.

KEY TERMS

Drug-dependent infants
Fetal alcohol effects (FAE)
Fetal alcohol syndrome (FAS)
Inborn errors of metabolism
Infant of diabetic mother (IDM)
Intrauterine growth retardation (IUGR)
Large for gestational age (LGA)
Phenylketonuria (PKU)
Postterm infant
Preterm infant
Small for gestational age (SGA)

Within the last 30 years, the field of neonatology has expanded greatly. Many levels of nursery care have evolved: special care; transitional care; and low- and high-risk care. The nurse is an important caregiver in all these nurseries. As a member of the multidisciplinary health care team, the nurse has contributed the high-touch human care necessary in a high-tech perinatal environment.

In addition to the availability of high-quality newborn care, other factors that influence the outcome for at-risk infants include birth weight, gestational age, type and length of newborn illness, environmental and maternal factors, and maternal-infant separation.

Identification of At-Risk Newborns

An at-risk newborn is one susceptible to illness (morbidity) or even death because of dysmaturity, immaturity, physical disorders, or complications of birth. In most cases, the infant is the product of a pregnancy involving one or more predictable risk factors, including

- Low socioeconomic level of the mother
- Exposure to environmental dangers such as toxic chemicals
- Preexisting maternal conditions such as heart disease or diabetes
- Pregnancy factors such as age or parity
- Medical conditions related to pregnancy such as prenatal maternal infection
- Pregnancy complications such as abruptio placentae

Various risk factors and their specific effects on the pregnancy outcome were listed in Table 8–1. Because these factors and the perinatal risks associated with them are known, the birth of many at-risk newborns can often be anticipated and prepared for through adequate prenatal care. The pregnancy can be closely monitored, treatment can be instituted as necessary, and arrangements can be made for birth to occur at a facility with appropriate equipment and personnel to care for both mother and baby.

Identification of at-risk infants cannot always be made before labor, since the course of labor and birth, or how the infant will withstand the stress of labor, is not known before the actual birth process. Thus during labor, fetal heart monitoring or contemporary fetoscope monitoring by the nurse has played a significant role in detecting fetuses in distress.

Immediately after birth the Apgar score is a useful tool for identifying the at-risk newborn, but it is difficult to predict long-term outcome based solely on Apgar scores. In general, the lower the Apgar score at 5 minutes after birth, the higher the incidence of neurologic abnormalities seen at 1 year of age.

The newborn classification and neonatal mortality risk chart is another useful tool for identifying newborns at risk. Before this classification tool was developed, birth weight of less than 2500 g was the sole criterion for determining immaturity. Eventually caregivers recognized that a newborn could weigh more than 2500 g and still be immature. Conversely, a newborn weighing less than 2500 g might be functionally at term or beyond. Thus birth weight and gestational age together became the criteria used to assess neonatal maturity and mortality risk.

According to the newborn classification and neonatal mortality risk chart, gestation is divided as follows:

- Preterm = 0–37 (completed) weeks
- Term = 38–41 (completed) weeks
- Postterm = greater than 42 weeks

As shown in Figure 22–11, large-for-gestational-age (LGA) newborns are those above the 90th percentile line. Appropriate-for-gestational-age (AGA) newborns are those between the lines labeled 10th percentile and 90th percentile. Small-for-gestational-age (SGA) newborns are those below the curved line labeled 10th percentile. A newborn is assigned to a category depending on birth weight and gestational age. For example, a newborn classified as Pr SGA is preterm and small for gestational age. The full-term newborn whose weight is appropriate for gestational age is classified F AGA.

Neonatal mortality risk is the chance of death within the neonatal period (within the first 28 days of life). The neonatal mortality risk decreases as both gestational age and birth weight increase. Infants who are preterm and small for gestational age have the highest neonatal mortality risk. The previously high mortality rates for LGA newborns have decreased at most perinatal centers because of improved management of diabetes in pregnancy and increased recognition of potential problems of LGA newborns.

Newborn morbidity can be anticipated based on birth weight and gestational age. In Figure 25–1 the infant's birth weight is located on the vertical axis, and the gestational age in weeks is found along the horizontal axis. The area where the two meet on the graph identifies commonly occurring problems. This tool assists in determining the needs of particular infants for special observation and care. For example, an infant of 2000 g at 40 weeks' gestation should be carefully assessed for evidence of fetal distress, hypoglycemia, congenital anomalies, congenital infection, and polycythemia.

Identification of the nursing care needs of the at-risk newborn depends on minute-to-minute observations of

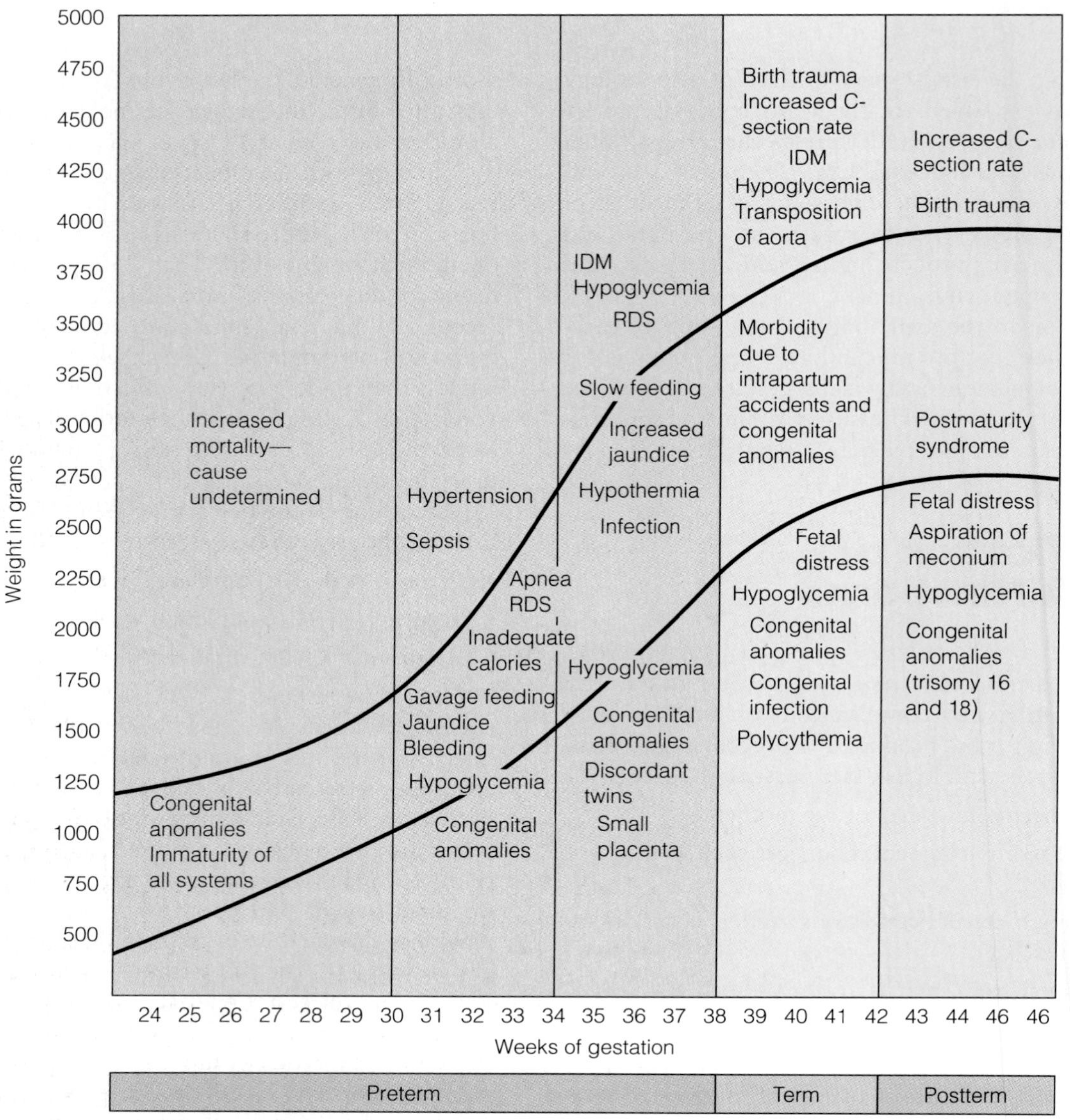

FIGURE 25–1 Neonatal morbidity by birth weight and gestational age.
Source: Lubchenco LO: *The High-Risk Infant.* Philadelphia: Saunders, 1976, p 122.

the changes in the newborn's physiologic status. It is essential to a baby's survival that the neonatal nurse understand the basic physiologic principles that guide nursing management of the at-risk newborn. The organization of nursing care must be directed toward

- Decreasing physiologically stressful situations
- Constantly observing for subtle signs of change in clinical condition
- Interpreting laboratory data and coordinating interventions
- Conserving the infant's energy, especially in frail, debilitated newborns
- Providing for developmental stimulation and sleep cycle
- Assisting the family in developing attachment behaviors
- Involving the family in the planning and provision of care

Care of the Small-for-Gestational-Age (SGA) Newborn

A **small-for-gestational-age (SGA)** newborn is any newborn who at birth is at or below the tenth percentile (intrauterine growth curves) on the newborn classification chart. It should be noted that intrauterine growth charts are influenced by altitude and ethnicity. There is a high correlation between increase in altitude and decrease in birth weight (Nagey and Viscardi 1993). When assigning SGA classification to a newborn, birth weight charts should be based on the local population into which the newborn is born (Creasy and Resnik 1994). An SGA newborn may be preterm, term, or postterm. Other terms used to designate a growth-retarded newborn include **intrauterine growth retarded (IUGR),** which describes the pregnancy circumstance of advanced gestation and limited fetal growth, and *dysmature*. We use SGA and IUGR interchangeably.

Small-for-gestational-age infants have a five times greater incidence of perinatal asphyxia and an eight times higher perinatal mortality than AGA infants (Ott 1995). The incidence of polycythemia and hypoglycemia also increases in this group of infants.

Factors Contributing to Intrauterine Growth Retardation (IUGR)

The causes of IUGR may be maternal, placental, or fetal factors and may not be apparent antenatally. Intrauterine growth is linear in the normal pregnancy from approximately 28 to 38 weeks' gestation. After 38 weeks, growth is variable, depending on the growth potential of the fetus and placental function. The most common causes of growth retardation are the following:

- *Maternal factors.* Primiparity, grand multiparity, smoking, lack of prenatal care, age extremes (<16 years or >40 years), and low socioeconomic class—which usually results in inadequate health care, inadequate education, and inadequate living conditions—affect SGA (Spinillo et al 1994). Before the third trimester, the nutritional supply to the fetus far exceeds its needs. Only in the third trimester is maternal malnutrition a limiting factor in fetal growth.
- *Maternal disease.* Maternal heart disease, substance abuse (drugs and alcohol), sickle cell anemia, phenylketonuria (PKU), and asymptomatic pyelonephritis are associated with SGA. Complications associated with pregnancy-induced hypertension (PIH), chronic hypertensive vascular disease, and advanced diabetes mellitus cause diminished blood flow to the uterus.
- *Environmental factors.* High altitude; x-rays; excessive exercise; hyperthermia; and maternal use of drugs that have teratogenic effects, such as antimetabolites, anticonvulsants, and trimethadione, affect IUGR (Cunningham 1993).
- *Placental factors.* Placental conditions such as small placenta, infarcted areas, abnormal cord insertions, placenta previa, or thrombosis may affect circulation to the fetus, which becomes more deficient with increasing gestational age (Harrington and Campbell 1993).
- *Fetal factors.* Congenital infections (rubella, toxoplasmosis) or malformations, multiple pregnancy (twins, triplets), sex of the fetus, chromosomal syndromes, and inborn errors of metabolism can predispose a fetus to IUGR (Creasy and Resnik 1994).

Antenatal identification of fetuses suffering IUGR is the first step in the detection of common disorders of the SGA infant. The perinatal history of maternal conditions, early serial ultrasound measurements, antepartal testing (NST, CST, BPP), the examination of the placenta (by pathology), gestational age assessment, and the physical and neurologic assessment of the newborn are also important (Gardosi et al 1995).

Patterns of IUGR

Intrauterine growth occurs by an increase in both cell number and cell size. If insult occurs early during the critical period of organ development in the fetus, fewer new cells are formed, organs are small, and organ weight is subnormal. In contrast, growth failure that begins later in pregnancy does not affect the total number of cells, only their size; the organs are normal, but their size is diminished. There are two clinical pictures of SGA newborns:

- *Symmetric (proportional) IUGR* is caused by long-term maternal conditions (such as chronic hypertension, severe malnutrition, chronic intrauterine infection, substance abuse, and anemia) or fetal genetic abnormalities (Gardosi et al 1995). Symmetric IUGR can be noted by ultrasound in the first half of the second trimester. In symmetric IUGR there is chronic prolonged retardation of growth in size of organs, weight, length, and, in severe cases, head circumference.
- *Asymmetric (disproportional) IUGR* is associated with an acute compromise of uteroplacental blood flow. Some associated causes are placental infarcts, PIH, and poor weight gain in pregnancy. The growth retardation is usually not evident before the third trimester because, although weight is decreased, length and head circumference remain appropriate for that gestational age. Birth weight is reduced below the tenth percentile, whereas head size may be between the 10th and 90th percentiles. Asymmetric SGA newborns are particularly at risk for perinatal asphyxia, pulmonary hemorrhage, hypocalcemia, and hypoglycemia in the newborn period.

Despite growth retardation, physiologic maturity develops according to gestational age. Therefore, the SGA newborn may be more physiologically mature than the preterm AGA newborn and less predisposed to complications of prematurity such as respiratory distress syndrome and hyperbilirubinemia. The SGA newborn's chances for survival are better because of organ maturity, although this newborn still faces many other potential difficulties.

Common Complications of the SGA Newborn

The complications occurring most frequently in the SGA newborn are

- *Perinatal asphyxia.* The SGA newborn suffers chronic hypoxia in utero, which leaves little reserve to withstand the demands of normal labor and birth. Thus, intrauterine asphyxia can occur with its potential systemic problems. Cesarean birth may be necessary.
- *Aspiration syndrome.* In utero hypoxia can cause the fetus to gasp during birth, resulting in aspiration of amniotic fluid into the lower airways. It can also lead to relaxation of the anal sphincter and passage of meconium. This results in aspiration of the meconium with the first breaths after birth.
- *Heat loss.* Diminished subcutaneous fat (used for survival in utero), depletion of brown fat in utero, and a large surface area decrease the IUGR newborn's ability to conserve heat. The effect of surface area is diminished somewhat because of the flexed position assumed by the term SGA newborn.
- *Hypoglycemia.* An increase in metabolic rate in response to heat loss and poor hepatic glycogen stores causes hypoglycemia. In addition, the newborn is compromised by inadequate supplies of enzymes to activate gluconeogenesis (conversion of nonglucogen sources such as fatty acids and proteins to glucose).
- *Hypocalcemia.* Decreased calcium levels occur secondary to birth asphyxia and preterm birth.
- *Polycythemia.* The number of red blood cells is increased in the SGA newborn. This finding is considered a physiologic response to in utero chronic hypoxic stress.

Newborns who have significant IUGR tend to have a poor prognosis, especially when born before 37 weeks' gestation. Factors contributing to poor outcome for these infants are

- *Congenital malformations.* Congenital malformations occur 10 to 20 times more frequently in SGA infants than in AGA infants. The more severe the IUGR, the greater the chance for malformation as a result of impaired mitotic activity and cellular hypoplasia.
- *Intrauterine infections.* When fetuses are exposed to intrauterine infections such as rubella and cytomegalovirus, they are profoundly affected by direct invasion of the brain and other vital organs by the offending virus, resulting in IUGR.
- *Continued growth difficulties.* It is generally agreed that SGA newborns tend to be shorter than newborns of the same gestational age (Ott 1995). Asymmetric IUGR infants can be expected to catch up at least in weight to normal-growth infants by 3 to 6 months of age. Symmetric SGA infants reportedly have varied growth potential but tend not to catch up to their peers (Ott 1995).
- *Learning difficulties.* Often SGA newborns exhibit poor brain development and subsequent failure to catch up, and learning disabilities are not uncommon. The disabilities are characterized by hyperactivity, short attention span, and poor fine motor coordination (reading, writing, and drawing) (Witter 1993). Poor scholastic performance is also a common problem (Creasy and Resnik 1994). Some hearing loss and speech defects also may occur.

Studies have determined that the quality of the home environment of an SGA infant predicts developmental outcome better than any single biologic risk factor (Sung et al 1993).

Medical Therapy

The goal of medical therapy is early recognition and implementation of the medical management of potential problems.

APPLYING THE NURSING PROCESS

Nursing Assessment

The nurse is responsible for assessing gestational age and identifying signs of potential complications associated with SGA infants.

All body parts of the symmetric IUGR infant are in proportion, but they are below normal size for the baby's gestational age. Therefore the head does not appear overly large or the length excessive in relation to the other body parts. These newborns are generally vigorous.

The asymmetric IUGR infant appears long, thin, and emaciated, with loss of subcutaneous fat tissue and muscle mass (Figure 25–2). The baby has loose skin folds; dry, desquamating skin; and a thin and often meconium-

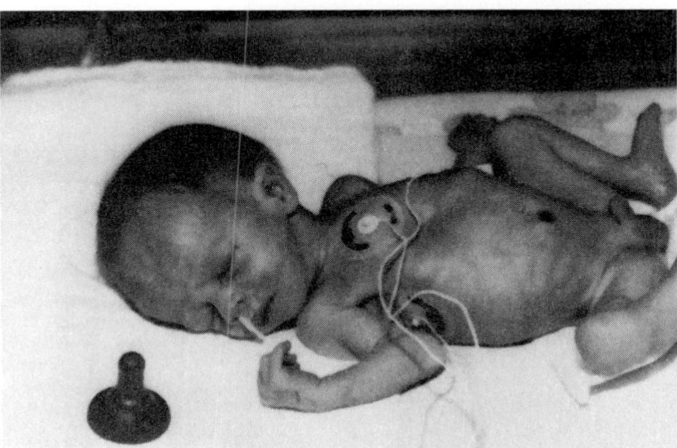

FIGURE 25–2 The infant with asymmetric IUGR appears long, thin, and emaciated. The gestational age of the infant shown here is 41 weeks; he weighed approximately 1560 g at birth.

stained cord. The head appears relatively large (although it approaches normal size) because the chest size and abdominal girth are decreased. The baby may have a vigorous cry and appear alert and wide eyed.

Nursing Diagnosis

Nursing diagnoses that may apply to the small-for-gestational-age newborn include the following:

- Impaired gas exchange related to aspiration of meconium
- Hypothermia related to decreased subcutaneous fat
- Risk for injury to tissues related to decreased glycogen stores and impaired gluconeogenesis
- Altered nutrition: less than body requirements related to SGA's increased metabolic rate
- Risk for altered tissue perfusion related to increased blood viscosity
- Risk for altered parenting related to prolonged separation of newborn from parents secondary to illness
- Knowledge deficit related to lack of information about care of newborn at home

Nursing Plan and Implementation

Hypoglycemia, the most common metabolic complication of IUGR, produces such sequelae as CNS abnormalities and mental retardation. Conditions such as asphyxia, hyperviscosity, and cold stress may also affect the baby's outcome. Meticulous attention to physiologic parameters is essential for immediate nursing management and reduction of long-term disorders (see Critical Pathway for Small-for-Gestational-Age Newborn on pp 622–623).

Community-Based Nursing Care

The long-term needs of the SGA newborn include careful follow-up evaluation of patterns of growth and possible disabilities that may later interfere with learning or motor functioning. Long-term follow-up care is especially necessary for those infants with congenital malformations, congenital infections, and obvious sequelae from physiologic problems. In addition, the parents of the IUGR newborn need support, because a positive atmosphere can enhance the baby's growth potential and the child's ultimate outcome.

Evaluation

Anticipated outcomes of nursing care include

- The small-for-gestational-age newborn is free from apnea.
- The small-for-gestational-age newborn maintains a stable temperature and glucose homeostasis.
- The small-for-gestational-age newborn gains weight and takes nipple feedings without developing physiologic distress or fatigue.
- The parents verbalize their concerns about their baby's health problems and understand the rationale behind management of their newborn.

Care of the Large-for-Gestational-Age (LGA) Newborn

A **large-for-gestational-age (LGA)** newborn is one whose birth weight is at or above the 90th percentile on the intrauterine growth curve (at any week of gestation). The classification of LGA may vary depending on the intrauterine growth curve chart used; the chart used should correlate with the characteristics of the client population (ACOG technical bulletin #159 1992; Harrington and Campbell 1993). Some LGA newborns have been incorrectly categorized as LGA because of miscalculation of the date of conception due to postconceptual bleeding. Careful gestational age assessment is essential to identify the potential needs and problems of such infants.

The best-known condition associated with excessive fetal growth is maternal diabetes (Classes A–C; see Table 12–2); however, only a minority of large newborns are born to diabetic mothers. The cause of the

Text continues on page 624

CRITICAL PATHWAY FOR SMALL-FOR-GESTATIONAL-AGE NEWBORNS

Category	Day of Birth—1st 4 Hours	Remaining Day of Birth
Referral	• Report from L&D, neonatal nurse practitioner • Check ID bands	• Check ID bands q shift → • Circumcision permit signed before procedure
Assessment	• Complete set of VS • Admission wt, length, head circumference • Check skin color • Gestational age assessment • Assess ongoing for hypoglycemia. If present, chemstrip should be done immediately. • Assess ongoing for polycythemia	• Assess mother/baby interaction, suck, color, respiratory status → • Assess temperature for hypothermia → • Monitor daily weights →
Comfort	• Admission activities performed at mother's bedside	
Nursing interventions and report	Diagnostic Tests • Blood type, Rh, Coombs on cord blood when applicable • Chemstrip within 1h of birth and q1h or q2h until feedings have been instituted → • Check chemstrip before at least two feedings or until condition appears to be stable (chemstrips > 40 mg/dL $\times 2$) • All SGA infants will have hematocrits performed per policy and procedure • Baer test	• VS q4h T/P/R → • Check for Baer test results • Newborn screen • Femoral pulse or BP 4 extremities if early discharge • Alcohol to cord q shift →
Activity	• Adjust and monitor radiant warmer to maintain skin temperature • Hep B form reviewed and/or signed (by nurse) • Tips for infant safety reviewed/signed with mother (by nurse) • Monitor infant activity → • Triple dye cord • Bath per policy	• Open crib → • Incubator if temp. instability → Adjust and monitor incubator to maintain skin temperature
Nutrition	• Initiate bottle feeding → • Initiate breast as soon as mother and baby condition allows → • Lavage and gavage prn → • Supplement breast only when medically indicated or ordered by MD with D_5W, sterile H_2O or 20 cal formula with iron • Feed SGA infants at 3–4 hours for first 24 hours → • Monitor feeding tolerance	• Continue feeding schedule (small frequent fdgs, high caloric formula, nutritional fortifiers) →
Elimination	• Note first void and stool color →	• Note all voids and color of stools q shift →
Medications	• Aquamephyton 1 mg IM • Ilotycin ophth ointment OU • Hep B vaccine if ordered by MD or signed by parent	
Discharge planning/ home care	• Evaluate for Social Services/home care/discharge planning needs → • Plan DC with parent/guardian in 1–3 days → • Car seat for DC	• Present birth certificate instructions • Car seat for DC • Baby pictures
Family involvement	• Evaluate additional psychosocial needs → • Evaluate parent teaching (bulb syringe, positioning, choking) → • Teen "Healthy Starts" Program	• Instruct mother on diapering, normal limits of void and stool, burping • Evaluate parent teaching →
Date		

CRITICAL PATHWAY continued

Category	Day #1	Day #2/#3 (if applicable)
Referral	• Check ID bands →	• Check ID bands q shift
Assessment	• Assess mother/baby interaction, suck, color, resp. status → • Assess thermoregulation → • Assess for potential complications: perinatal asphyxia, aspiration syndrome, hypoglycemia, hypocalcemia, polycythemia →	• Assess mother/baby interaction → • Assess color for jaundice • Assess for apnea
Comfort	• Assess for comfort needs →	• Assess for comfort needs →
Nursing interventions and report	• VS T/P/R. q4h → • Scalp treatment BID → • Daily weight • Check color q shift → • Check activity → • Check circumcision → • DC cord clamp • Alcohol cord q shift → • Total bilirubin level	• VS T/P/R q4h → • Daily weight → • Scalp treatment BID → • Color q shift → • Activity → • Circumcision care → • Alcohol to cord q shift → • Completion of Baer test • Completion of femoral pulses/BPs →
Activity	• Open crib → • Incubator if temp instability → • Adjust and monitor incubator to maintain skin temperature	• Open crib →
Nutrition	• Gavage prn → • Supplement breast only when medically indicate/policy or ordered by MD with D_5W, sterile H_2O, or 20 cal formula with iron • Encourage feeds at least q3–4h during day and more frequently as baby demands → • Bottle-feed q3–4h on demand → • Continue enhanced feeding regimen →	• Gavage prn • Supplement breast only when medically indicate/policy or ordered by MD with D_5W, sterile H_2O, or 20 cal formula with iron • Encourage feeds at least q3–4h during day and more frequently as baby demands • Bottle-feed q3–4h on demand
Elimination	• Note all voids and color of stools q shift →	• Note all voids and color of stools q shift
Medications	• Hep B vaccine at discharge	• Hep B vaccine at discharge
Discharge planning/ home care	• If vag birth, complete DC instructions • Complete Birth Certificate packet • Continue from "Remaining Day of Birth"	• Continue the completion of education from day #1 • If C/S birth complete DC instructions
Family involvement	• Bath and feeding class • Newborn Channel (if available) • Instruct parent on: bath, skin care, nail, cord care; use of thermometers, activity, sleep patterns, crying, soothing, reflexes, jaundice, growth patterns • Evaluate mother/parent teaching →	• Evaluate mother/parent teaching
Date		

majority of cases of LGA newborns is unclear, but the following factors or situations have been found to correlate with their birth:

- Prepregnancy weight and weight gain during pregnancy. Large parents tend to have large infants.
- Multiparous women have three times the number of LGA infants as primigravidas (ACOG technical bulletin #159 1992).
- Male infants are traditionally larger than female infants.
- Infants with erythroblastosis fetalis, Beckwith-Wiedemann syndrome (a genetic condition associated with neonatal hypoglycemia and hyperinsulinemia), or transposition of the great vessels are usually large.

The increase in the LGA infant's body size is characteristically proportional, although head circumference and body length are in the upper limits of intrauterine growth. The exception to this rule is the infant of the diabetic mother, whose body weight increases while length and head circumference may be in the normal range. Macrosomic infants are less competent motorically and have more difficulty in behavioral state regulation. LGA infants tend to be more difficult to arouse to a quiet alert state and may have feeding difficulties (Pressler 1991).

Common Complications of the LGA Newborn

Common disorders of the LGA newborn include

- *Birth trauma because of cephalopelvic disproportion (CPD).* Often these newborns have a biparietal diameter greater than 10 cm (4 inches) or are associated with a maternal fundal height measurement greater than 42 cm (16 inches) without the presence of hydramnios. Because of their excessive size, there are more breech presentations and shoulder dystocias. These complications may result in asphyxia, fractured clavicles, brachial palsy, facial paralysis, phrenic nerve palsy, depressed skull fractures, hematomas, and bleeding due to birth trauma.
- *Increased incidence of cesarean births and oxytocin-induced births due to fetal size.* These births are accompanied by all the risk factors associated with cesarean births (ACOG technical bulletin #159 1992).
- *Hypoglycemia, polycythemia, and hyperviscosity.* These disorders are most often seen in infants with diabetic mothers, erythroblastosis fetalis, and Beckwith-Wiedemann syndrome.

Nursing Care

The perinatal history, in conjunction with ultrasonic measurement of fetal skull and gestational age testing, is important in identifying an at-risk LGA newborn. Nursing care is directed toward early identification and immediate treatment of the common disorders. Essential components of the nursing assessment are monitoring vital signs, screening for hypoglycemia and polycythemia, and observing for signs and symptoms related to birth trauma. The nurse needs to address parental concerns about the visual signs of birth trauma (Pressler 1991) and the potential for continuation of the overweight pattern. The nursing care involved in the complications associated with LGA newborns applies to the care needed by the infant of a diabetic mother and will be discussed in the next section.

Care of the Infant of a Diabetic Mother (IDM)

Infants of diabetic mothers (IDMs) are considered at risk and require close observation the first few hours to the first few days of life. Mothers with severe diabetes or diabetes of long duration (type 1, or White's classes D–F, associated with vascular complications) may give birth to SGA infants. The typical IDM (type 1, or White's classes A–C), however, is LGA. He or she is fat, macrosomic, and ruddy (Figure 25–3). The cord and placenta are also large. There is a higher incidence of macrosomic infants born to certain ethnic groups (Homko et al 1995).

IDMs have decreased total body water, particularly in the extracellular spaces, and are therefore not edematous. Their excessive weight is due to increased weight of the visceral organs, cardiomegaly (hypertrophy), and increased body fat. The only organ not affected is the brain (Ogata 1994).

The excessive fetal growth of the IDM is caused by exposure to high levels of maternal glucose, which readily crosses the placenta. The fetus responds to these high glucose levels with increased insulin production and hyperplasia of the pancreatic beta cells. The main action of the insulin is to facilitate the entry of glucose into muscle and fat cells in a function similar to a cellular growth hormone. Once in the cells, glucose is converted to glycogen and stored. Insulin also inhibits the breakdown of fat to free fatty acids, thereby maintaining lipid synthesis, increasing the uptake of amino acids, and promoting protein synthesis. Insulin is an important regulator of fetal metabolism and has a "growth hormone" effect that results in increased linear growth (Warshaw 1994). There has been an association between IDM and childhood obesity (Dashier 1995).

Common Complications of the IDM

Although IDMs are usually large, they are immature in physiologic functions and exhibit many of the problems of the preterm infant. The complications most often seen in an IDM are

- *Hypoglycemia.* After birth the most common problem of an IDM is hypoglycemia. Even though the high maternal blood supply is lost, this newborn continues to produce high levels of insulin, which deplete the blood glucose within hours after birth. IDMs also have less ability to release glucagon and catecholamines, which normally stimulate glucagon breakdown and glucose release. The incidence of hypoglycemia in IDMs varies from 25–40 percent (Tyrala 1996). Incidence of hypoglycemia varies according to the degree of success in controlling the maternal diabetes, differences in maternal blood sugars at the time of birth, length of labor, the class of maternal diabetes, and early versus late feedings of the newborn.
- *Hypocalcemia.* Tremors are the obvious clinical sign of hypocalcemia. This may be due to the IDM's increased incidence of prematurity and to the stresses of difficult pregnancy, labor, and birth, which predispose any infant to hypocalcemia. Diabetic women also tend to have higher calcium levels at term, causing possible secondary hypoparathyroidism in their infants (Ogata 1994).
- *Hyperbilirubinemia.* This condition may be seen at 48 to 72 hours after birth. It may be caused by slightly decreased extracellular fluid volume, which increases the hematocrit level, and the presence of hepatic immaturity (Warshaw 1994). Enclosed hemorrhages resulting from complicated vaginal birth may also cause hyperbilirubinemia. There may also be an increase in rate of bilirubin production in the presence of polycythemia.
- *Birth trauma.* Since most IDMs are LGA, trauma may occur during labor and birth.
- *Polycythemia.* This condition may be caused by the decreased extracellular volume in IDMs. Fetal hyperglycemia and hyperinsulinism results in increased oxygen consumption, leading to fetal hypoxia (Warshaw 1994). Recent research centers on the fact that hemoglobin A_{1c} binds oxygen, which decreases the oxygen available to the fetal tissues. This tissue hypoxia stimulates increased erythropoietin production, which increases the hematocrit level.
- *Respiratory distress syndrome (RDS).* This complication occurs especially in newborns of diabetic mothers in White's classes A–C. It has been demonstrated that insulin antagonizes the cortisol-induced stimulation of lecithin synthesis that is necessary for lung maturation. Therefore, IDMs may have less mature lungs than expected for their gestational age. There is also a decrease in the phospholipid PG that stabilizes surfactant and thereby increases the incidence of RDS. RDS does not appear to be a problem for infants born of diabetic mothers in White's classes D–F; instead, the stresses of poor uterine blood supply may lead to increased production of steroids, which accelerates lung maturation.
- *Congenital birth defects.* These may include transposition of the great vessels, ventricular septal defect, patent ductus arteriosus, small left colon syndrome, and sacral agenesis (caudal regression) (Tyrala 1996). Early close control of maternal glucose before and during pregnancy decreases the risk of birth defects (Wyse et al 1994).

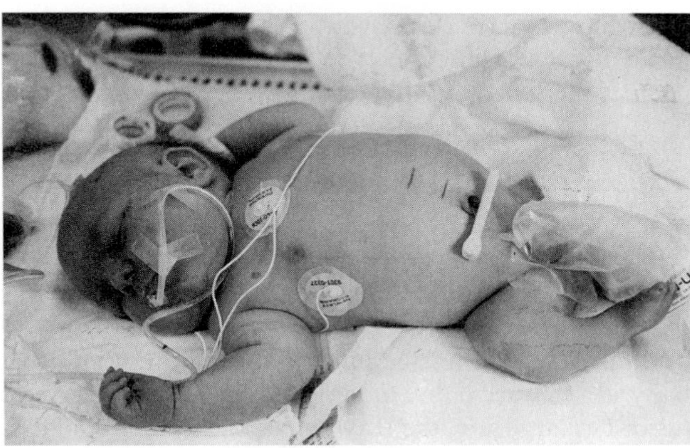

FIGURE 25–3 Macrosomic infant of diabetic mother. X-ray examination of this infant revealed caudal regression of the spine.

Medical Therapy

Key prenatal management is directed toward control of maternal hyperglycemia, which minimizes the common complications of IDMs.

Because the onset of hypoglycemia occurs between 1 and 3 hours after birth in IDMs (with a spontaneous rise to normal levels by 4–6 hours), blood glucose determinations should be done on cord blood hourly during the first 4 hours after birth and then at 4-hour intervals until the risk period (about 24 hours) has passed (Ogata 1994).

IDMs whose serum glucose falls below 40 mg/dL should have early feedings with formula or breast milk (colostrum). The infant may need to be gavage fed if lethargic. If normal glucose levels cannot be maintained with oral feedings or if seizures occur, an intravenous infusion of glucose will be necessary. Once the blood glucose has been stable for 24 hours, the infusion rate can be decreased as oral feedings are increased. The newborn's blood glucose levels must be carefully monitored.

Dextrose (25–50%) as a rapid infusion is contraindicated because it may lead to severe rebound hypoglycemia following an initial brief increase in glucose level.

APPLYING THE NURSING PROCESS

Nursing Assessment

The nurse should not be lulled into thinking that a big baby is a mature baby. In almost every case, because of his or her large size, the IDM will appear older than gestational age scoring indicates. You must consider both the gestational age and whether the baby is AGA or LGA in planning and providing safe care.

In caring for the IDM, the nurse assesses for signs of respiratory distress, hyperbilirubinemia, birth trauma, and congenital anomalies.

Nursing Diagnosis

Nursing diagnoses that may apply to IDMs include the following:

- Altered nutrition: less than body requirements related to increased glucose metabolism secondary to hyperinsulinemia
- Impaired gas exchange related to respiratory distress secondary to impaired production of surfactant
- Ineffective family coping: compromise related to the illness of the baby

Nursing Plan and Implementation

Nursing care of the IDM is directed toward early detection and ongoing monitoring of hypoglycemia (by doing glucose tests) and polycythemia (by obtaining central hematocrits). Specific nursing interventions for respiratory distress syndrome, hypoglycemia, hyperbilirubinemia, and polycythemia are presented in Chapter 26. In caring for the IDM, the nurse assesses for signs of birth trauma and congenital anomalies.

Education of parents is directed toward prevention of macrosomia and resulting fetal-neonatal problems by instituting early and ongoing diabetic control. Parents are advised that with early identification and care most IDMs' neonatal problems have no significant sequelae.

Evaluation

Anticipated outcomes of nursing care include

- The IDM's respiratory distress and metabolic problems are minimized.
- The parents understand the effects of maternal diabetes on the baby and preventive steps they can initiate to decrease its impact on subsequent fetuses.
- The parents verbalize their concerns about their baby's health problems and understand the rationale behind management of their newborn.

Care of the Postterm Infant

The **postterm infant** is any infant born after 42 weeks' gestation (product of a prolonged pregnancy). In the past, the terms *postterm* and *postmature* were used interchangeably. The term *postmaturity* is now used only when the infant is born after 42 weeks of gestation and also demonstrates characteristics of the postmaturity syndrome.

Postterm, or prolonged pregnancy, occurs in approximately 3–12 percent of all pregnancies (McMahon et al 1996). The cause of postterm pregnancy is not completely understood, but several factors are known to be associated with it, including primiparity, high multiparity mothers (five or more pregnancies), and a history of prolonged pregnancies. Many pregnancies classified as prolonged are thought to be due to inaccurate estimates of date of birth (EDB) (Spellacy 1994). A positive correlation exists between postterm pregnancy and Australian, Greek, and Italian ethnic groups (Iams and Zuspan 1990). Most babies born as a result of prolonged pregnancy are of normal size and health; some keep on growing after term and are over 4000 g, which supports the premise that the postterm fetus can remain well nourished (Harrington and Campbell 1993). Intrapartal problems for these healthy but large fetuses are cephalopelvic disproportion (CPD) and shoulder dystocia. Only about 5 percent of postterm newborns show signs of postmaturity syndrome (Iams and Zuspan 1990). The major portion of the following discussion will address the fetus who is not tolerating the prolonged pregnancy, is suffering from uteroplacental compromise to blood flow and resultant hypoxia, and is considered to have postmaturity syndrome.

Common Complications of the Newborn with Postmaturity Syndrome

The truly postmature infant is at high risk for morbidity and has a mortality rate two to three times greater than that of term infants. Although today the percentages are extremely low, the majority of deaths occur during labor, because oxygenation and nutrition transport are impaired in the placenta, leaving the fetus prone to hypoglycemia and asphyxia when the stresses of labor begin. The most common disorders of the postmature infant are

- Hypoglycemia, from nutritional deprivation and depleted glycogen stores.
- Meconium aspiration in response to in utero hypoxia. In the presence of oligohydramnios the danger of aspirating thick meconium increases. Severe meconium aspiration syndrome increases the baby's chance of developing persistent pulmonary hypertension, pneumothorax, and pneumonia.
- Polycythemia due to increased production of red blood cells (RBCs) in response to hypoxia.
- Congenital anomalies of unknown cause.
- Seizure activity because of hypoxic insult.
- Cold stress because of loss or poor development of subcutaneous fat.

The long-term effects of postmaturity syndrome are unclear. At present, studies do not agree on the effect of postmaturity syndrome on weight gain and IQ scores.

Prolonged pregnancy itself is not solely responsible for the postmaturity syndrome. The characteristics of the postmature newborn are primarily caused by a combination of advanced gestational age, placental aging and subsequent insufficiency, and continued exposure to amniotic fluid (Resnik 1994).

Medical Therapy

The aim of antenatal management is to differentiate the fetus who has postmaturity syndrome from the fetus who at birth is large, well-nourished, alert, and tolerating the prolonged (postterm) pregnancy.

Antenatal tests that can be done to evaluate fetal status and determine obstetric management include fetal ultrasound, fetal biophysical profile (refer to Table 14–4), measurement of serum placental hormones such as human chorionic gonadotropin (hCG) and human placental lactogen (hPL), and the nonstress and contraction stress tests (NST and CST). Chapter 19 discusses these tests and their use in postterm pregnancy in more depth.

If the amniotic fluid is meconium stained, the baby's nose and mouth should be suctioned by the clinician before birth of the chest and trunk and before the baby takes its first breath to minimize the chance of meconium aspiration syndrome. In some cases, direct suctioning of the trachea is needed. For detailed discussion of medical management and nursing assessments and care, see Chapter 26.

Hypoglycemia is monitored by serial glucose determinations. The baby may be placed on glucose infusions or given early feedings if respiratory distress is not present; but these measures must be instituted with caution because of the frequency of asphyxia in the first 24 hours (Cunningham 1993). Postmature newborns are often voracious eaters.

As with SGA infants, peripheral and central hematocrits are tested to assess the presence of polycythemia. Oxygen is provided for respiratory distress. A partial exchange transfusion may be necessary to prevent adverse sequelae such as hyperviscosity.

APPLYING THE NURSING PROCESS

Nursing Assessment

The newborn with postmaturity syndrome appears alert. This wide-eyed, alert appearance is not necessarily a positive sign because it may indicate chronic intrauterine hypoxia.

The infant has dry, cracking, parchmentlike skin without vernix or lanugo (Figure 25–4). Fingernails are long, and scalp hair is profuse. The infant's body appears long and thin. The wasting involves depletion of previously stored subcutaneous tissue, causing the skin to be loose. Fat layers are almost nonexistent. Postmature newborns frequently have meconium staining, which colors the nails, skin, and umbilical cord. The varying shades (yellow to green) of meconium staining can give some clue about whether the expulsion of meconium was a recent or chronic problem. Green coloring indicates a more recent event.

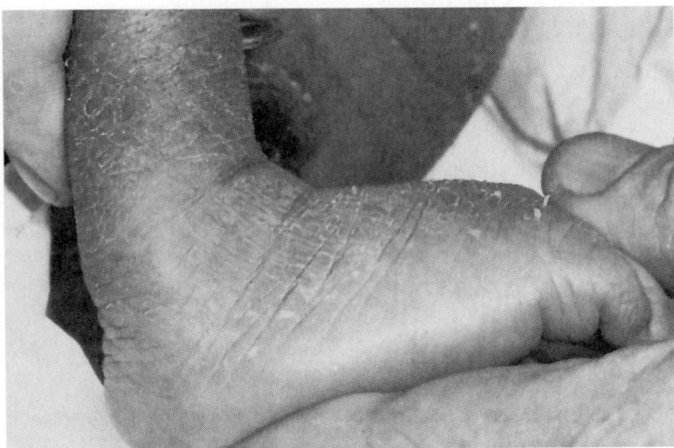

FIGURE 25–4 Postterm infant demonstrates deep cracking and peeling of skin.

Source: Dubowitz L, Dubowitz V: *The Gestational Age of the Newborn.* Redwood City, CA: Addison-Wesley, 1977. Reprinted by permission of V Dubowitz, MD, Hammersmith Hospital, London, England.

Nursing Diagnosis

Nursing diagnoses that may apply to the postmature newborn include the following:

- Hypothermia related to decreased liver glycogen and brown fat stores
- Altered nutrition: less than body requirements related to increased use of glucose secondary to in utero stress and decreased placenta perfusion
- Impaired gas exchange in the lungs and at the cellular level related to airway obstruction from potential meconium aspiration

Nursing Plan and Implementation

Promotion of Physical Well-Being

Nursing interventions are primarily supportive measures. They include

- Observation of cardiopulmonary status, since the stresses of labor are poorly tolerated and severe asphyxia can occur at birth
- Provision of warmth to counterbalance a poor response to cold stress and decreased liver glycogen and brown fat stores
- Frequent monitoring of blood glucose and initiation of early feeding (at 1 or 2 hours of age) or intravenous glucose per physician order
- Observation for the common disorders identified earlier and institution of nursing care and medical management as ordered

Provision of Emotional Support to the Parents

The nurse encourages parents to express their feelings and fears about the newborn's condition and potential long-term problems. The nurse gives careful explanations of procedures, includes the parents in the development of care plans for their baby, and encourages follow-up care as needed.

Evaluation

Anticipated outcomes of nursing care include

- The postterm newborn establishes effective respiratory function.
- The postmature baby is free of metabolic alterations (hypoglycemia) and maintains a stable temperature.

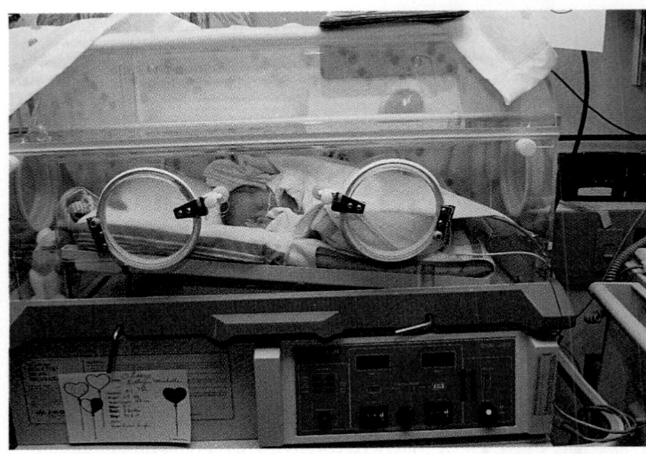

FIGURE 25–5 Preterm infant.

Care of the Preterm (Premature) Newborn

A **preterm infant** is any infant born before the end of 37 weeks' gestation. The length of gestation and thus the level of maturity vary even in the "premature" population. Figure 25–5 shows a preterm newborn.

The incidence of preterm births in the United States ranges from 7 percent of white newborns to 14–15 percent of nonwhites. A higher incidence of prematurity is also seen in single women and adolescents. Prematurity and low birth weight are two common outcomes of pregnancy in young mothers (Makinson 1985).

The causes of preterm labor are poorly understood, but more and more of the factors that influence preterm labor and birth are being identified. (See Chapter 19 for a discussion of preterm labor and birth.) With the help of modern technology, some babies under 500 g and between 23 and 26 weeks' gestation are surviving, but not without significant morbidity.

Physiologic Considerations

The major problem of the preterm newborn is variable immaturity of all systems. The degree of immaturity depends on the length of gestation. For example, newborns of 32 weeks' gestation can be expected to exhibit more immaturity than newborns of 36 weeks' gestation. Maintenance of the preterm newborn falls within narrow physiologic parameters. The preterm newborn must traverse the same complex, interconnected pathways from intrauterine to extrauterine life as the term newborn. Because of immaturity, the premature newborn is ill equipped to make this transition smoothly.

COMMUNITY IN FOCUS Follow-up Neonatal Home Care

Home care has played only a limited role in addressing the needs of preterm infants following discharge. Consequently the focus of nursing efforts to date has been on discharge preparation of the family. However, many preterm infants have continuing health needs following discharge. To address these needs and to provide a mechanism for early discharge for qualified infants, one Fort Worth, Texas community has designed an innovative approach using a home care model that represents a partnership between clinical nurse specialists (CNS) and neonatal intensive care unit (NICU) nurses.

The Harris Home Health program is directed by a clinical nurse specialist who works closely with both the Harris Hospital neonatal CNS and perinatal CNS to ensure a seamless system of follow-up care after discharge. Typically home care visits are planned for stable preterm infants who are feeding well and weigh more than 4 lb. The visits are made by specially selected, carefully educated NICU nurses who cared for the infant in the NICU. On average, the infants are visited twice a week until they have attained a weight of 7–8 lb.

Each pattern of visits is planned individually with the family based on their needs and those of their newborn. The initial home visit includes a thorough assessment of the infant including developmental and nutritional status, and of the family's environment, caregiving abilities, and areas of concern. At each subsequent visit the nurse completes a physical assessment of the infant including vital signs, length, and weight.

Parental education is an important aspect of each visit and focuses on a variety of topics such as infection prevention, IV infusion therapy procedures and maintenance, feeding issues, safety, growth and development, and the like. In addition, the home care nurse works with the insurance case manager when necessary to address coverage issues. Referral to community agencies is made as indicated. A home care nurse is available to families round the clock for consultation and guidance about problems or concerns.

The Harris Home Care CNS coordinates the program and orients the NICU nurses who participate. To be eligible, a nurse must have a minimum of one year NICU experience. The orientation program includes both a didactic portion and a home care clinical component under the supervision of the home care CNS or a designated RN preceptor. Ultimately, home care visits will become a part of each NICU nurse's job description.

The Harris Home Care CNS is responsible for modeling nursing expertise, assessing health care needs of the infants in the program, and networking in the community. In addition, the CNS is responsible for collecting outcomes data. These data will focus on three areas: infant outcomes, parent satisfaction and improved caregiving behaviors, and cost effectiveness. Such information should prove invaluable in assessing the effectiveness of this creative new program, which builds on the expertise of nurses in differing roles and is an innovative response to issues of cost containment.

Source: Christian A: Clinical nurse specialists: Creating new programs for neonatal home care. *J Perinatal Neonatal Nurs* 1996; 10(1):54.

Respiratory and Cardiac Physiology and Considerations

The preterm newborn's lungs are not fully mature and ready to take over the process of oxygen and carbon dioxide exchange without assistance until 35–36 weeks' gestation. Critical factors in the development of respiratory distress include the following:

1. The preterm infant is unable to produce adequate amounts of surfactant. (See Chapter 21 for discussion of respiratory adaptation and development.) When surfactant decreases, compliance (ability of the lung to fill with air easily) also lessens and the inspiratory pressure needed to expand the lungs with air increases. The collapsed (or atelectatic) alveoli will not facilitate an exchange of oxygen and carbon dioxide; the result is hypoxia, inefficient pulmonary blood flow, and depletion of the preterm newborns' available energy.
2. In the preterm infant, the muscular coat of pulmonary blood vessels is incompletely developed. Because of this, the pulmonary arterioles do not constrict as well in response to decreased oxygen levels (Whitsett et al 1994). Lower pulmonary vascular resistance leads to left-to-right shunting of blood through the ductus arteriosus back into the lungs.
3. The ductus arteriosus usually responds to rising oxygen levels by vasoconstriction; in the preterm infant, who has higher susceptibility to hypoxia, the ductus may remain open. A patent ductus increases the blood volume to the lungs, causing pulmonary congestion, increased respiratory effort, and higher oxygen use.

Thermoregulation and Considerations

Heat loss is a major problem that the nurse can do much to prevent in preterm infants. Two limiting factors in heat production, however, are the availability of glycogen in the liver (glycogen stores are primarily laid down during the third trimester) and the amount of brown fat available for metabolism (the preterm infant does not have a full supply of brown fat). If the baby is chilled after birth, both glycogen and brown fat stores are metabolized rapidly for heat production, leaving the newborn with no reserves in the event of future stress. Since the muscle mass is small in preterm infants, and muscular activity is diminished (they are unable to shiver), little heat is produced.

Heat loss occurs as a result of several physiologic and anatomic factors:

1. The preterm baby has a higher ratio of body surface to body weight. This means that the baby's ability to produce heat (body weight) is much less than the potential for losing heat (surface area). The loss of heat in a preterm infant weighing 1500 g is five times greater per unit of body weight than in an adult.
2. The preterm baby has very little subcutaneous fat, which is the human body's insulation. Without adequate insulation, heat is easily conducted from the core of the body (warmer temperature) to the surface of the body (cooler temperature). Heat is lost from the body as the blood vessels, which lie close to the skin surface in the preterm infant, transport blood from the body core to the subcutaneous tissues.
3. The preterm baby has thinner, more permeable skin than the term infant. This increased permeability contributes to a greater insensible water loss as well as heat loss.
4. The posture of the preterm baby is another important factor influencing heat loss. Flexion of the extremities decreases the amount of surface area exposed to the environment; extension increases the surface area exposed to the environment and thus increases heat loss. The gestational age of the infant influences the amount of flexion, from completely hypotonic and extended at 28 weeks to strong flexion displayed by 36 weeks.
5. The preterm baby has a decreased ability to vasoconstrict superficial blood vessels and conserve heat in the body core.

In summary, the more preterm a baby the less able he or she is to maintain heat balance. Prevention of heat loss by providing a neutral thermal environment is one of the most important considerations in nursing management of the preterm infant. Cold stress, with its accompanying severe complications, can be prevented (see Chapter 26).

Digestive Physiology and Considerations

The basic structure of the gastrointestinal (GI) tract is formed early in gestation. Maturation of the digestive and absorptive process is more variable, however, and occurs later in gestation.

As a result of GI immaturity, the preterm newborn has the following digestive and absorption problems:

- Limited ability to convert certain essential amino acids to nonessential amino acids. Certain amino acids, such as histidine, taurine, and cysteine, are essential to the preterm infant but not to the term infant.
- Kidney immaturity causes an inability to handle the increased osmolarity of formula protein. The preterm infant requires a higher concentration of whey protein than of casein.
- Difficulty absorbing saturated fats occurs because of decreased bile salts and pancreatic lipase. Severe illness of the newborn may also prevent intake of adequate nutrients.
- Lactose digestion may not be fully functional during the first few days of a preterm's life. The preterm newborn can digest and absorb most simple sugars.
- Deficiency of calcium and phosphorus may exist since two-thirds of these minerals are deposited in the last trimester. As a result the preterm infant is prone to rickets and significant bone demineralization.
- Fatigue associated with sucking may lead to increased basal metabolic rate, increased oxygen requirements, and necrotizing entercolitis (NEC).
- Feeding intolerance and NEC are caused by diminished blood flow to the intestinal tract because of shock or prolonged hypoxia at birth.

Renal Physiology and Considerations

The kidneys of the preterm infant are immature compared to those of the term infant. This situation poses clinical problems in the management of fluid and electrolyte balance. Specific characteristics of the preterm infant include the following:

1. The glomerular filtration rate (GFR) is lower due to decreased renal blood flow. Since the GFR is directly related to lower gestational age, the more preterm the newborn, the lower the GFR. The GFR also decreases in the presence of diseases or conditions that decrease the renal blood flow and oxygen content, such as severe respiratory distress and perinatal asphyxia. Anuria and oliguria may be observed in the preterm infant after severe asphyxia with associated hypotension.
2. The preterm infant's kidneys are limited in their ability to concentrate urine or to excrete excess amounts of fluid. This means that if excess fluid is administered, the infant is at risk for fluid retention and overhydration. If too little is administered, the infant will become dehydrated because of the inability to retain adequate fluid.
3. The kidneys of the preterm infant will begin excreting glucose (glycosuria) at a lower serum glucose level than occurs in the adult. Therefore, glycosuria with hyperglycemia is common.
4. The buffering capacity of the kidney is less, predisposing the infant to metabolic acidosis. Bicarbonate is excreted at a lower serum level, and excretion of acid is accomplished more slowly. Therefore, after

periods of hypoxia or insult, the kidneys require a longer time to excrete the lactic acid that accumulates. Sodium bicarbonate is frequently required to treat the metabolic acidosis.

5. The immaturity of the renal system affects the infant's ability to excrete drugs. Because excretion time is longer, many drugs are given over longer intervals in the preterm infant (that is, every 12 hours instead of every 8 hours). Urine output must be carefully monitored when the infant is receiving nephrotoxic drugs such as gentamicin, nafcillin, and others. In the event of poor urine output, drugs can become toxic in the infant much more quickly than in the adult.

Reactivity Periods and Behavioral States

The newborn infant's response to extrauterine life is characterized by two periods of reactivity, as discussed in Chapter 21. Because of the immaturity of all systems compared to those of the term newborn, the preterm infant's periods of reactivity are delayed. The very ill infant may be hypotonic and unreactive for several days, so these periods of reactivity may not be observed at all.

As the preterm newborn grows and the condition stabilizes, it becomes increasingly possible to identify behavioral states and traits unique to each infant. This is a very important part of nursing management of the high-risk infant. The nurse can help parents learn their infant's cues for interaction.

In general, stable preterm infants do not demonstrate the same behavioral states as term infants. Preterm infants tend to be more disorganized in their sleep-wake cycles and are unable to attend as well to the human face and objects in the environment. Neurologically, their responses (sucking, muscle tone, states of arousal) are weaker than full-term infants' responses.

By observing each infant's patterns of behavior and responses, especially sleep-wake states, the nurse can teach parents optimal times for interacting with their infant. The parents and nurse can plan nursing care around the times when the infant is alert and best able to attend. In addition, the more knowledge parents have about the meaning of their infant's responses and behaviors, the better prepared they will be to meet their newborn's needs and form a positive attachment with their child.

Management of Nutrition and Fluid Requirements

Providing adequate nutrition and fluids for the preterm infant is a major concern of the health care team. Early feedings are extremely valuable in maintaining normal metabolism and lowering the possibility of such complications as hypoglycemia, hyperbilirubinemia, hyperkalemia, and azotemia. However, the preterm infant is at risk for complications that may develop because of immaturity of the digestive system.

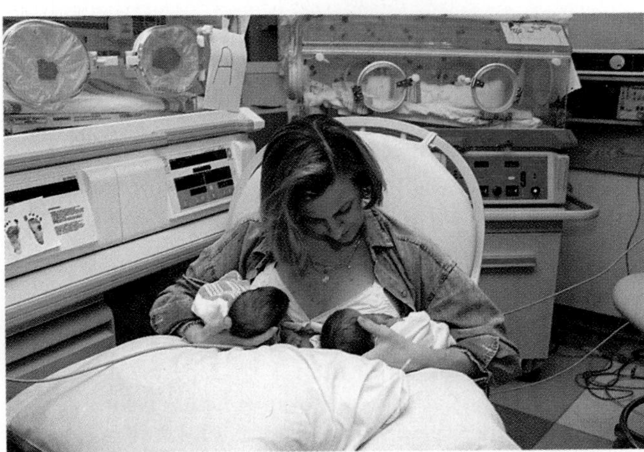

FIGURE 25–6 Mother visits intensive care unit to breastfeed her preterm twin infants.

Nutritional Requirements

Oral caloric intake necessary for growth in an uncompromised healthy preterm newborn is 110–130 kcal/kg/day (Bernbaum 1994). In addition to these relatively high caloric needs, the preterm newborn requires more protein (3–4 g/kg/day, as opposed to 2.0–2.5 g/kg/day for the term infant) (Fletcher 1994). To meet these needs, many institutions use breast milk or special preterm formulas. Besides breast milk's many benefits for the infant, breastfeeding allows the mother to actively contribute to the infant's well-being (Figure 25–6). The nurse should encourage mothers to breastfeed if they choose to do so. It is important for the nurse to be aware of the advantages of breastfeeding as well as the possible disadvantages if breast milk is the sole source of food for the preterm infant. See Chapter 24 for a detailed discussion of breastfeeding.

Whether breast milk or formula is used, feeding regimens are established based on the infant's weight and estimated stomach capacity. Initial formula feedings may be diluted to 12 cal/oz and gradually increased, as the infant tolerates them, to 24 cal/oz. In many instances it is necessary to supplement oral feedings with parenteral fluids to maintain adequate hydration and caloric intake until the baby is on full oral feeds.

In addition to a higher calorie and protein formula, it is recommended that preterm infants receive supplemental multivitamins and vitamin E. The requirement for vitamin E is increased by a diet high in polyunsaturated fats (which preterm infants tolerate best). Preterm infants fed iron-fortified formulas have higher red cell hemolysis and lower vitamin E concentrations and thus require additional vitamin E (Fletcher 1994). Preterm formulas also need to contain medium-chain triglycerides (MCT) and additional amino acids such as cysteine, as well as calcium and vitamin D supplements to increase mineralization of bones.

Nutritional intake is considered adequate when there is consistent weight gain of 20–30 g per day. Initially, no weight gain may be noted for several days, but total weight loss should not exceed 15 percent of the total birth weight or more than 1 to 2 percent per day. Some institutions add the criteria of head circumference growth and increase in body length of 1 cm per week, once the newborn is stable.

Methods of Feeding

The preterm infant is fed by various methods depending on the infant's gestational age, health and physical condition, and neurologic status. The three most common oral feeding methods are bottle, breast, and gavage.

Bottle Feeding Preterm infants who have a coordinated suck and swallow reflex and those showing continued weight gain (20–30 g/day) may be fed by bottle. To avoid excessive expenditure of energy, a soft, smaller nipple is usually used.

The feeding should take no longer than 15–20 minutes. A premature infant nipple or regular-sized nipple may be used, depending on the infant's strength and ability (nippling requires more energy than other methods). The infant is fed in a semisitting position and burped gently after each half ounce or ounce. Babies who are progressing from gavage feedings to bottle-feeding should start with one session of bottle-feeding a day and slowly increase the number of times a day a bottle is given until the baby tolerates all feedings from a bottle.

The infant's ability to suck is assessed. Sucking may be affected by age, asphyxia, sepsis, intraventricular hemorrhage, or other neurologic insult. Before initiating bottle feeding, observe for signs of stress, such as tachypnea (more than 60 respirations/minute), respiratory distress, or hypothermia, which may increase the risk of aspiration. During the feeding the nurse observes the infant for signs of feeding difficulty (tachypnea, cyanosis, bradycardia, lethargy, and uncoordinated suck and swallow). After the feeding, the nurse gently burps and positions the infant on the right side.

Breastfeeding Mothers who wish to breastfeed their preterm infants should be given the opportunity to put the infant to breast as soon as the infant has demonstrated a coordinated suck and swallow reflex, is showing consistent weight gain, and can control body temperature outside of the incubator, regardless of weight. Delaying transition from bottle to breast results in the infant's developing a sucking mechanism specific to the artificial nipple that impedes subsequent transfer to the breast (Auerbach and Walker 1994).

Even if the infant can't be put to the breast, mothers can pump their breasts, and the breast milk can be given via gavage. Use of the double pumping system produces higher levels of prolactin than sequential pumping of the breasts. Lactaids can also be used as adjuncts to the mother's breast milk to increase the amount of fluid the infant receives without becoming tired (Auerbach and Walker 1994). Studies have shown that preterm infants can maintain higher transcutaneous oxygen pressures and control their body temperature better when breastfeeding than when bottle-feeding (Meier 1988).

The infant is placed at the mother's breast. It has been suggested that the football hold is a convenient position for preterm babies. Feeding time may take up to 45 minutes, and babies should be burped as they alternate breasts.

The nurse should coordinate a flexible feeding schedule so babies can nurse during alert times and be allowed to set their own pace. A similar regimen should be used for the baby who is progressing from gavage to breastfeeding. The baby should begin with one feeding per day at the breast and then gradually increase the number of breastfeedings per day.

Gavage Feeding The gavage feeding method is used with preterm infants (less than 34 weeks' gestation) who lack or have a poorly coordinated suck and swallow reflex or are ill. Gavage feeding may be used as an adjunct to bottle feeding if the infant tires easily, or as an alternative if an infant is losing weight because of the energy expenditure required for nippling. See Procedure 25–1: Performing Gavage Feeding.

Transpyloric Feeding An alternative method of feeding is transpyloric feeding. This feeding method should be used only in specially equipped and staffed high-risk nurseries, since it can cause perforation of the stomach or intestines. Preterm infants who cannot tolerate any oral (enteral) feedings may be given nutrition by total parenteral nutrition (hyperalimentation).

Fluid Requirements

Calculation of fluid requirements takes into account the infant's weight and postnatal age. Recommendations for fluid therapy in the preterm infant are approximately 80–100 mL/kg/day for day 1; 100–120 mL/kg/day for day 2; and 120–150 mL/kg/day by day 3 of life. These amounts may be increased up to 200 mL/kg/day if the infant is very small, receiving phototherapy, or under a radiant warmer. The infant may need less fluid if a heat shield is used, the environment is more humid, or humidified oxygen is being provided.

PROCEDURE 25–1 Performing Gavage Feeding

Nursing Action	Rationale
Objective: Assemble and prepare the equipment.	
• No. 5 or no. 8 Fr. feeding tube. See the material below for guidelines for choosing tube size. • 10–30 mL syringe, for aspirating stomach contents • 1/4 in paper tape, to mark the tube for insertion depth and to secure the catheter during feeding • Stethoscope, for auscultating the rush of air into the stomach when testing the tube placement • Appropriate formula • Small cup of sterile water to test for tube placement and to act as lubricant	Equipment organization facilitates the procedure.
Objective: Explain the procedure to the parents.	
Objective: Insert the tube accurately into the stomach. See the material below for step-by-step instructions.	
Objective: Maximize the feeding pleasure of the infant.	
• Whenever possible, hold the infant during gavage feeding. If it is too awkward to hold the infant during feeding, be sure to take time for holding after the feeding.	Feeding time is important to the infant's tactile sensory input.
• Offer a pacifier to the infant during the feeding.	Sucking during feeding comforts and relaxes the infant, making the formula flow more easily. Infants can lose their sucking reflexes when fed by gavage for long periods.

Gavage Feeding Guidelines

Choosing a Catheter Size

When choosing the catheter size, consider the size of the infant, the area of insertion (oral or nasal), and the desired rate of flow. The size of the catheter will influence the rate of flow.

The very small infant (less than 1600 g) requires a 5 Fr. feeding tube; an infant greater than 1600 g may tolerate a larger tube.

Orogastric insertion is preferable to nasogastric because most infants are obligatory nose breathers. If nasogastric is used, a 5 Fr. catheter should be used to minimize airway obstruction.

Inserting and Checking the Tube

- Elevate the head of the bed and position the infant on the back or side to allow easy passage of the tube.
- Measure the distance from the tip of the ear to the nose to the xiphoid process, and mark the point with a small piece of paper tape (Figure 25–7) to ensure enough tubing to enter the stomach.

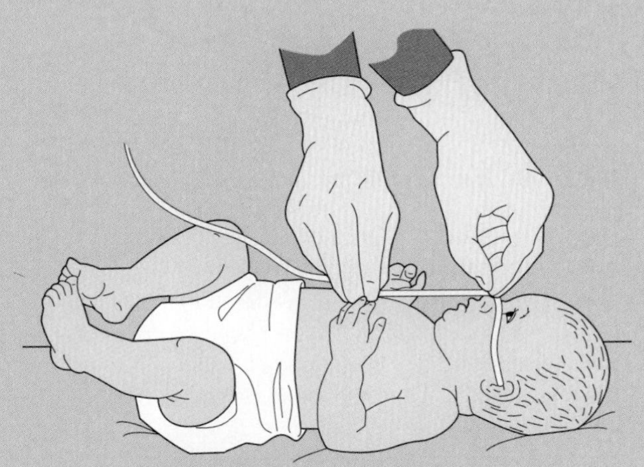

FIGURE 25–7 Measuring gavage tube length.

PROCEDURE 25–1 Performing Gavage Feeding continued

Inserting and Checking the Tube *continued*

- If inserting the tube nasally, lubricate the tip in a cup of sterile water. Use water instead of an oil-based lubricant, in case the tube is inadvertently passed into a lung. Shake any excess drops to prevent aspiration.
- If inserting the tube orally, the oral secretions are enough to lubricate the tube adequately.
- Stabilize the infant's head with one hand and pass the tube via the mouth (or nose) into the stomach to the point previously marked. If the infant begins coughing or choking or becomes cyanotic or phonic, remove the tube immediately as the tube has probably entered the trachea.
- If no respiratory distress is apparent, lightly tape the tube in position, draw up 0.5–1.0 mL of air in the syringe, and connect the syringe to the tubing. Place the stethoscope over the epigastrum and briskly inject the air (Figure 25–8). You will hear a sudden rush as the air enters the stomach.

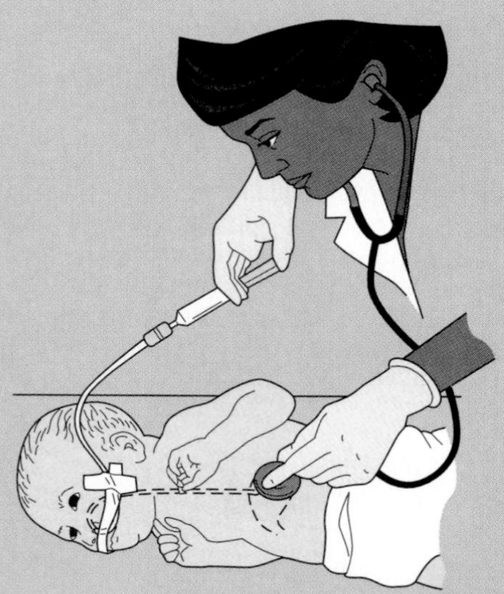

FIGURE 25–8 Auscultation for placement of gavage tube.

- Aspirate the stomach contents with the syringe, and note the amount, color, and consistency to evaluate the infant's feeding tolerance. Return the residual to the stomach unless you are asked to discard it. It is usually not discarded because of the potential for electrolyte imbalance.
- If the aspirated contents contain only a clear fluid or mucus and if it is unclear whether or not the tube is in the stomach, test the aspirate for pH. Stomach aspirate has a pH between 1 and 3.

Administering the Feeding

- Hold the infant for feeding, or position the infant on the right side, to decrease the risk of aspiration in case of emesis during feeding.
- Separate the syringe from the tube, remove the plunger from the barrel, reconnect the barrel to the tube, and pour the formula into the syringe.
- Elevate the syringe 6–8 inches over the infant's head and allow the formula to flow by gravity at a slow, even rate. You may need to initiate the flow of formula by inserting the plunger of the syringe into the barrel just until you see formula enter the feeding tube. Do not use pressure.
- Regulate the rate to prevent sudden stomach distention leading to vomiting and aspiration. Continue adding formula to the syringe until the infant has absorbed the desired volume.

Clearing and Removing the Tube

- Clear the tubing with a 2–3 mL sterile water or with air. This ensures that the infant has received all of the formula. If the tube is going to be left in place, clearing it will decrease the risk of clogging and bacterial growth in the tube.
- To remove the tube, loosen the tape, fold the tube over on itself, and quickly withdraw the tube in one smooth motion to minimize the potential for fluid aspiration as the tube passes the epiglottis. If the tube is to be left in, position it so that the infant is unable to remove it. Replace the tube every 24 hours.

Common Complications of Prematurity

The preterm newborn is at risk for many complications secondary to the immaturity of various body systems in addition to those already discussed. The most common of these complications are the following:

1. *Apnea.* Apnea of prematurity refers to cessation of breathing for 20 seconds or longer or for less than 20 seconds when associated with cyanosis, bradycardia, and limpness (Grisemer 1990). Apnea is a common problem in the preterm infant (less than 36 weeks' gestation) and is thought to be primarily a result of neuronal immaturity, a factor that contributes to the preterm infant's irregular breathing patterns. Factors that adversely affect brain nerve cells include hypoxia, acidosis, edema, intracranial bleeding, hyperbilirubinemia, hypoglycemia, hypocalcemia, and sepsis.
2. *Patent ductus arteriosus.* The ductus arteriosus fails to close because of decreased pulmonary arteriole musculature and hypoxemia.
3. *RDS.* Respiratory distress results from inadequate surfactant production.
4. *Intraventricular hemorrhage.* Intraventricular hemorrhage (IVH) is the most common type of intracranial hemorrhage in the small preterm infant, especially those weighing less than 1500 g or of less than 34 weeks' gestation. Up to 35 weeks' gestation the preterm's brain ventricles are lined by the germinal matrix, which is highly susceptible to hypoxic events such as respiratory distress, birth trauma, and birth asphyxia. The germinal matrix is very vascular, and these blood vessels rupture in the presence of hypoxia.
5. *Anemia.* The preterm infant is at risk for anemia of prematurity because of the rapid rate of growth required, shorter red-blood-cell life, excessive blood sampling, decreased iron stores, and deficiency of vitamin E.

Other common problems of preterm infants such as hypocalcemia, hypoglycemia, and NEC are discussed earlier in the physiologic sections. For discussion of hyperbilirubinemia and sepsis see Chapter 26.

Long-Term Needs and Outcome

The care of preterm infants and their families does not stop on discharge from the nursery. Follow-up care is extremely important because many developmental problems are not noted until an infant is older and begins to demonstrate motor delays or sensory disability.

Within the first year of life, low-birth-weight preterm infants face higher mortality than term infants. Causes of death include sudden infant death syndrome (SIDS) (which occurs about five times more frequently in the preterm infant), respiratory infections, and neurologic defects. Morbidity is also much higher among preterm infants, with those weighing less than 1500 g at highest risk for long-term complications.

The most common long-term problems observed in preterm infants include the following:

- *Retinopathy of prematurity (ROP).* Premature newborns are particularly susceptible to characteristic retinal changes known as retinopathy of prematurity (ROP). This disease has previously been known as retrolental fibroplasia (RLF). In spite of new technology and the ability to monitor arterial oxygen closely, ROP and resulting loss of eyesight continue to occur in the preterm infant (Bowen and Tasman 1993).
- *Bronchopulmonary dysplasia (BPD).* Long-term lung disease is a result of damage to the alveolar epithelium secondary to positive pressure respirator therapy and high oxygen concentration. These infants have long-term dependence on oxygen therapy and an increased incidence of respiratory infection during their first few years of life.
- *Speech defects.* The most frequently observed speech defects involve delayed development of receptive and expressive ability, which may persist into the school years.
- *Neurologic defects.* The most common neurologic defects include cerebral palsy, hydrocephalus, seizure disorders, lower IQ scores, and learning disabilities. However, the socioeconomic climate and family support systems are extremely important influences on the child's ultimate school performance in the absence of major neurologic defects. Families can be reminded that risk does not equal injury, injury does not equal damage, and description of damage does not allow a precise prediction about recovery or outcome.
- *Auditory defects.* Preterm infants have a 1 to 4 percent incidence of moderate to profound hearing loss and should have a formal audiologic exam before discharge and at 3–6 months (corrected age). The brain-stem auditory evoked response (BAER) is the best test; any infant with abnormal results on the BAER should be referred to speech-and-language specialists (Hulseman and Norman 1992).

When evaluating the infant's abilities and disabilities, it is important for parents to understand that developmental progress must be evaluated from the expected date of birth, not from the actual date of birth. Developmental level cannot be evaluated based on chronologic age. In addition, the parents need the consistent support of health care professionals in the long-term management of their infant to promote the highest quality of life possible.

APPLYING THE NURSING PROCESS

Nursing Assessment

Accurate assessment of the physical characteristics and gestational age of the preterm newborn is imperative to anticipate the special needs and problems of this baby. Physical characteristics vary greatly depending on gestational age, but the following characteristics are frequently present:

- Color is usually pink or ruddy but may be acrocyanotic. (Cyanosis, jaundice, or pallor, are abnormal and should be noted.)
- Skin is reddened and translucent, blood vessels are readily apparent, there is little subcutaneous fat.
- Lanugo is plentiful and widely distributed.
- Head size appears large in relation to body.
- Skull bones are pliable; fontanelle is smooth and flat.
- Ears have minimal cartilage and are pliable, folded over.
- Nails are soft, short.
- Genitals are small; testes may not be descended.
- Resting position is flaccid, froglike.
- Cry is weak.
- Reflexes (sucking, swallowing, and gag) are poor.
- Activity consists of jerky, generalized movements. (Seizure activity is abnormal.)

Determination of gestational age in preterm newborns requires knowledge and experience in administering gestational assessment tools. The tool used should be specific, reliable, and valid. For a discussion of gestational age assessment tools, see Chapter 22.

Nursing Diagnosis

Nursing diagnoses that may apply to the preterm newborn include the following:

- Impaired gas exchange related to immature pulmonary vasculature
- Ineffective breathing pattern: apnea related to immature central nervous system
- Altered nutrition: less than body requirements related to weak suck and swallow reflexes and decreased ability to absorb nutrients
- Fluid volume deficit related to high insensible water losses and inability of kidneys to concentrate urine
- Alteration in metabolic processes related to cold stress
- Ineffective family coping related to anger or guilt at having delivered a premature baby
- Grieving related to actual or perceived loss of a normal newborn

Nursing Plan and Implementation

Maintenance of Respiratory Function

There is increased danger of respiratory obstruction in preterm newborns because their bronchi and trachea are so narrow that mucus can obstruct the airway. The nurse must maintain patency through judicious suctioning.

Positioning of the newborn can also affect respiratory function. If the baby is in the supine position, the nurse should slightly elevate the infant's head to maintain the airway. Because the newborn has weak neck muscles and cannot control head movement, the nurse should ensure that this head position is maintained by placing a small roll under the shoulders. The nurse should avoid placing the infant in the supine position because the newborn has difficulty raising the chest because of weak chest and abdominal muscles. In contrast, the prone position splints the chest wall and decreases the amount of respiratory effort used to move it. The prone position therefore facilitates chest expansion and improves air entry and oxygenation. Weak or absent cough or gag reflexes increase the chance of aspiration in the premature newborn. The nurse should ensure that the infant's position facilitates drainage of mucus or regurgitated formula.

The nurse monitors heart and respiratory rates with cardiorespiratory monitors and observes the newborn to identify alterations in cardiopulmonary status. Nursery nurses must be alert to signs of respiratory distress, including

- Cyanosis—serious sign when generalized
- Tachypnea—sustained respiratory rate greater than 60/min after first 4 hours of life
- Retractions
- Expiratory grunting
- Flaring nostrils
- Apneic episodes
- Presence of rales or rhonchi on auscultation
- Diminished air entry
- Fatigue

The nurse who observes any of these alterations records and reports them for further evaluation. If respiratory distress occurs, the nurse administers oxygen per physician order to relieve hypoxemia. If hypoxemia is not treated immediately, it may result in patent ductus arteriosus or metabolic acidosis. If oxygen is administered to the newborn, the nurse monitors the oxygen concentration with devices such as the transcutaneous oxygen monitor (tcPO_2) or the pulse oximeter. Monitoring of oxygen concentration in the baby's blood is essential since hyperoxemia can lead to blindness (retinopathy of prematurity).

The nurse must also consider respiratory function during feeding. To prevent aspiration and increased energy expenditure and oxygen consumption, the nurse must ensure that the infant's gag and suck reflexes are intact before initiating oral feedings.

Maintenance of Neutral Thermal Environment

Provision of a neutral thermal environmental minimizes the oxygen consumption expended to maintain a normal core temperature; it also prevents cold stress and facilitates growth by decreasing the calories needed to maintain body temperature. The preterm infant's immature central nervous system provides poor temperature control, and stores of brown fat are decreased. A small infant (<1200 g) can lose 80 kcal/kg/day through radiation of body heat.

The nurse can minimize heat loss and temperature instability effects by taking the following measures:

1. Warm and humidify oxygen without blowing it over the face to minimize convective heat loss and increase oxygen consumption.
2. Place the baby in a double-walled incubator, and use a heat shield over small preterm infants.
3. Avoid placing the baby on cold surfaces such as metal treatment tables and cold x-ray plates; pad cold surfaces with diapers and use radiant warmers during procedures; and warm hands before handling the baby to prevent heat transfer via conduction.
4. Warm the blood before exchange transfusions.
5. Keep the skin dry and place a cap on the baby's head to prevent heat loss via evaporation. (The head makes up 25 percent of the total body size.)
6. Keep radiant warmers and cribs away from windows and cold external walls and out of drafts to prevent heat loss by radiation.
7. Use a skin probe to monitor the baby's skin temperature. Correlate ambient temperatures with the skin probe in the incubator. The temperature should be 36–37C (96.8–97.7F). Temperature fluctuations indicate hypothermia or hyperthermia.
8. Warm formula or stored breast milk before feeding.

The nurse begins the process of weaning to a crib when the premature infant is medically stable, doesn't require assisted ventilation, weighs approximately 1500 g, has 5 days of consistent weight gain, and is taking oral feedings and apnea and bradycardia episodes have stabilized. Once preterm infants are medically stable, they should be clothed with a double-thickness cap, cotton shirt, and diaper (Medoff-Cooper 1994).

Maintenance of Fluid and Electrolyte Status

Maintenance of hydration is accomplished by providing adequate intake based on the newborn's weight, gestational age, chronologic age, and volume of sensible and insensible water losses. Adequate fluid intake should provide sufficient water to compensate for increased insensible losses and to provide the amount needed for renal excretion of metabolic products. Insensible water losses can be minimized by providing a high ambient humidity, humidifying oxygen, using heat shields, covering the skin with plastic wrap, and placing the infant in a double-walled incubator.

The nurse evaluates the hydration status of the baby by assessing and recording signs of dehydration. Signs of dehydration include sunken fontanelle, loss of weight, poor skin turgor (skin returns to position slowly when squeezed gently), dry oral mucous membranes, decreased urine output, and increased specific gravity (>1.013). The nurse must also identify signs of overhydration by observing the newborn for edema or excessive weight gain and by comparing urine output with fluid intake.

The preterm infant should be weighed at least once daily at the same time each day. Weight change is one of the most sensitive indicators of fluid balance. Weighing diapers is also important for accurate input and output measurement. A comparison of intake and output measurements over an 8- or 24-hour period provides important information about renal function and fluid balance. Assessment of patterns and whether they show a net gain or loss over several days is also essential to fluid management. The nurse should monitor blood serum levels and pH to evaluate for electrolyte imbalances.

The nurse should maintain accurate hourly intake calculations when administering intravenous fluids. Since the preterm infant is unable to excrete excess fluid, it is important to maintain the correct amount of intravenous fluid to prevent fluid overload. This can be accomplished by using neonatal or pediatric infusion pumps. To prevent electrolyte imbalance and dehydration, the nurse must take care to give the correct IV solutions and volumes and concentrations of formulas. Urine specific gravity and pH are obtained periodically. Urine osmolality provides an indication of hydration, although this factor must be correlated with other assessments (for example, serum sodium). Hydration is considered adequate when the urine output is 1 to 3 mL/kg/hr.

Provision of Adequate Nutrition and Prevention of Fatigue During Feeding

The feeding method depends on the feeding abilities and health status of the preterm newborn; see the discussion of various feeding methods. All these methods are initially supplemented with intravenous therapy until oral intake is sufficient to support growth (110–130 kcal/kg/day). The first feedings are small amounts given every 2–3 hours. These small amounts are increased slowly by 1–2 mL. Formula or breast milk (with or without fortifiers to increase caloric content) is incorporated into the feedings slowly; initially it may be at quarter strength, then half strength, and so on. This is done to avoid overtaxing the digestive capacity of the preterm newborn.

The nurse should carefully watch for any signs of feeding intolerance, including

- Increasing gastric residuals
- Abdominal distention (measured routinely before feedings)
- Guaiac-positive stools (occult blood in stools)
- Glucose in the stools
- Vomiting
- Diarrhea

The nurse must be watchful for any signs of respiratory distress or fatigue during feedings. Before each feeding, the nurse measures abdominal girth and auscultates the abdomen to determine the presence and quality of bowel sounds. Such assessments promote early detection of abdominal distention and decreased peristaltic activity, which may indicate necrotizing enterocolitis (NEC) or paralytic ileus. The nurse also checks for residual formula in the stomach before feeding. This is done when the newborn is fed by gavage or transpyloric method or in the presence of abdominal distention in a fed newborn. The presence of residual formula is an indication of intolerance to the type or amount of feeding or the increase in amount of feeding. Residual formula is usually readministered because digestive processes have already been initiated.

Preterm newborns who are ill or fatigue easily with nipple feedings are usually fed by gavage or transpyloric feeding. The infant is essentially passive with these methods, thus conserving energy and calories. As the baby matures, gavage feedings are replaced with breast- or bottle-feedings (nipple-feedings) to assist in strengthening the sucking reflex and meeting oral and emotional needs. Nurses are key in the decision of when preterm infants are ready to start a nipple-feeding program. Factors used to indicate readiness are a strong gag reflex, presence of nonnutritive sucking, and rooting behavior. Kinneer and Beachy (1994) found that both low-birth-weight and preterm infants nipple-feed more effectively in a quiet state, so crying should not be used as a hunger cue. The nurse establishes a gradual nipple-feeding program, such as one nipple-feeding per day, then one nipple-feeding per shift, and then a nipple-feeding every other feeding. Daily weights are monitored because often there is a small weight loss when nipple-feedings are started. After feedings, the caregiver places the baby on the right side (with support to maintain this position) to enhance gastric emptying and decrease the chance of aspiration if regurgitation occurs. Gastroesophageal reflux is not uncommon in preterm newborns.

The nurse involves the parents in feeding their preterm baby. This is essential to the development of attachment between parents and infant. In addition, such involvement increases parental knowledge about the care of their infant and helps them cope with the situation.

Prevention of Infection

The nurse is responsible for minimizing the preterm newborn's exposure to pathogenic organisms. The preterm newborn is susceptible to infection because of an immature immune system and thin and permeable skin. Invasive procedures, techniques such as umbilical catheterization and mechanical ventilation, and prolonged hospitalization place the infant at greater risk for infection.

Strict hand washing, reverse isolation, and use of equipment for only one infant help minimize the preterm newborn's exposure to infectious agents. Many intensive care nurseries require a 2- to 3-minute scrub with iodined antibacterial solutions, which decrease growth of gram-positive cocci and gram-negative rod organisms. Other specific nursing interventions include limiting visitors; requiring visitors to wash their hands; and maintaining strict aseptic practices when changing intravenous tubing and solutions (IV solutions and tubing should be changed every 24 hours), administering parenteral fluids, and assisting with sterile procedures. If infection is detected, the infant is placed in an incubator or isolation room. Isolettes and radiant warmers should be changed weekly. Caregivers prevent pressure area breakdown by changing the baby's position, doing range-of-motion exercises, or using a sheepskin or a water bed. To avoid skin tears, a protective transparent covering can be applied over vulnerable joints (*Neonatal Skin Care* 1992). Nurses should avoid using chemical skin preps and tape, which may cause skin trauma.

If infection (sepsis) occurs in the preterm newborn, the nurse may be the first to identify the subtle clinical signs associated with infection. The nurse informs the clinician of the findings immediately and implements the treatment plan per clinician orders in the presence of infection. For specific nursing care required for the newborn with an infection, see Chapter 26.

Promotion of Parent-Infant Attachment

Preterm newborns are generally separated from their parents for prolonged periods. Illness or complications may be detected in the first few hours or days after birth. The resulting interruption in parent-newborn bonding necessitates intervention to ensure successful attachment of parent and infant.

Nurses should take measures to promote positive parental feelings toward the newborn. They can give photographs of the baby to parents to take home or to the mother if she is in a different hospital. They can place the infant's first name on the incubator as soon as it is known to help the parents feel that their infant is a unique and special person. They also send a weekly card with the baby's footprint, weight, and length to promote bonding. Parents are given the telephone number of the nursery or intensive care unit and the names of staff members so that they have access to information about their baby at any time of the day or night.

Early parental involvement in the care of and decisions about their baby, as well as early and frequent visits, provide parents with realistic expectations. Parents need education to develop caregiving skills and to understand the premature infant's behavioral characteristics (Haut et al 1994). The nurse provides opportunities for parents to touch, hold, talk to, and care for the baby. Skin-to-skin (kangaroo) holding has been shown to help parents feel close to their small intubated or nointubated infants even with parents at risk for attachment difficulties (Gale et al 1993) (Figure 25–9).

Some parents may progress easily to touching and cuddling their infant; others do not. Parents need to know that apprehension is normal and the acquaintance process moves slowly. Rooming-in provides a more private environment, but with help readily available, for the stable preterm infant and family to get acquainted (Cusson and Lee 1994).

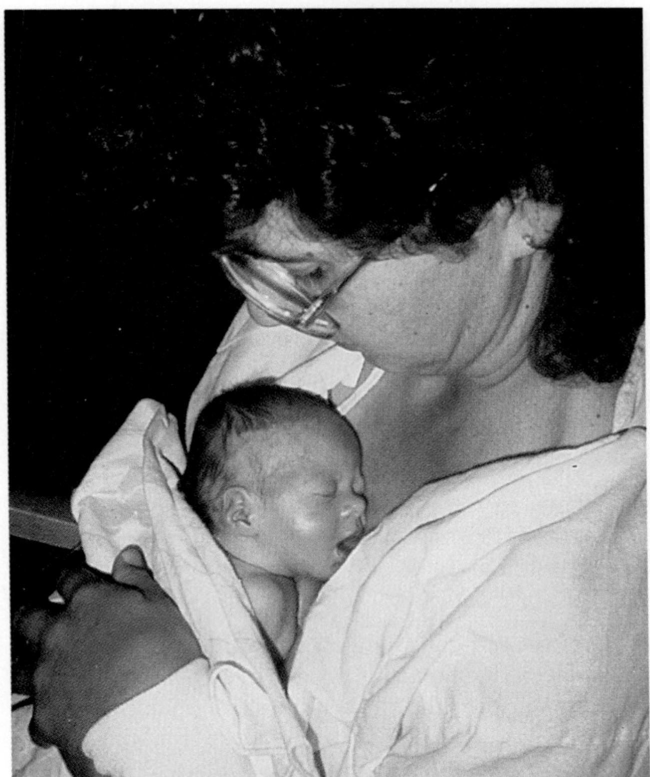

FIGURE 25–9 Kangaroo (skin-to-skin) care facilitates closeness and attachment between parents and their premature infant.

Source: Courtesy of Kadlac Medical Center Kangaroo Care Study and Carol Thompson, RNC, BSN, NNP.

Promotion of Developmentally Supportive Care

With prolonged separation and the neonatal intensive care unit (NICU) environment, individualized baby sensory stimulation programs are necessary. The nurse plays a key role in determining the appropriate type and amount of sensory (visual, tactile, and auditory) stimulation.

Research into the unique behavioral characteristics of the preterm infant highlights many responses that reflect disorganization of the autonomic system. This work suggests that some preterm infants are not developmentally able to deal with more than one sensory input at a time. The Assessment of Preterm Infant Behavior (APIB) scale (Als et al 1982) identifies individual preterm newborn behaviors according to five areas of development. The preterm baby's behavioral reactions to stimulation are observed, and developmental interventions are then based on reducing detrimental environmental stimuli to the lowest possible level and providing appropriate opportunities for development.

The NICU environment contains many detrimental stimuli that the nurse can help reduce. Noise levels can be reduced by responding to and silencing alarms quickly and keeping conversations away from the baby's bedside. Bright lights can be modified by shielding the baby's eyes with blankets over the top portion of the incubator. Dimming the lights may encourage infants to open their eyes and be more responsive to their parents (Cusson and Lee 1994). Nurses take actions designed to decrease the times infants are disturbed and promote uninterrupted sleep, such as displaying "Quiet Please" cards in the nursery (NANN Practice Committee 1993). Some other developmental supportive interventions include the following:

- Facilitate handling by using containment measures when turning or moving the infant or doing procedures such as suctioning. Containment is accomplished by using your hands to hold the infant's arms and legs, flexed, close to the midline of the body. This helps stabilize the infant's motor and physiologic subsystems during stressful activities.

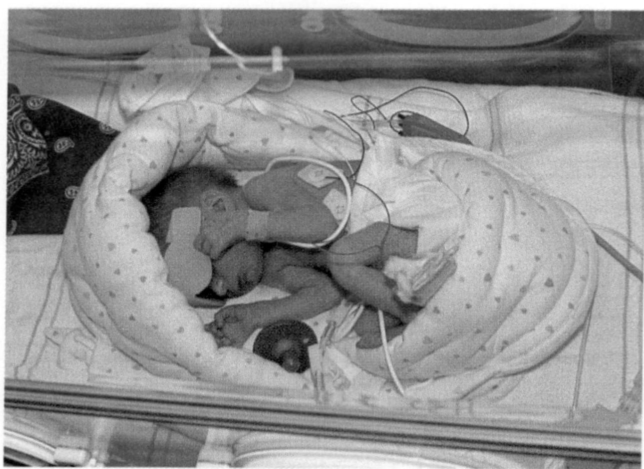

FIGURE 25–10 Infant is "nested." Hand to mouth behavior facilitates self-consoling and soothing activities.
Source: Courtesy of Theresa Kledzik, RN, Developmental Nurse, Memorial Hospital.

- Facilitate self-consoling and soothing activities such as placing blanket rolls or approved manufactured devices next to the infant's sides and against the feet to provide "nesting." Swaddle the infant with the extremities in a flexed position while ensuring that the hands can reach the face to do hand-to-mouth activities (Figure 25–10).
- Simulate the kinesthetic advantages of the intrauterine environment by using sheepskin or approved waterbeds.
- Provide opportunities for nonnutritive sucking with a pacifier. This improves oxygen saturation; decreases body movements; improves sleep, especially after feedings; and increases weight gain.

Teaching the parents to read behavioral cues will help them move at their infant's own pace when providing stimulation. Parents are ideally equipped to meet the baby's need for stimulation. Stroking, rocking, cuddling, quiet singing, and talking to the baby can all be an integral part of the baby's care. Visual stimulation in the form of *en face* interaction with caregivers and mobiles is also important.

Preparation for Home Care

Parents are often anxious when their premature infant is transferred out of the NICU or is discharged home. Parents of preterm babies should receive the same postpartal teaching as any parent taking a new infant home. In preparing for discharge, parents are encouraged to spend time caring directly for their baby. This familiarizes the parents with their baby's behavior patterns and helps them establish realistic expectations about the infant.

Discharge instruction includes breast- and bottle-feeding techniques, formula preparation (including bottle sterilization), and vitamin administration. Mothers of preterm babies desiring to breastfeed are taught to pump their breasts to keep the milk flowing and provide milk even before discharge. This activity (pumping) allows breastfeeding after discharge from the hospital. Nurses also give parents information on bathing, diapering, hygiene, and normal elimination patterns. Parents should be told to expect changes in the color of the baby's stool, number of bowel movements, and timing of elimination when the infant is switched from bottle- to breastfeeding. This information can prevent unnecessary concern by the parents. Normal growth and development patterns, reflexes, and activity for preterm infants are discussed. Emphasis should be placed on bonding behaviors and dealing with newborn crying. Care of the preterm infant with complications, prevention of infections, signs of a sick child, and the need for continued medical follow-up are emphasized.

Families with preterm infants usually do not need to be referred to community agencies, such as visiting nurse assistance. Referral may be necessary if the infant has severe congenital abnormalities, feeding problems, or complications with infections or respiratory problems, or if the parents seem unable to cope with an at-risk baby. Parents of preterm infants can benefit from meeting with others in a similar situation to share common experiences and concerns. Nurses can refer parents to support groups sponsored by the hospital or by others in the community.

Evaluation

Anticipated outcomes of nursing care include

- The preterm newborn is free of respiratory distress and establishes effective respiratory function.
- The preterm newborn gains weight and shows no signs of fatigue or aspiration during feedings.
- The parents are able to verbalize their anger and guilt feelings about the birth of a preterm baby and show attachment behavior such as frequent visits and growing confidence in their participatory care activities.

Care of the Newborn of a Substance-Abusing Mother

An infant of a substance-abusing mother (ISAM) was formerly called an infant of an addicted mother. The newborn of an alcoholic or drug-dependent woman will also be alcohol- or drug-dependent. After birth, when an infant's connection with the maternal blood supply is severed, the newborn suffers withdrawal. In addition, the drugs ingested by the mother may be teratogenic, resulting in congenital anomalies.

Drug Dependency

Drug-dependent infants are predisposed to a number of problems. Since almost all narcotic drugs cross the placenta and enter the fetal circulation, the fetus can develop problems in utero or soon after birth.

The greatest risks to the fetus of the drug-dependent mother include

- *Intrauterine asphyxia*—often a direct result of fetal withdrawal secondary to maternal withdrawal. Fetal withdrawal is accompanied by hyperactivity with increased oxygen consumption, which, if not adequately compensated, can lead to fetal asphyxia. Moreover, narcotic-addicted women tend to have a higher incidence of PIH, abruptio placentae, and placenta previa, resulting in placental insufficiency and fetal asphyxia.
- *Intrauterine infection*—particularly sexually transmitted disease and hepatitis—often connected with the pregnant addict's lifestyle. Such infections can involve the fetus.
- *Alterations in birth weight*—may depend on the type of drug the mother uses. Women using predominantly heroin have infants of lower birth weight who are SGA, whereas women maintained on methadone have higher-birth-weight infants, some of whom are LGA.
- *Low Apgar scores*—possibly related to the intrauterine asphyxia or the medication the woman received during labor. The use of a narcotic antagonist (nalorphine or naloxone) to reverse respiratory depression is contraindicated, as it may precipitate acute withdrawal in the infant.

Patterns of abuse of alcohol, marijuana, and heroin in childbearing women have changed very little, but the incidence of cocaine (especially "crack") use has risen dramatically (see Chapter 12 for more discussion of maternal substance abuse). Marijuana, alcohol, and nicotine are sometimes used in conjunction with cocaine. Therefore, the effects of secondary drugs on the newborn must also be taken into consideration. A high rate of perinatal complications has been noted for cocaine-exposed infants (see Chapter 12).

Common Complications of the Drug-Dependent Newborn

The newborn of a woman who abused drugs during her pregnancy is predisposed to the following problems:

- *Respiratory distress.* The heroin-addicted newborn frequently suffers respiratory stress, mainly meconium-aspiration pneumonia and transient tachypnea. Meconium aspiration is usually secondary to increased oxygen consumption and activity experienced by the fetus during intrauterine withdrawal. Transient tachypnea may develop secondary to the inhibitory effects of narcotics on the reflex responsible for clearing the lungs. Respiratory distress syndrome occurs less often in heroin-addicted newborns, even in the presence of prematurity, because they have tissue-oxygen unloading capabilities comparable to those of a 6-week-old term infant. In addition, heroin stimulates production of glucocorticoids via the anterior pituitary gland.
- *Jaundice.* Newborns of methadone-addicted women may develop jaundice due to prematurity. Heroin contributes to early maturity of the liver, leading to a lower incidence of hyperbilirubinemia for these babies (Wennberg et al 1994).
- *Congenital anomalies and growth retardation.* The incidence of anomalies of the genitourinary and cardiovascular systems is slightly increased in infants of heroin-addicted mothers. Infants of cocaine-addicted mothers exhibit congenital malformations involving bony skull defects such as microencephaly and symmetric intrauterine growth retardation (Jhaveri et al 1993).
- *Behavioral abnormalities.* Babies exposed to cocaine have poor state organization and decreased interactive behaviors when tested with the Brazelton Neonatal Behavioral Assessment Scale (Cole 1996). They have difficulty moving through the various sleep and awake states. Cocaine-exposed infants have difficulty attending to and actively engaging in auditory and visual stimuli.
- *Withdrawal.* The most significant postnatal problem of the drug-addicted newborn is that of narcotic withdrawal (usually from heroin or methadone). The onset of the withdrawal manifestations usually occurs within the first 72 hours after birth. For heroin-addicted newborns, a majority of withdrawal symptoms are seen within the first 24 to 48 hours. For newborns exposed to barbiturates, symptoms may be delayed for several days. Withdrawal for cocaine-addicted infants may occur 4 to 5 days after birth. For methadone-addicted infants, withdrawal symptoms may appear immediately after birth or within the first 48 hours of age (Frank et al 1993). In most cases, the withdrawal manifestations peak in the newborn about the third day and subside by the fifth to seventh day.

Long-Term Complications

During the first two years of life, many cocaine-exposed infants demonstrate deviant psychologic behavior. This is attributed to the irreversible damage to dopamine neurons caused by long-term administration of cocaine. This damage is manifested by susceptibility to behavior lability and the inability to express strong feelings such as pleasure, anger, or distress or even a strong reaction to being separated from their parents. Cocaine-exposed infants are at higher risk for motor development problems, a delay in expressive language skills, and feeding difficulties because of swallowing problems.

Infants of drug-addicted mothers often demonstrate a higher incidence of gastrointestinal and respiratory illnesses. It is believed these are related not to narcotic addiction but to lack of education about proper infant care, feeding, and hygiene.

Another important long-term complication is the high (15–20 per 1000 births) rate of sudden infant death syndrome (SIDS) in heroin- or methadone-exposed infants when compared to those in the general population (Frank et al 1993). Some studies have shown that infants of cocaine-addicted mothers have a SIDS rate of 8.5 per 1000 births and suggest that the rate may be even higher in those infants who have moderate to severe postnatal withdrawal (Bell and Lau 1995). After birth the infant born to a drug-dependent mother may also be subject to neglect or abuse (Scherling 1994).

Medical Therapy

The goal of medical therapy is prevention through prenatal management (see Chapter 12) and pharmacologic management of neonatal narcotic withdrawal. For optimal fetal and neonatal outcome, the narcotic-addicted woman should receive complete prenatal care as early as possible. She should be started on a methadone program with a reduction in dosage to 20 mg or less, if possible. The aim of methadone maintenance during pregnancy is the prevention of heroin use. The dose of methadone used for maintenance should be sufficient to ensure this goal even if the dose is greater than 20 mg. It is not recommended that the woman be withdrawn completely from narcotics while pregnant, since this induces fetal withdrawal with poor newborn outcomes.

Newborn treatment may include management of newborn complications; serologic tests for syphilis, HIV, and hepatitis B; drug screen and meconium analysis for cocaine; and social service referral (Ryan et al 1994).

About 50 percent of newborns of addicted mothers experience withdrawal symptoms severe enough to require treatment. Drugs to control withdrawal symptoms are phenobarbital or tincture of opium. Nutritional support is important in light of the increase in energy expenditure that withdrawal may entail. In 1989, the American Academy of Pediatrics began recommending use of a formula that supplies 24 calories per ounce to provide 150–250 kcal/kg/day if the infant has diarrhea and vomiting or if the infant is excessively active (Angelini and Knapp 1991).

APPLYING THE NURSING PROCESS

Nursing Assessment

Early identification of the newborn needing medical or pharmacologic interventions decreases the incidence of mortality and morbidity. During the newborn period, nursing assessment focuses on

- Discovering the mother's last drug intake and dosage level. This is accomplished through the perinatal history and laboratory tests. Because women may be reluctant to disclose this information, a nonjudgmental interview technique is essential.
- Assessing the complications related to intrauterine withdrawal such as SGA, intrauterine asphyxia, and prematurity.
- Identifying the signs and symptoms of newborn drug withdrawal or neonatal abstinence syndrome, which can be classified in five groups:
    1. Central nervous system signs
        - Hyperactivity
        - Hyperirritability (persistent high-pitched cry)
        - Increased muscle tone
        - Exaggerated reflexes
        - Tremors, seizures
        - Sneezing, hiccups, yawning
        - Short, unquiet sleep
        - Fever
    2. Respiratory signs
        - Tachypnea
        - Excessive secretions
    3. Gastrointestinal signs
        - Disorganized, vigorous suck
        - Vomiting
        - Drooling
        - Sensitive gag reflex
        - Hyperphagia
        - Diarrhea
        - Abdominal cramping
    4. Vasomotor signs
        - Stuffy nose, yawning, sneezing
        - Flushing
        - Sweating
        - Sudden, circumoral pallor
    5. Cutaneous signs
        - Excoriated buttocks, knees, elbows
        - Facial scratches
        - Pressure point abrasions

Although many of the signs and symptoms of narcotic withdrawal are similar to those seen with hypoglycemia and hypocalcemia, glucose and calcium values are reported to be within normal limits for these infants.

The severity of withdrawal can be assessed by a scoring system based on clinical manifestations. It evaluates the infant on potentially life-threatening signs such as

TABLE 25–1 Assessment of the Clinical Severity of Neonatal Narcotic Withdrawal

Symptom	Mild	Moderate	Severe
Vomiting	Spitting up	Extensive vomiting for three successive feedings	Vomiting associated with imbalance of serum electrolytes
Diarrhea	Watery stools < four times per day	Watery stools five to six times per day for 3 days; no electrolyte imbalance	Diarrhea associated with imbalance of serum electrolytes
Weight loss	<10% of birth weight	10%–15% of birth weight	>15%
Irritability	Minimal	Marked but relieved by cuddling or feeding	Unrelieved by cuddling or feeding
Tremors or twitching	Mild tremors when stimulated	Marked tremors or twitching when stimulated	Convulsions
Tachypnea	60–80 breaths/minute	80–100 breaths/minute	>100 breaths/minute; associated with respiratory alkalosis

Source: Ostrea EM, Chavez CJ, Stryker JS: *The Care of the Drug Dependent Woman and Her Infant.* Lansing, MI: Michigan Department of Public Health, 1978, p 33.

vomiting, diarrhea, weight loss, irritability, tremors, and tachypnea (Table 25–1). Drugs are used to treat severe clinical signs.

Nursing Diagnosis

Nursing diagnoses that may apply to drug-dependent newborns include the following:

- Altered nutrition and fluid requirements: less than body requirements related to vomiting and diarrhea, uncoordinated suck and swallow reflex, hypertonia secondary to withdrawal
- Sleep pattern disturbance related to CNS excitation related to drug withdrawal
- Altered parenting related to hyperirritable behavior of the infant
- Ineffective family coping related to drug abuse, poverty, and lack of education

Nursing Plan and Implementation

Promotion of Physical Well-Being

Care of the drug-dependent newborn is based on reducing withdrawal symptoms and promoting adequate respiration, temperature, and nutrition. See Critical Pathway for Newborn of a Substance-Abusing Mother on pp 644–646 for specific nursing measures. General nursery care measures include the following:

- Temperature regulation.
- Careful monitoring of pulse and respirations every 15 minutes until stable; stimulation if apnea occurs.
- Small frequent feedings, especially in the presence of vomiting, regurgitation, and diarrhea.
- Intravenous therapy as needed.
- Medications as ordered, such as phenobarbital, tincture of opium, diazepam (Valium), or chlorpromazine hydrochloride (Thorazine). Methadone should not be given because of possible neonatal addiction to it and paregoric is not recommended because of the additives of alcohol and camphor (D'Apolito and McRorie 1996).
- Proper positioning on the right side to avoid possible aspiration of vomitus or secretions.
- Noting frequency of diarrhea and vomiting and weighing infant every 8 hours during withdrawal (Ostrea 1993).
- Observation for problems of SGA or LGA newborns.
- Swaddling with hands near mouth to minimize injury and help achieve more organized behavioral state.
- Placing newborn in quiet, dimly lit area of nursery.

HOME CARE

Parents should be prepared for what they can expect for the first few months at home. At the time of discharge the mother should be instructed to anticipate mild jitteriness and irritability in the newborn, which may persist from 8 to 16 weeks, depending on the initial severity of the withdrawal. The nurse should help the mother learn feeding techniques and comforting measures. In one study, substance-abusing mothers tended either to become frustrated with their failure to engage their unresponsive infant and then to detach emotionally from them or to overstimulate the infant (Brooks-Gunn et al 1994). Parents are to be counseled regarding available resources, such as support groups, and signs and symptoms that indicate the need for further care. Ongoing evaluation is necessary because of the potential for long-term problems.

Text continues on page 647

CRITICAL PATHWAY FOR NEWBORN OF A SUBSTANCE-ABUSING MOTHER

Category	Day of Birth—1st 4 Hours	Remaining Day of Birth
Referral	• Report from L&D, neonatal nurse practitioner • Check ID bands →	• Check ID bands q shift → • Circumcision permit checked and initialed before procedure
Assessment	• Complete set of VS • Admission wt → • Length • Head circumference • Check color of skin and assess skin for breakdown or rashes • Monitor activity → • Gestational age assessment • Maternal history of drugs consumed during each month of pregnancy • Obtain prior history of addiction and treatment • Withdrawal symptoms: hyperactivity, jitteriness, irritability, shrill high-pitched cry, vomiting, diarrhea, weak suck, stuffy nose, frequent sneezing, yawning, tachycardia, hypertension, apnea. Cocaine withdrawal pattern may be unpredictable or may be asymptomatic with only subtle behavioral state organization problems.	• Assess mother/baby interaction, suck, color, respiratory status • Assess for hypothermia
Comfort	• Admission activities performed at mother's bedside	
Nursing interventions and reports	• Serum electrolytes to detect losses from vomiting/diarrhea • Blood type, Rh, Coombs on cord blood when applicable • Chemstrip → • Baer test • Maintain universal precautions until baby has had first bath • Phisonex bath immediately/triple dye cord • Hep B form reviewed and/or signed and administered if ordered after bath • Peripheral hematocrit per protocol • Toxicology screen to identify drug levels in infant • CBC and blood cultures to detect sepsis	• Check for Baer test results • Newborn screens • DC same day • Femoral pulse or BP all 4 extremities if early discharge • Temp q shift • VS q4h T/P/R • Daily wt → • Check color q shift → • Alcohol cord q shift

Activity	• Adjust and monitor radiant warmer to maintain skin temperature until stable then open crib
	• Provide calming techniques, including:
	  • Swaddling infant tightly in side-lying or prone position with small pillow supporting back
	  • Provide quiet, dim environment for rest
	  • Hold, rock and cuddle infant. Use touching, petting, smiling, and talking. Use infant snugglies for closeness
	  • Provide pacifier or position so that baby can get hand to mouth
		• Open crib

Nutrition	• Initiate bottle-feeding • Initiate breastfeeding as soon as mother and baby condition allows • Lavage and gavage prn → • Supplement breast only when medically indicated/policy or ordered by MD with D_5W, sterile H_2O, or 20 cal formula with iron → • Assess for increased nutritional needs because of gestational age, weight, uncoordinated suck and swallow, vomiting, diarrhea, and regurgitation	• Continue feeding schedule → • Encourage frequent feedings at least q3–4h during day → • More frequently as baby demands/nsg std → • Bottle-feed q3h–q4h on demand →
Elimination	• Note first void and stool color • Provide meticulous and frequent skin care, especially after voiding and stooling → • Urine specific gravity to detect dehydration	• Monitor stools for amount, type, consistency and any change in pattern • Monitor all voids q shift

CRITICAL PATHWAY continued

Category	Day of Birth—1st 4 Hours	Remaining Day of Birth
Medications	• Administer medications for withdrawal as ordered, such as paregoric, chlorpromazine, Valium, phenobarbital, tincture of opium, observe for effectiveness and side effects → • Aquamephyton 1mg IM—not administered until after bath • Ilotycin ophth ointment OU—not administered until after bath	
Discharge planning/ home care	• Evaluate for SS/VNS and DC planning needs • Plan DC with parent/guardian in 1–3 days • Car seat for DC →	• Present birth certificate instructions • Car seat • Baby pictures

Family involvement	• Evaluate additional psychosocial needs—provide time for expressions of concerns, determine parental understanding of substance abuse
	• Evaluate parent teaching
	• Teen "Healthy Starts" Program if applicable
	• Bulb syringe, choking, positioning
	• Identify mother's/family knowledge needs and readiness for learning
	• Provide information including
	  • Signs and symptoms of baby's withdrawal, current condition, and rationale for treatment
	  • Newborn capabilities and developmental behaviors
	  • Newborn's need for appropriate stimulation as well as rest, depending on cues
	  • Physical care needs such as feeding, bathing, clothing, and holding
	• Encourage and support positive mothering/parenting behaviors with infant
		• Instruct mother on diapering, normal limits of void and stool, burping
		• Evaluate parent teaching
		• Instruct parents of need after discharge for frequent position changes, thorough skin cleansing with each diaper change, and to report any sign of rash or skin breakdown and infections to health care provider

Date		

Category	Day #1	Day #2/#3 (if applicable)
Referral	• Check ID bands when the baby is leaving nursery	• Check ID bands q shift →
Assessment	• Assess: mother/baby interaction, suck, color, resp. status → • Assess temperature stability • Assess abdominal distension, gastric residuals • Assess altered sleep-wake cycle and rhythm at 24–48 h →	• Assess mother/baby interaction → • Assess abdominal distension, gastric residuals, wt gain
Comfort	• Assess for comfort needs	• Assess for comfort needs
Nursing interventions and reports	• Newborn screen • Femoral pulses or BPs 4 extremities before DC or 48 hours → • HSV culture (rapid & conventional) for 24–48 hours or at DC for maternal or paternal Hx of HSV • VS: temp q shift • Daily wt→ • Scalp treatment prn bid → • Check color q shift → • Check activity →	• Completion of femoral pulses and BPs → • Completion of Baer test • VS temp q shift • Daily wt → • Scalp treatment prn bid → • Color q shift → • Activity → • Circumcision → • Alcohol cord q shift →

›

CRITICAL PATHWAY FOR NEWBORN OF A SUBSTANCE-ABUSING MOTHER continued

Category	Day #1	Day #2/#3 (if applicable)
Nursing interventions and reports *continued*	• Circumcision → • Alcohol cord q shift → • DC cord clamp • Skin breakdown/rash • Adjust and monitor incubator to maintain skin temperature	• Skin breakdown/rash • Wear gloves for diaper changes in presence of diarrhea
Activity	• Open crib → • Incubator if temp instability	• Open crib →
Nutrition	• Provide appropriate nutrition: Initiate IV feedings until stable • Supplement oral or gavage feedings with intravenous intake per orders • Give small, frequent feedings of high-calorie formula (may start feedings at one-half strength q3h) • Check for residuals after oral or gavage feedings; reduce feeding volume if residuals are high. As hyperactivity decreases, increase feedings as tolerated. • Supplement breast only when medically indicated/policy or ordered by MD with D_5W, sterile H_2O, or 20 cal formula → • Bottle-feed at least q3–4h on demand →	• Gavage prn → • Supplement breast only when medically indicated/policy or ordered by MD with D_5W, sterile H_2O, or 20 cal formula → • Encourage frequent feeds at least q3–4h during day and more frequently as baby demands/nsg std → • Bottle-feed q3–4h on demand →
Elimination	• Monitor stools for amount, type, consistency and any change in pattern, occult blood, and reducing substances • Monitor all voids q shift	• Monitor stools for amount, type, consistency and any change in pattern, occult blood, and reducing substances • Monitor all voids q shift
Medications	• Hep B vaccine at DC • Administer medications for withdrawal as ordered, such as paregoric, chlorpromazine, Valium, phenobarbital, tincture of opium; observe for effectiveness and side effects →	• Hep B vaccine before DC
Discharge planning/ home care	• If vag birth, complete DC instructions • Complete birth certificate packet • Continuation from "Remaining Day of Birth"	• If C/S birth, complete DC summary → • Instruction on cleansing of baby's individual skin care items, toys

Family involvement	• Bath and feeding class (mother)
	• Mother/Newborn Channel
	• Instruct mother/parent on:
	  • Bath and skin care, nail and cord care
	  • Circumcised/uncirc penis, rashes
	  • Use of thermometer
	  • Infant abilities, developmental behaviors, crying/soothing responses
	  • Active/sleep status
	  • Need for appropriate stimulation and rest
	  • Infant's cues
	  • Reflexes, jaundice
	  • Special nutritional needs
	  • Monitoring weight gain, report feeding intolerance
	• Evaluate mother/parent teaching → Provide information about cause of AIDS, signs of HIV in infants, support groups and community resources
		• Continue the completion of education on Day 1 →
		• Eval mother/parent teaching →

Date		

Evaluation

Anticipated outcomes of nursing care include

- The newborn tolerates feedings, gains weight, and has a decreased number of stools.
- The parents learn ways to comfort their newborn.
- The parents are able to cope with their frustrations and begin to use outside resources as needed.

Alcohol Dependency

Infants born to alcohol-dependent mothers can suffer long-term complications in addition to suffering withdrawal symptoms.

The **fetal alcohol syndrome (FAS)** includes a series of malformations frequently found in infants born to women who have been severe alcoholics (Volpe 1995). It has been estimated that the complete FAS syndrome occurs in the range of 0.3–1.9 live births per 1000 (Coles 1993; Committee on Substance Abuse and Committee on Children with Disabilities 1993). FAS rates among American Indians and Alaska natives are estimated at 1.3–10.3 per 1000 live births because of increased alcohol consumption in these populations (Duimstra et al 1993). **Fetal alcohol effects (FAE)** are less severe effects of maternal alcohol use during pregnancy and include mild to moderate mental and physical growth retardation.

Controversy surrounds the exact cause of FAS. Although it is known that ethanol freely crosses the placenta to the fetus, it is still not known whether the alcohol alone or the break-down products of alcohol cause the damage. Chapter 12 discusses alcohol abuse in pregnancy. The effects of other substances often combined with alcohol, such as nicotine, diazepam (Valium), marijuana, and caffeine, as well as poor diet, enhance the likelihood of FAS.

Long-Term Complications

The long-term prognosis for the FAS newborn is less than favorable. Most infants with FAS are growth-deficient at birth and only a few infants demonstrate postnatal catch-up growth (Krishna and Phillips 1994). In fact, most FAS infants are evaluated for failure to thrive. Decreased adipose tissue is a constant feature of persons with FAS.

These infants have a delay in oral feeding development but have a normal progression of oral motor function. Many FAS infants nurse poorly and have persistent vomiting until 6–7 months of age. They have difficulty adjusting to solid foods and show little spontaneous interest in food.

Central nervous system dysfunctions are the most common and serious problem associated with FAS. Most children exhibiting FAS are mildly to severely mentally retarded. The more abnormal the facial features, the lower the IQ scores. However, cases of infants of chronic alcoholics in whom neurologic disturbance appeared to be the only apparent abnormality are well documented (Volpe 1995). Providing a better environment for FAS infants has not been found to have an influence on IQ, which indicates that the brain damage occurred prenatally. These children are often hyperactive and show a high incidence of speech and language abnormalities indicative of CNS disorders (Wekselman et al 1995).

Nursing Assessment

Newborns with FAS may show the following characteristics:

- *Abnormal structural development and CNS dysfunction,* including mental retardation, microcephaly, and hyperactivity.
- *Growth deficiencies.* Infants with FAS are often IUGR with weight, length, and head circumference being affected. These infants continue to show a persistent postnatal growth deficiency, with weight being more affected than linear growth.
- *Distinctive facial abnormalities.* These include short palpebral fissures, midfacial and maxillary hypoplasia, micrognathia (abnormally small lower jaw), hypoplastic upper lip, and diminished or absent philtrum (groove on upper lip).
- *Associated anomalies.* Abnormalities affecting cardiac (primarily septal), ocular, renal, and skeletal (especially involving joints, such as congenital dislocated hips) systems are often noted.

Withdrawal symptoms of the alcohol-dependent newborn have been documented in children with normal facial features, as well as in those with the typical features of FAS. These symptoms include tremors, seizures, sleeplessness, unconsolable crying, abnormal reflexes, activeness with little ability to maintain alertness and attentiveness to environment, abdominal distention, and exaggerated mouthing behaviors such as hyperactive rooting and increased nonnutritive sucking. Seizures are treated with phenobarbital or diazepam.

Signs and symptoms of withdrawal often appear within 6 to 12 hours and at least within the first 3 days of life. Seizures after the neonatal period are rare. Alcohol dependence in the infant is physiologic, not psychologic.

Nursing Care

The nurse's awareness of the signs and symptoms of fetal alcohol effects is important in structuring and

CRITICAL THINKING IN ACTION

Mrs Jean Corrigan, a 23-year-old G1P1, positive for HIV, has just given birth to a 7 lb 1 oz baby girl. As she watches you assessing her daughter in the birthing room, she asks why you are wearing gloves and whether her daughter will have to be in isolation. What will your response be?

Answers can be found in Appendix H.

guiding nursing care. Nursing care of the FAS newborn is aimed at avoiding heat loss, protecting the infant from injury during seizures, administering medications such as phenobarbital or diazepam to limit convulsions, monitoring intravenous fluid therapy, and reducing environmental stimuli. The FAS baby is most comfortable in a quiet, dimly lit environment. Because of their feeding problems, these infants require extra time and patience during feedings.

Mothers should be informed that breastfeeding is not contraindicated but that excessive alcohol consumption may intoxicate the newborn and inhibit the letdown reflex. The nurse must monitor the newborn's vital signs closely and observe for evidence of seizure activity and respiratory distress.

Infants affected by maternal alcohol abuse are also at risk psychologically. Restlessness, sleeplessness, agitation, resistance to cuddling or holding, and frequent crying can be frustrating to parents as their efforts to relieve the distress are unrewarded. Feeding dysfunction can also result in frustrations for the caregiver and digestive upsets for the infant. Frustration may cause the parents to punish the baby or result in the unconscious desire to stay away from the infant. Either outcome may create an unstable family environment and result in failure to thrive.

The nurse should focus on providing support for the parents and reinforcing positive parenting activity. Before discharge, parents are provided with opportunities to provide baby care so that they can feel confident in their interpretations of their baby's cues and ability to meet the baby's needs. Referring the family to social services and visiting nurse or public health nurse associations is essential for the well-being of the infant. Follow-up care and teaching can strengthen the parents' skill and coping abilities and help them create a stable, healthy environment for their family (Wekselman et al 1995).

Evaluation

Anticipated outcomes of nursing care include

- The FAS newborn is able to tolerate feedings and gain weight.
- The FAS infant's hyperirritability or seizures are controlled, and the baby has suffered no physical injuries.
- The parents are able to identify the special needs of their newborn and accept outside assistance as needed.

Care of the Newborn with AIDS

An increasing number of newborns are being born with or acquiring AIDS in the newborn period or early infancy. Perinatal and neonatal modes of transmission have been identified as transplacental, breastfeeding, and contaminated blood. Ongoing prospective studies indicate maternal-to-newborn vertical transmission rates of about 30–40 percent. Vertical transmission rates can be decreased to about 8 percent in mothers taking AZT during gestation (Kuhn and Stein 1995). For discussion of maternal/fetal AIDS characteristics see Chapter 12.

Early identification of babies with or at risk for AIDS is essential during the newborn period. The currently available HIV serologic tests (ELISA and Western blot test) cannot distinguish between maternal and infant antibodies; therefore, they are inappropriate for infants up to 15 months of age. It may take up to 15 months for infected infants to form their own antibodies to the HIV (Kellinger 1994). In infants under 15 months, HIV culture or viral p24 antigen detection can be used for diagnosing congenital AIDS. Diagnostic tests that detect the infant's specific antibody (IgG or IgM) response to HIV or tests for viral DNA are becoming generally more available (Sherwen 1995). Opportunistic diseases such as gram-negative sepsis and problems associated with prematurity are the primary causes of mortality in HIV-infected babies.

APPLYING THE NURSING PROCESS

Nursing Assessment

Many newborns with AIDS are premature or SGA and show failure to thrive during neonatal and infant life. They can show signs and symptoms of disease within days of birth. Signs that may be seen in the newborn period include failure to thrive, enlarged spleen and liver, swollen glands, interstitial pneumonia (rarely seen in adults), recurrent GI (diarrhea and weight loss) and urinary system infections, persistent or recurrent oral candidiasis, evidence of Epstein-Barr virus, developmental delays or failure to reach developmental milestones, and neurologic deficits (Kellinger 1994; Scott and Parks

TABLE 25–2 Issues for Caregivers of Infants at Risk for AIDS

Resuscitation	For suctioning use a bulb syringe, mucus extractor, or meconium aspirator with wall suction on low setting.
Admission care	To remove blood from baby's skin, give warm water, mild soap bath using gloves as soon as possible after admission.
Hand washing	Thorough hand washing is indicated before and after caring for infant. Hands must be washed immediately if contaminated with blood or body fluids. Wash hands after removal of gloves.
Gowns	Long-sleeved gowns are indicated when at bedside.
Gloves	Gloves are indicated when touching blood or body fluids. Gloves should also be worn when handling newborns before and during their initial baths, cord care, eye prophylactics, and vitamin K administration.
Mask	Not routinely needed. Masks are indicated if mouth is likely to come in contact with body fluids (eg, when caring for intubated or coughing infant who has copious secretions) or if caregiver feels she or he is infectious, thereby posing risk to infant.
Goggles	Not routinely needed. Goggles are indicated if eyes are likely to come in contact with body fluids (eg, when caring for intubated or coughing infant who has copious secretions). If glasses are worn, goggles are not necessary.
Needles and syringes	Care should be taken to avoid needle stick injuries. Used needles should not be recapped or bent; they should be placed in a prominently labeled, puncture-resistant plastic container designed specifically for such disposal and belonging specifically to that baby. After the newborn is discharged the container is discarded.
Specimens	Blood and other specimens should be double-bagged and/or sealed in an impervious container and labeled "blood/body fluids precautions."
Equipment and linen	Articles contaminated with blood or body fluids should be discarded or bagged according to isolation protocol or institution and labeled "blood/body fluids precautions" before being sent for decontamination and reprocessing.
Body fluid spills	Blood and body fluids should be cleaned promptly with a solution of 5.25% sodium hypochlorite (household bleach) diluted 1:10 with water.
Education and support	Provide education and psychologic support for family and staff. Caregivers who avoid contact with baby at risk or who overdress in unnecessary isolation garb subtly exacerbate an already difficult family situation. Information resources include the National AIDS Hotline (1-800-342-2437).
Exempted personnel	Immunologically compromised staff (pregnant women may be included in this group) and possibly infectious staff members should not care for these infants.

Sources: Adapted from Mendez H, Jule JE: Care of the infant born exposed to HIV. *Obstet Gynecol Clin North Am* 1990; 17(3):637; Berry RK: Home care of the child with AIDS. *Pediatr Nurs* July/August 1988; 14(4):341.

1994). Some cranial and facial stigmas have been associated with AIDS contracted in utero. However, these findings do not establish a diagnosis of HIV infection at birth.

Nursing Diagnosis

Nursing diagnoses that may apply to the newborn at risk for AIDS include the following:

- Altered nutrition: less than body requirements related to formula intolerance and inadequate intake
- Risk for impaired skin integrity related to chronic diarrhea
- Risk for infection related to perinatal exposure and immunoregulation suppression
- Altered parenting related to diagnosis of AIDS and fear of future outcome

Nursing Plan and Implementation

Nursing care of the newborn with AIDS calls for the normal care required for a newborn in an NICU. In addition, the nurse must include care for a newborn suspected of having a blood-borne infection, as with hepatitis B. Universal precautions should be used when caring for the newborn immediately after birth and when obtaining blood samples via vein puncture or heel stick. (The blood of *all* newborns must be considered potentially infectious because the status of the infant's blood is often not known until after the infant is discharged and there is a window of time before seroconversion occurs when the baby is still considered infectious.)

Nursing care involves providing for comfort; keeping the newborn well nourished and protected from opportunistic infections; and facilitating growth, development, and attachment. See Critical Pathway for Newborn at Risk for AIDS on pp 650–651 for specific nursing care measures. Also see Table 25–2, Issues for Caregivers of Infants at Risk for AIDS.

Community-Based Nursing Care

Hand washing is crucial when caring for newborns with AIDS. Parents should learn proper hand-washing technique. Nutrition is essential since failure to thrive and weight loss are common. Small, frequent feedings and food supplementation are helpful. The nurse should discuss sanitary formula preparation with parents. The baby should not be put to bed with juice or formula because of potential bacteria growth. Parents need to be alert to the signs of feeding intolerance, such as increasing regurgitation, abdominal distention, and loose stools. The newborn should be weighed three times a week.

Text continues on page 652

CRITICAL PATHWAY FOR NEWBORN AT RISK FOR AIDS

Category	Day of Birth—1st 4 Hours	Remaining Day of Birth
Referral	• Report from L&D, neonatal nurse practitioner • Check ID bands →	• Check ID bands q shift → • Circumcision permit initialed and checked before procedure
Assessment	• Complete set of VS • Admission wt → • Length • Head circumference • Check color of skin and assess skin for breakdown or rashes • Monitor activity → • Gestational age assessment • Maternal history of drug abuse or needle sharing • Check history of sexual partner or partners of the mother with a positive HIV antibody test or ELSA test	• Assess mother/baby interaction, suck, color, respiratory status • Thermoregulation
Comfort	• Admission activities performed at mother's bedside	
Nursing interventions and reports	• Blood type, Rh, Coombs on cord blood when applicable • Chemstrip → • Baer test • Maintain universal precautions until baby has had first bath • Phisohex bath immediately/triple dye cord • Hep B form reviewed and/or signed and administered if ordered after bath • Peripheral hematocrit per protocol	• Check for Baer test results • NBS for vaginal birth • DC same day • Femoral pulse or BP all 4 extremities if early discharge • Temp q shift • VS q4h T/P/R • Daily wt → • Check color q shift • Alcohol cord q shift
Activity	• Adjust and monitor radiant warmer to maintain skin temperature until stable then open crib	• Open crib
Nutrition	• Initiate bottle-feeding • Initiate breast as soon as mother and baby condition allows → • Lavage and gavage prn → • Supplement breast only when medically indicated/policy or ordered by MD with D_5W, sterile H_2O, or 20 cal formula with iron	• Continue feeding schedule → • Encourage frequent feedings at least q4h during day → • More frequently as baby demands/nsg std • Bottle-feed q3–6h on demand →
Elimination	• Note first void and stool color • Provide meticulous and frequent skin care, especially after voiding and stooling →	• Monitor stools for amount, type, consistency and any change in pattern • Monitor all voids q shift
Medications	• Aquamephyton 1 mg IM—not administered until after bath • Ilotycin ophth ointment OU—not administered until after bath	
Discharge planning/ home care	• Evaluate SS/VNS and DC planning needs • Plan DC with parent/guardian in 1–3 days • Car seat for DC	• Present birth certificate instructions • Car seat • Baby pictures
Family involvement	• Evaluate additional psychosocial needs—provide time for expressions of concerns, determine parental understanding of AIDS • Evaluate parent teaching • Teen "Healthy Starts" Program • Bulb syringe, choking, positioning	• Instruct mother on diapering, normal limits of void and stool, burping • Evaluate parent teaching • Instruct parents of need after discharge for frequent position changes, thorough skin cleansing with each diaper change, and to report any sign of rash or skin breakdown and infections to health care provider
Date		

CRITICAL PATHWAY continued

Category	Day #1	Day #2/#3 (if applicable)
Referral	• Check ID bands when the baby is leaving nursery	• Check ID bands q shift →
Assessment	• Assess mother/baby interaction, suck, color, resp. status → • Thermoregulation • Assess abdominal distension, gastric residuals	• Assess mother/baby interaction → • Assess abdominal distension, gastric residuals, wt gain
Comfort	• Assess for comfort needs	• Assess for comfort needs
Nursing interventions and reports	• Newborn screen for vag delivery • Femoral pulses or BPs all 4 extremities before DC or 48 hours → • HSV culture (rapid & conventional) for 24–48 hours or at DC for maternal or pateernal Hx of HSV • Adjust and monitor incubator to maintain skin temperature • VS: temp q shift → • Daily wt→ • Scalp treatment prn bid → • Check color q shift → • Check activity → • Circumcision → • Alcohol cord q shift → • DC cord clamp • Skin breakdown/rash	• Completion of femoral pulses/BPs → • Completion of Baer test • VS temp q shift • Daily wt → • Scalp treatment prn bid → • Color q shift → • Activity → • Circumcision → • Alcohol cord q shift → • Skin breakdown/rash • Wear gloves for diaper changes in presence of diarrhea
Activity	• Open crib → • Incubator if temp instability	• Open crib →
Nutrition	• Gavage prn → • Supplement breast only when medically indicated/policy or ordered by MD with D_5W, sterile H_2O, or 20 cal formula → • Encourage frequent small feeds at least q3–4h during day and more frequently as baby demands/nsg std → • Bottle-feed q3–4h on demand →	• Gavage prn • Supplement breast only when medically indicated/policy or ordered by MD with D_5W, sterile H_2O, or 20 cal formula → • Encourage frequent small feeds at least q3–4h during day and more frequently as baby demands/nsg std → • Bottle-feed q3–4h on demand →
Elimination	• Monitor stools for amount, type, consistency and any change in pattern, occult blood and reducing substances • Monitor all voids q shift • Provide meticulous and frequent skin care after each voiding and stooling • Change diapers frequently	• Monitor stools for amount, type, consistency and any change in pattern, occult blood and reducing substances • Monitor all voids q shift • Provide meticulous and frequent skin care after each voiding and stooling • Change diapers frequently
Medications	• Hep B vaccine at DC	• Hep B vaccine before DC
Discharge planning/ home care	• If vag birth, complete DC instructions • Complete birth certificate packet • Continue from "Remaining Day of Birth"	• If C/S birth, complete DC summary → • Instruction on cleansing of baby's individual skin care items, toys • Provide list of contact persons for available community resources • Instruct family on importance of keeping follow-up appointments
Family involvement	• Bath and feeding class (mother) • Mother/Newborn Channel education programs • Instruct mother/parent on: bath and skin care, nail and cord care; circumcised/uncirc penis, rashes; use of thermometer, infant abilities and stimuli; active/sleep status, crying/soothing responses; reflexes; jaundice; special nutritional needs; monitoring weight gain, report feeding intolerance • Evaluate mother/parent teaching → Provide information about cause of AIDS, signs of HIV in infants, support groups and community resources	• Continue the completion of education on Day 1 → • Eval mother/parent teaching →
Date		

Prompt diaper changing and perineal care can prevent or minimize diaper rash and promote comfort. It is important to remember that the diaper-changing area in the home should be separate from food preparation and serving areas. Disposable diapers are recommended over cloth diapers. The diapers are to be placed in plastic bags, sealed, and placed in the garbage can daily. Even though the American Academy of Pediatrics doesn't require gloves to be worn during routine diaper changes (American Academy of Pediatrics Committee on Fetus and Newborn 1992), most institutions recommend that their caregivers wear gloves during all diaper changes and examinations of babies. Disposable gloves are worn when changing diapers or cleaning the diaper area, especially in the presence of diarrhea, because blood may be in the stool. Good skin care is essential to prevent skin rashes.

The baby should have his or her own skin care items, towels, and washcloths. Most clothing and linens can be washed with other household laundry. Linen that is visibly soiled with blood or body fluids should be kept separate and washed separately in hot sudsy water with household bleach. Diaper-changing areas should be cleaned with a 1:10 dilution of household bleach after each diaper change. Toys should be kept as clean as possible, and they should not be shared with other children. Toys should be checked for sharp edges to prevent scratches.

Parents should be instructed on what signs of infection to be alert to and when to call their health care provider. The inability to feed without pain may indicate esophageal yeast. Topical mycostatin or Desitin ointment is used for diaper rashes and oral mycostatin for oral thrush. If diarrhea occurs, the baby requires frequent perineal care and fluid replacements. Antidiarrheal medications are often ineffective. Irritability may be the first sign of fever. Taking rectal temperatures should be avoided, as it may stimulate diarrhea. Fluids, antipyretics, and sponging with tepid water are of use in managing fever.

Parents and family members need to be reassured that there are no documented cases of people contracting AIDS from routine care of infected babies. Emotional support for family members is essential because of the stress and social isolation they may face. Because of these stresses, attachment may not occur and the infant may suffer from lack of sensory and tactile stimulation (Bastin et al 1992). Babies should be held for feedings and they will benefit from frequent, gentle touch. Auditory stimulation may also be provided by using music or tapes of parents' voices. Families should be informed about support groups, available counseling, and information resources. Current therapeutic information about HIV disease is available to both health care providers and families through the AIDS Clinical Trials Information Service (1-800-TRIALS-A) (Kellinger 1994). The CDC recommends that HIV-infected women not breastfeed, as HIV has been found to be transmitted via breast milk. If there is a viable alternative feeding method, it should be used (Kuhn and Stein 1995).

Preventive care for at-risk and HIV-infected infants is the same as for other infants and includes routine immunizations except that the live polio vaccine should be avoided. At 1 month of age the baby's physical exam should include a developmental assessment; complete blood count, including differential blood count, CD4 count, and IG (quantitative immunoglobulins); HIV test or PCR (polymerase chain reaction) test for HIV, if available, or p24 antigen test for HIV after 1 month of age; and a #2 dose of hepatitis vaccine (Kellinger 1994). Pediatric HIV disease raises many health care issues for the family. The parents, depending on their health status, may or may not be able to care for their infant, and they must deal with many psychosocial and economic issues.

Evaluation

Anticipated outcomes of nursing care include

- The parents are able to bond with their infant and have realistic expectations about the baby.
- Early identification and treatment of potential opportunistic infections is provided.
- The parents verbalize their concerns about their baby's existing and potential health problems and accept outside assistance as needed.

Care of the Newborn with Congenital Anomalies

The birth of a baby with a congenital defect places both newborn and family at risk. Many congenital anomalies can be life-threatening if not corrected within hours after birth; others are very visible and cause the families emotional distress. When one congenital anomaly is found, health care providers should look for other ones, particularly in body systems that develop at the same time during gestation. Table 25–3 identifies some of the more common anomalies and their early management and nursing care in the neonatal period.

Text continues on page 655

TABLE 25–3 Congenital Anomalies: Identification and Care in Newborn Period

Congenital Anomaly	Nursing Assessments	Nursing Goals and Interventions
Congenital hydrocephalus	Enlarged head Enlarged or full fontanelles Split or widened sutures "Setting sun" eyes Head circumference > 90% on growth chart	Assess presence of hydrocephalus: Measure and plot occipital-frontal baseline measurements; then measure head circumference once a day. Check fontanelle for bulging and sutures for widening. Assist with head ultrasound and transillumination. Maintain skin integrity: Change position frequently. Clean skin creases after feeding or vomiting. Use sheepskin pillow under head. Postoperatively, position head off operative site. Watch for signs of infection.
Choanal atresia	Occlusion of posterior nares Cyanosis and retractions at rest Snorting respirations Difficulty breathing during feeding Obstruction by thick mucus	Assess patency of nares: Listen for breath sounds while holding baby's mouth closed and alternately compressing each nostril. Assist with passing feeding tube to confirm diagnosis. Maintain respiratory function: Assist with taping airway in mouth to prevent respiratory distress. Position with head elevated to improve air exchange.
Cleft lip	Unilateral or bilateral visible defect May involve external nares, nasal cartilage, nasal septum, and alveolar process Flattening or depression of midfacial contour 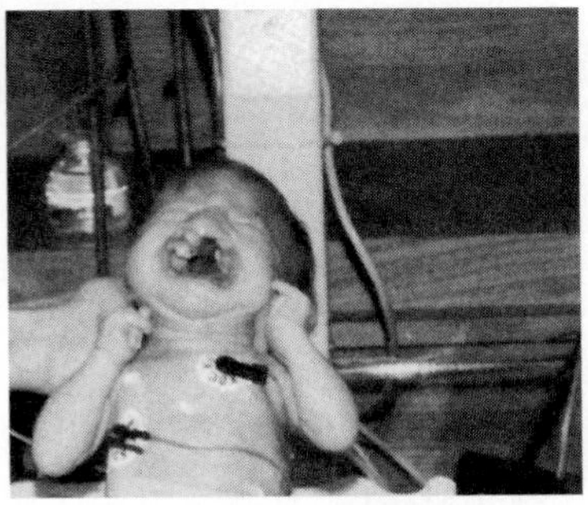	Provide nutrition: Feed with special nipple. Burp frequently (increased tendency to swallow air and reflex vomiting). Clean cleft with sterile water (to prevent crusting on cleft prior to repair). Support parental coping: Assist parents with grief over loss of idealized baby. Encourage verbalization of their feelings about visible defect. Provide role model in interacting with infant. (Parents internalize others' responses to their newborn.) (At left) Unilateral cleft lip with cleft abnormality involving both hard and soft palates.
Cleft palate	Fissure connecting oral and nasal cavity May involve uvula and soft palate May extend forward to nostril involving hard palate and maxillary alveolar ridge Difficulty in sucking Expulsion of formula through nose	Prevent aspiration/infection: Place prone or in side-lying position to facilitate drainage. Suction nasopharyngeal cavity (to prevent aspiration or airway obstruction) During newborn period feed in upright position with head and chest tilted slightly backward (to aid swallowing and discourage aspiration). Provide nutrition: Feed with special nipple that fills cleft and allows sucking. Also decreases change of aspiration through nasal cavity. Clean mouth with water after feedings. Burp after each ounce (tend to swallow large amounts of air). Thicken formula to provide extra calories. Plot weight gain patterns to assess adequacy of diet. Provide parental support: Refer parents to community agencies and support groups. Encourage verbalization of frustrations because feeding process is long and frustrating. Praise all parental efforts. Encourage parents to seek prompt treatment for upper respiratory infection (URI) and teach them ways to decrease URI.
Tracheoesophageal fistula (type 3)	History of maternal hydramnios Excessive mucous secretions Constant drooling Abdominal distention beginning soon after birth Periodic choking and cyanotic episodes Immediate regurgitation of feeding Clinical symptoms of aspiration pneumonia (tachypnea, retractions, rhonchi, decreased breath sounds, cyanotic spells) Failure to pass nasogastric tube	Maintain respiratory status and prevent aspiration: Withhold feeding until esophageal patency is determined. Quickly assess patency before putting to breast in birth area. Place on low intermittent suction to control saliva and mucus (to prevent aspiration pneumonia). Place in warmed, humidified incubator (liquefies secretions, facilitating removal). Elevate head of bed 20–40 degrees (to prevent reflux of gastric juices). Keep quiet (crying causes air to pass through fistula and to distend intestines, causing respiratory embarrassment). Maintain fluid and electrolyte balance: Give fluids to replace esophageal drainage and maintain hydration. Provide parent education: Explain staged repair—provision of gastrostomy and ligation of fistula, then repair of atresia. Keep parents informed; clarify and reinforce physician's explanations regarding malformation, surgical repair, pre- and postoperative care, and prognosis (knowledge is ego strengthening).

TABLE 25–3 Congenital Anomalies: Identification and Care in Newborn Period continued

Congenital Anomaly	*Nursing Assessments*	*Nursing Goals and Interventions*
Tracheoesophageal fistula (type 3) *continued*		Involve parents in care of infant and in planning for future; facilitate touch and eye contact (to dispel feelings of inadequacy, increase self-esteem and self-worth, and promote incorporation of infant into family).
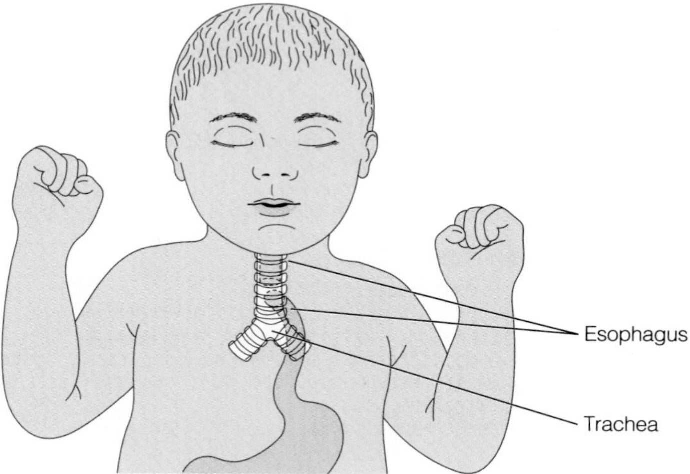		(At left) The most frequently seen type of congenital tracheoesophageal fistula and esophageal atresia.
Diaphragmatic hernia	Difficulty initiating respirations Gasping respirations with nasal flaring and chest retraction Barrel chest and scaphoid abdomen Asymmetric chest expansion Breath sounds may be absent Usually on left side Heart sounds displaced to right Spasmodic attacks of cyanosis and difficulty in feeding Bowel sounds may be heard in thoracic cavity	Nurse should never ventilate with bag and mask O_2 because the stomach will inflate, further compressing the lungs. Maintain respiratory status: Immediately administer oxygen. Initiate gastric decompression. Place in high semi-Fowler's position (to use gravity to keep abdominal organs' pressure off diaphragm). Turn to affected side to allow unaffected lung expansion. Carry out interventions to alleviate respiratory and metabolic acidosis. Assess for increased secretions around suction tube (denotes possible obstruction). Aspirate and irrigate tube with air or sterile water.
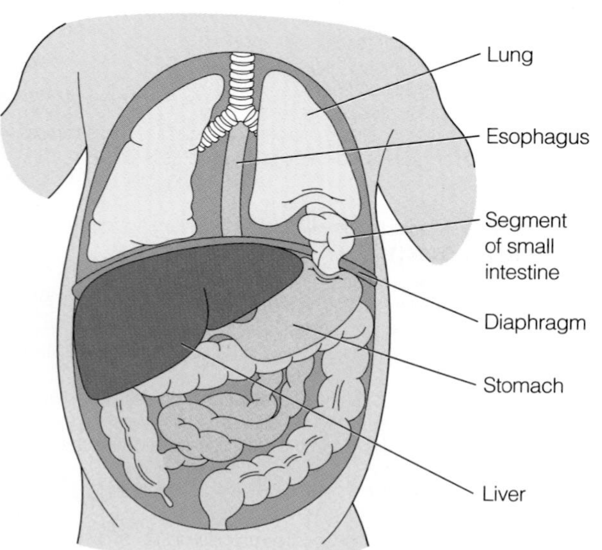		(At left) Diaphragmatic hernia. Note compression of the lung by the intestine on the affected side.

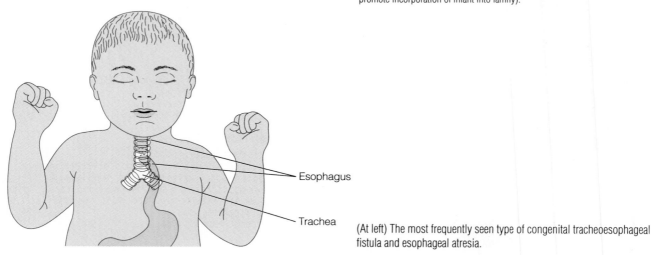

TABLE 25–3 continued

Congenital Anomaly	Nursing Assessments	Nursing Goals and Interventions
Myelomeningocele	Saclike cyst containing meninges, spinal cord, and nerve roots in thoracic and/or lumbar area Myelomeningocele directly connects to subarachnoid space so hydrocephalus often associated No response or varying response to sensation below level of sac May have constant dribbling of urine Incontinence or retention of stool Anal opening may be flaccid	Prevent trauma and infection. Position on abdomen or on side and restrain (to prevent pressure and trauma to sac). Meticulously clean buttocks and genitals after each voiding and defecation (to prevent contamination of sac and decrease possibility of infection). May put protective covering over sac (to prevent rupture and drying). Observe sac for oozing of fluid or pus. Credé bladder (apply downward pressure on bladder with thumbs, moving urine toward the urethra) as ordered to prevent urinary stasis. Assess amount of sensation and movement below defect. Observe for complications: Obtain occipital-frontal circumference baseline measurements; then measure head circumference once a day (to detect hydrocephalus). Check fontanelle for bulging. 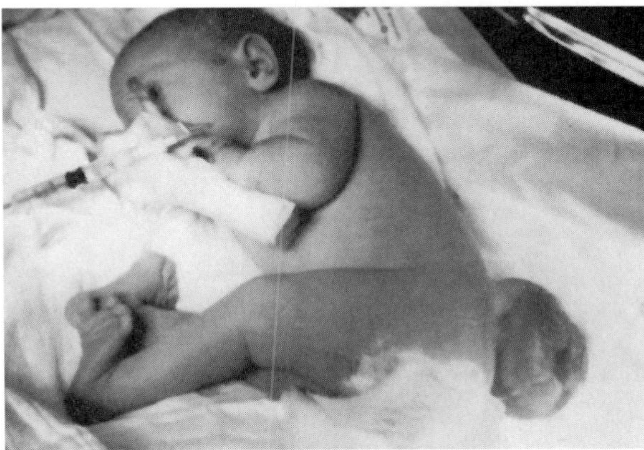 (At left) Newborn with lumbar myelomeningocele. Source: Courtesy of Dr. Paul Winchester.
Omphalocele	Herniation of abdominal contents into base of umbilical cord May have an enclosed transparent sac covering	Maintain hydration and temperature: Provide D_5LR and albumin for hypovolemia. Place infant in sterile bag up to and covering defect. Cover sac with moistened sterile gauze, and place plastic wrap over dressing (to prevent rupture of sac and infection). Initiate gastric decompression by insertion of nasogastric tube attached to low suction (to prevent distention of lower bowel and impairment of blood flow). Prevent infection and trauma to defect. Position to prevent trauma to defect. Administer broad-spectrum antibiotics.
Imperforate anus, congenital dislocated hip, and clubfoot	See discussion in Chapter 22, Anus and Extremities	Identify defect and initiate appropriate referral early.

Care of the Newborn with Congenital Heart Defect

The incidence of congenital heart defects is 4 to 5 per 1000 live births. They account for one-third of the deaths caused by congenital defects in the first year of life. Because accurate diagnosis and surgical treatment are now available, many such deaths can be prevented. It is now possible to do corrective surgery at an earlier age; for example, more than half the children undergoing surgery are less than 1 year of age, and one-fourth are less than 1 month old (Benson 1989). It is crucial for the nurse to have comprehensive knowledge of congenital heart disease to detect deviations from normal and initiate interventions. (See Table 25–4.)

Overview of Congenital Heart Defects

Factors that might influence development of congenital heart malformation can be classified as environmental or genetic. Infections of the pregnant woman, such as rubella, coxsackie B, and influenza, have been implicated. Thalidomide, steroids, alcohol, lithium, and some anticonvulsants have been shown to cause malformations of the heart. Seasonal spraying of pesticides has also been linked to an increase in congenital heart defects. Clinicians are also beginning to see cardiac defects in infants of mothers with phenylketonuria (PKU) who do not follow their diets.

Text continues on page 658

TABLE 25–4 Cardiac Defects of the Early Newborn Period

Congenital Heart Defect	Clinical Findings	Medical/Surgical Management
Acyanotic		
Patent ductus arteriosus (PDA) ↑ in females, maternal rubella, RDS, <1500 g preterm newborns, high-altitude births 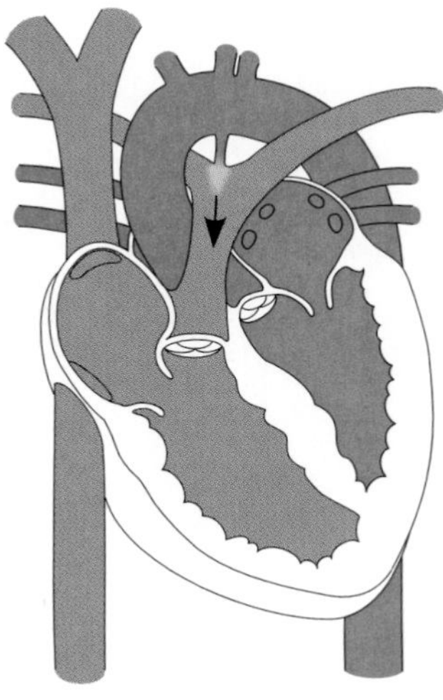	Harsh grade 2–3 machinery murmur upper left sternal border (LSB) just beneath clavicle ↑ difference between systolic and diastolic pulse pressure Can lead to right heart failure and pulmonary congestion ↑ left atrial (LA) and left ventricular (LV) enlargement, dilated ascending aorta ↑ pulmonary vascularity The patent ductus arteriosus is a vascular connection that, during fetal life, short-circuits the pulmonary vascular bed and directs blood from the pulmonary artery to the aorta. Postnatally, blood shunts through the ductus from the aorta to the pulmonary artery.	Indomethacin—0.2 mg/kg orally (prostaglandin inhibitor) Surgical ligation Use of O_2 therapy and blood transfusion to improve tissue oxygenation and perfusion Fluid restriction and diuretics
Atrial septal defect (ASD) ↑ in females and Down syndrome	Initially frequently asymptomatic Systolic murmur second left intercostal space (LICS) With large ASD, diastolic rumbling murmur lower left sternal (LLS) border Failure to thrive, upper respiratory infection (URI), poor exercise tolerance	Surgical closure with patch or suture
Ventricular septal defect (VSD) ↑ in males	Initially asymptomatic until end of first month or large enough to cause pulmonary edema Loud, blowing systolic murmur third–fourth intercostal space (ICS) pulmonary blood flow Right ventricular hypertrophy Rapid respirations, growth failure, feeding difficulties Congestive right heart failure at 6 weeks–2 months of age	Follow medically—some spontaneously close Use of lanoxin and diuretics in congestive heart failure (CHF) Surgical closure with Dacron patch
Coarctation of aorta Can be preductal or postductal 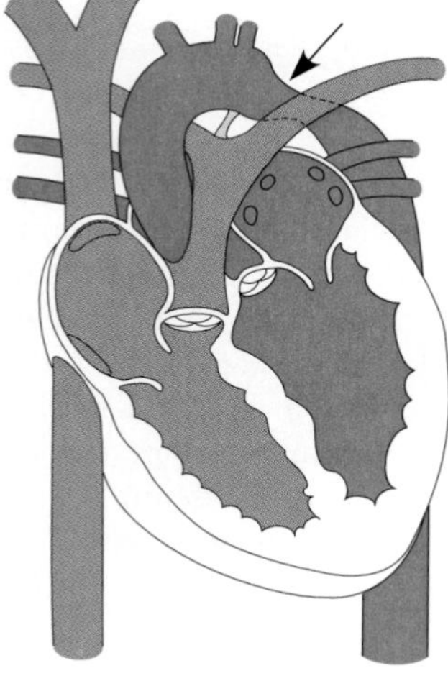	Absent or diminished femoral pulses Increased brachial pulses Late systolic murmur left intrascapular area Systolic BP in lower extremities Enlarged left ventricle Can present in CHF at 7–21 days of life Coarctation of the aorta is characterized by a narrowed aortic lumen. The lesion produces an obstruction to the flow of blood through the aorta, causing an increased left ventricular pressure and work load.	Surgical resection of narrowed portion of aorta Prostaglandin E_1 to maintain peripheral perfusion No afterload reducer drugs

TABLE 25–4 continued

Congenital Heart Defect	Clinical Findings	Medical/Surgical Management
Hypoplastic left heart syndrome	Normal at birth—cyanosis and shocklike congestive heart failure develop within a few hours to days Soft systolic murmur just left of the sternum Diminished pulses Aortic and/or mitral atresia Tiny, thick-walled left ventricle Large, dilated, hypertrophied right ventricle X-ray: cardiac enlargement and pulmonary venous congestion	PGE_1 until decision made Transplant Currently no effective corrective treatment
Cyanotic		
Tetralogy of Fallot (Most common cyanotic heart defect) Pulmonary stenosis Ventricular septal defect (VSD) Overriding aorta Right ventricular hypertrophy 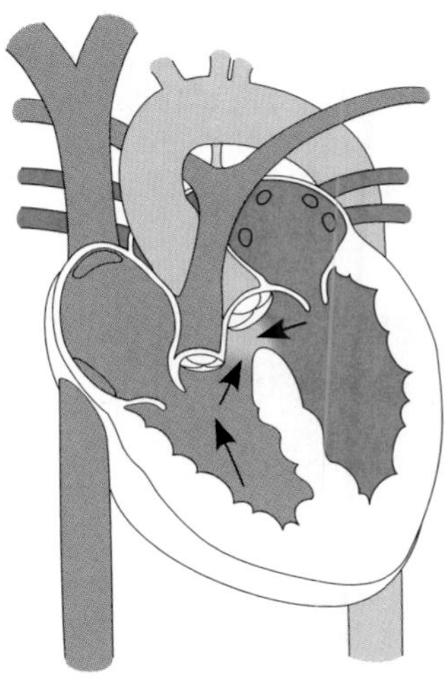	May be cyanotic at birth or within first few months of life Harsh systolic murmur LSB Crying or feeding increases cyanosis and respiratory distress X-ray: boot-shaped appearance secondary to small pulmonary artery Right ventricular enlargement In tetralogy of Fallot, the severity of symptoms depends on the degree of pulmonary stenosis, the size of the ventricular septal defect, and the degree to which the aorta overrides the septal defect.	Prevention of dehydration, intercurrent infections Alleviation of paroxysmal dyspneic attacks Palliative surgery to increase blood flow to the lungs Corrective surgery—resection of pulmonic stenosis, closure of VSD with Dacron patch
Transposition of great vessels (TGA) (↑ females, IDMs, LGAs) 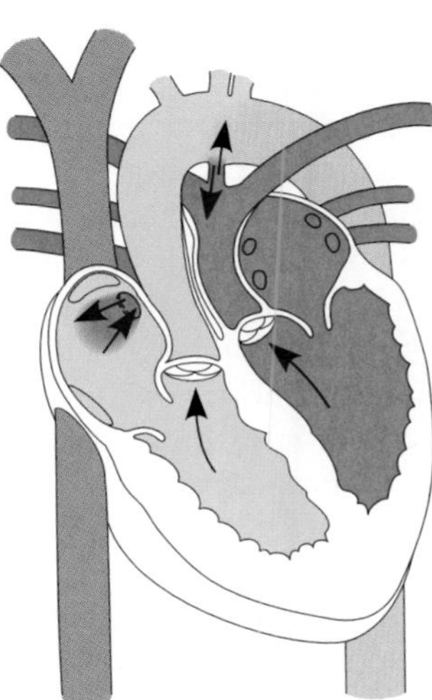	Cyanosis at birth or within 3 days Possible pulmonic stenosis murmur Right ventricular hypertrophy Polycythemia "Egg on its side" x-ray Complete transposition of great vessels is an embryonic defect caused by a straight division of the bulbar trunk without normal spiraling. As a result, the aorta originates from the right ventricle, and the pulmonary artery from the left ventricle. An abnormal communication between the two circulations must be present to sustain life.	Prostaglandin E to vasodilate ductus to keep it open Inotropic support Initial surgery to create opening between right and left side of heart if none exists Total surgical repair—usually the arterial switch procedure—done within first few days of life

Among infants with congenital heart disease, 12 percent were found to have chromosomal abnormalities (Lin and Garver 1988). Infants with Down syndrome and trisomy 13/15 and 16/18 frequently have heart lesions. Increased incidence and risk of recurrence of specific defects occur in families.

It is customary to describe congenital malformations of the heart as either *acyanotic* or *cyanotic*. If an opening exists between the right and left sides of the heart, blood will normally flow from the area of greater pressure (left side) to the area of lesser pressure (right side). This process is known as left-to-right shunt and does not produce cyanosis because oxygenated blood is being pumped out to the systemic circulation. If pressure in the right side of the heart, due to obstruction of normal flow, exceeds that in the left side, unoxygenated blood will flow from the right side to the left side of the heart and out into the systemic circulation. This right-to-left shunt causes cyanosis. If the opening is large, there may be a bidirectional shunt with mixing of blood in both sides of the heart, which also produces cyanosis.

The common cardiac defects seen in the first 6 days of life are left ventricular outflow obstructions (mitral stenosis, aortic stenosis, or atresia), hypoplastic left heart, coarctation of the aorta, patent ductus arteriosus (PDA, the most common defect, especially in premature infants), transposition of the great vessels, tetralogy of Fallot, and large ventricular septal defect or atrial septal defects (Table 25–4, pp 656–657).

The primary goal of the neonatal nurse is early identification of cardiac defects and initiation of referral to the physician. The three most common manifestations of cardiac defect are cyanosis, detectable heart murmur, and congestive heart failure signs (tachycardia, tachypnea, diaphoresis, hepatomegaly, and cardiomegaly). Nursing assessment of the following signs and symptoms assists in identifying the newborn with a cardiac problem:

- *Tachypnea*—reflects increased pulmonary blood flow
- *Dyspnea*—caused by increased pulmonary venous pressure and blood flow; can also cause chest retractions, wheezing
- *Color*—ashen, gray, or cyanotic because of decreased peripheral circulation or low oxygen saturation of the blood
- *Difficulty in feeding*—requires many rest periods before finishing even 1 or 2 ounces
- *Diaphoresis*—beads of perspiration over the upper lip and forehead; may accompany feeding fatigue
- *Stridor or choking spells*
- *Failure to gain weight*
- *Heart murmur*—may not be heard in left-to-right shunting defects since the pulmonary pressure in the newborn is greater than pressure in the left side of the heart in the early newborn period
- *Hepatomegaly*—in right-sided heart failure caused by venous congestion in the liver
- *Tachycardia*—pulse over 160, may be as high as 200
- *Cardiac enlargement*

After the baby is stabilized and gaining weight, decisions are made about ongoing care and surgical interventions. Table 25–4 presents the clinical manifestations and medical/surgical management of these specific cardiac defects.

The parents need careful and complete explanations and the opportunity to take part in decision making. They also require ongoing emotional support. Families with any baby born with a congenital anomaly also need genetic counseling about future conception. Parents need opportunities to verbalize their concerns about their baby's health maintenance and understand the rationale for follow-up care (Paul 1995).

Care of the Newborn with Inborn Errors of Metabolism

Inborn errors of metabolism are a group of hereditary disorders transmitted by mutant genes. Each causes an enzyme defect that blocks a metabolic pathway and leads to an accumulation of toxic metabolites. Most of the disorders are transmitted by an autosomal recessive gene, requiring two heterozygous parents to produce a homozygous infant with the disorder. Heterozygous parents carrying some inborn errors of metabolism disorders can be identified by special tests, and some inborn errors of metabolism can be detected in utero.

The detection of many inborn errors of metabolism is now accomplished neonatally through newborn screening programs. These programs principally test for disorders associated with mental retardation.

Phenylketonuria (PKU) is the most common of the amino acid disorders. Newborn screenings have set its incidence at about one in 12,000 live births worldwide (Seashore and Rinaldo 1993). The highest incidence is noted in white populations from northern Europe and the United States. It is less commonly observed in people of African, Chinese, or Japanese descent (American Academy of Pediatrics Committee on Pediatrics and Committee on Genetics 1996).

Phenylalanine is an essential amino acid used by the body for growth, and in the normal individual any excess is converted to tyrosine. The newborn with PKU lacks this converting ability, which results in an accumulation of phenylalanine in the blood. Phenylalanine produces two abnormal metabolites, phenylpyruvic acid and phenylacetic acid, which are eliminated in the urine, producing a musty odor. Excessive accumulation of phenylalanine and its abnormal metabolites in the brain tissue leads to progressive mental retardation.

Maple syrup urine disease (MSUD) is an inborn error of metabolism and, when untreated, is a rapidly progressing and often fatal disease caused by an enzymatic defect in the metabolism of the branched chain amino acids leucine, isoleucine, and valine.

Homocystinuria is a disorder caused by a deficiency of the enzyme cystathionine B synthase, which produces a block in the normal conversion of methionine to cystine.

Galactosemia is an inborn error of carbohydrate metabolism in which the body is unable to use the sugars galactose and lactose. Enzyme pathways in liver cells normally convert galactose and lactose to glucose. In galactosemia, one step in that conversion pathway is absent, either because of the lack of the enzyme galactose l-phosphate uridyl transferase, or because of the lack of the enzyme galactokinase. High levels of unusable galactose circulate in the blood, which causes cataracts, brain damage, and liver damage (American Academy of Pediatrics Committee on Pediatrics and Committee on Genetics 1996).

Another disorder frequently included in mandatory newborn screening blood tests is *congenital hypothyroidism*. An inborn enzymatic defect, lack of maternal dietary iodine, or maternal ingestion of drugs that depress or destroy thyroid tissue can cause congenital hypothyroidism.

The incidence of metabolic errors is relatively low, but these disorders pose a threat to survival for affected infants and their families, and they frequently require lifelong treatment.

Nursing Assessment

The clinical picture of a PKU baby involves a normal-appearing newborn, most often with blond hair, blue eyes, and fair complexion. Decreased pigmentation may be related to the competition between phenylalanine and tyrosine for the available enzyme, tyrosinase. Tyrosine is needed for the formation of melanin pigment and the hormones epinephrine and thyroxin. Without treatment, the infant fails to thrive, and develops vomiting and eczematous rashes. By about 6 months of age, the infant exhibits behaviors indicative of mental retardation and other CNS involvement, including seizures and abnormal electroencephalogram (EEG) patterns.

Newborns with MSUD have feeding problems and neurologic signs (seizures, spasticity, opisthotonus) during the first week of life. A maple syrup odor of the urine is noted and, when ferric chloride is added to the urine, its color changes to gray-green.

Homocystinuria varies in its presentation, but the more common characteristics are skeletal abnormalities, dislocation of ocular lenses, intravascular thromboses, and mental retardation. Abnormalities occur because of the toxic effects of the accumulation of methionine and the metabolite homocystine in the blood.

Clinical manifestations of galactosemia include vomiting, diarrhea, failure to thrive (Holton and Leonard 1994), hepatosplenomegaly, jaundice, and mental retardation. The condition is frequently associated with anemia, sepsis, and cataracts in the neonatal period. Except for cataracts and mental retardation, those findings are reversible when galactose is excluded from the diet. Mental retardation can be prevented by early diagnosis and careful dietary management.

A large tongue, umbilical hernia, cool and mottled skin, low hairline, hypotonia, and large fontanelles are frequently associated with congenital hypothyroidism. Early symptoms include prolonged neonatal jaundice, poor feeding, constipation, low-pitched cry, poor weight gain, inactivity, and delayed motor development.

Community-Based Nursing Care

Newborn screening for several inborn errors of metabolism is mandatory in many states. Some states simultaneously test all hospitalized newborns for MSUD, homocystinuria, and PKU during the first 3 to 4 days of life. Identification via newborn screening and early medical intervention for inborn errors of metabolism has become more difficult with the advent of early discharge of newborns. It is the nurse's responsibility to obtain the heel stick blood on the filter paper before discharge of the baby. The first filter paper test screens for PKU, homocystinuria, MSUD, galactosemia, and sickle cell anemia. A second blood specimen is often required but the nurse must remember that this second blood specimen tests only for PKU.

In most states, the Guthrie blood test for PKU is required for all newborns before discharge. The Guthrie test uses a drop of blood collected from a heel stick and placed on filter paper. The Guthrie test should be done at least 24 hours, but preferably 72 hours, after the initiation of feedings containing the usual amounts of breast milk or formula so phenylalanine metabolites can begin to build up in the PKU baby. Because it is possible to do the testing with early discharge on an infant with PKU before the phenylalanine concentration rises, and thus miss the diagnosis, some states routinely request a repeat test at 10 to 14 days (Sinai et al 1995). When the Guthrie blood test is performed early, during the first 3 to 4 days of life, a phenylalanine blood level of about

4 to 6 mg/dL is considered a presumptive positive; but only one in 20 to 30 infants with this level are true positives (Seashore and Rinaldo 1993).

High-risk newborns should be receiving a 60 percent milk intake with no more than 40 percent of their total intake coming from nonprotein intravenous fluids. The PKU testing of high-risk newborns should be deferred for at least 48 hours after hyperalimentation is initiated. It is vital that the parents understand the need for the screening procedure, and a follow-up check is necessary to confirm that the test was done.

Some clinicians have the parents perform a diaper test for PKU. At about 6 weeks of age, the parent should take a freshly wet diaper and press the prepared test stick against the wet area. They note the color of the test stick, record the color on the prepared sheet, and mail the form back to the physician. A green color reaction is positive and indicates probable PKU.

Treatment involves stringent restriction of phenylalanine intake. Once identified, an afflicted PKU infant can be treated by a special diet that limits ingestion of phenylalanine. Special formulas low in phenylalanine, such as Lofenalac, Phenyl-Free, PKU1, and PKU2 are available. Special food lists are helpful for parents of a PKU child (Bowe 1995). If treatment is begun before 3 months of age, CNS damage can be minimized. Because of the rigidity and severe limitations of the low phenylalanine diet, many clinicians terminate the special diet at 6 years of age. But myelination continues actively through adolescence and to some extent possibly through 40 years of age. Recent studies have shown loss of intellectual function some years after relaxation of dietary restriction (Acosta 1995). Most centers now recommend keeping blood phenylalanine levels below 20 mg/dL, or even below 15 mg/dL, for life. There is a 95 percent risk of producing a child with mental retardation if the mother with PKU is not on a low-phenylalanine diet during pregnancy. It is recommended that the woman reinstate her low phenylalanine diet a few months before becoming pregnant (Acosta 1995).

Diagnosis of MSUD is made by analyzing blood levels of leucine, isoleucine, and valine. Confirmation of the diagnosis depends on blood assay for the enzyme oxidative decarboxylase. Dietary management of MSUD must be initiated immediately with a formula that is low in the branched-chain amino acids leucine, isoleucine, and valine, which must be continued indefinitely. Dietary treatment prior to 12 days of life has been reported to result in normal intelligence (American Academy of Pediatrics Committee on Pediatrics and Committee on Genetics 1996).

In several states newborn screening includes an enzyme assay for galactose l-phosphate uridyl transferase; however, this test does not detect galactosemia if it is caused by a deficiency of the enzyme galactokinase. There appear to be ethnic differences in age of onset of symptoms and in severity of course. Caucasians have more severe symptoms and earlier onset (3 to 14 days) than people of African descent (14 to 28 days) (Wright et al 1992). Treatment involves a galactose-free diet. Galactose-free formulas include Nutramigen (a protein hydrolysate process formula), meat-base formulas, or soybean formulas. As the infant grows, parents must be educated not only to avoid giving their child milk and milk products but also to read all labels carefully and avoid any foods containing dry milk products. Even with early treatment, children may have learning disabilities, speech problems, and ovarian failure (Holton and Leonard 1994).

For hypothyroidism, immediate and appropriate thyroid replacement therapy is established based on newborn screening and laboratory data. Frequently, premature infants of less than 30 weeks' gestation have low T_4 or thyroid stimulating hormone (TSH) values when compared with normal values of term infants. This may reflect the premature infant's inability to bind thyroid. Management includes frequent laboratory monitoring and adjustment of thyroid medication to accommodate growth and development of the child. With adequate treatment, children remain free of symptoms, but if the condition is untreated, stunted growth and mental retardation occur.

Infants with homocystinuria are managed on a diet that is low in methionine but supplemented with cystine and pyridoxine (vitamin B_6). With early diagnosis and careful management, mental retardation may be prevented.

Parents of affected newborns should be referred to support groups. The nurse should also ensure that parents are informed about centers that can provide them with information about biochemical genetics and dietary management. With the passage of Public Law 100-290 many states provide funding for the special nutritional products (Committee on Nutrition 1994).

Evaluation

Anticipated outcomes of nursing care include

- The risk of inborn errors of metabolism is promptly identified, and early intervention is initiated.
- The parents verbalize their concerns about their baby's health problems, long-term care needs, and potential outcomes.
- The parents are aware of available community health resources and use them as indicated.

Care of Family with Birth of an At-Risk Newborn

The birth of a preterm or ill infant or an infant with a congenital anomaly is a serious crisis situation for a family. Acute grief reactions follow the loss of the perfect baby they have envisioned. In the case of a preterm birth, the mother is denied the last few weeks of pregnancy that seem to prepare her psychologically for the stress of birth and the attachment process. Attachment at this time is fragile, and interruption of the process by separation can affect the future mother-child relationship.

Feelings of guilt and failure often plague mothers of preterm newborns. They may ask themselves "Why did labor start? What did I do (or not do)?" A woman may have guilt fantasies, and wonder "Was it because I had sexual intercourse with my husband (a week, 3 days, a day) ago?" "Was it because I carried three loads of wash up from the basement?" "Am I being punished for something done in the past—even in childhood?"

The birth of the newborn with congenital abnormalities also engenders feelings of guilt and failure. As in the birth of a preterm infant, the woman may entertain ideas of personal guilt. "What did I do (or not do) to cause this?" "Am I being punished for something?"

Parental reactions and steps of attachment are altered by the birth of a preterm infant or one with a congenital anomaly. A variety of new feelings, reactions, and stresses must be recognized and dealt with before the family can work toward the establishment of a healthy parent-infant relationship.

Although reactions and steps of attachment are altered by the birth of these infants, a healthy parent-child relationship can occur. Kaplan and Mason (1974) have identified four psychologic tasks as essential for coping with the stress of an at-risk newborn and for providing a basis for the maternal-infant relationship:

1. Anticipatory grief as a psychologic preparation for possible loss of the child, while still hoping for his or her survival.
2. Acknowledgment of maternal failure to produce a term or perfect newborn expressed as anticipatory grief and depression and lasting until the chances of survival seem secure.
3. Resumption of the process of relating to the infant, which was interrupted by the threat of nonsurvival. This task may be impaired by continuous threat of death or abnormality, and the mother may be slow in her response of hope for the infant's survival.
4. Understanding of the special needs and growth patterns of the at-risk newborn, which are temporary and yield to normal patterns.

Most authorities agree that the birth of a preterm infant or a less-than-perfect infant does require major adjustments as the parents are forced to surrender the image they had nurtured for so long of their ideal child.

Solnit and Stark (1961) postulate that grief and mourning over the loss of the loved object—the idealized child—mark parental reactions to a child with abnormalities. Simultaneously, parents must adopt the imperfect child as the new love object. Parental responses to a child with health problems may be viewed as a five-stage process (Klaus and Kennell 1982):

1. *Shock* is felt at the reality of the birth of this child. This stage may be characterized by forgetfulness, amnesia about the situation, and a feeling of desperation.
2. There is disbelief *(denial)* of the reality of the situation, characterized by a refusal to believe the child is defective. This stage is exemplified by assertions that "It didn't really happen!" "There has been a mistake; it's someone else's baby."
3. *Depression* over the reality of the situation and a corresponding grief reaction follows acknowledgement of the situation. This stage is characterized by much crying and sadness. Anger may also occur at this stage. A projection of blame on others or on self and feelings of "not me" are characteristic of this stage.
4. *Equilibrium* and *acceptance* are characteristic of a decrease in the emotional reactions of the parents. This stage is variable and may be prolonged by a continuing threat to the infant's survival. Some parents experience chronic sorrow in relation to their child.
5. *Reorganization* of the family is necessary to deal with the child's problems. Mutual support of the parents facilitates this process, but the crisis of the situation may precipitate alienation between them.

These stages of parental adjustment are similar to the stages of dying and of grieving. Indeed, reorganization is necessary to deal with a crisis concerning a newborn at risk.

In the birth of either an infant with an anomaly or a preterm infant, the process of mourning is necessary for attachment to the less-than-perfect child. *Grief work*, the emotional reaction to a significant loss, must occur before adequate attachment to the actual child is possible. Parental detachment precedes parental attachment.

APPLYING THE NURSING PROCESS

Nursing Assessment

Development of a nurse-family relationship facilitates information gathering in areas of concern. A concurrent illness of the mother or other family members or other concurrent stress (lack of hospitalization insurance, loss of job, age of parents) may alter the family response to the baby. Feelings of apprehension, guilt, failure, and grief that are verbally or nonverbally expressed are important aspects of the nursing history. These observations enable all professionals to be aware of the parental state, coping behaviors, and readiness for attachment, bonding, and caretaking. Appropriate nursing observations during interviewing and relating to the family include:

1. *Level of understanding.* Observations concerning the ability to assimilate information given and to ask appropriate questions; the need for constant repetition of "the same" information.
2. *Behavioral responses.* Appropriateness of behavior in relation to information given; lack of response; "flat" affect.
3. *Difficulties with communication.* Deafness (reads lips only); blindness; dysphagia; understanding only of foreign language.
4. *Paternal and maternal education level.* Parents unable to read or write; only eighth grade completed; mother an MD, RN, or PhD; and so on.

Documentation of such information, obtained by the nurse through continuing contact and development of a therapeutic family relationship, enables all professionals to understand and use the nursing history in providing continuous individual care.

Visiting and caregiving patterns give an indication of the level or lack of parental attachment. A record of visits, caretaking procedures, affect (in relating to the newborn), and telephone calls is essential. Serial observations must be obtained, rather than just isolated instances of concern. Grant (1978) has developed a conceptual framework depicting adaptive and maladaptive responses to parenting of a preterm or less-than-perfect infant (Figure 25–11).

If a pattern of distancing behaviors evolves, appropriate intervention should be instituted. Follow-up studies have found that a statistically significant number of preterm, sick, and congenitally defective infants suffer from failure to thrive, battering, or other parenting disorders. Early detection and intervention will prevent these aberrations in parenting behaviors from leading to irreparable damage or death.

Nursing Diagnosis

Nursing diagnoses that may apply to the family of a newborn at risk include the following:

- Grief related to loss of idealized newborn
- Fear related to emotional involvement with an at-risk newborn
- Altered parenting related to impaired bonding secondary to feelings of inadequacy about caretaking activities

Nursing Plan and Implementation

Preparation of Parents for Initial Viewing of Newborn

Before parents see their child, the nurse must prepare them for the viewing. It is important that a positive, realistic attitude regarding the infant be presented to the parents rather than a pessimistic one. An overly negative, fatalistic attitude further alienates the parents from their infant and retards attachment behaviors. Instead of allowing attachment and bonding to develop, the parents will begin the process of anticipatory grieving, and once started, this process is difficult to reverse.

In preparing parents for the first view of their infant, it is important for a professional to have looked at the baby. The parents should be prepared to see both the deviations and the normal aspects of their infant. All infants exhibit strengths as well as deficiencies. The nurse may say, "Your baby is small, about the length of my two hands. She weighs 2 lb 3 oz but is very active and cries when we disturb her. She is having some difficulty breathing but is breathing without assistance and in only 35 percent oxygen."

The nurse should describe the equipment being used for the at-risk newborn and its purpose before the parents enter the intensive care unit. Many intensive care units have booklets for parents to read before entering. Through explanations and pictures, the parents can be better prepared to deal with the feelings they may experience when they see their infant for the first time.

Support of Parents During Their Initial Viewing of the Newborn

Upon entering the unit, parents may be overwhelmed by the sounds of monitors, alarms, and respirators, as well as by the unfamiliar language and "foreign" atmosphere. It is more reassuring when parents are prepared and accompanied to the unit by the same person(s). The primary nurse and physician caring for the newborn should be with the parents when they first visit their baby. Parental reactions are varied, but there is usually an element of initial shock. Provision of chairs and time to regain composure will assist the parents. Slow, complete, and simple explanations—first about the infant and then about the equipment—allay fear and anxiety.

As parents attempt to deal with the initial stages of shock and grief, they may fail to grasp new information. The parents may need repeated explanations to accept the reality of the situation, procedures, equipment, and the infant's condition on subsequent visits.

Misconceptions about equipment and its placement on the infant and about its potential harm are common.

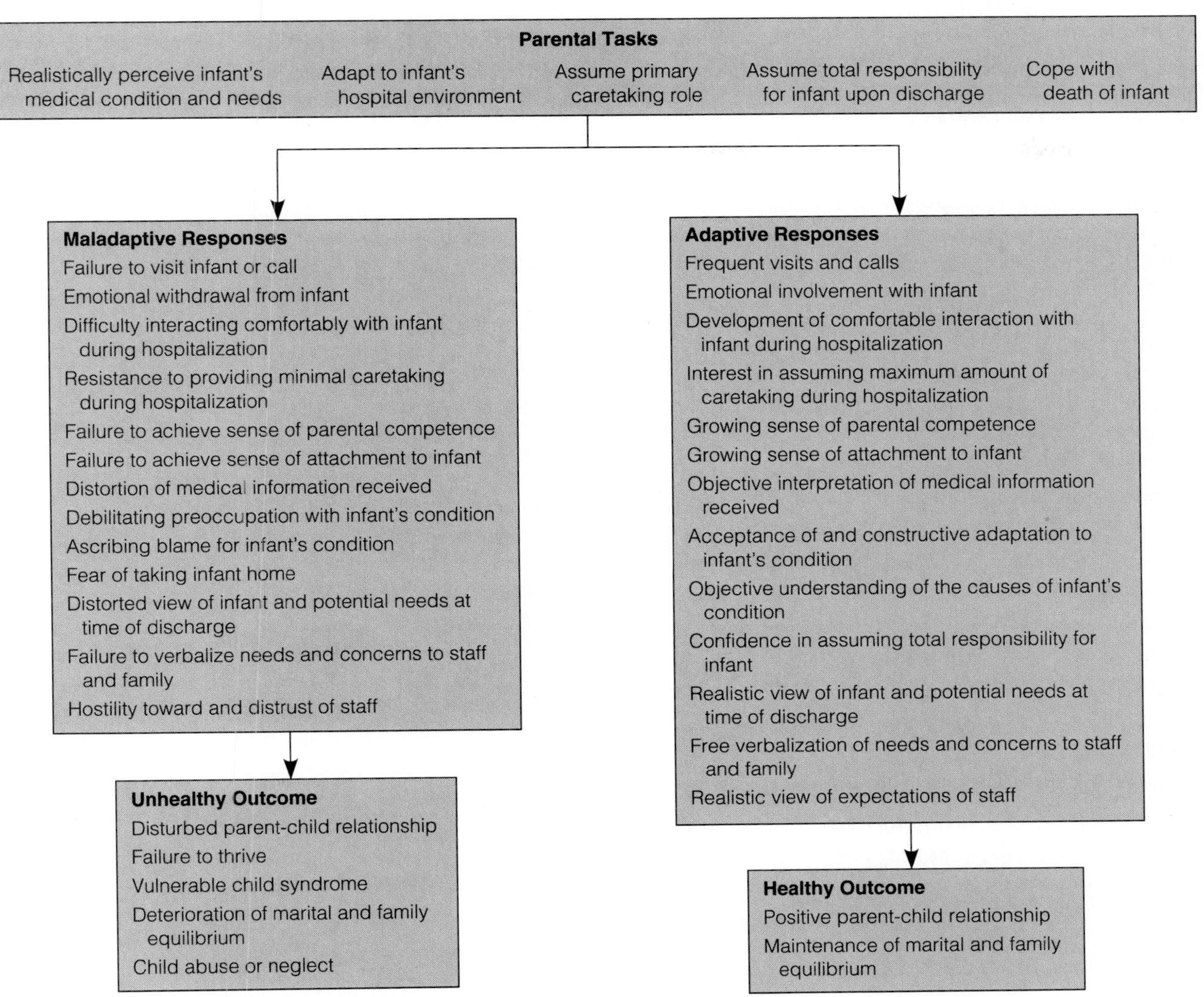

Parental Tasks
Realistically perceive infant's medical condition and needs
Adapt to infant's hospital environment
Assume primary caretaking role
Assume total responsibility for infant upon discharge
Cope with death of infant
Maladaptive Responses
Failure to visit infant or call
Emotional withdrawal from infant
Difficulty interacting comfortably with infant during hospitalization
Resistance to providing minimal caretaking during hospitalization
Failure to achieve sense of parental competence
Failure to achieve sense of attachment to infant
Distortion of medical information received
Debilitating preoccupation with infant's condition
Ascribing blame for infant's condition
Fear of taking infant home
Distorted view of infant and potential needs at time of discharge
Failure to verbalize needs and concerns to staff and family
Hostility toward and distrust of staff
Adaptive Responses
Frequent visits and calls
Emotional involvement with infant
Development of comfortable interaction with infant during hospitalization
Interest in assuming maximum amount of caretaking during hospitalization
Growing sense of parental competence
Growing sense of attachment to infant
Objective interpretation of medical information received
Acceptance of and constructive adaptation to infant's condition
Objective understanding of the causes of infant's condition
Confidence in assuming total responsibility for infant
Realistic view of infant and potential needs at time of discharge
Free verbalization of needs and concerns to staff and family
Realistic view of expectations of staff
Unhealthy Outcome
Disturbed parent-child relationship
Failure to thrive
Vulnerable child syndrome
Deterioration of marital and family equilibrium
Child abuse or neglect
Healthy Outcome
Positive parent-child relationship
Maintenance of marital and family equilibrium

FIGURE 25–11 Maladaptive and adaptive parental responses during crisis period, showing unhealthy and healthy outcomes.

Source: Grant P: Psychological needs of families of high-risk infants. *Fam Community Health* 1978; 1(3):93; with permission of Aspen Publisher, Inc., © 1978.

Such statements as "Does the fluid go into the brain?" "Does the white wire on the abdomen go into the stomach?" and "Does the monitor make the baby's heart beat?" imply much fear for the infant's safety and misconception about the machines. These worries are easily overcome by simple explanations of all equipment being used.

Concern about the infant's physical appearance is common, yet may remain unvoiced. Parents may express such concerns as "He looks so small and red—like a drowned rat." "Why do her genitals look so abnormal?" "Will that awful-looking mouth [cleft lip and palate] ever be normal?" Such questions need to be anticipated by the nurse and addressed. Use of pictures, such as of an infant after cleft lip repair, may be reassuring to doubting parents. Knowledge of the development of a "normal" preterm infant will allow the nurse to make reassuring statements such as "The baby's labia may look very abnormal to you, but they are normal for her maturity. As she grows, the outer lips of the labia will become larger and the clitoris will be covered and the genitals will then look as you expect them to. She is normal for her level of maturity."

The tone of the neonatal intensive care unit is set by the nursing staff. Development of a safe, trusting environment depends on viewing the parents as essential caregivers, not as visitors or nuisances in the unit. Provision of chairs, privacy when needed, and easy access to staff and facilities are all important in developing an open, comfortable environment. An uncrowded and welcoming atmosphere lets parents know "You are welcome here." However, even in crowded physical surroundings, an attitude of openness and trust can be conveyed by the nursing staff.

A trusting relationship is essential for collaborative efforts in caring for the infant. Nurses must therapeutically use their own responses to relate to the parents on a one-to-one basis. Each individual has different needs, different ways of adapting to crisis, and different means of support. Professionals must use techniques that are real and spontaneous to them and avoid words or actions that are foreign to them. Nurses must also gauge their interventions to match the parents' pace and needs.

Powell (1981) suggests several positive strategies that increase the effectiveness of nursing interventions with parents:

- Work on problem solving with the family rather than giving advice.
- View the baby as a total individual rather than emphasizing the problem.
- Observe the uniqueness of the newborn rather than stereotyping or labeling the newborn as slow, unmanageable, and so on.
- Avoid labeling parents as inadequate, rejecting, or angry.
- Stress the baby's similarities to other babies.
- Stress the strengths and competence of the parents.
- Help parents realize that they are in charge of their children and themselves.
- Be aware of the needs of all members of the family, including siblings.

Parental Support

It is essential that the mother be reunited with her infant as soon as possible after birth so that

1. She knows that her infant is alive.
2. She knows what the infant's real problems are. Early acquaintance between mother and infant allows a realistic perspective of the baby's condition.
3. She can begin the grief work over the loss of the idealized child and begin the process of attachment to the actual child.
4. She can share the experience of the infant's problems with the father, who may have already seen and touched the infant.

Facilitation of Attachment if Neonatal Transport Occurs

Small hospitals may be unable to care for sick infants. Transport to a regional referral center may be necessary.

STAGE I: Touching
Uses fingertips
Uses whole hand
Strokes child
Holds and studies child "en face"
Spontaneously lowers crib rails to fondle, hold, or talk to child

↓

STAGE II: Caretaking
Provides clean clothing, toys, grooming aids
Performs activities of daily living (bathing, diapering, feeding, dressing)
Performs caretaking tasks with proficiency and expresses pleasure in meeting infant's needs
Able to comfort child when distressed or crying
Able to meet child's special health needs (suctioning, cleaning stoma sites, treatments)

↓

STAGE III: Identity
Brings linens from home
Takes photographs
Brings individualized toys
Can make personalized observations about child
Offers suggestions and makes demands for personalized care
Demonstrates "advocacy" behavior
Feels he or she can care for child better than anyone else
Demonstrates consistent visiting and/or calling pattern
Questions focus on total child, not only physiologic parameters

FIGURE 25–12 Stages of parenting behavior toward infants in intensive care.

Source: Adapted from work of Rubin, Schaeffer, Jay, and Schraeder by Schraeder BD: Attachment and parenting despite lengthy intensive care. *MCN* January/February 1980; 5:38. Reprinted with permission from the American Journal of Nursing Company, 1980.

These centers may be as far as 500 miles from the parents' community; it is therefore essential that the mother see and touch her infant before the infant is transported. Facilitation of this important contact may be the responsibility of the referring hospital staff as well as the transport team.

Bringing the mother to the nursery or taking the infant in a warmed transport incubator to the mother's bedside will allow her to see the infant before transportation to the center. When the infant reaches the referral center, a staff member should call the parents with information about the infant's condition during transport, safe arrival at the center, and present condition.

Support of parents, with explanations from the professional staff, is crucial. Occasionally the mother may be unable to see the infant before transport, for example, if she is still under general anesthesia or experiencing complications such as shock, hemorrhage, or seizures. In these cases, before the infant is transported caregivers should take a photograph of the infant to give to the mother, along with an explanation of the infant's condition, problems, and a detailed description of the infant's characteristics. An additional photograph is also helpful for the father to share with siblings or extended family. With the increased attention to improved fetal outcome, prenatal maternal transports, rather than neonatal transports, are occurring more frequently. This practice gives the mother of an at-risk infant the opportunity to visit and care for her infant during the early postpartal period.

Promotion of Touching

Parents visiting a small or sick infant may need several visits to become comfortable and confident in their ability to touch the infant without injuring her or him. Barriers such as incubators, incisions, monitor electrodes, and tubes may delay the mother's confidence. Knowledge of this "normal" delay in touching behavior will help the nurse understand parental behavior.

Klaus and Kennell (1982) have demonstrated a significant difference in the amount of eye contact and touching behaviors of mothers of normal newborns and mothers of preterm infants. Whereas mothers of normal newborns progress within minutes to palm contact of the infant's trunk, the mother of a preterm infant is slower to progress from fingertip to palm contact and from the extremities to the trunk. The progression to palm contact with the infant's trunk may take several visits to the nursery.

Through support, reassurance, and encouragement, the nurse can facilitate the mother's positive feelings about her ability and her importance to her infant. Touching facilitates "getting to know" the infant and thus establishes a bond with the infant. Touching as well as seeing the infant helps the mother realize the "normals" and potentials of her baby (Figure 25–12).

The nurse can also encourage parents to meet their newborn's need for stimulation. Stroking, rocking, cuddling, singing, and talking should be an integral part of the parents' caretaking responsibilities.

Facilitation of Parental Caretaking

The nurse can facilitate bonding by encouraging parents to visit and become involved in their baby's care (Figure 25–13). When visiting is impossible, the parents should feel free to phone whenever they wish to receive information about their baby. A warm, receptive attitude on the part of the nurse is very supportive. Nurses can also facilitate parenting by personalizing a baby to the parents; this can be done by referring to the infant by name or by relating personal behavioral characteristics. Remarks such as "Jenny loves her pacifier" help make the infant more individual and unique.

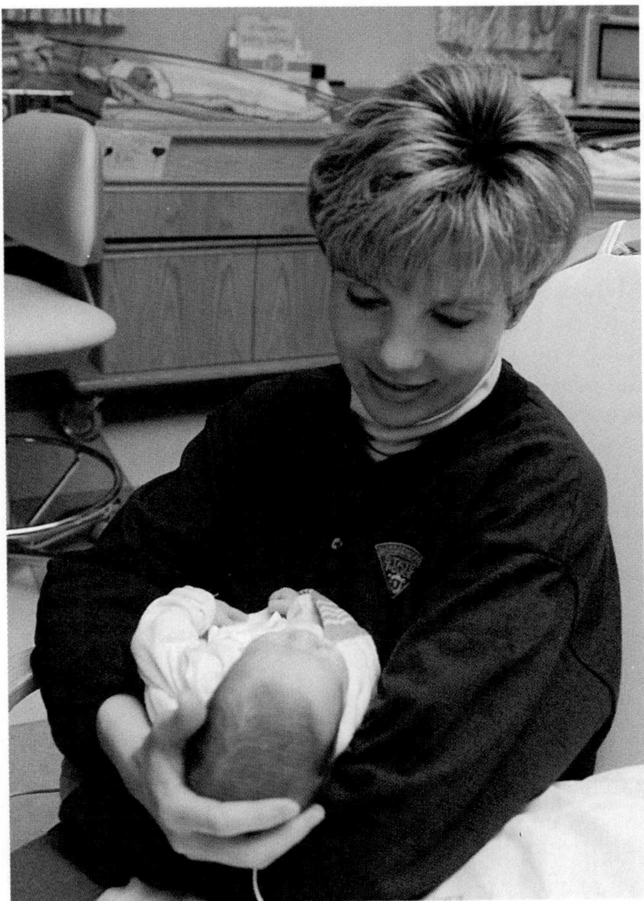

FIGURE 25–13 It is important that the parents of high-risk infants be given the opportunity to get acquainted with their children. Physical contact is extremely important in the bonding process and should be encouraged whenever possible.

Caretaking may be delayed for the mother of a preterm, defective, or sick infant. The variety of equipment needed for life support is hardly conducive to anxiety-free caretaking by the parents. However, even the sickest infant may be cared for, if only in a small way, by the parents. As a facilitator of parental caretaking, it is the nurse's responsibility to promote the parents' success. Demonstration and explanation, followed by support of the parents in initial caretaking behaviors, positively reinforce this behavior. Changing their infant's diaper, giving skin or oral care, or helping the nurse turn the infant may at first provoke anxiety, but the parents will become more comfortable and confident in caretaking and receive satisfaction from the baby's reactions and their ability "to do something." Complimenting the parents' competence in caretaking also increases their self-esteem, which has received recent "blows" of guilt and failure. It is vitally important that the parents never be given a task if there is any possibility that they will not be able to accomplish it.

Parents of high-risk infants often have ambivalent feelings toward the nurse. As they watch the nurse competently perform caretaking tasks, they feel both grateful for the nurse's abilities and expertise and jealous of the nurse's ability to care for their infant. These feelings may be acted out in criticism of the care being received by the infant, manipulation of staff, or personal guilt. Instead of fostering (by silence) these inferiority feelings of parents, nurses should recognize such feelings and intervene appropriately to enhance parent-infant attachment. The nurse needs to deal with ambivalent feelings that contribute to a competitive atmosphere. For example, the nurse should avoid making unfavorable comparisons between the baby's responses to parental caretaking and nursing care. During a quiet time it may help for the nurse to encourage the parents to talk about their hopes and fears and to facilitate their involvement in parent groups (Mercer 1990).

Nurses who are understanding and secure will be able to support the parents' egos instead of collecting rewards for themselves. To reinforce positive parenting behaviors, professionals must first believe in the importance of the parents. The nurse can hardly convince doubting parents of their importance to the infant unless the nurse really believes it. Both attitudes and words must say: "You are good parents. You have an important contribution to make to the care of your infant." Unless as much care is taken in facilitating parental attachment as in providing physiologic care, the outcome will not be a healthy family.

Verbalizations by the nurse that improve parental self-esteem are essential and easily shared. The nurse can point out that, in addition to physiologic use, breast milk is important because of the emotional investment of the mother. Pumping, storing, labeling, and delivering quantities of breast milk is time-consuming and a "labor of love" for mothers. Positive remarks regarding breast milk reinforce the maternal behavior of caretaking and providing for her infant: "Breast milk is something that only you can give your baby" or "You really have brought a lot of milk today" or "Look how rich this breast milk is" or "Even small amounts of milk are important, and look how rich it is."

If the infant begins to gain weight while being fed breast milk, it is important to point this out to the mother. Parents should also be advised that initial weight loss with beginning nipple-feedings is common because of the increased energy expended when the infant begins active rather than passive nutritional intake. Provision of care by the parents is appropriate even for very sick or defective infants who are likely to die. It has been found that detachment is easier after attachment, because the parents are comforted by the knowledge that they did all they could for their child while he or she was alive.

Provision of Continuity in Information Giving

During crisis, maintenance of interpersonal relationships is difficult. Yet in a newborn intensive care area, the parents are expected to relate to many different care providers. It is important that parents have as few professionals as possible relaying information to them. A primary nurse should coordinate and provide continuity in information given to parents. Care providers are individuals and thus will use different terms, inflections, and attitudes. These subtle differences are monumental to parents and only confuse, confound, and produce anxiety (Bass 1991). Relationships with a few trusted professionals minimize unnecessary anxiety and concern and facilitate open communication. The nurse not only functions as a liaison between the parents and the wide variety of professionals interacting with the infant and parents but also offers clarification, explanation, interpretation of information, and support to the parents.

Use of the Family's Support System

The parents should be encouraged to deal with the crisis with help from their support system. The support system attempts to meet the emotional needs and provide support for the family members in crisis and stress situations. Biologic kinship is not the only valid criterion for a support system; an emotional kinship is the most important factor. In our mobile society of isolated nuclear families, the support system may be a next-door neighbor, a best friend, or perhaps a school chum. The nurse must search out the significant others in the lives of the parents and help them understand the problems so that they can provide parental support.

Facilitation of Family Adjustment

The impact of the crisis on the family is individual and varied. Information about the family's ability to adapt to the situation is obtained through the nurse-family relationship. The birth of the infant (normal newborn, preterm infant, infant with congenital anomaly) should be viewed as it is defined by the family, and appropriate intervention can then be instituted.

Because the family is a unit composed of individuals who must deal with the situation, it is important to encourage open intrafamily communication. Secret-keeping should not be encouraged, especially between spouses, because secrets undermine the trust of their relationship. Well-meaning rationales such as "I want to protect her," "I don't want him to worry about it," and so on can be destructive to open communication and to the basic element of a relationship—trust.

The nurse should encourage open communication between family members, particularly between spouses. Open communication is especially important when the mother is hospitalized apart from the infant. In this situation, the father is the first to visit the infant and relays information about the infant's care and condition to the mother. The mother has had minimal contact, if any, with her infant. Because of her anxiety and isolation, she may mistrust all those who provide information (the father, nurse, physician, or extended family) until she can see the infant for herself. This can put tremendous stress on the relationship between spouses. The parents (and family) should be given information together. This practice helps overcome misunderstandings and misinterpretations and promotes mutual "working through" of problems.

The entire family—siblings as well as relatives—should be encouraged to visit and receive information about the baby. Methods of intervention in helping the family cope with the situation include providing support, confronting the crisis, and understanding the reality. The nurse should extend support, explanations, and the helping role to the kin network, as well as to the nuclear family, in an attempt to aid them in communication and support ties with the nuclear family.

The needs of siblings should not be overlooked. They have been looking forward to the new baby, and they too suffer a degree of loss. Young children may react with hostility and older ones with shame at the birth of an infant with an anomaly. Both reactions make them feel guilty. Parents, preoccupied with working through their own feelings, often cannot give the other children the attention and support they need. Sometimes another child becomes the focus of family tension. Anxiety thus directed can take the form of finding fault or of overconcern. This is a form of denial; the parents cannot face the real worry—the infant at risk. After assessing the situation, the observant nurse can see that another family member or friend steps in and gives the needed support to the siblings of the affected baby.

Desires and needs of the individuals must be respected and facilitated; differences are tolerable and should be able to exist side by side. Eliciting the parents' feelings is easily accomplished with the question: "How are you doing?" The emphasis is on "you," and the interest must be sincere.

Families with children in the newborn intensive care unit become friends and support one another. To encourage the development of these friendships and to provide support, many units have established parent groups. The core of the groups consists of parents who have previously had an infant in the intensive care unit. Most groups make contact with families within a day or two of the infant's admission to the unit, through either phone calls or visits to the hospital. Early one-on-one parent contacts help families work through their feelings better than discussion groups. This personalized method gives the grieving parents an opportunity to express personal feelings about the pregnancy, labor, and delivery of their "different than expected" infant with others who have experienced the same feelings and with whom they can identify (Ladden and Damato 1992).

Provision of Home Care Instruction

Predischarge planning begins once the infant's condition becomes stable and indications suggest the newborn will survive. Adequate predischarge teaching will help the parents transform their feelings of inadequacy and competition with the nurse into feelings of self-assurance and attachment. From the beginning the parents should be taught about their infant's special needs and growth patterns (Sudia Robinson 1991). This teaching and involvement are best facilitated by a nurse who is familiar with the infant and his or her family over a period of time and who has developed a comfortable and supportive relationship with them.

The nurse's responsibility is to provide home care instructions in an optimal environment for parental learning. Learning should take place over time, to avoid bombarding the parents with instructions in the day or hour before discharge.

Parents often enjoy doing minimal caretaking tasks with gradual expansion of their role. Many intensive care units provide facilities for parents to room-in with their infants for a few days before discharge. This allows parents a degree of independence in the care of their infant with the security of nursing help nearby. This practice is particularly helpful for anxious parents, parents who have not had the opportunity to spend extended time with their infant, or parents who will be giving complex physical care at home, such as tracheostomy care.

The following are the basic elements of home care instruction:

1. Teach parents routine well-baby care, such as bathing, temperature taking, formula preparation, and breastfeeding.
2. Train parents to do special procedures as needed by the newborn, such as gavage or gastrostomy feedings, tracheostomy or enterostomy care, medication administration, cardiopulmonary resuscitation (CPR), and operation of apnea monitor. Before discharge, the parents should be as comfortable as possible with these tasks and should demonstrate independence. Written tools and instruction are useful for parents to refer to once they are home with the infant, but these should not replace actual participation in the infant's care.

3. Refer parents to community health and support organizations. The Visiting Nurses' Association, public health nurses, or social services can assist the parents in the stressful transition from hospital to home by providing the necessary home teaching and support. Some intensive care nurseries have their own parent support groups to help bridge the gap between hospital and home care. Parents can also find support from a variety of community support organizations, such as mothers-of-twins groups, trisomy 13 clubs, the March of Dimes Birth Defects Foundation, handicapped children services, and teen mother and child programs. Each community has numerous agencies capable of assisting the family in adapting emotionally, physically, and financially to the chronically ill infant. The nurse should be familiar with community resources and help the parents identify which agencies may benefit them.
4. Help parents recognize the growth and development needs of their infant. A development program begun in the hospital can be continued at home, or parents may be referred to an infant development program in the community.
5. Arrange medical follow-up care before discharge. The infant may need to be followed up by a family pediatrician, a well-baby clinic, or a specialty clinic. The first appointment should be made before the infant is discharged from the hospital.
6. Evaluate the need for special equipment for infant care (such as a respirator, oxygen, apnea monitor) in the home. Any equipment or supplies should be placed in the home before the infant's discharge. The nurse can help the parents assess the newborn's needs and coordinate services.

Further evaluation after the infant has gone home is useful in determining whether the crisis has been resolved satisfactorily. The parents are usually given the intensive care nursery's telephone number to call for support and advice. It is suggested that the staff follow up each family with visits or telephone calls at intervals for several weeks to assess and evaluate the infant's (and parents') progress.

Evaluation

Anticipated outcomes of nursing care include

- The parents are able to verbalize their feelings of grief and loss.
- The parents verbalize their concerns about their baby's health problems, care needs, and potential outcome.
- The parents are able to participate in their infant's care and show attachment behaviors.

CHAPTER HIGHLIGHTS

- Early identification of potential high-risk fetuses through assessment of prepregnant, prenatal, and intrapartal factors facilitates strategically timed nursing observations and interventions.
- High-risk newborns, whether they are premature, SGA, LGA, postterm, or infant of a diabetic or substance-addicted mother, have many similar problems, although their problems are based on different physiologic processes.
- SGA newborns are associated with perinatal asphyxia and resulting aspiration syndrome, hypothermia, hypoglycemia, hypocalcemia, polycythemia, congenital anomalies, and intrauterine infections. Long-term problems include continued growth and learning difficulties.
- LGA newborns are at risk for birth trauma as a result of cephalopelvic disproportion, hypoglycemia, polycythemia, and hyperviscosity.
- IDMs are at risk for hypoglycemia, hypocalcemia, hyperbilirubinemia, polycythemia, and respiratory distress due to delayed maturation of their lungs.
- Postterm newborns frequently encounter the following intrapartal problems: CPD (shoulder dystocia) and birth traumas, hypoglycemia, polycythemia, meconium aspiration, cold stress, and possible seizure activity. Long-term complications may involve poor weight gain and low IQ scores.
- The common problems of the preterm newborn are a result of the baby's immature body systems. Potential problems include respiratory distress syndrome, patent ductus arteriosus, hypothermia and cold stress, feeding difficulties and necrotizing enterocolitis, marked insensible water loss and loss of buffering agents through the kidneys, infection, anemia of prematurity, apnea and intraventricular hemorrhage, retinopathy of prematurity, and behavioral state disorganization. Long-term needs and problems include bronchopulmonary dysplasia, speech defects, sensorineural hearing loss, and neurologic defects.
- Newborns of alcohol-dependent mothers are at risk for physical characteristic alterations and the long-term complications of feeding problems; CNS dysfunction, including lower IQ, hyperactivity, and language abnormalities; and congenital anomalies.
- Newborns born to drug-dependent mothers experience drug withdrawal as well as respiratory distress, jaundice, congenital anomalies, and behavioral abnormalities. With early recognition and intervention, the potential long-term physiologic and emotional consequences of these difficulties can be avoided or at least lessened in severity.

- Newborns born to mothers with AIDS require early recognition and treatment to lessen the severity of the physiologic and emotional consequences and to implement CDC guidelines.
- Cardiac defects are a significant cause of morbidity and mortality in the newborn period. Early identification and nursing and medical care of newborns with cardiac defects are essential to the improved outcome of these infants. Care is directed toward lessening the workload of the heart and decreasing oxygen and energy consumption.
- Inborn errors of metabolism such as galactosemia, PKU, homocystinuria, and maple syrup urine disease are usually included in a newborn screening program designed to prevent mental retardation through dietary management and medication.
- The nursing care of the newborn with special problems involves the understanding of normal physiology, the pathophysiology of the disease process, clinical manifestations, and supportive or corrective therapies. Only with this theoretical background can the nurse make appropriate observations about responses to therapy and development of complications.
- The nurse is the facilitator for interdisciplinary communication with the parents, identifying their understanding of their infant's care and their needs for emotional support.
- Parents of at-risk newborns need support from nurses and health care providers to understand the special needs of their baby, feel comfortable in an overwhelmingly strange environment, and feel confident in their ability to care for their children at home.

REFERENCES

Acosta PB: Nutrition support of maternal phenylketonuria. *Semin Perinatol* 1995; 19(3):182.

ACOG technical bulletin #159: Fetal macrosomia. *Int J Gynecol Obstet* 1992; 39:341.

Als H et al: Assessment of preterm infant behavior (APIB). In: *Theory and Research in Behavioral Pediatrics,* Vol. 1. Fitzgerald HE, Lester BM, Yogman MW (editors). New York: Plenum, 1982.

American Academy of Pediatrics Committee on Fetus and Newborn: *Guidelines for Perinatal Care,* 3rd ed. Elk Grove Village, IL: AAP, 1992.

American Academy of Pediatrics Committee on Pediatrics and Committee on Genetics: Newborn screening fact sheets. *Pediatrics* 1996; 98(3):473.

Angelini DJ, Knapp CM: Narcotic addiction in pregnancy. *Case Studies in Perinatal Nursing.* Rockville, MD: Aspen, 1991.

Auerbach KG, Walker M: When the mother of a premature infant uses a breast pump: What every NICU nurse needs to know. *Neonatal Network* 1994; 13(4):23.

Bass LS: What do parents need when their infant is a patient in the NICU? *Neonatal Network* 1991; 10(4):25.

Bastin N et al: Postpartum care of the HIV-positive woman and her newborn. Part 3. *JOGNN* 1992; 21(2):105.

Bell GL, Lau K: Perinatal and neonatal issues of substance abuse. *Pediatr Clin North Am* 1995; 42(2):261.

Benson DW: Changing profile of congenital heart disease. *Pediatrics* 1989; 83(5):790.

Bernbaum JC: Medical care after discharge. In: *Neonatology: Pathophysiology and Management of the Newborn,* 4th ed. Avery GB, Fletcher M, MacDonald MG (editors). Philadelphia: Lippincott, 1994.

Bowe K: Phenylketonuria: An update for pediatric community health nurses. *Pediatr Nurs* 1995; 21(2):191.

Bowen FW, Tasman W: Retinopathy of prematurity. In: *Neonatology for the Clinician.* Pomerance JJ, Richardson CJ (editors). Norwalk, CT: Appleton & Lange, 1993.

Brooks-Gunn J, McCarton C, Hawley T: Effects of in utero drug exposure on children's development. *Arch Pediatr Adolesc Med* 1994; 148(1):33.

Cole JG: Intervention strategies for infants with prenatal drug exposure. *Inf Young Children* 1996; 8(3):35.

Coles CD: Impact of prenatal alcohol exposure on the newborn and the child. *Clin Obstet Gynecol* 1993; 36(2):255.

Committee on Nutrition: Reimbursement for medical foods for inborn errors of metabolism. *Pediatrics* 1994; 93(5):860.

Committee on Substance Abuse and Committee on Children with Disabilities: Fetal alcohol syndrome and fetal alcohol effects. *Pediatrics* 1993; 89(1):1004.

Creasy RK, Resnik R: Intrauterine growth restriction. In: *Maternal Fetal Medicine: Principles and Practice,* 3rd ed. Philadelphia: Saunders, 1994.

Cunningham MD: Special problems in the fetus and neonate. In: *Gellis & Kagan's Current Pediatric Therapy,* Vol. 14. Burg FD, Inglefinger JR, Wald ER (editors). Philadelphia: Saunders, 1993.

Cusson RM, Lee AL: Parental intervention and the development of the preterm infant. *JOGNN* 1994; 23(1):60.

D'Apolito KC, McRorie TI: Pharmacologic management of neonatal abstinence syndrome. *J Perinatal Neonatal Nurs* 1996; 9(4):70.

Dashier S: What happens to the offspring of diabetic pregnancies? *MCN* 1995; 20(1):25.

Duimstra C et al: A fetal alcohol syndrome surveillance pilot project in American Indian communities in the northern plains. *Pub Health Rep* 1993; 198(2):225.

Fletcher AB: Nutrition. In: *Neonatology: Pathophysiology and Management of the Newborn,* 4th ed. Avery GB, Fletcher M, MacDonald MG (editors). Philadelphia: Lippincott, 1994.

Frank DA, Bresnahan K, Zuckerman BS: Maternal cocaine use: Impact on child health and development. *Adv Pediatr* 1993; 40:65.

Gale G, Franck L, Lund C: Skin-to-skin (kangaroo) holding of the intubated premature infant. *Neonatal Network* 1993; 12(6):49.

Gardosi JO, Mongellii JM, Mul T: Intrauterine growth retardation. *Clin Obstet Gynecol* 1995; 9(3):445.

Grant P: Psychosocial needs of families of high-risk infants. *Fam Comm Health* November 1978; 1:91.

Grisemer AN: Apnea of prematurity: Current management and nursing implications. *Pediatr Nurs* 1990; 16(6):606.

Harrington K, Campbell S: Fetal size and growth. *Cur Op Obstet Gynecol* 1993; 5:186.

Haut C, Peddicord K, O'Brien E: Supporting parental bonding in the NICU: A care plan for nurses. *Neonatal Network* 1994; 13(8):19.

Holton JB, Leonard JV: Clouds still gathering over galactosaemia. *Lancet* 1994; 344(5):1242.

Homko CJ et al: The interrelationship between ethnicity and gestational diabetes in fetal macrosomia. *Diabetes Care* 1995; 18(11):1442.

Hulseman ML, Norman LA: The neonatal ICU graduate: Part I. Common problems. *Am Fam Physician* 1992; 45(3):1301.

Iams JD, Zuspan FP: *Manual of Obstetrics and Gynecology,* 2nd ed. St Louis: Mosby, 1990.

Jhaveri MK et al: Perinatal cocaine/crack exposure in infants: A different perspective. *Neonatal Int Care* May/June 1993; 18.

Kaplan DM, Mason EA: Maternal reactions to premature birth viewed as an acute emotional disorder. In: *Crisis Interventions.* Parad HJ (editor). New York: Family Services Association of America, 1974.

Kaplan P et al: Intellectual outcome in children with maple syrup urine disease. *J Pediatr* 1991; 119:46.

Kellinger KG: Providing primary care to the HIV-at-risk and infected child. *Nurse Pract* 1994; 19(8):48.

Kinneer MD, Beachy P: Nipple feeding premature in the neonatal intensive-care unit: Factors and decisions. *JOGNN* 1994; 23(2):105.

Kinsey KK: "But I know my man!" HIV/AIDS risk appraisals and heuristical reasoning patterns among childbearing women. *Holistic Nurs Pract* 1994; 8(2):79.

Klaus MH, Kennell JH: *Maternal-Infant Bonding,* 2nd ed. St Louis: Mosby, 1982.

Krishna A, Phillips LS: Fetal alcohol syndrome and insulin-like growth factors. *J Lab Clin Med* 1994; 124(2):149.

Kuhn L, Stein ZA: Mother-to-infant HIV transmission: Timing, risk factors and prevention. *Pediatr Perinatol Epidemiol* 1995; 9:1.

Ladden M, Damato E: Parenting and supportive programs. *NAACOG's Clinical Issues* 1992; 3(1):174.

Lin AE, Garver KL: Genetic counseling for congenital heart defects. *J Pediatr* 1988; 113(6):1105.

McMahon, MJ, Kuller JA, Yankowitz J: Assessment of the postterm pregnancy. *Am Fam Physician* 1996; 54(2):631.

Makinson C: The health consequences of teenage fertility. *Fam Plan Perspect* 1985; 17:132.

Medoff-Cooper B: Transition of the preterm infant to an open crib. *JOGNN* 1994; 23(4):329.

Meier P: Bottle and breast feeding: Effects on transcutaneous oxygen pressure and temperature in preterm infants. *Nurs Res* 1988; 37(1):36.

Mercer R: *Parents at Risk.* New York: Springer, 1990.

Nagey DA, Viscardi RM: Retarded intrauterine growth. In: *Neonatology for the Clinician.* Pomerance JJ, Richardson CJ (editors). Norwalk, CT: Appleton & Lange, 1993.

NANN Practice Committee: *Infant Development Care Guidelines.* Petaluma, CA: National Association of Neonatal Nurses, 1993.

Neonatal Skin Care. OGN Nursing Practice Resource. NAACOG, January 1992.

Ogata ES: Carbohydrate homeostasis. In: *Neonatology: Pathophysiology and Management of the Newborn,* 4th ed. Avery GB, Fletcher M, MacDonald MG (editors). Philadelphia: Lippincott, 1994.

Ostrea EM: Infants of drug-dependent mothers. In: *Gellis & Kagan's Current Pediatric Therapy,* Vol 14. Burg FD, Ingelfinger JR, Wald ER (editors). Philadelphia: Saunders, 1993.

Ott WJ: Small for gestational age fetus and neonatal outcome: Reevaluation of the relationship. *Am J Perinatol* 1995; 12(6):396.

Paul KE: Recognition, stabilization and early management of infant with critical heart disease presenting in the first days of life. *Neonatal Network* 1995; 14(5):13.

Powell ML: *Assessment and Management of Developmental Changes and Problems in Children,* 2nd ed. St Louis: Mosby, 1981.

Pressler JL: Strategies useful in caring for macrosomic newborn. *J Pediatr Nurs* 1991; 6(3):149.

Resnik R: Post-term pregnancy. In: *Maternal Fetal Medicine: Principles and Practice,* 3rd ed. Creasy RK, Resnik R (editors). Philadelphia: Saunders, 1994.

Ryan RM et al: Meconium analysis for improved identification of infants exposed to cocaine in utero. *J Pediatr* 1994; 125(3):435.

Scherling D: Prenatal cocaine exposure and childhood psychopathology: A developmental analysis. *Am J Orthopsychiat* 1994; 64(1):9.

Scott GB, Parks WP: Pediatric AIDS. In: *Principles and Practice of Pediatrics,* 2nd ed. Oski FA et al (editors). Philadelphia: Lippincott, 1994.

Seashore MR, Rinaldo P: Metabolic disease of the neonate and young infant. *Semin Perinatol* 1993; 17(5):318.

Sherwen, LN: Human immunodeficiency virus infection during the perinatal period. *J Perinatol* 1995; 15(1):54.

Sinai LN et al: Phenylketonuria screening: Effects of early newborn discharge. *Pediatrics* 1995; 96(4):605.

Solnit A, Stark M: Mourning and the birth of a defective child. *Psychoanal Study Child* 1961; 16:505.

Spellacy WN: Postdate pregnancy. In: *Danforth's Obstetrics and Gynecology,* 7th ed. Scott JR et al (editors). Philadelphia: Lippincott, 1994.

Spinillo A et al: Maternal high-risk factors and severity of growth deficit in small for gestational age infants. *Early Hum Dev* 1994; 38:35.

Sudia Robinson TM: Discharge teaching in the NICU. *Neonatal Network* 1991; 10(4):77.

Sung I, Vohr B, Oh W: Growth and neurodevelopmental outcome of very low birth weight infants with intrauterine growth retardation. *J Pediatr* 1993; 123(4):618.

Tyrala EE: The infant of the diabetic mother. *Obstet Gynecol Clin North Am* 1996; 23(1):221.

Volpe JJ: *Neurology of the Newborn,* 3rd ed. Philadelphia: Saunders, 1995.

Warshaw JB: Infant of the diabetic mother. In: *Principles and Practice of Pediatrics,* 2nd ed. Oski FA et al (editors). Philadelphia: Lippincott, 1994.

Wekselman K et al: Fetal alcohol syndrome from infancy through childhood: A review of the literature. *J Pediatr Nurs* 1995; 10(5):296.

Wennberg RP et al: Fetal cocaine exposure and neonatal bilirubinemia. *J Pediatr* 1994;125(4):613.

Whitsett JA et al: Acute respiratory disorders. In: *Neonatology: Pathophysiology and Management of the Newborn,* 4th ed. Avery GB, Fletcher MA, MacDonald MG (editors). Philadelphia: Lippincott, 1994.

Witter FR: Perinatal mortality and intrauterine growth retardation. *Cur Op Obstet Gynecol* 1993; 5:56.

Wright L, Brown A, Davidson-Mundt A: Newborn screening: The miracle and the challenge. *J Pediatr Nurs* 1992; 17(1):26.

Wyse LJ, Jones M, Mandel F: Relationship of glycosylated hemoglobin, fetal macrosomia, and birthweight macrosomia. *J Perinatol* 1994; 11(4):260.

Chapter 26 The Newborn at Risk: Birth-Related Stressors

OBJECTIVES

- Discuss how to identify infants in need of resuscitation and the appropriate method of resuscitation based on the labor record and observable physiologic indicators.
- Differentiate the various types of respiratory distress (respiratory distress syndrome, transient tachypnea of the newborn, and meconium aspiration syndrome) in the newborn based on clinical manifestations.
- Identify the components of nursing care for a newborn with respiratory distress syndrome.
- Discuss selected metabolic abnormalities (including cold stress and hypoglycemia), their effects on the newborn, and the nursing implications.
- Differentiate between physiologic and pathologic jaundice based on onset, cause, possible sequelae, and specific management.
- Explain the set of circumstances that must be present for the development of erythroblastosis and ABO incompatibility.
- Summarize the nurse's role in the care of an infant with hemolytic disease.
- Identify nursing responsibilities in caring for the newborn receiving phototherapy or an exchange transfusion.
- Discuss selected hematologic problems such as anemia and polycythemia and the nursing implications associated with each problem.
- Describe the nursing assessment that would lead the nurse to suspect newborn sepsis.
- Relate the consequences of selected maternally transmitted infections such as maternal syphilis, gonorrhea, herpesvirus, or chlamydia, to the management of the infant in the neonatal period.

KEY TERMS

Cold stress
Erythroblastosis fetalis
Hemolytic disease of the newborn
Hydrops fetalis
Hyperbilirubinemia
Hypoglycemia
Jaundice
Kernicterus
Meconium aspiration syndrome (MAS)
Phototherapy
Physiologic anemia
Polycythemia
Respiratory distress syndrome (RDS)
Sepsis neonatorum

Marked homeostatic changes occur during the transition from fetal to neonatal life. The most rapid anatomic and physiologic changes of this period occur in the cardiopulmonary system. Problems frequently seen in the newborn include asphyxia, respiratory distress, cold stress, jaundice, hemolytic disease, and anemia. Ideally, problems are anticipated and identified prenatally, and appropriate intervention measures are begun at that time or immediately after birth. See Essential Precautions for Practice: At-Risk Newborns.

Care of the Newborn at Risk Due to Asphyxia

Neonatal asphyxia results in circulatory, respiratory, and biochemical changes.

Circulatory patterns that accompany asphyxia indicate an inability to make the transition to extrauterine circulation—in effect a return to fetal circulatory patterns. Failure of lung expansion and establishment of respiration rapidly produces hypoxia (decreased Pa_{O_2}), acidosis (decreased pH), and hypercarbia (increased P_{CO_2}). These biochemical changes cause pulmonary vasoconstriction with retention of high pulmonary vascular resistance, hypoperfusion of the lungs, and a large right-to-left shunt through the ductus arteriosus. The foramen ovale opens (as right atrial pressure exceeds left atrial pressure), and blood flows from right to left.

Biochemical changes that occur in asphyxia contribute to these circulatory changes. The most serious biochemical abnormality is a change from aerobic to anaerobic metabolism in the presence of hypoxia. This change results in the accumulation of lactates and the development of metabolic acidosis. Simultaneous respiratory acidosis may also occur due to a rapid increase in P_{CO_2} during asphyxia. In response to hypoxia and anaerobic metabolism, the amounts of free fatty acids (FFA) and glycerol in the blood increase. Glycogen stores are also mobilized to provide a continuous glucose source for the brain. Rapid use of hepatic and cardiac stores of glycogen may occur during an asphyxial attack.

The newborn is supplied with several protective mechanisms against hypoxial insults. These mechanisms include a relatively immature brain and a resting metabolic rate lower than that of adults, an ability to mobilize substances within the body for anaerobic metabolism and use the resulting energy more efficiently, and an intact circulatory system that is able to redistribute lactate and hydrogen ions in tissues still being perfused. Unfortunately, severe prolonged hypoxia will overcome these protective mechanisms, resulting in brain damage or death of the newborn.

The newborn who is apneic at birth requires immediate resuscitative efforts. The need for resuscitation can be anticipated if specific risk factors are present during the pregnancy or labor and birth period.

Risk Factors Predisposing to Asphyxia

The need for resuscitation may be anticipated if the mother demonstrates the antepartal and intrapartal risk factors described in Tables 7–1 and 16–1. Neonatal risk factors for resuscitation are

- Nonreassuring fetal heart rate pattern
- Difficult birth
- Fetal blood loss
- Apneic episode unresponsive to tactile stimulation
- Inadequate ventilation
- Prematurity
- Structural lung abnormality (congenital diaphragmatic hernia, lung hypoplasia)
- Cardiac arrest

ESSENTIAL PRECAUTIONS FOR PRACTICE

At-Risk Newborns

Examples of times when disposable gloves should be worn include the following:

- Handling baby prior to first bath when all blood and amniotic fluid has been removed
- Suctioning oral and nasal secretions
- During resuscitation, with use of bag and mask ventilation
- Administering vitamin K injection, eye prophylaxis, and cord care
- Carrying out routine heel stick blood work (ie, glucose, hematocrit)
- Inserting umbilical catheter lines—umbilical artery (UAC) and umbilical vein (UVC)—and any other invasive lines
- Flushing and blood drawing from umbilical catheter lines (UAC, UVC)

All invasive procedures require sterile gloves and should be carried out over thoroughly cleansed areas of skin. At times, goggles and protective gowns or aprons may be required.

REMEMBER to wash your hands before putting on the disposable gloves and AGAIN immediately after you remove the gloves.

For further information, consult OSHA and CDC guidelines.

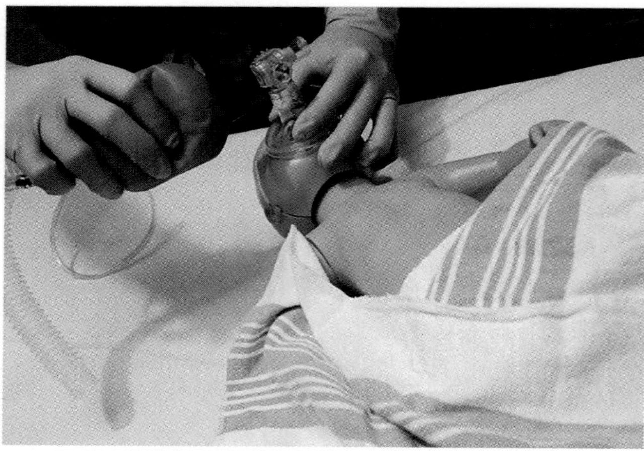

FIGURE 26–1 Demonstration of resuscitation of an infant with bag and mask. Note that the mask covers the nose and mouth, and the head is in a neutral position. The resuscitating bag is placed to the side of the baby so that chest movement can be seen.

At times no risk factors may be apparent prenatally. Particular attention must be paid to all at-risk pregnancies during the intrapartal period. Certain aspects of labor and birth challenge the oxygen supply to the fetus, and often the at-risk fetus has less tolerance to the stress of labor and birth.

Medical Therapy

The initial goal of medical management is to identify the fetus at risk for asphyxia, so that resuscitative efforts can begin at birth.

Fetal biophysical assessment (see Chapter 14), monitoring fetal and maternal pH and blood gases and fetal heart rate, during the intrapartal period may help identify fetal distress. If fetal distress is present, appropriate measures can be taken to deliver the fetus immediately, before major damage occurs, and to treat the asphyxiated newborn.

The fetal biophysical profile improves the ability to predict an abnormal perinatal outcome. In addition, fetal scalp blood sampling may indicate asphyxic insult and the degree of fetal acidosis, when considered in relation to the stage of labor, uterine contractions, and nonreassuring fetal heart rate (FHR) patterns. The test is done by using a microscalpel, collecting blood in a capillary tube, and analyzing it for pH values. Normal fetal pH ranges from 7.3 to 7.35. The pH falls gradually during the first stage of labor, and continues to decrease during second stage and birth. The stress of labor causes an intermittent decrease in exchange of gases in the placental intervillous space, which causes the fall in pH and fetal acidosis. The acidosis is primarily metabolic.

During labor, a fetal pH of 7.25 or higher is considered normal. A pH value of 7.20 or less is considered an ominous sign of fetal asphyxia (Jepson et al 1991). However, low fetal pH without associated hypoxia can be caused by maternal acidosis secondary to prolonged labor, dehydration, and maternal lactate production.

The treatment of fetal or newborn asphyxia is resuscitation. The goal of resuscitation is to provide an adequate airway with expansion of the lungs, to decrease the P_{CO_2} and increase the P_{O_2}, to support adequate cardiac output, and to minimize oxygen consumption by reducing heat loss.

Initial resuscitative management of the newborn is extremely important. Caregivers should keep the infant in a head-down position before the first gasp to avoid aspiration of the oropharyngeal secretions and must suction the oropharynx and nasopharynx immediately. Clearing the nasal and oral passages of fluid that may obstruct the airway establishes a patent airway. Suction is always performed before resuscitation so that the infant doesn't aspirate mucus, blood, and meconium.

After the first few breaths, the nurse places the newborn in a level position under a radiant heat source and dries the baby quickly with towels to maintain skin temperature at about 36.5C (97.7F). Drying is also a good stimulation to breathing. Heat loss through evaporation is tremendous during the first few minutes of life. The temperature of a wet 1500 g baby in a 16C (62F) birthing room drops 1C every 3 minutes. Hypothermia increases oxygen consumption. In an asphyxiated infant, it increases the hypoxic insult, and may lead to severe acidosis and development of respiratory distress.

Assessment of the newborn's need for resuscitation begins at the time of birth. The nurse should note the time of the first gasp, first cry, and onset of sustained respirations in the order of occurrence.

Breathing is established by employing the simplest form of resuscitative measures initially, with progression to more complicated methods as required. For example

1. Simple stimulation is provided by rubbing the back or flicking the feet.
2. If respirations have not been initiated or are inadequate (gasping or occasional respirations), the lungs must be inflated with positive pressure. The mask is positioned securely on the face (over nose and mouth, avoiding the eyes) with the infant's head in "sniffing" or neutral position (Figure 26–1). Hyperextension of the infant's neck will obstruct the trachea. An airtight connection is made between the baby's face and the mask (thus allowing the bag to inflate). The lungs are inflated rhythmically by squeezing the bag. Oxygen can be delivered at 100 percent with an anesthesia or Laerdal bag with manometer and adequate liter flow. The self-inflating bag delivers only 40 percent oxygen unless it

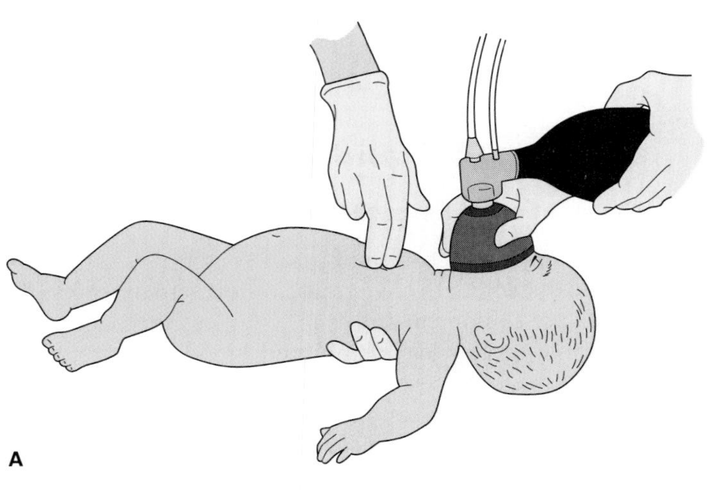

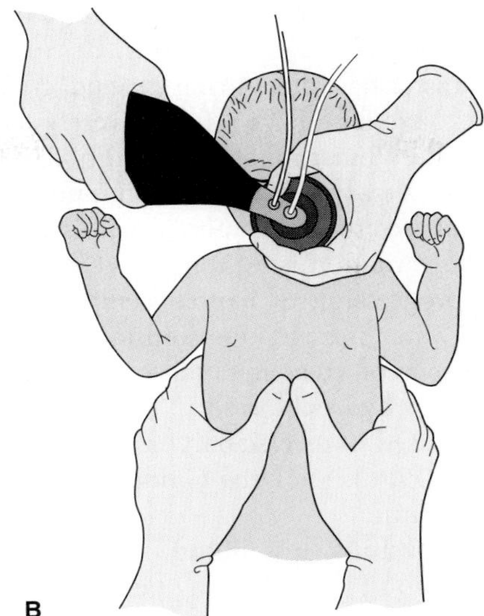

FIGURE 26–2 External cardiac massage. The lower third of the sternum is compressed with two fingertips or thumbs at a rate of 90 beats/minute. ***A*** The two-fingers method uses the tips of two fingers of one hand to compress the sternum and the other hand or a firm surface to support the infant's back. ***B*** The thumb method uses the fingers to support the infant's back and uses both thumbs to compress the sternum.

has been adapted with oxygen reservoirs so it can deliver 90–100 percent oxygen. In a crisis situation it is crucial that 100 percent oxygen be delivered with adequate pressure.

3. The rise and fall of the chest is observed for proper ventilation. Air entry and heart rate are checked by auscultation. Manual resuscitation is coordinated with any voluntary efforts. The rate of ventilation should be between 40 and 60 breaths per minute. Pressure should be adequate to move the chest wall. The pressure gauge (manometer) must be in place to avoid overdistention of the newborn's lungs and other problems such as pneumothorax or abdominal distention. In newborns with normal lungs, 15–25 cm H_2O may be adequate. If the newborn has lung disease, 20–40 cm H_2O may be necessary. If the newborn has not taken a first breath after birth, pressures of 30–40 cm H_2O may be transiently required to expand collapsed alveoli. If ventilation is adequate, the chest moves with each inspiration, bilateral breath sounds are audible, and the lips and mucous membranes become pink. If color and heart rate fail to respond to ventilatory efforts, poor or improper placement of an endotracheal tube may be the cause. If the baby is intubated properly, pneumothorax, diaphragmatic hernia, or hypoplastic lungs (Potter's syndrome) may exist. Distention of the stomach is controlled by inserting a nasogastric tube for decompression.
4. Endotracheal intubation may be needed. However, most newborns, except for very-low-birth-weight (VLBW) infants, can be resuscitated by bag and mask ventilation.

Once breathing has been established, the heart rate should increase to over 100 beats per minute. If the heart rate is less than 60 beats per minute or between 60 and 80 beats per minute and is not increasing despite 15–30 seconds of ventilation with 100 percent oxygen, external cardiac massage (chest compression) is begun. Chest compressions are started immediately if there is no detectable heartbeat.

1. The infant is positioned properly on a firm surface.
2. The resuscitator may use the two-finger method (Figure 26–2) or may stand at the foot of the infant and place both thumbs over the lower third of the sternum, (just below an imaginary line drawn between the nipples) with the fingers wrapped around and supporting the back.
3. The sternum is depressed approximately two-thirds of the distance to the vertebral column (1–2 cm or ½ to ¾ in) at a rate of 90 compressions per minute (Bloom and Cropley 1994).

Drugs that should be available in the birthing area include those needed in the treatment of shock, cardiac arrest, and narcosis. Oxygen, because of its effective use in ventilation, is the drug most often used.

If, after 30 seconds of ventilation and cardiac compression, the newborn has not responded with spontaneous respirations and a heart rate above 80 beats per minute, it is necessary to administer resuscitative medications. The most accessible route for administering medications is the umbilical vein. If bradycardia is present, epinephrine (0.1–0.3 mL/kg of a 1:10,000 solution) is given through the umbilical vein catheter, the peripheral IV, or the endotracheal tube (if an IV has not yet been started). Give 2 to 3 times the IV dose of epinephrine followed immediately by 1 mL of normal saline when administering epinephrine by endotracheal tube (Young and Mangum 1996). In a severely asphyxiated newborn, sodium bicarbonate (1–2 mEq/kg of 4.2% solution) is given slowly over at least 2 minutes, at a rate of 1 mEq/kg/min, to correct metabolic acidosis, but only after effective ventilation is established. Dextrose is given to prevent progression of hypoglycemia. A 10 percent dextrose in water intravenous solution is usually sufficient to prevent or treat hypoglycemia in the birthing area. Naloxone hydrochloride (0.1 mg/kg), a narcotic antagonist, is used to reverse narcotic depression (Young and Mangum 1996). See Drug Guide: Naloxone Hydrochloride (Narcan).

If shock develops (low blood pressure or poor peripheral perfusion), the baby may be given a volume expander such as 5 percent albumin or lactated Ringer's in a dose of 10 mL/kg. Whole blood, fresh frozen plasma, plasminate, and packed red blood cells can also be used for volume expansion and treatment of shock. In some instances of prolonged resuscitation associated with shock and poor response to resuscitation, dopamine (5 μg/kg/minute) may be necessary (Osborne and Kassity 1993).

APPLYING THE NURSING PROCESS

Nursing Assessment

Communication between the physician's office or clinic and the birthing area nurse facilitates the identification of potential newborns in need of resuscitation. When the woman arrives in the birthing area, the nurse should have the antepartal record and should note any contributory perinatal history factors and assess present fetal status. As labor progresses, nursing assessments include ongoing monitoring of FHR and fetal heart rate response to contractions, assisting with fetal scalp blood sampling, and observing for the presence of meconium in the amniotic fluid to assess for fetal asphyxia. In addition, the nurse should alert the resuscitation team and the practitioner responsible for care of the newborn of any potential high-risk laboring women.

Nursing Diagnosis

Nursing diagnoses that may apply to the newborn with asphyxia include the following:

- Ineffective breathing pattern related to lack of spontaneous respirations at birth secondary to in utero asphyxia
- Decreased cardiac output related to impaired oxygenation
- Ineffective family coping related to baby's lack of spontaneous respirations at birth and fear of losing their newborn

Nursing Plan and Implementation

Preparation of Resuscitation Equipment

Following identification of possible high-risk situations, the next step in effective resuscitation is to assemble the necessary equipment and ensure proper functioning. It is desirable to provide for pH and blood gas determination as well. Necessary equipment includes a radiant warmer that provides an overhead radiant heat source (a thermostatic mechanism that is taped to the infant's abdomen triggers the radiant warmer to turn on or off to maintain a level of thermoneutrality), and an open bed for easy access to the newborn. It is essential that the nurse keep the newborn warm. To do so the nurse dries the newborn quickly with warmed towels or blankets to prevent evaporative heat loss and places him or her under the radiant warmer with the servocontrol set at 36.5C.

Resuscitative equipment in the birthing room must be sterilized after each use. In the high-risk nursery the need for resuscitation may occur at any time. Equipment reliability must be maintained at all times. The nurse inspects all equipment—bag and mask, oxygen and flow meter, laryngoscope, and suction machines—for damaged or nonfunctioning parts before a birth or when setting up an admission bed. A systematic check of the emergency cart and equipment is a routine responsibility of each shift.

Provision and Documentation of Resuscitation

Training and knowledge about resuscitation are vital to personnel in the birth setting for both normal and high-risk births. Since resuscitation is at least a two-person effort, the nurse should call for assistance so that there is adequate staff available. The resuscitative efforts should be recorded on the newborn's chart so that all members of the health care team will have access to the information.

Parent Education

Birthing room resuscitation is particularly distressing for the parents. If the need for resuscitation is anticipated, the parents should be assured that a team will be present at the birth to care specifically for their newborn. As soon as the infant is stable, a member of the interdisciplinary team should discuss the newborn's condition with the parents. The parents may have many fears about the reasons for resuscitation and the condition of their baby after resuscitation.

DRUG GUIDE Naloxone Hydrochloride (Narcan)

Overview of Neonatal Action

Naloxone hydrochloride (Narcan) is used to reverse respiratory depression due to acute narcotic toxicity. It displaces morphinelike drugs from receptor sites on the neurons; therefore the narcotics can no longer exert their depressive effects. Naloxone reverses narcotic-induced respiratory depression, analgesia, sedation, hypotension, and pupillary constriction.

Route, Dosage, Frequency

Intravenous dose is 0.1 to 0.2 mg/kg (0.25 to 0.5 mL/kg of 0.4 mg/mL) concentration at birth, including premature infants. This drug is usually given through the umbilical vein or endotracheal tube, although naloxone can be given intramuscularly or subcutaneously. The use of neonatal naloxone (Narcan 0.02 mg/mL) is no longer recommended by the American Academy of Pediatrics Committee on Drugs because of the extremely large fluid volumes.

Reversal of drug depression occurs within 1 to 2 minutes after IV administration. The duration of action is variable (minutes to hours) and depends on the amount of the drug present and the rate of excretion. Dose may be repeated in 3–5 minutes. If there is no improvement after two or three doses, discontinue naloxone administration. If initial reversal occurs, repeat dose as needed.

Neonatal Contraindications

Should not be administered to infants of narcotic-addicted mothers because it may precipitate acute withdrawal syndrome (increased HR and BP, vomiting, tremors).

Respiratory depression resulting from nonmorphine drugs such as sedatives, hypnotics, anesthetics, or other nonnarcotic CNS depressants.

Neonatal Side Effects

Excessive doses may result in irritability, increased crying, and possible prolongation of partial thromboplastin time (PTT).

Tachycardia.

Nursing Considerations

Monitor respirations closely—rate and depth.

Assess for return of respiratory depression when naloxone effects wear off and effects of longer-acting narcotics reappear.

Have resuscitative equipment, O_2, and ventilatory equipment available.

Monitor bleeding studies.

Note that naloxone is incompatible with alkaline solutions.

Store at room temperature and protect from light.

Compatible with heparin.

Evaluation

Anticipated outcomes of nursing care include

- The risk of asphyxia is promptly identified, and intervention is started early.
- The newborn's metabolic and physiologic processes are stabilized, and recovery is proceeding without complications.
- The parents can verbalize the reason for resuscitation and what was done to resuscitate their newborn.
- The parents can verbalize their fears about the resuscitation process and potential implications for their baby's future.

Care of the Newborn with Respiratory Distress

One of the severest conditions to which the newborn may fall victim is respiratory distress—an inappropriate respiratory adaptation to extrauterine life. The nursing care of a baby with respiratory distress requires understanding of the normal pulmonary and circulatory physiology (Chapter 21), the pathophysiology of the disease process, clinical manifestations, and supportive and corrective therapies. Only with this knowledge can the nurse make appropriate observations about responses to therapy and development of complications. Unlike the verbalizing adult client, the newborn communicates needs only by behavior. The neonatal nurse interprets this behavior as clues about the individual baby's condition.

Idiopathic Respiratory Distress Syndrome (Hyaline Membrane Disease)

Respiratory distress syndrome (RDS), also referred to as *hyaline membrane disease* (HMD), is a complex disease that affects approximately 40,000 infants a year in the United States; these are primarily preterm infants (Nugent 1991). RDS accounts for approximately 7000 deaths per year in the United States alone or 20 percent of all newborn deaths (Glomella 1994). The syndrome occurs more frequently in premature white infants than in black infants and almost twice as often in males as in females.

The factors precipitating the pathologic changes of RDS have not been determined, but two main factors are associated with its development:

1. *Prematurity.* All preterm newborns—whether AGA, SGA, or LGA—and especially IDMs are at risk for RDS. The incidence of RDS increases with the degree of prematurity, with most deaths occurring in newborns weighing less than 1500 g. The maternal

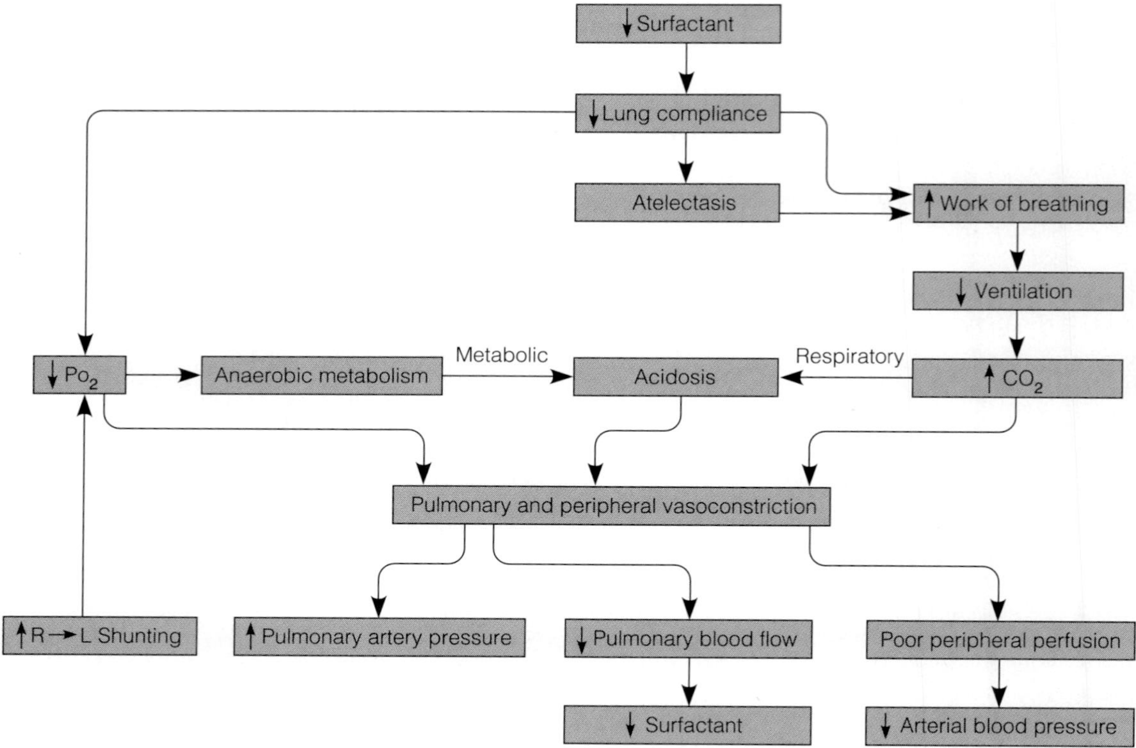

FIGURE 26–3 Cycle of events of RDS leading to eventual respiratory failure.
Source: Modified from Gluck L, Kulovich MV: Fetal lung development. *Pediatr Clin North Am* 1973; 20:375.

and fetal factors resulting in preterm labor and birth, complications of pregnancy, cesarean birth (indications for), and familial tendency are all associated with RDS.

2. *Surfactant deficiency disease.* Normal pulmonary adaptation requires adequate surfactant, a lipoprotein that coats the inner surface of the alveoli. Surfactant provides alveolar stability by decreasing the alveoli's surface tension and tendency to collapse. In the normal or mature newborn lung, it is continuously synthesized, oxidized during breathing, and replenished. Adequate surfactant levels lead to better lung compliance and permit breathing with less work. Respiratory distress syndrome is due to alterations in surfactant quantity, composition, function, or production (Verma 1995).

Development of RDS indicates a failure to synthesize surfactant, which is required to maintain alveolar stability (see Chapter 21). Upon expiration this instability increases atelectasis, which causes hypoxia and acidosis because of the lack of gas exchange. These conditions further inhibit surfactant production and cause pulmonary vasoconstriction. The resulting lung instability causes the biochemical problems of hypoxemia (decreased Po_2), hypercarbia (increased Pco_2), and acidemia (decreased pH) primarily metabolic, which further increases pulmonary vasoconstriction and hypoperfusion. The cycle of events of RDS leading to eventual respiratory failure is diagrammed in Figure 26–3.

Because of these pathophysiologic conditions, the newborn must expend increasing amounts of energy to reopen the collapsed alveoli with every breath, so that each breath becomes as difficult as the first. The progressive expiratory atelectasis upsets the physiologic homeostasis of the pulmonary and cardiovascular systems and prevents adequate gas exchange. Lung compliance decreases, which accounts for the difficulty of inflation, labored respirations, and increased work of breathing.

The physiologic alterations of RDS produce the following complications:

1. *Hypoxia.* As a result of hypoxia, the pulmonary vasculature constricts, pulmonary vascular resistance increases, and pulmonary blood flow is reduced. Increased pulmonary vascular resistance may precipitate a return to fetal circulation as the ductus opens and blood flow is shunted around the lungs. This increases the hypoxia and further decreases pulmonary perfusion. Hypoxia also causes impairment or absence of metabolic response to cold, reversion to anaerobic metabolism resulting in lactate accumulation (acidosis), and impaired cardiac output, which decreases perfusion to vital organs.

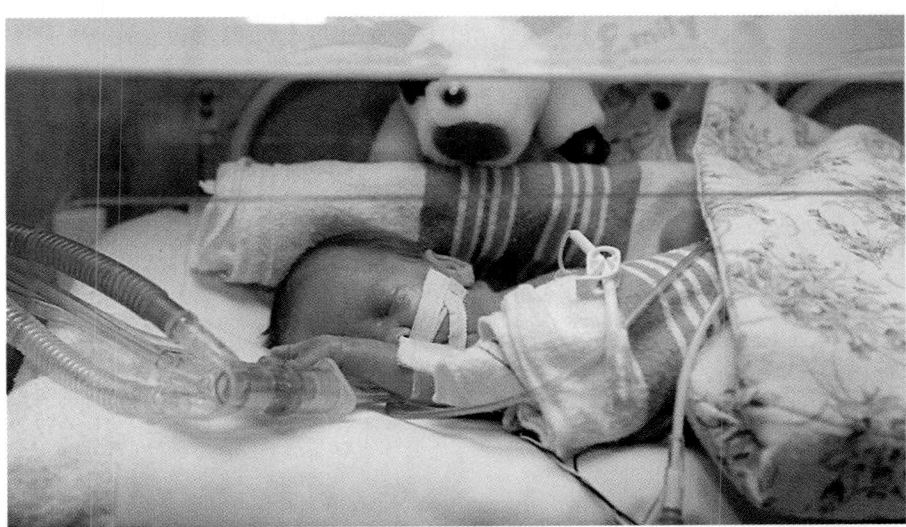

FIGURE 26–4 Infant on a mechanical ventilator.

2. *Respiratory acidosis.* Increased PCO_2 and decreased pH are results of alveolar hypoventilation, whereas persistently rising PCO_2 and decrease in pH are poor prognostic signs of pulmonary function and adequacy.
3. *Metabolic acidosis.* Because of the lack of oxygen at the cellular level, the newborn begins an anaerobic pathway of metabolism, with an increase in lactate levels and a resulting base deficit (loss of bicarbonate). As the lactate levels increase, the pH becomes acidotic (decreased pH), and the buffer base decreases in an attempt to compensate and maintain acid-base homeostasis.

The classic radiologic picture of RDS is diffuse reticulogranular density that occurs bilaterally, with portions of the air-filled tracheobronchial tree (air bronchogram) outlined by the opaque ("white-out") lungs and widespread atelectasis (Hicks 1995). The progression of x-ray findings parallels the pattern of resolution, which usually occurs in 4 to 7 days, and the time of surfactant reappearance, unless surfactant replacement therapy has been used. Echocardiography is a valuable tool in diagnosing vascular shunts that move blood either away from or toward the lungs.

Medical Therapy

The primary goal of prenatal management is the prevention of preterm birth through aggressive treatment of preterm labor and possible administration of glucocorticoids to enhance fetal lung development (see Chapter 13). The goals of postnatal therapy are maintenance of adequate oxygenation and ventilation, correction of acid-base abnormalities, and provision of the supportive care required to maintain homeostasis.

Supportive medical management consists of ventilation therapy, transcutaneous oxygen and carbon dioxide monitoring or pulse oximetry correction of acid-base imbalance, environmental temperature regulation, adequate nutrition, and protection from infection. Ventilation therapy is directed toward prevention of hypoventilation and hypoxia. Mild cases of RDS may require only increased humidified oxygen concentrations. Use of continuous positive airway pressure (CPAP) may be required in moderately afflicted infants. Babies with severe RDS require mechanical ventilation, with positive end-expiratory pressure (PEEP) (Figure 26–4). Surfactant replacement therapy is now available for infants to decrease the severity of RDS in low-birth-weight newborns (Verma 1995). Extracorporeal membrane oxygenation (ECMO) and high-frequency ventilation have been tried in cases where conventional ventilator therapy has not been successful (Verma 1995).

APPLYING THE NURSING PROCESS

Nursing Assessment

Increasing cyanosis, tachypnea, grunting respirations, nasal flaring, and significant retractions are characteristics of the disease. Table 26–1 reviews clinical findings associated with respiratory distress. The Silverman-Andersen index (Figure 26–5) may be helpful in evaluating the signs of respiratory distress used in the birthing area.

In babies with respiratory distress syndrome who are on ventilators, increased urination (determined by weighing diapers) may be an early clue that the baby's

TABLE 26–1 Clinical Assessments Associated with Respiratory Distress

Clinical Picture	Significance
Skin Color	
Pallor or mottling	These represent poor peripheral circulation due to systemic hypotension and vasoconstriction and pooling of independent areas (usually in conjunction with severe hypoxia).
Cyanosis (bluish tint)	Depending on hemoglobin concentration, peripheral circulation, intensity and quality of viewing light, and acuity of observer's color vision, this is frankly visible in advanced hypoxia. Central cyanosis is most easily detected by examination of mucous membranes and tongue.
Jaundice (yellow discoloration of skin and mucous membranes due to presence of unconjugated [indirect] bilirubin)	Metabolic alterations (acidosis, hypercarbia, asphyxia) of respiratory distress predispose to dissociation of bilirubin from albumin-binding sites and deposition in the skin and central nervous system.
Edema (presents as slick, shiny skin)	This is characteristic of preterm infants because of low total protein concentration with decrease in colloidal osmotic pressure and transudation of fluid. Edema of hands and feet is frequently seen within first 24 hours and resolved by fifth day in infants with severe RDS.
Respiratory System	
Tachypnea (normal respiratory rate 30–60/minute, elevated respiratory rate 60+/minute)	Increased respiratory rate is the most frequent and easily detectable sign of respiratory distress after birth. This compensatory mechanism attempts to increase respiratory dead space to maintain alveolar ventilation and gas exchange in the face of an increase in mechanical resistance. As a decompensatory mechanism it increases work load and energy output by increasing respiratory rate, which causes increased metabolic demand for oxygen and thus increases alveolar ventilation of an already overstressed system. During shallow, rapid respirations, there is an increase in dead space ventilation, thus decreasing alveolar ventilation.
Apnea (episode of nonbreathing for more than 20 seconds; periodic breathing, a common "normal" occurrence in preterm infants, is defined as apnea of 5–10 seconds alternating with 10–15 seconds of ventilation)	This poor prognostic sign indicates cardiorespiratory disease, CNS disease, metabolic alterations, intracranial hemorrhage, sepsis, or immaturity. Physiologic alterations include decreased oxygen saturation, respiratory acidosis, and bradycardia.
Chest	Inspection of the thoracic cage includes shape, size, and symmetry of movement. Respiratory movements should be symmetrical and diaphragmatic; asymmetry reflects pathology (pneumothorax, diaphragmatic hernia). Increased anteroposterior diameter indicates air trapping (meconium aspiration syndrome).
Labored respirations (Silverman-Anderson chart in Figure 26–5 indicates severity of retractions, grunting, and nasal flaring, which are signs of labored respirations)	Indicates marked increase in the work of breathing.
Retractions (inward pulling of soft parts of the chest cage—suprasternal, substernal, intercostal, subcostal—at inspiration)	These reflect the significant increase in negative intrathoracic pressure necessary to inflate stiff, noncompliant lungs. Infants attempt to increase lung compliance by using accessory muscles. Lung expansion markedly decreases. Seesaw respirations are seen when the chest flattens with inspiration and the abdomen bulges. Retractions increase the work of breathing and O_2 need so that assisted ventilation may be necessary due to exhaustion.
Flaring nares (inspiratory dilation of nostrils)	This compensatory mechanism attempts to lessen the resistance of the narrow nasal passage.
Expiratory grunt (Valsalva maneuver in which the infant exhales against a closed glottis, thus producing an audible moan)	This increases transpulmonary pressure, which decreases or prevents atelectasis, thus improving oxygenation and alveolar ventilation. Intubation should not be attempted unless the infant's condition is rapidly deteriorating, because it prevents this maneuver and allows the alveoli to collapse (Lapido 1989).
Rhythmic body movement with labored respirations (chin tug, head bobbing, retractions of anal area)	This is a result of using abdominal and other respiratory accessory muscles during prolonged forced respirations.
Auscultation of chest reveals decreased air exchange with harsh breath sounds or fine inspiratory rales; rhonchi may be present	Decrease in breath sounds and distant quality may indicate interstitial or intrapleural air or fluid.
Cardiovascular System	
Continuous systolic murmur may be audible	Patent ductus arteriosus is a common occurrence with hypoxia, pulmonary vasoconstriction, right-to-left shunting, and congestive heart failure.
Heart rate usually within normal limits (fixed heart rate may occur with a rate of 110–120/minute)	A fixed heart rate indicates a decrease in vagal control.
Point of maximal impulse usually located at fourth to fifth intercostal space, left sternal border	Displacement may reflect dextrocardia, pneumothorax, or diaphragmatic hernia.
Hypothermia	This is inadequate functioning of metabolic processes that require oxygen to produce necessary body heat.
Muscle Tone	
Flaccid, hypotonic, unresponsive to stimuli	These may indicate deterioration in the newborn's condition and possible CNS damage due to hypoxia, acidemia, or hemorrhage.
Hypertonia and/or seizure activity	

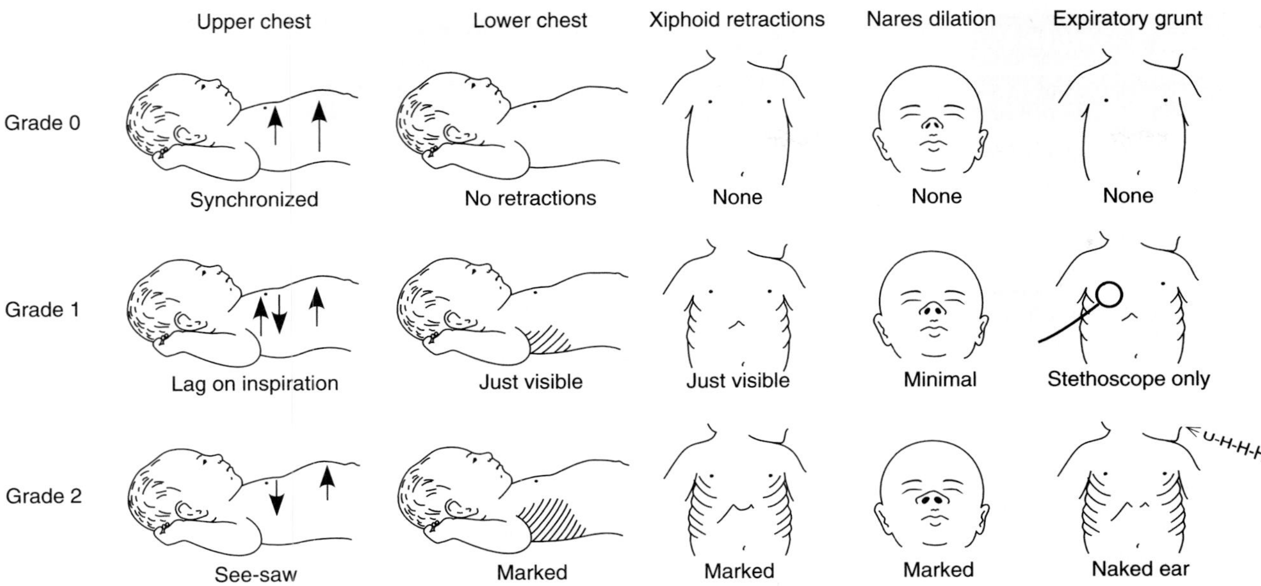

FIGURE 26–5 Evaluation of respiratory status using the Silverman-Andersen index. The baby's respiratory status is assessed. A grade of 0, 1, or 2 is determined for each area, and a total score is charted in the baby's record or on a copy of this tool and placed in the chart.

Source: Ross Laboratories, Nursing Aid No. 2. Columbus, OH: Silverman WA, Andersen DH: *Pediatrics* 1956; 17:1. Copyright 1956, American Academy of Pediatrics.

condition is improving. As fluid moves out of the lungs into the bloodstream, alveoli open, and kidney perfusion increases, which results in increased voiding. At this point the nurse must monitor chest expansion closely. If chest expansion is increasing, ventilator settings may have to be decreased. Too high a ventilator setting may "blow the lungs," resulting in pneumothorax.

Nursing Diagnosis

Nursing diagnoses that may apply to the newborn with respiratory distress syndrome include the following:

- Impaired gas exchange related to inadequate lung surfactant
- Altered nutrition: less than body requirements related to increased metabolic needs of stressed infant
- Risk for infection related to invasive procedures

Nursing Plan and Implementation

Based on clinical parameters, the neonatal nurse implements therapeutic approaches to maintain physiologic homeostasis and provides supportive care to the newborn with RDS. See Critical Pathway for Care of Newborn with Respiratory Distress (p 683).

Nursing interventions and criteria for instituting mechanical ventilation are done according to institutional protocol. Methods of oxygen monitoring and nursing interventions are included in Table 26–2. The nursing care of infants on ventilators or with umbilical artery catheters will not be discussed here. These infants have severe respiratory distress and are cared for in intensive care nurseries by nurses with advanced knowledge and training.

Evaluation

Anticipated outcomes of nursing care include

- The risk of RDS is promptly identified and early intervention is initiated.
- The newborn is free of respiratory distress and metabolic alterations.
- The parents verbalize their concerns about their baby's health problem and survival and understand the rationale behind the management of their newborn.

Transient Tachypnea of the Newborn

Some newborns, primarily AGA preterm and near-term infants, develop progressive respiratory distress that resembles classic RDS. These infants have usually had some intrauterine or intrapartal asphyxia caused by maternal oversedation, cesarean birth, maternal bleeding,

TABLE 26–2 Oxygen Monitors

Type	Function and Rationale	Nursing Interventions
Transcutaneous Oxygen Monitor—$TcPo_2$		
Measures oxygen diffusion across the skin Clark electrode is heated to 43C (preterm) or 44C (term) to warm the skin beneath the electrode and promote diffusion of oxygen across the skin surface. Po_2 is measured when oxygen diffuses across the capillary membrane, skin, and electrode membrane (Poets and Southall 1994).	When transcutaneous monitors are properly calibrated and electrodes are appropriately positioned, they will provide reliable, continuous, noninvasive measurements of Po_2, Pco_2, and oxygen saturation. Readings vary when skin perfusion is decreased. Reliable as trend monitor. Frequent calibration necessary to overcome mechanical drift. Following membrane change, machine must "warm up" 1 hour prior to initial calibration; otherwise, after turning it on, it must equilibrate for 30 minutes prior to calibration. When placed on infant, values will be low until skin is heated; approximately 15 minutes required to stabilize.	Use $TcPo_2$ to monitor trends of oxygenation with routine nursing care procedures. Clean electrode surface to remove electrolyte deposits; change solution and membrane once a week. Allow machine to stabilize before drawing arterial gases; note reading when gases are drawn, and use values to correlate. Ensure airtight seal between skin surface and electrode; place electrodes on clean, dry skin on upper chest, abdomen, or inner aspect of thigh; avoid bony prominences.
	Second-degree burns are rare but can occur if electrodes remain in place too long. Decreased correlations noted with older infants (related to skin thickness); with infants with low cardiac output (decreased skin perfusion); and with hyperoxic infants.	Change skin site and recalibrate at least every 4 hours; inspect skin for burns; if burns occur, use lowest temperature setting and change position of electrode more frequently.
	The adhesive that attaches the electrode may abrade the fragile skin of the preterm infant. May be used for both pre- and postductal monitoring of oxygenation for observations of shunting.	Adhesive disks may be cut to a smaller size, or skin prep may be used under the adhesive circle only; allow membrane to touch skin surface at center.
Pulse Oximetry—SaO_2		
Monitors beat-to-beat arterial oxygen saturation. Microprocessor measures saturation by the absorption of red and infrared light as it passes through tissue. Changes in absorption related to blood pulsation through vessel determine saturation and pulse rate (Poets and Southall 1994).	Calibration is automatic. Less dependent on perfusion than $TcPo_2$ and $TcPco_2$; however, functions poorly if peripheral perfusion is decreased due to low cardiac output. Much more rapid response time than $TcPo_2$—offers "real-time" readings. Can be located on extremity, digit, or palm of hand, leaving chest free; not affected by skin characteristics. Requires understanding of oxyhemoglobin dissociation curve. Pulse oximeter reading of 85% to 90% reflects clinically safe range of saturation. Extreme sensitivity to movement; decreases if average of 7th or 14th beat is selected rather than beat to beat. Poor correlation with extreme hyperoxia.	Understand and use oxyhemoglobin dissociation curve. Monitor trends over time and correlate with arterial blood gases (Hanna 1995). Check disposable sensor at least q8h. Use disposable cuffs (reusable cuffs allow too much ambient light to enter, and readings may be inaccurate).

prolapsed cord, breech birth, or maternal diabetes. The resultant effect on the newborn is failure to clear the airway of lung fluid, mucus, and other debris, or an excess of fluid in the lungs due to aspiration of amniotic or tracheal fluid.

Usually the newborn experiences little or no difficulty at the onset of breathing. However, shortly after birth, expiratory grunting, flaring of the nares, and mild cyanosis may be noted in the newborn breathing room air. Tachypnea is usually present by 6 hours of age, with respiratory rates as high as 100–140 breaths per minute.

Medical Therapy

The goal of medical management is to identify the type of respiratory distress present and to start treatment.

Initial x-ray findings may be identical to those showing RDS within the first 3 hours. However, radiographs of infants with transient tachypnea usually reveal a generalized overexpansion of the lungs (hyperaeration of alveoli), which is identified principally by flattened contours of the diaphragm. Dense perihilar streaks (increased vascularity) radiate from the hilar region and represent engorgement of the lymphatics, which clear alveolar fluid upon initiation of air breathing.

Text continues on page 686

CRITICAL PATHWAY FOR CARE OF NEWBORN WITH RESPIRATORY DISTRESS

Category	Day of Birth–1st 4 Hours	Remaining Day of Birth
Referral	• Report from L&D, Neonatal Nurse Practitioner • Check ID bands →	• Check ID bands q shift →

Assessment	• Assess development of signs of distress, such as:
	  • Initially tachypnea (>60 respirations/min)
	  • Expiratory grunting (audible) or subcostal/intercostal retractions, followed by flaring of nares on inspiration
	  • Cyanosis and pallor
	  • Signs of increased air hunger (apneic spells, hypotonus), rhythmic movement of body and labored respirations, and chin tug
	  • Arterial blood gases (indicating respiratory failure): $Pa{O_2}$ less than 50 mm Hg, and $P{CO_2}$ above 60 mm Hg
	• Auscultation:
	  • Initially breath sounds may be normal; then decreased air exchange occurs with harsh breath sounds and, upon deep inspiration, rales
	  • Later a low-pitched systolic murmur indicates patent ductus arteriosus
	• Determine baseline of respiratory effort and ventilatory adequacy:
	  • Observe chest wall movement
	  • Assess skin, mucous membranes for color
	  • Estimate degree and equality of air entry by auscultation
	  • Assess arterial blood gases and pH
	• Increasing O_2 concentration requirements to maintain adequate $P{O_2}$ levels
	• VS: temp (ax), pulse, resp →
	• Admission wt, length, head circumference →
	• Check color and perfusion of skin
	• Gestational age assessment (preterm birth)
	• Gestational history: including recent episodes of fetal or intrapartal stress (maternal hypotension, bleeding, maternal and resultant fetal oversedation), or severe fetal lung circulation compromise
	• Lung profile to determine lung maturity is done on amniotic fluid
	• Newborn history, including birth asphyxia resulting in acute hypoxia,hypothermia, low Apgar score, and bag and mask resuscitation in birthing area
	• Monitor activity →
		• Assess color, respiratory status, mother/baby interaction
		• Observe infant for temperature instability and signs of increased oxygen consumption and metabolic acidosis

Comfort	• Provide minimal stimulation/handling • Sedation as warranted	• Provide minimal stimulation/handling • Sedation as warranted
Nursing interventions and report	• Admission/activities performed with parents present if possible • Blood type, Rh, Coombs on cord blood when applicable • Chemstrip for hypoglycemia • Hep B form reviewed and/or signed • Peripheral hematocrit and blood cultures per protocol • Monitor electrolytes and blood gases as needed → • Administer antibiotics as ordered and monitor drug levels → • Provide for infection control by cleaning and replacing nebulizers/humidifiers at least q24h → • Use sterile tubing and replace q24h → • Use sterile distilled water • Manage route of IV administration	• Check for Baer test results • VS q4h: T/P/R • Daily wt → • Check color q shift → • Alcohol cord q shift
Activity	• Change position prn →	

CRITICAL PATHWAY FOR CARE OF NEWBORN WITH RESPIRATORY DISTRESS continued

Category	Day of Birth–1st 4 Hours	Remaining Day of Birth

Nutrition	• Provide total parenteral nutrition (TNP) when indicated
	• Provide adequate caloric intake: consider amount of intake, route of administration, need for supplementation of intake by other routes, type of formula
	• Gavage prn →
	• Maintain IV rate at prescribed levels via infusion pump, usually 60–80 mL/kg/day
	  • Record type and amount of fluid infused hourly
	  • Observe VS for signs of too rapid infusion
		• Advance, based on tolerance, from intravenous to gastrointestinal feedings. Gavage or nipple feedings are used, and IV is used as supplement (discontinue when oral intake is sufficient)
		• Initiate bottle-feeding if applicable
		• Initiate breastfeeding as soon as condition of mother and baby allows →
		• Supplement breastfeeding only when medically indicated/policy or ordered by physician with D_5W, sterile water, or 20 cal formula with iron →

Elimination	• Note first void and stool color • Provide meticulous and frequent skin care, especially after voiding and stooling →	• Monitor stools for amount, type, consistency, and any change in pattern • Monitor all voids q shift • Maintain normal urine output (1–3 mL/kg/h) • Maintain specific gravity of urine between 1.006 and 1.012
Medications	• Aquamephyton, 1 mg IM—not administered until after bath • Ilotycin ophth ointment OU—not administered until after bath	
Discharge planning/ home care	• Eval Social Services/Visiting Nurse/DC planning needs • Plan DC with parent/guardian	• Present birth certificate instructions
Family involvement	• Eval additional psychosocial needs—provide time for expressions of concerns, determine parent's understanding of respiratory distress syndrome • Eval parent teaching	• Instruct mother on diapering, normal limits of void and stool, burping, bulb syringe, choking, positioning • Eval parent teaching • Instruct parents of need after DC for frequent position changes, thorough skin cleansing with each diaper change, and reporting any sign of rash or skin breakdown to health care provider
Date		

Category	Day 1 After Birth	Day 2/3 (if applicable) After Birth
Referral		
Assessment	• Assess respiratory effort and ventilatory adequacy • Assess mother/baby interaction • Thermoregulation • Assess abdominal distention, gastric residuals • Monitor blood gases, capillary refill, O_2 saturations	• Assess respiratory effort and level of distress • Assess mother/baby interaction → • Assess abdominal distention, gastric residuals, wt gain • Monitor blood gases, capillary refill, O_2 saturation
Comfort	• Provide minimal stimulation/handling • Sedation as warranted	• Provide minimal stimulation/handling • Sedation as warranted

CRITICAL PATHWAY continued

Category	Day 1 After Birth	Day 2/3 (if applicable) After Birth

Nursing interventions and report	• Maintain on respiratory and cardiac monitors:
	  • Check and calibrate all monitoring and measuring devices q8h →
	  • Calibrate oxygen devices to 21% and 100% O_2 concentrations →
	• Provide warmed air 31.7–33.9C (89–93F) and humidified (40–60%) oxygen
	• Monitor oxygen concentrations at least q1h
	• Femoral pulses or BPs 4 extremities before DC or 48 h →
	• VS q4h
	• Daily wt →
	• Check color q shift →
	• Isolette if temp instability
	  • Adjust and monitor to maintain skin temp
	• Use servocontrol to maintain constant temp regulation →
	• Use heat shields for small infants
	• Check activity →
	• Administer antibiotics as ordered →
	• Skin breakdown/rash
		• Newborn screen for vag delivery if stable
		• Completion of Baer test
		• VS: temp q shift
		• Administer O_2 by oxygen hood
		  • Avoid hood touching infant's face
		• Monitor O_2 concentration q1–4 h
		• Daily wt →
		• Scalp R_x prn bid →
		• Check color q shift →
		• Check activity →
		• Circumcision →
		• Alcohol cord q shift if needed →
		• Administer antibiotics as ordered →
		• Monitor antibiotic levels →
		• Skin breakdown/rash
		• Wear gloves for diaper changes in presence of diarrhea
		• HSV culture (rapid and conventional) for 24–48 h or at DC for maternal or paternal history of HSV
		• Open crib →

Activity	• Change position prn →	• Change position prn →
Nutrition	• Gavage prn → • Provide supplemental breastfeeding as indicated/policy or ordered by physician with D_5W, sterile water, or 20 cal formula → • Encourage frequent feedings as tolerated → • Bottle-feed q3–4h on demand →	• Gavage prn → • Provide supplemental breastfeeding as indicated/policy or ordered by physician with D_5W, sterile water, or 20 cal formula → • Encourage frequent feedings, at least q3–4h during day and more frequently as baby demands/nsg std → • Bottle-feed q3–4h on demand →
Elimination	• Monitor stools for amount, type, consistency, and any change in pattern, occult blood, and reducing substances • Monitor all voids q shift	• Monitor stools for amount, type, consistency, and any change in pattern, occult blood, and reducing substances • Monitor all voids q shift
Medications	• Hep B vaccine at DC	• Hep B vaccine before DC
Discharge/ planning home care	• If vag delivery, complete DC summary • Complete Birth Certificate packet • Continuation from "Remaining Day of Birth"	• If C/S delivery, complete DC summary • Instruction on cleaning of baby's individual skin care items, toys • Car seat for discharge →

Family involvement	• Bath and feeding class (mother)
	• Channel 13 films (mother) Newborn Channel
	• Instruct mother/parent on:
	  • Bath and skin care, nail and cord care
	  • Circumcised/uncirc penis
	  • Rashes; jaundice
	  • Use of thermometer; infant abilities and stimuli
	  • Active/sleep status; crying/soothing responses
	  • Reflexes
	  • Special nutritional needs
	  • Monitoring wt gain, report feeding intolerance
	• Eval mother/parent teaching →
	• Teen "Healthy Starts" program
		• Continue the completion of education on Day 1 →
		• Eval mother/parent teaching →

Date		

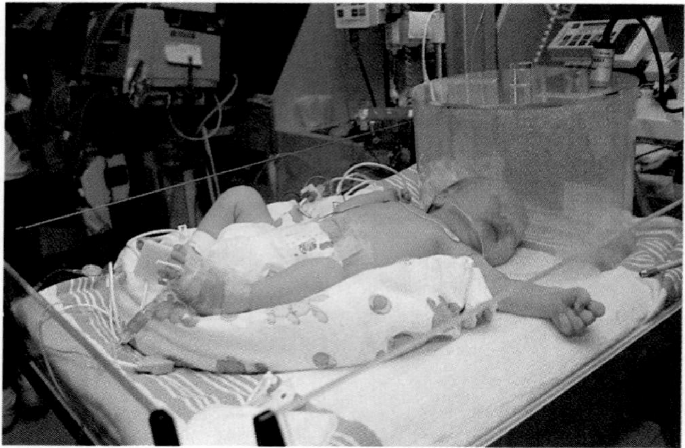

FIGURE 26–6 An infant under an oxyhood.

Ambient oxygen concentrations of 30 to 50 percent, usually under an oxyhood, may be required initially to correct the hypoxemia (Figure 26–6). The oxygen requirements of these infants usually decrease over the first 48 hours, unlike those of infants with RDS, whose oxygen needs increase during this time.

The infant should be improving by 24 to 48 hours, except for modest O_2 dependence (less than 30%). The duration of the clinical course of transient tachypnea is approximately 4 days (96 hours). Early acidosis, both respiratory and metabolic (with moderate elevations of P_{CO_2}), is easily corrected. Ventilation assistance is rarely needed, and most of these infants survive.

If progressive deterioration occurs to the extent that assisted ventilation is required, a diagnosis of superimposed sepsis must be considered and treatment measures initiated.

Nursing Care

For nursing actions, see the Critical Pathway for Care of Newborn with Respiratory Distress.

CRITICAL THINKING IN ACTION

You are caring for baby girl Linn, who is a 39-week, AGA female born by repeat cesarean birth to a 34-year-old, G3 now P3 mother. Baby Linn's Apgar scores were 7 and 9 at 1 and 5 minutes. At 2 hours of age, an elevated respiratory rate of 70–80 and mild cyanosis were noted. She is now receiving 30% oxygen and has a respiratory rate of 100–120. The baby's clinical course, chest x-ray, and lab work are all consistent with transient tachypnea of the newborn. Her mother calls you to ask about her baby. She tells you that her last child was born at 30 weeks' gestation, had respiratory distress syndrome requiring ventilator support, and was hospitalized for 6 weeks. She asks you, "Is this the same respiratory distress?" What will you tell her?

Answers can be found in Appendix H.

Care of Newborn with Meconium Aspiration Syndrome

The presence of meconium in amniotic fluid indicates an asphyxial insult to the fetus. The physiologic response to asphyxia is increased intestinal peristalsis, relaxation of the anal sphincter, and passage of meconium into the amniotic fluid.

Approximately 10 percent of all pregnancies will have meconium-stained fluid (Greenough 1995). This fluid may be aspirated into the tracheobronchial tree in utero or during the first few breaths taken by the newborn. This is called **meconium aspiration syndrome (MAS).** This syndrome primarily affects term, SGA, and postterm newborns, and those that have experienced a prolonged labor.

Presence of meconium in the lungs produces a ball-valve action (air is allowed in but not exhaled), so that alveoli overdistend; rupture with pneumomediastinum or pneumothorax is a common occurrence. The meconium also initiates a chemical pneumonitis in the lung with oxygen and carbon dioxide trapping and hyperinflation. Secondary bacterial pneumonia is common. Clinical manifestations of MAS include: (a) fetal hypoxia in utero a few days or a few minutes before birth, indicated by a sudden increase in fetal activity followed by diminished activity, slowing of fetal heart rate or weak and irregular heartbeat, and meconium staining of amniotic fluid; and (b) presence of signs of distress at birth, such as pallor, cyanosis, apnea, slow heartbeat, and low Apgar scores (below 6) at 1 and 5 minutes. As the victims of intrauterine asphyxia, meconium-stained newborns, or newborns who have aspirated meconium, are often depressed at birth and require resuscitation to establish adequate respiratory effort.

After the initial resuscitation, the severity of clinical symptoms correlates with the extent of aspiration. Mechanical ventilation is frequently required from birth because of immediate signs of distress (generalized cyanosis, tachypnea, and severe retractions). Later an overdistended, barrel-shaped chest with increased anteroposterior diameter is common. Auscultation reveals diminished air movement with prominent rales and rhonchi. Abdominal palpation may reveal a displaced liver due to diaphragmatic depression secondary to the overexpansion of the lungs. Yellowish staining of the skin, nails, and umbilical cord is usually present.

Medical Therapy

The combined efforts of the maternity and pediatric team are needed to prevent MAS. The most effective form of preventive management is outlined as follows:

1. After the head of the newborn is born and the shoulders and chest are still in the birth canal, first

the baby's oropharynx then the nasopharynx are suctioned. (The same procedure is followed with a cesarean birth.) To decrease the possibility of acquired immunodeficiency syndrome (AIDS) transmission, low-pressure wall suction is used.

2. If the infant is vigorous and there is thick meconium in the amniotic fluid, the glottis is visualized and meconium is suctioned from the trachea.
3. If the infant is vigorous and there is only thin meconium in the amniotic fluid, no subsequent special resuscitation is indicated.
4. For any depressed infant (heart rate less than 100 beats per minute or poor respiratory effort with meconium staining), the glottis is visualized and the trachea suctioned (Greenough 1995).

If the newborn's head is not adequately suctioned on the perineum, the respiratory or resuscitative efforts will push meconium into the airway and into the lungs. Stimulation of the newborn is avoided to minimize respiratory movements. Further resuscitative efforts as indicated follow the same principles mentioned earlier in this chapter. Resuscitated newborns should be immediately transferred to the nursery for closer observation. An umbilical arterial line may be used for direct monitoring of arterial blood pressures; blood sampling for pH and blood gases; and infusion of intravenous fluids, blood, or medications.

Treatment usually involves delivery of high ambient oxygenation and controlled ventilation, preferably at low positive end-expiratory pressures (PEEP) to avoid air leaks. Unfortunately, high pressures may be needed to cause sufficient expiratory expansion of obstructed terminal airways or to stabilize airways that are weakened by inflammation so that the most distal atelectatic alveoli are ventilated.

Surfactant replacement therapy if started early has shown promise in improving oxygenation and decreasing incidence of air leaks (Findlay et al 1996). Systemic blood pressure and pulmonary blood flow must be maintained. If pulmonary hypertension occurs as a result of this disorder, pulmonary vasodilators such as tolazoline (Priscoline) or isoproterenol (Isuprel) may be used to increase the pulmonary blood flow by overcoming the arterioles' vasoconstriction and pulmonary vasospasm, which has created a right-to-left cardiopulmonary shunt. Tolazoline must be used with extreme caution because it can cause dramatic falls in blood pressure and gastrointestinal hemorrhage. Tolazoline is usually used in conjunction with dopamine or dobutamine and/or volume expanders to maintain systemic blood pressure.

Full-term newborns over 3.17 kg (7 lb) with respiratory failure who are not responding to ventilator therapy may require treatment with ECMO, a form of heart-lung bypass. This treatment has proven successful for newborns with meconium aspiration, pneumonia, and PPHN who are not responding to traditional treatment modalities (Findlay et al 1996).

Treatment also includes chest physiotherapy (chest percussion, vibration, and drainage) to remove debris. Prophylactic antibiotics are frequently given. Bicarbonate may be necessary for several days for severely ill newborns. Mortality in term or postterm infants with MAS is very high, because the cycle of hypoxemia and acidemia is difficult to break.

APPLYING THE NURSING PROCESS

Nursing Assessment

During the intrapartal period, the nurse should observe for signs of fetal hypoxia and meconium staining of amniotic fluid. At birth, the nurse assesses the newborn for signs of distress. During the ongoing assessment of the newborn, the nurse carefully observes for complications such as pulmonary air leaks; anoxic cerebral injury manifested by cerebral edema and/or convulsions; anoxic myocardial injury evidenced by congestive heart failure or cardiomegaly; disseminated intravascular coagulation (DIC) resulting from hypoxic hepatic damage with depression of liver-dependent clotting factors; anoxic renal damage demonstrated by hematuria, oliguria, or anuria; fluid overload; sepsis secondary to bacterial pneumonia; and any signs of intestinal necrosis from ischemia, including gastrointestinal obstruction or hemorrhage.

Nursing Diagnosis

Nursing diagnoses that may apply to the newborn with MAS include the following:

- Ineffective gas exchange related to aspiration of meconium and amniotic fluid during birth
- Altered nutrition: less than body requirements related to respiratory distress and increased energy requirements
- Ineffective family coping related to life-threatening illness in term newborn

Nursing Plan and Implementation

Initial interventions are aimed primarily at prevention of the aspiration by assisting with the removal of the meconium from the infant's oropharynx and nasopharnyx prior to the first extrauterine breath.

When significant aspiration occurs, therapy is supportive with the primary goals of maintaining appropriate gas exchange and minimizing complications. Nursing interventions after resuscitation should include maintenance of adequate oxygenation and ventilation, temperature regulation, glucose strip test at 2 hours of age to check for hypoglycemia, observation of intravenous fluids, calculation of necessary fluids (which may be restricted in the first 48–72 hours due to cerebral edema), and provision of caloric requirements.

Evaluation

Anticipated outcomes of nursing care include

- The risk of MAS is promptly identified and early intervention is initiated.
- The newborn is free of respiratory distress and metabolic alterations.
- The parents verbalize their concerns about their baby's health problem and survival and understand the rationale behind the management of their newborn.

Care of the Newborn with Cold Stress

Cold stress is excessive heat loss resulting in the use of compensatory mechanisms (such as increased respirations and nonshivering thermogenesis) to maintain core body temperature. Heat loss that results in cold stress occurs in the newborn through the mechanisms of evaporation, convection, conduction, and radiation. (See Chapter 21 for types of heat loss.) Heat loss at birth that leads to cold stress can play a significant role in the severity of RDS and the ultimate outcome for the infant.

The amount of heat lost by an infant depends to a large extent on the actions of the nurse or caregiver. Both preterm and SGA newborns are at risk for cold stress because they have decreased adipose tissue, brown fat stores, and glycogen available for metabolism.

As discussed in Chapter 21, the newborn infant's major source of heat production in nonshivering thermogenesis (NST) is brown fat metabolism. The infant's ability to respond to cold stress by NST is impaired in the presence of several conditions:

- Hypoxemia (PO_2 less than 50 torr)
- Intracranial hemorrhage or any CNS abnormality
- Hypoglycemia (blood glucose < 40 mg/dL)

When these conditions occur, the infant's temperature should be monitored more closely and the neutral thermal environment conscientiously maintained. It is important for the nurse to recognize these conditions and treat them as soon as possible. The metabolic consequences of cold stress can be devastating and potentially fatal to an infant. Oxygen requirements rise, glucose use increases, acids are released into the bloodstream, and surfactant production decreases. The effects are graphically depicted in Figure 26–7.

Nursing Care

The nurse observes for signs of cold stress. These include increased respirations, decrease in skin temperature, decrease in peripheral perfusion, appearance of hypoglycemia, and the possible development of metabolic acidosis.

Skin temperature assessments are used because initial response to cold stress is vasoconstriction, resulting in a decrease in skin temperature; therefore, monitoring rectal temperature is not satisfactory. A decrease in rectal temperature represents long-standing cold stress with decompensation in the newborn's ability to maintain core body temperature.

If a decrease in skin temperature is noted, the nurse determines whether hypoglycemia is present. Hypoglycemia is a result of the metabolic effects of cold stress and is suggested by glucose strip values below 45 mg/dL, tremors, irritability or lethargy, apnea, or seizure activity.

If cold stress occurs, the following nursing interventions should be initiated:

- Warm the newborn slowly since rapid temperature elevation may cause apnea.
- Monitor skin temperature every 15 minutes to determine if the newborn's temperature is increasing.
- Place and maintain the newborn in a neutral thermal environment.

The presence of anaerobic metabolism is assessed and interventions initiated for the resulting metabolic acidosis. Attempts to burn brown fat increase oxygen consumption, lactic acid levels, and metabolic acidosis. Hypoglycemia may be reversed by adequate glucose intake, as described in the following section.

Care of the Newborn with Hypoglycemia

Hypoglycemia is the most common metabolic disorder occurring in IDM, SGA, and preterm AGA infants. The pathophysiology differs for each classification.

AGA preterm infants have not been in utero a sufficient time to store glycogen and fat. Therefore, they have very low glycogen and fat stores and a decreased ability to carry out gluconeogenesis. This situation is further aggravated by increased use of glucose by the tissues (especially the brain and heart) during stress and illness (chilling, asphyxia, sepsis, and RDS).

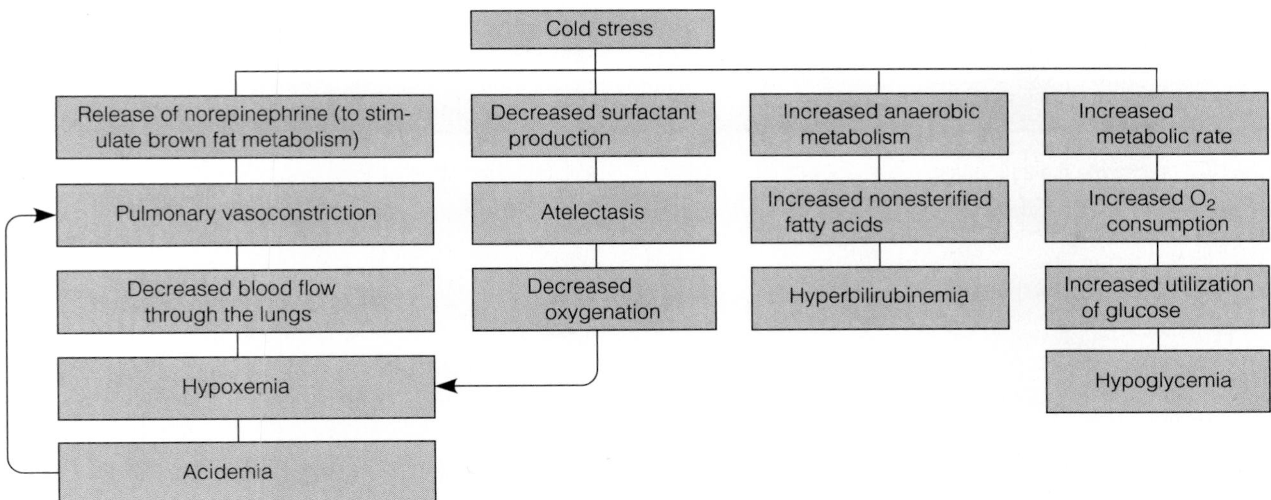

FIGURE 26–7 Cold stress chain of events. The hypothermic, or cold-stressed, newborn attempts to compensate by conserving heat and increasing heat production. These physiologic compensatory mechanisms initiate a series of metabolic events that result in hypoxemia and altered surfactant production, metabolic acidosis, hypoglycemia, and hyperbilirubinemia.

Infants of White's Class A–C or type 1 diabetic mothers have increased stores of glycogen and fat (see Chapter 25). Circulating insulin and insulin responsiveness are also higher when compared to other newborns. Because the high in utero glucose loads stop at birth, the newborn experiences rapid and profound hypoglycemia. The SGA infant has used up glycogen and fat stores because of intrauterine malnutrition and has a blunted hepatic enzymatic response with which to produce and use glucose. Any newborn who is stressed at birth (from asphyxia or cold) also quickly uses up available glucose stores and becomes hypoglycemic.

A recent study, reporting the incidence of hypoglycemia in AGA term newborns to be 7.9 percent after vaginal birth and 15.7 percent after cesarean section (without labor), suggests that epidural anesthesia may alter maternal-fetal glucose homeostasis, resulting in hypoglycemia (Cole and Peevy 1994).

Hypoglycemia is defined for all newborns as a blood glucose below 40 mg/dL (Brooks 1997). It may also be defined as a glucose oxidase reagent strip below 45 mg/dL, but only when corroborated with laboratory blood glucose. (See Procedure 26–1: Performing a Heelstick for Glucose Testing). Glucose reagent strips should not be used by themselves to screen and diagnose hypoglycemia because their results depend on the baby's hematocrit, and there is a wide variance (5–15 mg/dL) when compared to laboratory determinations, especially with blood glucose values of less than 40–50 mg/dL (Brooks 1997). Newer techniques, such as using a glucose oxidase analyzer or an optical bedside glucose analyzer, are more reliable for bedside screening but must also be validated with laboratory chemical analysis. A definitive diagnosis of hypoglycemia is made based on at least two successive values that are significantly low.

Medical Therapy

The goal of management includes early identification of hypoglycemia through observation and screening of newborns at risk. The newborn may be asymptomatic, or any of the following may occur:

- Lethargy, jitteriness
- Poor feeding
- Vomiting
- Pallor
- Apnea, irregular respirations, respiratory distress, cyanosis
- Hypotonia, possible loss of swallowing reflex
- Tremors, jerkiness, seizure activity
- High-pitched cry

Differential diagnosis of a newborn with nonspecific hypoglycemic symptoms includes determining if the newborn has any of the following:

- CNS disease
- Sepsis
- Metabolic aberrations
- Polycythemia
- Congenital heart disease
- Drug withdrawal
- Temperature instability
- Hypocalcemia

Aggressive treatment is recommended after a single low blood-glucose value if the infant shows any of these symptoms. In high-risk infants, routine screening should be carried out at 2, 4, 6, 12, 24, and 48 hours of age or whenever any of the noted clinical manifestations appear.

PROCEDURE 26–1 Performing a Heelstick for Glucose Testing

Nursing Action	Rationale
Objective: Assemble the equipment.	Equipment organization facilitates the procedure.
• Microlancet (do not use a needle)	A needle may nick the periosteum.
• Alcohol swabs	
• 2 x 2 sterile gauze squares	
• Small bandage	
• Transfer pipette	
• Glucose reagent strips or reflectance meters	
• Gloves	Gloves are used to implement universal precautions and prevent nosocomial infections.
Objective: Prepare the infant's heel for the procedure.	
• Use a warm wet wrap or specially designed chemical heat pad to warm the infant's heel for 5–10 seconds to facilitate blood flow.	
• Select a clear, previously unpunctured site.	The selection of a previously unpunctured site minimizes the risk of infection and excessive scar formation.
• Clean the site by rubbing vigorously with 70% isopropyl alcohol swab, followed by a dry gauze square.	Friction produces local heat, which aids vasodilation.
• Blot the site dry completely before lancing.	Alcohol is irritating to injured tissue and it may also produce hemolysis.
Objective: Lance the infant's heel and ensure accurate blood sampling. See the step-by-step instructions below.	
Objective: Prevent excessive bleeding.	
• Apply a folded gauze square to the puncture site and secure it firmly with a bandage.	
• Check the puncture site frequently for the first hour after sampling.	
Objective: Record the findings on the infant's chart.	
• Report immediately any results under 45 mg/dL or over 175 mg/dL.	Recording the results helps identify possible complications.

Performing the Heelstick

The infant's lateral heel is the site of choice because it precludes damaging the posterior tibial nerve and artery, plantar artery, and the important longitudinally oriented fat pad of the heel, which in later years could impede walking (Figure 26–8). This is especially important for infants undergoing multiple heel stick procedures. Toes are acceptable sites if necessary.

Lancing the Heel

- Grasp the infant's lower leg and foot so as to impede venous return slightly. This will facilitate extraction of the blood sample.
- With a quick, piercing motion, puncture the lateral heel with a microlancet. Be careful not to puncture too deeply. Optimal penetration is 4 mm (Figure 26–9).

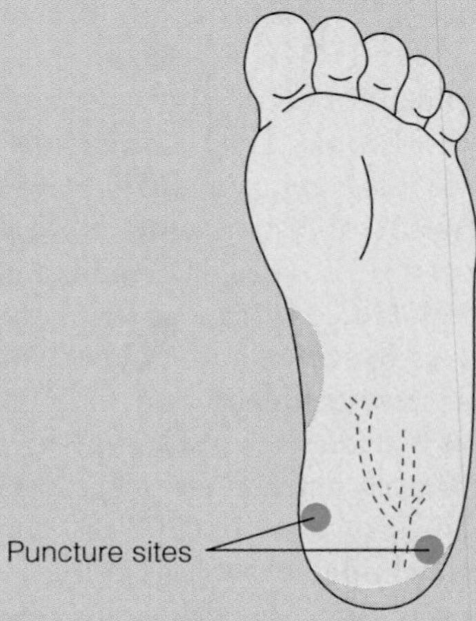

FIGURE 26–8 Potential sites for hell sticks. Avoid shaded areas in order to avoid injury to arteries and nerves in the foot.

PROCEDURE 26–1 continued

Collecting the Blood Sample

- Allow the first drop of blood to touch both test pads on the Chemstrip. Make sure you cover both yellow and white squares completely (Figure 26–10).
- If you are using a Dextrostix reagent strip, discard the first drop of blood as it tends to be minutely diluted with tissue fluid from the puncture.
- Use of transfer pipette to place drop of blood on glucose reflectance meter.

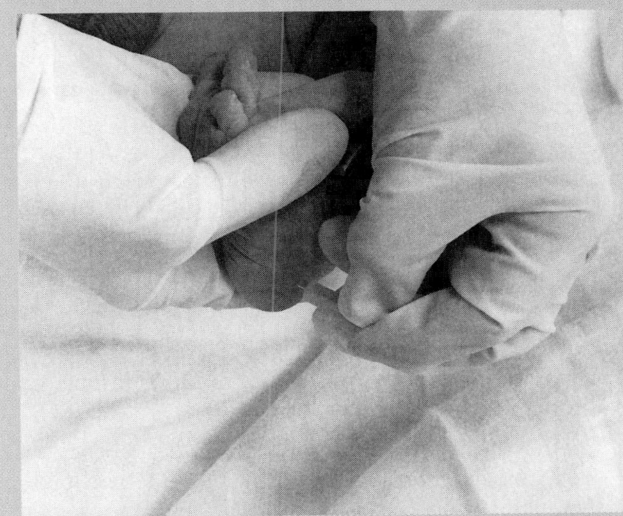

FIGURE 26–9 Puncturing the lateral heel.

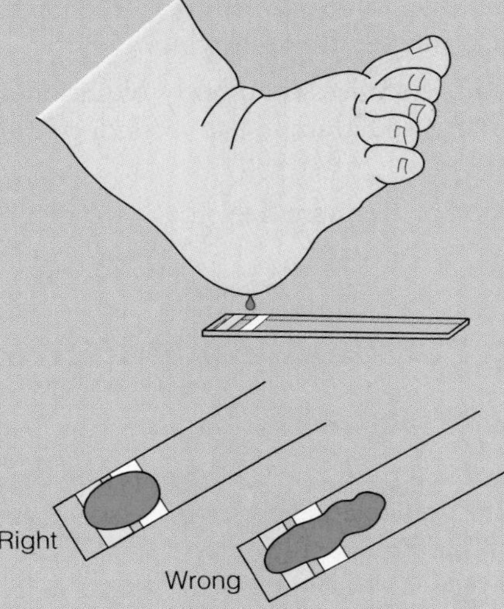

FIGURE 26–10 Application of drop of blood to glucose strip.

Provision of adequate caloric intake is important. Early formula feeding or breastfeeding is one of the major preventive approaches. If early feeding or intravenous glucose is started to meet the recommended fluid and caloric needs, the blood glucose is likely to remain above the hypoglycemic level. During the first hours after birth, nurses may give asymptomatic newborns oral glucose and then obtain another plasma glucose measurement 30–60 minutes after feeding. Intravenous infusions of a dextrose solution (5% to 10%) begun immediately after birth should prevent hypoglycemia. Plasma glucose levels are obtained when the parenteral infusion is started. However, in the very small AGA infant, infusions of 10 percent dextrose solution may cause *hyperglycemia* to develop, requiring an alteration in the glucose concentration. Infants require 6–8 mg/kg/min of glucose to maintain normal glucose concentrations. Therefore, an intravenous glucose solution should be calculated based on the infant's body weight, with blood glucose tests to determine adequacy of the infusion treatment (Sunnehag et al 1994).

A rapid infusion of 25 percent to 50 percent dextrose is contraindicated because it may lead to profound rebound hypoglycemia following an initial brief increase. In prolonged hypoglycemic periods, corticosteroids may be administered. It is thought that steroids enhance gluconeogenesis from noncarbohydrate protein sources (Brooks 1997).

The prognosis for untreated hypoglycemia is poor. It may result in permanent, untreatable CNS damage or death.

APPLYING THE NURSING PROCESS

Nursing Assessment

The objective of assessment is to identify newborns at risk. For newborns who are diagnosed as having hypoglycemia, assessment is ongoing with careful monitoring of glucose values. Glucose strips, urine dipsticks, and urine volume (monitor only if above 1–3 mL/kg/hr) are evaluated frequently for osmotic diuresis and glycosuria.

Nursing Diagnosis

Nursing diagnoses that may apply to the newborn with hypoglycemia include the following:

- Altered nutrition: less than body requirements related to increased glucose use secondary to physiologic stress
- Pain related to frequent heel sticks for glucose monitoring

Nursing Plan and Implementation

Monitoring of Glucose Levels

When caring for a preterm AGA infant, the nurse should monitor blood glucose levels using glucose strips or in combination with reflectance meter, or laboratory determinations every 4–8 hours for the first day of life and daily or as necessary thereafter. The IDM should be monitored hourly for the first several hours after birth, as this is the time when precipitous falls in glucose are most likely. In the SGA newborn, symptoms usually appear between 24 and 72 hours of age; occasionally they begin as early as 3 hours of age. Infants who are below the tenth percentile on the intrauterine growth curve should have blood sugar assessments at least every 8 hours until 4 days of age and more frequently if any symptoms develop. Once an infant's blood sugar is stable, glucose testing every 2–4 hours, or prior to feedings, adequately monitors glucose levels (Brooks 1997).

Calculation of glucose requirements and maintenance of intravenous glucose will be necessary for any symptomatic infant with low serum glucose levels. Careful attention to glucose monitoring is again required during the transition from intravenous to oral feedings. Titration of intravenous glucose may be required until the infant is able to take adequate amounts of formula or breast milk to maintain a normal blood sugar level. This titration is accomplished by decreasing the concentration of parenteral glucose gradually to 5 percent, then reducing the rate of infusion to 6 mg/kg/minute, then to 4 mg/kg/minute, and slowly discontinuing it over 4–6 hours.

Decreasing Physiologic Stress

The method of feeding greatly influences glucose and energy requirements. In addition, the therapeutic nursing measure of *nonnutritive sucking* (giving the newborn a pacifier) during gavage feedings has been reported to increase the baby's daily weight gain and lead to earlier bottle- or breastfeeding and discharge. Nonnutritive sucking may also lower activity levels, which allows newborns to conserve their energy stores. Activity can increase energy requirements; crying alone can double the baby's metabolic rate. Establishment and maintenance of a neutral thermal environment has a potent influence on the newborn's metabolism. The nurse pays careful attention to environmental conditions, physical activity, and organization of care, and integrates these factors into delivery of nursing care. The nurse identifies any discrepancies between the baby's caloric requirements and received calories and weighs the newborn daily at consistent times, preferably before a feeding. Only then can findings of unusual losses or gains, as well as the pattern of weight gain, be considered reliable.

Evaluation

Anticipated outcomes of nursing care include

- The risk of hypoglycemia is promptly identified, and intervention is started early.
- The newborn's metabolic and physiologic processes are stabilized, and recovery is proceeding without sequelae.
- The parents verbalize their concerns about their baby's health problem and understand the rationale behind the management of their newborn.

Care of the Newborn with Jaundice

The most common abnormal physical finding in newborns is **jaundice** (icterus neonatorium). Jaundice develops from deposit of the yellow pigment *bilirubin* in lipid tissues. Fetal unconjugated (indirect) bilirubin is normally cleared by the placenta in utero, so total bilirubin at birth is usually less than 3 mg/dL unless an abnormal hemolytic process has been present. Postnatally, the infant must conjugate bilirubin (convert a lipid-soluble pigment into a water-soluble pigment) in the liver.

The rate and amount of conjugation of bilirubin depends on the rate of hemolysis, the bilirubin load, the maturity of the liver, and the presence of albumin-binding sites. See Chapter 21 for discussion of conjugation of bilirubin. A normal term infant's liver is usually mature enough and producing enough glucuronyl transferase that the total serum bilirubin does not reach a pathologic level (above 12 mg/dL in the blood). However, physiologic jaundice remains a common problem for the term newborn and may require treatment with phototherapy. Physiologic jaundice is due to the newborn's shorter red cell life span, slower uptake by the liver, lack of intestinal bacteria, and poorly established hydration.

Pathophysiology

Serum albumin–binding sites are usually sufficient to meet the normal demands. However, certain conditions tend to decrease the sites available. Fetal or neonatal asphyxia decreases the binding affinity of bilirubin to albumin, as acidosis impairs the capacity of albumin to hold bilirubin. Hypothermia and hypoglycemia release free fatty acids that dislocate bilirubin from albumin. Maternal use of sulfa drugs or salicylates interferes with conjugation or with serum albumin–binding sites by competing with bilirubin for these sites.

A number of bacterial and viral infections (such as cytomegalic inclusion disease, toxoplasmosis, herpes, and syphilis) can affect the liver and produce jaundice. **Hyperbilirubinemia** (elevation of bilirubin level) may also result from blood disorders such as polycythemia (twin-to-twin transfusion, large placental transfer of blood), or enclosed hemorrhage (cephalhematoma, bleeding into internal organs, ecchymoses). Increased hemolysis due to conditions such as sepsis, hemolytic disease of the newborn, or an excessive dose of vitamin K may also cause elevated bilirubin levels.

The bilirubin level at which an infant is harmed varies, but at that level the infant may suffer neurologic defects and eventually death. While the mechanism of bilirubin-produced neuronal injury is uncertain, evidence indicates that high concentrations of total bilirubin can be neurotoxic (Gartner 1994). Unconjugated bilirubin has a high affinity for extravascular tissue such as fatty tissue (subcutaneous tissue) and the brain. Thus bilirubin not bound to albumin can cross the blood-brain barrier, damage the cells of the CNS, and produce kernicterus. **Kernicterus** (meaning "yellow nucleus") refers to the deposition of indirect or unconjugated bilirubin in the basal ganglia of the brain and to the symptoms of neurologic damage that follow untreated hyperbilirubinemia. The classic bilirubin encephalopathy of kernicterus most commonly found with blood group incompatibility is virtually unknown today due to aggressive treatment with phototherapy and exchange transfusions.

Kernicterus, usually associated with total bilirubin levels of over 20 mg/dL in normal term infants and over 10 mg/dL in sick preterm newborns, has been noted at autopsy in both types of babies at lower levels. The risk of kernicterus at lowered bilirubin levels has been associated with asphyxia, acidosis, and low serum albumin levels. Current therapy can reduce the incidence of kernicterus encephalopathy but cannot distinguish all infants who are at risk.

Causes of Hyperbilirubinemia

A primary cause of hyperbilirubinemia is **hemolytic disease of the newborn** secondary to Rh incompatibility. All the pregnant women who are Rh-negative or who have blood type O (possible ABO blood incompatibility) should be asked about outcomes of any previous pregnancies and history of blood transfusion. Prenatal amniocentesis with spectrophotographic examination may be indicated in some cases. Cord blood from newborns is evaluated for bilirubin level, which should not exceed 5 mg/dL. Newborns of Rh-negative and O blood-type mothers are carefully assessed for appearance of jaundice and levels of serum bilirubin.

Isoimmune hemolytic disease, also known as **erythroblastosis fetalis,** occurs after transplacental passage of a maternal antibody that predisposes fetal and neonatal red blood cells to early destruction. Jaundice, anemia, and compensatory erythropoiesis result. **Hydrops fetalis,** the most severe form of erythroblastosis fetalis, occurs when maternal antibodies attach to the Rh site on the fetal red blood cells, making them susceptible to destruction. The fetal system responds by increased production of immature red blood cells that do not have the functional capabilities of mature cells and cause multiorgan system failure.

If anemia is severe, as seen in hydrops fetalis, cardiomegaly with severe cardiac decompensation and hepatosplenomegaly occur. Severe generalized massive edema *(anasarca)* and generalized fluid effusion into the pleural cavity (hydrothorax), pericardial sac, and peritoneal cavity (ascites) develop. Jaundice is not present initially because the bilirubin pigments are excreted through the placenta into the maternal circulation. The hydropic hemolytic disease process is also characterized by hyperplasia of the pancreatic islets, which predisposes the infant to neonatal hypoglycemia similar to that of IDMs. These infants also have increased bleeding tendencies due to associated thrombocytopenia and hypoxic damage to the capillaries. Hydrops is a frequent cause of intrauterine death among infants with Rh disease.

ABO incompatibility (the mother is blood type O and the baby is blood type A or B) may result in jaundice, although it rarely results in hemolytic disease severe enough to be clinically diagnosed and treated. Hepatosplenomegaly may be found occasionally in newborns with ABO incompatibility, but hydrops fetalis and stillbirth are rare.

The best treatment for hemolytic disease is prevention. Prenatal identification of the fetus at risk for Rh or

ABO incompatibility will allow prompt treatment. See Chapter 13 for discussion of in utero management of this condition.

Certain prenatal and perinatal factors predispose the newborn to hyperbilirubinemia. During pregnancy, maternal conditions that predispose to neonatal hyperbilirubinemia include hereditary spherocytosis, diabetes, intrauterine infections, and gram-negative bacilli infections that stimulate production of maternal isoimmune antibodies, drug ingestion (such as sulfas, salicylates, novobiocin, diazepam), and oxytocin.

Certain newborn conditions predispose to hyperbilirubinemia: polycythemia (central hematocrit 65% or more), pyloric stenosis, obstruction or atresia of the biliary duct or of the lower bowel, low-grade urinary tract infection, sepsis, hypothyroidism, enclosed hemorrhage (cephalhematoma, large bruises), asphyxia neonatorum, hypothermia, acidemia, and hypoglycemia. Hepatitis from intrauterine infections or metabolic liver disease elevates the level of conjugated bilirubin.

The prognosis for a newborn with hyperbilirubinemia depends on the extent of the hemolytic process and the underlying cause. Severe hemolytic disease results in fetal and early neonatal death from the effects of severe anemia—cardiac decompensation, edema, ascites, and hydrothorax. Hyperbilirubinemia that is not aggressively treated may lead to kernicterus. The resultant neurologic damage is responsible for death, cerebral palsy, possible mental retardation, or hearing loss or, to a lesser degree, perceptual impairment, delayed speech development, hyperactivity, muscle incoordination, or learning difficulties (Gartner 1994).

Medical Therapy

When one or more of the predisposing factors for jaundice is present, laboratory determination should be made of the maternal and neonatal blood types for Rh or ABO incompatibility. Other necessary laboratory evaluations are Coombs' test, serum bilirubin levels (direct, indirect, and total), hemoglobin, reticulocyte percentage, and white cell count.

Neonatal hyperbilirubinemia of any origin must be considered pathologic if any of the following criteria are met (Taeusch et al 1991):

1. Clinically evident jaundice in the first 24 hours of life
2. Serum bilirubin concentration rising by more than 5 mg/dL per day
3. Total serum bilirubin concentrations exceeding 12.9 mg/dL in term infants or 15 mg/dL in preterm babies (since preterm newborns have less subcutaneous fat, bilirubin may reach higher levels before it is visible)
4. Conjugated bilirubin concentrations greater than 2 mg/dL
5. Persistence of clinical jaundice beyond 7 days in term infants or beyond 14 days in preterm infants

Initial diagnostic procedures are aimed at differentiating jaundice resulting from increased bilirubin production, impaired conjugation or excretion, increased intestinal reabsorption, or a combination of these factors. The Coombs' test is performed to determine whether jaundice is due to Rh or ABO incompatibility.

If the hemolytic process is due to Rh sensitization, laboratory findings reveal the following: (a) an Rh-positive neonate with a positive Coombs' test; (b) increased erythropoiesis with many immature circulating red blood cells (nucleated blastocysts); (c) anemia, in most cases; (d) elevated levels (5 mg/dL or more) of bilirubin in cord blood; and (e) a reduction in albumin-binding capacity. Maternal data may include an elevated anti-Rh titer and spectrophotometric evidence of fetal hemolytic process.

The indirect Coombs' test measures the amount of Rh-positive antibodies in the mother's blood. Rh-positive red blood cells are added to the maternal blood sample. If the mother's serum contains antibodies, the Rh-positive red blood cells will agglutinate (clump) when rabbit immune antiglobulin is added, a positive result.

The direct Coombs' test reveals the presence of antibody-coated (sensitized) Rh-positive red blood cells in the newborn. Rabbit immune antiglobulin is added to the specimen of neonatal blood cells. If the neonatal red blood cells agglutinate, they have been coated with maternal antibodies, a positive result.

If the hemolytic process is due to ABO incompatibility, laboratory findings reveal an increase in reticulocytes. The resulting anemia is usually not significant during the newborn period and is rare later on. The direct Coombs' test may be negative or mildly positive, while the indirect Coombs' test may be strongly positive. Infants with a direct Coombs' positive test have increased incidence of jaundice with bilirubin levels in excess of 10 mg/dL. Increased numbers of spherocytes (spherical, plump, mature erythrocytes) are seen on a peripheral blood smear. Increased numbers of spherocytes are not seen on blood smears from Rh disease infants.

Regardless of the cause of hyperbilirubinemia, treatment is directed toward

- Alleviating the anemia
- Removing maternal antibodies and sensitized erythrocytes
- Increasing serum albumin levels
- Reducing the levels of serum bilirubin
- Minimizing the consequences of hyperbilirubinemia

Early discharge of newborns from birthing centers has significantly influenced the diagnosis and management of neonatal jaundice, increasing the emphasis on outpatient and home care management (Gartner 1994).

Therapeutic management of hyperbilirubinemia includes phototherapy, exchange transfusion, infusion of albumin, and drug therapy. If hemolytic disease is present, it may be treated with phototherapy, exchange transfusion, and drug therapy. When determining the appropriate management of hyperbilirubinemia due to hemolytic disease, the three variables that must be taken into account are the newborn's (1) serum bilirubin level, (2) birth weight, and (3) age in hours. If a newborn has hemolysis with an unconjugated bilirubin level of 14 mg/dL, weighs less than 2500 g (birth weight), and is 24 hours old or less, an exchange transfusion may be the best management. However, if that same newborn is over 24 hours of age, phototherapy may be the treatment of choice to prevent the possible complication of kernicterus (Figure 26–11).

Phototherapy

Phototherapy is the exposure of the newborn to high-intensity light. It may be used alone or in conjunction with exchange transfusion to reduce serum bilirubin levels. Exposure of the newborn to high-intensity light (a bank of fluorescent light bulbs or bulbs in the blue-light spectrum) decreases serum bilirubin levels in the skin by facilitating biliary excretion of unconjugated bilirubin. This occurs when light absorbed by the tissue converts unconjugated bilirubin into two isomers called photobilirubin. The photobilirubin moves from the tissues to the blood by a diffusion mechanism. In the blood it is bound to albumin and transported to the liver. It moves into the bile and is excreted into the duodenum for removal with feces without requiring conjugation by the liver. In addition, the photodegradation products formed when light oxidizes bilirubin can be excreted in the urine.

Phototherapy plays an important role in preventing a rise in bilirubin levels but does not alter the underlying cause of jaundice, and hemolysis may continue to produce anemia. Currently there is no evidence that healthy term infants without a pathologic cause for the jaundice are at risk for brain damage, even at levels in the 20–24 mg/dL range (Newman and Maisels 1992).

It is generally accepted that phototherapy should be started at 4 to 5 mg/dL below the calculated exchange level for each infant. Sick newborns of less than 1000 g should have phototherapy instituted at a bilirubin concentration of 5 mg/dL. Many authors have recommended initiating phototherapy "prophylactically" in the first 24 hours of life in high-risk, very-low-birth-weight infants (Dennery et al 1995). Sick preterm infants who are at least 1500 g should have phototherapy instituted when the bilirubin level is 10 mg/dL. Any

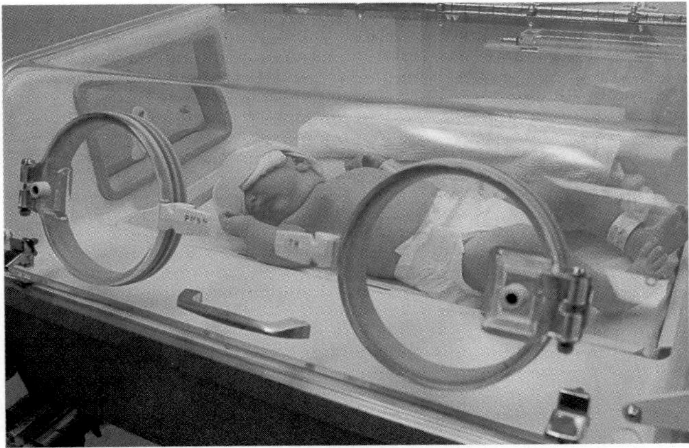

FIGURE 26–11 Infant receiving phototherapy. The phototherapy light is positioned over the incubator. Bilateral eye patches are always used to protect the baby's eyes during phototherapy.

newborn with a bilirubin level of 20 mg/dL or above may need an exchange transfusion if illness or associated conditions are present (Dennery et al 1995) (see Table 26–3).

An effective alternative method of delivering phototherapy to the term newborn is to place a fiberoptic blanket attached to a halogen light source around the trunk of the newborn (American Academy of Pediatrics 1994). The light stays on at all times, and the newborn is accessible for care, feeding, and diaper changes. The eyes are not covered. Fluid and weight loss are not complications of this system. Furthermore, it makes the infant accessible to the parents and is less alarming to parents than standard phototherapy (Tan 1994). Many institutions and pediatricians are using the blanket for home care.

APPLYING THE NURSING PROCESS

Nursing Assessment

Assessment is aimed at identifying prenatal and perinatal factors that predispose to development of jaundice and the jaundice as soon as it is apparent. Clinically, ABO incompatibility presents as jaundice and occasionally as hepatosplenomegaly. Hydrops is rare. Hemolytic disease of the newborn is suspected if the placenta is enlarged, if the newborn is edematous with pleural and pericardial effusion plus ascites, if pallor or jaundice is noted during the first 24 to 36 hours, if hemolytic anemia is diagnosed, or if the spleen and liver are enlarged. The nurse carefully notes changes in behavior and observes for evidence of bleeding. If laboratory tests indicate elevated bilirubin levels, the nurse checks the newborn for jaundice about every 2 hours and records observations.

TABLE 26–3 Management of Jaundice in Low-Birth-Weight Infants

	Indirect Bilirubin Concentrations					
Birth Weight	***5–6 mg/dL***	***7–9 mg/dL***	***10–12 mg/dL***	***12–15 mg/dL***	***15–20 mg/dL***	***>20 mg/dL***
≦1000 g	Phototherapy	→	Exchange transfusion*	→	→	→
1001–1500 g	Observe and repeat BR	Phototherapy	→	Exchange transfusion	→	→
1501–2000 g	Observe and repeat BR	→	Phototherapy	→	Exchange transfusion	→
>2000 g	Observe	Observe and repeat BR	Phototherapy (<2500 g)	Phototherapy (>2500 g)	→	Exchange transfusion

*Exchange if albumin binding is saturated or if serum indirect BR continues to rise. BR = bilirubin

Source: Cashore W, Stern L: The management of hyperbilirubinemia. *Clin Perinatol* June 1984; 11(2):353.

To check for jaundice, the nurse should blanch the skin over a bony prominence (forehead, nose, or sternum) by pressing firmly with the thumb. After pressure is released, if jaundice is present, the area appears yellow before normal color returns. The nurse should check oral mucosa and the posterior portion of the hard palate and conjunctival sacs for yellow pigmentation in darker-skinned babies. Assessment in daylight gives the best results, as pink walls and surroundings may mask yellowish tints and yellow light makes differentiation of jaundice difficult. The nurse records and reports the time of onset of jaundice. If jaundice appears, careful observation of the increase in depth of color and of the newborn's behavior is mandatory.

The newborn's behavior is assessed for neurologic signs of kernicterus, which are rare but may include hypotonia, diminished reflexes, lethargy, seizures, or opisthotonic posturing.

Nursing Diagnosis

Nursing diagnoses that may apply to care of a newborn with jaundice include the following:

- Fluid volume deficit related to increased insensible water loss and frequent loose stools
- Risk for injury related to use of phototherapy
- Sensory/perceptual alterations related to neurologic damage secondary to kernicterus
- Risk for altered parenting related to parenting a newborn with jaundice

Nursing Plan and Implementation

Promotion of Effective Phototherapy and Exchange Transfusion

See the Critical Pathway for Care of Newborn with Hyperbilirubinemia. Ideally the entire skin surface of the newborn is exposed to the light. Genitals are covered with a drape, since phototherapy may produce DNA strand breaks and possible mutations (Page 1989). Phototherapy success is measured every 12 hours or with daily serum bilirubin levels. The lights must be turned off while drawing blood to ensure accurate serum bilirubin levels. Because it is not known if phototherapy injures the delicate eye structures, particularly the retina, the nurse should apply eye patches over the newborn's closed eyes before beginning exposure (see Figure 26–11). The nurse discontinues phototherapy and removes the eye patches at least once per shift to assess the eyes for conjunctivitis. Patches are also removed to allow eye contact during feeding (social stimulation) or when parents are visiting (parental attachment).

The irradiance level at the skin determines the effectiveness of the phototherapy. The desired level is 5–6 microwatts per square centimeter per nanometer. Most phototherapy units will provide this level of irradiance 42–45 cm below the lamps. The nurse uses a photometer to measure and maintain desired irradiance levels.

The newborn's temperature is monitored to prevent hyperthermia or hypothermia. The newborn requires additional fluids to compensate for the increased water loss through the skin and loose stools. Loose stools and increased urine output are the results of increased bilirubin excretion. The nurse must observe the infant for signs of dehydration and perianal excoriation.

A transient bronze discoloration of the skin may occur with phototherapy when the infant has elevated direct serum bilirubin levels or liver disease. As a side effect of phototherapy, some newborns develop a maculopapular rash. In addition to assessing the newborn's skin color for jaundice and bronzing, the nurse examines the skin for developing pressure areas. The newborn should be repositioned at least every 2 hours to permit the light to reach all skin surfaces, to prevent pressure areas, and to vary the stimulation to the infant. The nurse keeps track of the number of hours each lamp is used so that it can be replaced before its effectiveness is lost.

CRITICAL PATHWAY FOR CARE OF NEWBORN WITH HYPERBILIRUBINEMIA

Category	Day 1	Day 2/Discharge
Referral	• Lactation specialist	• Lactation specialist
Assessment	• CBC, Rh, Coombs-direct • Retic count • Bili level ± Fractionated bili level • Baer screen if bili ≥ 18 • Obtain maternal/paternal history • Obtain birth history and history of newborn • Assess sclera and skin color for jaundice	• Bili level AM and PM • Assess for s/sx of dehydration • Assess sclera and skin color for progression of jaundice
Comfort	• Cuddle during feedings	• Cuddle during feedings
Nursing interventions and report	• VS q4h Ax temps • Monitor thermoregulation • Wt daily • Phototherapy • Maintain bili mask over eyes • Genitals covered • Check eyes for discharge, excessive pressure, corneal abrasions • Expose as much skin surface as possible • Administer thorough perianal cleansing with each stool • Bilimeter reading q shift • Note and document skin color q shift • Observe for abnormal neuro s/sx • No use of lotion or ointment • Turn off bili lights during lab draws • Reposition q2–3h • Assess neuro status, ongoing—report any changes (hypotonia lethargy, poor sucking reflex)	• VS q4h Ax temps • Monitor thermoregulation • Wt daily • Phototherapy • Maintain bili mask over eyes • Genitals covered • Check eyes for drainage, conjunctivitis, corneal abrasions, excessive pressure • Expose as much skin surface as possible • Administer thorough perianal cleansing with each stool • Reposition q2–3h • Bilimeter reading q shift • Note and document skin color q shift • Observe for abnormal neuro s/sx • No use of lotion or ointment • Turn off bili lights during lab draws • Assess neuro status, ongoing—report any changes (hypotonia lethargy, poor sucking reflex)
Activity	• Bassinet • Turn q2h reposition • Remove from lights only for feedings	• Bassinet • Turn q2h reposition • Remove from lights only for feedings

The nurse's responsibilities during *exchange transfusion* (withdrawal and replacement of the newborn's blood with donor blood) are to assemble equipment, prepare the baby, assist the physician during the procedure, and maintain a careful record of all events. After the procedure the nurse observes the newborn for complications from the transfusion and clinical signs of hyperbilirubinemia and neurologic damage.

Provision of Parental Support for Phototherapy in the Birthing Room or at Home

The terms *jaundice, hyperbilirubinemia, exchange transfusion,* and *phototherapy* may sound frightening and threatening. Some parents may feel guilty about their baby's condition and think they have caused the problem. Under stress, parents may not be able to understand the physician's first explanations. The nurse must expect that the parents will need explanations repeated and clarified and that they may need help in voicing their questions and fears. Eye and tactile contact with the newborn is encouraged. The nurse can coach parents when they visit with the baby. After the mother's discharge, parents are kept informed of their infant's condition and are encouraged to return to the hospital or telephone at any time so that they can be fully involved in the care of their infant. (See the Critical Pathway for Care of Newborn with Hyperbilirubinemia.)

While the mother is still hospitalized, phototherapy can also be carried out in the parents' room if the only problem is hyperbilirubinemia. The parents must be willing to keep the baby in the room for 24 hours a day, be able to take emergency action (eg, for choking) if necessary, and complete instruction checklists. Some institutions require that parents sign a consent form. The

CRITICAL PATHWAY FOR CARE OF NEWBORN WITH HYPERBILIRUBINEMIA continued

Category	Day 1	Day 2/Discharge
Nutrition	• Breast- or bottle-feed q2–3h • Supp with D_5W or formula—replace water loss • Remove newborn from under phototherapy and remove eye patches during feedings	• Breast- or bottle-feed q2–3h • Supp with D_5W or formula—replace water loss • Remove newborn from under phototherapy and remove eye patches during feedings
Elimination	• Record urine color and frequency • Specific gravity each void • Record quantity and characteristics each stool • I/O strict—weigh diapers before discarding	• Record urine color and frequency • Specific gravity each void • Record quantity and characteristics each stool • I/O strict—weigh diapers before discarding
Medications	• Eval routine meds • Eval needs for IV fluids	• Eval routine meds • Eval needs for IV fluids
Discharge planning/ home care	• Eval Social Services/Visiting Nurse/DC planning needs • Possible home phototherapy • Follow-up bili level as outpatient • Follow-up visit with health care provider	• Offer CPR film/review • Give CPR booklet
Family involvement	• Eval additional psychosocial needs • Orient to room, unit, and equipment • Discuss possible side effects of phototherapy (stooling, increased fluid loss, increased/decreased temp, slight lethargy, rash, altered sleep/wake patterns) • Safety precautions (per age) • Discuss lab draws • Review illness and recovery • Circ care • Cord care • Placement of bili mask over eyes - close eyes • Clear nares • I/O • Meals for mom • Role of pumping breasts if necessary • Demos understanding of above	• Encourage parents to provide tactile stimulation during feeding and diaper changes • Provide cuddling and eye contact during feedings and talk to baby frequently • Provide opportunities for parents to express feelings • Demos understanding of above
Date		

nurse gives the instructions to the parents but also continues to monitor the infant's temperature, activity, intake and output, and positioning of eye patches at regular intervals (Table 26–4).

If the baby is to receive phototherapy at home, the nurse teaches the parents to record the infant's temperature, weight, fluid intake and output, stools, and feedings and to use the phototherapy equipment. In addition, if phototherapy lights are being used, parents must agree that the baby will be exposed to the lights for long periods of time; that they will hold the baby for only short periods for feedings, comforting, and cleansing of the perineal area; and that the room temperature will be regulated to minimize heat loss. Fiberoptic phototherapy blankets eliminate the need for eye patches, decrease heat loss because the baby is clothed, and provide more opportunities for interaction between the baby and parents. The best method of home phototherapy depends on the cause of the hyperbilirubinemia and the rate of progression of the jaundice.

Evaluation

Anticipated outcomes of nursing care include

- The risks for development of hyperbilirubinemia are identified and action is taken to minimize the potential impact of hyperbilirubinemia.
- The baby does not have any corneal irritation or drainage, skin breakdown, or major fluctuations in temperature.

TABLE 26–4 Instructional Checklist for In-Room Phototherapy

Explain and demonstrate the placement of eye patches and explain that they must be in place when the infant is under the lights.
Explain the clothing to be worn (diaper under lights, dress and wrap when away from the lights).
Explain the importance of taking the infant's temperature regularly.
Explain the importance of adequate fluid intake.
Explain the charting flow sheet (intake, output, eyes covered).
Explain how to position the lights at a proper distance.
Explain the need to keep the infant under phototherapy except during feeding and diaper changes.

- Parents understand the rationale for, goal of, and expected outcome of therapy.
- Parents verbalize their concerns about their baby's condition and identify how they can facilitate their baby's improvement.

Care of the Newborn with Hemorrhagic Disease

Several transient coagulation-mechanism deficiencies normally occur in the first several days of a newborn's life. Foremost among these is a slight decrease in the level of prothrombin, resulting in a prolonged clotting time during the initial week of life. Vitamin K is required for the liver to form prothrombin (factor II) and proconvertin (factor VII) for blood coagulation. Vitamin K, a fat-soluble vitamin, may be obtained from food, but it is usually synthesized by bacteria in the colon, and consequently a dietary source is unnecessary. However, since intestinal flora are practically nonexistent in newborns, they are unable to synthesize vitamin K.

Bleeding due to vitamin K deficiency generally occurs on the second or third day of life, but it may occur earlier in babies of mothers treated with phenytoin sodium (Dilantin) or phenobarbital. These drugs impair vitamin K activity, and bleeding may be seen at birth. Coumarin compounds are vitamin K antagonists that can cross the placenta. The baby exposed to maternal coumarin may manifest bleeding in the first 24 hours of life. Bleeding may also occur in babies receiving parenteral nutrition without adequate vitamin K additives (1 mg/week).

Bleeding from the nose, umbilical cord, circumcision site, gastrointestinal tract, and scalp may be seen, as well as generalized ecchymoses. Internal hemorrhage may occur.

This disorder can be completely prevented by a prophylactic injection of vitamin K. A dose of 1 mg of AquaMEPHYTON is given as part of newborn care immediately after birth, and consequently the disease is rarely seen today (see Drug Guide: Vitamin K_1 in Chapter 23). Larger doses are contraindicated because they may result in the development of hyperbilirubinemia (Snapp 1996).

Care of the Newborn with Anemia

Neonatal anemia is often difficult to recognize by clinical evaluation alone. The hemoglobin concentration in a term newborn is 15–20 g/dL, slightly higher than in prematures, in whom the mean hemoglobin is 14–18 g/dL. Infants with hemoglobin values of less than 14 g/dL (term) and 13 g/dL (preterm) are usually considered anemic. The most common causes of neonatal anemia are blood loss, hemolysis, and impaired red blood cell production.

Blood loss (hypovolemia) occurs in utero from placental bleeding (placenta previa or abruptio placentae). Intrapartal blood loss may be fetomaternal, fetofetal, or the result of umbilical cord bleeding. Birth trauma to abdominal organs or the cranium may produce significant blood loss, and cerebral bleeding may occur because of hypoxia.

Excessive hemolysis of red cells is usually a result of blood group incompatibilities but may be due to infections. The most common cause of impaired red cell production is a deficiency in G-6-PD, which is genetically transmitted. Anemia and jaundice are the presenting signs.

A condition known as **physiologic anemia** exists as a result of the normal gradual drop in hemoglobin for the first 6–12 weeks of life. Theoretically, the bone marrow stops production of red blood cells as a response to the elevated oxygenation of extrauterine respirations. When the amount of hemoglobin becomes lower, reaching levels of 10–11 g/dL at about 6–12 weeks of age, the bone marrow begins production of RBCs again, and the anemia disappears.

Anemia in preterm newborns occurs earlier and reversal by bone marrow is initiated at lower levels of hemoglobin (7–9 g/dL). The preterm baby's hemoglobin reaches a low sooner (4–8 weeks after birth) than does a term newborn's (6–12 weeks) because a preterm infant's red blood cell survival time is shorter than a term newborn's. This is due to two factors: The preterm infant's growth rate is relatively rapid, and a vitamin E deficiency is common in small preterm newborns.

Medical Therapy

Hematologic problems can be anticipated based on the pregnancy history and clinical manifestations. The age at which anemia is first noted is also of diagnostic value. Clinically, anemic infants are very pale in the absence of other symptoms of shock and usually have abnormally low red blood cell counts. In acute blood loss, symptoms of shock may be present, such as pallor, low arterial blood pressure, and a decreasing hematocrit value. The initial laboratory workup should include hemoglobin and hematocrit measurements, reticulocyte count, examination of peripheral blood smear, bilirubin determinations, direct Coombs' test of infant's blood, and examination of maternal blood smear for fetal erythrocytes (Kleihauer-Betke test). Medical management depends on the severity of the anemia and whether blood loss is acute or chronic. The baby should be placed on constant cardiac and respiratory monitoring. Mild or slow chronic anemia may be treated adequately with iron supplements alone or with iron-fortified formulas. Frequent determinations of hemoglobin, hematocrit, and bilirubin levels (in hemolytic disease) are essential. In severe cases of anemia, transfusions are the treatment of choice. Management of anemia of prematurity includes recombinant human erythropoietin, supplemental iron, and blood transfusions (Shannon 1995).

Nursing Care

The nurse assesses the newborn for symptoms of anemia (pallor). If the blood loss is acute, the baby may exhibit signs of shock. Continued observations will be necessary to identify physiologic anemia as the preterm newborn grows. Signs of compromise include poor weight gain, tachycardia, tachypnea, and apneic episodes. The nurse promptly reports any symptoms indicating anemia or shock. The amount of blood drawn for all laboratory tests should be recorded so that total blood removed can be assessed and replaced by transfusion when necessary. If the newborn exhibits signs of shock, the nurse may need to initiate interventions.

Care of the Newborn with Polycythemia

Polycythemia is a condition in which blood volume and hematocrit values increase. A common problem in low-risk nurseries, polycythemia affects 0.4 to 12 percent of newborns. It is commonly observed in SGA and term infants with delayed cord clamping, maternofetal and twin-to-twin transfusions, or chronic intrauterine hypoxia (Werner 1995).

An infant is considered polycythemic when the central venous hematocrit value is greater than 65 to 70 percent, or the venous hemoglobin level is greater than 22 g/dL during the first week of life.

Other conditions that present with polycythemia are chromosomal anomalies such as trisomy 21, 18, and 13; endocrine disorders such as hypoglycemia and hypocalcemia; and births at altitudes over 5000 feet.

Medical Therapy

The goal of therapy is to reduce the central venous hematocrit to a range of 50–55 percent in symptomatic infants. Treatment of asymptomatic infants is more controversial, but most authorities agree that these newborns benefit from a prophylactic exchange (Werner 1995). To decrease the red cell mass, the symptomatic infant receives a partial exchange transfusion in which blood is removed from the infant and replaced millimeter for millimeter with fresh plasma, plasmonate, or 5% albumin. Supportive treatment of presenting symptoms is required until resolution. This usually occurs spontaneously following the partial exchange transfusion.

Nursing Care

The nurse does an initial screening of the newborn's hematocrit on admission to the nursery. It is important to remember that if a capillary hematocrit is done, warming the heel before obtaining the blood helps to decrease falsely high values. Peripheral venous hematocrit samples are usually obtained from the antecubital fossa.

Many infants are asymptomatic, but symptomatic newborns have a characteristic plethoric (ruddy) appearance. The most common symptoms observed include

- Tachycardia and congestive heart failure due to the increased blood volume
- Respiratory distress with grunting, tachypnea, and cyanosis; increased oxygen need; or respiratory hemorrhage due to pulmonary venous congestion, edema, and hypoxemia
- Hyperbilirubinemia due to increased numbers of hemolysed red blood cells
- Decrease in peripheral pulses, discoloration of extremities, alteration in activity or neurologic depression, renal vein thrombosis with decreased urine output, hematuria, or proteinuria due to thromboembolism
- Seizures due to decreased perfusion of the brain and increased vascular resistance secondary to sluggish blood flow, which can result in neurologic or developmental problems

The nurse must observe closely for the signs of distress or change in vital signs during the partial exchange. The nurse must also assess carefully for potential complications resulting from the exchange such as transfusion overload (may result in congestive heart failure), irregular cardiac rhythm, bacterial infection, hypovolemia, and anemia.

Parents need specific explanations about polycythemia and its treatment. The newborn needs to be reunited with the parents as soon as the baby's status permits.

Care of the Newborn with Infection

Newborns up to 1 month of age are particularly susceptible to infection, referred to as **sepsis neonatorum,** by organisms that do not cause significant disease in older children. Once any infection occurs in the newborn, it can spread rapidly through the bloodstream, regardless of its primary site. The incidence of primary neonatal sepsis ranges from 7.3 to 16 per 1000 live births (Askin 1995). Nosocomial infection frequency ranges from 0.6–1.7 percent in normal newborn infants and from 0.9–18.2 percent in infants in the NICU (Payne et al 1994).

One predisposing factor is prematurity. Prematurity and low birth weight are associated with nosocomial infection rates up to 15 times higher than average (Payne et al 1994). The general debilitation and underlying illnesses often associated with prematurity necessitate invasive procedures such as umbilical catheterization, intubation, resuscitation, ventilator support, monitoring, and parenteral alimentation (especially lipid emulsions); and prior broad-spectrum antibiotic therapy. However, even full-term infants are susceptible, because their immunologic systems are immature. They lack the complex factors involved in effective phagocytosis and the ability to localize infection or to respond with a well-defined recognizable inflammatory response.

Most nosocomial infections in the NICU present as bacteremia/sepsis, urinary tract infections, meningitis, or pneumonia. Maternal antepartal infections such as rubella, toxoplasmosis, cytomegalic inclusion disease, and herpes may cause congenital infections and resulting disorders in the newborn. Intrapartal maternal infections, such as amnionitis and those resulting from premature rupture of membranes and precipitous birth, are also sources of neonatal infection (see Chapter 13 for more detailed information). Passage through the birth canal and contact with the vaginal flora (β-hemolytic streptococci, herpes, listeria, and gonococci) expose the infant to infection (Table 26–5). With infection anywhere in the fetus or newborn, the adjacent tissues or organs are very easily penetrated, and the blood-brain barrier is ineffective. Septicemia is more common in males, except for those infections caused by group B β-hemolytic streptococcus.

At present, gram-negative organisms (especially *E coli, Enterobacter, Proteus,* and *Klebsiella*) and the gram-positive organism β-hemolytic streptococcus are the most common causative agents. Pseudomonas is a common fomite contaminant of ventilator support and oxygen therapy equipment. Gram-positive bacteria, especially coagulase-negative staphylococci, are common pathogens in nosocomial bacteremias, pneumonias, and urinary tract infections. Other gram-positive bacteria frequently isolated are enterococci and *Staphylococcus aureus* (Gaynes et al 1996).

Protection of the newborn from infections starts prenatally and continues throughout pregnancy and birth. Prenatal prevention should include maternal screening for sexually transmitted infections and monitoring of rubella titers in women who are negative. Intrapartally, sterile technique is essential, smears from genital lesions are taken, and placenta and amniotic fluid cultures are obtained if amnionitis is suspected. If genital herpes is present toward term, cesarean birth may be indicated. Local eye treatment with silver nitrate or an antibiotic ophthalmic ointment is given to all newborns to prevent damage from gonococcal infection. Prophylactic antibiotic therapy, for asymptomatic GBS-culture-positive women during the intrapartum period, has been shown to be beneficial in preventing early-onset sepsis (Clay 1996).

Medical Therapy

Infants with a history of possible exposure to infection in utero (for example, premature rupture of membranes [PROM] more than 24 hours before birth or questionable maternal history of infection) should have cultures (gastric aspirate and ear canal) taken as soon after birth as possible. Cultures are obtained before antibiotic therapy is begun.

1. Two blood cultures are obtained from different peripheral sites. They are taken from a peripheral rather than an umbilical vessel, because catheters have yielded false positives resulting from contamination. The skin is prepared by cleaning with an antiseptic solution, such as one containing iodine, and allowed to dry; the specimen is obtained with a sterile needle and syringe.
2. Spinal fluid culture is done following a spinal tap.
3. The specimen for urine culture is best obtained by a suprapubic bladder aspiration.
4. Skin cultures are taken of any lesions or drainage from lesions or reddened areas.
5. Nasopharyngeal, rectal, ear canal, and gastric aspirate cultures may be obtained.

Other laboratory investigations include a complete blood count, chest x-ray examination, serology, and

TABLE 26–5 Maternally Transmitted Newborn Infections

Infection	Nursing Assessment	Nursing Plan and Implementation
Group B Streptococcus 1% to 2% colonized with one in ten developing disease. Early onset—usually within hours of birth or within first week. Late onset—1 week to 3 months.	Severe respiratory distress (grunting and cyanosis). May become apneic or demonstrate symptoms of shock. Meconium-stained amniotic fluid seen at birth.	Early assessment of clinical signs necessary. Assist with x-ray—shows aspiration pneumonia or hyaline membrane disease. Immediately obtain blood, gastric aspirate, external ear canal and nasopharynx cultures. Administer antibiotics, usually aqueous penicillin or ampicillin combined with gentamicin, as soon as cultures are obtained. Early assessment and intervention are essential to survival. Initiate referral to evaluate for blindness, deafness, learning or behavioral problems.
Syphilis Spirochetes cross placenta after 16th–18th week of gestation.	Check perinatal history for positive maternal serology. Assess infant for: Elevated cord serum IgM and FTA-ABS IgM Rhinitis (snuffles) Fissures on mouth corners and excoriated upper lip Red rash around mouth and anus Copper-colored rash over face, palms, and soles Irritability Generalized edema, particularly over joints; bone lesions; painful extremities Hepatosplenomegaly, jaundice Congenital cataracts SGA and failure to thrive	Initiate isolation techniques until infants have been on antibiotics for 48 hours. Administer penicillin. Provide emotional support for parents because of their feelings about mode of transmission and potential long-term sequelae.
Gonorrhea Approximately 30–35% of newborns born vaginally to infected mothers acquire the infection.	Assess for: Ophthalmia neonatorum (conjunctivitis) Purulent discharge and corneal ulcerations Neonatal sepsis with temperature instability, poor feeding response, and/or hypotonia, jaundice	Administer 1% silver nitrate solution or ophthalmic antibiotic ointment (see Drug Guide: Erythromycin [Ilotycin] Ophthalmic Ointment in Chapter 23) or, in lieu of silver nitrate, penicillin. Initiate follow-up referral to evaluate any loss of vision.
Herpes Type 2 1 in 7500 births (Lott 1994). Usually transmitted during vaginal birth; a few cases of in utero transmission have been reported.	Small cluster vesicular skin lesions over all the body. Check perinatal history for active herpes genital lesions. Disseminated form—DIC, pneumonia, hepatitis with jaundice, hepatosplenomegaly, and neurologic abnormalities. Without skin lesions, assess for fever or subnormal temperature, respiratory congestion, tachypnea, and tachycardia.	Carry out careful hand washing and gown and glove isolation with linen precautions. Administer intravenous vidarabine (Vira A) or acyclovir (Zovirax). Initiate follow-up referral to evaluate potential sequelae of microcephaly, spasticity, seizures, deafness, or blindness. Encourage parental rooming-in and touching of their newborn. Show parents appropriate hand-washing procedures and precautions to be used at home if mother's lesions are active. Obtain throat, conjunctiva, cerebral spinal fluid (CSF), blood, urine, and lesion cultures to identify herpesvirus type 2 antibiotics in serum IgM fraction. Cultures positive in 24–48 hours.
Oral Candidal Infection (Thrush) Acquired during passage through birth canal.	Assess newborn's buccal mucosa, tongue, gums, and inside the cheeks for white plaques (seen 5 to 7 days of age). Check diaper area for bright red, well-demarcated eruptions. Assess for thrush periodically when newborn is on long-term antibiotic therapy.	Differentiate white plaque areas from milk curds by using cotton tip applicator (if it is thrush, removal of white areas causes raw, bleeding areas). Maintain cleanliness of hands, linen, clothing, diapers, and feeding apparatus. Instruct breastfeeding mothers on treating their nipples with nystatin. Administer gentian violet (1% to 2%) swabbed on oral lesions 1 hour after feeding or nystatin instilled in baby's oral cavity and on mucosa. Swab skin lesions with topical nystatin. Discuss with parents that gentian violet stains mouth and clothing. Avoid placing gentian violet on normal mucosa; it causes irritation.
Chlamydia Trachomatis Acquired during passage through birth canal.	Assess for perinatal history of preterm birth. Symptomatic newborns present with pneumonia—conjunctivitis after 3–4 days. Chronic follicular conjunctivitis (corneal neovascularization and conjunctival scarring).	Instill ophthalmic erythromycin (see Drug Guide: Erythromycin [Ilotycin] Ophthalmic Ointment in Chapter 23). Initiate follow-up referral for eye complications and late development of pneumonia at 4–11 weeks postnatally.

TABLE 26–6 Neonatal Sepsis Antibiotic Therapy

Drug	Dose (mg/kg) Total Daily Dose	Schedule for Divided Doses	Route	Comments
Ampicillin	50–100 mg/kg	Every 12 hours* Every 8 hours†	IM or IV	Effective against gram-positive microorganisms, *Haemophilus influenzae,* and majority of *E coli* strains. Higher doses indicated for meningitis. Used with aminoglycoside for synergy.
Cefotaxime	50 mg/kg 100–150 mg/kg/day	Every 12 hours* Every 8 hours†	IM or IV	Active against most major pathogens in infants; effective against aminoglycoside-resistant organisms; achieves CSF bactericidal activity; lack of ototoxicity and nephrotoxicity; wide therapeutic index (levels not required); resistant organisms can develop rapidly if used extensively; ineffective against pseudomonas, listeria.
Gentamicin	2.5–3 mg/kg 5.0–7.5 mg/kg/day	Every 12–24 hours* § Every 8–24 hours†	IM or IV	Effective against gram-negative rods and staphylococci; may be used instead of kanamycin against penicillin-resistant staphylococci and *E coli* strains and *Pseudomonas aeruginosa.* May cause ototoxicity and nephrotoxicity. Need to follow serum levels. Must never be given as IV push. Must be given over at least 30–60 minutes. In presence of oliguria or anuria, dose must be decreased or discontinued. In infants less than 1000 g or 29 weeks, lower dosage 2.5–3.0 mg/kg/day. Monitor serum levels before administration of second dose. Peak 5–10 μg/mL Trough 1–2 μg/mL
Methicillin	25–50 mg/dose 50–100 mg/kg/day	Every 12 hours* Every 6–8 hours†	IM or IV	Effective against penicillinase-resistant staphylococci. Monitor CBC and UA. Slow IV push.
Nafcillin	25–50 mg/kg 50–100 mg/kg/day	Every 8–12 hours* Every 6–8 hours†	IM or IV	Effective against penicillinase-resistant staphylococci. Caution in presence of jaundice.
Penicillin G (aqueous crystalline)	25,000–50,000 IU/kg 50,000–125,000 IU/kg/day	Every 12 hours* Every 8 hours†	IM or IV	Initial sepsis therapy effective against most gram-positive microorganisms except resistant staphylococci; can cause heart block in infants.
Vancomycin	10–20 mg/kg 30 mg/kg/day	Every 12–24 hours* § Every 8 hours†	IV	Effective for methicillin-resistant strains *(S epidermidis);* must be administered by slow intravenous infusion to avoid prolonged cutaneous eruption. For smaller infants <1200 g; <29 weeks, smaller dosages and longer intervals between doses. Nephrotoxic, especially when given in combination with aminoglycosides. Slow IV infusion over 60 minutes. Peak 25–40 μg/mL Trough 5–10 μg/mL

*Up to seven days of age.
†Greater than seven days of age.
§Dependent on GA.

gram stains of cerebrospinal fluid, urine, skin exudate, and umbilicus. White blood count (WBC) with differential may indicate the presence or absence of sepsis. A level of 30,000 WBC may be normal in the first 24 hours of life, while a low WBC may be indicative of sepsis. A low neutrophil count and a high band (immature white cells) count indicate that an infection is present. Stomach aspirate should be sent for culture and smear if a gonococcal infection or amnionitis is suspected. C-reactive protein may or may not be elevated. Serum IgM levels are elevated (normal level less than 20 mg/dL) in response to transplacental infections. If available, counterimmuno-electrophoresis tests for specific bacterial antigens are done.

Evidence of congenital infections may be seen on skull x-ray films for cerebral calcifications (cytomegalovirus, toxoplasmosis), on bone x-ray films (syphilis, cytomegalovirus), and in serum-specific IgM levels (rubella). Cytomegalovirus infection is best diagnosed by urine culture.

Because neonatal infection causes high mortality, therapy is instituted before results of the septic workup are obtained. A combination of two broad spectrum antibiotics, such as ampicillin and gentamicin, is given in large doses until culture with sensitivities is obtained.

After the pathogen and its sensitivities are determined, appropriate specific antibiotic therapy is begun. Combinations of penicillin or ampicillin and kanamycin have been used in the past, but new kanamycin-resistant enterobacteria and penicillin-resistant staphylococcus necessitate increasing use of gentamicin.

Rotating aminoglycosides has been suggested to prevent development of resistance. Use of cephalosporins and, in particular, cefotaxime, has emerged as an alternative to aminoglycoside therapy in the treatment of neonatal infections. Duration of therapy varies from 7 to 14 days (Table 26–6). If cultures are negative and symptoms subside, antibiotics may be discontinued after 3 days. Supportive physiologic care may be required to maintain respiratory, hemodynamic, nutritional, and metabolic homeostasis.

APPLYING THE NURSING PROCESS

Nursing Assessment

Symptoms are most often noticed by the nurse during daily care of the newborn rather than during the infant's sporadic contact with the physician. The infant may deteriorate rapidly in the first 12 to 24 hours after birth if β-hemolytic streptococcal infection is present, with signs and symptoms mimicking RDS. On the other hand, the onset of sepsis may be more gradual with more subtle signs and symptoms. The most common signs observed include the following:

1. Subtle behavioral changes—the infant "isn't doing well" and is often lethargic or irritable (especially after first 24 hours) and hypotonic. Color changes may include pallor, duskiness, cyanosis, or a "shocky" appearance. Skin is cool and clammy.
2. Temperature instability, manifested by either hypothermia (recognized by a decrease in skin temperature) or hyperthermia (elevation of skin temperature) necessitating a corresponding increase or decrease in Isolette temperature to maintain neutral thermal environment.
3. Poor feeding, evidenced by a decrease in total intake, abdominal distention, vomiting, poor sucking, lack of interest in feeding, and diarrhea.
4. Hyperbilirubinemia.
5. There is initially tachycardia, followed by spells of apnea/bradycardia.

Signs and symptoms may suggest CNS disease (jitteriness, tremors, seizure activity), respiratory system disease (tachypnea, labored respirations, apnea, cyanosis), hematologic disease (jaundice, petechial hemorrhages, hepatosplenomegaly), or gastrointestinal disease (diarrhea, vomiting, bile-stained aspirate, hepatomegaly). A differential diagnosis is necessary because of the similarity of symptoms to other more specific conditions.

Nursing Diagnosis

Nursing diagnoses that may apply to the infant with sepsis neonatorum include the following:

- Infection: high risk related to immature immunologic system
- Fluid volume deficit related to feeding intolerance
- Ineffective family coping related to present illness resulting in prolonged hospital stay for the newborn

Nursing Plan and Implementation

Prevention of Infection

In the nursery, environmental control and prevention of acquired infection are the responsibilities of the neonatal nurse. The nurse must promote strict hand-washing technique for all who enter the nursery, including nursing colleagues; physicians; laboratory, x-ray, and respiratory therapists; and parents. The nurse must be prepared to assist in the aseptic collection of laboratory specimens. Scrupulous care of equipment—changing and cleaning of incubators at least every 7 days, removal and sterilization of wet equipment every 24 hours, prevention of cross-use of linen and equipment, and special care with the open radiant warmers (access without prior hand washing is much more likely than with the closed incubator)—will prevent fomite contamination or contamination through improper hand washing. An infected newborn can be effectively isolated in an incubator and receive close observation. Visiting the nursery area by unnecessary personnel should be discouraged.

Provision of Antibiotic Therapy

The nurse administers antibiotics as ordered by the clinician. The nurse is responsible to be knowledgeable about

- The proper dose to be administered, based on the weight of the newborn and desired peak and trough levels
- The appropriate route of administration, as some antibiotics cannot be given intravenously
- Admixture incompatibilities, since some antibiotics are precipitated by intravenous solutions or by other antibiotics
- Side effects and toxicity

Provision of Supportive Care

In addition to antibiotic therapy, physiologic supportive care is essential in caring for a septic infant (Askin 1995). The nurse should

- Observe for resolution of symptoms or development of other symptoms of sepsis
- Maintain neutral thermal environment with accurate regulation of humidity and oxygen administration
- Provide respiratory support by administering oxygen and observing and monitoring respiratory effort
- Provide cardiovascular support by observing and monitoring pulse and blood pressure and observing for hyperbilirubinemia, anemia, and hemorrhagic symptoms
- Provide adequate calories, because oral feedings may be discontinued because of increased mucus, abdominal distention, vomiting, and aspiration

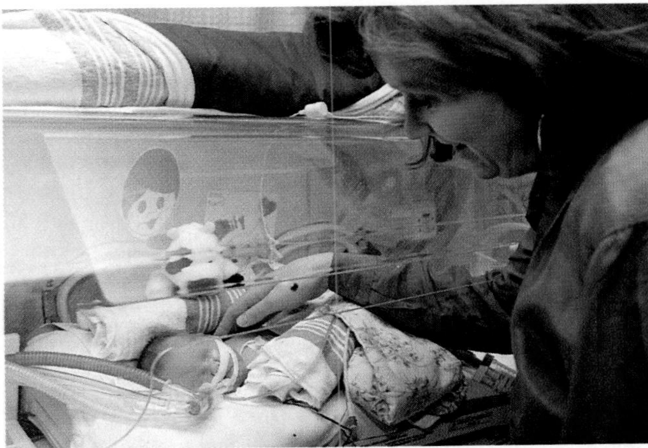

FIGURE 26–12 When parents participate in their baby's care, they tend to have realistic expectations about the child's long-term developmental needs.

- Provide fluids and electrolytes to maintain homeostasis and monitor weight changes, urine output, and urine specific gravity
- Detect and treat metabolic disturbances, which are common
- Observe for the development of hypoglycemia, hyperglycemia, acidosis, hyponatremia, and hypocalcemia

Restriction of parent visits has not been shown to have any effect on the rate of infection and may indeed be harmful for the newborn's psychologic development. With instruction and guidance from the nurse, both parents should be allowed to handle the baby and participate in daily care. Support of the parents is crucial. They need to be informed of the newborn's prognosis as treatment continues and to be involved in care as much as possible (Figure 26–12). They also need to understand how infection is transmitted.

Evaluation

Anticipated outcomes of nursing care include

- The risks for development of sepsis are identified early, and immediate action is taken to minimize the development of the illness.
- Appropriate use of aseptic technique protects the newborn from further exposure to illness.
- The baby's symptoms are relieved, and the infection is treated.
- The parents verbalize their concerns about their baby's illness and understand the rationale behind the management of their newborn.

CHAPTER HIGHLIGHTS

- The sick newborn—whether preterm, term, or postterm—must be managed within narrow physiologic parameters.
- These parameters (respiratory and thermal regulation) will maintain physiologic homeostasis and prevent introduction of iatrogenic stress to the already stressed infant.
- The nursing care of the newborn with special problems involves the understanding of normal physiology, the pathophysiology of the disease process, clinical manifestations, and supportive or corrective therapies. Only with this theoretical background can the newborn nurse make appropriate observations concerning responses to therapy and development of complications.
- Asphyxia results in significant circulatory, respiratory, and biochemical changes in the newborn that make the successful transition to extrauterine life difficult. Asphyxia requires early identification and resuscitative management.
- Newborn conditions that commonly present with respiratory distress and require oxygen and ventilator assistance are respiratory distress syndrome, meconium aspiration syndrome, and transient tachypnea of the newborn.
- Cold stress sets up the chain of physiologic events of hypoglycemia, pulmonary vasoconstriction, hyperbilirubinemia, respiratory distress, and metabolic acidosis. Nurses are responsible for early detection and initiation of treatment for hypoglycemia.
- Differentiation between pathologic and physiologic jaundice is the key to early and successful intervention.
- Anemia (decreased amount of red blood cell volume) or polycythemia (excess amount) place the newborn at risk for alterations in blood flow and the oxygen-carrying capacity of the blood.
- Nursing assessment of the septic newborn involves identification of very subtle clinical signs that are also seen in other clinical disease states.
- The nurse is the facilitator for interdisciplinary communication with the parents, identifying their understanding of their infant's care and their needs for emotional support.
- Parents of at-risk newborns need support from nurses and health care providers to understand the special needs of their baby and to feel comfortable in an overwhelmingly strange environment.

REFERENCES

American Academy of Pediatrics: Practice parameter: Management of hyperbilirubineamia in the healthy term newborn. *Pediatrics* 1994; 94(4):558.

Askin DF: Bacterial and fungal infections in the neonate. *JOGNN* 1995; 24(7):635.

Bloom RS, Cropley C: *Textbook of Neonatal Resuscitation.* Elk Grove Village, IL: American Heart Association and American Academy of Pediatrics, 1994.

Brooks C: Neonatal hypoglycemia. *Neonatal Network* 1997; 16(2):15.

Cole MD, Peevy K: Hypoglycemia in normal neonates appropriate for gestational age. *J Perinatol* 1994; 14(2):118.

Connolly AM, Volpe JJ: Clinical features of bilirubin encephalopathy. *Clin Perinatol* 1990; 17(2):371.

Dennery PA, Rhine WD, Stevenson DK: Neonatal jaundice: What now? *Clin Pediatr* February 1995:103.

Ennever JF: Blue light, green light, white light, more light: treatment of neonatal jaundice. *Clin Perinatol* 1990; 17(2):467.

Findlay RD, Taeusch HW, Walther FJ: Surfactant replacement therapy for meconium aspiration syndrome. *Pediatrics* 1996; 97(1):48.

Gartner LM: Neonatal jaundice. *Pediatr in Rev* 1994; 15(11):422.

Gaynes RP et al: Nosocomial infections among neonates in high risk nurseries in the United States. *Pediatrics* 1996; 98(3):357.

Gill NE et al: Effect of nonnutritive sucking on behavioral state in preterm infants before feeding. *Nurs Res* 1988; 37(8):344.

Glomella TL: *Neonatology: Management, Procedures, On-Call Problems, Diseases, and Drugs,* 3rd ed. Norwalk, CT: Appleton and Lange, 1994.

Greenough A: Meconium aspiration syndrome: Prevention and treatment. *Early Hum Develop* 1995; 41:183.

Hanna D: Guidelines for pulse oximetry use in pediatrics. *J Pediatr Nurs* 1995; 10(2):124.

Hicks MA: A systematic approach to neonatal pathophysiology: Understanding respiratory distress syndrome. *Neonatal Network* 1995; 14(1):29.

Jepson HA, Talashek ML, Tichy AM: The Apgar score: Evolution, limitations, and scoring guidelines. *Birth* 1991; 18(2):83.

Krause K, Younger V: Nursing diagnoses as guidelines in the care of the neonatal ECMO patient. *JOGNN* 1992; 21(3):169.

Merenstein GB, Gardner SL: *Handbook of Neonatal Intensive Care,* 3rd ed. St Louis: Mosby, 1993.

Newman TB, Maisels MJ: Evaluation and treatment of jaundice in the term newborn: A kinder, gentler approach. *Pediatrics* 1992; 89(5):809.

Nugent J: *Acute Respiratory Care of the Neonate.* Petaluma, CA: NICU Ink, 1991.

Osborne SE, Kassity NA: Neonatal resuscitation program update. *Neonatal Intensive Care* 1993; 6(7): 32.

Page S: Rh hemolytic disease of the newborn. *Neonatal Network* 1989; 7(6):31.

Payne NR, Schilling CG, Steinberg S: Selecting antibiotics for nosocomial bacterial infections in patients requiring neonatal intensive care. *Neonatal Network* 1994; 13(3):41.

Poets CF, Southall DP: Noninvasive monitoring of oxygenation in infants and children: Practical considerations and areas of concern. *Pediatrics* 1994; 3(5):737.

Shannon K: Recombinant human erythropoietin in neonatal anemia. *Clin Perinatol* 1995; 22(3):627.

Snapp B: Hemorrhagic disease of the newborn and vitamin K. *Mother Baby J* 1996; 1(4):17.

Sunnehag A, Gustafsson, Ewald U: Very immature infants (<30 wk) respond to glucose infusion with incomplete suppression of glucose production. *Pediatr Res* 1994; 36(4):550.

Taeusch HW, Ballard RA, Avery ME (editors): *Schaffer Avery's Diseases of the Newborn,* 6th ed. Philadelphia: Saunders, 1991.

Tan KL: Comparison of the efficacy of fiberoptic and conventional phototherapy for neonatal hyperbilirubinemia. *J Pediatr* 1994; 125(4):607.

Verma RP: Respiratory distress syndrome of the newborn infant. *Obstet Gynecol Surv* 1995; 50(7):542.

Werner EJ: Neonatal polycythemia and hyperviscosity. *Clin Perinatol* 1995; 22(3):693.

Young TE, Mangum OB: *Neofax®: A Manual of Drugs Used in Neonatal Care,* 9th ed. Raleigh, NC: Acorn Publishing, 1996.

Part Five | Postpartum

I had heard about the negatives—the fatigue, the loneliness, loss of self. But nobody told me about the wonderful parts: holding my baby close to me, seeing her first smile, watching her grow and become more responsive day by day. . . . For the first time I cared about somebody else more than myself, and I would do anything to nurture and protect her.

—The New Our Bodies, Ourselves—

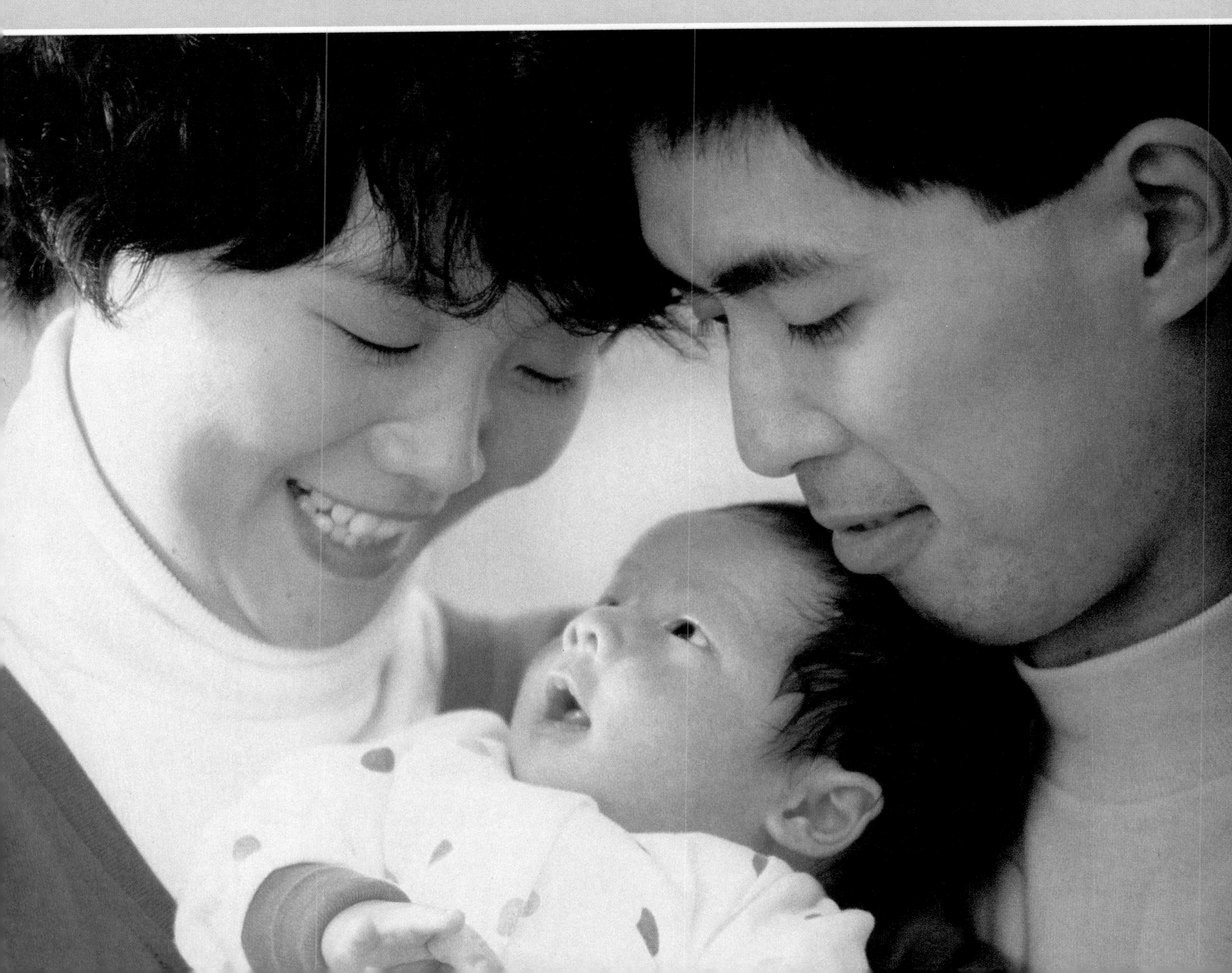

Chapter 27 Postpartal Adaptation and Nursing Assessment

OBJECTIVES

- Describe the basic physiologic changes that occur in the postpartal period as a woman's body returns to its prepregnant state.
- Discuss the psychologic adjustments that normally occur during the postpartal period.
- Summarize the factors that influence the development of parent-infant attachment.
- Delineate a normal postpartal assessment.
- Discuss the physical and developmental tasks that the mother must accomplish during the postpartal period.

KEY TERMS

Afterpains
Boggy uterus
Diastasis recti abdominis
En face
Engrossment
Fundus
Involution
Lochia
Lochia alba
Lochia rubra
Lochia serosa
Postpartum blues
Puerperium
Reciprocity

The **puerperium,** or postpartal period, is the period during which the woman adjusts, physically and psychologically, to the process of childbirth. It begins immediately after birth and continues for approximately 6 weeks or until the body has returned to a near prepregnant state. This chapter describes the physiologic and psychologic changes that occur postpartally and the basic aspects of a thorough postpartal assessment.

Postpartal Physical Adaptations

Comprehensive nursing assessment is based on a sound understanding of the normal anatomic and physiologic processes of the puerperium. These processes involve the reproductive organs and other major body systems.

Reproductive Organs

Involution of the Uterus

The term **involution** is used to describe the rapid reduction in size and the return of the uterus to a nonpregnant state.

Following separation of the placenta, the decidua of the uterus is irregular, jagged, and varied in thickness. The spongy layer of the decidua is cast off as lochia, while the inner layer forms the basis for the development of new endometrium. Except at the placenta attachment site, this process takes about 3 weeks. Bleeding from the larger uterine vessels of the placenta site is controlled by compression of the retracted uterine muscle fibers. The clotted blood is gradually absorbed by the body. Some of these vessels are eventually obliterated and replaced by new vessels with smaller lumens.

Rather than forming a fibrous scar in the decidua, the placenta site heals by a process of exfoliation. In this process, the site is undermined by the growth of the endometrial tissue both from the margins of the site and from the fundi of the endometrial glands left in the basal layer of the site. The infarcted superficial tissue then becomes necrotic and is sloughed off.

Exfoliation is a very important aspect of involution. If healing of the placenta site left a fibrous scar, the area available for future implantation would be limited, as would the number of possible pregnancies.

The uterus gradually decreases in size as the cells grow smaller and the hyperplasia of pregnancy reverses. Protein material in the uterine wall is broken down and absorbed. The process is basically one of cell size reduction rather than a radical decrease in cell number.

Factors that slow uterine involution include prolonged labor, anesthesia or excessive analgesia, difficult birth, grandmultiparity, a full bladder, and incomplete expulsion of all of the placenta or fragments of the membranes. Factors that enhance involution include an uncomplicated labor and birth, complete expulsion of the placenta or membranes, breastfeeding, and early ambulation.

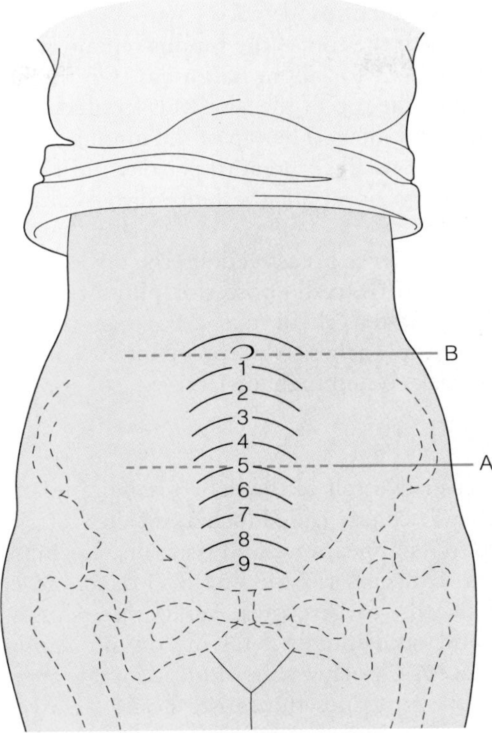

FIGURE 27–1 Involution of the uterus. ***A*** Immediately after delivery of the placenta, the top of the fundus is in the midline and approximately halfway between the symphysis pubis and the umbilicus. ***B*** About 6 to 12 hours after birth, the fundus is at the level of the umbilicus. The height of the fundus then decreases about one fingerbreadth (approximately 1 cm) each day.

Changes in Fundal Position

Immediately following the birth of the placenta, the uterus contracts to the size of a large grapefruit. The **fundus,** or top portion of the uterus, is situated in the midline midway between the symphysis pubis and the umbilicus (Figure 27–1). The walls of the contracted uterus are in close proximity, and the uterine blood vessels are firmly compressed by the myometrium. Within 6 to 12 hours after birth, the fundus of the uterus rises to the level of the umbilicus. A fundus that is above the umbilicus and is **boggy** (feels soft and spongy rather than firm and well contracted) is associated with excessive uterine bleeding. As blood collects and forms clots within the uterus, the fundus rises and firm contractions of the uterine muscles are interrupted. When the fundus is higher than expected on palpation and is not in the midline (usually deviated to the right), distention of the bladder should be suspected.

After birth the top of the fundus remains at the level of the umbilicus for about half a day. On the first postpartum day, the top of the fundus is located about 1 cm below the umbilicus. The top of the fundus descends approximately one fingerbreadth per day until it descends into the pelvis on about the tenth day (Blackburn and Loper 1992).

If the mother is breastfeeding, the release of endogenous oxytocin from the posterior pituitary in response to suckling hastens this process. Barring complications, the uterus approaches its prepregnant size and location by 5–6 weeks (Cunningham 1997).

Lochia

The uterus rids itself of the debris remaining after birth through a discharge called **lochia,** which is classified according to its appearance and contents. **Lochia rubra** is dark red. It occurs for the first 2–3 days and contains epithelial cells, erythrocytes, leukocytes, shreds of decidua, and occasionally fetal meconium, lanugo, and vernix caseosa. Lochia should not contain large (plum-sized) clots; if it does the cause should be investigated without delay. **Lochia serosa** is a pinkish color. It follows from about the third until the tenth day. Lochia serosa is composed of serous exudate (hence the name), shreds of degenerating decidua, erythrocytes, leukocytes, cervical mucus, and numerous microorganisms. Gradually the red blood cell component decreases, and **lochia alba,** a creamy or yellowish discharge, persists for an additional week or two. This final discharge is composed primarily of leukocytes, decidual cells, epithelial cells, fat, cervical mucus, cholesterol crystals, and bacteria. When the lochia stops, the cervix is considered closed, and chances of infection ascending from the vagina to the uterus decrease.

Like menstrual discharge, lochia has a musty, stale odor that is not offensive. Foul-smelling lochia suggests infection and should be assessed promptly.

The total volume of lochia is about 240–270 mL, and the volume gradually declines with each passing day. The amount of discharge is greater in the morning due to pooling in the vagina and uterus while the mother lies sleeping. The amount of lochia may also be increased by exertion or breastfeeding.

Evaluation of lochia is necessary not only to determine the presence of hemorrhage but also to assess uterine involution. The type, amount, and consistency of lochia determine the stage of healing of the placenta site, and a progressive change from bright red at birth to dark red to pink to white/clear discharge should be observed. Persistent discharge of lochia rubra or a return to lochia rubra indicates subinvolution or late postpartal hemorrhage (see Chapter 30).

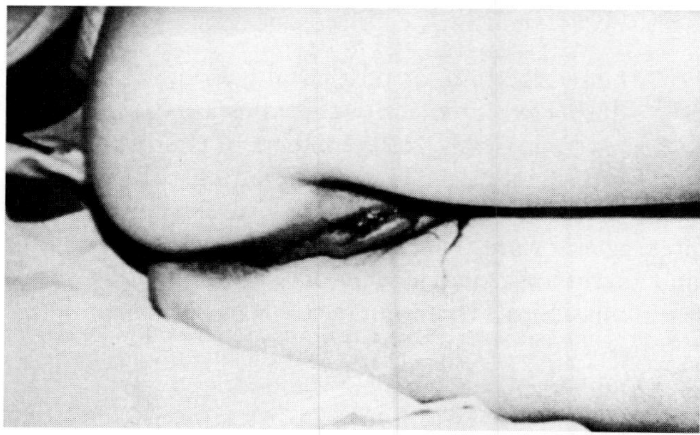

FIGURE 27–2 Bruising and edema of the vulva and perineum in a primipara 3 days after a forceps delivery.

Source: Bennett VR and Brown LK: *Myles Textbook for Midwives,* 11th ed. Edinburgh: Churchill Livingstone, 1989. Page 235, Figure 16–2.

Cervical Changes

Following birth the cervix is flabby and formless and may appear bruised. The external os is markedly irregular and closes slowly. It admits two fingers for a few days following birth, but by the end of the first week it will admit only a fingertip.

The shape of the external os is permanently changed by the first childbearing. The characteristic dimplelike os of the nullipara changes to the lateral slit (fish-mouth) os of the multipara. After significant cervical laceration or several lacerations, the cervix may appear lopsided.

Vaginal Changes

Following birth the vagina appears edematous and may be bruised. Small superficial lacerations may be evident, and the rugae have been obliterated. The apparent bruising is due to pelvic congestion and will quickly disappear. The hymen, torn and jagged, heals irregularly, leaving small tags called the carunculae myrtiformes.

The size of the vagina decreases and rugae return within 3 weeks. This facilitates the gradual return to smaller, although not nulliparous, dimensions. By 6 weeks the nonlactating woman's vagina usually appears normal. The lactating woman is in a hypoestrogenic state because of ovarian suppression, and her vaginal mucosa may be pale and without rugae. This may lead to dyspareunia (painful intercourse) (Zlatnik 1994). Tone and contractility of the vaginal orifice may be improved by perineal tightening exercises such as Kegel's (see Chapter 9). The labia majora and labia minora are more flaccid in the woman who has born a child than in the nullipara.

Perineal Changes

During the early postpartal period the soft tissue in and around the perineum may appear edematous with some bruising (Figure 27–2). If an episiotomy is present, the edges should be drawn together. Occasionally ecchymosis occurs, and this may delay healing.

Recurrence of Ovulation and Menstruation

The return of menstruation and ovulation varies for each postpartal woman. Menstruation generally returns in nonnursing mothers between 6 and 10 weeks after birth, and 50 percent of the first cycles are anovulatory (Blackburn and Loper 1992). Overall, 40 percent of nonnursing mothers resume menstruation by 6 weeks, while 90 percent resume within 24 weeks after birth.

The return of menstruation and ovulation in nursing mothers is usually prolonged and is associated with the length of time the woman breastfeeds and whether formula supplements are used. If a nursing mother breastfeeds for less than 1 month, the return of menstruation and ovulation is similar to that of the nonnursing mother. In women who continue to breastfeed, the average time for the return of menstruation is 30–36 weeks, and 17–28 weeks for the return of ovulation (Blackburn and Loper 1992).

Abdomen

Following birth the stretched abdominal wall appears loose and flabby, but it will respond to exercise within 2–3 months. In the grandmultipara, in the woman in whom overdistention of the abdomen has occurred, or in the woman with poor muscle tone before pregnancy, the abdomen may fail to regain good tone and will remain flabby. **Diastasis recti abdominis**, a separation of the abdominal muscle, may occur with pregnancy, especially in women with poor abdominal muscle tone. If diastasis occurs, part of the abdominal wall has no muscular support but is formed only by skin, subcutaneous fat, fascia, and peritoneum. If rectus muscle tone is not regained, support may be inadequate during future pregnancies. This may result in a pendulous abdomen and increased maternal backache. Fortunately, diastasis responds well to exercise and abdominal muscle tone can improve significantly. (See Figure 28–1 for a discussion of postpartal exercises.)

Striae (stretch marks), which are caused by stretching and rupture of the elastic fibers of the skin, are red to purple at the time of birth. These gradually fade and after a time appear as silver or white streaks.

Lactation

During pregnancy, breast development in preparation for lactation results from the influence of both estrogen and progesterone. After birth, the interplay of maternal hormones leads to milk production. For further details, see the section on breastfeeding in Chapter 25.

Gastrointestinal System

Hunger following birth is common, and the mother may enjoy a light meal. She may also be quite thirsty and will drink large amounts of fluid. This helps replace fluids lost in labor, in the urine, and through perspiration.

The bowels tend to be sluggish following birth because of the lingering effects of progesterone and decreased abdominal muscle tone. Women who have had an episiotomy may tend to delay elimination for fear of increasing their pain or in the belief that their stitches will be torn if they bear down. In refusing or delaying the bowel movement, the woman may cause increased constipation and more pain when bowel elimination finally occurs.

The woman with a cesarean birth may receive clear liquids shortly after surgery and, once bowel sounds are present, the diet is quickly advanced to solid food. The woman may experience some initial discomfort from flatulence. This is relieved by early ambulation and use of antiflatulent medications. It may take a few days for the bowel to regain its tone, especially if general anesthesia was used.

Urinary Tract

The postpartal woman has an increased bladder capacity, swelling and bruising of the tissue around the urethra, decreased sensitivity to fluid pressure, and a decreased sensation of bladder filling. Consequently, she is at risk for overdistention, incomplete emptying, and a buildup of residual urine. Women who have had an anesthetic block have inhibited neural functioning of the bladder and are more susceptible to bladder distention, difficulty voiding, and bladder infections.

Puerperal diuresis causes rapid filling of the bladder. Thus adequate bladder elimination is an immediate concern. Stasis increases the chances that a urinary tract infection will develop. A full bladder may also increase the tendency toward uterine relaxation by displacing the uterus and interfering with contractility, all of which may lead to hemorrhage.

In the absence of infection, the dilated ureters and renal pelves will return to prepregnant size by the end of the sixth week.

Vital Signs

A temperature of up to 38C (100.4F) may occur after birth as a result of the exertion and dehydration of labor. After the first 24 hours, the woman should be afebrile, and any temperature of 38C (100.4F) or greater suggests infection. (See discussion in Chapter 30.)

Blood pressure readings should remain stable after birth. A decrease may indicate physiologic readjustment to decreased intrapelvic pressure, or it may be related to uterine hemorrhage. Blood pressure elevations, especially when accompanied by headache, suggest pregnancy-induced hypertension (PIH), and the woman should be evaluated further.

Puerperal bradycardia with rates of 50–70 beats per minute commonly occurs during the first 6–10 days of the postpartal period. It may be related to decreased cardiac effort, the decreased blood volume following placental separation and contraction of the uterus, and increased stroke volume. Tachycardia occurs less frequently and is related to increased blood loss or difficult, prolonged labor and birth.

Blood Values

Blood values should return to the prepregnant state by the end of the postpartal period. Pregnancy-associated activation of coagulation factors may continue for variable amounts of time within the postpartal period. This condition, in conjunction with trauma, immobility, or sepsis, predisposes the woman to development of thromboembolism.

Leukocytosis often occurs, with white blood counts of 15,000–20,000/mL. Hemoglobin and hematocrit levels may be difficult to interpret in the first 2 days after birth because of the changing blood volume. In general, a decrease of two percentage points from the hematocrit done on admission to the birthing unit indicates a blood loss of 500 mL (Varney 1987).

Hemoglobin and hematocrit values should approximate or exceed prelabor values within 2–6 weeks as normal concentrations are reached. As extracellular fluid is excreted, hemoconcentration coincides with a rise in hematocrit.

Weight Loss

An initial weight loss of about 10–12 lb occurs as a result of the birth of infant, placenta, and amniotic fluid. Puerperal diuresis accounts for the loss of an additional 5 lb during the early puerperium. By the sixth to eighth week after birth, many women have returned to approximately prepregnant weight if they gained the average 25–30 lb. For others, a return to prepregnant weight takes longer.

Postpartal Chill

Frequently the mother experiences a shaking chill immediately after birth, which is related to a nervous response or to vasomotor changes. If not followed by fever, this chill is of no clinical concern, but it is uncomfortable for the woman. The woman's comfort may be increased by covering her with a warmed blanket and encouraging her to relax. Some women may also find a warm beverage helpful. Later in the puerperium, chill and fever indicate infection and require further evaluation.

Postpartal Diaphoresis

The elimination of excess fluid and waste products via the skin during the puerperium produces greatly increased perspiration. Diaphoretic (sweating) episodes frequently occur at night, and the woman may awaken drenched with perspiration. This perspiration is not significant clinically, but the mother should be protected from chilling.

Afterpains

Afterpains more commonly occur in multiparas than primiparas and are caused by intermittent uterine contractions. Although the uterus of the primipara usually remains consistently contracted, the lost tone of the multiparous uterus results in alternate contraction and relaxation. This phenomenon also occurs if the uterus has been markedly distended, as with a multiple pregnancy or hydramnios, or if clots or placental fragments were retained. These afterpains may cause the mother severe discomfort for 2–3 days after birth. The administration of oxytocic agents stimulates uterine contraction and increases the discomfort of the afterpains. Because endogenous oxytocin is released when the infant suckles, breastfeeding also increases the severity of the afterpains. The nursing mother may find it helpful to take a mild analgesic approximately 1 hour before feeding her infant. The nurse can assure the nursing mother that the prescribed analgesics are not harmful to the newborn and help improve the quality of the breastfeeding experience. An analgesic is also helpful at bedtime if the afterpains interfere with the mother's rest.

Postpartal Psychologic Adaptations

Maternal Role

The postpartal period is a time of readjustment and adaptation for the entire childbearing family, but especially for the mother. The woman experiences a variety of responses as she adjusts to a new family member, postpartum discomforts, changes in her body image, and the reality that she is no longer pregnant. During the first day or two after birth, the woman tends to be passive and somewhat dependent. She follows suggestions, hesitates to make decisions, and is still rather preoccupied with her needs. She may have a great need to talk about her perceptions of her labor and birth. This helps her work through the process, sort out the reality from her fantasized experience, and clarify anything that she did not understand. Food and sleep are major focuses. In her early work, Rubin (1961) labeled this the *taking-in* period.

By the second or third day after birth, the new mother is ready to resume control over her life. She may be concerned about controlling her bodily functions such as elimination. If she is breastfeeding, she may worry about the quality of her milk and her ability to nurse her baby. If her baby spits up after a feeding, she may view it as a personal failure. She may also feel that the nurse handles her baby more proficiently than she does. She requires assurance that she is doing well as a mother. Rubin (1961) labeled this the *taking-hold* period.

Today's mothers seem to be more independent and to adjust more rapidly. Ament (1990) found that women did exhibit behavior characteristic of "taking-in" and "taking-hold" but found that the time periods were shorter than those cited by Rubin.

Postpartally the woman must adjust to a changed body image. Women often express dissatisfaction about their appearance and concern about the return of their weight and figure to normal. Multiparas tend to be more positive than primiparas. This may be because the multipara's previous experience has prepared her for the fact that the body does not immediately return to a prepregnant state.

The psychologic outcomes of the postpartal period are far more positive when the parents have access to a support network. Women and their partners may find that family relationships become increasingly important, but the increased family interaction can be a source of stress. The new parents may also have increasing contact with other parents of small children while contact with coworkers declines. Of great concern are women and their partners who have no family or friends to form a social network. Isolation when the woman feels an increased need for support can result in tremendous stress and is often a contributing factor in situations of child neglect or abuse.

Recent nursing research has focused on the attainment of the maternal role. *Maternal role attainment* is the process by which a woman learns mothering behaviors and becomes comfortable with her identity as a mother. Formation of a maternal identity occurs with each child a woman bears. As the mother grows to know this child and forms a relationship, the mother's maternal identity gradually, systematically evolves and she "binds in" to the infant (Rubin 1984).

Maternal role attainment occurs in four stages (Mercer 1995). (The formal and informal stages of maternal attainment correspond with the taking-in and taking-hold stages previously identified by Rubin [1961].)

1. The *anticipatory stage* occurs during pregnancy. The woman looks to role models, especially her own mother, for examples of how to mother.
2. The *formal stage* begins when the child is born. The woman is still influenced by the guidance of others and tries to act as she believes others expect her to act.
3. The *informal stage* begins when the mother begins to make her own choices about mothering. The woman begins to develop her own style of mothering and finds ways of functioning that work well for her.
4. The *personal stage* is the final stage of maternal role attainment. When the woman reaches this stage, she is comfortable with the notion of herself as "mother."

In most cases maternal role attainment occurs within 3–10 months after birth. Social support, the woman's age and personality traits, the temperament of her infant, and the family's socioeconomic status all influence the woman's success in attaining the maternal role.

The postpartum woman faces a number of challenges as she adjusts to her new role (Mercer 1995):

- For many women, finding time for themselves is one of the greatest challenges. It is often difficult for the new mother to find time to read a book, talk to her partner, or even eat a meal without interruption!
- Women also report feelings of incompetence because they have not mastered all aspects of the mothering role. Often they are unsure of what to do in a given situation.
- The next greatest challenge involves fatigue resulting from sleep deprivation. The demands of nighttime care are tremendously draining, especially if the woman has other children.
- One challenge faced by the new mother involves the feeling of responsibility that having a child brings. Women experience a sense of lost freedom, an awareness that they will never again be quite as carefree as they were before becoming mothers.
- Mothers sometimes cite the infant's behavior as a problem, especially when the child is about 8 months old. Stranger anxiety develops, the infant begins crawling and getting into things, teething may cause fussiness, and the baby's tendency to put everything in his or her mouth requires constant vigilance by the parent.

All too often postpartum nurses are unaware of the long-term adjustments and stresses that the childbearing family faces as its members adjust to new and different roles. Nurses can help by providing anticipatory guidance about the realities of being a mother. Agencies should have literature available for reference at home. Ongoing parenting groups give parents an opportunity to discuss problems and become comfortable in new roles.

Postpartum Blues

The **postpartum blues** consist of a transient period of depression that often occurs during the first few days of the puerperium. It may be manifested by tearfulness, anorexia, difficulty in sleeping, and a feeling of letdown. This depression frequently occurs while the woman is still hospitalized, but it may occur at home too. Psychologic adjustments and hormonal factors are thought to be the main cause, although fatigue, discomfort, and overstimulation may play a part.

Development of Parent-Infant Attachment

A mother's first interaction with her infant is influenced by many factors, including participation in her family of origin, her relationships, the stability of her home environment, the communication patterns she developed, and the degree of nurturing she received as a child. These factors have shaped the self she has become. Certain characteristics of that self are also important:

- *Level of trust.* What level of trust has this mother developed in response to her life experiences? What is her philosophy of childrearing? Will she be able to treat her infant as a unique individual with changing needs that should be met as much as possible?
- *Level of self-esteem.* How much does she value herself as a woman and as a mother? Does she feel generally able to cope with the adjustments of life?
- *Capacity for enjoying oneself.* Is the mother able to find pleasure in everyday activities and human relationships?
- *Interest in and adequacy of knowledge about childbearing and childrearing.* What beliefs about the course of pregnancy, the capacities of newborns, and the nature of her emotions may influence her behavior at first contact with her infant and later?
- *Her prevailing mood or usual feeling tone.* Is the woman predominantly content, angry, depressed, or anxious? Is she sensitive to her own feelings and those of others? Will she be able to accept her own needs and to obtain support in meeting them?
- *Reactions to the present pregnancy.* Was the pregnancy planned? Did it go smoothly? Were there ongoing life events that enhanced her pregnancy or depleted her reserves of energy?

By the time of birth each mother has developed an emotional orientation of some kind to the baby based on these factors, as well as a physical awareness of the fetus within her and her fantasy images and perceptions.

Initial Attachment Behavior

New mothers demonstrate a fairly regular pattern of maternal behaviors at first contact with a normal newborn. In a progression of touching activities, the mother proceeds from fingertip exploration of the newborn's extremities toward palmar contact with larger body areas and finally to enfolding the infant with the whole hand and arms. The time taken to accomplish these steps varies from minutes to days, depending, it appears, on the timing of the first contact, the clothing barriers present, and the physical condition of the baby. Maternal excitement and elation tend to increase during the time of the initial meeting. The mother also increases the proportion of time spent in the **en face** position (Figure 27–3). She arranges herself or the newborn so that she has direct face-to-face and eye-to-eye contact. There is an intense interest in having the infant's eyes open. When the eyes are open, the mother characteristically greets the newborn and talks in high-pitched tones to him or her.

In most instances the mother relies heavily on her senses of sight, touch, and hearing in getting to know what her baby is really like. She tends also to respond verbally to any sounds emitted by the newborn, such as cries, coughs, sneezes, and grunts. The sense of smell may also be involved, although this possibility has not yet been adequately studied.

In addition to acting on and interacting with the newborn, the mother is undergoing her own emotional reactions to the whole happening and, more specifically, to the baby as she perceives him or her. The frequency of the "I can't believe" reaction leads to speculation that human gains as well as losses may initially be met with a degree of shock, disbelief, and denial. A feeling of emotional distance from the newborn is quite common: "I felt he was a stranger." On the other hand, feelings of connectedness between the newborn and the rest of the family can be expressed in positive or negative terms: "She's got your cute nose, Daddy" or "Oh, no! He looks just like the first one, and he was an impossible baby." A mother's facial expressions or the frequency and content of her questions may demonstrate concerns about the infant's general condition or normality, especially if her pregnancy was complicated or if a previously delivered baby was not normal.

What are the characteristic behaviors of a newborn? Unless care is taken to effect a gentle birth, a number of harsh stimuli assault the senses of the newborn at birth. The newborn is probably suctioned, held with head down somewhat, exposed to bright lights and cool air, and in some way cleansed. The infant usually responds by crying. In fact, caregivers typically stimulate the newborn to cry to reassure themselves that the baby is well and normal. When newborns no longer need to concentrate most of their energy on physical and physiologic responses to the immediate crisis of birth, they are able

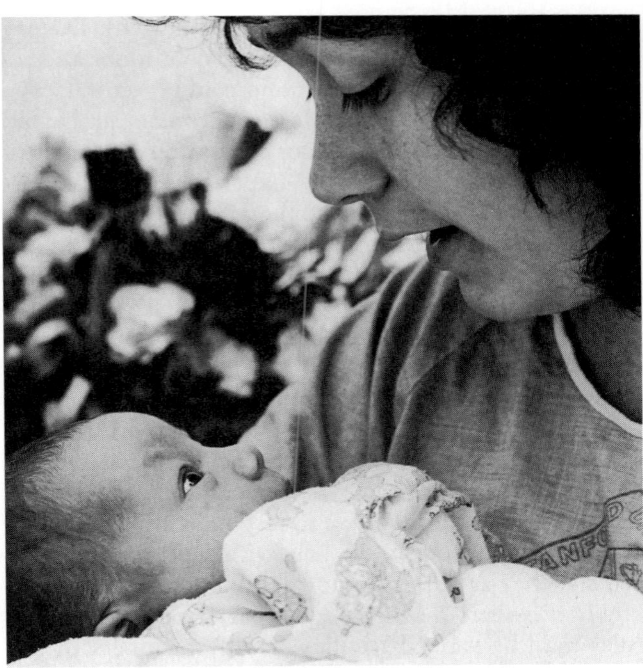

FIGURE 27–3 The mother has direct face-to-face and eye-to-eye contact in the *en face* position.

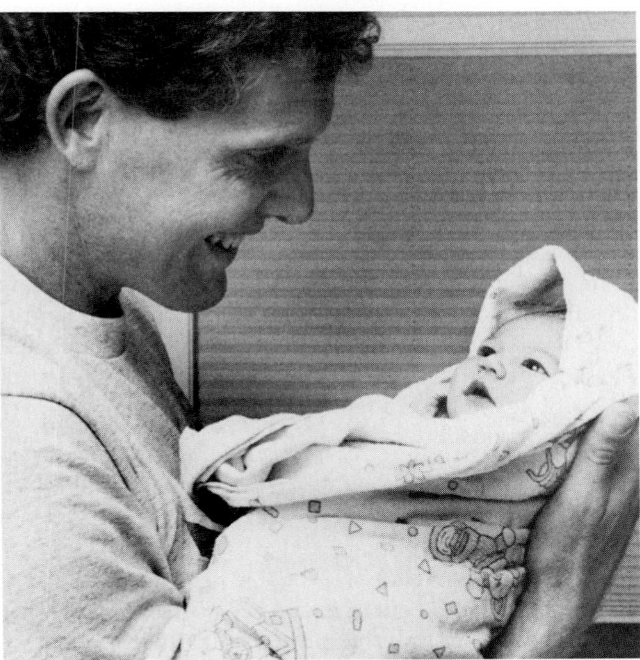

FIGURE 27–4 The father experiences strong feelings of attraction during engrossment.

to lie quietly with eyes open, looking about, moving their limbs occasionally, making sucking motions, possibly attempting to get hand to mouth. Placed in appropriate proximity to the mother, the newborn appears to focus briefly on her face and attend to her voice in the first moments of life.

During the first few days after her child's birth, the new mother applies herself to the task of getting to know her baby. This is termed the *acquaintance phase*. If the infant gives clear behavioral cues about needs, the infant's responses to mothering will be predictable, which will make the mother feel effective and competent. Other behaviors that make an infant more attractive to caretakers are smiling, grasping a finger, nursing eagerly, cuddling, and being easy to console.

During this time the newborn is also becoming acquainted. Within a few days after birth, infants show signs of recognizing recurrent situations and responding to changes in routine. To the extent that their mother is their world, it can be said that they are actively acquainting themselves with her.

During the *phase of mutual regulation,* mother and infant seek to deal with the issue of the degree of control to be exerted by each partner in their relationship. In this phase of adjustment, a balance is sought between the needs of the mother and the needs of the infant. The most important consideration is that each should obtain a good measure of enjoyment from the interaction. During the mutual adjustment phase negative maternal feelings are likely to surface or intensify. Because "everyone knows that mothers love their babies," these negative feelings often go unexpressed and are allowed to build up. If they are expressed, the response of friends, relatives, or health care personnel is often to deny the feelings to the mother: "You don't mean that." Some negative feelings are normal in the first few days after birth, and the nurse should be supportive when the mother vocalizes these feelings.

When mutual regulation arrives at the point where both mother and infant primarily enjoy each other's company, reciprocity has been achieved. **Reciprocity** is an interactional cycle that occurs simultaneously between mother and infant. It involves mutual cuing behaviors, expectancy, rhythmicity, and synchrony. The mother develops a new relationship with an individual who has a unique character and evokes a response entirely different from the fantasy response of pregnancy. When reciprocity is synchronous, the interaction between mother and infant is mutually gratifying and is sought and initiated by both partners. They find pleasure and delight in each other's company and grow in mutual love.

Father-Infant Interactions

Traditionally in Western cultures the primary role of the expectant father has been one of support for the pregnant woman. Commitment to family-centered maternity care, however, fostered interest in understanding the feelings and experiences of the new father. Evidence suggests that the father has a strong attraction to his newborn and that the feelings he experiences are similar to the mother's feelings of attachment (Figure 27–4). The characteristic sense of absorption, preoccupation, and interest in the infant demonstrated by fathers during early contact has been termed **engrossment.**

Siblings and Others

Recent work with infants has shown that they are capable of maintaining a number of strong attachments without loss of quality. These attachments may include siblings, grandparents, aunts, and uncles. The social setting and personality of the individual seem to be significant factors in the development of multiple attachments. The advent of open visiting hours and rooming-in permits siblings and grandparents to participate in the attachment process.

Cultural Influences in the Postpartal Period

The new mother's beliefs about her postpartal care are influenced by her culture and personal values. Her expectations about food, fluids, rest, hygiene, medications and relief measures, support and counsel, and other aspects of her life will be influenced by the beliefs and values of her family and cultural group. Sometimes, a new mother's wishes will differ from what the physician or nurse expects.

Nurses also belong to a particular culture, as well as to the health care cultural group. As part of the health care cultural group, nurses may take on some practices that support the general beliefs, such as offering food in the recovery period after birth, providing iced fluids, expecting the woman to ambulate as soon as possible, and assuming the woman will want to shower and perhaps wash her hair soon after birth. It is important for nurses to recognize that they are approaching their client's care from their own perspective and that, in order to individualize care for each mother, they need to offer and support individual choices.

Although listing particular practices of differing cultural groups always involves some generalization, it is helpful for nurses to understand some of the possible differences in beliefs and practices. The woman of European heritage may expect to eat a full meal and have large amounts of iced fluids after the birth, in the belief that the food restores energy and the fluids help replace fluid lost during the labor. She may want to ambulate shortly after the birth and shower, wash her hair, and put on a fresh gown. She may expect a short stay in the hospital and may or may not be interested in educational classes.

Many cultures emphasize certain postpartal routines or rituals for mother and baby that are designed to restore the harmony, or the hot-cold balance, of the body. Some women of Mexican, African, and Asian cultures may avoid cold after birth. This prohibition includes cold air, wind, and all water (even if heated). Dietary changes also reflect the need to avoid cold foods and restore the balance between hot and cold (Spector 1991). For instance, a traditional Mexican woman may avoid eating "hot" foods such as pork just after the birth of her baby (considered a "hot" experience). It is important to note that each individual may define hot and cold conditions and foods differently. The nurse should ask each woman what she can eat and what foods she thinks would be helpful for healing (Spector 1991). The nurse may encourage family members to bring preferred food and drink.

In many cultures the extended family frequently plays an essential role during the puerperium. The grandmother is often the primary helper to the mother and newborn. She brings wisdom and experience, allowing the new mother time to rest and giving her ready access to someone who can help with problems and concerns as they arise. It is important to ensure access of all family members during the postpartal period. Visiting rules may be waived to allow family members or authority figures access to the mother and newborn. These practices show respect and foster a blending of old and new behaviors to meet the goals of all concerned.

Postpartal Nursing Assessment

Comprehensive care is based on a thorough assessment that identifies individual needs or potential problems. See the accompanying Postpartal Assessment Guide: First 24 Hours After Birth.

Risk Factors

Ongoing assessment and client education during the puerperium is designed to meet the needs of the childbearing family and to detect and treat possible complications. Table 27–1, on p 720, identifies factors that may place the new mother at risk during the postpartal period. The nurse uses this knowledge during the assessment and is particularly alert for possible complications associated with identified risk factors.

Physical Assessment

The nurse should remember several principles in preparing for and completing the assessment of the postpartal woman.

- Select the time that will provide the most accurate data. Palpating the fundus when the woman has a

Text continues on page 720

POSTPARTAL ASSESSMENT GUIDE | First 24 Hours After Birth

Physical Assessment/ Normal Findings	Alterations and Possible Causes*	Nursing Responses to Data[†]
Vital Signs		
Blood pressure (BP): Should remain consistent with baseline BP during pregnancy.	High BP (PIH, essential hypertension, renal disease, anxiety). Drop in BP (may be normal; uterine hemorrhage).	Evaluate history of preexisting disorders and check for other signs of PIH (edema, proteinuria). Assess for other signs of hemorrhage (↑ pulse, cool clammy skin).
Pulse: 50–90 beats/minute. May be bradycardia of 50–70 beats/minute.	Tachycardia (difficult labor and birth, hemorrhage).	Evaluate for other signs of hemorrhage (↓ BP, cool clammy skin).
Respirations: 16–24/minute.	Marked tachypnea (respiratory disease).	Assess for other signs of respiratory disease.
Temperature: 36.2–38C (98–100.4F).	After first 24 hours temperature of 38C (100.4F) or above suggests infection.	Assess for other signs of infection; notify physician/certified nurse-midwife.
Breasts		
General appearance: Smooth, even pigmentation, changes of pregnancy still apparent; one may appear larger.	Reddened area (mastitis).	Assess further for signs of infection.
Palpation: Depending on postpartal day, may be soft, filling, full, or engorged.	Palpable mass (caked breast, mastitis). Engorgement (venous stasis). Tenderness, heat, edema (engorgement, caked breast, mastitis).	Assess for other signs of infection: If blocked duct, consider heat, massage, position change for breastfeeding. Assess for further signs. Report mastitis to physician/certified nurse-midwife.
Nipples: Supple, pigmented, intact; become erect when stimulated.	Fissures, cracks, soreness (problems with breastfeeding), not erectile with stimulation (inverted nipples).	Reassess technique; recommend appropriate interventions.
Abdomen		
Musculature: Abdomen may be soft, have a "doughy" texture; rectus muscle intact.	Separation in musculature (diastasis recti abdominis).	Evaluate size of diastasis; teach appropriate exercises for decreasing the separation.
Fundus: Firm, midline; following expected schedule of involution.	Boggy (full bladder, uterine bleeding).	Massage until firm; assess bladder and have woman void if needed; attempt to express clots when firm. If bogginess remains or recurs, report to physician/certified nurse-midwife.
May be tender when palpated.	Constant tenderness (infection).	Assess for evidence of endometritis.
Lochia		
Scant to moderate amount, earthy odor; no clots.	Large amount, clots (hemorrhage). Foul-smelling lochia (infection).	Assess for firmness, express additional clots; begin peripad count. Assess for other signs of infection; report to physician/certified nurse-midwife.

*Possible causes of alterations are placed in parentheses.

[†]This column provides guidelines for further assessment and initial nursing actions.

POSTPARTAL ASSESSMENT GUIDE | First 24 Hours After Birth continued

Physical Assessment/ Normal Findings	Alterations and Possible Causes*	Nursing Responses to Data†
Normal progression: First 1–3 days: rubra. Days 3–10: serosa (alba seldom seen in hospital).	Failure to progress normally or return to rubra from serosa (subinvolution).	Report to physician/certified nurse-midwife.
Perineum		
Slight edema and bruising in intact perineum.	Marked fullness, bruising, pain (vulvar hematoma).	Assess size; apply ice glove or ice pack; report to physician/certified nurse-midwife.
Episiotomy: No redness, edema, ecchymosis, or discharge; edges well approximated.	Redness, edema, ecchymosis, discharge, or gaping stitches (infection).	Encourage sitz baths; review perineal care, appropriate wiping techniques.
Hemorrhoids: None present; if present, should be small and nontender.	Full, tender, inflamed hemorrhoids.	Encourage sitz baths, side-lying position; tucks pads, anesthetic ointments, manual replacement of hemorrhoids, stool softeners, increased fluid intake.
Costo-Vertebral Angle (CVA) Tenderness		
None.	Present (kidney infection).	Assess for other symptoms of urinary tract infection (UTI); obtain clean-catch urine; report to physician/certified nurse-midwife.
Lower Extremities		
No pain with palpation; negative Homan's sign.	Positive findings (thrombophlebitis).	Report to physician/certified nurse-midwife.
Elimination		
Urinary output: Voiding in sufficient quantities at least every 4–6 hours; bladder not palpable.	Inability to void (urinary retention). Symptoms of urgency, frequency, dysuria (UTI).	Employ nursing interventions to promote voiding; if not successful, obtain order for catheterization. Report symptoms of UTI to physician/certified nurse-midwife.
Bowel elimination: Should have normal bowel movement by second or third day after birth.	Inability to pass feces (constipation due to fear of pain from episiotomy, hemorrhoids, perineal trauma).	Encourage fluids, ambulation, roughage in diet; sitz baths to promote healing of perineum; obtain order for stool softener.

Cultural Assessment‡	Variations to Consider	Nursing Responses to Data†
Determine customs and practices regarding postpartum care.	Individual preference may include:	Provide for specific request if possible. If woman is unable to provide specific information, the nurse may draw from general information regarding cultural variation.
Ask the mother if she would like fluids, and ask what temperature she prefers.	Receiving room temperature or warmed fluids rather than iced drinks.	
Ask the mother what foods or fluids she would like.	Inclusion of special foods or fluids to hasten healing after childbirth.	Mexican women may want food and fluids that restore hot-cold balance to the body. Women of European background may ask for iced fluids.

‡These are only a few suggestions. It is not our intent to imply this is a comprehensive cultural assessment.

*Possible causes of alterations are placed in parentheses.

†This column provides guidelines for further assessment and initial nursing actions.

POSTPARTAL ASSESSMENT GUIDE continued

Cultural Assessment[‡]	Variations to Consider	Nursing Responses to Data[†]
Ask the mother if she would prefer to be alone during breastfeeding.	Some women may be hesitant to have someone with them when their breast is exposed.	

Psychosocial Assessment/ Normal Findings	Variations to Consider	Nursing Responses to Data
Psychologic Adaptation		
During first 24 hours: Passive; preoccupied with own needs; may talk about her labor and birth experience; may be talkative, elated, or very quiet.	Very quiet and passive; sleeps frequently (fatigue from long labor; feelings of disappointment about some aspect of the experience; may be following cultural expectation).	Provide opportunities for adequate rest; provide nutritious meals and snacks that are consistent with what the woman desires to eat and drink; provide opportunities to discuss birth experience in nonjudgmental atmosphere if the woman desires to do so.
By 24–48 hours: Beginning to assume responsibility; some women eager to learn; easily feels overwhelmed.	Excessive weepiness, mood swings, pronounced irritability (postpartum blues, feelings of inadequacy; culturally prescribed behavior).	Explain postpartum blues; provide supportive atmosphere; determine support available for mother; consider referral for evidence of profound depression.
Attachment		
En face position; holds baby close; cuddles and soothes; calls by name; identifies characteristics of family members in infant; may be awkward in providing care.	Continued expressions of disappointment in sex, appearance of infant; refusal to care for infant; derogatory comments; lack of bonding behaviors (difficulty in attachment, following expectations of cultural/ethnic group).	Provide reinforcement and support for infant caretaking behaviors; maintain nonjudgmental approach and gather more information if caretaking behaviors are not evident.
Initially may express disappointment over sex or appearance of infant but within 1–2 days demonstrates attachment behaviors.		
Client Education		
Has basic understanding of self-care activities and infant care needs; can identify signs of complications that should be reported.	Unable to demonstrate basic self-care and infant care activities (knowledge deficit; postpartum blues; following prescribed cultural behavior and will be cared for by grandmother or other family member).	Determine whether woman understands English and provide interpreter if needed; provide reinforcement of information through conversation and through written material (remember that some women and their families may not be able to understand written materials due to language difficulties or inability to read); provide information regarding infant care skills that are culturally consistent; give woman opportunity to express her feelings; consider social service home referral for women who have no family or other support, are unable to take in information about self-care and infant care, and demonstrate no caretaking activities.

[‡]These are only a few suggestions. It is not our intent to imply this is a comprehensive cultural assessment.

[†]This column provides guidelines for further assessment and initial nursing actions.

TABLE 27–1 Postpartal High-Risk Factors

Factor	Maternal Implication
PIH	↑ Blood pressure ↑ CNS irritability ↑ Need for bed rest → ↑ risk thrombophlebitis
Diatebes	Need for insulin regulation Episodes of hypoglycemia or hyperglycemia ↓ Healing
Cardiac disease	↑ Maternal exhaustion
Cesarean birth	↑ Healing needs ↑ Pain from incision ↑ Risk of infection ↑ Length of hospitalization
Overdistention of uterus (multiple gestation, hydramnios)	↑ Risk of hemorrhage ↑ Risk of anemia ↑ Stretching of abdominal muscles ↑ Incidence and severity of afterpains
Abruptio placentae, placenta previa	Hemorrhage → anemia ↓ Uterine contractility after birth → ↑ infection risk
Precipitous labor (<3 hours)	↑ Risk of lacerations to birth canal → hemorrhage
Prolonged labor (>24 hours)	Exhaustion ↑ Risk of hemorrhage Nutritional and fluid depletion ↑ Bladder atony and/or trauma
Difficult birth	Exhaustion ↑ Risk of perineal lacerations ↑ Risk of hematomas ↑ Risk of hemorrhage → anemia
Extended period of time in stirrups at birth	↑ Risk of thrombophlebitis
Retained placenta	↑ Risk of hemorrhage ↑ Risk of infection

ESSENTIAL PRECAUTIONS FOR PRACTICE

During Postpartal Assessment

Examples of times when disposable gloves should be worn include

- Assessing the breast if there is leakage of colostrum or milk
- Assessing the perineum and lochia
- Changing perineal pads or chux
- Handling clothing, chux, perineal pads, and/or bedding contaminated with lochia
- Handling used breast pads

REMEMBER to wash your hands before putting on the disposable gloves and AGAIN immediately after you remove the gloves.

For further information consult OSHA and CDC guidelines.

full bladder, for example, may give false information about the progress of involution.

- Explain the purpose of regular assessment.
- The woman should be relaxed, and the procedures should be done as gently as possible to avoid unnecessary discomfort.
- The data obtained should be recorded and reported as clearly as possible.
- Take care to protect yourself from exposure to bodily fluids (see Essential Precautions for Practice: During Postpartal Assessment).

While performing the physical assessment, the nurse should also be teaching the woman. For example, when assessing the breasts of a nursing woman, the nurse can discuss breast milk production, the letdown reflex, and breast self-examination. Mothers may be very receptive to instruction on postpartal abdominal tightening exercises when the nurse assesses the woman's fundal height and diastasis. The assessment also provides an excellent time to provide information about the body's postpartal physical and anatomic changes as well as danger signs to report. (See Key Facts to Remember: Common Postpartal Concerns.) Since the time the woman spends in the postpartum unit is often limited, nurses should use every available opportunity for client education about self-care. One of the best opportunities comes during the normal postpartal assessment. To assist nurses in recognizing these opportunities, examples of client teaching during the assessment have been provided throughout the following discussion.

Vital Signs

The nurse may choose to organize the physical assessment in a variety of ways. Many nurses begin by assessing vital signs because the findings will be more accurate when they are obtained with the woman at rest. In addition, establishing whether the vital signs are within the expected normal range will assist the nurse in determining other assessments that might be needed. For instance, if the temperature is elevated, the nurse considers the time since birth and gathers information to determine whether the woman is dehydrated or an infection is present.

Alterations in vital signs may indicate complications, so the nurse assesses them at regular intervals. The blood pressure should remain stable, while the pulse often shows a characteristic slowness that is no cause for alarm. Pulse rates return to prepregnant norms very quickly unless complications arise.

Temperature elevations (less than 38C [100.4F]) due to normal processes should last for only a few days and should not be associated with other clinical signs of infection. The nurse should evaluate any elevation in light of other signs and symptoms and should carefully review the woman's history to identify other factors, such as premature rupture of membranes (PROM) or prolonged labor, which might increase the incidence of infection in the genital tract.

The nurse informs the woman of the results of the vital signs assessment and provides information about the normal changes in blood pressure and pulse. This may be an opportunity to assess whether the mother knows how to assess her own and her infant's temperature and how to read a thermometer.

Auscultation of Lungs

The breath sounds are auscultated and should be clear. Women who have been treated for preterm labor or PIH are especially at risk for pulmonary edema (see Chapter 13 for further discussion).

Breasts

The nurse can first assess the fit and support provided by the bra. The nurse provides information about how to select a supportive bra. A properly fitting bra provides support to the breasts and helps maintain breast shape by limiting stretching of supporting ligaments and connective tissue. If the mother is breastfeeding, the straps of the bra should be cloth, not elastic, and easily adjustable. The back should be wide and have at least three rows of hooks to adjust for fit. Traditional nursing bras have a fixed inner cup and a separate half cup that can be unhooked for breastfeeding while continuing to support the breast. Purchasing a nursing bra one size too large during pregnancy will usually result in a good fit because the breasts increase in size with milk production.

The bra is then removed so the breasts can be examined. The nurse notes the size and shape of the breasts and any abnormalities, reddened areas, or engorgement. The breasts are also lightly palpated for softness, slight firmness associated with filling, firmness associated with engorgement, warmth, or tenderness. The nipples are assessed for fissures, cracks, soreness, or inversion. The nurse teaches the woman the characteristics of the breast and explains how to recognize problems such as fissures or cracks.

The nonnursing mother is assessed for evidence of breast discomfort, and relief measures are taken if necessary. (See discussion of lactation suppression in the nonnursing mother in Chapter 28.) Breast assessment findings for a nursing woman may be recorded as follows: Breasts soft, filling, no evidence of nipple tenderness or cracking.

Abdomen and Fundus

Before examination of the abdomen, the woman should void. This practice assures that a full bladder is not causing displacement of the uterus or any uterine atony; if atony is present, other causes must be investigated.

The nurse determines the relationship of the fundus to the umbilicus and also assesses the firmness of the fundus. The nurse notes whether the fundus is in the midline or displaced to either side of the abdomen. Because the most common cause of displacement is a full bladder, this finding requires further assessment. The nurse should then record the results of the assessment. (See Procedure 27–1.)

While completing the assessment, the nurse teaches the woman about fundal position. The mother can be assisted in gently massaging her fundus to determine firmness.

In the woman who has had a cesarean birth, the abdominal incision is exquisitely tender. The fundus is therefore palpated with extreme care. The nurse also inspects the abdominal incision for any signs of infection, including drainage, foul odor, or redness. During the assessment, the nurse teaches the woman about her incision. Characteristics of normal healing may be reviewed and signs of infection discussed.

KEY FACTS TO REMEMBER

Common Postpartal Concerns

Several postpartal occurrences cause special concern for mothers. The nurse will frequently be asked about the following events:

Source of Concern	Explanation
Gush of blood that sometimes occurs when she first arises.	Due to normal pooling of blood in vagina when the woman lies down to rest or sleep. Gravity causes blood to flow out when she stands.
Night sweats.	Normal physiologic occurrence that results as body attempts to eliminate excess fluids that were present during pregnancy. May be aggravated by plastic mattress pad.
Afterpains.	More common in multiparas. Due to contraction and relaxation of uterus. Increased by oxytocin, breastfeeding. Relieved with mild analgesics and time.
"Large stomach" after birth and failure to lose all weight gained during pregnancy.	The baby, amniotic fluid, and placenta account for only a portion of the weight gained during pregnancy. The remainder takes approximately 6 weeks to lose. Abdomen also appears large due to ↓ muscle tone. Postpartal exercises will help.

PROCEDURE 27–1 Assessing the Fundus Following Vaginal Birth

Nursing Action	Rationale
Objective: Prepare the woman.	
• Explain the procedure.	Explanation decreases anxiety and increases cooperation.
• Ask the woman to void.	A full bladder will cause uterine atony.
• Position the woman flat in bed with her head comfortable on a pillow. If the procedure is uncomfortable, the woman may flex her legs.	The supine position prevents falsely high assessment of fundal height. Flexing the legs relaxes the abdominal muscles.
Objective: Determine uterine firmness.	
• Gently place one had on the lower segment of the uterus. Using the side of the other hand, palpate the abdomen until you locate the top of the fundus.	This position provides support for the uterus and a larger surface for palpation.
• Determine whether the fundus is firm. If it is not firm, massage the abdomen lightly until the fundus is firm.	A firm fundus indicates that the muscles are contracted and bleeding will not occur.
Objective: Determine the height of the fundus.	
• Measure the top of the fundus in fingerbreadths above, below, or at the umbilicus (Figure 27–5).	Fundal height gives information about the progress of involution.

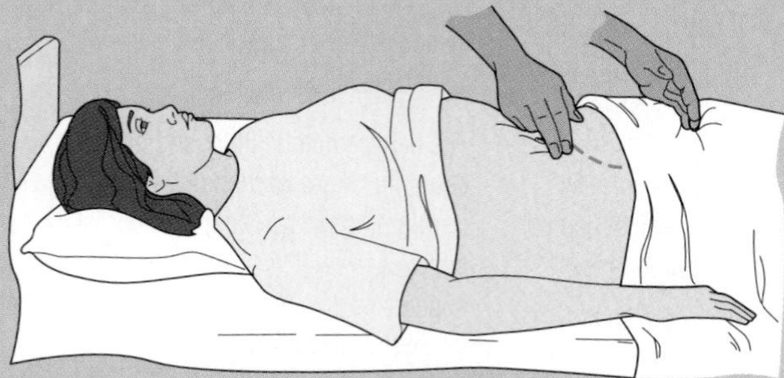

FIGURE 27–5 Measurement of descent of fundus for the woman with vaginal birth. The fundus is located two fingerbreadths below the umbilicus.

Nursing Action	Rationale
Objective: Ascertain the position of the fundus.	
• Determine whether the fundus has deviated from the midline. If it is not in the midline, locate the position. Evaluate the bladder for distention.	The fundus may be deviated when the bladder is full.
• Measure urine output for the next few hours until normal elimination status is established.	
Objective: Correlate the uterine status with lochia.	
• Observe the amount, color, and odor of the lochia and the presence of clots.	As normal involution occurs, the lochia decreases and changes from rubra to serosa. Increased amounts of lochia may be associated with uterine relaxation; failure to progress to the next type of lochia may indicate uterine relaxation or infection.
Objective: Record the findings.	Provides a permanent record.
• Fundal height is recorded in fingerbreadths; for example, "2 FB ↓ U; 1 FB ↑ U."	
• If massage was necessary: "Uterus: Boggy ⟶ firm c̄ light massage."	

Lochia

The next aspect to be evaluated is the lochia, which is assessed for character, amount, odor, and the presence of clots. Disposable gloves must be worn when assessing the perineum and lochia. Nurses may put on the gloves before beginning the assessment, just before assessing the abdomen and fundus, or when they are ready to assess the perineum and lochia. (See Essential Precautions for Practice: During Postpartal Assessment.) During the first 1–3 days the lochia should be rubra. A few small clots are normal and occur as a result of blood pooling in the vagina. However, the passage of numerous or large clots is abnormal, and the cause should be investigated immediately. After 2–3 days, the lochia becomes serosa.

Lochia should never exceed a moderate amount, such as four to eight partially saturated perineal pads daily, with an average of six. However, because this is influenced by an individual woman's pad-changing practices, as well as the absorbency of the pad, she should be questioned about the length of time the current pad has been in use, whether the amount is normal, and whether any clots were passed before this examination, such as during voiding. If heavy bleeding is reported but not seen, the woman is asked to put on a clean perineal pad and is then reassessed in 1 hour (Figure 27–6). Clots and heavy bleeding may be caused by uterine relaxation (atony) or retained placental fragments and may require further assessment. Because of the evacuation of the uterine cavity during cesarean birth, women with such surgery usually have less lochia after the first 24 hours than mothers who give birth vaginally. If the woman is at increased risk for bleeding, or is actually experiencing heavy flow of lochia rubra, the physician may also order methylergonovine maleate (Methergine). See Drug Guide: Methylergonovine Maleate (Methergine) in Chapter 28.

The odor of the lochia is nonoffensive and never foul. If foul odor is present, so is an infection. The amount of lochia is charted first, followed by character. For example:

- Lochia: moderate rubra
- Lochia: small rubra/serosa

Client teaching during assessment of the lochia may center on normal changes that can be expected in the amount and color of the flow. The nurse can review hygienic measures if appropriate. The nurse should approach the teaching of hygienic practices delicately and with the goals of promoting comfort, enhancing tissue healing, and preventing infection, and avoid value-laden statements about the need for cleanliness or control of body odor.

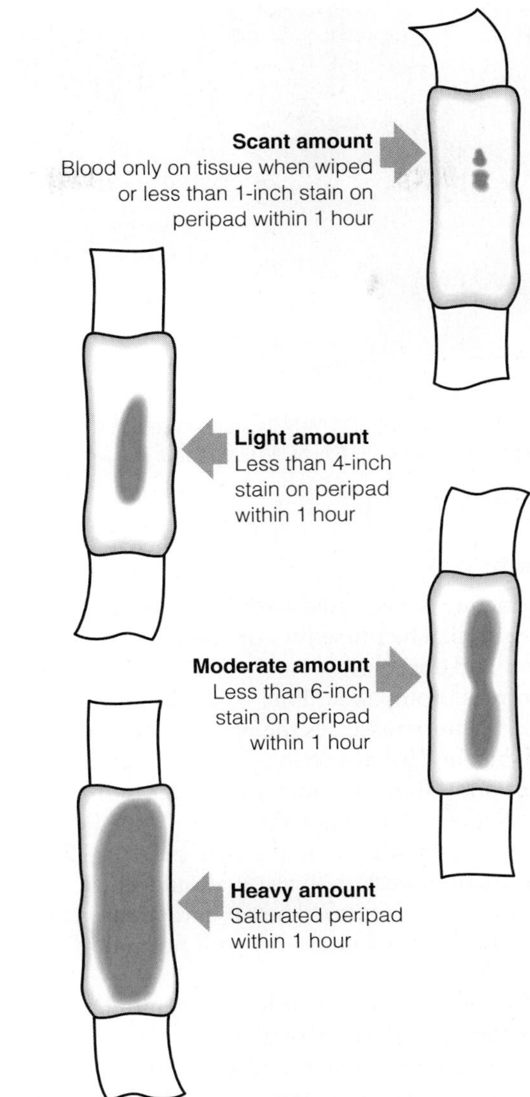
Scant amount
Blood only on tissue when wiped or less than 1-inch stain on peripad within 1 hour
Light amount
Less than 4-inch stain on peripad within 1 hour
Moderate amount
Less than 6-inch stain on peripad within 1 hour
Heavy amount
Saturated peripad within 1 hour

FIGURE 27–6 Suggested guideline for assessing lochia volume.

Source: Jacobson H: A standard for assessing lochia volume. *MCN* May/June 1985; 10:175. New York: The American Journal of Nursing Company, 1985.

CRITICAL THINKING IN ACTION

You have completed your assessment of Patty Clark, a 24-year-old, G2P2, woman who is 24 hours past birth. The fundus is just above the umbilicus, and slightly to the right. Lochia rubra is present, and a pad is soaked every 2 hours. What would you do?

Answers can be found in Appendix H.

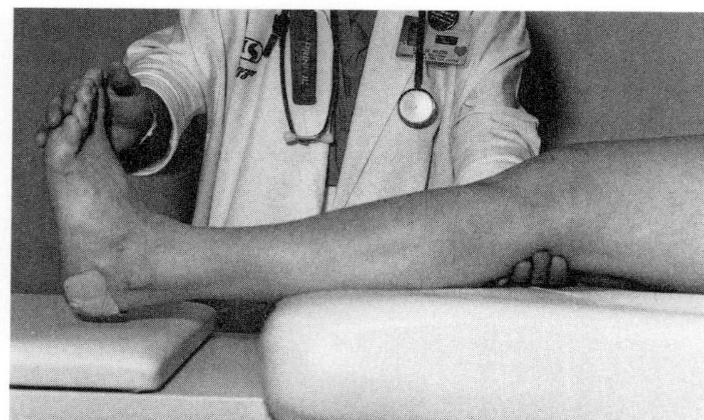

FIGURE 27–7 Homan's sign: With the woman's knee flexed, the nurse dorsiflexes the foot. Pain in the foot or leg is a positive Homan's sign.

Perineum

The perineum is inspected with the woman lying in a Sims' position. The nurse lifts the buttock to expose the perineum and anus.

If an episiotomy was done or a laceration required suturing, the nurse assesses the wound and evaluates the state of healing by observing for ecchymosis and approximation. After 24 hours some edema may still be present, but the skin edges should be "glued" together (well approximated) so that gentle pressure does not separate them. Gentle palpation should elicit minimal tenderness and there should be no hard areas suggesting infection. Ecchymosis interferes with normal healing, as does infection.

Foul odors associated with drainage indicate infection. Further observation of the incision for warmth, redness, tenderness, edema, and separation should also be made. The nurse next assesses whether hemorrhoids are present around the anus. If present, they are assessed for size, number, and pain or tenderness.

During the assessment, the nurse talks with the woman to determine the effectiveness of comfort measures that have been used. The nurse provides teaching about the episiotomy. Some women do not thoroughly understand what and where an episiotomy is, and they may believe that the stitches must be removed as with other types of surgery. Frequently, when women fear that the stitches must be removed manually, they are afraid to ask about them. While explaining the findings of the assessment, the nurse provides information about the episiotomy, its location, and the signs that are being assessed. In addition, the nurse can casually add that the sutures are special and will dissolve slowly over the next few weeks as the tissues heal. By the time the sutures are dissolved the tissues are strong and the incision edges will not separate. This is also an opportunity to teach comfort measures (see Chapter 29).

An example of charting a perineal assessment might be: Midline episiotomy; no edema, tenderness, or ecchymosis present. Skin edges well approximated. Patient reports pain relief measures are controlling discomfort.

Lower Extremities

If thrombophlebitis occurs, the most likely site will be in the woman's legs. To assess for this, her legs should be stretched out straight and relaxed with the knees flexed. The nurse grasps the foot and sharply dorsiflexes it. No discomfort or pain should be present. If pain is elicited, the nurse notifies the certified nurse-midwife/physician that the woman has a positive Homan's sign (Figure 27–7). The pain is caused by inflammation of the vessel. The nurse also evaluates the legs for edema by comparing both legs, since usually only one leg is involved. Any areas of redness, tenderness, and increased skin temperature should also be noted.

Early ambulation is an important aspect in the prevention of thrombophlebitis. Most women are able to be up shortly after birth. The cesarean birth client requires range-of-motion exercises until she is ambulating more freely.

Client teaching associated with assessment of the lower extremities focuses on the signs and symptoms of thrombophlebitis. In addition, the nurse may review self-care measures to promote circulation, and measures to prevent thrombophlebitis, such as ambulation and avoiding pressure behind the knees, using the knee gatch on the bed, and crossing the legs.

Elimination

During the hours after birth the nurse carefully monitors a new mother's bladder status. A boggy uterus, a displaced uterus, or a palpable bladder are signs of bladder distention and require nursing intervention.

The postpartal woman should be encouraged to void every 4–6 hours. The nurse should assess the bladder for distention until the woman demonstrates complete emptying of the bladder with each voiding. The nurse may employ techniques to facilitate voiding, such as helping the woman out of bed to void or pouring warm water on the perineum. Catheterization is required when the bladder is distended and the woman cannot void or no voiding has occurred in 8 hours. The cesarean birth mother may have an indwelling catheter inserted prophylactically. The same assessments should be made in evaluating bladder emptying once the catheter is removed.

During the physical assessment, the nurse elicits information from the woman about the adequacy of her fluid intake, whether she feels she is emptying her bladder completely when she voids, and any signs of urinary tract infection (UTI) she may be experiencing.

In the same way, the nurse obtains information about the new mother's intestinal elimination and any concerns she may have about it. Many mothers fear that the first bowel movement will be painful and possibly even damaging if an episiotomy has been done. Stool softeners may be ordered to increase bulk and moisture in the fecal material and to allow more comfortable and complete evacuation. Constipation is avoided to prevent pressures on sutures that may increase discomfort. Encouraging ambulation, forcing fluids (up to 2000 mL/day or more), and providing fresh fruits and roughage in the diet enhance bowel elimination and help the woman reestablish her normal bowel pattern.

During the assessment, the nurse may provide information about postpartum diuresis and why the woman may be emptying her bladder so frequently. The need for additional fluid intake with suggestions of specific amounts may be helpful. The woman should drink at least eight 8-oz glasses of water or juice per day in addition to other fluids. The nurse discusses signs of retention and overflow voiding and may review symptoms of UTI if it seems an appropriate moment for teaching. The nurse can also review methods of assisting bowel elimination and provide opportunities for the woman to ask questions.

Rest and Sleep Status

As part of the postpartal assessment, the nurse evaluates the amount of rest a new mother is getting. If the woman reports difficulty sleeping at night, the nurse should try to determine the cause. If it is simply the strange environment, a warm drink, backrub, or mild sedative may prove helpful. Appropriate nursing measures are indicated if the woman is bothered by normal postpartal discomforts such as afterpains, diaphoresis, or episiotomy or hemorrhoidal pain.

The nurse should encourage a daily rest period and schedule hospital activities to allow time for napping. The nurse can also provide information about the fatigue new mothers experience and the impact it can have on a woman's emotions and sense of control.

Nutritional Status

Determination of postpartal nutritional status is based primarily on information provided by the mother and on direct assessment. During pregnancy the daily recommended dietary allowances call for increases in calories, proteins, and most vitamins and minerals. After birth, the nonnursing mother's dietary requirements return to prepregnancy levels (Food and Nutrition Board 1989).

Visiting the mother during mealtime provides an opportunity for unobtrusive nutritional assessment and counseling. The nonnursing mother should be advised about the need to reduce her caloric intake by about 300 kcal and to return to prepregnancy levels for other nutrients. The nursing mother, on the other hand, should increase her caloric intake by about 200 kcal over the pregnancy requirements, or a total of 500 kcal over the nonpregnant requirement. Basic discussion will prove helpful, followed by referral as needed. In all cases, literature on nutrition should be provided, so that the woman will have a source of information after discharge.

KEY FACTS TO REMEMBER

Encouraging Healthful Nutrition

Encourage the woman to have daily

- 2–3 servings of milk, yogurt, and cheese group
- 2–3 servings of meat or protein group
- 3–5 servings of vegetable group
- 4 servings of whole grain
- 2–4 servings of fruit group
- 6–11 servings of bread, cereal, rice, and pasta group
- Fats, oils, and sweets sparingly

The dietitian should be informed of any mother who is a vegetarian or whose cultural or religious beliefs require specific foods. Appropriate meals can then be prepared for her. Many women, especially those who gained excessively, are interested in losing weight after birth. The dietitian can design weight-reduction diets to meet nutritional needs and food preferences. The nurse may also refer women with unusual eating habits or numerous questions about good nutrition to the dietitian.

New mothers are also advised that it is common practice to prescribe iron supplements for 4–6 weeks after birth. The hematocrit is then checked at the postpartal visit to detect any anemia.

As part of the nutritional assessment, the nurse can provide teaching about the nutritional needs of the woman during the postpartal period. See Key Facts to Remember: Encouraging Healthful Nutrition, as well as the discussion in Chapter 11.

Psychologic Assessment

Adequate assessment of the mother's psychologic adjustment is an integral part of postpartal evaluation. This assessment focuses on the mother's general attitude, feelings of competence, available support systems, and caregiving skills. It also evaluates her fatigue level, sense of satisfaction, and ability to accomplish her developmental tasks.

Fatigue is often a highly significant factor in a new mother's apparent disinterest in her newborn. Frequently the woman is so tired from a long labor and birth that everything seems to be an effort. To avoid inadvertently classifying a very tired mother as one with a potential attachment problem, the nurse should do the psychologic assessment on more than one occasion. After a nap the new mother is often far more receptive to her baby and her surroundings.

Some new mothers have little or no experience with newborns and may feel totally overwhelmed. They may show these feelings by asking questions and reading all available material or by becoming passive and quiet because they simply cannot deal with their feelings of inadequacy. Unless a nurse questions the woman about her plans and previous experience in a supportive, nonjudgmental way, one might conclude that the woman was disinterested, withdrawn, or depressed.

Problem clues might include excessive continued fatigue, marked depression, excessive preoccupation with physical status or discomfort, evidence of low self-esteem, lack of support systems, marital problems, inability to care for or nurture the newborn, and current family crises (illness, unemployment, and so on). These characteristics frequently indicate a potential for maladaptive parenting, which may lead to child abuse or neglect (physical, emotional, intellectual) and cannot be ignored. Referrals to public health nurses or other available community resources may provide greatly needed assistance and alleviate potentially dangerous situations.

Assessment of Early Attachment

If attachment is accepted as a desired outcome of nursing care, a nurse in any of the various postpartal settings can periodically observe and note progress toward attachment. The following questions can be addressed in the course of nurse-client interaction:

1. Is the mother attracted to her newborn? To what extent does she seek face-to-face contact and eye contact? Has she progressed from fingertip touch, to palmar contact, to enfolding the infant close to her own body? Is attraction increasing or decreasing? If the mother does not exhibit increasing attraction, why not? Do the reasons lie primarily within her, in the baby, or in the environment?
2. Is the mother inclined to nurture her infant? Is she progressing in her interactions with her infant?
3. Does the mother act consistently? If not, is the source of unpredictability within her or her infant?
4. Is her mothering consistently carried out? Does she seek information and evaluate it objectively? Does she develop solutions based on adequate knowledge of valid data? Does she evaluate the effectiveness of her maternal care and make appropriate adjustments?
5. Is she sensitive to the newborn's needs as they arise? How quickly does she interpret her infant's behavior and react to cues? Does she seem happy and satisfied with the infant's responses to her efforts? Is she pleased with feeding behaviors? How much of this ability and willingness to respond is related to the baby's nature, and how much to her own?
6. Does she seem pleased with her baby's appearance and sex? Is she experiencing pleasure in interaction with her infant? What interferes with the enjoyment? Does she speak to the baby frequently and affectionately? Does she call him or her by name? Does she point out family traits or characteristics she sees in the newborn?
7. Are there any cultural factors that might modify the mother's response? For instance, is it customary for the grandmother to assume most of the child care responsibilities while the mother recovers from childbirth?

When the nurse has addressed these questions and assembled the facts, the nurse's intuition and formal background of knowledge should combine to answer three more questions: Is there a problem in attachment? What is the problem? What is its source? The nurse can then devise a creative approach to the problem as it presents itself in the context of a unique, developing mother-infant relationship.

Assessment of Physical and Developmental Tasks

During the first several postpartal weeks, the woman must accomplish certain physical and developmental tasks:

- Restoring physical condition
- Developing competence in caring for and meeting the needs of her infant
- Establishing a relationship with her new child
- Adapting to altered lifestyles and family structure resulting from the addition of a new member

The new mother may have an inadequate or incorrect understanding of what to expect during the early postpartal weeks. She may be concerned with restoring her figure and surprised because of continuing physical discomfort from sore breasts, episiotomy, or hemorrhoids. Fatigue is perhaps her greatest yet most underestimated problem during the early weeks. This may be aggravated if she has no extended family support or there are other young children at home (Lederman 1996).

Developing skill and confidence in caring for an infant may be especially anxiety-provoking for a new mother. As she struggles to establish a mutually acceptable pattern with her baby, small unanticipated concerns may seem monumental. The woman may begin to feel inadequate and, if she lacks support systems, isolated.

Nurses have been in the forefront of health care providers in attempting to improve the care currently existing during the postpartal period. Many obstetricians and nurse practitioners now routinely see all postpartal women 1 to 2 weeks after birth in addition to the routine 6 week checkup. This extra visit provides an opportunity for physical assessment as well as assessment of the mother's psychologic and informational needs.

Postdischarge Care

Postdischarge care for the postpartal woman may be accomplished by home visits or follow-up phone calls. A home visit 1 to 3 days after discharge provides opportunities for further assessment and teaching.

The follow-up telephone call is usually initiated by a nurse from the postpartal unit of the agency where the mother gave birth. It is made soon after discharge and is designed to provide assessment and care if necessary, to reinforce knowledge and provide additional teaching, and to make referrals if indicated.

Postpartal Home Care

The routine physical assessment, which can be made rapidly, focuses on the woman's general appearance, breasts, reproductive tract, bladder and bowel elimination, and any specific problems or complaints. (See the Postpartal Assessment Guide: First Home Visit and Anticipated Progress at Six Weeks, in Chapter 29.) In addition, the nurse should talk with the mother about her diet, fatigue level, family adjustment, and psychologic status. The nurse explores any problems with child care, refers the mother to a pediatric nurse practitioner or pediatrician if needed, and mentions available community resources, telephone information lines (Valaitis et al 1996), including public health department follow-up visits, when appropriate. If not already discussed, teaching about family planning is appropriate at this time, and the nurse can provide information about birth control methods.

In ideal situations a family approach involving the father, infant, and possibly other siblings permits a total evaluation and provides an opportunity for all family members to ask questions and express concerns. Such an approach also promotes diagnosis and treatment of disturbed family patterns to prevent future problems of neglect or abuse.

CHAPTER HIGHLIGHTS

- The uterus involutes rapidly, primarily through a reduction in cell size.
- Involution is assessed by measuring fundal height. The fundus is at the level of the umbilicus within a few hours after childbirth and should decrease by approximately one fingerbreadth per day.
- The placental site heals by a process of exfoliation, so no scar formation occurs.
- Lochia progresses from rubra to serosa to alba and is assessed in terms of type, quantity, and characteristics.
- The abdomen may be flabby initially. Diastasis recti should be measured.
- Constipation may develop postpartally due to decreased tone, limited diet, and denial of the urge to defecate due to fear of pain.
- Decreased bladder sensitivity, increased capacity, and postpartal diuresis may lead to problems with bladder elimination. Frequent assessment and prompt intervention are indicated. A fundus that is boggy but does not respond to massage, is higher than expected, or deviates to the side usually indicates a full bladder.
- Postpartally a healthy woman should be normotensive and afebrile. Bradycardia is common.
- Postpartally the WBC is often elevated. Activation of clotting factors predisposes the woman to thrombus formation.
- Psychologic adaptations include maternal role attainment and attachment to the newborn.
- In consideration of the client's background, the nurse should recognize and respect cultural variations and individual preferences.
- Postpartal assessment should be completed in a systematic way, usually cephalocaudally. It provides a tremendous opportunity for informal teaching.
- In the weeks following birth, the woman's physical condition returns to a nonpregnant state and she gains competence and confidence in herself as a parent.

REFERENCES

Ament LA: Maternal tasks of the puerperium reidentified. *JOGNN* July/August 1990; 19:330.

Blackburn ST, Loper DL: *Maternal, Fetal and Neonatal Physiology.* Philadelphia: Saunders, 1992.

Cunningham FG et al: *Williams Obstetrics,* 19th ed. Norwalk, CT: Appleton and Lange, 1993.

Food and Nutrition Board, National Academy of Sciences—National Research Council: *Recommended Dietary Allowances,* 10th ed. Washington, DC: 1989.

Lederman, RP: *Psychosocial Adaptation in Pregnancy,* 2nd ed. New York: Springer, 1996.

Mercer RT: *Becoming a Mother.* New York: Springer, 1995.

Rubin R: Puerperal change. *Nurs Outlook* 1961; 9:753.

Rubin R: *Maternal Identity and the Maternal Experience.* New York: Springer, 1984.

Spector RE: *Cultural Diversity in Health and Illness.* Norwalk, CT: Appleton & Lange, 1991.

Varney H: *Nurse Midwifery,* 2nd ed. Boston: Blackwell Scientific Publications, 1987.

Valaitis R, Tuff K, Swanson L: Meeting parent's postpartal needs with a telephone information line. *MCN* 1996; 21:90.

Zlatnik FJ: The puerperium: Normal and abnormal. In: *Danforth's Obstetrics and Gynecology,* 7th ed. Scott JB et al (editors). Philadelphia: Lippincott, 1994.

Chapter 28 The Postpartal Family: Needs and Care

OBJECTIVES

- Relate the use of nursing diagnoses to the findings of the "normal" postpartum assessment and analysis.
- Delineate nursing responsibilities for client education during the early postpartum period.
- Discuss appropriate nursing interventions to meet identified nursing goals for the childbearing family.
- Explore the nursing needs of the woman and family who experience a cesarean birth.
- Summarize the nursing needs of the childbearing adolescent during the postpartum period.
- Discuss the nursing needs of a woman with an unwanted pregnancy.
- Describe possible approaches to follow-up nursing care for the childbearing family.

KEY TERMS

Engorgement
Patient-controlled analgesia (PCA)

Certain premises form the basis of effective nursing care during the postpartal period.

- The best postpartal care is family centered; incorporates the family's needs, desires, and values as much as possible; and disrupts the family unit as little as possible. This approach uses the family's resources to support an early and smooth adjustment to the newborn by all family members.
- Knowledge of the range of normal physiologic and psychologic adaptations occurring during the postpartal period allows the nurse to recognize alterations and initiate interventions early. Communicating information about postpartal adaptations to the family facilitates their adjustment to their situation.
- Nursing care is aimed at accomplishing specific goals that are intended to ultimately meet individual and family needs. These goals are formulated after careful assessment, consultation with the woman and her family, and consideration of factors that could influence the outcome of care.

Chapter 27 provided a thorough discussion of postpartal assessment. This chapter describes how the nurse can use the remaining steps of the nursing process effectively to plan and provide care. Specific nursing responses to the mother's physical needs and the family's psychosocial needs are described at length. The Postpartal Critical Pathway begins on p 733.

Nursing Diagnosis During the Postpartal Period

For most postpartal women, physical recovery goes smoothly and is considered a healthy process. Because of this perception, it is all too common for caregivers to think that the woman and her family have no "real" needs and that no care plan is needed. Nothing could be further from the truth. Every member of the family has needs, although they may not be obvious, especially if they are psychologic or educational.

The postpartal family's needs, which should be identified during assessment, are the basis for developing nursing diagnoses. Once a nursing diagnosis is made and recorded, systematic action, as delineated in a nursing care plan, can be taken to meet the identified need.

Many nurses have suggested that nursing diagnoses are difficult to make in a wellness setting because of their emphasis on "problems." Nurses involved in the effort to formulate standardized diagnoses recognize this difficulty and continue working to develop nursing diagnoses that are more congruent with wellness settings.

Many agencies that use nursing diagnoses prefer to use only the NANDA list. Consequently, physiologic alterations form the basis of many postpartal diagnoses. Examples of such diagnoses include

- Constipation related to fear of tearing stitches or pain
- Altered patterns of urinary elimination related to dysuria

Diagnoses related to family coping or instructional needs are also used frequently. Examples of these diagnoses include

- Knowledge deficit related to a lack of understanding about infant behavior
- Family coping: potential for growth related to successful adjustment to new baby

After completing the assessment and diagnosis steps of the nursing process, the nurse identifies expected outcomes and selects nursing interventions that will help the family meet the expected outcomes.

KEY FACTS TO REMEMBER

Position of the Uterine Fundus Following Birth

- Immediately after birth: The top of the fundus is in the midline about midway between the symphysis pubis and umbilicus.
- Six to twelve hours after birth: The top of the fundus is in the midline at the level of the umbilicus.
- One day after birth: The top of the fundus is in the midline and one finger-breadth below the umbilicus.
- Second day after birth and thereafter: The top of the fundus remains in the midline and descends about one finger-breadth per day.

Nursing Plan and Implementation During the Postpartal Period

Promotion of Maternal Physical Well-Being

Maternal physical well-being is promoted and restored by monitoring: the status of the uterus, vital signs, cardiovascular status, elimination patterns, nutritional needs, sleep and rest, and support and educational needs. In addition, medications may be needed to promote comfort, treat anemia, provide immunity to rubella, and prevent development of antigens in the nonsensitized Rh-negative woman.

Monitoring Uterine Status

The nurse completes an assessment of the uterus as discussed in Chapter 27. The assessment interval is usually

DRUG GUIDE | Methylergonovine Maleate (Methergine)

Overview of Action

Methylergonovine maleate is an ergot alkaloid that stimulates smooth muscle tissue. Because the smooth muscle of the uterus is especially sensitive to this drug, it is used postpartally to stimulate the uterus to contract in order to decrease blood loss by clamping off uterine blood vessels and to promote the involution process. In addition the drug has a vasoconstrictive effect on all blood vessels, especially the larger arteries. This may result in hypertension, particularly in a woman whose blood pressure is already elevated.

ROUTE, DOSAGE, AND FREQUENCY

Methergine has a rapid onset of action and may be given intramuscularly, orally, or intravenously.

Usual IM dose: 0.2 mg following delivery of the placenta. The dose may be repeated every 2–4 hours if necessary.

Usual oral dose: 0.2 mg every 4 hours (six doses).

Usual IV dose: Because the adverse effects of Methergine are far more severe with IV administration, this route is seldom used.

MATERNAL CONTRAINDICATIONS

Pregnancy, hepatic or renal disease, cardiac disease, and hypertension contraindicate this drug's use.

MATERNAL SIDE EFFECTS

Hypertension (particularly when administered IV), nausea, vomiting, headache, bradycardia, dizziness, tinnitus, abdominal cramps, palpitations, dyspnea, chest pain, and allergic reactions may be noted.

EFFECTS ON FETUS OR NEONATE

Because Methergine has a long duration and action and can thus produce tetanic contractions, it **should never be used during pregnancy or in labor,** when it may result in fetal trauma or death.

Nursing Considerations

1. Monitor fundal height and consistency and the amount and character of the lochia.
2. Assess the blood pressure before and routinely throughout drug administration.
3. Observe for adverse effects or symptoms of ergot toxicity.

every 15 minutes for the first hour after childbirth, every 30 minutes for the next hour, and then hourly for approximately 2 hours. After that, the nurse monitors uterine status every 8 hours or more frequently if problems arise such as bogginess, positioning out of midline, heavy lochia flow, or the presence of clots. See Key Facts to Remember: Position of the Uterine Fundus Following Birth on the previous page.

Occasionally medications need to be ordered to promote uterine contractions. See Drug Guide: Oxytocin (Pitocin), section on postpartal use in Chapter 20, and Methylergonovine Maleate (Methergine) above.

The nurse monitors amount, consistency, color, and odor of the lochia on an ongoing basis. See Key Facts to Remember: Normal Characteristics of Lochia. Changes in lochia that need to be assessed further, documented, and reported to the physician/certified nurse-midwife appear in Table 28–1.

Promotion of Comfort and Relief of Pain

Discomfort may be present to varying degrees in the postpartal woman. Potential sources of discomfort include an edematous perineum; an episiotomy, perineal laceration, or extension; vaginal hematoma; engorged hemorrhoids; or engorged breasts with sore nipples.

Relief of Perineal Discomfort

There are many nursing interventions for the relief of perineal discomfort. Before selecting a method, the nurse needs to assess the perineum to determine the degree of edema and so on. It is also important to ask the woman if there are special measures that she feels will be particularly effective and to offer her choices when possible. It is important for the nurse to use disposable gloves while applying all relief measures and to complete a handwashing before and after using the gloves. (See Essential Precautions for Practice: During Postpartal Care on p 732.) At all times, it is important to remember hygienic practices, such as moving from the front (area of the symphysis pubis) to the back (area around the anus) of the perineum. This is important to remember while placing ice packs and perineal pads and applying topical anesthetics or pain relief products. Avoiding contamination between the anal area and the urethral/vaginal area is important to prevent infection.

Ice Pack If an episiotomy is done at the time of birth, an ice pack is generally applied to reduce edema and

KEY FACTS TO REMEMBER

Normal Characteristics of Lochia

- Lochia rubra is red and is present for the first 2–3 days.
- Lochia serosa is pinkish red and is present from the 3rd to the 10th day.
- Lochia alba is creamy white and is present from the 11th to about the 21st day.

TABLE 28–1 Changes in Lochia That Cause Concern

Change	Possible Problem	Nursing Action
Presence of clots	Inadequate uterine contractions that allow bleeding from vessels at the placental site.	Assess location and firmness of fundus. Assess voiding pattern. Record and report findings.
Persistent lochia rubra	Inadequate uterine contractions; retained placental fragments; infection.	Assess location and firmness of fundus. Assess activity pattern. Assess for signs of infection. Record and report findings.

provide numbing of the tissues, which promotes comfort. In some agencies, chemical ice bags are used. These are usually activated by folding both ends toward the middle. Inexpensive ice bags may be made by filling a disposable glove with ice chips or crushed ice and then taping the top of the glove. To protect the perineum from burns caused by contact with such an ice pack, the glove needs to be rinsed under running water to remove any powder and then wrapped in an absorbent towel or washcloth before placing it against the perineum. To attain the maximum effect of this cold treatment, the ice pack should remain in place for approximately 20 minutes and then be removed for about 10 minutes before replacing it. Usually ice packs are needed for the first 24 hours. The nurse provides information about the purpose of the ice pack, anticipated effects, benefits, and possible problems, and how to prepare an ice pack for home use if edema is present and early discharge is planned.

ESSENTIAL PRECAUTIONS FOR PRACTICE

During Pospartal Care

Examples of times when disposable gloves should be worn include

- Assessing the perineum and lochia
- Changing perineal pads and chux
- Assessing the breast if there is leakage of colostrum or milk
- Handling used breast pads
- Handling used clothing, chux, perineal pads, and/or bedding contaminated with lochia
- Applying ice packs or topical anesthetic sprays to the perineum. (Although an ice pack or anesthetic spray could be applied in such a manner that contact with the perineum and a perineal pad is avoided, it is best to have gloves on so that you can assist with removal of the pad if needed.)

REMEMBER to wash your hands before putting on the disposable gloves and again immediately after you remove them.

For further information consult OSHA and CDC guidelines.

Sitz Bath The warmth of the water in the sitz bath provides comfort, decreases pain, and promotes circulation to the tissues, which promotes healing and reduces the incidence of infection. Sitz baths may be ordered TID and PRN. The nurse prepares the sitz bath by cleaning the sitz tub or portable sitz and adding water at 102–105F. The woman is encouraged to remain in the sitz bath for 20 minutes. Care needs to be taken during the first sitz bath as the warm moist heat and warm environment may cause the woman to faint. Placing a call bell well within reach and checking on the woman at frequent intervals will increase her comfort and maintain safety. The woman needs to be observed at frequent intervals for signs that she may faint, such as dizziness, a floaty or spacy feeling, or difficulty hearing. It is important for the woman to have a clean unused towel to pat dry her perineum after the sitz and to have a clean perineal pad to apply.

Recently cool sitz baths have gained popularity because they are effective in reducing perineal edema. Until definite research supports one temperature (warm or cold) as more effective, it may be best to offer the woman a choice. The nurse provides information about the purpose and use of the sitz bath; anticipated effects, benefits, and possible problems; and safety measures to prevent injury from fainting, slipping, or excessive water temperature. Home use of sitz baths may be recommended for the woman with an extensive episiotomy, and the woman may use a portable sitz or her bathtub. It is important for the nurse to emphasize that in using a bathtub, the woman draws only 4–6 inches of water, assesses the temperature of the water, and uses the water only for the sitz and not for bathing. If the woman takes a tub bath, she should release the water, have a helper clean the tub, and draw new water prior to the sitz to prevent infection.

CRITICAL THINKING IN ACTION

Ellen Baker is 24 hours past birth. She tells you that she is passing clots and asks you if this is normal. Would you tell her that this is normal?

Answers can be found in Appendix H.

POSTPARTAL CRITICAL PATHWAY

Category	1–4 Hours Postpartum	4–8 Hours Postpartum	8–24 Hours Postpartum
Referral	Report from labor nurse if not continuing in an LDR room	Lactation consultation if needed	Home nursing referral if indicated
Assessment	Postpartum assessments q$\frac{1}{2}$h × 2, q1h × 2, then q4h. Includes: • Fundus firm, in midline, at or below umbilicus • Lochia rubra <1 pad/h; no free flow or passage of clots with massage • Bladder: voids large amts urine spontaneously; bladder not palpable following voiding • Perineum: sutures intact; no bulging or marked swelling; no c/o severe pain. Minimal bruising may be present. If hemorroids present, no tenseness or marked engorgement; <2 cm diameter • Breasts: soft, colostrum present Vital signs: • BP WNL; no hypotension; not >30 mm systolic or 15 mm diastolic over baseline • Temperature: <38C (100.4F) • Pulse: bradycardia normal; consistent with baseline • Respirations: 12–20/min; quiet; easy Comfort level: <3 on scale of 1 to 10	Continue postpartum assessment q4h × 2, then q8h Breast: evaluate nipple status; should be no evidence of cracks or bruising Observe feeding technique with newborn Vital signs assessment q8h: all WNL; report temperature >38C (100.4F) Continue assessment of comfort level	Continue postpartum assessment q8h Breasts: nipples should remain free of cracks, fissures, bruising Feeding technique with newborn: should be good or improving Vital signs assessment q8h: all WNL; report temperature >38C (100.4F) Continue assessment of comfort level
Comfort	Institute comfort measures: • Perineal discomfort: peri-care, sitz baths, topical analgesics • Hemorrhoids: sitz baths, topical analgesics, digital replacement of external hemorrhoids; side-lying or prone position • Afterpains: prone with sm. pillow under abdomen; warm shower or sitz baths; ambulation • Administer pain medication________	Continue with pain management techniques	Continue with pain management techniques
Teaching/ psychosocial	Explain postpartum assessments Teach self-massage of fundus & expected findings Instruct to call for assistance first time OOB and prn Demonstrate peri-care, surgigator, sitz bath prn Explain comfort measures Begin newborn teaching: bulb suctioning, positioning, feeding, diaper change, cord care Orient to room if transferred from LDR room Provide information on early postpartum period	Discuss psychologic changes of postpartum period Stress need for frequent rest periods Continue newborn teaching: soothing/comforting techniques, swaddling; return demonstrations indicate woman's understanding Provide opportunities for questions and review; reinforce previous teaching Breastfeeding: nipple care: air-drying, lanolin; proper latch-on technique; tea bags Bottle feeding: supportive bra, ice bags, breast binder	Reinforce previous teaching; answer questions Discuss involution; anticipated physical changes in first 2 weeks postpartum; postpartum exercises; need to limit visitors Discuss postpartum nutrition: balanced diet, nutritionally rich Breastfeeding: • Increase calories by 500 kcal over nonpregnant state (200 kcal over pregnant intake) • Explain milk production, let-down reflex, use of supplements, breast pumping, and milk storage Bottle feeding: • Return to normal caloric intake for nonpregnant state • Explain formula preparation and storage Discuss sibling rivalry. Mother should have plan for supporting siblings at home Teaching evaluation completed

POSTPARTAL CRITICAL PATHWAY continued

Category	1–4 Hours Postpartum	4–8 Hours Postpartum	8–24 Hours Postpartum
Therapeutic nursing interventions and reports	Ice pack to perineum to ↓ swelling & ↑ comfort Straight cath. prn × 1 if distented or voiding small amts If continues unable to void or voiding sm. amts, insert Foley catheter and notify CNM/physician	Sitz baths prn If woman Rh$^-$ and infant Rh$^+$, RhoGAM work up; obtain consent; complete teaching Obtain consent for rubella vaccine if indicated; explain purpose, procedure, implications Obtain hematocrit Determine rubella status	Continue sitz baths prn May shower if ambulating s̜ difficulty DC buffalo cap (hep lock) if present
Activity	Assistance when OOB first time, then prn Ambulate ad lib Rests comfortably between checks	Encourage rest periods Ambulate ad lib; may leave birthing unit	Up ad lib
Nutrition	Regular diet Fluid intake ≥2000 mL/day	Continue diet and fluids	Continue diet and fluids
Elimination	Voiding large amts straw-colored urine	Voiding large quantities May have bowel movement	Same
Medications	Methergine 0.2 mg q4h prn if ordered Stool softener______________ Tucks pads prn	Continue meds Lanolin to nipples PRN; tea bags to nipples if tender; heparin flush to buffalo cap (if present) q8h or as ordered	Continue medications May take own prenatal vitamins RhoGAM administered if indicated Rubella vaccine administered if indicated
Discharge planning/ home care	Evaluate knowledge of normal postpartum, newborn care Evaluate support systems	Discuss typical newborn schedule; plan for periods of rest Birth certificate paperwork completed Evaluate plans for transporting newborn; car seat available	Review discharge instruction sheet and checklist Describe postpartum warning signs and when to call CNM/physician Provide prescriptions. Gift pack given to woman Arrangements made for baby pictures if desired Postpartum visit scheduled Newborn check scheduled
Family involvement	Identify available support persons Assess family perceptions of birth experience Parenting: demonstrates culturally expected early parenting behaviors	Involve support persons in care, teaching; answer questions Evidence of parental bonding behaviors apparent	Continue to involve support persons in teaching Evidence of parental bonding behaviors present Plans made for providing support to mother following discharge. Support persons verbalize understanding of need for woman to rest, eat nutritionally, recover

Topical Agents Topical anesthetics such as Dermoplast aerosol spray or Americain spray may be used to relieve perineal discomfort. The woman is advised to apply the anesthetic after a sitz bath or perineal care. Witch hazel compresses may be used to relieve perineal discomfort and edema. Nupercainal ointment or Tucks may be ordered for relief of hemorrhoidal pain. It is important for the nurse to emphasize the need for the woman to wash her hands before and after using the topical treatments.

The nurse provides information about the anesthetic spray or topical agent. The woman needs to understand the purpose, use, anticipated effects and benefits, and possible problems associated with the product. The nurse can combine a demonstration of application with teaching. A return demonstration is a useful method of evaluating the woman's understanding.

Perineal Care Perineal care after each elimination cleanses the perineum and helps promote comfort. Many agencies provide "peri bottles" that the woman can use to squirt warm tap water over her perineum following elimination. To cleanse her perineum, the woman should use moist antiseptic towelettes or toilet paper in a blotting (patting) motion and should be taught to start at the front (area just under the symphysis pubis) and proceed toward the back (area around the anus), to prevent contamination from the anal area. In addition, to prevent contamination the perineal pad should be applied from front to back (place the front portion against the perineum first).

The nurse demonstrates how to cleanse the perineum and assists the woman as necessary. Additional information regarding the use of perineal pads may be offered. The pads need to be placed snugly against the perineum but should not produce pressure. If the pad is worn too loosely, it may rub back and forth, irritating perineal tissues and causing contamination between the anal area and vaginal area. Many women have never used a perineal pad or belt and will need additional assistance in using them during the postpartal period.

Relief of Hemorrhoidal Discomfort

Some mothers experience hemorrhoidal pain after giving birth. Relief measures include the use of sitz baths, anesthetic ointments, rectal suppositories, or witch hazel pads applied directly to the anal area. The woman may be taught to digitally replace external hemorrhoids in her rectum. She may also find it helpful to maintain a side-lying position when possible and to avoid prolonged sitting. The mother is encouraged to maintain an adequate fluid intake, and stool softeners are administered to ensure greater comfort with bowel movements. The hemorrhoids usually disappear a few weeks after birth if the woman did not have them before her pregnancy.

Afterpains

Afterpains are the result of intermittent uterine contractions. A primipara may not experience afterpains because her uterus is able to maintain a contracted state. Multiparous women and those who have had a multiple pregnancy or hydramnios frequently experience discomfort from afterpains as the uterus intermittently contracts. Breastfeeding women are also more likely to experience afterpains than bottle-feeding women because of the release of oxytocin when the infant suckles. The nurse can suggest the woman lie prone with a small pillow under the lower abdomen. The woman needs to be told that the discomfort may feel intensified for about 5 minutes but then will diminish greatly if not completely. The prone position applies pressure to the uterus and therefore stimulates contractions. When the uterus maintains a constant contraction, the afterpains cease. Additional nursing interventions include a sitz bath (for warmth), positioning, ambulation, or administration of an analgesic agent. For breastfeeding mothers, a mild analgesic administered an hour before feeding will promote comfort and enhance maternal-infant interaction (Table 28–2).

The nurse provides information about the cause of afterpains and methods to decrease discomfort. The nurse explains any medications that are ordered, expected effect and benefits and possible side effects, and any special considerations such as the possibility of dizziness or sleepiness with particular medications.

Discomfort from Immobility

Discomfort may also be caused by immobility. The woman who has been in stirrups for any length of time may experience muscular aches from such extreme positioning. It is not unusual for women to experience joint pains and muscular pain in both arms and legs, depending on the effort they exerted during the second stage of labor.

Early ambulation is encouraged to help reduce the incidence of complications such as constipation and thrombophlebitis. It also helps promote a feeling of general well-being.

The nurse assists the woman the first few times she gets up during the postpartal period. Fatigue, effects of medications, loss of blood, and possibly even lack of food intake may cause feelings of dizziness or faintness when the woman stands up. Because this may be a problem during the woman's first shower, the nurse should remain in the room, check the woman frequently, and have a chair close by in case she becomes faint. During this first shower the nurse instructs the woman in the use of the emergency call button in the bathroom; if she becomes faint during a future shower, she can call for assistance.

The nurse provides information about ambulation and the importance of monitoring any signs of dizziness

TABLE 28–2 Essential Information for Common Postpartum Drugs

EMPIRIN #3 (325 mg aspirin and 30 mg codeine)

Drug class: Narcotic analgesic.
Dose/Route: Usual adult dose: 1–2 tablets PO every 4 hours PRN.
Indication: For relief of mild to moderate pain.
Adverse Effects: Aspirin: Nausea, dyspepsia, epigastric discomfort, dizziness. Codeine: Respiratory depression, apnea, light-headedness, dizziness, nausea, sweating, dry mouth, constipation, facial flushing, suppression of cough reflex, ureteral spasm, urinary retention, pruritus.
Nursing Implications: Determine if woman is sensitive to aspirin or codeine; has history of impaired hepatic or renal function.
Monitor bowel sounds, respirations, urine output.
Administer with food or after meals if GI upset occurs; encourage woman to drink one full glass (240 mL) with the tablet to reduce the risk of the tablet lodging in the esophagus.

Client Teaching: Inform client about name of drug, expected action, possible side effects, that it is secreted in breast milk (Note: Some physicians/certified nurse-midwives may avoid ordering this medication for nursing mothers), and review safety measures (assess for dizziness, use side rails, call for assistance when getting out of bed and ambulating, report to nurse any signs of adverse effects); ask if she has any questions.

Nursing Diagnoses Related to Drug Therapy: Knowledge deficit related to lack of information regarding the drug therapy.
Potential for injury related to dizziness secondary to effect of drug.

PERCOSET (325 mg acetaminophen and 5 mg oxycodone)

Drug Class: Narcotic analgesic.
Dose/Route: 1–2 tablets PO every 4 hours PRN.
Indication: For moderate to moderately severe pain. Can be used in aspirin-sensitive women.
Adverse Effects: Acetaminophen: Hepatotoxicity, headache, rash, hypoglycemia. Oxycodone: Respiratory depression, apnea, circulatory depression, euphoria, facial flushing, constipation, suppression of cough reflex, ureteral spasm, urinary retention.
Nursing Implications: Determine if woman is sensitive to acetaminophen or codeine; has bronchial asthma, respiratory depression, convulsive disorder.
Observe woman carefully for respiratory depression if given with barbiturates or sedative/hypnotics. Consider that postcesarean-birth woman may have depressed cough reflex, so teaching and encouragement to deep breathe and cough is needed.
Monitor bowel sounds, urine and bowel elimination.

Client Teaching: Teaching should include name of drug, expected effect, possible adverse effects, that drug is secreted in the breast milk, encouragement to report any signs of adverse effects immediately.

Nursing Diagnoses Related to Drug Therapy: Altered breathing patterns related to depression.
Constipation related to slowed gastrointestinal activity.

RUBELLA VIRUS VACCINE, LIVE (Meruvax 2)

Dose/Route: Single dose vial, inject subcutaneously in outer aspect of the upper arm.
Indication: Stimulate active immunity against rubella virus.
Adverse Effects: Burning or stinging at the injection site; about 2–4 weeks later may have rash, malaise, sore throat, or headache.
Nursing Implications: Determine if woman has sensitivity to neomycin (vaccine contains neomycin); is immunosuppressed, or has received blood transfusions (not to be administered within 3 months of blood transfusion, plasma transfusion, or serum immune globulin).
Note: If a woman is to receive both RhoGAM and rubella, there is a possibility that the formation of antibodies to rubella may be suppressed by the RhoGAM injection. Most physicians will go ahead and order both injections and retest for maternal rubella immune status in about 3 months (Varney 1987).

Client Teaching: Name of drug, expected effect, possible adverse effects, possible comfort measures to use if adverse effects occur; rubella titer will be assessed in about 3 months. Instruct woman to AVOID PREGNANCY FOR 3 MONTHS following vaccination. Provide information regarding contraceptives and their use.

Nursing Diagnoses Related to Drug Therapy: Knowledge deficit regarding drug therapy. Knowledge deficit regarding types and use of contraceptives.
Pain related to rash and malaise.

RhoGAM (Rh immune globulin specific for D antigen)

Dose/Route: Postpartum: One vial IM within 72 hours of birth. Antepartal: One vial microdose RhoGAM IM at 28 weeks in Rh-negative women; after amniocentesis, spontaneous or therapeutic abortion, or ectopic pregnancy.
Indication: Prevention of sensitization to the Rh factor in Rh-negative women and to prevent hemolytic disease in the newborn in subsequent pregnancies. Mother must be Rh-negative, not previously sensitized to Rh factor. Infant must be Rh-positive, direct antiglobulin negative.
Adverse Effects: Soreness at injection site.
Nursing Implications: Confirm criteria for administration are present. Assure correct vial is used for the client (each vial is cross-matched to the specific woman and must be carefully checked).
Inject entire contents of vial.

Client Teaching: Name of drug, expected action, possible side effects; report soreness at injection site to nurse; woman should carry information regarding Rh status and dates of RhoGAM injections with her at all times; explain use of RhoGAM with subsequent pregnancies.

Nursing Diagnoses Related to Drug Therapy: Knowledge deficit related to the need for RhoGAM and future implications.
Pain related to soreness at injection site.

SECONAL SODIUM (secobarbital sodium)

Drug Class: Sedative, short-acting barbiturate.
Dose/Route: 100 mg PO at bedtime.
Indication: Promote sleep.
Adverse Effects: Somnolence, confusion, ataxia, vertigo, nightmares, hypoventilation, bradycardia, hypotension, nausea, vomiting, rashes.
Nursing Implications: Determine if woman has sensitivity to barbiturates, or respiratory distress. Monitor respirations, blood pressure, pulse. Modify environment to increase relaxation and promote sleep.
Monitor for drug interaction if woman also is taking tranquilizers or TACE.

Client Teaching: Name of drug, expected effect, possible adverse effects, safety measures (siderails, use call bell, ask for assistance when out of bed); medication is secreted in breast milk.

Nursing Diagnoses Related to Drug Therapy: Potential for injury related to possible ataxia or vertigo.
Altered thought processes related to drug-induced confusion.
Knowledge deficit related to lack of information regarding drug therapy.

or weakness. If dizziness occurs, the mother should sit down and call for assistance.

Postpartal Diaphoresis

Postpartal diaphoresis (excessive perspiration) may cause discomfort for new mothers. The nurse can offer a fresh dry gown and bed linens to enhance comfort. Some women may feel refreshed by a shower. It is important to consider cultural practices and realize that some women of Hispanic or Asian cultural background may prefer not to shower in the first few days following birth. Because diaphoresis may also increase thirst, the nurse can offer fluids as the woman desires. Again, it is important to consider cultural practices. Women of Western European background may prefer iced water, while Asian women may prefer water at room temperature. It is important to ascertain the woman's wishes rather than operate solely from one's own value or cultural belief system.

The nurse provides information about the normal physiologic occurrence of the diaphoresis and methods to increase comfort.

Suppression of Lactation in the Nonnursing Mother

For the woman who chooses not to breastfeed, lactation may be suppressed by mechanical inhibition. Although signs of engorgement do not usually occur until the second or third postpartum day, prevention of engorgement is best accomplished by beginning mechanical inhibition of lactation as soon as possible after birth. Ideally this involves having the woman begin wearing a supportive, well-fitting bra within 6 hours after birth. The bra is worn continuously until lactation is suppressed (usually about 5–7 days) and is removed only for showers. The bra provides support and eases the discomfort that can occur with tension on the breasts because of fullness. Ice packs should be applied over the axillary area of each breast for 20 minutes four times daily. This, too, should be begun soon after birth. Ice is also useful in relieving discomfort if engorgement occurs. Breast **engorgement** may be a source of pain for the postpartal woman. Specific nursing interventions for pain in the bottle-feeding mother are discussed in Chapter 25.

The mother is advised to avoid any stimulation of her breasts by her baby, herself, breast pumps, or her sexual partner until the sensation of fullness has passed (usually about 5–7 days). Such stimulation will increase milk production and delay the suppression process. Heat is avoided for the same reason, and the mother is encouraged to let shower water flow over her back rather than her breasts.

Promotion of Rest and Graded Activity

Following birth a woman may feel exhausted and in need of rest. In other cases she may be euphoric and full of psychic energy immediately after birth, ready to relive the experience of birth repeatedly. The nurse can provide a period for airing of feelings and then encourage a period of rest.

Physical fatigue often affects other adjustments and functions of the new mother. For example, fatigue can reduce milk flow, thereby increasing problems with establishing breastfeeding. Energy is also needed to make the psychologic adjustments to a new infant and to assume new roles. Adjustments are most smoothly accomplished when adequate rest is obtained. Nurses can encourage rest by organizing their activities to avoid frequent interruptions for the woman.

Although most mothers feel fatigued, if they have perceived the pregnancy and birth as a natural process, they tend to view themselves as healthy and well. Some mothers view the postpartal period as a time of sickness. For instance, some Korean women and their families view the mother as sick and in need of care by the mother-in-law and the father. A Korean mother may take on some activity but for the most part, it will be for activities such as picking up the baby from the nursery rather than activity directed toward herself (Schneiderman 1996).

Postpartal Exercises

The woman should be encouraged to begin simple exercises while in the birthing unit and continue them at home. She is advised that increased lochia or pain means she should reevaluate her activity and make necessary alterations. Most agencies provide a booklet describing suggested postpartal activities. (Exercise routines vary for women undergoing cesarean birth or tubal ligation after childbirth.) See Figure 28–1 for a description of some commonly used exercises.

Resumption of Activities

Ambulation and activity may gradually increase after birth. The new mother should avoid heavy lifting, excessive stair climbing, and strenuous activity. One or two daily naps are essential and are most easily achieved if the mother sleeps when her baby does.

By the second week at home, light housekeeping may be resumed. Although it is customary to delay returning to work for 6 weeks, most women are physically able to resume practically all activities by 4 to 5 weeks. Delaying the return to work until after the final postpartal examination will minimize the possibility of problems.

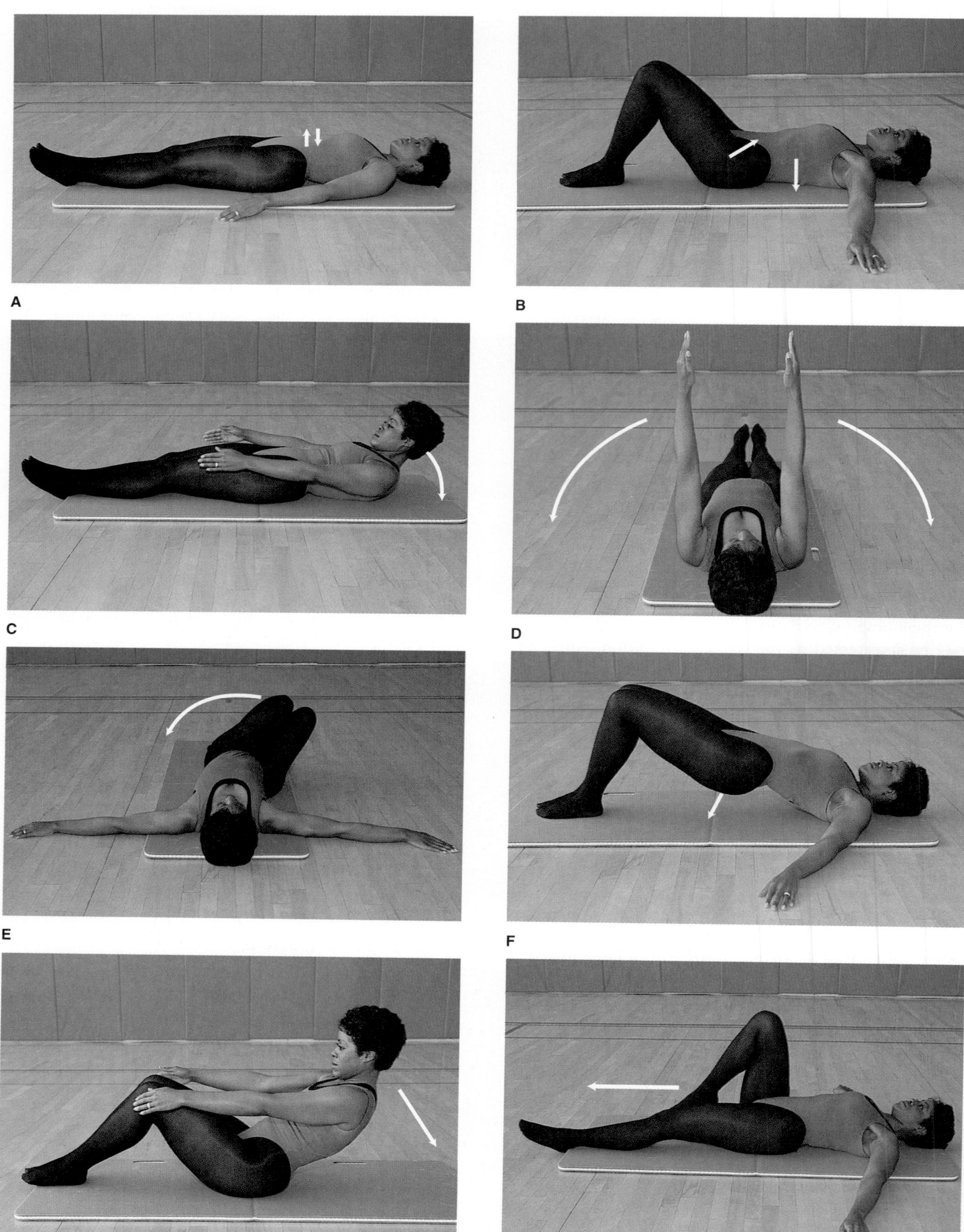
A
B
C
D
E
F
G
H

Pharmacologic Interventions

Rubella Vaccine

Women who have a rubella titer of less than 1:10, or are ELISA antibody-negative, are usually given rubella vaccine in the postpartal period (Cunningham 1997). (See Table 28–2.)

The nurse needs to ensure that the woman understands the purpose of the vaccine and that she must avoid becoming pregnant in the next 3 months. To ensure that the woman understands, an informed consent is obtained before administration. Because the avoidance of pregnancy is so important, counseling regarding contraception is suggested.

RhoGAM

All Rh-negative women who meet specific criteria should receive RhIgG (RhoGAM) within 72 hours after childbirth to prevent sensitization from the fetomaternal transfusion of the Rh-positive fetal red blood cells. See discussion of criteria in Procedure 12–2.

The Rh-negative woman needs to understand the implications of her Rh-negative status in future pregnancies. The nurse provides opportunities for questions.

Promotion of Maternal Psychologic Well-Being

The birth of a child, with the changes in role and the increased responsibilities it produces, is a time of emotional stress for the new mother. During the early postpartum period the mother may be emotionally labile, and mood swings and tearfulness are common.

Initially the mother may repeatedly discuss her experiences of labor and birth. This allows the mother to integrate her experiences. If she feels that she did not cope well with labor, she may have feelings of inadequacy and may benefit from reassurance that she did well. Some women feel that they did not have any perception of time during the labor and birth and want to know how long it really lasted, or they may not remember the entire experience. In this case, it is helpful for the nurse to talk with her and provide information that the mother is missing and desires (Waldenstrom et al 1996).

During this time the new mother must also adjust to the loss of her fantasized child and accept the child she has borne. This may be more difficult if the child is not of the desired sex or if he or she has birth defects.

Immediately after the birth (the taking-in period) the mother is focused on bodily concerns and may not be fully ready to learn about personal and infant care. Following the initial dependent period, the mother becomes very concerned about her ability to be a successful parent (the taking-hold period). During this time the mother requires reassurance that she is effective. She also tends to be more receptive to teaching and demonstration designed to assist her in mothering successfully. The depression and weepiness and "let-down feeling" that characterize the "postpartum blues" are often a surprise for the new mother. She requires reassurance that these feelings are normal, an explanation about why they occur, and a supportive environment that permits her to cry without feeling guilty (Mercer 1995).

FIGURE 28–1 (at left) Postpartal exercises. Begin with five repetitions two or three times daily and gradually increase to ten repetitions. First day: ***A*** Abdominal breathing. Lying supine, inhale deeply using the abdominal muscles. The abdomen should expand. Then exhale slowly through pursed lips, tightening the abdominal muscles. ***B*** Pelvic rocking. Lying supine with arms at sides, knees bent, and feet flat, tighten abdomen and buttocks and attempt to flatten back on floor. Hold for a count of ten, then arch the back, causing the pelvis to "rock." On second day add: ***C*** Chin to chest. Lying supine with no pillow, legs straight, raise head and attempt to touch chin to chest. Slowly lower head. ***D*** Arm raises. Lying supine, arms extended perpendicular to body, raise arms until hands touch. Lower slowly. On fourth day add: ***E*** Knee rolls. Lying supine with knees bent, feet flat, arms extended to the side, roll knees slowly to one side, keeping shoulders flat. Return to original position and roll to opposite side. ***F*** Buttocks lift. Lying supine, arms at sides, knees bent, feet flat, slowly raise the buttocks and arch the back. Return slowly to starting position. On sixth day add: ***G*** Abdominal tighteners. Lying supine, knees bent, feet flat, slowly raise head toward knees. Arms should extend along either side of legs. Return slowly to original position. ***H*** Knee to abdomen. Lying supine, arms at sides, bend one knee and thigh until foot touches buttocks. Straighten leg and lower it slowly. Repeat with other leg. After 2–3 weeks, more strenuous exercises such as side leg raises may be added as tolerated. Kegel exercises, begun antepartally, should be done many times daily during postpartum to restore vaginal and perineal tone.

Promotion of Effective Parent Education

Meeting the educational needs of the new mother and her family is one of the primary challenges facing the postpartum nurse. Each woman's educational needs vary based on age, background, experience, and expectations. In addition, the brief period of time that the mother is in the postpartal area makes it even more difficult to address all individual characteristics and informational needs (Barnes 1996). The steps of the nursing process provide a useful tool for identifying and meeting educational needs after childbirth.

The nurse first assesses the learning needs of the new mother through observation and tactfully phrased questions. For example, "What plans have you made for handling things when you get home?" will elicit a response of several words and may provide the opportunity for some information sharing and guidance. Some agencies also use checklists of common concerns for new mothers. The woman can check those that are of interest to her.

The nurse should then plan and implement teaching to provide learning experiences in a logical, nonthreatening way based on knowledge and respect of the family's cultural values and beliefs. For example, some Korean women will look to the mother-in-law for information regarding all aspects of self- and infant care (Schneiderman 1996). The nurse needs to recognize this and explore the care that is planned. Unless there is an activity that the nurse believes would be harmful, most cultural customs can be supported and encouraged. Postpartal units use a variety of approaches, including handouts, formal classes, videotapes, and individual interaction. Regardless of the technique, timing is important. The new mother is more receptive to teaching after the first 24–48 hours when she is ready to assume responsibility for her own care and that of her newborn. Unfortunately, many women are discharged during the first 24 hours after birth. Because of this, many units provide printed material for new mothers to consult if questions arise at home.

Teaching should include information on role change and psychologic adjustments as well as skills. Anticipatory guidance can help prepare new parents for the many changes they experience with a new family member.

Information is also essential for women with specialized educational needs: the mother who has had a cesarean birth, the parents of twins, the parents of an infant with congenital anomalies, and so on. Nurses who are attuned to these individual problems can begin providing guidance as soon as possible.

Evaluation may take several forms: return demonstrations, question-and-answer sessions, and even formal evaluation tools. Follow-up phone calls after discharge provide additional evaluative information and continue the helping process for the family.

Promotion of Family Wellness

The promotion of family wellness involves several areas of concern. These include a satisfactory maternity experience, the need for follow-up care for mother and infant, and birth control. The new or expanding family may also have needs for information about adjustment of siblings and resuming sexual relations.

Family-centered care may be supported with postpartal care that is focused on keeping the mother and baby together as much as the mother desires. This type of care is called "mother-baby care" and provides increased opportunities for parent-child interaction as the newborn shares the mother's unit and they are cared for together. This enables the mother to have time to bond with her baby and learn to care for her or him in a supportive environment. Mother-baby care is especially conducive to a self-demand feeding schedule for both breast- and bottle-feeding babies. It also allows the father, siblings, and friends to participate in the care of the new baby.

Mother-baby unit policies must be flexible enough to permit the mother to return the baby to the nursery if she finds it necessary because of fatigue or physical discomfort. Some mother-baby units also return the newborns to a central nursery at night so the mothers can get more rest. Mother-baby care provides excellent opportunities for family bonds to grow as the father, mother, newborn, and often siblings can begin functioning as a family unit immediately.

Reactions of Siblings

Sibling visitation helps meet the needs of both the siblings and their mother. A visit to the mother-baby unit reassures children that their mother is well and still loves them. It also provides an opportunity for the children to become familiar with the new baby. For the mother the pangs of separation are lessened as she interacts with her children and introduces them to the newest family member (Figure 28–2).

Although the parents have prepared their children for the presence of a new brother or sister, the actual arrival of the infant in the home requires some adjustments. If small children are waiting at home, it is helpful if the father carries the baby inside. This practice keeps the mother's arms free to hug and touch her older children. Many mothers bring a doll home with them for an older child. Caring for the doll alongside mother or father helps the child identify with the parents. This identification helps decrease anger and the need to regress for attention.

Parents may also provide supervised times when older children can hold the new baby and perhaps even help with a bottle-feeding. The older children feel a sense of accomplishment and learn tenderness and caring—qualities appropriate for both males and females. The nurse can help the parents come up with ways to show the other children that they, too, are valued and have their own places in the family.

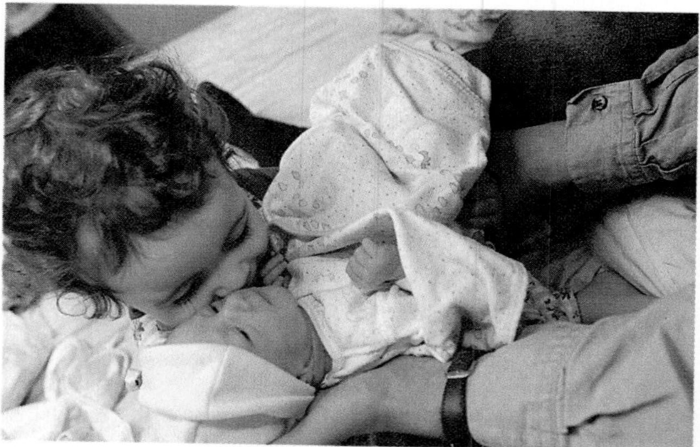

FIGURE 28–2 The sister of this newborn becomes acquainted with the new family member during a nursing assessment.

Resumption of Sexual Relations

Previously couples were discouraged from engaging in sexual intercourse until 6 weeks postpartum. Currently the couple is advised to abstain from intercourse until the episiotomy has healed and the lochial flow has stopped (usually by the end of the third week). Because the vaginal vault is "dry" (hormone poor), some form of lubrication such as K-Y jelly may be necessary during intercourse. The female-superior or sidelying coital positions may be preferable because they allow the woman to control the depth of penile penetration.

Breastfeeding couples should be forewarned that during orgasm milk may spurt from the nipples due to the release of oxytocin. Some couples find this pleasurable, others choose to have the woman wear a bra during sex. Nursing the baby before lovemaking may reduce the chance of milk release.

Other factors may serve as deterrents to fully satisfactory sexual experience: the baby's crying may "spoil the mood"; the woman's changed body may seem unattractive to her or her partner; maternal sleep deprivation may interfere with a mutually satisfying experience; and the woman's physiologic response to sexual stimulation may be changed due to hormonal changes (this lasts about 3 months). With anticipatory guidance during the prenatal and postpartal periods, the couple can be forewarned of potential temporary problems. Anticipatory guidance is enhanced if the couple can discuss their feelings and reactions as they are experienced. See Teaching Guide: Resumption of Sexual Activity After Childbirth.

Promotion of Parent-Infant Attachment

Nursing interventions to enhance the quality of parent-infant attachment should be designed to promote feelings of well-being, comfort, and satisfaction. Following are some suggestions for ways of achieving this.

1. Determine the childbearing and childrearing goals of the infant's mother and father and adapt them wherever possible in planning nursing care for the family. This includes giving the parents choices about their labor and birth experience and their initial time with their new infant.
2. Postpone eye prophylaxis for one hour after birth to facilitate eye contact between parents and their newborn (eye ointment further clouds the newborn's vision and makes eye contact difficult for the baby).
3. Provide time in the first hour after birth for the new family to become acquainted, with as much privacy as possible.
4. Arrange the health care setting so that the individual nurse-client relationship can be developed and maintained. A primary nurse can develop rapport and assess the mother's strengths and needs.
5. Encourage the parents to involve the siblings in integrating the infant into the family by bringing them to the birthing center for sibling visits.
6. Use anticipatory guidance from conception through the postpartal period to prepare the parents for expected problems of adjustment.
7. Include parents in any nursing intervention, planning, and evaluation. Give choices whenever possible.
8. Initiate and support measures to alleviate fatigue in the parents.
9. Help parents identify, understand, and accept both positive and negative feelings related to the overall parenting experience.
10. Support and assist parents in determining the personality and unique needs of their infant.

Whenever possible, mother-baby care should be available. This practice gives the mother a chance to learn her newborn's normal patterns and develop confidence in caring for him or her. It also allows the father more uninterrupted time with his infant in the first days of life. If mother and baby are doing well, help is available for the mother at home and the family and certified nurse-midwife/physician agree, early discharge may be advantageous.

The beginnings of parent-newborn attachment may be observed in the first few hours after birth. Continued assessments may occur in home visits after discharge. As the nurse assesses attachment, it is important to remember that cultural values, beliefs, and practices will direct the child-care activities and self-care practices. For example, some Mexican-American women treat the umbilical stump by placing a coin or belly band over it. Some Mexican-American women or women from Southeast Asia may not want the baby to receive compliments or any attention because of their belief that this may bring on unwanted attention of evil spirits (AWHONN 1996) (Table 28–3).

Nursing Plan and Implementation After Cesarean Birth

After a cesarean birth the new mother has postpartal needs similar to those of her counterparts who gave birth vaginally. Because she has undergone major abdominal surgery, the woman's nursing care needs are also similar to those of other surgical clients.

The chances of pulmonary infection are increased due to immobility after the use of narcotics and sedatives, and because of the altered immune response in

TEACHING GUIDE Resumption of Sexual Activity After Childbirth

Assessment

The nurse recognizes that couples, especially if they have become parents for the first time, may have questions about resuming sexual activity. Although the woman may initiate this discussion, often the nurse can best assess the woman's (and her partner's) understanding by providing some general information followed by some tactful questions.

Nursing Diagnosis

The key nursing diagnosis will probably be: Knowledge deficit related to lack of information about changes in sexual activity that commonly occur postpartally.

Nursing Plan and Implementation

For the teaching plan to be effective the nurse must first establish rapport with the couple and should promote an environment that is conducive to teaching and discussion. It is helpful to provide privacy during the session so that the couple feels free to ask questions without fear of interruption. The format is generally a question and answer or discussion approach.

Client Goals

At the completion of the teaching the couple will be able to

1. Discuss the changes in the woman's body that affect sexual activity.
2. Formulate alternative approaches to sexual activity based on an understanding of these changes.
3. Identify the length of time it is advisable to wait before resuming sexual activity.
4. Discuss information needed to make contraceptive choices.

Teaching Plan

Content	Teaching Method
Present information about changes that may affect sexual activity, including the following: • Tenderness of the vagina and perineum • Presence of lochia and the healing process • Dryness of the vagina • Breast engorgement and tenderness • Escape of milk during sexual activity	Discussion is a logical approach. It may be useful to make a universal statement and link it with a question to determine a couple's initial level of knowledge. For example, "Many women experience vaginal dryness when they resume intercourse for the first several weeks after childbirth. Are you familiar with this change and the cause for it?" Use the information gained during this discussion to determine the depth to which to cover the material.
The nurse discusses healing at the placental site and stresses that the presence of lochia indicates that healing is not yet complete. The nurse points out that because the vagina is "hormone-poor" postpartally, vaginal dryness may be problematic. This can be avoided by using a water-soluble lubricant. Escape of milk during sexual activity can be minimized by having the breastfeeding mother nurse immediately beforehand.	Provide printed information to clarify content and serve as a resource for the couple following discharge.
Discuss the importance of contraception even during the early postpartal period. Provide information on the advantages and disadvantages of different methods. The woman's body needs adequate time to heal and recover from the stress of pregnancy and childbirth. Couples who are opposed to contraception may choose abstinence at this time.	Have samples of different types of contraceptives available. Provide literature on specific contraceptive methods.
Discuss impact of fatigue and the new baby's schedule on the woman's feelings of desire. Refer to physician/certified nurse-midwife for additional information if needed.	Many couples are unprepared for the impact of fatigue and the baby on lovemaking. Information enables the couple to anticipate this impact.

Evaluation

The nurse determines the couple's learning by providing time for discussion and questions. If the couple indicates that they plan to use a particular contraceptive method, the nurse may ask them about aspects of the method to ascertain that they have correct and complete information.

TABLE 28–3 Parent Attachment Behaviors

Assessment Area	Attachment	Behavior Requiring Assessment and Information
Caretaking	Talks with baby. Demonstrates and seeks eye-to-eye contact. Touches and holds baby. Changes diapers when needed. Baby is clean. Clothing is appropriate for room temperature. Feeds baby as needed and baby is gaining weight. Positions baby comfortably and checks on baby.	Does not refer to baby. Completes activities without addressing the baby or looking at the baby. Lack of interaction. Does not recognize need for or demonstrate concern for baby's comfort or needs. Feeding occurs intermittently. Baby does not gain weight. Waits for baby to cry and then hesitates to respond.
Perception of the baby	Has knowledge of expected child development. Understands that the baby is dependent and cannot meet parent's needs. Accepts sex of child and characteristics.	Has unrealistic expectations of the baby's abilities and behaviors. Expects love and interaction from the baby. Believes that the baby will fulfill parent's needs. Is strongly distressed over sex of baby or feels that some aspect of the baby is unacceptable.
Support	Has friends who are available for support. Seems to be comfortable with being a parent. Has realistic beliefs of parenting role.	Is alone or isolated. Is on edge, tense, anxious, and hesitant with the baby. Demonstrates difficulty incorporating parenting with own wants and needs.

Please note: These are a few of the behaviors that may be associated with attachment. It is vitally important for the nurse to observe the parents on more than one occasion and to take into consideration individual characteristics, values, beliefs, and customs.

postoperative patients. For this reason, the woman is encouraged to cough and deep breathe every 2–4 hours while awake until she is ambulating frequently.

Leg exercises are also encouraged every 2 hours until the woman is ambulating. These exercises increase circulation, help prevent thrombophlebitis, and also aid intestinal motility by tightening abdominal muscles.

Promotion of Comfort and Relief of Pain

Monitoring and management of the woman's pain experience is carried out during the postpartum period. Sources of pain include incisional pain, gas pain, referred shoulder pain, periodic uterine contractions (afterbirth pains), and pain from voiding, defecation, or constipation.

Nursing interventions are oriented toward preventing or alleviating pain or helping the woman cope with pain. The nurse should undertake the following measures:

- Administer analgesics as needed, especially during the first 24–72 hours. Use of analgesics will relieve the woman's pain and enable her to be more mobile and active.
- Offer comfort through proper positioning, backrubs, oral care, and the reduction of noxious stimuli such as noise and unpleasant odors.
- Encourage visits by significant others, including the newborn. This provides distraction from the painful sensations and helps reduce the woman's fear and anxiety.
- Encourage the use of breathing, relaxation, and distraction (for example, stimulation of cutaneous tissue) techniques taught in childbirth preparation class.

Epidural analgesia administered just after the cesarean birth is an effective method of pain relief for most women in the first 24 hours following birth (see Drug Guide: Postpartum Epidural Morphine).

The physician may order **patient-controlled analgesia (PCA)**. With this approach the woman is given a bolus of analgesia, usually morphine or meperidine, at the beginning of therapy. Using a special IV pump system, the woman presses a button to self-administer small doses of the medication as needed. For safety, the pump is preset with a time lock-out so that the woman cannot deliver another dose until a specified period of time has elapsed. The use of a PCA helps women feel a greater sense of control and less dependence on nursing staff. The frequent, smaller doses help the woman experience rapid pain relief without grogginess and a drugged feeling, and also avoid the discomfort associated with injections.

If a general anesthetic was used, abdominal distention may produce marked discomfort for the woman during the first few postpartal days. Measures to prevent or minimize abdominal distention include leg exercises, abdominal tightening, ambulation, avoiding carbonated or very hot or cold beverages, avoiding the use of straws, and providing a high-protein, liquid diet for the first 24–48 hours until bowel sounds return. Medical intervention for gas pain includes using rectal suppositories and enemas to stimulate passage of flatus and stool and encouraging the woman to lie on her left side. Lying on the left side allows the gas to rise from the descending colon to the sigmoid colon so that it can be expelled more readily.

DRUG GUIDE Postpartum Epidural Morphine

Overview of Obstetric Action

Epidural morphine is used to provide relief of pain associated with cesarean birth, extensive episiotomies (mediolaterals), or third- and fourth-degree lacerations. Epidural morphine pain relief results directly from its effect on the opiate receptors in the spinal cord (it depresses pain impulse transmission). Morphine binds opiate receptors, thereby altering both the perception of and emotional response to pain. Women experience little or no discomfort or pain during recovery and for up to 24 hours afterward. There is no motor or sympathetic block or associated hypotension. Onset of analgesia is slower, but duration is longer.

Route, Dosage, Frequency

Five to seven and one-half mg of morphine is injected through a catheter into the epidural space, providing pain relief for about 24 hours (Datta 1995).

Maternal Contraindications

Allergy to morphine, narcotic addition, or chronic debilitating respiratory disease.

Maternal Side Effects

Late onset respiratory depression (rare but may occur 8–12 hours after administration), nausea and vomiting (occurring between 4 and 7 hours after injection), itching (begins within 3 hours and lasts up to 10 hours), urinary retention, and, rarely, somnolence. Side effects can be managed with naloxone.

Neonatal Effects

No adverse effects since medication is injected after birth of baby.

Nursing Considerations

Assess client's sensitivity to narcotics on admission.

Monitor and evaluate analgesic effect. Ask client about comfort level and notify anesthesiologist of inadequate pain relief.

Check catheter for obvious knots, breaks, and leakage at insertion site and catheter hub.

Assess for pruritus (scratching and rubbing, especially around face and neck).

Administer comfort measures for narcotic-induced pruritus, such as: lotion, back rubs, cool/warm packs, or diversional activities. If the itching can be tolerated, naloxone should be avoided, especially since it counteracts the pain relief.

If allergic reaction (urticaria, edema, or respiratory difficulties) occurs, administer naloxone or diphenhydramine per physician order.

Provide comfort measures for nausea/vomiting, such as frequent oral hygiene or gradual increase of activity; administer naloxone, trimethobenzamide (Tigan), or metoclopramide HCl per physician order.

Assess postural blood pressure and heart rate before ambulation.

Assist client with her first ambulation and then as needed.

Assess respiratory function every hour for 24 hours, then q2–8 hrs as needed. Also assess level of consciousness and mucous membrane color. May need to monitor client via apnea monitor for 24 hours.

Monitor urinary output and assess bladder for distention. Assist client to void.

The nurse can minimize discomfort and promote satisfaction as the mother assumes the activities of her new role. Instruction and assistance in assuming comfortable positions when holding or breastfeeding the infant will do much to increase the mother's sense of competence and comfort.

The cesarean birth mother usually does extremely well postoperatively. Most women are ambulating by the day after the surgery. Usually by the second postpartal day the incision can be covered with plastic wrap so the woman can shower, which seems to provide a mental as well as physical lift. Most women are discharged by the third day after birth.

Promotion of Parent-Infant Interaction After Cesarean Birth

Signs of depression, anger, or withdrawal may indicate a grief response to the loss of the fantasized birth experience. Fathers as well as mothers may experience feelings of "missing out," guilt, or even jealousy toward another couple who had a vaginal birth. The cesarean birth couple may need the opportunity to tell their story repeatedly to work through these feelings. The nurse can provide factual information about their situation and support the couple's effective coping behaviors.

By the second or third day the cesarean birth mother moves into the "taking-hold period" and is usually receptive to learning how to care for herself and her infant. Special emphasis should be given to home management. She should be encouraged to let others assume responsibility for housekeeping and cooking. Fatigue not only prolongs recovery but also interferes with breastfeeding and mother-infant interaction.

Many factors associated with cesarean birth may hinder successful and frequent maternal-infant interaction. These include the physical condition of the mother and newborn and maternal reactions to stress, anesthesia, and medications. The mother and her infant may be separated after birth because of birthing unit routines, prematurity, or neonatal complications. A healthy infant born by uncomplicated cesarean is no more fragile than one born vaginally. However, some agencies automatically place cesarean-birth infants in the high-risk nursery for a time. If this occurs it may cause anxiety for the parents and interfere with early parent-infant interaction.

The presence of the father or significant other during the birth process positively influences the woman's perception of the birth event. Not only does his or her presence reduce the woman's fears, but it also enhances her sense of control and enables the couple to share feelings and respond to one another with touch and eye contact. Later, they have the opportunity to relive the experience and fill in any gaps or missing pieces. This is especially valuable if the mother has had general anesthesia. The father or significant other can take pictures, hold the baby, and foster the discovery process by directing the mother's attention to the details of the newborn.

The perception of and reactions to a cesarean birth experience depend on how the woman defines that experience. Her reality is what she perceives it to be. If the woman's attitude is more positive than negative, successful resolution of subsequent stressful events is more likely. Because the definition of events is transitory, the possibility of change and growth is present. Often the mothering role is perceived as an extension of the childbearing role. Inability to fulfill expected childbearing behavior (vaginal birth) may lead to parental feelings of role failure and frustration. The nurse can help families alter their negative definitions of cesarean birth, and bolster and encourage positive perceptions.

Nursing Plan and Implementation for the Postpartal Adolescent

The adolescent mother has special postpartal needs, depending on her level of maturity, support systems, and cultural background. The nurse needs to assess maternal-infant interaction, roles of support people, plans for discharge, knowledge of childrearing, and plans for follow-up care. It is imperative to have a community health service be in touch with the adolescent shortly after discharge.

Contraception counseling is an important part of teaching. The incidence of repeat pregnancies during adolescence is high. The younger the adolescent, the more likely she is to become pregnant again.

The nurse has many opportunities for teaching the adolescent about her newborn in the postpartal unit. Because the nurse is a role model, the manner in which she handles the newborn greatly influences the young mother. The father should be included in as much of the teaching as possible.

A newborn examination done at the bedside gives the adolescent information about her baby's health and shows her possible positions for handling a baby. Because adolescent mothers tend to focus their interaction in the physical domain, they need to learn the importance of verbal, visual, and auditory stimulation as well. The nurse can also use this time to give information about newborn and infant behavior. Parents who have some idea of what to expect from their infant will be less frustrated with the newborn's behavior.

The adolescent mother appreciates positive feedback about her newborn and her developing maternal responses. This praise and encouragement will increase her confidence and self-esteem.

Group classes for adolescent mothers should include infant care skills, how to take the baby's temperature and clear the nose and mouth, information about growth and development, infant feeding, well-baby care, and danger signals in the ill newborn.

Ideally, teenage mothers should visit adolescent clinics where the mother and newborn are assessed for several years after birth. In this way, the adolescent's enrollment in classes on parenting, need for vocational guidance, and school attendance can be supported and followed closely. School systems offering classes for young mothers are an excellent way of helping adolescents finish school and learn how to parent at the same time.

Nursing Plan and Implementation for the Woman Who Is Relinquishing Her Baby

Sometimes a woman is unable to keep her baby. The woman may be single, an adolescent, or economically restricted, or the pregnancy may be the result of incest or rape. She may feel that she is not emotionally ready for the responsibilities of parenthood. Her partner may strongly disapprove of the pregnancy. These and many other reasons may cause the woman to continue to reject the idea of her pregnancy. An emotional crisis arises as she attempts to resolve the problem. She may choose to have an abortion, to carry the fetus to term and keep the baby, or to have the baby and relinquish it for adoption.

Many mothers who choose to give their infants up for adoption are young and/or unmarried. More young women choose to keep a child than to give it up, however. Approximately two-thirds of children born to single women are raised by their mothers alone.

The decision of a mother to relinquish her infant is an extremely difficult one. There are social pressures against giving up one's child. Some women may want to prove to themselves that they can manage on their own by keeping their baby.

The mother who chooses to let her child be adopted usually experiences intense ambivalence. These feelings may heighten just before birth and upon seeing her baby. After childbirth, the mother will need to complete a grieving process to work through her loss.

The mother who decides to relinquish the child has usually made considerable adjustments in her lifestyle to give birth to this child. She may not have told friends and relatives about the pregnancy and so lacks an extended support system. During the prenatal period, the nurse can help her by encouraging her and providing opportunities to express her grief, loneliness, guilt, and other feelings.

When the relinquishing mother is admitted to the birthing unit, the nurse should be informed about the mother's decision to relinquish the baby. The nurse should respect any special requests for the birth and encourage the woman to express her emotions. After the birth the mother should have access to the baby; she will decide whether she wants to see the newborn. Seeing the newborn often aids the grieving process. When the mother sees her baby, she may feel strong attachment and love. The nurse needs to assure the woman that these feelings do not mean that her decision to relinquish the child is a wrong one; relinquishment is often a painful act of love (Arms 1990). Postpartal nursing care also includes arranging ongoing care for the relinquishing mother.

In the event that a woman decides to keep an unwanted child, the nurse should be aware of the potential for parenting problems. Families with unwanted children are more crisis prone than others, although in many cases, parents grow to love their child after attachment occurs. The nurse should be ready to initiate crisis strategies or make appropriate referrals as the need arises.

Nursing Plan and Implementation for Discharge Information

Ideally, preparation for discharge begins at the moment a woman enters the birthing unit to give birth. Nursing efforts should be directed toward assessing the parents' knowledge, expectations, and beliefs and then providing anticipatory guidance and teaching accordingly. Since teaching is one of the primary responsibilities of the postpartum nurse, many agencies have elaborate teaching programs and videos. Before the actual discharge, however, the nurse should spend time with the parents to determine if they have any last-minute questions. In general, discharge teaching includes at least the following information:

1. The signs of possible complications (see Key Facts to Remember: Signs of Postpartal Complications) and encouragement to contact her caregiver if she develops any of them.
2. Review of literature she has received that explains recommended postpartum exercises, the need for adequate rest, the need to avoid overexertion initially, and the recommendation to abstain from sexual intercourse until lochia has ceased. The woman may take either a tub bath or shower and may continue sitz baths at home. If the family desires information about birth control methods, the nurse can provide such information at this time.
3. The phone number of the mother-baby unit and encouragement to call if she has any questions or concerns.
4. Information on local agencies and/or support groups, such as La Leche League and Mothers of Twins, that might be of particular assistance to her.
5. Information geared to the specific nutritional needs of breastfeeding or bottle-feeding mothers. If the mother has been receiving vitamins and/or iron supplements, encourage her to continue until the first postpartal examination.
6. When to schedule the first appointment for her postpartal examination and for her newborn's first well-baby examination.
7. The procedure for obtaining copies of her infant's birth certificate.
8. How to provide basic care for the infant; when to anticipate that the cord will fall off; when the infant can have a tub bath; when the infant will need her or his first immunizations; and so on. Parents should also be comfortable feeding and handling the baby, and should be aware of basic

KEY FACTS TO REMEMBER

Signs of Postpartal Complications

After discharge, a woman should contact her physician/certified nurse-midwife if any of the following develop:

- Sudden persistent or spiking fever
- Change in the character of the lochia—foul smell, return to bright red bleeding, excessive amount, passage of large clots
- Evidence of mastitis, such as breast tenderness, reddened areas, malaise
- Evidence of thrombophlebitis, such as calf pain, tenderness, redness
- Evidence of urinary tract infection, such as urgency, frequency, burning on urination
- Continued severe or incapacitating postpartal depression

safety considerations, including the need to use a car seat whenever the infant is in a car.

9. The signs and symptoms that indicate possible problems in the infant and who they should contact about them.
10. Plans for home care visits so that the parents know when to expect the visit and what it will entail (see Chapter 29).

The nurse can also use this final opportunity to reassure the couple of their ability to be successful parents. She can stress the infant's need to feel loved and secure. She can also urge parents to talk to each other and work together to solve any problems that arise.

The ideal teaching situation is a family approach involving the father, infant, and possibly other siblings. This permits a total evaluation and provides opportunities for all family members to ask questions and express concerns. It also promotes diagnosis and treatment of disturbed family patterns to prevent future problems of neglect or abuse.

Community-Based Nursing Care

Resources to assist and support the new parents are usually available in most cities. County Health Departments are a valuable source of care with visits from community health nurses; community education programs; well-baby clinics; Women, Infants and Children (WIC); and parenting programs. Other care may be provided by the Visiting Nurses Association and home care agencies centered in hospitals or free standing.

As the length of the postpartum stay has shortened, home care has become more readily available (see discussion in Chapter 29). In this time of rapid change in the health care setting and funding bases and downsizing of facilities, more and more agencies and groups are joining to address and meet the needs of new parents and their children.

Evaluation

As a result of comprehensive nursing care the postpartal family will achieve the following outcomes:

- The mother is reasonably comfortable and has learned pain-relief measures.
- The mother is rested and understands how to add more activity over the next few days and weeks.
- The mother's physiologic and psychologic well-being have been supported.
- The mother verbalizes her understanding of self-care measures.
- The new parents demonstrate how to care for their baby.
- The new parents have had opportunities to form attachment with their baby.
- The cesarean birth mother has been supported and received safe care.

CHAPTER HIGHLIGHTS

- Nursing diagnoses can be used effectively in caring for women postpartally.
- Postpartum discomfort may be due to a variety of factors, including engorged breasts, an edematous perineum, an episiotomy or extension, engorged hemorrhoids, or hematoma formation. Various self-care approaches are helpful in promoting comfort.
- Lactation suppression may be accomplished by mechanical techniques.
- The new mother requires opportunities to discuss her childbirth experience with an empathic listener.
- In the first day or two after birth maternal behaviors are more dependent and comfort oriented. Then the woman becomes more independent and ready to assume responsibility.
- Mother-baby care provides the childbearing family with opportunities to interact with their new member during the first hours and days of life. This enables the family to develop some confidence and skill in a "safe" environment.
- Sexual intercourse may resume once the episiotomy has healed and lochia has ceased. Couples should be forewarned of possible changes; for example, the vagina may be "dry," desire may be reduced by fatigue, or the woman's breasts may leak milk during orgasm.
- After a cesarean birth, the woman has the nursing care needs of an abdominal surgical client in addition to her needs as a postpartum client. She may also require assistance in working through her feelings if the cesarean birth was unexpected.
- Postpartally the nurse evaluates the adolescent mother in terms of her level of maturity, available support systems, cultural background, and existing knowledge and then plans care accordingly.
- The mother who decides to relinquish her baby needs emotional support. She should be able to decide

whether to see and hold her baby and should have any special requests regarding the birth honored.

- Prior to discharge the couple should be given any information necessary for the woman to provide appropriate self-care. Parents should have a beginning skill in caring for their newborn and should be familiar with warning signs of possible complications for mother or baby. Printed information is valuable in helping couples deal with questions that may arise at home.
- Because of the trend toward early discharge, follow-up care is more important than ever. Many approaches are used, especially home visits and telephone follow-up.

REFERENCES

Arms S: *Adoption: A Handbook of Hope.* Berkeley, CA: Celestial Arts, 1990.

AWHONN: *Compendium of Postpartum Care.* Skillman, NJ: Johnson & Johnson Consumer Products, 1996.

Barnes LP: Meeting the challenge of early postpartum discharge. *MCN* 1996; 21:129.

Cunningham et al: *Williams Obstetrics,* 20th ed. Stamford, CT: Appleton & Lange, 1997.

Datta S: *The Obstetric Anesthesia Handbook,* 2nd ed. St Louis: Mosby, 1995.

Mercer RT: *Becoming a Mother.* New York: Springer, 1995.

Schneiderman JU: Postpartum nursing for Korean mothers. *MCN* 1996; 21:155.

Varney H: *Nurse Midwifery,* 2nd ed. Boston: Blackwell Scientific Publications, 1987.

Waldenstrom U, Borg IM, Skold M, Wall S: The childbirth experience: A study of 295 new mothers. *Birth* 1996; 23(3):144.

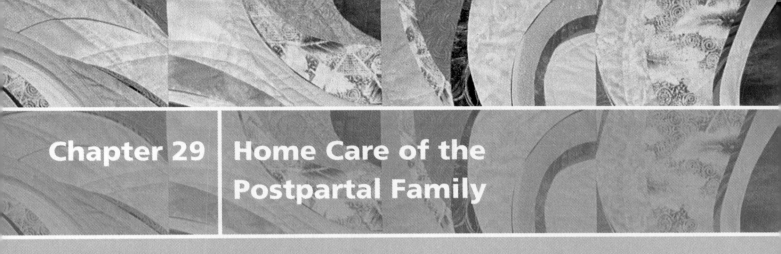

Chapter 29 Home Care of the Postpartal Family

OBJECTIVES

- Discuss the components of postpartal home care.
- Delineate aspects of fostering a caring relationship in the home.
- Describe assessment, care of the newborn, and reinforcement of parent teaching in the home.
- Discuss maternal and family assessment and anticipated progress after birth.

KEY TERMS

Active awake state
Crying state
Quiet alert state
Quiet sleep
Postpartal home care
Short stay

Home care has become essential as the length of stay in the birth setting has steadily decreased over the past few years. The length of time in the hospital or birthing center after birth has been referred to as **short stay;** however, there is no agreement about how long this period should be. The short stay has been fueled by efforts to contain health care costs rather than by well-developed research studies that validate the efficacy and safety of this practice (Bravemen et al 1995) or cooperative decision making between health care professionals and families (Committee on Fetus and Newborn 1995). A short stay following an uncomplicated vaginal birth may range from less than 24 hours in some areas to 48 hours in others, and a short stay after a cesarean birth may be no more than 72 hours (Evans 1995; Soskolne et al 1996).

As the length of stay declined, a number of new issues developed. The shortened stay (less than 48 hours) raises issues for the newborn because many conditions such as jaundice, ductal dependent cardiac lesions, and gastrointestinal obstructions may require a longer period of time to develop, and identification of these problems depends on a skilled, experienced professional (Committee on Fetus and Newborn 1995; Soskolne et al 1996). Catz (1995) found that in one year, 1–4 percent (up to 110,000 newborns) of term newborns with less than a 48-hour stay were readmitted and in 85 percent of the cases it was because of jaundice. There are also implications for the mother. The stability of her health, availability of support systems, and opportunities to become comfortable with her new baby may be compromised, and less than 48 hours is too little time to establish breastfeeding (Committee on Fetus and Newborn 1995). Furthermore, in the first 24 hours after birth, the mother is in the taking-in phase, which is not conducive to learning (Evans 1995; Soskolne et al 1996). The Committee on Fetus and Newborn (1995) has developed minimum criteria to guide the timing of early discharge in order to enhance excellence in maternal-newborn care (Table 29–1).

Because of concern for maternal-newborn and family health and safety, some states have passed legislation mandating at least a 48-hour stay after vaginal birth and 96 hours after cesarean birth, and other states are considering enacting similar legislation (Bowers 1995). Many of the legislative efforts state that if the stay is less than 48 or 96 hours, the discharge must be the result of a cooperative decision between the physician and the parent(s), and the mother can request up to three home visits (Lynch 1996a).

As the length of stay decreases, nursing professionals in the birthing center are pressed to complete essential assessments, assure holistic care (physiologic, psychologic, and spiritual) and provide opportunities for education about maternal self-care and newborn care. The new family, eager to learn about important aspects of care, also need to rest and spend time with their newborn. The needs of the family and the goals of the health care provider can be addressed through the development of postpartal home care.

Home care for the postpartal family is focused more on assessment, teaching, and counseling than on physical care. **Postpartal home care** provides opportunities for enhancing information and self- and infant care techniques initially presented in the birth setting. In addition, the home setting provides an opportunity for the nurse and family to interact in a more relaxed environment in which the family has control of the setting. In some instances, the challenges of assessing and enhancing self-care and infant care may be unique in the home, and the nurse will have many opportunities to exercise critical thinking to develop creative options with the family.

TABLE 29–1 Minimal Criteria for Discharge of Newborns

1. Uncomplicated prenatal, intrapartal, and postpartal course and vaginal birth.
2. A single baby who is term, 38–42 weeks, and AGA (average weight for gestational age).
3. The newborn's vital signs are within normal limits and have been stable for the 12 hours preceding discharge. (Respirations < 60/min; apical pulse 100–160 beats per minute; axillary temperature of 36.1–37C in an open crib with appropriate clothing)
4. The newborn has passed at least one stool and has urinated.
5. At least two feedings have been successfully completed, and the baby's ability to coordinate sucking, swallowing, and breathing has been observed and documented.
6. No physical abnormalities have been found that require continued hospitalization.
7. If a circumcision has been done, no excessive bleeding has been evident for at least two hours before discharge.
8. There has been no significant jaundice in the first 24 hours of life.
9. The mother has received education about breast- or bottle-feeding; the newborn's expected stool and urinary patterns; care of circumcision; cord, skin, and genital care; ways to recognize signs of illness or distress and common infant problems; signs of jaundice and who to contact if it develops; infant safety, including positioning of baby after feeding and for sleep; and use of a car seat.
10. Review of pertinent laboratory data including maternal syphilis and hepatitis B surface antigen status; cord or infant blood type.
11. Completion of screening tests (eg: PKU).
12. First hepatitis B vaccine has been administered or appointment for administration has been scheduled within the first week.
13. Method and schedule for continuing care has been ascertained and planned, and the family is aware of the plan.
14. Family assessment has been completed for social and environmental risk factors such as history of previous child abuse or neglect; spousal or partner abuse either preceding or beginning during the pregnancy; parental substance abuse; lack of support within the family or community; lack of funds, shelter, or food; mental illness of one of the parents that impairs ability to care for self and newborn; single first-time mother without social support.

Source: Committee on Fetus and Newborn: Hospital stay for healthy term newborns. *Pediatrics* 1995; 96(4):788.

Considerations for the Home Visit

In planning a home visit the nurse should clearly understand the purpose of the visit and the maximum content to be addressed. Other important considerations include ways of creating and fostering relationships with families, techniques for preplanning and executing the visit while maintaining safety, documentation of the visit, and telephone follow-up.

Because of the established guidelines for early discharge of the mother and baby (refer to Table 29–1) the nurse can logically expect certain levels of health and wellness. However, because the status of the mother and newborn can change, the nurse should stay alert for deviations from the norm.

Purpose of the Home Visit

The postpartal home visit has many purposes. It provides an opportunity to assess the mother and infant's status after birth for signs of any complications and to complete follow-up blood work if needed. The nurse also assesses current informational needs and provides additional information as needed. The home visit also provides time to cover additional information in a more relaxed setting. In addition, the nurse assesses adaptation of the family to the new baby and adjustment of any siblings, answers questions about breastfeeding, provides support and encouragement, and addresses the need for referrals (Lowdermilk 1995).

The postpartal home visit differs from community health visits in that only one or two postpartal visits are typically planned and long-term follow-up by the postpartal nurse is not anticipated. Although the postpartal home visit is comprehensive, it is more specifically focused on postpartal family needs and care.

The postpartal home visit usually occurs within 24–48 hours of discharge and is conducted by a registered nurse who is experienced in postpartal maternal and newborn care (Barnes 1996).

Fostering a Caring Relationship with the Family

Although the nurse in the birthing center strives to enhance family autonomy and control, the inherent atmosphere of the institutional environment may cause the new mother and family to feel unempowered. It is important for the professional nurse to recognize that the parameters of the home visit are different in many ways from those of the hospital or birthing center environment. In the home, the family has control of their environment and the nurse is an invited visitor. The nurse can rely on the same characteristics of a caring relationship that have been integral to hospital-based practice—regard for clients, genuineness, empathy, and establishment of trust and rapport—but the relationship may take on new elements as the nurse moves into the home setting for the first time (see Key Facts to Remember: Fostering a Caring Relationship).

KEY FACTS TO REMEMBER

Fostering a Caring Relationship

Evidence of genuineness and empathy, coupled with the establishment of trust and rapport, form the foundation for a caring relationship.

Demonstrated Goal	Approaches to Achieve Goal
Regard	Introduce yourself to the family. Call the family members by their surnames until you have been invited to use the given or a less formal name. Ask to be introduced to other members of the family who are present. Allow the mother or spokesperson to assume this role. Use active listening. Maintain objectiveness. Ask permission before sitting.
Genuineness	Mean what you say. Make sure that your verbal and nonverbal messages are congruent. Be nonjudgmental. Don't make assumptions about individuals or settings. Always strive to demonstrate caring behaviors. Be prepared for the visit, honestly answer questions and provide information, and be truthful. If you don't know the answer to a question, tell the client you will find the information and report back.
Empathy	Listen to the mother and family where "they are" without judgment. Be attentive to what the birthing experience is for them so that you will understand from their perspective. Remember empathy denotes understanding, not sympathy.
Trust and rapport	Do what you say you will do. Be prepared for the visit and be on time. Follow-up on any areas that are needed.

Planning the Home Visit

Prior to the home visit, the nurse prepares by identifying the purpose of the home visit and gathering anticipated materials and equipment. A personal contact while the woman is still in the birth setting or a previsit telephone call is used to arrange the appointment with the woman and her family. During the previsit contact, it is important for the nurse to identify clearly the purpose and goals of the visit and to begin establishing rapport.

Maintaining Safety

In the past nurses were received as a mainstay of communities and could move in most settings without fear or concern for safety. However, in current times some communities are not safe for visiting nurses. It is important for the nurse to follow some basic safety rules such as

- Know the specific address, and ask for directions during the previsit contact.
- Trace out the route on a map before leaving for the visit and take the map along.
- Notify an instructor or supervisor when leaving for a visit and check in as soon as the visit is completed.
- Carry a cellular phone or another method of communication.
- Carry enough change to make a call from a pay phone if needed.
- Wear a name tag.
- Don't wear expensive jewelry.
- If a situation arises in which you feel unsafe, terminate the visit.
- If the visit is in an area that seems very unsafe, it may be wise for two nurses to go together. Avoid entering areas where violence is in progress. In such cases, return to the car and contact the appropriate facility, such as 911.

Most people are more comfortable in familiar settings and have some hesitation in entering other residential areas. It is always important to be aware of one's surroundings and the people who are nearby. First home visits may feel uncomfortable because they are unfamiliar but with experience comfort increases (Figure 29–1).

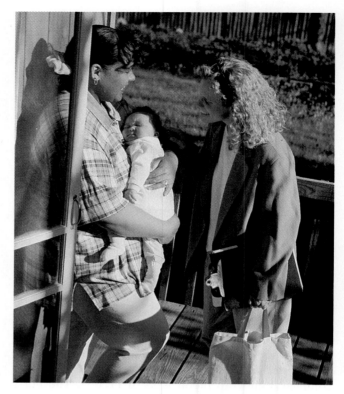

FIGURE 29–1 Nurse arriving for a home visit.

Carrying Out the Home Visit

When the door is answered, the nurse should introduce herself or himself and confirm that the location is correct. If a place to sit is not indicated, the nurse may inquire "Where is the best place to sit so that we can talk for awhile?" In some homes, the mother or family may offer refreshments and this may be an important aspect of welcoming a visitor. In this case, it is beneficial to the relationship to accept the refreshment graciously.

The aspects that will be assessed and addressed during the home visit are discussed in the following sections.

Home Care: The Newborn

Positioning and Handling

The nurse demonstrates methods of positioning and handling the newborn as needed. As the family provides care, the nurse can instill confidence by giving them positive feedback. If the family encounters problems, the nurse can suggest alternatives and serve as a role model.

After the newborn is out of the crib, one of the following holds can be used (Figure 29–2). The *cradle hold* is frequently used during feeding. It provides a sense of warmth and closeness, permits eye contact, frees one of the adult's hands, and provides security because the cradling protects the newborn's body. Extra security is provided by gripping the thigh with the hand while the arm supports the newborn's body. The *upright position* provides security and a sense of closeness and is ideal for burping. One hand should support the neck and shoulders, while the other hand holds the buttocks or is

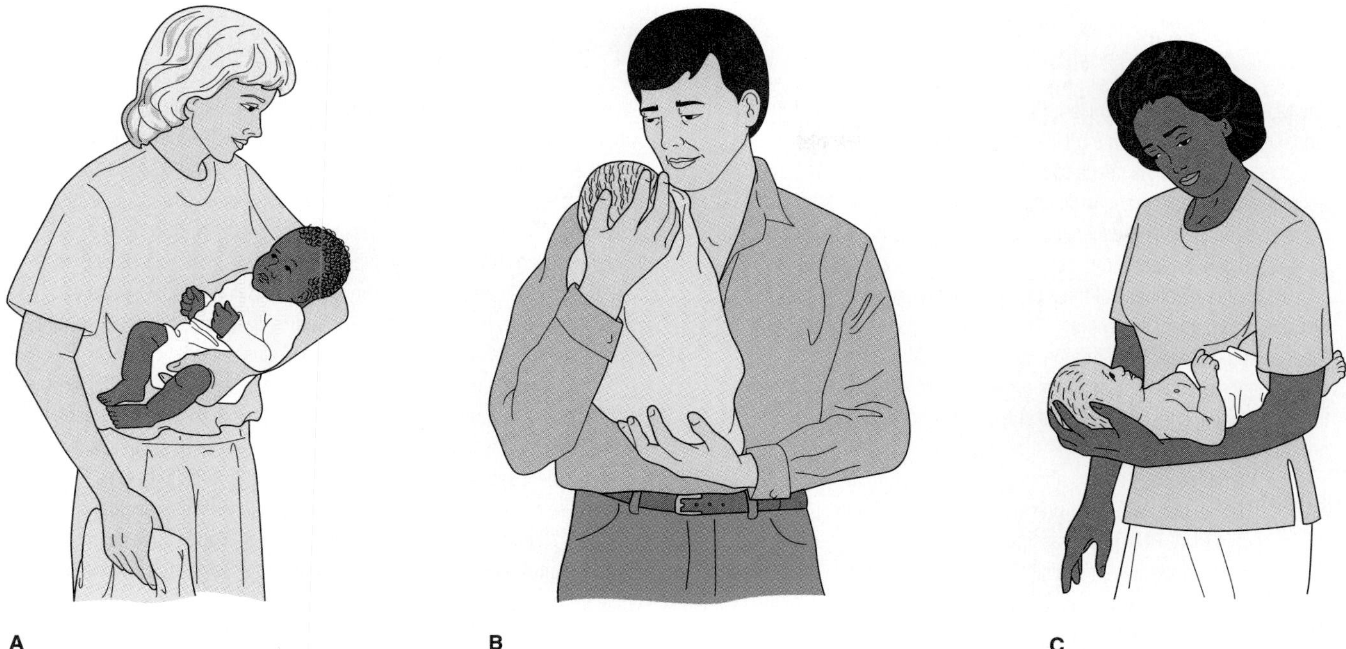

FIGURE 29–2 Various positions for holding an infant. ***A*** Cradle hold. ***B*** Upright position. ***C*** Football hold.

placed between the newborn's legs. The newborn may also be held upright in a cloth sling carrier that gently holds the baby against the mother or father's chest and frees their hands for other tasks. The *football hold* frees one of the caregiver's hands and permits eye contact. This hold is ideal for shampooing, carrying, or breastfeeding. It frees the caregiver to talk on the telephone, answer the door, or do the myriad tasks that await attention at this busy time.

The newborn is most frequently positioned on his or her side with a rolled blanket or diaper behind the back for support and to prevent rolling (Figure 29–3). The side-lying position aids drainage of mucus and allows air to circulate around the cord. It is also more comfortable for the newly circumcised male. After feeding, the newborn is placed on the right side to aid digestion and to prevent aspiration of regurgitated feedings; this position makes it easier to expel air bubbles from the stomach.

A firm, flat mattress without pillows should be provided for the newborn. Recent studies have shown an increased incidence of sudden infant death syndrome (SIDS) in infants who sleep on their stomachs. There is no evidence that sleeping on the back or side is harmful to healthy infants. Certain infants may need to be placed on their stomachs, including premature infants with respiratory distress (severe breathing problems); infants with symptoms of gastroesophageal reflux (severe spitting up); and infants with certain upper airway abnormalities. There may be other valid reasons for infants to be placed on their stomachs for sleep. Parents should discuss their individual circumstances with their care provider. Although the risk of SIDS for infants who sleep on their stomachs may be higher than for those who sleep on their sides or backs, the actual risk of SIDS when placing infants on their stomachs is still extremely low *(Infant Sleep Position and SIDS Position Statement* 1992*)*. The infant's position should be changed periodically during the early months of life, because skull bones are soft, and permanently flattened areas may develop if the newborn consistently lies in one position. A newborn in the first days of life should not be left in a supine position when unattended, because of the danger of aspiration.

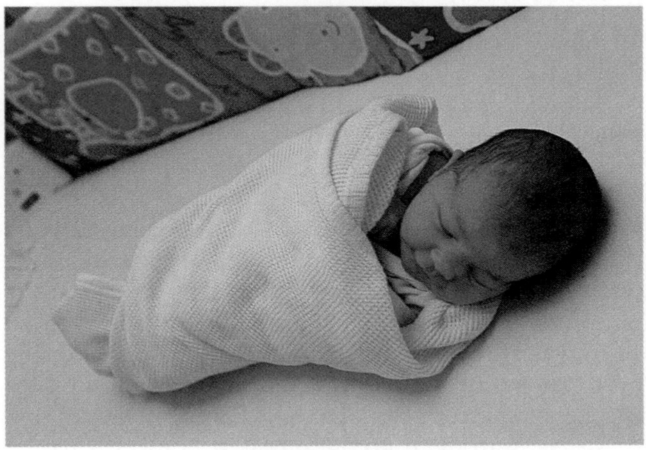

FIGURE 29–3 The most common sleeping position of the newborn is on the side. A rolled blanket may be placed behind the back to provide additional support.

COMMUNITY IN FOCUS **Postpartum Home Care Program**

The Maternity and Newborn Home Visit Program, a joint effort of Professional Nurse Associates, Inc (PNA) and Kaiser Permanente of Ohio, is designed to address the needs of childbearing families following their hospital stay. The program, which has been in effect since 1989, is an example of an effective partnership between a private nursing practice and a managed care organization.

The program consists of three phases: the prenatal phase, referral process, and home visit program. The prenatal phase is educationally focused and includes waiting room videotapes, childbirth classes, and educational mailings. The mailings provide information on a variety of topics including the short length of stay and the home follow-up visit program.

The referral process begins about one month before the woman's expected date of birth when her prenatal history and demographic information is sent to PNA. PNA in turn assigns a nurse case manager who will complete the postpartum home visit. The actual home visit is initiated by a hospital nurse or discharge planner who completes a summary of the woman's hospital stay and forwards it to PNA.

As initially designed, the postpartum home visit program, implemented by registered nurses, was provided for women discharged on the first postpartum day following vaginal birth or the third postpartum day following cesarean birth. Because of the positive outcomes demonstrated by the program, a home visit is currently provided to all postpartum families regardless of length of stay. The home visit program includes a previsit phone call to the family, case management from PNA, and a home visit within 72 hours of discharge if a problem that requires immediate attention (such as poor infant feeding) is identified. Additional home visits may also be scheduled if a need is identified by the home visit nurse or medical providers. PNA nurses make necessary referrals to a variety of community resources such as WIC, parent support groups, domestic violence prevention programs. In addition, a 24-hour PNA help line, staffed by clinical nurse specialists, is also available for families with questions, concerns, or problems. Over half the families served make use of it.

On the average, home visits last approximately 97 minutes; the average number of phone contacts per family is 2.4. Despite the shortened length of stay, the readmission rate for both mothers and newborns is less than 1 percent. Client satisfaction is measured via a survey mailed with a stamped self-addressed envelope after the case is closed. Response rates approach 75 percent and reflect an impressive 99 percent satisfaction rate. Equally impressive is the cost benefit, which is estimated at one million dollars each year since 1991.

This program is a wonderful example of innovative approaches to limited resources. It also exemplifies the best of entrepreneurial nursing practice.

Sources: Personal communication with Lenore R. Williams, Director, Professional Nurse Associates, Inc; Williams LR, Cooper MK: A new paradigm for postpartum care. *JOGNN* 1996; 25(9):745; Williams LR, Cooper MK: Nurse-managed postpartum home care. *JOGNN* 1993; 22(1):25.

Bathing

An actual bath demonstration is the best way for the nurse to provide information to parents. Because excess bathing and use of soap removes natural skin oils and dries out the newborn's sensitive skin, bathing should be done every other day or twice a week. Sponge baths are recommended for the first 2 weeks or until the umbilical cord completely falls off and the umbilicus has healed. Some agencies use a tub bath for the bath demonstration and apply alcohol to the cord after the bath to facilitate drying.

Supplies can be kept in a plastic bag or some type of container to eliminate the necessity of hunting for them each time (Table 29–2). At home, the family may want to use a small plastic tub, a clean kitchen or bathroom sink, or a large bowl as the baby's tub. Expensive baby tubs are not necessary, but some prefer to purchase them. Some nurses recommend spreading a beach towel out on the floor and placing a small plastic dishpan on the towel. If the mother or father is comfortable sitting on the floor for the bath, this arrangement provides a spacious work surface.

Before starting, if no one else is at home, the parent may want to take the phone off the hook and put a sign on the door to prevent being disturbed. Having someone home during the first few baths will be helpful, because that person can get forgotten items, attend to interruptions, and provide moral support. The room should be warm and free of drafts.

Sponge Bath

After the supplies are gathered, the tub (or any of the containers mentioned) is filled with water that is warm to the touch. Even though the newborn won't be placed in the tub, the bath giver carefully tests the water temperature with an elbow or forearm. Families may also choose to purchase a thermometer to help them determine when the bath water is at approximately 37.8C (100F) and safe to use. Soap should not be added to the water. The newborn should be wrapped in a blanket, with a T-shirt and diaper on, to keep her or him warm and secure.

To start the bath, the adult wraps a washcloth around the index finger once. Each eye is gently wiped from inner to outer corner. This direction prevents the potential for clogging the tear duct at the inner corner, where the eye naturally drains. A different portion of the washcloth is used for each eye to prevent cross-contamination. Cotton balls can also be used for this purpose, using a new one for each eye. Some swelling and drainage may be present the first few days after birth as a result of the eye prophylaxis.

The bath giver washes the ears next by wrapping the washcloth once around an index finger and gently cleaning the external ear and behind the ear. Cotton swabs are never used in the ear canal because it is possible to put the swab too far into the ear and damage the ear drum. In addition, the swab may back any discharge farther down into the ear canal.

The caregiver then wipes the remainder of the baby's face with the soap-free washcloth. Many babies start to cry at this point. The face should be washed every day and the mouth and chin wiped off after each feeding.

The neck is washed carefully but thoroughly with the washcloth. Soap may now be used. Formula or breast milk and lint collect in the skin folds of the neck, so it may be helpful to sit the newborn up, supporting the neck and shoulders with one hand while washing the neck with the other hand.

The bath giver now unwraps the blanket, removes the T-shirt, and wets the chest, back, and arms with the washcloth. The bath giver may then lather the hands with soap and wash the baby's chest, back, and arms. Wetting the cord is avoided, if possible, because it delays drying. Soap is rinsed off with the wet washcloth, and the upper part of the body is dried with a towel or blanket. The newborn's upper body is then wrapped with a clean, dry blanket to prevent a chill.

Next the bath giver unwraps the newborn's legs, wets them with the washcloth, and lathers, rinses, and dries them well. If the newborn has dry skin, a small amount of unscented lotion or ointment (petroleum jelly or A and D ointment) may be used. Ointments are thought to be better than lotions for dry, cracked feet and hands. Baby oil is not recommended, as it clogs skin pores. Powders are not currently recommended. Some believe they aggravate dry skin and others avoid powders because of the possible danger of inhalation.

Families should be warned that baby powder can cause serious respiratory problems if inhaled. If parents want to use powder, they should be advised to use one that is talc free. The powder should be shaken into the hand and then placed on the newborn rather than shaken directly onto the baby.

The genital area is cleansed daily with soap and water, and with water after each wet or dirty diaper. Females are washed from the front of the genital area toward the rectum to avoid fecal contamination of the urethra and thus the bladder. Newborn females often have a thick, white mucous discharge or a slight bloody discharge from their vaginal area. This discharge is normal for the first 1 to 2 weeks of age and should be wiped off with a damp cloth during diaper changes.

Parents of uncircumcised males should cleanse the penis daily. Even minimal retraction of the foreskin is not advised (see in-depth discussion of care of uncircumcised male babies in Chapter 23). Males who have been circumcised also need daily gentle cleansing. A very wet washcloth is rubbed over a bar of soap. The washcloth is squeezed above the baby's penis, letting the soapy water run over the circumcision site. The area is rinsed off with plain warm water and lightly patted dry. A small amount of petroleum jelly, A and D, or bactericidal ointment may be put on the circumcised area, but excessive amounts may block the meatus and should be avoided. It is important to avoid using ointments if a Plastibell is in place. Use of ointments may cause the Plastibell ring to slip off the penis too early. The Plastibell usually falls off within 5 to 8 days. If it doesn't, the family needs to call the health care provider.

TABLE 29–2 Bath Supplies

Washcloths (2)	Petroleum jelly or A and D ointment
Towels (2)	Rubbing alcohol
Blankets (2)	Cotton balls
Unperfumed mild soap (eg, Castile, Neutrogena)	Diapers
Shampoo	Clean clothes

It is important to cleanse the diaper area with each diaper change to prevent diaper rash. Although this cleansing is done on a routine basis, a diaper rash may occasionally occur. Baby powder (or cornstarch) is not recommended for diaper rash. Baby powder may cake with urine and irritate the perineal area. Cornstarch may promote fungal infection. Ointments that provide a barrier, such as zinc oxide, A and D ointment, or petroleum jelly are more effective for diaper rash. If the ointment does not help the rash, families using single-use (disposable) diapers should try another brand. If they use cloth diapers, a different detergent or fabric softener, more thorough rinsing, and hanging them in the sun to dry may alleviate the problem. If the rash persists, parents should discuss the problem with their nurse practitioner or physician, because it may be due to a yeast or fungal infection.

The umbilical cord should be kept clean and dry. The close proximity of the umbilical vessels makes the cord a common entry area for infection. At discharge, most parents are advised to cleanse the area around the cord with a cotton ball and alcohol (70% isopropyl) 2 to 3 times a day until the cord falls off and the umbilicus is healed. The cord stump generally falls off in 7 to 14 days. The diaper should be folded down to allow air to circulate around the cord. The parents should consult their health care provider if redness, bright red bleeding, or puslike drainage with foul odor appears around the umbilicus, or if the area remains unhealed 2 to 3 days after the cord stump has sloughed off. See Teaching Guide: What to Tell Families About Home Cord Care in Chapter 23.

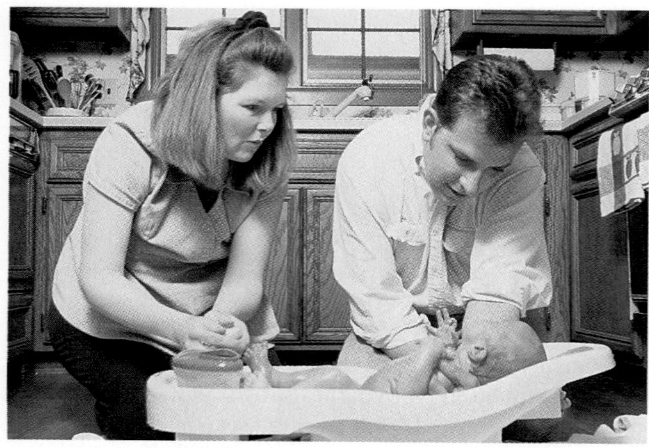

FIGURE 29–4 When bathing the newborn, it is important to support the head. Wet babies are very slippery.

The last step in bathing is washing the hair (some suggest doing this step first). The newborn is swaddled in a dry blanket, leaving only the head exposed, and held in the football hold with the head tilted slightly downward to prevent water running in the eyes. Water should be brought to the head by a cupped hand. The hair is moistened and lathered with a small amount of shampoo. A very soft brush may be used to massage the shampoo over the entire head, including the soft spots. The hair is then rinsed and toweled dry. Oils or lotions are not used on the newborn's head unless there is evidence of cradle cap. Moistening the scaly area with lotion or mineral oil a half an hour or more before shampooing softens the crusts or scales and makes it easier to remove them with a soft brush during the shampoo.

Tub Baths

The baby may be put in a small tub after the cord has fallen off and the circumcision site is healed (approximately 2 weeks) (Figure 29–4). Newborns usually enjoy a tub bath more than a sponge bath, although some cry during either type.

Only 3 or 5 inches of water is needed in the tub. To prevent slipping, a washcloth is placed in the bottom of the tub or sink or the newborn can be brought into a tub with the parent.

The face is washed in the same manner as for a sponge bath. The parent then places the newborn in the tub using the cradle hold and grasping the distal thigh. The neck is supported by the parent's elbow in the cradle position. An alternative hold is to support the newborn's head and neck with the forearm while grasping the distal shoulder and arm.

Because wet newborns are slippery, some parents pull a cotton sock (with the holes cut out for the fingers) over the supporting arm to provide a "nonskid" surface. The newborn's body may be washed with a soapy washcloth or hand. To wash the back, the bath giver places his or her noncradling hand on the newborn's chest with the thumb under the newborn's arm closest to the adult. Gently tipping the newborn forward onto the supporting hand frees the cradling arm to wash the back. After the bath, the newborn is lifted out of the tub in the cradle position, dried well, and wrapped in a dry blanket. The hair can then be washed in the same way as for a sponge bath.

Nail Care

The nails of the newborn are seldom cut in the birthing center. During the first days of life, the nails may adhere to the skin of the fingers, and cutting is contraindicated. Within a week the nails separate from the skin and frequently break off. If the nails are long or if the newborns are scratching themselves, the nails may be trimmed. This is most easily done while they are asleep. Nails should be cut straight across using adult cuticle scissors or blunt-ended infant cuticle scissors.

Dressing the Newborn

Newborns need to wear a T-shirt, diaper (diaper cover or plastic pants if using cloth diapers), and a sleeper. On a fairly cool day, they should be wrapped in a light blanket while being fed. Newborns may be covered with a blanket in air-conditioned buildings. The blanket should be unwrapped or removed when inside a warm building.

At home, the amount of clothing the newborn wears is determined by the temperature. Families who maintain their home at 60–65F should dress the infant more warmly than those who maintain a temperature of 70–75F.

Newborns should wear head coverings outdoors to protect their sensitive ears from drafts. A blanket can be wrapped around the baby, leaving one corner free to place over the head while outdoors or in crowds for added protection. Families must also be advised of the ease with which a newborn's skin can burn when exposed to the sun. To prevent sunburn, the newborn should remain shaded, wear a light layer of clothing, or be protected with sunscreen.

Diaper shapes vary and are subject to personal preference (Figure 29–5). Prefolded and disposable diapers are usually rectangular. Cloth diapers may also be triangular or kite-folded. Extra material is placed in front for males and toward the back for females to increase absorbency.

Baby clothing should be laundered separately with a mild soap or detergent. Diapers may be presoaked before washing. All clothing should be rinsed twice to remove soap and residue and to decrease the possibility of rash. Some newborns may not tolerate clothing treated with fabric softeners added to the washer or dryer.

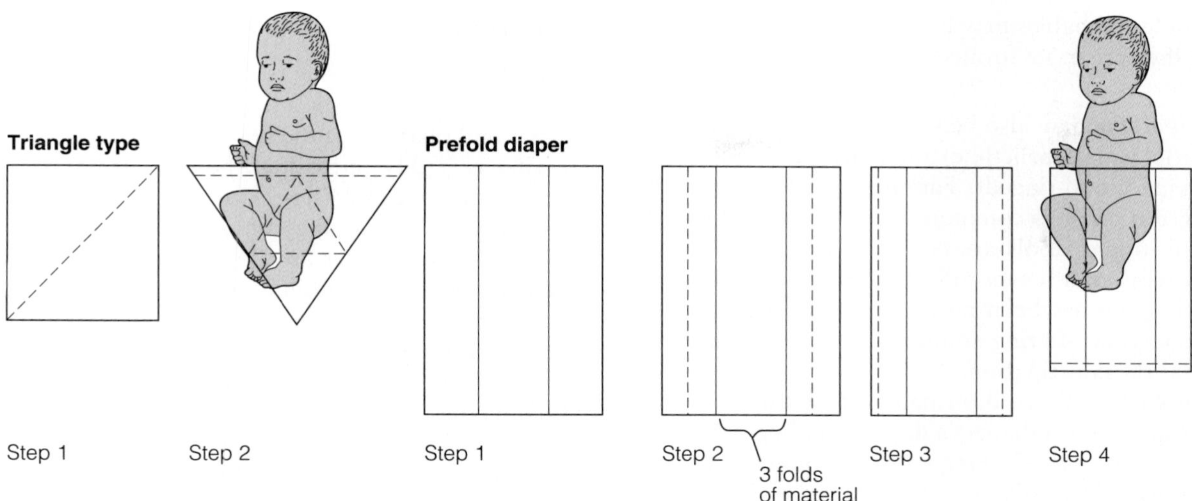

FIGURE 29–5 Two basic cloth diaper shapes. Dotted lines indicate folds.

Temperature Assessment

As the nurse prepares to teach parents about taking their baby's temperature, it is important to provide opportunities for discussion and demonstration. Bordman and Holzman (1996) found that even with individual teaching in the hospital setting, more than half the mothers in their study were unsure of how to take their baby's temperature, and almost half of them were unsure of when to call their primary health care provider. The study provides further encouragement to create opportunities for questions and to pose questions to the parents about what they would do in different situations. This can be accomplished only after a supportive relationship has been established.

The nurse shows the family how to take an axillary temperature and discusses the different types of thermometers. It is important that parents understand the differences and how to select the appropriate one. If the parents are planning to use a glass thermometer, they need information about shaking the mercury down (the mercury needs to be below 94F on the thermometer), reading the thermometer, and making sure that the thermometer bulb is underneath the armpit. To take an axillary temperature, the thermometer is placed under one of the newborn's arms and held in place 3 to 4 minutes. It is important to hold the baby's arm still, because friction between the arm and chest creates heat and can make the thermometer record an inaccurate temperature. Parents should not take the temperature rectally because this method can be both irritating and unsafe for the baby. When taken properly, the axillary method is an accurate way to measure the baby's temperature.

Parents need to take the newborn's temperature only when the signs of illness are present. They should call their physician or pediatric nurse practitioner immediately if any signs of illness are present. See Key Facts to Remember: When Parents Should Call Their Health Care Provider in Chapter 23. Parents should also check with their clinician for advice about over-the-counter medications to be kept in the medicine cabinet.

When parents find their newborn has a temperature, they may expect to give an antipyretic such as Tylenol (acetaminophen). They should not give any form of aspirin for an illness that may be viral; use of aspirin in viral illnesses has been linked to Reye's syndrome in children. They should discuss management of flu, colds, teething, constipation, diarrhea, and other common ailments with their clinician before they occur. When analgesic or antipyretic medication is needed, clinicians frequently recommend acetaminophen drops.

Stools and Urine

The appearance and frequency of a newborn's stools can cause concern for parents. The nurse prepares them by discussing and showing pictures of meconium stools and transitional stools and by describing the difference between breast milk and formula stools. Although each baby develops his or her own stooling patterns, parents can get an idea what to expect (see Figure 21–8).

- Breastfed newborns may have 6 to 10 small, semiliquid, yellow stools per day by the third or fourth day, since milk production is established, unless the mother is having problems with her milk supply. Once breastfeeding is well established, usually by 1 month, the newborn may have only 1 stool every few days because of the increased digestibility of breast milk or still may have several daily. Constipation is unlikely to occur in newborns receiving only breast milk. Infrequent stooling in the first few weeks may indicate inadequate milk intake.

- Formula-fed babies may have only 1 or 2 stools a day; they are more formed and yellow or yellow-brown.

The parents may also be shown pictures of a constipated stool (small, pelletlike) and diarrhea (loose, green, or perhaps blood-tinged). Families should understand that a green color is common in transitional stools, so that transitional stools are not confused with diarrhea the first week of a newborn's life. Constipation may indicate that the newborn needs additional fluid intake. Parents may try offering additional water in an attempt to reverse the constipation.

Babies normally void (urinate) 5 to 8 times per day. Fewer than 6–8 wet diapers a day may indicate the newborn needs more fluids. Frequency of voiding is easy to assess with cloth diapers. Parents who use superabsorbent single-use disposable diapers may have difficulty determining voiding patterns because the surface of the diaper feels dry. The liquid is pooling inside the filling of the diaper.

Sleep and Activity

The newborn demonstrates several different sleep-wake states after the initial periods of reactivity described in Chapter 27. It is not uncommon for a newborn to sleep almost continuously for the first 2 to 3 days following birth, awakening only for feedings every 3 to 4 hours. Some newborns bypass this stage of deep sleep and require only 12–16 hours of sleep. The parents need to know that this is normal.

Quiet sleep is characterized by regular breathing and no movement except for sudden body jerks. During this sleep state, normal household noise will not awaken the infant. In the active sleep state, the newborn has irregular breathing and fine muscular twitching. The newborn may cry out during sleep, but this does not mean he or she is uncomfortable or awake. Unusual household noise may awaken the newborn more easily in this state; however, he or she will quickly go back to sleep.

Quiet alert is a state in which newborns are quietly involved with the environment. They watch a moving mobile, smile, and, as they become older, discover and play with their hands and feet. When newborns become uncomfortable due to wet diapers, hunger, or cold, they enter the **active awake** and **crying state.** In these states, parents should identify and eliminate the cause of the crying. Sometimes families are frustrated as they try to identify the external or internal stimuli that are causing the angry, hurt crying. Parents need to be told that the state may be changed from crying to quiet alert by moving the newborn toward an upright position where scanning and exploration are possible (Klaus and Klaus 1985). See Table 29–3 for the characteristics of the various states.

Crying

For the newborn, crying is the only means of expressing needs vocally. Families learn to distinguish different tones and qualities of the newborn's cry. The amount of crying is highly individual. Some will cry as little as 15–30 minutes in 24 hours, or as long as 2 hours every 24 hours. When crying continues after causes such as discomfort or hunger are eliminated, the newborn may be comforted by swaddling or by rocking and other reassuring activities. There is some indication that newborns who are held more tend to be calmer and cry less when not being held. Some parents may be afraid that holding may "spoil" the newborn and will need reassurance that that is not the case. Picking the babies up when they cry teaches them that adults try to meet their needs and are responsive to them. This helps build a sense of trust in humankind. Excessive crying should be noted and assessed, taking other factors into consideration. After the first 2 or 3 days, newborns settle into individual patterns.

Safety Considerations

Newborns should not have pillows or stuffed animals in the crib while they sleep; these items could cause suffocation. Mattresses should fit snugly in a crib to prevent entrapment and suffocation, and the crib should be inspected regularly to determine whether it is in safe working order. Crib slats should be no more than 2⅜ inches apart. Parents can be encouraged to attend infant cardiopulmonary resuscitation (CPR) classes, especially if there is a family history of SIDS or the infant requires special care.

Newborn Screening and Immunization Program

Before the newborn and mother are discharged from the hospital, parents are informed about the normal screening tests for newborns and told when to return for further tests if needed. Newborn screening tests detect disorders that cause mental retardation, physical handicaps, or death if left undiscovered. Inborn errors of metabolism that can usually be detected from a drop of blood obtained by a heel stick on the second or third day include galactosemia, hemocystinuria, hypothyroidism, maple syrup urine disease, phenylketonuria (PKU), and sickle cell anemia. Parents should be instructed that a second blood specimen will be required from the newborn after 7–14 days (American Academy of Pediatrics Committee on Genetics 1992). In some states, the second blood specimen is not recommended if the first specimen is obtained after 48 hours of age. However, it must be clarified that an abnormal test result is not diagnostic. More definitive tests must be performed to verify the results. It is important to follow

TABLE 29–3 Infant State* Chart (Sleep and Awake States)

Sleep States	Characteristics of State: Body Activity	Eye Movement	Facial Movement	Breathing Pattern	Level of Response	Implications for Caregiving
Deep sleep	Nearly still except for occasional startle or twitch	None	Without facial movements, except for occasional sucking movement at regular intervals	Smooth and regular	Only very intense and disturbing stimuli will arouse infants.	Caregivers trying to feed infant in deep sleep will probably find the experience frustrating. Infants will be unresponsive, even if caregivers use disturbing stimuli (flicking feet) to arouse infants. Infants may arouse only briefly and then become unresponsive as they return to deep sleep. If caregivers wait until infants move to a higher, more responsive state, feeding or caregiving will be much more pleasant.
Light sleep	Some body movements	Rapid eye movement (REM): fluttering of eyes beneath closed eyelids	May smile and make brief fussy or crying sounds	Irregular	Infants are more responsive to internal and external stimuli. When these stimuli occur, infants may remain in light sleep or move to drowsy state.	Light sleep makes up the highest proportion of newborn sleep and usually precedes awakening. Caregivers who are not aware that the brief fussy or crying sounds made during this state occur normally may think it is time for feeding and may try to feed infants before they are ready to eat.
Drowsy	Activity level variable, with mild startles interspersed from time to time; movements usually smooth	Eyes open and close occasionally; are heavy-lidded with dull, glazed appearance	May have some facial movements; often are none and the face appears still	Irregular	Infants react to sensory stimuli although responses are delayed. State change after stimulation frequently noted.	From the drowsy state infants may return to sleep or awaken further. In order to wake them, caregivers can provide something for infants to see, hear, or suck. This may arouse them to a quiet alert state, a more responsive state. Infants left alone without stimuli may return to a sleep state.
Quiet alert	Minimal	Brightening and widening of eyes	Faces have bright, shining, sparkling looks	Regular	Infants attend most to environment, focusing attention on any stimuli that are present.	Infants in this state provide much pleasure and positive feedback for caregivers. Providing something for infants to see, hear, or suck will often maintain a quiet alert state in the first few hours after birth. Most newborns commonly experience a period of intense alertness before going into a long sleeping period.
Active alert	Much body activity; may have periods of fussiness	Eyes open with less brightening	Much facial movement; faces not as bright as in alert state	Irregular	Infants are increasingly sensitive to disturbing stimuli (hunger, fatigue, noise, excessive handling).	Caregivers may intervene at this stage to console and to bring infants to a lower state.
Crying	Increased motor activity with color changes	Eyes may be tightly closed or open	Grimaces	More irregular	Infants are extremely responsive to unpleasant external or internal stimuli.	Crying is the infant's communication signal. It is a response to unpleasant stimuli from the environment or from within infants (fatigue, hunger, discomfort). Crying tells us infants have been reached. Sometimes infants can console themselves and return to lower states. At other times they need help from caregivers.

* *State* is a group of characteristics that regularly occur together: body activity, eye movements, facial movements, breathing pattern, and level of response to external stimuli (eg, handling) and internal stimuli (eg, hunger).

Source: Blackburn S, Kang R: Early Parent-Infant Relationships, 2nd ed, module 3, series 1. *The First Six Hours After Birth.* White Plains, NY: March of Dimes Birth Defects Foundation, 1991. Reprinted with permission of the copyright holder.

protocols that incorporate state laws about newborn testing.

If additional tests are positive, treatment is initiated. These conditions may be treated by dietary means or by administration of missing hormones. The inborn conditions cannot be cured, but they can be treated. They are not contagious, but they may be inherited (Chapter 25).

Follow-up Care

Each newborn will have variations in normal physiologic responses and growth-and-development patterns. Parents need to learn to interpret these changes in their child. To help parents care for their newborn at home, some physicians encourage prenatal pediatric visits to establish this contact before the birth. Public health nurses have long been involved as guides in newborn care and parent education. Birthing units are now expanding their primary-care functions to the new family to include one home visit by the nurse who cared for the family in the birthing unit. The birthing unit nursery staff may also make themselves available as a 24-hour telephone resource for the new family that needs additional support and consultation during the first few days at home with their newborn.

Routine well-baby visits should be scheduled with the clinic, pediatric nurse practitioner, or physician.

The family should be taught all necessary caregiving methods before discharge. A checklist may be helpful to see if the teaching has been completed. The nurse needs to review with the couple all areas for understanding and any outstanding questions, taking time to answer all queries. The mother should have the certified nurse-midwife/nurse practitioner/physician's and lactation consultant's phone number, address, and any specific instructions. Having the nursery phone number is also reassuring to a new family. They are encouraged to call with questions.

Home Care: The Mother and Family

During the first few postpartal weeks many changes are occurring. The family adjusts to incorporating a new family member and siblings become familiar with new roles and responsibilities. During this period the woman must accomplish a variety of physical and developmental tasks, including

- Restoring physical condition
- Developing competence in caring for and meeting the needs of her infant
- Establishing a relationship with her new child
- Adapting to altered lifestyles and family structure resulting from the addition of a new member

Assessment of the Mother and Family

During the first home visit, the nurse completes a physical and psychologic assessment. The physical assessment focuses on maternal physical adaptation, which is assessed by focusing on vital signs, breasts, abdominal musculature, elimination patterns, reproductive tract, and laboratory values. The nurse should also talk with the mother about her diet, fatigue level, ability to rest and sleep, pain management, and signs of postpartal complications. Before completing the assessment the nurse should ensure privacy.

The psychologic assessment focuses on attachment, adjustment to the parental role, sibling adjustment, and educational needs. When appropriate the nurse mentions available community resources, including public health department follow-up visits. If not already discussed, teaching about family planning is appropriate at this time, and the nurse provides information about birth control methods. In ideal situations a family approach involving the presence of the father and any siblings provides an opportunity to observe family interactions and opportunities for all family members to ask questions and express concerns. In addition, any questionable family interaction pattern such as one suggestive of abuse or neglect may be evident and further referral could be considered if needed. See Postpartal Assessment Guide: First Home Visit and Anticipated Progress at Six Weeks.

Follow-Up

Telephone Follow-Up

The nurse usually makes a follow-up telephone call a few days after the home visit. During the call, the nurse can provide additional information, address questions or areas of confusion, and make referrals if indicated.

Help Lines for Parents

Many communities have established 24-hour help lines for new parents to call when they have questions or need support. In areas where help lines are not available, parents may be directed to call the birthing center. In either case, the nurse may provide the number so that it is readily accessible for the family.

Postpartal Classes and Support Groups

Postpartal classes are becoming more common as caregivers recognize the continuing needs of the childbearing family. In many instances, classes are prepared to meet the specific needs of a variety of families so that, for example, single mothers and adolescent mothers can attend class with peers. A series of structured classes may focus on topics such as parenting, postpartal exercise, or nutrition, or there may be loosely structured group sessions that address mothers' concerns as they arise. Such classes offer chances for the new mother to socialize, share her concerns, and receive encouragement. Because babysitting arrangements may be difficult or expensive, it is desirable to provide child care for newborns and siblings; in some instances infants may remain with mothers in the class.

Text continues on page 765

POSTPARTAL ASSESSMENT GUIDE First Home Visit and Anticipated Progress at Six Weeks

Physical Assessment/ Normal Findings	Alterations and Possible Causes*	Nursing Responses to Data[†]
Vital Signs		
Blood pressure: Return to normal prepregnant level.	Elevated blood pressure (anxiety, essential hypertension, renal disease).	Review history, evaluate normal baseline; refer to physician/certified nurse-midwife if necessary.
Pulse: 60–90 beats/minute (or prepregnant normal rate).	Increased pulse rate (excitement, anxiety, cardiac disorders).	Count pulse for full minute, note irregularities; marked tachycardia or beat irregularities require additional assessment and possible physician/certified nurse-midwife referral.
Respirations: 16–24/minute.	Marked tachypnea or abnormal patterns (respiratory disorders).	Evaluate for respiratory disease; refer to physician/certified nurse-midwife if necessary.
Temperature: 36.2C–37.6C (98F–99.6F).	Increased temperature (infection).	Assess for signs and symptoms of infection or disease state.
Weight		
2 days: Possible weight loss of 12–20+ lb.	Minimal weight loss (fluid retention, PIH).	Evaluate for fluid retention, edema, deep tendon reflexes and blood pressure elevation.
6 weeks: Returning to normal prepregnant weight.	Retained weight (excessive caloric intake).	Determine amount of daily exercise. Provide dietary teaching. Refer to dietitian if necessary for additional dietary counseling.
	Extreme weight loss (excessive dieting, inadequate caloric intake).	Discuss appropriate diets; refer to dietitian for additional counseling if necessary.
Breasts		
Nonnursing: 2 days: May have mild tenderness; small amount of milk may be expressed. 6 weeks: Soft, with no tenderness; return to prepregnant size.	Some engorgement (incomplete suppression of lactation). Redness; marked tenderness (mastitis). Palpable mass (tumor).	Engorgement may be seen in nonnursing mothers. Advise client to wear a supportive, well-fitted bra, avoid very warm showers, use ice packs for comfort; evaluate for signs and symptoms of mastitis (rare in nonnursing mothers).
Nursing: Full, with prominent nipples; lactation established.	Cracked, fissured nipples (feeding problems). Redness, marked tenderness, or even abscess formation (mastitis). Palpable mass (full milk duct, tumor).	Counsel about nipple care. Evaluate client condition, evidence of fever; refer to physician/certified nurse-midwife for initiation of antibiotic therapy, if indicated. Opinion varies as to value of breast examination for nursing mothers; some feel a nursing mother should examine her breasts monthly, after feeding, when breasts are empty; if palpable mass is felt, refer to physician for further evaluation.

*Possible causes of alterations are placed in parentheses.

[†]This column provides guidelines for further assessment and initial nursing actions.

POSTPARTAL ASSESSMENT GUIDE — First Home Visit and Anticipated Progress at Six Weeks continued

Physical Assessment/ Normal Findings	Alterations and Possible Causes*	Nursing Responses to Data[†]
Breasts *continued*		For breast inflammation instruct the mother to 1. Keep breast empty by frequent feeding. 2. Rest when possible. 3. Take prescribed pain relief med. 4. Force fluids. If symptoms persist for more than 24 hours, instruct her to call her physician/certified nurse-midwife.
Abdominal Musculature		
2 days: Improved firmness, although "bread dough" consistency is not unusual, especially in multipara. Striae pink and obvious.	Marked relaxation of muscles.	Evaluate exercise level; provide information on appropriate exercise program.
Cesarean incision healing.	Drainage, redness, tenderness, pain, edema (infection).	Evaluate for infection; refer to physician/ certified nurse-midwife if necessary.
6 weeks: Muscle tone continues to improve; striae may be beginning to fade, may not achieve a silvery appearance for several more weeks; linea nigra fading.		
Elimination Pattern		
Urinary tract: Return to prepregnant urinary elimination routine.	Urinary incontinence, especially when lifting, coughing, laughing, and so on (urethral trauma, cystocele).	Assess for cystocele; instruct in appropriate muscle tightening exercises; refer to physician/certified nurse-midwife.
	Pain or burning when voiding, urgency and/or frequency, pus or white blood cells (WBC) in urine, pathogenic organisms in culture (urinary tract infection).	Evaluate for urinary tract infection; obtain clean-catch urine; refer to physician/certified nurse-midwife for treatment if indicated.
Routine urinalysis within normal limits (proteinuria disappeared).	Sugar or ketone in urine—may be some lactose present in urine of breastfeeding mothers (diabetes).	Evaluate diet; assess for signs and symptoms of diabetes; refer to physician/certified nurse-midwife.
Bowel habits: 2 days: May be some discomfort with defecation, especially if client had severe hemorrhoids or third- or fourth-degree extension.	Severe constipation or pain when defecating (trauma or hemorrhoids).	Discuss dietary patterns; encourage fluid, adequate roughage. Continue use of stool softener if necessary to prevent pain associated with straining; continue sitz baths, periods of rest for severe hemorrhoids; assess healing of episiotomy and/or lacerations; severe constipation may require administration of laxatives, stool softeners, and an enema.

*Possible causes of alterations are placed in parentheses.

[†]This column provides guidelines for further assessment and initial nursing actions.

POSTPARTAL ASSESSMENT GUIDE continued

Physical Assessment/ Normal Findings	Alterations and Possible Causes*	Nursing Responses to Data†
Elimination Pattern *continued*		
Bowel habits *continued*		
6 weeks: Return to normal prepregnancy bowel elimination.	Marked constipation.	See above.
	Fecal incontinence or constipation (rectocele).	Assess for evidence of rectocele; instruct in muscle tightening exercises; refer to physician/certified nurse-midwife.
Reproductive Tract		
Lochia:		
2 days: Lochia rubra or lochia serosa, scant amounts, fleshy odor.	Excessive amounts (nonfirm uterus), foul odor (infection).	Assess for evidence of infection and/or failure of the uterus to decrease in size; refer to physician/certified nurse-midwife.
6 weeks: No lochia, or return to normal menstruation pattern.	See above.	See above.
Fundus and perineum:		
2 days: Uterine fundus is at least two fingerbreadths below the umbilicus; uterine muscles still somewhat lax; introitus of vagina lacks tone—gapes when intra-abdominal pressure is increased by coughing or straining.	Uterus not decreasing in size appropriately (infection).	Assess fundus for firmness and/or signs of infection; refer to physician/certified nurse-midwife if indicated.
Episiotomy and/or lacerations healing; no signs of infection.	Evidence of redness, tenderness, poor tissue approximation in episiotomy and/or laceration (wound infection).	
6 weeks: Uterus almost returned to prepregnant size with almost completely restored muscle tone.	Continued flow of lochia, failure to decrease appropriately in size (subinvolution).	Assess for evidence of subinvolution and/or infection; refer to physician for further evaluation and for dilatation and curettage if necessary.
Hemoglobin and Hematocrit Levels		
6 weeks: Hb 12 g/dL. Hct 37% $\pm$ 5%.	Hb $<$ 12 g/dL. Hct 32% (anemia).	Assess nutritional status, begin (or continue) supplemental iron; for marked anemia (Hb $\leq$ 9 g/dL) additional assessment and/or physician/certified nurse-midwife referral may be necessary.

Psychosocial Assessment/ Normal Findings	Alterations and Possible Causes*	Nursing Responses to Data†
Attachment		
Bonding process demonstrated by soothing, cuddling, and talking to infant; appropriate feeding techniques; eye-to-eye contact; calling infant by name.	Failure to bond demonstrated by lack of behaviors associated with bonding process, calling infant by nickname that promotes ridicule, inadequate infant weight gain, infant is dirty, hygienic measures are not being maintained, severe diaper rash, failure to obtain adequate supplies to provide infant care (malattachment).	Provide counseling; talk with the woman about her feelings regarding the infant; provide support for the caretaking activities that are being performed; refer to public health nurse for continued home visits.

*Possible causes of alterations are placed in parentheses.

†This column provides guidelines for further assessment and initial nursing actions.

POSTPARTAL ASSESSMENT GUIDE First Home Visit and Anticipated Progress at Six Weeks continued

Psychosocial Assessment/ Normal Findings	Alterations and Possible Causes*	Nursing Responses to Data†
Attachment *continued*		
Parent interacts with infant and provides soothing, caretaking activities.	Parent is unable to respond to infant needs (inability to recognize needs, inadequate education and support, fear, family stress).	Provide support for caretaking activities observed; provide information regarding caretaking activities, such as responding to infant cry; methods of wrapping infant; methods of soothing the infant such as swaddling, rocking, increasing stimuli by singing to the infant or decreasing stimuli by putting infant to rest in quiet room; methods of holding the infant; differences in the cry. Identify support system such as friends, neighbors; provide information regarding community resources and support groups.
Parents express feelings of comfort and success with the parent role.	Evidence of stress and anxiety (difficulty moving into or dealing with the parent role).	Provide support and encouragement; provide information regarding progression into parent role and assist parents in talking through their feelings; refer to community resources and support groups.
Woman is in the informal or personal stage of maternal role attainment.	Woman is still greatly influenced by others, has not developed an image or style of her own (woman remains in the anticipatory stage).	Provide role modeling for the woman in working through problem solving with the infant; provide encouragement as she thinks through decisions and develops her sense of problem solving; encourage her to make decisions regarding infant care.
Adjustment to Parental Role		
Parents are coping with new roles in terms of division of labor, financial status, communication, readjustment of sexual relations, and adjusting to new daily tasks.	Inability to adjust to new roles (immaturity, inadequate education and preparation, ineffective communication patterns, inadequate support, current family crisis).	Provide counseling; refer to parent groups.
Education		
Mother understands self-care measures.	Inadequate knowledge of self-care (inadequate education).	Provide education and counseling.
Parents are knowledgeable regarding infant care.	Inadequate knowledge of infant care (inadequate education).	
Siblings are adjusting to new baby.	Excessive sibling rivalry.	
Parents have a method of contraception.	Birth control method not chosen.	

*Possible causes of alterations are placed in parentheses.

†This column provides guidelines for further assessment and initial nursing actions.

Some cities offer support groups through birthing centers, hospitals, or as a community effort. Once again, the support group provides an opportunity for parents to interact with one another and share information and experiences.

Return Visits

If the mother and family and physician/certified nurse-midwife have chosen discharge earlier than 48 hours after vaginal birth, in some states, the mother may request a total of three visits. In such cases the nurse would schedule the first visit about 24 hours after discharge and then space out the other two visits over the next week. In other instances the nurse may schedule additional home visits based on the findings of the first home visit and the follow-up phone call.

CHAPTER HIGHLIGHTS

- The overall goal of postpartal home visits is to enhance opportunities for smooth transition of the new family. The home visit provides opportunities for assessment, teaching, and fostering a caring relationship with new families.
- Professional nursing has a role in establishing and maintaining excellence in care for the new family after discharge from the birthing center.
- Nursing goals during home visits include reinforcement of daily newborn care, maintenance of neutral thermal environment, promotion of adequate hydration and nutrition, prevention of complications, promotion of safety, and enhancement of attachment and family knowledge of child care.
- Essential care during a home visit includes assessments of the vital signs, weight, overall color, intake/output, umbilical cord and circumcision, newborn nutrition, parent education, and attachment.
- The physician or pediatric nurse practitioner should be notified if there is evidence of redness around the umbilicus or bright red bleeding or puslike drainage near the cord stump or if the umbilicus remains unhealed.
- Following a circumcision, the newborn must be observed closely for inability to void and signs of infection.
- Signs of illness in newborns include temperature above 38.4C (101F) or below 36.1C (97F), more than one episode of forceful vomiting, refusal of two feedings in a row, lethargy, cyanosis with or without a feeding, and absence of breathing for longer than 15 seconds.
- Newborn screening for galactosemia, hemocystinuria, hypothyroidism, maple syrup urine disease, phenylketonuria, and sickle cell anemia is done on all newborns in the first 1–3 days, with a second blood specimen drawn after 7–14 days.
- Signs of illness in mothers include mastitis, excessive or foul-smelling lochia, failure of fundus to descend at anticipated rate; temperature of 101.4F or above, elevation of blood pressure, and tenderness, redness, or pain in the legs.

REFERENCES

Barnes LP: Meeting the challenge of early postpartum discharge. *MCN* 1996; 21:129.

Braveman P et al: Problems associated with early discharge of newborn infants: Early discharge of newborns and mothers: A critical review of the literature. *Pediatrics* 1995; 96(4):716.

Brown L, Towne S, York R: Controversial issues surrounding early postpartum discharge. *Nurs Clin North Am* 1996; 31(2):333.

Bordman B, Holzman C: Infant care knowledge of primiparous urban mothers. *J Perinatology* 1996; 16(2), pt 1:107.

Bowers S: Legislative action. *Perinatal Home Care News* 1995; 1(1):1.

Catz C et al: Summary of workshop: Early discharge and neonatal hyperbilirubinemia. *Pediatrics* 1995; 96(4):743.

Committee on Fetus and Newborn: Hospital stay for healthy term newborns. *Pediatrics* 1995; 96(4):788.

Evans CJ: Postpartum home care in the United States. *JOGNN* 1995; 24(2):180.

Infant Sleep Positioning and SIDS Position Statement. Evanston, IL: American Academy of Pediatrics, 1992.

Klaus M, Klaus P: *The Amazing Newborn.* Menlo Park, CA: Addison-Wesley, 1985.

Lowdermilk D: *AWHONN Perinatal Home Care Guidelines: An Overview.* Perinatal Home Care Conference. AWHONN and Mosby. New Orleans, LA. December 14–15, 1995.

Lynch AM: Controversies in practice: Discharge decisions and dollars. *House Calls* 1996a; 1(1):12.

Lynch AM: Postpartum home care. *House Calls* 1996b; 1(1):1.

Soskolne E et al: The effect of early discharge and other factors on readmission rates of newborns. *Arch Pediatr Adolesc Med* 1996; 150:373.

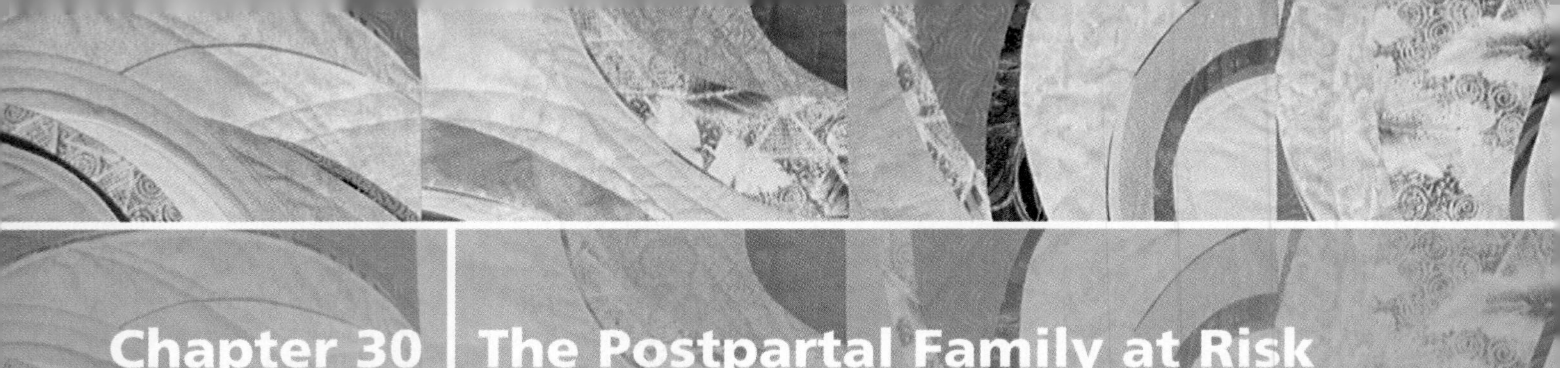

Chapter 30 The Postpartal Family at Risk

OBJECTIVES

- Describe assessment of the postpartum woman for predisposing factors, signs, and symptoms of various postpartum complications to facilitate early and effective management of complications.
- Incorporate preventive measures for various complications of the postpartum period into nursing care of the postpartum woman.
- List the causes of and appropriate nursing interventions for hemorrhage during the postpartal period.
- Develop a nursing care plan that reflects a knowledge of etiology, pathophysiology, and current medical management for the woman experiencing postpartum hemorrhage, reproductive tract infection, thromboembolic disease, urinary tract infection, mastitis, or a postpartal psychiatric disorder.
- Evaluate the mother's knowledge of self-care measures, signs of complications to be reported to the primary care provider, and measures to prevent recurrence of complications.
- Describe the role of telephone follow-up and home visits in the extended care of postpartum families at risk.

KEY TERMS

Early postpartal hemorrhage
Endometritis
Late postpartal hemorrhage
Mastitis
Oophoritis
Pelvic cellulitis (parametritis)
Peritonitis
Puerperal morbidity
Pulmonary embolism
Salpingitis
Subinvolution
Thrombophlebitis
Uterine atony

The postpartal period is often thought of as a smooth, uneventful transition time—and it usually is. However, the nurse must be aware of problems that may develop postpartally and their implications for the childbearing family.

Home Care of Postpartal Women

Early postpartum discharge (within 24 to 48 hours of birth) is becoming increasingly common. Health care outreach services can be especially valuable for clients at risk for postpartum complications, sometimes enabling the family to remain at home together rather than being separated by the mother's readmission to the hospital.

Comprehensive nursing assessment of postpartum clients assumes particular importance when early discharge is anticipated. Systematic data collection allows the nurse to note the normality of findings and identify early signs of complications that would necessitate a longer hospital stay. Data collected before hospital discharge provide baseline findings against which subsequent data, collected by telephone or home visits, can be judged.

Signs and symptoms of many postpartum complications (late hemorrhage, mastitis, thromboembolic disease, and major depression) typically occur only after the woman has returned home, despite the fact that she met criteria for early discharge. Telephone or home visit follow-up may facilitate early recognition of such complications and help the mother get earlier intervention from her primary provider.

Telephone or home visit follow-up care by a professional nurse may also be initiated or extended in response to referral from a physician who has diagnosed a postpartal complication. In either event the nurse continues systematic assessment and plans and implements strategies in collaboration with the physician and family.

Postpartal Assessment by Telephone or During Home Visit

Because 92 percent of all American homes are accessible by telephone, this outreach method is reasonable for extending services to the postpartum family (Donaldson 1988). The telephone follow-up option is explained to families before discharge from the hospital, and a mutually agreeable time is set for the call, usually within 3 to 7 days after discharge, or earlier if desired. Calls typically last about 20 minutes and are preplanned and goal directed. The initial goal is assessment, albeit indirect, of the woman's perception of her current circumstances, her recovery from childbirth, her and her partner's adjustment to parenthood, the newborn's condition, family-newborn bonding, and any problems or concerns that have arisen since homecoming.

A home visit has the advantage of allowing direct assessment to identify postpartum families at risk. The initial visit, planned in collaboration with the family, is usually made within the first 24–72 hours after discharge. The visiting nurse performs a systematic assessment of mother and newborn, family members' adjustment to their new life situation and its inherent role changes, maternal self-care, and newborn care. When the father and other children are present, the nurse has an excellent opportunity to assess the family dynamics within the security of their home. The nurse is also able to assess the residence for adequacy of resources and evidence of safety hazards and to plan interventions accordingly. See Chapter 29 for an in-depth discussion of home care.

Care of the Woman with Postpartal Hemorrhage

Hemorrhage in the postpartal period is described as either early or late postpartal hemorrhage. Early postpartal hemorrhage (or immediate postpartal hemorrhage) occurs in the first 24 hours after birth. Late postpartal hemorrhage (delayed postpartal hemorrhage) occurs after the first 24 hours. Postpartal hemorrhage has traditionally been defined as loss of greater than 500 mL of blood after the end of the third stage of labor. That definition is being questioned in light of recent quantitative studies indicating that blood loss during normal birth is 500 to 600 mL. Furthermore, blood loss during both vaginal and cesarean births is commonly underestimated by half. As the amount of blood loss increases, as in the case of hemorrhage, estimates are likely to be even less accurate (Andersen and Hopkins 1996).

Early Postpartal Hemorrhage

The main causes of **early postpartal hemorrhage** are uterine atony (relaxation of the uterus), lacerations of the genital tract, retained placental fragments, and blood coagulation problems. Certain factors predispose to hemorrhage:

- Overdistention of the uterus due to hydramnios, a large infant, or multiple gestation
- Grand multiparity
- Use of anesthetic agents (especially halothane) to relax the uterus

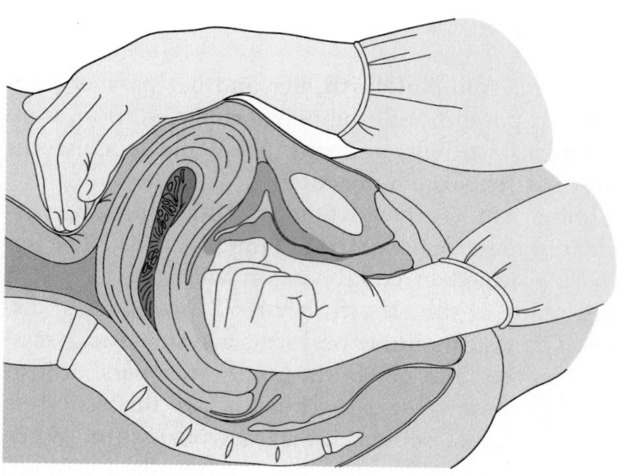

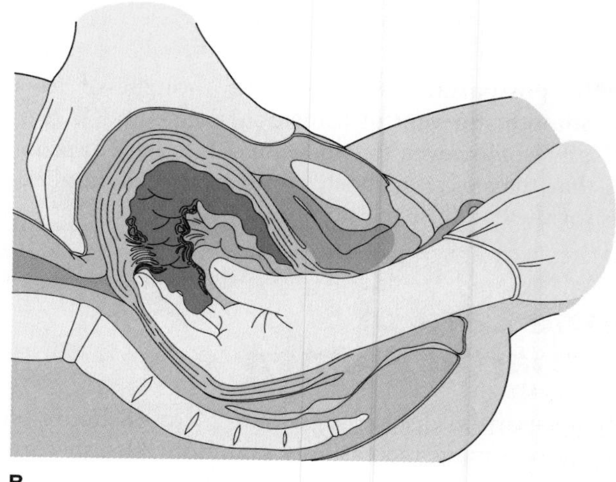

FIGURE 30–1 ***A*** Manual compression of the uterus and massage with the abdominal hand usually will effectively control hemorrhage from uterine atony. ***B*** Manual removal of placenta. The fingers are alternately abducted, adducted, and advanced until the placenta is completely detached. Both procedures are performed only by the medical clinician.

Source: Adapted from Cunningham FG, MacDonald PC, Gant NF [editors]: *Willams Obstetrics,* 18th ed. Norwalk, CT: Appleton & Lange, 1989, pp 417–418.

- Trauma due to procedures such as midforceps-assisted birth, intrauterine manipulation, or forceps rotation
- A prolonged or very rapid labor
- Use of oxytocin to induce or augment labor
- Uterine infection
- Maternal malnutrition, anemia, pregnancy-induced hypertension (PIH), history of hemorrhage, or history of blood coagulation problems

Uterine Atony

Uterine atony, the relaxation of the uterus (or insufficient contractions) following birth, can frequently be anticipated in the presence of

- Overdistention of the uterus
- Dysfunctional labor that has already indicated the uterus is contracting abnormally
- Oxytocin use during labor
- Use of anesthesia or other drugs, like magnesium sulfate, that produce uterine relaxation

Hemorrhage from uterine atony may be slow and steady rather than sudden and massive. The blood may escape the vagina or collect in the uterus. Because of the increased blood volume associated with pregnancy, changes in maternal blood pressure and pulse may not occur until blood loss has been significant.

In most cases the clinician can predict when a woman is at risk for hemorrhage. The key to successful management is prevention. Prevention begins with adequate nutrition, good prenatal care, and early diagnosis and management of any complications. Traumatic procedures should be avoided, and birth should take place in a facility that has blood immediately available. Any woman at risk should be typed and crossmatched for blood and have intravenous lines in place. Excellent labor management and childbirth technique is imperative. After expulsion of the placenta, the fundus should be palpated to assure that it is firm and well contracted. If it is not firm (if it is boggy), fundal massage should be performed until the uterus contracts. If bleeding is excessive, the physician undertakes bimanual uterine compression (Figure 30–1*A*) while ordering the administration of intravenous oxytocin (Pitocin) at a rapid rate. (An undiluted bolus of oxytocin *should not* be given because it can cause hypotension.) Because of longer-lasting effects, methylergonovine maleate (Methergine) may be ordered for the immediate management of uterine atony. (See Drug Guide: Methylergonovine Maleate in Chapter 28.) Oxygen is also administered by mask. The combination of bimanual compression and oxytocin is usually effective in treating uterine atony.

If bleeding persists, the cervix and vagina should be inspected for lacerations. The physician may manually examine the uterine cavity for retained placental fragments or may perform a curettage. If the atony does not respond to these measures, 250 μg of 15-methyl prostaglandin $F_{2\alpha}$ (Prostin 15M) may be administered intramuscularly (Andersen and Hopkins 1996). The dose may be repeated at 15- to 20-minute intervals, if necessary. The side effects, such as nausea, vomiting, and diarrhea, are unpleasant and are often treated with medication. Other side effects include fever, flushing, and elevated diastolic blood pressure.

If hemorrhage continues despite these measures, therapy may include inspection for uterine rupture, blood coagulation studies, curettage, bilateral internal iliac artery ligation, angiographic embolization, or hysterectomy.

Lacerations of the Reproductive Tract

Early postpartum hemorrhage is associated with lacerations of the perineum, vagina, or cervix in 20 percent of cases (Kapernick 1994). Several factors predispose women to higher risk of reproductive tract lacerations:

- Nulliparity
- Epidural anesthesia
- Precipitous birth
- Forceps-assisted birth
- Macrosomia

Thorough inspection of the reproductive tract by the birth attendant facilitates recognition and timely repair of most lacerations. Lacerations are suspected when bright red bleeding persists in the presence of a firmly contracted uterus. The nurse who suspects a laceration on the basis of these findings notifies the physician so that immediate suturing can be done to control the hemorrhage and repair the integrity of the reproductive tract.

Retained Placenta

Hemorrhage may also occur if the placenta is only partially separated. The most common cause of partial separation is massage of the fundus before placental separation, so this practice should be avoided. Management of hemorrhage due to a partial separation, once it has occurred, includes uterine massage and manual removal of the placenta (Figure 30–1*B*). After expulsion of the placenta, the consistency of the fundus is assessed. Rarely, placenta accreta, an abnormal adherence of the placenta to the uterine wall, is the cause of the hemorrhage; it may require curettage or emergency hysterectomy.

Late Postpartal Hemorrhage

Late postpartal hemorrhage generally occurs 1 to 2 weeks after delivery and is most often the result of abnormal involution of the placental site or retained placental fragments. In the case of retained placenta, fragments may become necrosed, and fibrin may be deposited, forming a placental polyp.

Medical Therapy

To prevent late postpartal hemorrhage from retained placental fragments, the placenta should be inspected after expulsion for evidence of missing pieces or cotyledons. The uterine cavity may also be checked for retained placental fragments or membranes.

ESSENTIAL PRECAUTIONS FOR PRACTICE

During Postpartal Hemorrhage

The same basic precautions that apply in caring for any woman during the postpartal period apply when caring for a woman experiencing postpartal hemorrhage. In addition, remember the following specifics:

- Wear gloves when assessing the perineum and when changing or disposing of peripads, chux, or linens soiled with blood or body fluids.
- Place blood-soaked disposable material in appropriate waste containers. Store blood-soaked bedding in an appropriate receptacle for the laundry according to agency procedure.
- Wear a splash apron when changing very soiled bedding or helping a clinician control severe hemorrhage.

For further information consult OSHA and CDC guidelines.

Often a boggy uterus is the first indication of the possibility of late postpartal hemorrhage. Bleeding is controlled by intravenous oxytocin, methylergonovine-maleate (Methergine) (usual dosage is 0.2 mg every four hours for six doses), ergotrate, or prostaglandins. Antibiotics are also used to prevent infection. Sonography is used to determine the presence of retained placental fragments. Curettage, formerly the standard treatment, is now thought to traumatize the implantation site and thereby increase bleeding (Cunningham et al 1997).

APPLYING THE NURSING PROCESS

Nursing Assessment

Careful evaluation of the woman's prenatal history and ongoing assessment during labor and birth will help identify factors that put the woman at risk for postpartal hemorrhage. Periodic assessment for evidence of vaginal bleeding is a major nursing responsibility during the postpartal period. This is done by visual assessment, pad counts, weighing the perineal pads, vital signs every 15 minutes, and perhaps mean arterial pressure readings. See Essential Precautions for Practice: During Postpartal Hemorrhage.

Nursing Diagnosis

Nursing diagnoses that may apply to a woman experiencing postpartal hemorrhage include the following:

- Knowledge deficit related to lack of information about signs of delayed postpartal hemorrhage

KEY FACTS TO REMEMBER

Signs of Postpartal Hemorrhage

Excessive or bright red bleeding

A boggy fundus that does not respond to massage

Abnormal clots

Any unusual pelvic discomfort or backache

Persistent bleeding in the presence of a firmly contracted uterus

Rise in the level of the fundus of the uterus

Increased pulse or decreased BP

Hematoma formation or bulging/shiny skin in the perineal area

Decreased level of consciousness

- Fluid volume deficit related to blood loss secondary to uterine atony, lacerations, or retained placental fragments

Nursing Plan and Implementation

Regular assessment of fundal height and firmness will alert the nurse to the possible development or recurrence of hemorrhage. A soft, boggy uterus is massaged until firm. If the uterus is not contracting well and appears larger than anticipated, the nurse may express clots during fundal massage. Once clots are removed, the uterus tends to contract more effectively.

If the woman seems to have a slow, steady, free flow of blood, the nurse begins to weigh the perineal pads (500 mL fluid weighs approximately 1 lb or 454 g) and monitors the woman's vital signs closely to detect the development of hypovolemic shock. If the fundus is displaced upward or to one side due to a full bladder, the nurse encourages the woman to empty her bladder—or catheterizes her if she is unable to void—to allow for efficient uterine contractions.

The nurse assesses the woman for signs of anemia, such as fatigue, pallor, headache, thirst, and orthostatic changes in pulse or blood pressure, and reviews the results of all hematocrit determinations. The nurse also monitors and evaluates the effectiveness of all medical interventions, intravenous infusions, blood transfusions, oxygen therapy, and medications such as methylergonovine maleate. Urinary output should be monitored to determine adequacy of fluid replacement and renal perfusion. The nurse also encourages the woman to obtain adequate rest and helps her plan activities so that rest is possible. With this in mind the nurse should find ways to promote maternal-infant attachment while accommodating the health needs of the mother. In addition to helping the mother as needed in caring for the newborn, the nurse can work with the woman's partner and family to find ways to help the mother cope.

Due to current trends, the mother may be discharged as early as 4 hours after birth. Because hemorrhage may develop after discharge, she and her support persons should receive clear, preferably written, explanations of the normal postpartum course the signs of complications. Instructions for the prevention of bleeding should include fundal massage, ways to assess the fundal height and consistency, and inspection of any episiotomy and lacerations. The woman and her family are advised to contact her caregiver if any of the signs of postpartal hemorrhage occur. See Key Facts to Remember: Signs of Postpartal Hemorrhage.

Community-Based Nursing Care

The woman may continue to need help with self-care for a time. She should be advised to rise slowly to minimize the likelihood of orthostatic hypotension. Until she regains strength, she should be seated when holding the newborn.

The person who will assume responsibility for grocery shopping and meal preparation will need advice about the importance of including iron-rich foods in the daily menus. Including the client's selection of preferences from a list of such foods will facilitate compliance with the diet. The nurse also explains the rationale for continuing medications containing iron.

The woman should continue to count perineal pads for several days to watch out for any recurring problems with excessive blood loss. The debilitated condition and anemia associated with hemorrhage increase the woman's risk of puerperal infection. She and her caregivers should use good hand washing and minimize exposure to infection in the home. The nurse should give them a list of the signs of infection and emphasize the importance of alerting the physician should any signs occur.

A sense of emergency often exists in the event of late postpartal hemorrhage. Quick decisions about child care arrangements must often be made so that the mother can return to the hospital. Both mother and father are likely to be alarmed by the excessive bleeding and concerned about her prognosis. There will be additional worries about separation from the newborn, especially when the mother is breastfeeding. The father may be in the unenviable position of being torn between the needs of the mother and those of the newborn. Ideally, arrangements can be made to minimize separation of the family members.

Evaluation

Anticipated outcomes of nursing care include

- Signs of postpartal hemorrhage are detected quickly and managed effectively.
- Maternal-infant attachment is maintained successfully.
- The woman is able to identify abnormal changes that might occur following discharge and understands the importance of notifying her caregiver if they develop.

Hematomas

Hematomas are usually the result of injury to a blood vessel without noticeable trauma to the superficial tissue. Hematomas occur following spontaneous as well as forceps-assisted births. Hematomas may be vulvar, vaginal (especially in the area of the ischial spines), or subperitoneal. The most frequently observed hematomas are of the vagina and vulva. The soft tissue in the area offers no resistance, and hematomas containing 250–500 mL of blood may develop rapidly. Signs and symptoms vary somewhat with the type of hematoma.

Medical Therapy

Small vulvar hematomas may be treated with the application of ice packs and continued observation. Large hematomas or those increasing in size require surgical intervention to evacuate the clot and achieve hemostasis by ligating the bleeding point. Antibiotics, replacement of blood and coagulation factors, and vaginal packing may also be indicated. When large amounts of vaginal packing are necessary, voiding may be difficult, if not impossible, because of pressure on the urethra. An indwelling catheter is often necessary until the vaginal packing is removed. Infrequently, a pelvic hematoma that is extensive or difficult to control may require angiographic embolization or additional surgery (Zlatnik 1994).

APPLYING THE NURSING PROCESS

Nursing Assessment

Often the woman complains of severe vulvar pain (pain that seems out of proportion or excessive, usually from her "stitches") or of severe rectal pressure. On examination, the large hematoma appears as a unilateral, tense, fluctuant, bulging mass at the introitus or within the labia majora. With smaller hematomas the nurse may note unilateral bluish or reddish discoloration of the skin of the perineum. The area feels firm and is painful to the touch. The nurse should estimate the size of the hematoma so that increasing size will be quickly noted. Frequent visualization of the perineum in women who are still under the effects of regional anesthesia is especially important.

Hematomas can also develop in the upper portion of the vagina. In these cases, besides pain the woman may have difficulty voiding because of pressure on the urethra or meatus. Diagnosis is confirmed through careful vaginal examination.

Hematomas that occur upward into the broad ligament may be more difficult to detect. The woman may complain of severe lateral uterine pain, flank pain, or abdominal distention. Occasionally the hematoma can be discovered with high rectal examination or with abdominal palpation, although these procedures may be quite uncomfortable for the woman. If the bleeding continues, signs of anemia may be noted.

Signs and symptoms of shock in the presence of a well-contracted uterus and no visible vaginal blood loss should also alert the nurse to the possibility of a hematoma.

Nursing Diagnosis

Nursing diagnoses that may apply when a woman develops a hematoma postpartally include the following:

- Risk for injury related to tissue damage secondary to prolonged pressure from a large vaginal hematoma
- Pain related to tissue trauma secondary to hematoma formation

Nursing Plan and Implementation

If birth was long or traumatic or if forceps or a vacuum extractor was used, the nurse can promote comfort and decrease the possibility of hematoma formation by applying an ice pack to the woman's perineum during the first hour after birth and intermittently thereafter for the next 8–12 hours. The discomfort experienced by a woman who develops a hematoma cannot be overlooked. If a hematoma develops despite preventive measures, a sitz bath after the first 24 hours will aid fluid absorption once the bleeding has stopped and will promote comfort, as will the judicious use of analgesics.

Evaluation

Anticipated outcomes of nursing care include

- Hematoma formation is avoided; if it does occur, it is detected quickly and managed successfully.
- The woman's discomfort is relieved effectively.
- Tissue damage is avoided or minimized.

Subinvolution

Subinvolution of the uterus occurs when the uterus fails to follow the normal pattern of involution (decrease in size of about 1 cm/day) and remains enlarged. Retained placental fragments and infection are the most frequent causes. With subinvolution the fundus is higher in the abdomen than expected. In addition, lochia often fails to progress from rubra to serosa to alba. Lochia rubra that persists longer than 2 weeks postpartum is highly suggestive of subinvolution (Cunningham et al 1997). Leukorrhea and backache may occur if infection is the cause. Subinvolution is most commonly diagnosed during the routine postpartal examination at 4 to 6 weeks. The woman may relate a history of irregular or excessive bleeding, or describe the symptoms listed previously. Diagnosis is made when an enlarged, softer-than-normal uterus is palpated with bimanual examination. Treatment involves oral administration of methylergonovine (Methergine) 0.2 mg every 3 to 4 hours for 24 to 48 hours. When metritis (inflammation of the uterus) is present, antibiotics are also administered. If this treatment is not effective or the cause is believed to be retained placental fragments, curettage is indicated (Cunningham et al 1997).

Care of the Woman with a Postpartal Reproductive Tract Infection

Puerperal infection is an infection of the reproductive tract associated with childbirth that can occur any time from birth to 6 weeks postpartum. The most common infection is metritis/endometritis and is limited to the uterine cavity. However, infection can spread by way of the lymphatics and blood vessels to become a progressive disease resulting in peritonitis or pelvic cellulitis.

The standard definition of **puerperal morbidity** established in the 1930s by the Joint Committee on Maternal Welfare is a temperature of 100.4F (38C) or higher, with the temperature (taken by mouth by a standard technique at least four times a day) occurring on any two of the first ten postpartum days, exclusive of the first 24 hours. However, serious infections can occur in the first 24 hours or may cause only persistent low-grade temperatures. Therefore, careful assessment of all postpartum women with elevated temperatures is essential.

Causative Factors and Infectious Agents

The vagina and cervix of pregnant women usually contain pathogenic bacteria sufficient to cause infection. Generally other factors must be present, however, for infection to occur. Premature rupture of membranes (PROM) allows organisms to ascend into the uterus and is a major factor in the development of infection postpartally. Bacterial contamination of the amniotic fluid with the membranes still intact is more common than previously believed and may contribute to preterm labor. The placental site, episiotomy, lacerations, abrasions, and any operative incisions are all potential portals for bacterial entrance and growth. Hematomas are easily infected and enhance the possibility of sepsis. Tissue that has been compromised through trauma is less able to combat infection. Other factors predisposing the woman to infection include frequent vaginal examinations, lapses in aseptic technique, urethral catheterization, anemia, malnutrition, intrauterine manipulation, hemorrhage, cesarean birth, retained placental fragments, and faulty perineal care.

Group B streptococcus, other streptococci, and *Gardnerella vaginalis* are among the most common aerobic bacteria found in women with postpartal infection. Other aerobic bacteria implicated in puerperal infections include *Escherichia coli* and *Staphylococcus aureus* (associated with an increasing number of cases of postpartum toxic shock). *E coli* may be introduced as a result of contamination of the vulva or reproductive tract from feces during labor and birth. Group A β-hemolytic streptococci, a less common cause (Hamadeh et al 1995), may be transmitted from the skin or nasopharynx of the woman herself or more probably from an external source such as personnel and equipment. Aseptic technique is essential to avoid this.

Anaerobic bacteria most frequently isolated from women with postpartal infection include *Bacteroides* species, *Peptostreptococcus* species, and, occasionally, *Clostridium perfringens*. Genital mycoplasmas, *Ureaplasma urealyticum* and *Mycoplasma hominis,* are found in women with postpartal endometritis, but their role in the infection is unclear because the endometritis responds to antibiotics that are not effective against these particular organisms (Cunningham 1997).

Late postpartal endometritis is most commonly associated with the genital mycoplasmas and *Chlamydia trachomatis. C. trachomatis* has a longer replication time and latency period than other bacteria and is not consistently eradicated by antibiotics used for early postpartum infections.

Types of Infections

Localized Infections

A less severe complication of the puerperium is a localized infection of the episiotomy or of lacerations to the perineum, vagina, or vulva. Early signs are hip pain, perineal pain, erythema, edema, and induration at the episiotomy site with later development of skin discoloration and systemic shock. Treatment includes intravenous and oral antibiotics and aggressive surgical debridement (Hamadeh et al 1995). Wound infection of the abdominal incision site after cesarean birth is also possible. The skin edges become reddened, edematous, firm, and painful. The skin edges then separate, and purulent material, sometimes mixed with sanguineous liquid, drains from the wound. The woman may complain of localized pain and dysuria and may have a low-grade fever (less than 101F or 38.3C). If the wound develops an abscess or is unable to drain, high temperature and chills may result.

Endometritis (Metritis)

Endometritis, an inflammation of the endometrium, may occur postpartally. After expulsion of the placenta, the placental site provides an excellent culture medium for bacterial growth. The remaining portion of the decidua is also susceptible to pathogenic bacteria because of its thinness (approximately 2 mm) and its large blood supply. The cervix may also be a bacterial breeding ground because of the multiple small lacerations attending normal labor and birth.

In mild cases of endometritis the woman will generally have discharge that is scant (or profuse), bloody, and foul smelling. In more severe cases, the symptoms may include uterine tenderness and jagged, irregular temperature elevation, usually between 38.3C (101F) and 40C (104F). Tachycardia, chills, and evidence of subinvolution may be noted. Although foul-smelling lochia is cited as a classic sign of endometritis, with infection caused by β-hemolytic streptococcus the lochia may be scant and odorless (Cunningham et al 1997).

Salpingitis and Oophoritis

Occasionally bacteria spreads into the lumen of the fallopian tubes, producing infection in the tubes (**salpingitis**) and ovaries (**oophoritis**). Such infections are most often caused by a gonorrheal infection, *Chlamydia trachomatis,* anerobic baccilli and cocci, and gram-negative aerobes. Symptoms include bilateral (or unilateral) lower abdominal and pelvic pain, fever, chills, possible adnexal mass (if abscess develops), and tachycardia. Approximately 50–60 percent of women with salpingitis severe enough to cause infertility from tubal obstruction have never had a recognized episode of salpingitis (Eschenbach 1994). If tubal closure results, sterility may ensue.

Pelvic Cellulitis (Parametritis) and Peritonitis

Pelvic cellulitis (parametritis) is infection involving the connective tissue of the broad ligament or, in more severe forms, the connective tissue of all the pelvic structures. It is generally spread by way of the lymphatics in the uterine wall but may also occur if pathogenic organisms invade a cervical laceration that extends upward into the connective tissue of the broad ligament. This laceration then serves as a direct pathway for the pathogens already in the cervix to spread into the pelvis. **Peritonitis** is infection involving the peritoneum and is a major, life-threatening infection.

A pelvic abscess may form in the case of puerperal peritonitis and is most commonly found in the uterine ligaments, cul-de-sac of Douglas, and the subdiaphragmatic space. Pelvic cellulitis may be a secondary result of pelvic vein thrombophlebitis. This condition occurs when the clot becomes infected and the wall of the vein breaks down from necrosis, spilling the infection into the connective tissues of the pelvis.

A woman suffering from parametritis may demonstrate a variety of symptoms, including marked high temperature (102–104F or 38.9–40C), chills, malaise, lethargy, abdominal pain, subinvolution of the uterus, tachycardia, and local and referred rebound tenderness. If peritonitis develops, the woman will be acutely ill with severe pain, marked anxiety, high fever, rapid, shallow respirations, pronounced tachycardia, excessive thirst, abdominal distention, nausea, and vomiting.

Medical Therapy

Diagnosis of the infection site and causative pathogen is accomplished by careful history and complete physical examination, blood work, cultures of the lochia (although this may be of limited value since multiple organisms are usually present), and urinalysis to rule out urinary tract infection. When a localized infection develops, it is treated with antibiotic creams, sitz baths, and analgesics as necessary for pain relief. If an abscess has developed or a stitch site is infected, the suture is removed and the area is allowed to drain.

Metritis is treated by aggressive administration of antibiotics. The route and dosage are determined by the severity of the infection. Severe infection warrants administration of parenteral antibiotics. Careful monitoring is also necessary to prevent the development of a more serious infection.

Parametritis and peritonitis are treated with intravenous antibiotics. Broad-spectrum antibiotics effective against the most commonly occurring causative organisms are chosen initially, pending the results of culture and sensitivity reports. If multiple organisms are present, the approach to antibiotic therapy is continued unless no improvement is observed, in which case the antibiotic is changed.

The development of an abscess is frequently heralded by the presence of a palpable mass and may be confirmed with ultrasound. An abscess usually requires incision and drainage to avoid rupture into the peritoneal cavity and the possible development of peritonitis. Following drainage of the abscess, the cavity may be packed with iodoform gauze to promote drainage and facilitate healing.

The woman with a severe systemic infection is acutely ill and may require care in an intensive care unit. Supportive therapy will include maintenance of adequate hydration with intravenous fluids, analgesics, ongoing assessment of the infection, and possibly continuous nasogastric suctioning if paralytic ileus develops.

APPLYING THE NURSING PROCESS

Nursing Assessment

The woman's perineum should be inspected every 8–12 hours for signs of early developing infection. The REEDA scale helps the nurse remember to consider redness, edema, ecchymosis, discharge, and approximation. Any degree of induration (hardening) should be immediately reported to the clinician.

Fever, malaise, abdominal pain, foul-smelling lochia, tachycardia, and other signs of infection should be noted and reported immediately so that treatment can be instituted.

Nursing Diagnosis

Nursing diagnoses that may apply to the women with a puerperal infection include the following:

- Risk for injury related to the spread of infection
- Pain related to the presence of infection
- Knowledge deficit related to lack of information about condition and its treatment
- Risk for altered parenting related to delayed parent-infant attachment secondary to woman's malaise and other symptoms of infection

Nursing Plan and Implementation

During the puerperium the nurse teaches the woman self-care measures that are helpful in preventing infection. The woman should understand the importance of perineal care, good hygiene practices to prevent contamination of the perineum (including wiping from front to back and changing perineal pads after going to the bathroom), and thorough hand washing. Once edema and perineal pain are under control, the nurse can also encourage sitz baths, which are cleansing and promote healing. Adequate fluid intake and a diet high in protein and vitamin C, which are necessary for wound healing, also help prevent infection.

If the woman is seriously ill, the nurse administers antibiotics as ordered, regulates the intravenous fluid, monitors the woman's vital signs and intake and output, and meets her comfort and hygiene needs. Ongoing assessment is indicated to detect subtle changes in the woman's condition. The nurse also promotes maternal-infant attachment, which may be difficult when the woman is acutely ill. Pictures and information about the newborn as well as brief visits help promote attachment. See the Critical Pathway for the Woman with a Puerperal Infection on pp 775–777 for specific nursing care measures.

Community-Based Nursing Care

The woman with a puerperal infection needs assistance when she is discharged from the hospital. If the family cannot provide this home assistance, a referral to home care services is needed. Home care services should be contacted as soon as puerperal infection is diagnosed so that the nurse can meet with the woman for a family and home assessment and development of a home care plan.

The family needs instruction in the care of a newborn, including feeding, bathing, cord care, immunizations, and significant observations that should be reported. A well baby appointment should be scheduled. Breastfeeding mothers should be instructed to inspect the infant's mouth for signs of thrush and to report the finding to their physician.

The mother should be instructed regarding activity, rest, medications, diet, and signs and symptoms of complications, and she should be scheduled for a return medical visit. She needs to know the importance of taking the entire course of prescribed antibiotics even though she may begin to feel better before the bottle is empty. She also needs to be informed about the importance of pelvic rest. That is, she should not use tampons or douches or have intercourse until she has been examined by the physician and told it is safe to resume those activities.

Evaluation

Anticipated outcomes of nursing care include

- The infection is quickly identified and treated successfully without further complications.
- The woman understands the infection and the purpose of therapy; she cooperates with ongoing antibiotic therapy after discharge.
- Maternal-infant attachment is maintained.

CRITICAL PATHWAY FOR THE WOMAN WITH A PUERPERAL INFECTION

Category	1–4 Hours Postpartum	4–8 Hours Postpartum	8–24 Hours Postpartum
Referral	Report from labor nurse if not continuing in an LDR room	Lactation consultation if needed	Home nursing referral if indicated
Assessment	• Postpartum assessments q½h ×2, q1h ×2, then q4h. Includes: • Fundus firm, in midline, at or below umbilicus • Lochio rubra <1 pad/h; no free flow or passage of clots with massage • Bladder: voids large amts urine spontaneously; bladder not palpable following voiding • Perineum: sutures intact; no bulging or marked swelling; no c/o severe pain. Minimal bruising may be present. If hemorrhoids present, no tenseness or marked engorgement; <2 cm diameter. • Breasts: soft, colostrum present • Vital signs: • BP WNL; no hypotension; not >30 mm systolic or 15 mm diastolic over baseline • Temperature: <38C (100.4F) • Pulse: Bradycardia normal; consistent with baseline • Respirations: 12–20/min; quiet; easy • Comfort level: <3 on scale of 1 to 10	• Continue postpartum assessment q4h ×2, then q8h • Assess for bowel sounds • Assess lochia for color, odor, amount • Breasts: evaluate nipple status; should be no evidence of cracks or bruising • Observe feeding technique with newborn • Assess VS q8h; all WNL; report temp >38C (100.4F) • Continue assessment of comfort level q3–4h	• Continue postpartum assessment q8h • Breasts: nipples should remain free of cracks, fissures, bruising • Feeding technique with newborn should be good or improving • Assess VS q4h; report temp >38C (100.4F) • Continue assessment of comfort level q3–4h • Continue s/sx of infection (ie, episiotomy, endometritis, pelvic cellulitis, or puerperal peritonitis) • Inspect incision/episiotomy for redness, approximation, and drainage • Assess for signs of progressive infection (ie, uterine subinvolution, foul-smelling lochia, uterine tenderness, severe lower abdominal pain, fever, elevated WBC, malaise, chills, lethargy, tachycardia, nausea and vomiting, abdominal rigidity)
Comfort	• Institute comfort measures: • Perineal discomfort: peri-care, sitz baths, topical analgesics • Hemorrhoids: sitz baths, topical analgesics, digital replacement of external hemorrhoids, side-lying or prone position • Afterpains: prone with small pillow under abdomen; warm shower or sitz baths; ambulation • Administer pain medication__________	• Continue with pain management techniques	• Continue with pain management techniques • Promote comfort by: • Ensuring adequate periods of rest • Minimizing disturbing environmental stimuli • Judicious use of analgesics and antipyretics • Providing emotional support • Using supportive nursing measures (ie, back rubs, instruction in relaxation techniques, maintenance of cleanliness, provision of diversional activities)
Teaching/ psychosocial	• Explain postpartum assessments • Teach self-massage of fundus and expected findings • Instruct to call for assistance first time OOB and prn • Demonstrate peri-care, surgigator, sitz baths prn • Explain comfort measures • Begin newborn teaching (bulb suctioning, positioning, feeding, diaper change, cord care) • Orient to room if transferred from LDR room • Provide information on early postpartum period • If breastfeeding mother is unable to nurse, assist her in pumping her breasts to maintain adequate milk supply	• Discuss psychologic changes of postpartum period • Stress need for frequent rest periods • Continue newborn teaching: soothing/comforting techniques, swaddling; return demonstrations indicate woman's understanding • Provide opportunities for questions and review; reinforce previous teaching • Breastfeeding: nipple care; air-drying, lanolin; proper latch-on technique; tea bags • Bottle feeding: supportive bra; ice bags, breast binder	• Reinforce previous teaching: answer questions • Discuss need to take antibiotics until course completed • Discuss involution; anticipated physical changes in first 2 weeks postpartum; postpartum exercises; need to limit visitors • Breastfeeding/bottle feeding: • Explain milk production, let-down reflex, use of supplements, breast pumping, and milk storage • If cannot breastfeed, assist mother with pumping her breasts • Explain formula preparation and storage • Discuss sibling rivalry; mother should have plan for supporting siblings at home • Teaching evaluation completed

CRITICAL PATHWAY FOR THE WOMAN WITH A PUERPERAL INFECTION continued

Category	1–4 Hours Postpartum	4–8 Hours Postpartum	8–24 Hours Postpartum
Therapeutic nursing interventions and reports	• Ice pack to perineum to decrease swelling and increase comfort • Straight cath prn × 1 if distended or voiding small amts • If continues unable to void or voiding small amts, insert Foley catheter and notify CNM/physician	• Sitz baths prn • If woman Rh− and infant Rh+, RhoGAM work up; obtain consent; complete teaching • Obtain consent for rubella vaccine if indicated; explain purpose, procedure, implications • Obtain hematocrit • Determine rubella status	• Continue sitz baths 2–3 times/day or surgigator • May shower if ambulating without difficulty • Obtain blood cultures per dr order if temp elevated • Obtain wound culture and assist with wound drainage and packing • Use principles of medical asepsis in handwashing and disposal of contaminated material by client and caregiver • Promote normal wound healing by pericare, wiping front to back after each voiding, frequent changing of pads
Activity	• Assistance when OOB first time, then prn • Ambulate ad lib • Rests comfortably between checks	• Encourage rest periods • Ambulate ad lib; may leave birthing unit	• Up ad lib
Nutrition	• Regular diet, high in vit C and protein • Fluid intake ⩾2000 mL/day	• Continue diet and fluids	• Continue diet and fluids • Increase calories by 500 kcal over nonpregnant state (200 kcal over pregnant intake) if breastfeeding • Return to normal caloric intake for nonpregnant state if bottle feeding
Elimination	• Voiding large amts straw-colored urine	• Voiding large quantities • May have bowel movement, assess bowel sounds	• Monitor I/O, urine specific gravity, and level of hydration
Medications	• Methergine 0.2 mg q4h prn if ordered • Stool softener__________________ • Tucks pads prn	• Continue meds • Lanolin to nipples prn; tea bags to nipples if tender; heparin flush to buffalo cap (if present) q8h or as ordered	• IV antibiotics • Continue meds • May take own prenatal vitamins • RhoGAM administered if indicated • Rubella vaccine administered if indicated
Discharge planning/ home care	• Evaluate knowledge of normal postpartum, newborn care • Evaluate support systems	• Discuss typical newborn schedule; plan for periods of rest • Birth certificate paperwork completed • Evaluate plans for transporting newborn; car seat available	• Provide information regarding predisposing factors, s/sx, and treatment • Discuss the value of a nutritious diet in promoting healing • Review hygiene practice (ie, correct wiping after voiding, and hand washing, to prevent the spread of infection) • Discuss home care routines to be used following postpartal infection • Review discharge instruction sheet and checklist • Describe postpartum and infection warning signs and when to call CNM/physician • Provide prescriptions; gift pack given to woman • Arrangements made for baby pictures if desired • Postpartum visit scheduled • Newborn check scheduled

CRITICAL PATHWAY continued

Category	1–4 Hours Postpartum	4–8 Hours Postpartum	8–24 Hours Postpartum

Family involvement	• Identify available support persons
	• Assess family perceptions of birth experience
	• Parenting: demonstrates culturally expected early parenting behaviors
		• Involve support persons in care, teaching; answer questions
		• Evidence of parental bonding behaviors apparent
		• Provide and maintain mother-infant interaction:
		  • Provide opportunities for the mother to see and hold her infant
		  • Encourage partner or support person to discuss infant with woman and to become involved in infant's care if the woman is not able to do so
			• Continue to involve support persons in teaching
			• Evidence of parental bonding behaviors continued
			• Plans made for providing support to mother following discharge. Support persons verbalize understanding of need for woman to rest, eat nutritionally, recover

Date			

Care of the Woman with Postpartal Thromboembolic Disease

Although thrombosis may occur antepartally, it is generally considered a postpartal complication. *Venous thrombosis* refers to thrombus formation in a superficial or deep vein with the accompanying risk that a portion of the clot might break off and result in pulmonary embolism. When the thrombus is formed in response to inflammation in the vein wall, it is termed **thrombophlebitis.** In this type of thrombosis, the clot tends to be more firmly attached and therefore is less likely to result in embolism. In *noninflammatory venous thrombosis* (also called phlebothrombosis) the clot tends to be more loosely attached and the risk of embolism is greater. The main factor responsible for noninflammatory deep vein thrombosis is venous stasis (Cunningham et al 1997).

Factors contributing directly to the development of thromboembolic disease postpartally include (a) increased amounts of certain blood clotting factors; (b) postpartal thrombocytosis (increased quantity of circulating platelets) and their increased adhesiveness; (c) release of thromboplastin substances from the tissue of the decidua, placenta, and fetal membranes; and (d) increased amounts of fibrinolysis inhibitors. Predisposing factors are (a) obesity, increased maternal age, and high parity; (b) anesthesia and surgery with possible vessel trauma and venous stasis due to prolonged inactivity; (c) previous history of venous thrombosis; (d) maternal anemia, hypothermia, or heart disease; (e) use of estrogen for suppression of lactation; (f) endometritis; and (g) varicosities.

Superficial Vein Leg Disease

Superficial thrombophlebitis is far more common postpartally than during pregnancy. Often the clot involves the saphenous veins. This disorder is more common in women with preexisting varices, although it is not limited to these women. The symptoms—tenderness in a portion of the vein, some local heat and redness, absent or low-grade fever, and occasionally slight elevation of the pulse—usually become apparent about the third or fourth postpartal day. Treatment involves application of local heat, elevation of the affected limb, bed rest and analgesics, and the use of elastic support hose. Anticoagulants are usually not necessary unless complications develop. Pulmonary embolism is rare. Occasionally the involved veins have incompetent valves, and as a result, the problem may spread to the deeper leg veins, such as the femoral vein.

Deep Vein Thrombosis (DVT)

Deep vein thrombosis (DVT) is more frequently seen in women with a history of thrombosis. Certain obstetric complications, such as hydramnios, PIH, and operative birth, are associated with an increased incidence. Clinical manifestations may include edema of the ankle and leg, and an initial low-grade fever often followed by high temperature and chills. Depending on the vein involved, the woman may complain of pain in the popliteal and lateral tibial areas (popliteal vein), entire lower leg and foot (anterior and posterior tibial veins), inguinal tenderness (femoral vein), or pain in the lower abdomen (iliofemoral vein). The Homan's sign (refer to Figure 27–7) may or may not be positive, but calf pressure often produces pain. Because of reflex arterial spasm, sometimes the limb is pale and cool to the touch—the so-called milk leg or *phlegmasia alba dolens*—and peripheral pulses may be decreased.

Septic Pelvic Thrombophlebitis

Septic pelvic thrombophlebitis may develop in conjunction with infections of the reproductive tract and is more common in women who have had a cesarean birth (Hamadeh et al 1995). The classic sign is fever of unknown origin. However, when the ovarian vein is involved, lower abdominal pain also occurs. If untreated, tachycardia, nausea, ileus, and elevated white count usually develop.

Medical Therapy

Because cases are seldom clear-cut, diagnosis involves a variety of approaches, such as client history and physical examination, occlusive cuff impedence plethysmography (IPG), Doppler ultrasonography (increased circumference of affected extremity), pelvic CT scan or MRI, and contrast venography. In questionable cases, contrast venography provides the most accurate diagnosis of deep vein thrombophlebitis. Unfortunately, venography is not practical for multiple examinations or prospective screening and may itself induce phlebitis.
Treatment involves the administration of intravenous heparin, using an infusion pump to permit continuous, accurate infusion of medication. Strict bed rest and elevation of the leg are required, and analgesics are given as necessary to relieve discomfort. The woman is often given antibiotic therapy if fever is present. In most cases thrombectomy is not necessary.

Once the symptoms have subsided (usually in several days), the woman may begin ambulation while wearing elastic support stockings. Intravenous heparin is continued, and treatment with sodium warfarin (Coumadin) is begun. Because osteoporosis may occur with prolonged heparin therapy (Cosico et al 1993), the heparin is discontinued when prothrombin time reaches 1.5 to 1.7. The woman will continue on Coumadin for 2 to 6 months at home. While on warfarin, prothrombin times are assessed periodically to maintain correct dosage levels.

CRITICAL THINKING IN ACTION

Lei Chang, G1P1, had a cesarean birth after a prolonged labor and failure to progress. You notice that, as she is walking in the hallway with her husband, Lei is limping slightly, and you comment on that observation. Lei responds that she is having pain in her right lower leg. She says, "Maybe I pulled a muscle during labor." What would you do?

Answers can be found in Appendix H.

APPLYING THE NURSING PROCESS

Nursing Assessment

The nurse carefully assesses the woman's history for factors predisposing to thrombophlebitis. In addition, the nurse is alert to any complaints of pain in the legs, inguinal area, or lower abdomen because such pain may indicate deep vein thrombosis. The nurse also assesses the woman's legs for evidence of edema, temperature change, or pain with palpation.

Nursing Diagnosis

Nursing diagnoses that may apply to the woman with a thrombolic disease include the following:

- Altered tissue perfusion in periphery related to obstructed venous return
- Pain related to tissue hypoxia and edema secondary to vascular obstruction
- Risk for altered parenting related to decreased maternal-infant interaction secondary to bed rest and IVs
- Altered family processes related to illness of family member
- Knowledge deficit related to lack of information about the DVT/thrombophlebitis, its treatment, preventive measures, and the medication (warfarin)

Nursing Plan and Implementation

Women with varicosities should be evaluated for need of support hose during labor and the postpartum period. Adequate fluid intake is necessary during labor to avoid dehydration. Because trauma is often a factor in the development of thrombophlebitis, the nurse avoids keeping the woman's legs elevated in stirrups for prolonged periods. If stirrups are used, they should be comfortably padded and adjusted to provide correct support and prevent pressure on popliteal vessels. In addition the nurse encourages early ambulation after birth and avoids using the knee gatch on the bed. Women confined to bed following a cesarean birth are encouraged to do regular leg exercises to promote venous return.

Once the diagnosis of deep venous thrombosis is made, the nurse maintains the heparin therapy, provides appropriate comfort measures, and monitors the woman closely for signs of pulmonary embolism. The nurse also assesses for evidence of bleeding related to heparin and keeps the antagonist for heparin, protamine sulfate, readily available.

The woman is instructed to avoid prolonged standing or sitting because they contribute to venous stasis. She is also instructed to avoid crossing her legs because of the pressure it causes. Walking is acceptable because it promotes venous return. The woman is reminded to identify her history of thrombosis/thrombophlebitis to her physician during subsequent pregnancies so that preventive measures can be instituted early.

Women who are discharged on warfarin must understand the purpose of the medication and be alert for signs of bleeding such as bleeding gums, epistaxis, petechiae or ecchymosis, or evidence of blood in the urine or stool. Because careful monitoring is important, the woman should clearly understand the need to keep scheduled appointments for prothrombin time assessment. Certain medications such as aspirin and nonsteroidal anti-inflammatory drugs increase anticoagulant activity and should be avoided. In fact, the woman should check for possible medication interaction before taking any medication while on warfarin. She should also have vitamin K available in case bleeding occurs, and may choose to wear a MedicAlert bracelet in case of emergency.

Warfarin is excreted in the breast milk and thus may present problems for infants of breastfeeding mothers. Women who wish to continue nursing may be maintained at home on low doses of subcutaneous heparin since heparin is not excreted in breast milk. See the Critical Pathway for the Woman with Thromboembolic Disease on pp 780–783 for specific nursing care measures.

Community-Based Nursing Care

Because the mother with postpartum thromboembolic disease will depend on others for much of her initial home care, it is helpful for the father to be involved in preparations for discharge. The nurse should provide ample opportunities for questions to be answered and instructions clarified, verbally and in writing. The nurse will evaluate the extent to which both mother and father have understood instructions regarding the plan of care. It is especially important to assess the couple's plans to ensure complete bed rest for the mother. They might explore ways for her to maintain bed rest and still spend quality time with her newborn and any other children. For example, young children can sit on the bed for storytelling or play quiet games, and the newborn's crib can be placed next to the mother's bed.

Signs of postpartum thrombophlebitis may not occur until after discharge from the hospital. Consequently all couples must be taught to recognize its signs and symptoms and appreciate the importance of reporting them immediately and of not massaging the affected leg. Should signs and symptoms occur after discharge, a short readmission may be required. In that case every effort is made to allow mother, father, and newborn to remain together.

Evaluation

Anticipated outcomes of nursing care include

- If thrombophlebitis develops, it is detected quickly and managed successfully without further complications.
- At discharge the woman is able to explain the purpose, dosage regimen, and necessary precautions associated with any prescribed medications such as anticoagulants.
- The woman can discuss self-care measures and ongoing therapies (such as the use of elastic stockings) that are indicated.
- The woman has bonded successfully with her newborn and is able to care for her baby effectively.

Pulmonary Embolism

A sudden onset of dyspnea accompanied by sweating, pallor, cyanosis, confusion, systemic hypotension, cough (with or without hemoptysis), tachycardia, shortness of breath, fever, and increased jugular pressure may indicate **pulmonary embolism.** Chest pain that mimics heart attack, coupled with the woman's verbalized fear of imminent death and complaint of pressure in the bowel and rectum, should alert the nurse to the extensive size of the embolus. A friction rub and evidence of atelectasis may be noted upon auscultation. A gallop (heart) rhythm may be present even if respiratory inspiration is normal, although smaller emboli may present with only transient syncope, tightness of the chest, or unexplained fever.

Even x-ray films, EKG changes, and laboratory data are not always reliable. If a case of pulmonary embolism is suspected, prompt treatment should begin even in the absence of corroborative data. If the embolism is small and heparin therapy is begun quickly, the chance of survival is excellent. However, when a large thrombus occludes a major pulmonary vessel, death may occur before therapy can even begin.

Therapy involves the administration of a variety of intravenous medications, such as meperidine hydrochloride to relieve the pain, lidocaine to correct any arrhythmias, and drugs such as papaverine hydrochloride and aminophylline to reduce spasms of the bronchi and coronary and pulmonary vessels. Oxygen is administered and heparin infusion begun. In severe cases an embolectomy may be necessary, although thrombolytic therapy with medications (such as streptokinase) that break up clots may be tried first (Eftychiou 1996).

Text continues on page 783

CRITICAL PATHWAY FOR THE WOMAN WITH THROMBOEMBOLIC DISEASE*

Category	Antepartal Management	Intrapartal Management	Postpartal Management
Referral	Perinatologist Internist Social worker Psych clinical nurse practitioner Dietary/nutrionist Infectious disease consult	Obtain prenatal record	Home nursing referral if indicated

Assessment	• Obtain hx of present pregnancy
	• Assess estimated gestational age
	• Assess any sensitivity to medications
	• Obtain complete physical examination to include:
	  • Fetal size, fetal status (FHR), and fetal maturity
	  • Signs of fatigue, weakness, recurrent diarrhea, pallor, night sweats
	  • Present weight and amount of weight gain or weight loss
	• Obtain diagnostics studies:
	  • Ultrasound
	  • Fetal maturity studies (L/S ratio, PG creatinine)
	  • Hemoglobin, hematocrit, platelet count
	  • WBC and differential
	  • HIV-I
	  • CD4+ T lymphocyte count
	  • ESR
			• Monitor daily Hct
			• Continue normal postpartum assessment q8h
			• Feeding technique with newborn: should be good or improving
			• TPR assessment: q8h; all WNL; report temperature >38C (100.4F)
			• Continue assessment of comfort level
			• Assess for superficial thrombophlebitis:
			  • Tenderness along involved vein
			  • Areas of palpable thrombosis
			  • Warmth and redness in the involved area
			• Deep venous thrombosis (DVT):
			  • Positive Homan's sign (pain occurs when foot is dorsiflexed while leg is extended)
			  • Tenderness and pain in affected area
			  • Fever (initially low, followed by high fever and chills)
			  • Edema in affected extremity
			  • Pallor and coolness in affected limb
			  • Diminished peripheral pulses
			  • Increased potential for pulmonary embolus
			• Immediately report the development of any signs of pulmonary embolism, including the following:
			  • Sudden onset of severe chest pain, often located substernally
			  • Apprehension and sense of impending catastrophe
			  • Cough (may be accompanied by hemoptysis)
			  • Tachycardia
			  • Fever
			  • Hypotension
			  • Diaphoresis, pallor, weakness
			  • Shortness of breath
			  • Neck engorgement
			  • Friclion rub and evidence of atelectasis upon auscultation

Comfort			• Continue with pain management techniques. No aspirin or ibuprofen. Acetaminophen may be ordered. • Provide supportive nursing comfort measures such as rubs, provision of quiet time for sleep, diversional activities • Maintain warm moist soaks as ordered with legs elevated

*All of the interventions for a normal labor and delivery and postpartum patient may be found in those appropriate critical pathways.

CRITICAL PATHWAY continued

Category	Antepartal Management	Intrapartal Management	Postpartal Management
Teaching/ psychosocial	• Room orientation • Explain s/sx of labor • Increase pt awareness of fetal monitoring • Evaluation of client teaching	Tour of ICN Discuss with woman: • Mode of childbirth • Postpartum expectation	Implement normal postpartum teaching and psychosocial support (see Chapter 28) • Maintain mother/infant attachment; when mother is on bed rest provide frequent contacts for mother and infant; modified rooming-in is possible if the crib is placed close to the mother's bed and nurse checks often to help mother lift or move infant
Therapeutic nursing interventions and reports	• Assess emotional response so that support and teaching can be planned accordingly • Weigh woman • Obtain food history • Establish rapport • Provide opportunities to talk without interruption • Monitor for signs of infection • Maintain appropriate isolation precautions	• Ongoing monitoring of blood pressure • Electronic fetal monitoring in place • Try to have same nurses caring for woman during her hospitalization • Monitor for signs of infection	• Continue sitz baths prn • May shower if ambulating without difficulty • DC buffalo cap (heparin lock) if present • Monitor for signs of infection • For DVT obtain prothrombin time (PT) and review prior to beginning warfarin. Repeat periodically per physician order
Activity	Decreased stimulation in room including visitors		• Maintain bed rest and limb in elevated position • Initiate progressive ambulation following the acute phase; provide properly fitting elastic stockings prior to ambulation for management of superficial thrombophlebitis and DVT
Nutrition	Plan high-protein, high-calorie diet		Continue diet and fluids
Elimination			

Medications		Continuous IV infusion	• May take own prenatal vitamins
			• RhoGAM administered if indicated
			• Rubella vaccine administered if indicated
			• For DVT administer intravenous heparin as ordered by continuous intravenous drip, heparin lock, or subcutaneously, including the following:
			  • Monitor IV or heparin lock site for signs of infiltration
			  • Obtain Lee-White clotting times or partial thromboplastin time (PTT) per physician order, and review prior to administering heparin
			  • Observe for signs of anticoagulant overdose with resultant bleeding, including the following: hematuria, epistaxis, ecchymosis, and bleeding gums
			  • Provide protamine sulfate per physician order to combat bleeding problems related to heparin overdosage

CRITICAL PATHWAY FOR THE WOMAN WITH THROMBOEMBOLIC DISEASE continued

Category	Antepartal Management	Intrapartal Management	Postpartal Management

Discharge planning/ home care	• Assess home care needs
	• Provide support and counseling
			• Discuss ways of avoiding circulatory stasis such as avoiding prolonged standing, sitting, and crossing legs
			• Review need to wear support stockings and to plan for rest periods with legs elevated
			• In the presence of DVT, discuss the following:
			  • The use of warfarin, its side effects, possible interactions with other medications, and need to have dosage assessed through periodic checks of the prothrombin time
			  • Signs of bleeding, which may be associated with warfarin sodium and which need to be reported immediately, including the following: hematuria, epislaxis, ecchymosis, bleeding gums, and rectal bleeding
			  • Monitor menstrual flow: bleeding may be heavier
			  • Review need for woman to eat a consistent amount of leafy green vegetables (lettuce, cabbage, brussels sprouts, broccoli) every day (high in Vit K so affects dose of warfarin and PT balance)
			  • Instruct the woman to report any bleeding that continues more than 10 minutes
			  • Instruct the woman to do the following:
			    • Routinely inspect the body for bruising
			    • Carry MedicAlert card indicating she is on anticoagulant therapy
			    • Use electric razor to avoid scratching skin
			    • Use soft bristle toothbrush
			    • Avoid alcohol intake or keep intake at minimum
			    • Avoid taking any other drugs without checking with the physician
			    • Note that stools may change color to pink, red, or black as a result of anticoagulant use
			    • Advise all health providers, including dentists, that she is taking anticoagulants
			• Review discharge instruction sheet and checklist
			  • Provide list or make appropriate referrals to available community resources
			• Describe postpartum warning signs and when to call CNM/physician
			• Provide prescriptions: Gift pack given to woman
			• Arrangements made for baby pictures if desired
			• Postpartum visit scheduled
			• Newborn check scheduled

CRITICAL PATHWAY continued

Category	Antepartal Management	Intrapartal Management	Postpartal Management
Family involvement	Assess support systems	Encourage family member to stay with the woman as long as possible throughout labor and childbirth	• Continue to involve support persons in teaching • Plans made for providing support to mother following discharge. Support persons verbalize understanding of need for woman to rest, eat nutritionally, recover • Encourage woman to express her concerns to her partner. Assist couple in planning ways to manage while woman is hospitalized and after her discharge • Encourage partner or support person to bring other children to hospital to visit mother and meet new sibling • Encourage partner or support person to bring in family pictures. Encourage phone calls • Contact social services if indicated to obtain additional assistance for family if needed
Date			

Care of the Woman with a Urinary Tract Infection (UTI)

The postpartal woman is at increased risk of developing urinary tract problems due to the normal postpartal diuresis, increased bladder capacity, decreased bladder sensitivity from stretching and/or trauma, and possible inhibited neural control of the bladder following the use of general or regional anesthesia.

Emptying the bladder is vital. Women who have not sufficiently recovered from the effects of anesthesia cannot void spontaneously, and catheterization is necessary. However, retention of residual urine, bacteria introduced at the time of catheterization, and a bladder traumatized by birth combine to provide an excellent environment for the development of cystitis.

Overdistention of the Bladder

Overdistention occurs postpartally when, as a result of the predisposing factors previously identified, the woman is unable to empty her bladder.

Medical Therapy

Overdistention, if discovered in the recovery room, is often managed by draining the bladder with a straight catheter as a one-time measure. If the overdistention recurs or is diagnosed later in the postpartal period, an indwelling catheter is generally ordered for 24 hours.

APPLYING THE NURSING PROCESS

Nursing Assessment

The overdistended bladder appears as a large mass, reaching sometimes to the umbilicus and displacing the uterine fundus upward and to the right. There is increased vaginal bleeding, the fundus is boggy, and the woman may complain of cramping as the uterus attempts to contract. Some women also experience backache and restlessness.

Nursing Diagnosis

Nursing diagnoses that may apply when a woman experiences overdistention include the following:

- Risk for infection related to urinary stasis secondary to overdistention
- Urinary retention related to decreased bladder sensitivity and normal postpartal diuresis

Nursing Plan and Implementation

Diligent monitoring of the bladder during the recovery period and preventive health measures greatly reduce the chances for overdistention of the bladder. Encouraging the mother to void spontaneously and helping her use the toilet, if possible, or the bedpan, if she has received conductive anesthesia, prevent the largest percentage of overdistention. Before she attempts to void, the woman should be medicated if she is experiencing pain. Perineal ice packs applied after birth help minimize edema that may interfere with voiding. Pouring warm water over the perineum or having the woman void in the sitz bath may also be effective.

If catheterization becomes necessary, meticulous aseptic technique should be employed during catheter insertion. The vagina and vulva are traumatized to some degree by vaginal birth, and edema is common. This edema may obscure the urinary meatus; therefore the nurse needs to be extremely careful in cleansing the vulva and inserting the catheter. It is imperative to discard a catheter that has inadvertently been introduced into the vagina and thus contaminated. Because catheterization is an uncomfortable procedure due to the postpartal trauma and edema of the tissue, the nurse should be careful and gentle not only in inserting the catheter but also in handling and cleaning the perineal area.

If the amount of urine drained from the bladder reaches 900–1000 mL, the nurse should clamp the catheter, inflate the Foley balloon, and tape the catheter to the woman's leg. The procedure, including taking the woman's vital signs before and after the procedure and noting her responses, should be carefully charted. After an hour the nurse may unclamp the catheter and place it on gravity drainage. This technique protects the bladder and avoids rapid intra-abdominal decompression. The physician should be notified. When the indwelling catheter is removed, a urine specimen is often sent to the lab. The tip of the catheter may also be removed and sent for culture.

Evaluation

Anticipated outcomes of nursing care include

- The woman voids adequately to meet the demands of the increased fluid shifts during the postpartal period.
- The woman does not develop infection due to stasis of urine.
- The woman actively incooperates self-care measures to decrease bladder overdistention.

Cystitis (Lower Urinary Tract Infection)

E coli causes 73–90 percent of the cases of postpartal cystitis (bladder inflammation) and pyelonephritis. In most cases the infection ascends the urinary tract from the urethra to the bladder and then to the kidneys because vesiculoureteral reflux (backward flow of urine) forces contaminated urine into the renal pelvis.

When cystitis is suspected in the puerperium, a clean-catch midstream urine sample is obtained for microscopic examination, culture, and sensitivity tests. The specimen may require collection by the nurse with the woman on a bedpan because few postpartal women can collect a true midstream, clean-catch specimen without contaminating the specimen with lochia. A catheterized specimen is avoided when possible because of the increased risk of infection. When the bacterial concentration is greater than 100,000 microorganisms per milliliter of fresh urine, infection is generally present; counts between 10,000 and 100,000 are suggestive, particularly if clinical symptoms are noted.

Treatment is theoretically delayed until urine culture and sensitivity reports are available. In the clinical setting, however, antibiotic therapy is often begun immediately using one of the short-acting sulfonamides, or in the case of sulfa allergy, ampicillin. The antibiotic is begun immediately and can be changed later if indicated by the results of the sensitivity report (Cunningham et al 1997). Antispasmodics may be given to relieve discomfort.

Pyelonephritis (Upper Urinary Tract Infection)

Pyelonephritis is an inflammation of the renal pelvis that is usually the result of infection. In most cases the infection has ascended from the lower urinary tract. It occurs more commonly on the right, although both kidneys may be affected. If untreated, the renal cortex may be damaged and kidney function impaired.

Medical Therapy

With pyelonephritis, bed rest, forced fluids, and broad-spectrum antibiotics are prescribed immediately. The antibiotics can be changed if the culture so indicates. Bed rest and careful monitoring of intake and output are necessary to detect the development of bacterial shock. If nausea and vomiting are severe, fluids are given intravenously. Antispasmodics and analgesics are given to relieve discomfort. The woman usually continues to take antibiotics for 2–4 weeks after clinical and bacteriologic response. A clean-catch urine culture should be obtained 2 weeks after completion of therapy and then periodically for the next 2 years. An intravenous pyelogram may be ordered in 2–4 months to identify any residual renal damage.

Continuation of breastfeeding during therapy is limited only by the degree of the mother's malaise and clinical discomfort. For the breastfeeding mother the antibiotic should be selected carefully to avoid problems for the infant via the milk.

APPLYING THE NURSING PROCESS

Nursing Assessment

Symptoms of cystitis often appear 2–3 days after birth, after the woman has been discharged. Initial symptoms may include frequency, urgency, dysuria, and nocturia. Hematuria and suprapubic pain may be present. A slightly elevated temperature may occur, but systemic symptoms are often absent.

When a UTI progresses to pyelonephritis, systemic symptoms usually occur, and the woman becomes acutely ill. Symptoms include chills, high fever, flank pain (unilateral or bilateral), nausea, and vomiting, in addition to all the signs of lower UTI. Costovertebral pain may also be elicited. Urine culture and sensitivity are obtained to identify the causative organism.

Nursing Diagnosis

Nursing diagnoses that may apply if a woman develops a UTI postpartally include the following:

- Knowledge deficit related to a lack of information about the long-term effects of pyelonephritis
- Knowledge deficit related to lack of information about self-care measures to prevent UTI

Nursing Plan and Implementation

Screening for asymptomatic bacteriuria in pregnancy should be routine. The nurse should encourage frequent emptying of the bladder during labor and the postpartum period to prevent overdistention and trauma to the bladder. Catheterization technique and nursing actions to prevent overdistention that were discussed earlier also apply. The woman with pyelonephritis must understand the importance of follow-up care after discharge to prevent recurrence or further complications.

Teaching for Self-Care

The postpartal woman should be advised to continue good perineal hygiene after discharge. She is also advised to maintain a good fluid intake and to empty her bladder whenever she feels the urge to void, but at least every 2 to 4 hours while awake. The new mother should void before sexual intercourse (to prevent bladder trauma) and after intercourse (to wash contaminents from the vicinity of the urinary meatus). Wearing cotton crotch underwear to facilitate air circulation also reduces the risk of urinary tract infection.

Evaluation

Anticipated outcomes of nursing care include

- Signs of UTI are detected quickly and the condition is treated successfully.
- The woman incorporates self-care measures to prevent the recurrence of UTI as part of her personal hygiene routine.
- The woman cooperates with any long-term therapy or follow-up.
- Maternal-infant attachment is maintained and the woman is able to care for her newborn effectively.

Care of the Woman with Mastitis

Mastitis refers to an inflammation of the breast generally caused by *Staphylococcus aureus* and primarily seen in breastfeeding mothers. Because symptoms seldom occur before the second to fourth week after birth, nurses often are not fully aware of how uncomfortable and acutely ill the woman may be. The infection usually begins when bacteria invade the breast tissue. Often the tissue has been traumatized in some way (fissured or cracked nipples, overdistention, manipulation, or milk stasis) and is especially susceptible to pathogenic invasion. The most common sources of the bacteria are the infant's nose and throat, although other sources include the hands of the mother or birthing unit personnel or the woman's circulating blood.

Thomsen, Esperson, and Maigaard (1984) have suggested a classification of inflammatory symptoms of the breast based on leukocytes and bacterial counts per milliliter of breast milk: (1) milk stasis; (2) noninfectious inflammation of the breast; and (3) infectious mastitis. Milk stasis is a relatively mild, short-lived condition, usually without fever and not requiring antibiotics. Noninfectious inflammation of the breast presents with more severe inflammatory symptoms that last for several days. Infectious mastitis is a more serious infection with fever, headache, flulike symptoms, and a warm, reddened, painful area of the breast (Figure 30–2).

In other cases *Candida albicans* is the causative organism of mastitis, entering the breast through a small fissure or abrasion on the nipple. Signs include late-onset nipple pain, followed by shooting pain during and between feedings. Eventually, the skin of the affected breast will become pink, flaking, and pruritic.

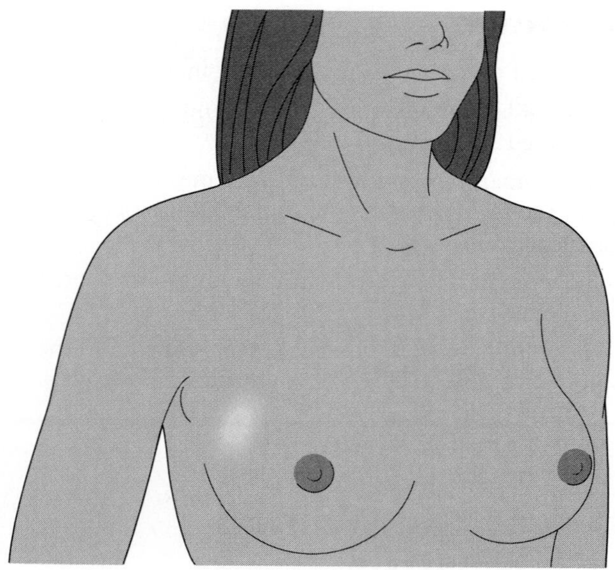

FIGURE 30–2 Mastitis. Erythemia and swelling are present in the upper outer quadrant of the breast. Axillary lymph nodes are enlarged and tender.

Medical Therapy

Diagnosis is usually based on symptoms and physical examination, even while waiting for laboratory results. The need for culture and antibody sensitivity of the breast milk remains controversial, although most authors agree on the need for cultures if there is a recurrence of the mastitis. Treatment involves bed rest, increased fluid intake, a supportive bra, feeding the baby frequently, local application of heat, and analgesics for discomfort. Early treatment may prevent the progression of milk stasis and nonfectious inflammation to mastitis. Treatment of mastitis includes all the measures mentioned previously plus a 10-day course of antibiotics (usually a penicillinase-resistant penicillin) (Cunningham et al 1997). Improved outcome, decreased duration of symptoms, and decreased incidence of breast abscess result if the breasts continue to be emptied by either nursing or pumping. Whether to continue nursing or not has been controversial in the past but most experts now recommend continued nursing in most cases. The woman should be contacted within 24 hours of initiation of treatment to ensure that symptoms are subsiding (Lawrence 1994).

Occasionally the process of mastitis may continue and a frank abscess develops. The mother's milk and any drainage from the nipple should be cultured and antibiotic therapy instituted. In addition, it is usually necessary to incise surgically and drain the abscessed area. If multiple abscesses are present, multiple incisions will be necessary, usually under general anesthesia. After incision and drainage, the area is packed with sterile gauze. The packing is gradually decreased to permit proper healing.

Often the breast is covered with a sterile surgical dressing and access to the breast is temporarily inhibited, making breastfeeding impossible. If possible, the dressing should be applied so that the woman can continue to breastfeed or pump her breast, thereby avoiding engorgement and maintaining lactation. A recent study recommended ultrasonically guided percutaneous treatment for acute puerperal breast abscesses (Karstrup et al 1993). This method allows continued breastfeeding.

APPLYING THE NURSING PROCESS

Nursing Assessment

Daily assessment of breast consistency, skin color, surface temperature, and nipple condition is essential to detect early signs of problems that may predispose to mastitis. The mother should be observed nursing her baby to ensure use of proper breastfeeding technique. If an infection has developed, the nurse should assess for contributing factors such as cracked nipples, poor hygiene, engorgement, supplemental feedings, change in routine or infant feeding pattern, abrupt weaning, or lack of proper breast support so that these factors can be corrected as part of the treatment plan.

Nursing Diagnosis

Nursing diagnoses that may apply to the woman with mastitis include the following:

- Knowledge deficit related to lack of information about appropriate breastfeeding practices
- Ineffective breastfeeding related to pain secondary to development of mastitis

Nursing Plan and Implementation

Prevention of Mastitis

Prevention of mastitis is far simpler than therapy. Ideally mothers should be instructed in proper breastfeeding technique prenatally. If not, instruction should begin as soon as possible in the postpartal period. The nurse should assist the mother to breastfeed soon after birth and should review correct technique. All women, even those not breastfeeding, are encouraged to wear a good supportive bra at all times to avoid milk stasis, especially in the lower lobes.

Meticulous hand washing by all personnel is the primary measure in preventing epidemic nursery infections and subsequent maternal mastitis. Prompt attention to

TABLE 30–1 Comparison of Findings of Engorgement, Plugged Duct, and Mastitis

	Engorgement	Plugged Duct	Mastitis
Onset	Gradual, immediately postpartum	Gradual, after feedings	Sudden, after 10 days
Site	Bilateral	Unilateral	Usually unilateral
Swelling and heat	Generalized	May shift, little or no heat	Localized, red, hot, and swollen
Pain	Generalized	Mild but localized	Intense but localized
Body temperature	<38.4C	<38.4C	>38.4C
Systemic symptoms	Feels well	Feels well	Flulike symptoms

Source: Lawrence RA: *Breastfeeding—A Guide for the Medical Profession.* St Louis: Mosby, 1994, p 261.

mothers who have blocked milk ducts eliminates stagnant milk as a growth medium for bacteria. If the mother finds that one area of her breast feels distended, she can rotate the position of her infant for nursing, manually express milk remaining in the breast after nursing (usually necessary only if the infant is not sucking well), or massage the caked area toward the nipple as the infant nurses. Early identification and intervention for sore nipples are also essential.

Education for Self-Care

The nurse stresses to the breastfeeding woman the importance of adequate breast and nipple care to prevent the development of cracks and fissures, a common portal for bacterial entry. For a detailed discussion of breastfeeding, see Chapter 24.

The woman should be aware of the importance of regular, complete emptying of the breasts to prevent engorgement and stasis. She should also understand the role of let-down in successful breastfeeding and the principle of supply and demand. Mothers who will be breastfeeding and returning to work need information about how to do so successfully. Since mastitis tends to develop after discharge, it is important to include information about signs and symptoms in the discharge teaching (Table 30–1). All flulike symptoms should be considered a sign of mastitis until proved otherwise. If symptoms develop, the woman should contact her caregiver immediately because prompt treatment helps to avoid abscess formation.

Community-Based Nursing Care

The woman who develops mastitis may need to temporarily discontinue breastfeeding. In that case she will need to learn techniques for bottle-feeding and formula preparation, including sterilization, if necessary. The home care nurse can help the mother obtain an appropriate breast pump to help her maintain lactation and can provide opportunities for demonstration and return demonstration of pumping. Referral to a lactation consultant or to La Leche League can be invaluable to the woman's physical and emotional adjustment to mastitis.

Evaluation

Anticipated outcomes of nursing care include

- The woman is aware of the signs and symptoms of mastitis.
- The woman's mastitis is detected early and treated successfully.
- The woman can continue breastfeeding if she chooses.
- The woman understands self-care measures she can employ to prevent the recurrence of the mastitis.

Care of the Woman with a Postpartal Psychiatric Disorder

Many types of psychiatric problems may occur in the postpartum period. The classification of postpartum psychiatric disorders is a subject of some controversy. The *Diagnostic and Statistical Manual of Mental Disorders,* 4th edition (DSM-IV), has added a postpartum onset specifier to the mood disorder diagnostic category of psychiatric disorders. It is proposed that postpartum psychiatric disorders be considered one diagnosable syndrome with three subclasses: (1) adjustment reaction with depressed mood, (2) postpartum psychosis, and (3) postpartum major mood disorder. The incidence, etiology, symptoms, treatment, and prognosis vary with each subclass.

Adjustment reaction with depressed mood is also known as postpartum, maternal, or "baby" blues. It occurs in as many as 50–80 percent of mothers and is characterized by mild depression interspersed with happier feelings. Postpartum blues typically occur within a few days after the baby's birth and is self-limiting, lasting from a few hours to 10 days (Horowitz et al 1995). It is more severe in primiparas and seems related to the rapid alteration of estrogen, progesterone, and prolactin levels after birth. New mothers experiencing postpartum blues commonly report feeling overwhelmed, unable to cope, fatigued, anxious, irritable, and oversensitive. A key feature is episodic tearfulness, often without an identifiable reason.

Validating the existence of this phenomenon, labeling it as a real but normal adjustment reaction, and providing reassurance can offer a measure of relief. Assistance with self- and infant care, information, and family support aids recovery. The partner should be encouraged to watch for and report signs that the new mother is not returning to a more normal mood but slipping into a deeper depression.

Postpartum psychosis, which has an incidence of 1 to 2 per 1000, usually becomes evident within the first 3 months postpartum. Symptoms include agitation, hyperactivity, insomnia, mood lability, confusion, irrationality, difficulty remembering or concentrating, poor judgment, delusions, and hallucinations. Treatment may include hospitalization, antipsychotics, sedatives, electroconvulsive therapy, removal of the infant, social support, and psychotherapy.

Postpartum major mood disorder, also known as postpartum depression, develops in about 10 percent of all postpartum women (Horowitz et al 1995). Although it may occur at any time during the first postpartum year, the greatest risks occur around the fourth week, just before the initiation of menses, and upon weaning.

Risk factors for postpartum depression include

- Primiparity
- Ambivalence about maintaining the pregnancy
- History of postpartum depression or bipolar illness
- Lack of social support
- Lack of a stable relationship with parents or partner
- The woman's dissatisfaction with herself
- Lack of a supportive relationship with her parents, especially her father, as a child (Horowitz et al 1995)

Certain other factors that have been highly correlated with postpartum depression may be assessed via screening questions for the disorder: (1) history of infertility, (2) early menarche (before age 11), (3) unrealistic expectations of parenthood, and (4) adverse emotional reactions (irritability or depression) resulting from earlier use of oral contraceptives (Horowitz et al 1995).

Medication, individual or group psychotherapy, and practical assistance with child care and other demands of daily life are common treatment measures. Support groups have proven to be successful adjuncts to such treatment. Within a support group of postpartal women and their partners, a couple may feel consolation that they are not alone in their experience. Moreover, the group provides a forum for exchanging information about postpartum depression, learning stress reduction measures, and experiencing renewed self-esteem and support (Logsdon et al 1994).

APPLYING THE NURSING PROCESS

Nursing Assessment

The nurse observes the woman for signs of depression, which may be manifested by tearfulness, exhaustion, anxiety, poor concentration, sleep difficulties, appetite change, and statements indicating feelings of failure and self-accusation. Severity and duration of symptoms should be noted. Behavior and verbalizations that are bizarre or seem to indicate a potential for violence against herself or others, including the infant, should be reported as soon as possible for further evaluation.

The nurse needs to be aware that many normal physiologic changes of the puerperium are similar to symptoms of depression (lack of sexual interest, appetite change, and fatigue). It is essential that observations be as specific and as objective as possible and that they be carefully documented (Horowitz et al 1996; Beck 1995).

Nursing Diagnosis

Possible nursing diagnoses that may apply to a woman with a postpartum psychiatric disorder include the following:

- Ineffective individual coping related to postpartum depression
- Risk for altered parenting related to postpartal mental illness

Nursing Plan and Implementation

The nurse should alert the mother, spouse, and other family members to the possibility of postpartum blues in the early days after birth and reassure them of the short-term nature of the condition. Symptoms of postpartum depression should be described and the mother encouraged to call her health care provider if symptoms become severe, if they fail to subside quickly, or if at any time she feels she is unable to function.

Community-Based Nursing Care

Home visits, especially for early-discharge families, are essential to fostering positive adjustments for the new family. Telephone follow-up at 3 weeks postpartum to ask if the mother is experiencing difficulties is also helpful (Ruchala and Halstead 1994).

Women with a history of depression or postpartum psychosis should be referred to a mental health professional for counseling and biweekly visits between the second and sixth week postpartum for evaluation of depression. Medication, social support, and assistance with child care may also be necessary (Mowbray et al 1995).

In all women the presence of three symptoms or one symptom for 3 days may signal serious depression. Referral to a mental health professional should be made immediately. Immediate referral should also be made if rejection of the infant or threatened or actual aggression against the infant has occurred. In such cases the newborn is never left unattended with the mother.

A diagnosis of postpartum depression or other psychiatric disorder will pose major problems for the family, especially the father. The symptoms of these disorders are difficult to witness and may be harder to understand than physical problems like hemorrhage or infection. The father may feel hurt by his partner's hostility, worry that she is becoming insane, or be baffled by her mood swings and lack of concern about herself, the newborn, or household responsibilities. There may be very real practical matters to handle—running the household; managing the children, including the totally dependent newborn; and caring for the mother—added to his usual routines and work responsibilities. Information, emotional support, and assistance in providing or obtaining care for the infant may be needed. Postpartum follow-up is especially important, as well as visits from a psychiatric home health nurse.

Evaluation

Anticipated outcomes of nursing care include

- Signs of potential postpartal disorders are detected quickly and therapy is implemented.
- The newborn is cared for effectively by the father or another support person until the mother is able to do her share.

CHAPTER HIGHLIGHTS

- The main causes of early postpartal hemorrhage are uterine atony, lacerations of the vagina and cervix, and retained placental fragments.
- The most common postpartal infection is endometritis, which is limited to the uterine cavity.
- Thromboembolic disease originating in the veins of the leg, thigh, or pelvis may occur in the antepartum or postpartum periods and carries with it the potential for creating a pulmonary embolus.
- A postpartal woman is at increased risk for developing urinary tract problems due to normal postpartal diuresis, increased bladder capacity, decreased bladder sensitivity from stretching or trauma, and, possibly, inhibited neural control of the bladder following the use of anesthetic agents.
- Mastitis is an inflammation of the breast caused by *Staphylococcus aureus* and is primarily seen in breastfeeding women. Symptoms seldom occur before the second to fourth week after birth.
- Although many different types of psychiatric problems may be encountered in the postpartal period, depression is the most common. Episodes occur frequently in the week after childbirth and are typically transient.
- Telephone calls and home visits are effective measures for extending comprehensive care into the home setting of the postpartum family at risk.

REFERENCES

American Psychiatric Association: *Diagnostic and Statistical Manual of Mental Disorders: DSM-IV,* 4th ed. Washington DC: APA, 1994.

Andersen HF, Hopkins M: Postpartum hemorrhage. In: *Gynecology and Obstetrics, Vol 2.* Sciarra JJ (editor). Philadelphia: Harper & Row, 1996.

Barger MK (editor): *Protocols for Gynecologic and Obstetric Health Care.* Orlando, FL: Grune & Stratton, 1988.

Beck CT: Screening methods for postpartum depression. *JOGNN* 1995; 24(4):308.

Cosico JN et al: Indications, management and patient education for anticoagulation therapy during pregnancy. *MCN* 1993; 17(3):130.

Cunningham FG, MacDonald PC, Gant NF (editors): *Williams Obstetrics,* 20th ed. Stamford, CT: Appleton & Lange, 1997.

Donaldson NE: Effect of telephone postpartum follow-up: A clinical trial. *Diss Abstr Int* 49:2567B. University Microfilms International DA8809495, 1988.

Eftychiou V: Clinical diagnosis and management of the patient with deep venous thromboembolism and acute pulmonary embolism. *Nurs Pract* 1996; 21(3):50.

Eschenbach DA: Pelvic infections and sexually transmitted diseases. In: *Danforth's Obstetrics and Gynecology,* 7th ed. Scott JR et al (editors). Philadelphia: Lippincott, 1994.

Hamadeh G, Dedmon C, Mozley PD: Postpartum fever. *Am Fam Pract* 1995; 52(2):531.

Horowitz JA et al: Identification of symptoms of postpartum depression: Linking research to practice. *J Perinatol* 1996; 16(5):360.

Horowitz JA et al: Postpartum depression: Issues in clinical assessment. *J Perinatol* 1995; 15(4):268.

Kapernick PS: Postpartum hemorrhage and the abnormal puerperium. In: *Current Obstetric and Gynecologic Diagnosis and Treatment,* 8th ed. Pernoll ML (editor). Norwalk, CT: Appleton & Lange, 1994.

Karstrup S et al: Acute puerperal breast abscesses: US-guided drainage. *Radiology* 1993; 188(3):807.

Lawrence RA: *Breastfeeding: A Guide for the Medical Profession,* 4th ed. St Louis: Mosby, 1994.

Logsdon M, McBride A, Berkimer J: Social support and postpartum depression. *Res Nurs Health* 1994; 17:449.

Mowbray CT et al: Motherhood for women with serious mental illness: Pregnancy, childbirth, and the postpartum period. *Am J Orthopsychiat* 1995; 65(1):21.

Ruchala PL, Halstead L: The postpartum experience of low-risk women: A time of adjustment and change. *Matern Child Nurs J* 1994; 22(3):83.

Thomsen AC, Esperson T, Maigaard S: Course and treatment of milk stasis, noninfectious inflammation of the breast, and infectious mastitis in nursing women. *Am J Obstet Gynecol* 1984; 149(5):492.

Zlatnik FJ: The normal and abnormal peurperium. In: *Danforth's Obstetrics and Gynecology,* 7th ed. Scott JR et al (editors). Philadelphia: Lippincott, 1994.

APPENDICES

APPENDIX A COMMON ABBREVIATIONS IN MATERNAL-NEWBORN AND WOMEN'S HEALTH NURSING

accel	Acceleration of fetal heart rate
AC	Abdominal circumference
AFAFP	Amniotic fluid α-fetoprotein
AFP	α-fetoprotein
AFV	Amniotic fluid volume
AGA	Average for gestational age
AID or AIH	Artificial insemination donor (H designates mate is donor)
ARBOW	Artificial rupture of bag of waters
AROM	Artificial rupture of membranes
BAT	Brown adipose tissue (brown fat)
BBT	Basal body temperature
BL	Baseline (fetal heart rate baseline)
BOW	Bag of waters
BPD	Biparietal diameter *or* Bronchopulmonary dysplasia
BPP	Biophysical profile
BSE	Breast self-examination
BSST	Breast self-stimulation test
CC	Chest circumference *or* Cord compression
C–H	Crown-to-heel length
CID	Cytomegalic inclusion disease
CMV	Cytomegalovirus
CNM	Certified nurse-midwife
CNS	Clinical nurse specialist
CPAP	Continuous positive airway pressure
CPD	Cephalopelvic disproportion *or* Citrate-phosphate-dextrose
CRL	Crown-rump length
C/S	Cesarean section (or C-section)
CST	Contraction stress test
CVA	Costovertebral angle
CVS	Chorionic villus sampling
D&C	Dilatation and curettage
decels	Deceleration of fetal heart rate
DFMR	Daily fetal movement response
dil	Dilatation
DRG	Diagnostic related groups
DTR	Deep tendon reflexes
ECMO	Extracorporal membrane oxygenator
EDB	Estimated date of birth
EDC	Estimated date of confinement
EDD	Estimated date of delivery
EFM	Electronic fetal monitoring
EFW	Estimated fetal weight
EIA	Enzyme immunoassay
ELF	Elective low forceps
ELISA	Enzyme-linked immunosorbent assay
epis	Episiotomy
ERT	Estrogen replacement therapy
FAD	Fetal activity diary
FAE	Fetal alcohol effects
FAS	Fetal alcohol syndrome
FBD	Fibrocystic breast disease
FBM	Fetal breathing movements
FBS	Fetal blood sample *or* Fasting blood sugar test
FECG	Fetal electrocardiogram
FHR	Fetal heart rate
FHT	Fetal heart tones
FL	Femur length
FM	Fetal movement
FPG	Fasting plasma glucose test
FSH	Follicle-stimulating hormone
FSHRH	Follicle-stimulating hormone–releasing hormone
G or grav	Gravida
GDM	Gestational diabetes mellitus
GIFT	Gamete intrafallopian transfer
GnRF	Gonadotropin-releasing factor
GnRH	Gonadotropin-releasing hormone
GTD	Gestational trophoblastic disease
GTPAL	Gravida, term, preterm, abortion, living children; a system of recording maternity history
HA	Head-abdominal ratio
HAI	Hemagglutination-inhibition test
HC	Head compression
hCG	Human chorionic gonadotropin
hCS	Human chorionic somatomammotropin (same as hPL)
HMD	Hyaline membrane disease
hMG	Human menopausal gonadotropin
hPL	Human placental lactogen
HPV	Human papilloma virus
HVH	Herpesvirus hominis
IDM	Infant of a diabetic mother
IPG	Impedance phlebography
IU	International units
IUD	Intrauterine device
IUFD	Intrauterine fetal death
IUGR	Intrauterine growth restriction
IVF	In vitro fertilization
LADA	Left-acromion-dorsal-anterior
LADP	Left-acromion-dorsal-posterior
LBW	Low birth weight
LDR	Labor, delivery, and recovery room
LGA	Large for gestational age
LH	Luteinizing hormone
LHRH	Luteinizing hormone–releasing hormone
LMA	Left-mentum-anterior
LML	Left mediolateral (episiotomy)
LMP	Last menstrual period *or* Left-mentum-posterior
LMT	Left-mentum-transverse
LOA	Left-occiput-anterior
LOF	Low outlet forceps
LOP	Left-occiput-posterior
LOT	Left-occiput-transverse
L/S	Lecithin/sphingomyelin ratio
LSA	Left-sacrum-anterior
LSP	Left-sacrum-posterior
LST	Left-sacrum-transverse

MAS	Meconium aspiration syndrome
mec	Meconium
mec st	Meconium stain
ML	Midline (episiotomy)
MSAFP	Maternal serum α-fetoprotein
MUGB	4-methylumbelliferyl quanidinobenzoate
multip	Multipara
NEC	Necrotizing enterocolitis
NGU	Nongonococcal urethritis
NP	Nurse practitioner
NSCST	Nipple stimulation contraction stress test
NST	Nonstress test *or* Nonshivering thermogenesis
NSVD	Normal sterile vaginal delivery
NTD	Neural tube defects
OA	Occiput anterior
OC	Oral contraceptives
OCT	Oxytocin challenge test
OF	Occipito-frontal diameter of fetal head
OFC	Occipito-frontal circumference
OGTT	Oral glucose tolerance test
OM	Occipitomental (diameter)
OP	Occiput posterior
p	Para
Pap smear	Papanicolaou smear
PDA	Patent ductus arteriosus
PEEP	Positive end-expiratory pressure
PG	Phosphatidylglycerol *or* Prostaglandin
PI	Phosphatidylinositol
PID	Pelvic inflammatory disease
PIH	Pregnancy-induced hypertension
Pit	Pitocin
PKU	Phenylketonuria
PMS	Premenstrual syndrome
PPHN	Persistent pulmonary hypertension
Preemie	Premature infant
primip	Primipara
PROM	Premature rupture of membranes
PSI	Prostaglandin synthesis inhibitor
PUBS	Percutaneous umbilical blood sampling
RADA	Right-acromion-dorsal-anterior
RADP	Right-acromion-dorsal-posterior
RDS	Respiratory distress syndrome
REM	Rapid eye movements
RIA	Radioimmunoassay
RLF	Retrolental fibroplasia
RMA	Right-mentum-anterior
RMP	Right-mentum-posterior
RMT	Right-mentum-transverse
ROA	Right-occiput-anterior
ROM	Rupture of membranes
ROP	Right-occiput-posterior *or* Retinopathy of prematurity
ROT	Right-occiput-transverse
RRA	Radioreceptor assay
RSA	Right-sacrum-anterior
RSP	Right-sacrum-posterior
RST	Right-sacrum-transverse
SET	Surrogate embryo transfer
SFD	Small for dates
SGA	Small for gestational age
SIDS	Sudden infant death syndrome
SMB	Submentobregmatic diameter
SOB	Suboccipitobregmatic diameter
SPA	Sperm penetration assay
SRBOW	Spontaneous rupture of the bag of waters
SROM	Spontaneous rupture of membranes
STI	Sexually transmitted infection
STH	Somatotropic hormone
STS	Serologic test for syphilis
SVE	Sterile vaginal exam
TC	Thoracic circumference
TCM	Transcutaneous monitoring
TDI	Therapeutic Donor Insemination
TNZ	Thermal neutral zone
TOL	Trail of labor
TORCH	Toxoplasmosis, rubella, cytomegalovirus, herpesvirus hominis type 2
TSS	Toxic shock syndrome
ū	Umbilicus
UA	Uterine activity
UAC	Umbilical artery catheter
UAU	Uterine activity units
UC	Uterine contraction
UPI	Uteroplacental insufficiency
US	Ultrasound
VBAC	Vaginal birth after cesarean
VDRL	Venereal Disease Research Laboratories
VLBW	Very low birth weight
WIC	Supplemental food program for Women, Infants, and Children
ZIFT	Zygote intrafallopian transfer

APPENDIX B CONVERSIONS AND EQUIVALENTS

TEMPERATURE CONVERSION

(Fahrenheit temperature − 32) × 5/9 = Celsius temperature

(Celsius temperature × 9/5) + 32 = Fahrenheit temperature

SELECTED CONVERSIONS TO METRIC MEASURES

Known value	Multiply by	To find
inches	2.54	centimeters
ounces	28	grams
pounds	454	grams
pounds	0.45	kilogram

SELECTED CONVERSIONS FROM METRIC MEASURES

Known value	Multiply by	To find
centimeters	0.4	inches
grams	0.035	ounces
grams	0.0022	pounds
kilograms	2.2	pounds

CONVERSION OF POUNDS AND OUNCES TO GRAMS

	Ounces															
S (Pounds)	0	1	2	3	4	5	6	7	8	9	10	11	12	13	14	15
0	—	28	57	85	113	142	170	198	227	255	283	312	340	369	397	425
1	454	482	510	539	567	595	624	652	680	709	737	765	794	822	850	879
2	907	936	964	992	1021	1049	1077	1106	1134	1162	1191	1219	1247	1276	1304	1332
3	1361	1389	1417	1446	1474	1503	1531	1559	1588	1616	1644	1673	1701	1729	1758	1786
4	1814	1843	1871	1899	1928	1956	1984	2013	2041	2070	2098	2126	2155	2183	2211	2240
5	2268	2296	2325	2353	2381	2410	2438	2466	2495	2523	2551	2580	2608	2637	2665	2693
6	2722	2750	2778	2807	2835	2863	2892	2920	2948	2977	3005	3033	3062	3090	3118	3147
7	3175	3203	3232	3260	3289	3317	3345	3374	3402	3430	3459	3487	3515	3544	3572	3600
8	3629	3657	3685	3714	3742	3770	3799	3827	3856	3884	3912	3941	3969	3997	4026	4054
9	4082	4111	4139	4167	4196	4224	4252	4281	4309	4337	4366	4394	4423	4451	4479	4508
10	4536	4564	4593	4621	4649	4678	4706	4734	4763	4791	4819	4848	4876	4904	4933	4961
11	4990	5018	5046	5075	5103	5131	5160	5188	5216	5245	5273	5301	5330	5358	5386	5415
12	5443	5471	5500	5528	5557	5585	5613	5642	5670	5698	5727	5755	5783	5812	5840	5868
13	5897	5925	5953	5982	6010	6038	6067	6095	6123	6152	6180	6209	6237	6265	6294	6322
14	6350	6379	6407	6435	6464	6492	6520	6549	6577	6605	6634	6662	6690	6719	6747	6776
15	6804	6832	6860	6889	6917	6945	6973	7002	7030	7059	7087	7115	7144	7172	7201	7228
16	7257	7286	7313	7342	7371	7399	7427	7456	7484	7512	7541	7569	7597	7626	7654	7682
17	7711	7739	7768	7796	7824	7853	7881	7909	7938	7966	7994	8023	8051	8079	8108	8136
18	8165	8192	8221	8249	8278	8306	8335	8363	8391	8420	8448	8476	8504	8533	8561	8590
19	8618	8646	8675	8703	8731	8760	8788	8816	8845	8873	8902	8930	8958	8987	9015	9043
20	9072	9100	9128	9157	9185	9213	9242	9270	9298	9327	9355	9383	9412	9440	9469	9497
21	9525	9554	9582	9610	9639	9667	9695	9724	9752	9780	9809	9837	9865	9894	9922	9950
22	9979	10007	10036	10064	10092	10120	10149	10177	10206	10234	10262	10291	10319	10347	10376	10404

APPENDIX C THE PREGNANT PATIENT'S BILL OF RIGHTS*

The Pregnant Patient has the right to participate in decisions involving her well-being and that of her unborn child, unless there is a clearcut medical emergency that prevents her participation. In addition to the rights set forth in the American Hospital Association's "Patient's Bill of Rights," the Pregnant Patient, because she represents two patients rather than one, should be recognized as having the additional rights listed below.

1. *The Pregnant Patient has the right,* prior to the administration of any drug or procedure, to be informed by the health professional caring for her of any potential direct or indirect effects, risks or hazards to herself or her unborn or newborn infant which may result from the use of a drug or procedure prescribed for or administered to her during pregnancy, labor, birth or lactation.
2. *The Pregnant Patient has the right,* prior to the proposed therapy, to be informed, not only of the benefits, risks and hazards of the proposed therapy but also of known alternative therapy, such as available childbirth education classes which could help to prepare the Pregnant Patient physically and mentally to cope with the discomfort or stress of pregnancy and the experience of childbirth, thereby reducing or eliminating her need for drugs and obstetric intervention. She should be offered such information early in her pregnancy in order that she may make a reasoned decision.
3. *The Pregnant Patient has the right,* prior to the administration of any drug, to be informed by the health professional who is prescribing or administering the drug to her that any drug which she receives during pregnancy, labor and birth, no matter how or when the drug is taken or administered, may adversely affect her unborn baby, directly or indirectly, and that there is no drug or chemical which has been proven safe for the unborn child.
4. *The Pregnant Patient has the right,* if cesarean birth is anticipated, to be informed prior to the administration of any drug, and preferably prior to her hospitalization, that minimizing her and, in turn, her baby's intake of nonessential preoperative medicine will benefit her baby.
5. *The Pregnant Patient has the right,* prior to the administration of a drug or procedure, to be informed of the areas of uncertainty if there is NO properly controlled follow-up research which has established the safety of the drug or procedure with regard to its direct and/or indirect effects on the physiological, mental and neurological development of the child exposed, via the mother, to the drug or procedure during pregnancy, labor, birth or lactation—(this would apply to virtually all drugs and the vast majority of obstetric procedures).
6. *The Pregnant Patient has the right,* prior to the administration of any drug, to be informed of the brand name and generic name of the drug in order that she may advise the health professional of any past adverse reaction to the drug.
7. *The Pregnant Patient has the right* to determine for herself, without pressure from her attendant, whether she will accept the risks inherent in the proposed therapy or refuse a drug or procedure.
8. *The Pregnant Patient has the right* to know the name and qualifications of the individual administering a medication or procedure to her during labor or birth.
9. *The Pregnant Patient has the right* to be informed, prior to the administration of any procedure, whether that procedure is being administered to her for her or her baby's benefit (medically indicated) or as an elective procedure (for convenience, teaching purposes or research).
10. *The Pregnant Patient has the right* to be accompanied during the stress of labor and birth by someone she cares for, and to whom she looks for emotional comfort and encouragement.
11. *The Pregnant Patient has the right,* after appropriate medical consultation, to choose a position for labor and for birth which is least stressful to her baby and to herself.
12. *The Obstetric Patient has the right* to have her baby cared for at her bedside if her baby is normal, and to feed her baby according to her baby's needs rather than according to the hospital regimen.

*Prepared by Doris Haire, Chair, Committee on Health Law and Regulation, International Childbirth Education Association, Inc, Rochester, NY.

13. *The Obstetric Patient has the right* to be informed in writing of the name of the person who actually delivered her baby and the professional qualifications of that person. This information should also be on the birth certificate.

14. *The Obstetric Patient has the right* to be informed if there is any known or indicated aspect of her or her baby's care or condition which may cause her or her baby later difficulty or problems.

15. *The Obstetric Patient has the right* to have her and her baby's hospital medical records complete, accurate and legible and have their records, including Nurses' Notes, retained by the hospital until the child reaches at least the age of majority, or to have the records offered to her before they are destroyed.

16. *The Obstetric Patient, both during and after her hospital stay, has the right* to have access to her complete hospital medical records, including Nurses' Notes, and to receive a copy upon payment of a reasonable fee and without incurring the expense of retaining an attorney.

It is the Obstetric Patient and her baby, not the health professional, who must sustain any trauma or injury resulting from the use of a drug or obstetric procedure. The observation of the rights listed above will not only permit the Obstetric Patient to participate in the decisions involving her and her baby's health care, but will help to protect the health professional and the hospital against litigation arising from resentment or misunderstanding on the part of the mother.

APPENDIX D AWHONN'S (NAACOG'S) STANDARDS FOR THE NURSING CARE OF WOMEN AND NEWBORNS*

Standard I: Nursing Practice

Comprehensive nursing care for women and newborns focuses on helping individuals, families, and communities achieve their optimum health potential. This is best achieved within the framework of the nursing process.

The nurse is responsible for decisions and actions within the domain of nursing practice, which may include

- integration of the nursing process components of assessment, planning, implementation, and evaluation in all areas of nursing practice;
- individualization and prioritization of nursing care to meet the physical, psychological, spiritual, and social needs of patients;
- collaboration with the individual, family, and other members of the health-care team;
- promotion of a safe and therapeutic environment for both the recipients and providers of nursing care;
- demonstration and validation of competence in nursing practice;
- acquisition of specialized knowledge and skills and additional formal education to provide specialized care; and
- provision for complete and accurate documentation of care.

The written or computerized patient record is the documented means of communication among all members of the health-care team. It also promotes continuity of care and provides a mechanism for evaluating care. The record should contain accurate and complete recordings of the patient's history and physical examination as well as the nursing plan of care, including goals, interventions, health education, and evaluation of patient and family responses. Additional documentation may include planned follow-up and appropriate referrals. All information contained in the patient record and related to the care of the patient and family is confidential and should be released only according to institutional policy.

Note: To apply this universal standard to a specific area of gynecologic, obstetric, or neonatal nursing practice, refer directly to the specialty-specific nursing practice standards section.

*From *NAACOG Standards for the Nursing Care of Women and Newborns,* 4th ed, Washington, DC: NAACOG, 1991. NAACOG is now known as AWHONN (Association of Women's Health, Obstetric, and Neonatal Nurses).

Standard II: Health Education and Counseling

Health education for the individual, family, and community is an integral part of comprehensive nursing care. Such education encourages participation in, and shared responsibility for, health promotion, maintenance, and restoration.

Comprehensive health education includes

- identification of the needs and abilities of the learner;
- collaboration with the patient and other health-care providers in design, content, and follow-up of the educational plan;
- provision of accurate and current information;
- provision of information based on educationally sound principles of teaching and learning;
- recognition of patient rights, responsibilities, and alternative choices;
- utilization of available educational resources to provide health education information to individuals/ families in the community; and
- documentation and evaluation of health education including patient response.

The nurse participates in and/or coordinates the health education and counseling process. It begins with the initial patient contact or admission to the unit or service and is an ongoing, continuous process.

Note: To apply this universal standard to a specific area of gynecologic, obstetric, or neonatal nursing practice, refer directly to the specialty-specific nursing practice standards section.

Standard III: Policies, Procedures, and Protocols

Written policies, procedures, and protocols clarify the scope of nursing practice and delineate the qualifications of personnel authorized to provide care to women and newborns within the health-care setting.

The components of policies, procedures, and protocols are based on

- recognition of the organization's philosophy;
- recognition of the unit's philosophy;
- coordination with the overall mission of the organization;

- assessment of the practice setting and determination of types of services to be provided;
- incorporation of a multidisciplinary approach in their development;
- identification of specific areas of practice to be addressed;
- reflection of current practice, standards, and local regulations; and
- anticipated use as references for health-care providers, orientation of new personnel and students, quality assurance activities, and/or guiding nursing actions in emergency situations.

The development of policies, procedures, and protocols should include consideration of staff availability, skill, and licensure; the physical plant and equipment; effects on other departments; and fiscal impact. Policies, procedures, and protocols should be reviewed and revised at least on an annual basis or more frequently as science/technology changes.

Note: To apply this universal standard to a specific area of gynecologic, obstetric, or neonatal nursing practice, refer directly to the specialty-specific nursing practice standards section.

Standard IV: Professional Responsibility and Accountability

Comprehensive nursing care for women and newborns is provided by nurses who are clinically competent and accountable for professional actions and legal responsibilities inherent in the nursing role.

Responsibility and accountability for knowledge and competence in nursing practice for women and newborns include

- awareness of changing practices and professional and ethical issues;
- knowledge and clinical skills gained through in-service education, professional continuing education, research data, and professional literature;
- implementation of newly acquired knowledge and skills;
- collaboration through networking and sharing with other professionals;
- participation in the development of standards and policies, procedures, and protocols;
- participation with professional committees within the institution;
- participation in periodic peer- and self-evaluations; and
- recognition of certification as one mechanism for the demonstration of special knowledge within a specialty area of practice.

Legal accountability extends to the

- nurse practice acts;
- parameters of professional practice established by professional organizations;
- institutional standards;
- legislative changes that affect practice; and
- policies, procedures, and protocols within the practice environment.

Standard V: Utilization of Nursing Personnel

Nursing care for women and newborns is conducted in practice settings that have qualified nursing staff in sufficient numbers to meet patient-care needs.

Each practice setting should have sufficient nursing personnel to meet patient-care requirements. Nursing staff who provide direct care to women and newborns should be supervised by registered nurses who are clinically proficient in the specialty area of practice. The patient-care unit or service is managed by a professional nurse who is prepared educationally and clinically to assume a leadership position. In all practice settings, the nurse may practice independently or collaboratively with other health-care team members. It is essential that nurses know both the responsibilities and the limitations of professional nursing practice specific to the practice setting.

Many variables are considered in determining both the number and type of nursing staff needed for a practice setting. Among these variables are those related to the patient, practice, organization, and personnel. Patient-related variables may include

- patient demographics and acuity of patients served;
- length of stay;
- educational needs;
- cultural factors and level of comprehension;
- communication barriers; and
- discharge or home-care needs.

Practice-related variables may include

- difference in educational and experiential level of nursing staff;
- nursing philosophy;
- type of nursing-care delivery system;
- use of assistive personnel;
- use of nurses in expanded roles; and
- participation in teaching programs.

Organizational variables may include

- scope of services provided;
- availability of support services;

- patient volume;
- mission or philosophy of the organization;
- risk-management concerns;
- quality assurance programs;
- policies, procedures, and protocols;
- physical plant;
- marketing strategies; and
- fiscal considerations.

Personnel variables relate to the type and number of professional and nonprofessional staff and may include

- education, skill, and experience of the nursing leadership;
- educational preparation, skill, and experience of staff;
- types and mix of nursing staff;
- availability of qualified alternative staff to deal with emergencies or unanticipated volumes;
- distribution of staff, eg, temporary reassignment, floating, on-call, cross-training, and supplemental staffing;
- responsibilities for orientation, precepting, or students;
- turnover rates; and
- clerical and technical support.

Competency-based job descriptions should be available for each level of nursing staff. Orientation for all personnel should include a general overview of the organization and specific information about the individual practice setting. Performance evaluations for all personnel should be conducted, documented, and discussed on a regular basis with input from the individual, colleagues, and supervisory staff.

Standard VI: Ethics

Ethical principles guide the process of decision making for nurses caring for women and newborns at all times and especially when personal or professional values conflict with those of the patient, family, colleagues, or practice setting.

The nurse should have the opportunity to participate in the ethical decision-making process. To participate actively, nurses should

- clarify their own personal and professional values;
- recognize the difficulty in selecting a course of action that is morally and ethically acceptable to all parties;
- communicate openly and assertively;
- identify options; and
- seek consultations.

Nurses must carefully examine their own value systems since values influence the decision-making process. Opportunities should be provided in the practice setting for discussion of potential ethical issues. Each practice setting should have a framework for decision making regarding bioethical dilemmas. Ethical dilemmas generally arise when there is a conflict between loyalties, rights, duties, or values.

For nurses, most ethical dilemmas occur when there is a real or perceived requirement to act in a manner contrary to personal values or when care ordered or provided does not seem compatible with the best interest of the patient. Common areas of concern may include

- nursing autonomy and decision making;
- maternal interests versus fetal interests;
- issues of duty, obligation, and loyalty (for example, employer to employee, professional to public, professional to professional);
- patients' rights to resources, privacy, confidentiality, information, participation in decision making, and refusal of therapy;
- the right to live or die;
- life cycle concerns, including contraception, sterilization, pregnancy termination, genetic manipulation, infanticide, sexuality and choices of life style, and euthanasia;
- fetal or neonatal conditions incompatible with life;
- fetal tissue use; and
- biomedical intervention.

The bioethics literature can provide nurses with strategies to cope with or resolve decisions in situations when conflicts of values occur. For ethical decision-making frameworks to be applied to practice situations, working relationships must be established in which individuals may express their own points of view. All persons potentially affected by an ethical decision have the right to participate in the decision-making process.

Standard VII: Research

Nurses caring for women and newborns utilize research findings, conduct nursing research, and evaluate nursing practice to improve the outcomes of care.

Knowledge of the research process and participation in scientific inquiry are necessary to

- conduct or participate in the conduct of research according to ethical guidelines;
- use research findings to provide appropriate and safe nursing care;
- use research findings as a basis for validating standards of nursing care;

- evaluate the relevance and application of research findings from nursing and related disciplines; and
- validate the effect of nursing practice on patient outcomes.

Standard VIII: Quality Assurance

Quality and appropriateness of patient care are evaluated through a planned assessment program using specific, identified clinical indicators.

Each unit or service should have a written quality assurance plan that reflects a philosophy that is coordinated with the organization's mission and overall quality assurance program. Objectives of the unit-based or service-based quality assurance plan should include

- assurance of consistent quality patient outcomes;
- identification and correction of potential nursing practice deficiencies;
- promotion of professional nursing practice based on appropriate nursing standards; and
- education and participation of staff in quality assurance activities.

The unit nurse manager is responsible for developing and implementing the unit-based quality assurance plan. The plan should include

- responsibilities of all personnel in the quality assurance process;
- the scope of service provided;
- important aspects of care or service involving high-risk, high-volume, and problem-prone patients or activities;
- clinical indicators or measurable standards that affect the aspects of care and service that have been identified as important;
- specific criteria and thresholds for use in monitoring clinical indicators;
- methods for the collection and analysis of data, including reference to collection tools, sample size, time frame, and staff responsibility;
- determination of appropriate corrective action, when indicated, that will fall into one of three categories: educational, organizational, or behavioral change;
- follow-up assessment of identified problems;
- documentation of all aspects of the quality assurance program, including results; and
- a process for communication related to quality assurance activities within the total organization.

CLINICAL ESTIMATION OF GESTATIONAL AGE

An Approximation Based on Published Data*

Examination First Hours

Physical findings		Weeks gestation	Finding
Vernix		20–24	Appears
		24–38	Covers body, thick layer
		38–40	On back, scalp, in creases
		40–42	Scant, in creases
		42–48	No vernix
Breast tissue and areola		20–34	Areola & nipple barely visible; no palpable breast tissue
		34–36	Areola raised
		36–38	1-2 mm nodule
		38–39	3-5 mm
		39–40	5-6 mm
		40–44	7-10 mm
		44–48	?12 mm
Ear	Form	20–34	Flat, shapeless
		34–36	Beginning incurving superior
		36–39	Incurving upper 2/3 pinnae
		39–48	Well-defined incurving to lobe
	Cartilage	20–32	Pinna soft, stays folded
		32–36	Cartilage scant, returns slowly from folding
		36–40	Thin cartilage, springs back from folding
		40–48	Pinna firm, remains erect from head
Sole creases		20–32	Smooth soles ∓ creases
		32–35	1-2 anterior creases
		35–36	2-3 anterior creases
		36–38	Creases anterior 2/3 sole
		38–42	Creases involving heel
		42–48	Deeper creases over entire sole
Skin	Thickness & appearance	20–32	Thin, translucent skin, plethoric, venules over abdomen, edema
		32–36	Smooth, thicker, no edema
		36–40	Pink, few vessels
		40–42	Some desquamation, pale pink
		42–48	Thick, pale, desquamation over entire body
	Nail plates	20–21	Appear
		21–42	Nails to finger tips
		42–48	Nails extend well beyond finger tips
Hair		20–23	Appears on head
		23–28	Eye brows & lashes
		28–37	Fine, woolly, bunches out from head
		37–42	Silky, single strands, lays flat
		42–48	?Receding hairline or loss of baby hair, short, fine underneath
Lanugo		20–21	Appears
		21–33	Covers entire body
		33–38	Vanishes from face
		38–42	Present on shoulders
		42–48	No lanugo
Genitalia	Testes	28–36	Testes palpable in inguinal canal
		36–42	In upper scrotum
		42–48	In lower scrotum
	Scrotum	28–36	Few rugae
		36–40	Rugae, anterior portion
		40–42	Rugae cover
		42–48	Pendulous
	Labia & clitoris	30–36	Prominent clitoris, labia majora small, widely separated
		36–40	Labia majora larger, nearly covered clitoris
		40–48	Labia minora & clitoris covered
Skull firmness		20–28	Bones are soft
		28–35	Soft to 1" from anterior fontanelle
		35–38	Spongy at edges of fontanelle, center firm
		38–42	Bones hard, sutures easily displaced
		42–48	Bones hard, cannot be displaced
Posture	Resting	20–26	Hypotonic, lateral decubitus
		26–29	Hypotonic
		29–32	Beginning flexion thigh
		32–34	Stronger hip flexion
		34–36	Frog-like
		36–38	Flexion all limbs
		38–42	Hypertonic
		42–48	Very hypertonic
	Recoil - leg	20–32	No recoil
		32–38	Partial recoil
		38–48	Prompt recoil
	Arm	20–34	No recoil
		34–36	Begin flexion, no recoil
		36–40	Prompt recoil, may be inhibited
		40–48	Prompt recoil after 30" inhibition

*Brazie JV and Lubchenco LO. The estimation of gestational age chart. In Kempe, Silver and O'Brien, *Current Pediatric Diagnosis and Treatment,* ed 3. Los Altos, Calif. Lange Medical Publications, 1974, ch 4.
Form courtesy of Mead Johnson Laboratories, Evansville, IN.

APPENDIX F ACTIONS AND EFFECTS OF SELECTED DRUGS DURING BREASTFEEDING*

Anticholinergics
Atropine: May cause hyperthermia in the newborn; may decrease maternal milk supply

Anticoagulants
Coumarin derivatives (Warfarin, Dicumarol): Only small amount in breast milk; check PTT
Heparin: Relatively safe to use; check PTT
Phenindione (Hedulin): Not used in USA; passes easily into breast milk; neonate may have increased prothrombin time and PTT

Anticonvulsants
Phenytoin (Dilantin), phenobarbital: Generally considered safe; if high doses of phenobarbital are ingested, may cause drowsiness; short-acting phenobarbiturates (secobarbital) preferred, as they appear in lower concentration in milk

Antihistamines
Diphenhydramine (Benadryl), pheniramine (Dimetane), Coricidin, Drixoral: May cause decreased milk supply; infant may become drowsy, irritable, or have tachycardia

Antimetabolites Unknown, probably long-term anti-DNA effect on the infant; potentially very toxic

Antimicrobials
Aminoglycosides: May cause ototoxicity or nephrotoxicity if given for more than 2 weeks
Ampicillin: Skin rash, candidiasis; diarrhea
Chloramphenicol: Possible bone marrow suppression; too low a dose for Gray syndrome; refusal of breast
Methacycline: Possible inhibition of bone growth; may cause discoloration of the teeth; use should be avoided
Metronidazole (Flagyl): Possible neurologic disorders or blood dyscrasias; delay breastfeeding for 12 hours after dose
Penicillin: Possible allergic response; candidiasis
Quinolones (synthetic antibiotics): Can cause arthropathies
Sulfonamides: May cause hyperbilirubinemia; use contraindicated until infant over 1 week old
Tetracycline: Long-term use and large doses should be avoided; may cause tooth staining or inhibition of bone growth

Antithyroids
Thiouracil: Contraindicated during lactation; may cause goiter or agranulocytosis
Propylthiouracil: Safe; monitor infant thyroid function

Barbiturates
Phenothiazines: May produce sedation

Bronchodilators
Aminophylline: May cause insomnia or irritability in the infant
Ephedrine, cromolyn (Intal): Relatively safe

Caffeine Excessive consumption may cause jitteriness or wakefulness

Cardiovascular
Methyldopa: Increase in milk volume
Propranolol (Inderal): May cause hypoglycemia; possibility of other blocking effects, especially if infant has renal or liver dysfunction
Quinidine: May cause arrhythmias in infant
Reserpine (Serpasil): Nasal stuffiness, lethargy, or diarrhea in infant

Corticosteroids Adrenal suppression may occur with long-term administration of doses greater than 10 mg/day

Diuretics
Furosemide (Lasix): Not excreted in breast milk
Thiazide diuretics (Esidrix, Hydrodiuril, Oretic): Safe but can cause dehydration, reduce milk production

Heavy metals
Gold: Potentially toxic; gold salts—compatible with nursing
Mercury: Excreted in the milk and hazardous to infant

Hormones
Androgens: Suppress lactation
Thyroid hormones: May mask hypothyroidism

Laxatives
Cascara: May cause diarrhea in infant
Milk of magnesia: Relatively safe

Narcotic analgesics
Codeine: Accumulation may lead to neonatal depression
Meperidine: May lead to neonatal depression
Morphine: Long-term use may cause newborn addiction

Nonnarcotic analgesics, NSAIDs
Acetaminophen (Tylenol): Relatively safe for short-term analgesia
Ibuprofen (Motrin): Safe
Propoxyphene (Darvon): May cause sleepiness and poor nursing in infant
Salicylates (aspirin): Safe after first week of life; monitor protime

Oral contraceptives
Combined estrogen/progestin pills: Significantly decrease milk supply; may alter milk composition; may cause gynecomastia in male infants

*Based on data from Kacew S: Adverse effects of drugs and chemicals in breast milk on the nursing infant. *J Clin Pharmacol* 1993; 33:213–221; Riordan J, Auerbach KG: *Breastfeeding and Human Lactation.* Boston: Jones and Bartlett, 1993, pp 135–166. Fanaroff AA, Martin RJ: *Neonatal-Perinatal Medicine: Diseases of the Fetus and Infant.* 6th ed. Vol 1, 1997 p 148–152. St Louis: Mosby. Briggs GG, Freeman RK, Yaffe SJ: *Drugs in Pregnancy and Lactation* 4th ed. 1994, Baltimore: Williams & Wilkins Committee on Drugs, American Academy of Pediatrics. The transfer of drugs and other chemicals into human milk. *Pediatrics* 1994; 93:137–50.

Progestin only: Safe if started after lactation is established

Radioactive materials for testing

Gallium citrate (^{67}G): Insignificant amount excreted in breast milk; no nursing for 2 weeks

Iodine: Contraindicated; may affect infant's thyroid gland

^{125}I: Discontinue nursing for 48 hours

^{131}I: Nursing should be discontinued until excretion is no longer significant; nursing may be resumed after 10 days

Technetium-99m: Discontinue nursing for 3 days (half-life = 6 hours)

Sedatives/Tranquilizers

Diazepam (Valium): May accumulate to high levels; may increase neonatal jaundice; may cause lethargy and weight loss

Lithium carbonate: Contraindicated; may cause neonatal flaccidity and hypotonia

Substance Abuse

Alcohol: Potential motor developmental delay; mild sedative effect

Amphetamines: Controversial; may cause irritability, poor sleeping

Cocaine, crack: Extreme irritability, tachycardia, vomiting, apnea

Marijuana: Drowsiness

APPENDIX G PROJECTED RECOMMENDATIONS FOR ISOLATION PRECAUTIONS (CDC 1995)

The guidelines established by the Centers for Disease Control and Prevention (CDC) in 1995 have two levels of prevention—standard precautions, designed to be used with all clients, and transmission-based precautions, designed to be used with clients with suspected or confirmed infections with epidemiologically important organisms transmitted by airborne or droplet route or by direct contact with contaminated surfaces or dry skin. Section A of this Appendix describes the projected 1995 CDC guidelines, and section B summarizes the 1991 OSHA Bloodborne Pathogen Standard, which is an integral part of the Standard Precautions (CDC 1995).

Section A Projected Recommendations for Isolation Precautions (CDC 1995)

Type of Precaution	Handwashing	Gloves	Gown	Mask, Eye Protection, Face Shield	Room Assignment of Client
Standard precautions *To be used with all clients	Between all client contacts; immediately after removing gloves; after any contact with bodily fluids or secretions; or after any contact with contaminated items.	Nonsterile gloves worn when coming in contact with any bodily substances (saliva, urine, feces, blood, etc), mucous membranes, or nonintact skin.	Nonsterile, clean gown used during procedures in which splashing of bodily fluids is anticipated. Gown is discarded after tasks are finished.	Mask and eye protection or face shield worn whenever splashing or spraying of bodily fluids is probable.	Private room preferred if client is unable to maintain own hygiene or environmental control of room; otherwise room with multiple clients is acceptable.
Transmission-based precautions:					
Droplet *To be used for clients with known or suspected infections with microorganisms > 5 microns known to be transmitted by droplets from sneezing, talking, coughing, etc.	Same as above.	Same as above.	Same as above.	A mask is worn when working within three feet of the client.	Private room preferred if possible; if not possible a spatial separation of at least three feet must be maintained between client and other individuals such as other clients, visitors, etc.
Airborne *To be used for clients with known or suspected infection with microorganisms (≤ 5 microns) that can remain in the air or be dispersed widely by air currents.	Same as above.	Same as above.	Same as above.	A special mask (particulate respirator) is recommended for entering the rooms of clients with tuberculosis. Individuals who have never had varicella or rubeola should not enter the rooms of clients diagnosed with or suspected of having these infections.	Client room should have the following: • monitored negative air pressure • at least 6 air exchanges per hour • appropriate discharge of air from room. In addition, the door to room should be kept closed at all times. Client may be in a semi-private room with another client who has the same diagnosis.

Contact *To be used for clients with known or suspected infection with epidemiologically important microorganisms that can be transmitted by direct contact with the client or by indirect contact (for example, by touching objects or equipment in the client's room).	Same as above.	Use nonsterile, clean gloves in providing direct client care or during contact with potentially contaminated items.	Clean, nonsterile gown is recommended if contact with bodily substances, equipment, or surfaces is anticipated.	Same as for standard precautions.	Private room if possible.

Note: CDC Guidelines are extrapolated from: Draft guideline for isolation precautions in hospitals: notice of comment period. *Federal Register* 59(214):55552-55570. November 7, 1994. The final version of the guidelines may differ. Reviewed by Marguerite McMillan Jackson RN, Doctoral Candidate, CIC, FAAN. Administrative Director Medical Center Epidemiology Unit, University of California San Diego.

Section B Occupational Safety and Health Administration (OSHA) Bloodborne Pathogens Standard (1991)

The Bloodborne Pathogens Standard (1991) will be an integral part of the Standard Precautions (CDC 1995). This standard is to be used to prevent contact with blood or other materials that are potentially infectious. If the circumstance arises that body fluids are difficult to differentiate, all body fluids are considered potentially infectious. The essential elements of the Bloodborne Pathogens Standard are as follows:

- Handwashing guidelines should include:
  - Washing hands with soap and water prior to and immediately after contact with all clients and/or any contaminated items.
  - Hands are to be washed immediately after removing gloves.
  - Handwashing materials are to be made readily available in each work setting.
- Nonsterile, disposable gloves are to be worn whenever contact with blood or other potentially infectious body fluids may be anticipated. Gloves should be replaced if they are punctured or torn. Disposable gloves are to be used only once.
- Masks, eye protection, and face shields are to be worn whenever potentially contaminated material may be splashed, sprayed or spattered on the face, eyes, nose or mouth.
- Special care is to be taken when using or discarding sharp instruments (needles, scalpels or other sharp devices).
  - Needles are never to be recapped using two hands.
  - If the needle needs to be recapped, a one-handed 'scoop' technique may be used, or a special device for recapping may be used.
  - Used needles should not be removed from the syringe by hand.
  - Needles should not be manipulated, twisted or broken by hand.
  - All sharps (needles, scalpels, and sharp disposable instruments) should be placed in an appropriate puncture-resistant container. The container should be clearly marked and/or color-coded, be leakproof on the sides and bottom, be located as close to the client as possible, be maintained in an upright position, and have a lid so spillage is not possible.
- During resuscitation, special disposable devices should be used as an alternative to the direct mouth-to-mouth method.

From: Department of Labor, Occupational Safety and Health Administration: *Federal Register* 56:64003-64182, Dec 6, 1991. Reviewed by Marguerite McMillan Jackson RN, Doctoral Candidate, CIC, FAAN. Administrative Director Medical Center, University of California San Diego.

APPENDIX H SUGGESTED ANSWERS TO CRITICAL THINKING IN ACTION QUESTIONS

Chapter 8

Elena's height and prepregnancy weight are normal. Her weight gain during pregnancy as been appropriate but not excessive. Research indicates that assessment of fundal height is more accurate between 22–24 and 34 weeks' gestation. At 33 weeks Elena's baby was growing normally. Thus this finding is not abnormal by itself and may simply be a reflection of decreased accuracy of the procedure late in pregnancy. It may also reflect variations in growth of the baby. To make your best assessment you need further information about the results of this week's examination. If during her examination there are no indicators of problems such as decreased fetal activity, maternal urinary tract infection, maternal hypertension, and so forth, you can reassure Elena that this finding is probably a normal variation.

Chapter 9

Competing in the marathon is not recommended. Even though Constance is in excellent shape, we do not know what impact prolonged participation in such a strenuous event might have on her fetus. Uterine blood flow is decreased during exercise as blood is shunted to the muscles, and the normal fetus seems able to withstand this. We don't know, however, whether this decreased blood flow to the fetus interferes with the fetus's ability to dissipate heat, especially since the fetus is not able to decrease temperature via perspiration or respiration (Fishbein & Phillips, 1990). With this in mind, ACOG guidelines recommend that, during pregnancy, competitive athletes avoid competition, and all women exercise for shorter intervals (no longer than 15 minutes at a time).

Chapter 10

Cindy has only recently turned 15. She may not be aware of good nutrition, and probably has minimal knowledge about how her nutritional habits impact the growing fetus. The nurse can begin by showing Cindy and her boyfriend pictures of the uterus, placenta, and umbilical cord, and discussing how the fetus is nourished. She then needs to help Cindy understand good nutritional habits and which of her favorite foods in the different food groups will also be healthy for her fetus. The use of audiovisual aids is important in teaching young teenagers. The nurse needs to determine food practices in Cindy's home. Who is cooking and preparing the food? How much control does Cindy have? If the mother prepares the food, the nurse and Cindy can discuss ways of sharing information about good nutrition with Cindy's mother. Evaluation of nutritional habits and reinforcement for positive changes throughout her pregnancy will be important. Since this was a planned pregnancy with a supportive boyfriend, compliance in health behaviors to produce a healthy baby is likely.

Expected weight gain in pregnancy also needs to be discussed. Body image is a concern in the teen years. Knowing a specific amount of weight that needs to be gained each trimester for normal growth of a healthy fetus, and that this weight will be lost after pregnancy, will be important for both Cindy and her boyfriend.

Chapter 11

Although Jane's intake is supporting an appropriate weight gain, her diet is not nutritionally adequate. Comparing her diet to the Food Guide Pyramid shows that she lacks servings from the grain and dairy groups and that she has a high intake from the meat group.

Grain group	Jane should not restrict her intake from this group. Breads, pasta, and other grain products will not cause weight gain unless they are prepared with large amounts of fat or eaten in excessive quantities.
Meat group	The number of servings from this group exceeds the recommended intake. This contributes to Jane's fat and calorie intake even though she may be selecting lean cuts of meat. The number of servings should be decreased and each portion size should be about 2–3 ounces.
Dairy group	A restricted dairy intake has decreased Jane's calcium intake. The items she does consume from this group tend to have a high fat content. She could use dairy products that have a reduced fat content in order to limit her calorie intake but maintain the calcium level in her diet.
Vegetable group	Broccoli and green leafy vegetables such as beet greens, collards, and kale will provide calcium to the diet but must be consumed in amounts

	greater than usual serving sizes in order to obtain adequate calcium (Table 17–5). Most salad greens contain very little calcium.
Beverages	The total amount of fluid consumed is adequate. The consumption of soda should be limited because it would increase the calorie intake without contributing to the nutrient content of the diet.

Chapter 12

It is not unusual for women to be upset and frustrated with news that they may have newly diagnosed glucose intolerance during pregnancy. It has been described that women with gestational diabetes approach the new diagnosis as a crisis or anxiety-provoking situation. These women may experience more difficulty with coping and learning than do women with chronic diabetes who become pregnant (Keohane 1991).

It is important for the nurse to first assess the woman's knowledge about gestational diabetes before attempting to provide any teaching. The woman will benefit most from discussions that build on her current knowledge level. It will usually take several sessions to ensure that the new information is accurately understood and retained.

The nurse can reassure Mrs Chang that the baby should be fine, and can stress the importance of keeping her glucose levels in a normal range. Women with gestational diabetes usually require treatment with diet therapy alone, but occasionally may need insulin administration to control hyperglycemia.

It is felt that gestational diabetes does not cause birth defects because it occurs later in pregnancy, after the baby's organs are formed. The two most common risks to the baby are macrosomia, potentially causing a problem in labor and birth, and hypoglycemia.

Chapter 18

We hope you would encourage her to take medication if she felt she needed it. There are many types of analgesic agents and many types of regional blocks that can help her if she decides she needs them. Sometimes, giving permission for someone to ask relieves her anxiety and decreases the need for intervention.

Chapter 19

The pattern described is within normal limits. No further action is needed because the pattern is reassuring.

Chapter 20

Once uterine contractions reach the desired characteristics (frequency of every 2–3 minutes, duration of 40–60 seconds, and moderate to strong intensity), and cervical dilitation is 5–6 cm, the infusion rate can be decreased by increments similar to those by which it was increased. In this case you should decrease the rate to the step it was just prior to 6 mU/min (36 mL/hr).

Chapter 22

The unique behavioral and temperament characteristics of newborn infants should be discussed. Additionally, aspects of the Brazelton exam may be helpful to show Mrs Reyes how her infant changes state with different stimuli and intervention. Teaching her how to console her newborn may also be helpful.

Chapter 23a

Reassure mother that you will help her baby as you carry out the following activities:

- Position the infant with her head lowered and to the side.
- Bulb suction the nares and mouth repeatedly until the airway is cleared.
- Hold and comfort the infant when normal respirations are restored.
- Reassure the mother, and review this procedure with her.

Note: If bulb suctioning alone does not clear the airway, use DeLee wall suction and administer oxygen as needed to restore normal respirations.

Chapter 23b

We hope you would first examine the infant's genitalia and wipe between the labia to verify the source of bleeding. If there were no external lacerations, you would explain to the mother that a small amount of bleeding, called pseudomenstruation, sometimes occurs in newborn girls because of maternal hormone levels. This is considered normal and generally resolves in a few days. The tissue she observes is a vaginal skin tag, also a normal finding. It usually disappears in a few weeks.

Chapter 24

Acknowledge Ann's frustration and pain. Tell her you are glad she called and ask how you may be of help. Let her ventilate about how she feels. Explain that her breasts are engorged, which is a problem that many women encounter. It is not unusual for infants to refuse to nurse when the breast is hard and the nipple difficult to grasp.

Identify methods to relieve the engorgement.

a. Warm or cool soaks, whichever she prefers, for comfort and to stimulate let-down.
b. Express a small amount of milk.
c. Put the baby to breast after stimulating let-down and expressing a little milk. (The breast will be softer and it will be easier to grasp the nipple.)
d. Use analgesics. (If taken immediately before nursing, less medication will go to the baby.)

Explain to Ann that her emotional upheaval is probably the "baby blues" or "postpartum blues" and that they usually subside in 24–72 hours. Instruct her to call her physician if the blues do not subside, or if she develops symptoms of depression.

Ask why she started supplemental feedings. Upon questioning, Ann tells you that she had started supplementing her baby with formula after each feeding because her mother-in-law told her that the baby was nursing too frequently (every 1–3 hours, sometimes clustering 3–4 feedings in one 2–3 hour period). She told Ann that the baby was obviously not getting enough breast milk. After receiving supplemental feedings, the baby began feeding once every 3–5 hours.

Tactfully explain that although Ann's mother-in-law meant well, her comments indicate a lack of information about breastfeeding; that is,

a. Breast milk digests faster than formula, so breastfeeding babies feed more frequently.
b. On average, babies nurse 8–12 times in 24 hours.
c. After lactation is well established, the baby will nurse less frequently. During growth spurts, however, all babies nurse more frequently for a few days.

Explain that Ann may still breastfeed successfully, and if she desires to continue breastfeeding, she should stop supplementing with formula.

Chapter 25

We hope that you would tell her that nurses always wear gloves during the initial assessment of a newborn, during all admission procedures until the newborn has its first bath, and sometimes during diaper changes. You should also tell her that her baby will not be isolated from the other babies when in the nursery, and that her baby can remain with her if she wishes. It is important to recognize the concern that Mrs Corrigan may have about people knowing that her baby may have HIV, and to assess her own feelings of social isolation.

Chapter 26

It is important to give this mother clear, factual information regarding the type, cause, and usual course of the baby's respiratory problem. You see that Linn's laboratory tests, chest x-ray, and clinical course so far are indicative of transient tachypnea of the newborn. Respiratory distress syndrome is probably not the problem since Linn is not premature and didn't have any asphyxia at birth. You recognize that prior experience with a premature newborn with respiratory distress and prolonged hospitalization will add to this mother's fear and anxiety regarding her new baby. Therefore, in addition to giving factual information regarding the baby's condition, it is important for you to see whether the mother can be brought to the nursery to see her baby, or to have the mother receive a picture of the baby for reassurance. Before the mother visits the baby, clearly describe the oxygen and monitoring equipment that is helping Linn so that the mother will not be alarmed upon seeing her daughter.

Chapter 27

These findings are not within the normal range. At 24 hours past birth the fundus should be approximately one finger-breadth below the umbilicus and located in the midline. A uterus that is deviated to the right may indicate that the bladder is full and the woman needs to urinate. You should determine whether she is having difficulty urinating and emptying her bladder; if so, you can try some nursing measures to help her void. The lochia will still be rubra, but the amount is excessive and may be related to a boggy uterus.

Chapter 28

Clots are a sign of a problem in any postpartal woman. You will need to obtain further information regarding the size of the clots, obtain the mother's vital signs, assess the uterus for position and firmness, and assess the amount of lochial flow. The clot may be associated with uterine relaxation and fundal massage may be needed. It is important to first obtain more information.

Chapter 30

You should have Lei return to her room via wheelchair. Assess her leg for warmth, edema, redness, tenderness, and Homan's sign. Discuss with Lei that she should not massage her leg or get out of bed until you consult with the primary provider concerning your findings. Notify her primary health care provider and document your assessment findings.

GLOSSARY

Abdominal effleurage Gentle stroking used in massage.

Abortion Loss of pregnancy before the fetus is viable outside the uterus; miscarriage.

Abruptio placentae Partial or total premature separation of a normally implanted placenta.

Abstinence Refraining voluntarily, especially from indulgence in food, alcoholic beverages, or sexual intercourse.

Acceleration Periodic increase in the baseline fetal heart rate.

Acini cells Secretory cells in the human breast that create milk from nutrients in the bloodstream.

Acme Peak or highest point; time of greatest intensity (of a uterine contraction).

Acrocyanosis Cyanosis of the extremities.

Acrosomal reaction Breakdown of the hyaluronic acid in the corona radiata by enzymes from the heads of sperm; allows one spermatozoon to penetrate the ovum zona pellucida.

Active acquired immunity Formation of antibodies by the pregnant woman in response to illness or immunization.

Adnexa Adjoining or accessory parts of a structure, such as the uterine adnexa: the ovaries and fallopian tubes.

Adolescence Period of human development initiated by puberty and ending with the attainment of young adulthood.

Afterbirth Placenta and membranes expelled after the birth of the infant, during the third stage of labor. Also called secundines.

Afterpains Cramplike pains due to contractions of the uterus that occur after childbirth. They are more common in multiparas, tend to be most severe during nursing, and last 2 to 3 days.

AIDS (Acquired immune deficiency syndrome) A sexually transmitted viral disease that so far has proved fatal in 100% of cases.

Allele One of a series of alternative genes at the same locus; one form of a gene.

Alveoli Small units of the breast tissue in which milk is synthesized by the alveolar secretory epithelium.

Amenorrhea Suppression or absence of menstruation.

Amniocentesis Removal of amniotic fluid by insertion of a needle into the amniotic sac; amniotic fluid is used to assess fetal health or maturity.

Amnion The inner of the two membranes that form the sac containing the fetus and the amniotic fluid.

Amnionitis Infection of the amniotic fluid.

Amniotic fluid The liquid surrounding the fetus in utero. It absorbs shocks, permits fetal movement, and prevents heat loss.

Amniotic fluid embolism Amniotic fluid that has leaked into the chorionic plate and entered the maternal circulation.

Amniotomy The artificial rupturing of the amniotic membrane.

Ampulla The outer two-thirds of the fallopian tube; fertilization of the ovum by a spermatozoon usually occurs here.

Androgen Substance producing male characteristics, such as the male hormone testosterone.

Android pelvis Male-type pelvis.

Antepartum Time between conception and the onset of labor; usually used to describe the period during which a woman is pregnant.

Anterior fontanelle Diamond-shaped area between the two frontal and two parietal bones just above the newborn's forehead.

Anthropoid pelvis Pelvis in which the anteroposterior diameter is equal to or greater than the transverse diameter.

Apgar score A scoring system used to evaluate newborns at 1 minute and 5 minutes after birth. The total score is achieved by assessing five signs: heart rate, respiratory effort, muscle tone, reflex irritability, and color. Each of the signs is assigned a score of 0, 1, or 2. The highest possible score is 10.

Apnea A condition that occurs when respirations cease for more than 20 seconds, with generalized cyanosis.

Areola Pigmented ring surrounding the nipple of the breast.

Artificial rupture of membranes (AROM) Use of a device such as an amnihook or allis forceps to rupture the amniotic membranes.

Artificial insemination Introduction of viable semen into the vagina by artificial means for the purpose of impregnation.

Assisted reproductive technology (ART) Term used to describe the highly technologic approaches used to produce pregnancy.

Attachment Enduring bonds or relationship of affection between persons.

Attitude Attitude of the fetus refers to the relationship of the fetal parts to each other.

Autosome A chromosome that is not a sex chromosome.

Babinski reflex Reflex found normally in infants under 6 months of age in which the great toe dorsiflexes when the sole of the foot is stimulated.

Bacterial vaginosis A bacterial infection of the vagina, formerly called *Gardnerella vaginalis* or *Hemophilus vaginalis,* characterized by a foul-smelling, grayish vaginal discharge that exhibits a characteristic fishy odor when 10% potassium hydroxide (KOH) is added. Microscopic examination of a vaginal wet prep reveals the presence of "clue cells" (vaginal epithelial cells coated with gram-negative organisms).

Bag of waters (BOW) The membrane containing the amniotic fluid and the fetus.

Ballottement A technique of palpation to detect or examine a floating object in the body. In obstetrics, the fetus, when pushed, floats away and then returns to touch the examiner's fingers.

Barr body Deeply staining chromatin mass located against the inner surface of the cell nucleus. It is found only in normal females. Also called sex chromatin.

Basal body temperature (BBT) The lowest waking temperature.

Baseline rate The average fetal heart rate observed during a 10-minute period of monitoring.

Baseline variability Changes in the fetal heart rate that result from the interplay between the sympathetic and the parasympathetic nervous systems.

Battledore placenta Placenta in which the umbilical cord is inserted on the periphery rather than centrally.

Bimanual palpation Examination of the pelvic organs by placing one hand on the abdomen and one or two fingers of the other hand into the vagina.

Biophysical profile Assessment of five variables in the fetus that help to evaluate fetal risk: breathing movement, body movement, tone, amniotic fluid volume, and fetal heart rate reactivity.

Birth center A setting for labor and birth that emphasizes a family-centered approach rather than obstetric technology and treatment.

Birth plan Decisions made by the expectant couple about aspects of the childbearing experience that are most important to them.

Birth rate Number of live births per 1000 population.

Birthing room A room for labor and birth with a relaxed atmosphere.

Bishop score A prelabor scoring system to assist in predicting whether an induction of labor may be successful. The total score is achieved by assessing five components: cervical dilatation, cervical effacement, cervical consistency, cervical position, and fetal station. Each of the components is assigned a score of 0 to 3, and the highest possible score is 13.

Blastocyst The inner solid mass of cells within the morula.

Blended family Families established through remarriage; may include children from previous marriages of each spouse as well as children of the current marriage.

Bloody show Pink-tinged mucous secretions resulting from rupture of small capillaries as the cervix effaces and dilates.

Body stalk Future umbilical cord; structure that attaches the embryo to the yolk sac and contains blood vessels that extend into the chorionic villi.

Boggy uterus A term used to describe the uterine fundus when it is not firmly contracted after the birth of the baby and in the early postpartum period; excessive bleeding occurs from the placental site and maternal hemorrhage may occur.

Bonding Process of parent-infant attachment occurring at or soon after birth.

Brachial palsy Partial or complete paralysis of portions of the arm resulting from trauma to the brachial plexus during a difficult birth.

Bradley method Partner-coached natural childbirth.

Braxton Hicks contractions Intermittent painless contractions of the uterus that may occur every 10 to 20 minutes. They occur more frequently toward the end of pregnancy and are sometimes mistaken for true labor signs.

Brazleton's neonatal behavioral assessment A brief examination used to identify the infant's behavioral states and responses.

Breasts Mammary glands.

Breast self-examination Recommended monthly procedure by which women may detect changes or abnormalities in their breasts.

Breech presentation A birth in which the buttocks and/or feet are presented instead of the head.

Broad ligament The ligament extending from the lateral margins of the uterus to the pelvic wall; keeps the uterus centrally placed and provides stability within the pelvic cavity.

Bronchopulmonary dysplasia (BPD) Chronic pulmonary disease of multifactorial etiology characterized initially by alveolar and bronchial necrosis, which results in bronchial metaplasia and interstitial fibrosis. Appears in x-ray films as generalized small, radiolucent cysts within the lungs.

Brown adipose tissue (BAT) Fat deposits in neonates that provide greater heat-generating activity than ordinary fat. Found around the kidneys, adrenals, and neck; between the scapulas; and behind the sternum. Also called brown fat.

Calorie Amount of heat required to raise the temperature of 1 kg of water 1 degree Celsius.

Capacitation Removal of the plasma membrane overlying the spermatozoa's acrosomal area with the loss of seminal plasma proteins and the glycoprotein coat. If the glycoprotein coat is not removed, the sperm will not be able to penetrate the ovum.

Caput succedaneum Swelling or edema occurring in or under the fetal scalp during labor.

Cardinal ligaments The chief uterine supports, suspending the uterus from the side walls of the true pelvis.

Cardinal movements of labor The positional changes of the fetus as it moves through the birth canal during labor and birth. The positional changes are descent, flexion, internal rotation, extension, restitution, and external rotation.

Cardiopulmonary adaptation Adaptation of the neonate's cardiovascular and respiratory systems to life outside the womb.

Cephalhematoma Subcutaneous swelling containing blood found on the head of an infant several days after birth, which usually disappears within a few weeks to 2 months.

Cephalic presentation Birth in which the fetal head is presenting against the cervix.

Cephalopelvic disproportion (CPD) A condition in which the fetal head is of such a shape or size, or in such a position, that it cannot pass through the maternal pelvis.

Certified nurse-midwife (CNM) An RN who has received special training and education in the care of the family during childbearing and the prenatal, labor and birth, and postpartal periods. After a period of formal education, the nurse-midwife takes a certification test to become a CNM.

Cervical cap A cup-shaped device placed over the cervix to prevent pregnancy.

Cervical dilatation Process in which the cervical os and the cervical canal widen from less than a centimeter to approximately 10 cm, allowing birth of the fetus.

Cervix The "neck" between the external os and the body of the uterus. The lower end of the cervix extends into the vagina.

Cesarean birth Birth of the fetus by means of an incision into the abdominal wall and the uterus.

Chadwick's sign Violet bluish color of the vaginal mucous membrane caused by increased vascularity; visible from about the fourth week of pregnancy.

Chemical conjunctivitis Irritation of the mucus membrane lining of the eyelid; may be due to instillation of silver nitrate ophthalmic drops.

Child abuse Nonaccidental physical or threatened harm, including mental or emotional injury, sexual abuse, and sexual exploitation.

Child neglect Failure by parents or other custodians to meet the medical, emotional, physical, or supervisory needs of a child.

Chloasma Brownish pigmentation over the bridge of the nose and the cheeks during pregnancy and in some women who are taking oral contraceptives. Also called mask of pregnancy.

Chorioamnionitis An inflammation of the amniotic membranes stimulated by organisms in the amniotic fluid, which then becomes infiltrated with polymorphonuclear leukocytes.

Chorion The fetal membrane closest to the intrauterine wall that gives rise to the placenta and continues as the outer membrane surrounding the amnion.

Chorionic villus sampling Procedure in which a specimen of the chorionic villi is obtained from the edge of the developing placenta at about 8 weeks' gestation. The sample can be used for chromosomal, enzyme, and DNA tests.

Chromosomes The threadlike structures within the nucleus of a cell that carry the genes.

Chronic grief Grief response involving a denial of the reality of the loss, which prevents any resolution.

Circumcision Surgical removal of the prepuce (foreskin) of the penis.

Circumoral cyanosis Bluish appearance around the mouth.

Circumvallate placenta A placenta with a thick white fibrous ring around the edge.

Cleavage Rapid mitotic division of the zygote; cells produced are called blastomeres.

Client advocacy An approach to client care in which the nurse educates and supports the client and protects the client's rights.

Climacteric The period of time that marks the cessation of a woman's reproductive function; the "change of life" or menopause.

Clitoris Female organ homologous to the male penis; a small oval body of erectile tissue situated at the anterior junction of the vulva.

Coitus Sexual intercourse between a male and female.

Coitus interruptus Method of contraception in which the male withdraws his penis from the vagina prior to ejaculation.

Cold stress Excessive heat loss resulting in compensatory mechanisms (increased respirations and nonshivering thermogenesis) to maintain core body temperature.

Colostrum Secretion from the breast before the onset of true lactation; contains mainly serum and white blood corpuscles. It has a high protein content, provides some immune properties, and cleanses the neonate's intestinal tract of mucus and meconium.

Colposcopy The use of an instrument inserted into the vagina to examine the cervical and vaginal tissues by means of a magnifying lens.

Conception Union of male sperm and female ovum; fertilization.

Conceptional age The number of complete weeks since the moment of conception. Because the moment of conception is almost impossible to determine, conceptional age is estimated at 2 weeks less than gestational age.

Condom A rubber sheath that covers the penis to prevent conception or disease.

Conduction Loss of heat to a cooler surface by direct skin contact.

Condyloma Wartlike growth of skin, usually seen on the external genitals or anus. There are two types, a pointed variety and a broad, flat form usually found with syphilis.

Conjugate Important diameter of the pelvis, measured from the center of the promontory of the sacrum to the back of the symphysis pubis. The diagonal conjugate is measured and the true conjugate is estimated.

Conjugate vera The true conjugate, which extends from the middle of the sacral promontory to the middle of the pubic crest.

Contraception The prevention of conception or impregnation.

Contraction Tightening and shortening of the uterine muscles during labor, causing effacement and dilatation of the cervix; contributes to the downward and outward descent of the fetus.

Contraction stress test A method of assessing the reaction of the fetus to the stress of uterine contractions. This test may be utilized when contractions are occurring spontaneously or when contractions are artificially induced by OCT (oxytocin challenge test) or BSST (breast self-stimulation test).

Convection Loss of heat from the warm body surface to cooler air currents.

Coombs' test A test for antiglobulins in the red cells. The indirect test determines the presence of Rh-positive antibodies in maternal blood; the direct test determines the presence of maternal Rh-positive antibodies in fetal cord blood.

Cornua The elongated portions of the uterus where the fallopian tubes open.

Corpus The upper two-thirds of the uterus.

Corpus luteum A small yellow body that develops within a ruptured ovarian follicle; it secretes progesterone in the second half of the menstrual cycle and atrophies about 3 days before the beginning of menstrual flow. If pregnancy occurs, the corpus luteum continues to produce progesterone until the placenta takes over this function.

Cotyledon One of the rounded portions into which the placenta's uterine surface is divided, consisting of a mass of villi, fetal vessels, and an intervillous space.

Couvade In some cultures, the male's observance of certain rituals and taboos to signify the transition to fatherhood.

Crack A form of free base cocaine that is smoked.

Crisis intervention Actions taken by the nurse to help the client deal with an impending, potentially overwhelming crisis, regain his or her equilibrium, grow from the experience, and improve coping skills.

Critical thinking Intellectual processes that include separating fact from opinion, identifying prejudices and stereotypes that may influence interpretation of information, exploring differing ideas and views, and arriving at conclusions or insights.

Crowning Appearance of the presenting fetal part at the vaginal orifice during labor.

Deceleration Periodic decrease in the baseline fetal heart rate.

Decidua Endometrium or mucous membrane lining of the uterus in pregnancy that is shed after childbirth.

Decidua basalis The part of the decidua that unites with the chorion to form the placenta. It is shed in lochial discharge after childbirth.

Decidua capsularis The part of the decidua surrounding the chorionic sac.

Decidua vera (parietalis) Nonplacental decidua lining the uterus.

Decrement Decrease or stage of decline, as of a contraction.

Depo-Provera A long acting, injectable progestin contraceptive.

Descriptive statistics Statistics that describe or summarize a set of data.

Desquamation Shedding of the epithelial cells of the epidermis.

Diagonal conjugate Distance from the lower posterior border of the symphysis pubis to the sacral promontory; may be obtained by manual measurement.

Diaphragm A flexible disk that covers the cervix to prevent pregnancy.

Diastasis recti abdominis Separation of the recti abdominis muscles along the median line. In women, it is seen with repeated childbirths or multiple gestations. In the newborn, it is usually caused by incomplete development.

Dilatation and curettage (D and C) Stretching of the cervical canal to permit passage of a curette, which is used to scrape the endometrium to empty the uterine contents or to obtain tissue for examination.

Dilatation of the cervix Expansion of the external os from an opening a few millimeters in size to an opening large enough to allow the passage of the infant.

Diploid number of chromosomes Containing a set of maternal and a set of paternal chromosomes; in humans, the diploid number of chromosomes is 46.

Dissociation relaxation A pattern of active relaxation in which the woman learns to tighten one area of the body and then relax other areas simultaneously. This relaxation pattern is very effective for some women during labor.

Doula A supportive companion who accompanies a laboring woman to provide emotional, physical, and informational support and acts as an advocate for the woman and her family.

Down syndrome An abnormality resulting from the presence of an extra chromosome number 21 (trisomy 21); characteristics include mental retardation and altered physical appearance. Formerly called mongolism.

Drug-dependent infant The newborn of an alcoholic or drug-addicted woman.

Ductus arteriosus A communication channel between the main pulmonary artery and the aorta of the fetus. It is obliterated after birth by rising PO_2 and changes in intravascular pressure in the presence of normal pulmonary functioning. It normally becomes a ligament after birth but sometimes remains patent (patent ductus arteriosus, a treatable condition).

Ductus venosus A fetal blood vessel that carries oxygenated blood between the umbilical vein and the inferior vena cava, bypassing the liver; it becomes a ligament after birth.

Duncan's mechanism Occurs when the maternal surface of the placenta presents upon delivery rather than the shiny fetal surface.

Duration The time length of each contraction, measured from the beginning of the increment to the completion of the decrement.

Dysmenorrhea Painful menstruation.

Dyspareunia Painful intercourse.

Dystocia Difficult labor due to mechanical factors produced by the fetus or the maternal pelvis, or due to inadequate uterine or other muscular activity.

Early decelerations Periodic change in fetal heart rate pattern caused by head compression; deceleration has a uniform appearance and early onset in relation to maternal contraction.

Early postpartal hemorrhage See *Postpartal hemorrhage.*

Eclampsia A major complication of pregnancy. Its cause is unknown; it occurs more often in the primigravida and is accompanied by elevated blood pressure, albuminuria, oliguria, tonic and clonic convulsions, and coma. It may occur during pregnancy (usually after the 20th week of gestation) or within 48 hours after childbirth.

Ectoderm Outer layer of cells in the developing embryo that gives rise to the skin, nails, and hair.

Ectopic pregnancy Implantation of the fertilized ovum outside the uterine cavity; common sites are the abdomen, fallopian tubes, and ovaries. Also called oocyesis.

Effacement Thinning and shortening of the cervix that occurs late in pregnancy or during labor.

Effleurage A light stroking movement of the fingertips over the abdominal area during labor; used to provide distraction during labor contractions.

Ejaculation Expulsion of the seminal fluids from the penis.

Embryo The early stage of development of the young of any organism. In humans the embryonic period is from about 2 to 8 weeks of gestation, and is characterized by cellular differentiation and predominantly hyperplastic growth.

Embryonic membranes The amnion and chorion.

Endoderm The inner layer of cells in the developing embryo that give rise to internal organs such as the intestines.

Endometriosis Ectopic endometrium located outside the uterus in the pelvic cavity. Symptoms may include pelvic pain or pressure, dysmenorrhea, dispareunia, abnormal bleeding from the uterus or rectum, and sterility.

Endometritis Infection of the endometrium.

Endometrium The mucous membrane that lines the inner surface of the uterus.

En face An assumed position in which one person looks at another and maintains his or her face in the same vertical plane as that of the other.

Engagement The entrance of the fetal presenting part into the superior pelvic strait and the beginning of the descent through the pelvic canal.

Engorgement Vascular congestion or distention. In obstetrics, the swelling of breast tissue brought about by an increase in blood and lymph supply to the breast, preceding true lactation.

Engrossment Characteristic sense of absorption, preoccupation, and interest in the infant demonstrated by fathers during early contact with their infants.

Entrainment Phenomenon in which a newborn moves in rhythm to adult speech.

Epidural block Regional anesthesia effective through the first and second stages of labor.

Episiotomy Incision of the perineum to facilitate birth and to avoid laceration of the perineum.

Epstein's pearls Small, white blebs found along the gum margins and at the junction of the hard and soft palates; commonly seen in the newborn as a normal manifestation.

Erb-Duchenne palsy Paralysis of the arm and chest wall as a result of a birth injury to the brachial plexus or a subsequent injury to the fifth and sixth cervical nerves.

Erythema toxicum Innocuous pink papular rash of unknown cause with superimposed vesicles; it appears within 24 to 48 hours after birth and resolves spontaneously within a few days.

Erythroblastosis fetalis Hemolytic disease of the newborn characterized by anemia, jaundice, enlargement of the liver and spleen, and generalized edema. Caused by isoimmunization due to Rh incompatibility or ABO incompatibility.

Estimated date of birth (EDB) During a pregnancy, the approximate date when childbirth will occur; the "due date."

Estrogen replacement therapy (ERT) Use of estrogen and a progestin to decrease the symptoms of menopause and to help prevent osteoporosis.

Estrogens The hormones estradiol and estrone, produced by the ovary.

Ethnocentrism An individual's belief that the values and practices of his or her own culture are the best ones.

Evaporation Loss of heat incurred when water on the skin surface is converted to a vapor.

Exchange transfusion The replacement of 70% to 80% of circulating blood by withdrawing the recipient's blood and injecting a donor's blood in equal amounts, for the purpose of preventing the accumulation of bilirubin or other by-products of hemolysis in the blood.

External os The opening between the cervix and the vagina.

External (cephalic) version Procedure involving external manipulation of the maternal abdomen to change the presentation of the fetus from breech to cephalic.

Fallopian tubes Tubes that extend from the lateral angle of the uterus and terminate near the ovary; they serve as a passageway for the ovum from the ovary to the uterus and for the spermatozoa from the uterus toward the ovary. Also called oviducts and uterine tubes.

False labor Contractions of the uterus, regular or irregular, that may be strong enough to be interpreted as true labor but that do not dilate the cervix.

False pelvis The portion of the pelvis above the linea terminalis; its primary function is to support the weight of the enlarged pregnant uterus.

Family-centered care An approach to health care based on the concept that a hospital can provide professional services to mothers, fathers, and infants in a homelike environment that would enhance the integrity of the family unit.

Female condom A thin, disposable polyurethane sheath with a flexible ring at each end which is placed inside the vagina and serves to prevent sperm from entering the cervix, thus preventing conception.

Female reproductive cycle (FRC) The monthly rhythmic changes in sexually mature women.

Ferning Formation of a palm-leaf pattern by the crystallization of cervical mucus as it dries at mid-menstrual cycle. Helpful in determining time of ovulation. Observed via microscopic examination of a thin layer of cervical mucus on a glass slide. This pattern is also observed when amniotic fluid is allowed to air dry on a slide and is a useful and quick test to determine whether amniotic membranes have ruptured.

Fertility awareness methods Natural family planning.

Fertility rate Number of births per 1000 women aged 15 to 44 in a given population per year.

Fertilization Impregnation of an ovum by a spermatozoon; conception.

Fetal acoustic stimulation test (FAST) A fetal assessment test that uses sound from a speaker, bell, or artificial larynx to stimulate acceleration of the fetal heart; may be used in conjunction with the nonstress test.

Fetal activity diary (FAD) A method for tracking fetal activity taught to pregnant women.

Fetal alcohol effects (FAE) The less severe fetal manifestations of maternal alcohol ingestion, including mild to moderate cognitive problems and physical growth retardation.

Fetal alcohol syndrome (FAS) Syndrome caused by maternal alcohol ingestion and characterized by microcephaly, intrauterine growth retardation, short palpebral fissures, and maxillary hypoplasia.

Fetal attitude Relationship of the fetal parts to one another. Normal fetal attitude is one of moderate flexion of the arms onto the chest and flexion of the legs onto the abdomen.

Fetal blood sampling Blood sample drawn from the fetal scalp (or from the fetus in breech position) to evaluate the acid-base status of the fetus.

Fetal bradycardia A fetal heart rate less than 120 beats per minute during a 10-minute period of continuous monitoring.

Fetal death Death of the developing fetus after 20 weeks' gestation. Also called fetal demise.

Fetal distress Evidence that the fetus is in jeopardy, such as a change in fetal activity or heart rate.

Fetal heart rate (FHR) The number of times the fetal heart beats per minute; normal range is 120 to 160.

Fetal lie Relationship of the cephalocaudal axis (spinal column) of the fetus to the cephalocaudal axis (spinal column) of the woman. The fetus may be in a longitudinal or transverse lie.

Fetal movement record See *Fetal activity diary.*

Fetal position Relationship of the landmark on the presenting fetal part to the front, sides, or back of the maternal pelvis.

Fetal presentation The fetal body part that enters the maternal pelvis first. The three possible presentations are cephalic, shoulder, or breech.

Fetal tachycardia A fetal heart rate of 160 beats per minute or more during a 10-minute period of continuous monitoring.

Fetoscope An adaptation of a stethoscope that facilitates auscultation of the fetal heart rate.

Fetoscopy A technique for directly observing the fetus and obtaining a sample of fetal blood or skin.

Fetus The child in utero from about the seventh to ninth week of gestation until birth.

Fibrocystic breast disease Benign breast disorder characterized by a thickening of normal breast tissue and the formation of cysts.

Fimbria Any structure resembling a fringe; the fringelike extremity of the fallopian tubes.

Folic acid An important vitamin directly related to the outcome of pregnancy and to maternal and fetal health.

Follicle-stimulating hormone (FSH) Hormone produced by the anterior pituitary during the first half of the menstrual cycle, stimulating development of the graafian follicle.

Fontanelle In the fetus, an unossified space or soft spot consisting of a strong band of connective tissue lying between the cranial bones of the skull.

Foramen ovale Special opening between the atria of the fetal heart. Normally, the opening closes shortly after birth; if it remains open, it can be repaired surgically.

Forceps Obstetric instrument occasionally used to aid in childbirth.

Foremilk Breast milk obtained at the beginning of the breastfeeding episode.

Fourth trimester First several postpartal weeks during which the woman returns to an essentially prepregnant state and becomes competent in caring for her newborn.

Frequency The time between the beginning of one contraction and the beginning of the next contraction.

Fundus The upper portion of the uterus between the fallopian tubes.

Galactorrhea Nipple discharge.

Gamete Female or male germ cell; contains a haploid number of chromosomes.

Gamete intrafallopian transfer (GIFT) Retrieval of oocytes by laparoscopy; immediately combining oocytes with washed, motile sperm in a catheter; and placement of the gametes into the fimbriated end of the fallopian tube.

Gametogenesis The process by which germ cells are produced.

Genotype The genetic composition of an individual.

Gestation Period of intrauterine development from conception through birth; pregnancy.

Gestational age The number of complete weeks of fetal development, calculated from the first day of the last normal menstrual cycle.

Gestational age assessment tools Systems used to evaluate the newborn's external physical characteristics and neurologic and/or neuromuscular development to accurately determine gestational age. These replace or supplement the traditional calculation from the woman's last menstrual period.

Gestational diabetes mellitus A form of diabetes of variable severity with onset or first recognition during pregnancy.

Gestational trophoblastic disease (GTD) Disorder classified into two types: benign (hydatidiform mole) and malignant.

Gonadotropin-releasing hormone (GnRH) A hormone secreted by the hypothalamus that stimulates the anterior pituitary to secrete FSH and LH.

Goodell's sign Softening of the cervix that occurs during the second month of pregnancy.

Graafian follicle The ovarian cyst containing the ripe ovum; it secretes estrogens.

Grasping reflex Normal newborn reflex elicited by stimulating the palm with a finger or object, resulting in newborn firmly holding on to the finger or object.

Gravida A pregnant woman.

Grief work The inner process of working through or managing the bereavement.

Gynecoid pelvis Typical female pelvis in which the inlet is round instead of oval.

Habituation Infant's ability to diminish innate responses to specific repeated stimuli.

Haploid number of chromosomes Half the diploid number of chromosomes. In humans there are 23 chromosomes, the haploid number, in each germ cell.

Harlequin sign A rare color change that occurs between the longitudinal halves of the newborn's body, such that the dependent half is noticeably pinker than the superior half when the newborn is placed on one side; it is of no pathologic significance.

Hegar's sign A softening of the lower uterine segment found upon palpation in the second or third month of pregnancy.

HELLP syndrome A cluster of changes including *h*emolysis, *e*levated *l*iver enzymes, and *l*ow *p*latelet count; sometimes associated with severe preeclampsia.

Hemolytic disease of the newborn *Hyperbilirubinemia* secondary to Rh incompatibility.

Heterozygous A genotypic situation in which two different alleles occur at a given locus on a pair of homologous chromosomes.

Hindmilk Breast milk released after initial letdown reflex; high in fat content.

Homozygous A genotypic situation in which two similar genes occur at a given locus on homologous chromosomes.

Hormone replacement therapy (HRT) Administration of hormones, usually estrogen and a progestin, to alleviate the symptoms of menopause.

Huhner test Postcoital examination to evaluate sperm and cervical mucus.

Human chorionic gonadotropin (hCG) A hormone produced by the chorionic villi and found in the urine of pregnant women. Also called prolan.

Human placental lactogen (hPL) A hormone synthesized by the syncytiotrophoblast that functions as an insulin antagonist and promotes lipolysis to increase the amounts of circulating free fatty acids available for maternal metabolic use.

Hydatidiform mole Degenerative process in chorionic villi, giving rise to multiple cysts and rapid growth of the uterus with hemorrhage.

Hydramnios An excess of amniotic fluid, leading to overdistention of the uterus. Frequently seen in diabetic pregnant women, even if there is no coexisting fetal anomaly. Also called polyhydramnios.

Hydrops fetalis See *Erythroblastosis fetalis*.

Hyperbilirubinemia Excessive amount of bilirubin in the blood; indicative of hemolytic processes due to blood incompatibility, intrauterine infection, septicemia, neonatal renal infection, and other disorders.

Hyperemesis gravidarum Excessive vomiting during pregnancy, leading to dehydration and starvation.

Hypnoreflexogenous method A combination of hypnosis and conditioned reflexes used during childbirth.

Hypoglycemia Abnormally low level of sugar in the blood.

Hysterectomy Surgical removal of the uterus.

Hysterosalpingogram Result of testing by instillation of radiopaque substance into the uterine cavity to visualize the uterus and fallopian tubes.

Hysteroscopy Use of a special endoscope to examine the uterus.

In vitro fertilization (IVF) Procedure during which oocytes are removed from the ovary, mixed with spermatozoa, fertilized, and incubated in a glass petri dish; then up to four viable embryos are placed in the woman's uterus.

Inborn error of metabolism A hereditary deficiency of a specific enzyme needed for normal metabolism of specific chemicals.

Incompetent (dysfunctional) cervix The premature dilatation of the cervix, usually in the second trimester of pregnancy.

Increment Increase or addition; to build up, as of a contraction.

Induction of labor The process of causing or initiating labor by use of medication or surgical rupture of membranes.

Infant A child under 1 year of age.

Infant mortality rate Number of deaths of infants under 1 year of age per 1000 live births in a given population per year.

Infant of a diabetic mother (IDM) At-risk infant born to a woman previously diagnosed as diabetic, or who develops symptoms of diabetes during pregnancy.

Inferential statistics Statistics that allow an investigator to draw conclusions about what is happening between two or more variables in a population and to suggest or refute casual relationships between them.

Infertility Diminished ability to conceive.

Informed consent A legal concept that protects a person's rights to autonomy and self-determination by specifying that no action may be taken without that person's prior understanding and freely given consent.

Infundibulopelvic ligament Ligament that suspends and supports the ovaries.

Innominate bone The hip bone, ilium, ischium, and pubis.

Intensity The strength of a uterine contraction during acme.

Internal os An inside mouth or opening; the opening between the cervix and the uterus.

Internal version Procedure used to vaginally deliver a second twin. The obstetrician inserts a hand into the uterus, grasps the feet of the fetus, and changes the fetus from a transverse to a breech presentation.

Intrapartum The time from the onset of true labor until the birth of the infant and delivery of the placenta.

Intrauterine catheter A catheter that can be placed through the cervix into the uterus to measure uterine pressure during labor. Some types of catheters may be inserted for the purpose of infusing warmed saline to add additional intrauterine fluid when oligohydramnios is present.

Intrauterine device (IUD) Small metal or plastic form that is placed in the uterus to prevent implantation of a fertilized ovum.

Intrauterine fetal surgery Surgery performed on a fetus to correct anatomic lesions that are not compatible with life if left untreated.

Intrauterine growth restriction (IUGR) Fetal undergrowth due to any etiology, such as intrauterine infection, deficient nutrient supply, or congenital malformation. Formerly called intrauterine growth retardation.

Introitus Opening or entrance into a cavity or canal such as the vagina.

Involution Rolling or turning inward; the reduction in size of the uterus following childbirth.

Ischial spines Prominences that arise near the junction of the ilium and ischium and jut into the pelvic cavity; used as a reference point during labor to evaluate the descent of the fetal head into the birth canal.

Isthmus The straight, narrow part of the fallopian tube with a thick muscular wall and an opening (lumen) 2–3 mm in diameter; the site of tubal ligation. Also a constriction in the uterus that is located above the cervix and below the corpus.

Jaundice Yellow pigmentation of body tissues caused by the presence of bile pigments. See also *Physiologic jaundice*.

Karyotype The set of chromosomes arranged in a standard order.

Kegel's exercises Perineal muscle tightening that strengthens the pubococcygeus muscle and increases its tone.

Kernicterus An encephalopathy caused by deposition of unconjugated bilirubin in brain cells; may result in impaired brain function or death.

Kilocalorie (kcal) Equivalent to 1000 calories, it is the unit used to express the energy value of food.

Klinefelter syndrome A chromosomal abnormality caused by the presence of an extra X chromosome in the male; characteristics include tall stature, sparse pubic and facial hair, gynecomastia, small firm testes, and absence of spermatogenesis.

Labor The process by which the fetus is expelled from the maternal uterus. Also called childbirth, confinement, or parturition.

Lactation The process of producing and supplying breast milk.

Lacto-ovovegetarians Vegetarians who include milk, dairy products, and eggs in their diets, and occasionally fish, poultry, and liver.

Lactose intolerance A condition in which an individual has difficulty digesting milk and milk products.

Lactovegetarians Vegetarians who include dairy products but no eggs in their diets.

La Leche League Organization that provides information on and assistance with breastfeeding.

Lamaze method A method of childbirth preparation. See also *Psychoprophylaxis.*

Lanugo Fine, downy hair found on all body parts of the fetus, with the exception of the palms of the hands and the soles of the feet, after 20 weeks' gestation.

Laparoscopy Procedure that enables direct visualization of pelvic organs.

Large for gestational age (LGA) Excessive growth of a fetus in relation to the gestational time period.

Last menstrual period (LMP) The last normal menstrual period experienced by the woman prior to pregnancy; sometimes used to calculate the infant's gestational age.

Late decelerations Periodic change in fetal heart rate pattern caused by uteroplacental insufficiency; deceleration has a uniform shape and late onset in relation to maternal contraction.

Late postpartal hemorrhage See *Postpartal hemorrhage.*

Leboyer method Birthing technique that eases the newborn's transition to extrauterine life wherein lights in the birthing room are dimmed and noise is kept to a minimum.

Lecithin/sphingomyelin (L/S) ratio Lecithin and sphingomyelin are phospholipid components of surfactant; their ratio changes during gestation. When the L/S ratio reaches 2:1, the fetal lungs are thought to be mature and the fetus will have a low risk of respiratory distress syndrome if born at that time.

Leiomyoma A benign tumor of the uterus, composed primarily of smooth muscle and connective tissue. Also referred to as a myoma or a fibroid.

Leopold's maneuvers A series of four maneuvers designed to provide a systematic approach whereby the examiner may determine fetal presentation and position.

Letdown reflex Pattern of stimulation, hormone release, and resulting muscle contraction that forces milk into the lactiferous ducts, making it available to the infant. Also called milk ejection reflex.

Leukorrhea Mucous discharge from the vagina or cervical canal that may be normal or pathologic, as in the presence of infection.

Lie Relationship of the long axis of the fetus and the long axis of the pregnant woman. The fetal lie may be longitudinal, transverse, or oblique.

Lightening Moving of the fetus and uterus downward into the pelvic cavity.

Linea nigra The line of darker pigmentation extending from the umbilicus to the pubis noted in some women during the later months of pregnancy.

Local anesthesia Injection of an anesthetic agent into the subcutaneous tissue in a fanlike pattern.

Lochia Maternal discharge of blood, mucus, and tissue from the uterus; may last for several weeks after birth.

Lochia alba White vaginal discharge that follows lochia serosa and that lasts from about the 10th to the 21st day after birth.

Lochia rubra Red, blood-tinged vaginal discharge that occurs following birth and lasts 2 to 4 days.

Lochia serosa Pink, serous, and blood-tinged vaginal discharge that follows lochia rubra and lasts until the seventh to tenth day after birth.

Long-term variability (LTV) Large rhythmic fluctuations of the FHR that occur from two to six times per minute.

Luteinizing hormone (LH) Anterior pituitary hormone responsible for stimulating ovulation and for development of the corpus luteum.

Macrosomia A condition seen in neonates of large body size and high birth weight, as those born of prediabetic and diabetic mothers.

Malposition An abnormal position of the fetus in the birth canal.

Malpresentation A presentation of the fetus into the birth canal that is not "normal," that is, brow, face, shoulder, or breech presentation.

Mammogram A soft tissue radiograph of the breast without the injection of a contrast medium.

Mastitis Inflammation of the breast.

Maternal mortality The number of maternal deaths from any cause during the pregnancy cycle per 100,000 live births.

Mature milk Breast milk that contains 10% solids for energy and growth.

McDonald's sign A probable sign of pregnancy characterized by an ease in flexing the body of the uterus against the cervix.

Meconium Dark green or black material present in the large intestine of a full-term infant; the first stools passed by the newborn.

Meconium aspiration syndrome (MAS) Respiratory disease of term, postterm, and SGA newborns caused by inhalation of meconium or meconium-stained amniotic fluid into the lungs; characterized by mild to severe respiratory distress, hyperexpansion of the chest, hyperinflated alveoli, and secondary atelectasis.

Meiosis The process of cell division that occurs in the maturation of sperm and ova that decreases their number of chromosomes by one-half.

Menarche Beginning of menstrual and reproductive function in the female.

Mendelian inheritance A major category of inheritance whereby a trait is determined by a pair of genes on homologous chromosomes. Also called single gene inheritance.

Menopause The permanent cessation of menses.

Menorrhagia Excessive or profuse menstrual flow.

Menstrual cycle Cyclic buildup of the uterine lining, ovulation, and sloughing of the lining occurring approximately every 28 days in nonpregnant females.

Mentum The chin.

Mesoderm The intermediate layer of germ cells in the embryo that gives rise to connective tissue, bone marrow, muscles, blood, lymphoid tissue, and epithelial tissue.

Metrorrhagia Abnormal uterine bleeding occurring at irregular intervals.

Mifepristone (RU 486) Experimental postcoital contraceptive.

Milia Tiny white papules appearing on the face of a neonate as a result of unopened sebaceous glands; they disappear spontaneously within a few weeks.

Milk/plasma ratio Comparison of the concentration of substances in the breast milk and the maternal blood serum.

Miscarriage See *Spontaneous abortion.*

Mitosis Process of cell division whereby both daughter cells have the same number and pattern of chromosomes as the original cell.

Molding Shaping of the fetal head by overlapping of the cranial bones to facilitate movement through the birth canal during labor.

Mongolian spot Dark, flat pigmentation of the lower back and buttocks noted at birth in some infants; usually disappears by the time the child reaches school age.

Moniliasis Yeastlike fungal infection caused by *Candida albicans.*

Mons pubis Mound of subcutaneous fatty tissue covering the anterior portion of the symphysis pubis.

Moro reflex Flexion of the newborn's thighs and knees accompanied by fingers that fan, then clench, as the arms are simultaneously thrown out and then brought together, as though embracing something. This reflex can be elicited by startling the newborn with a sudden noise or movement. Also called the startle reflex.

Morula Developmental stage of the fertilized ovum in which there is a solid mass of cells.

Mosaicism Condition of an individual who has at least two cell lines with differing karotypes.

Mottling Discoloration of the skin in irregular areas; may be seen with chilling, poor perfusion, or hypoxia.

Mucous plug A collection of thick mucus that blocks the cervical canal during pregnancy. Also called operculum.

Multigravida Woman who has been pregnant more than once.

Multipara Woman who has had more than one pregnancy in which the fetus was viable.

Multiple pregnancy More than one fetus in the uterus at the same time.

Myometrium Uterine muscular structure.

Nägele's rule A method of determining the estimated date of birth (EDB): after obtaining the first day of the last menstrual period, subtract 3 months and add 7 days.

Natural childbirth Prepared childbirth, in which the couple attends a prenatal education program and learns exercises and breathing patterns that are used during labor and childbirth.

Neonatal mortality rate Number of deaths of infants in the first 28 days of life per 1000 live births.

Neonatal mortality risk The chance of death within the newborn period.

Neonatal transition The first few hours of life in which the newborn stabilizes its respiratory and circulatory functions.

Neonate Infant from birth through the first 28 days of life.

Neonatology The specialty that focuses on the management of high-risk conditions of the newborn.

Nevus flammeus Large port-wine stain.

Nevus vasculosus "Strawberry mark": raised, clearly delineated, dark red, rough-surfaced birthmark commonly found in the head region.

Newborn screening tests Tests that detect inborn errors of metabolism that, if left untreated, cause mental retardation and physical handicaps.

Nidation Implantation of a fertilized ovum in the endometrium.

Nipple A protrusion about 0.5 to 1.3 cm in diameter in the center of each mature breast.

Nipple preparation Prenatal activities designed to toughen the nipple in preparation for breastfeeding.

Non-Mendelian (multifactorial) inheritance The occurrence of congenital disorders that result from an interaction of multiple genetic and environmental factors.

Nonstress test (NST) An assessment method by which the reaction (or response) of the fetal heart rate to fetal movement is evaluated.

Norplant A subdermal progestin contraceptive which is implanted in a woman's arm and provides contraceptive protection for up to 5 years.

Nuchal cord Term used to describe the umbilical cord when it is wrapped around the neck of the fetus.

Nulligravida A woman who has never been pregnant.

Nullipara A woman who has not delivered a viable fetus.

Obstetric conjugate Distance from the middle of the sacral promontory to an area approximately 1 cm below the pubic crest.

Oligohydramnios Decreased amount of amniotic fluid, which may indicate a fetal urinary tract defect.

Oocyte Early primitive ovum before it has completely developed.

Oogenesis Process during fetal life whereby the ovary produces oogenia, cells that become primitive ovarian eggs.

Oophoritis Infection of the ovaries.

Ophthalmia neonatorum Purulent infection of the eyes or conjunctiva of the newborn, usually caused by gonococci.

Oral contraceptives "Birth control pills" that work by inhibiting the release of an ovum and by maintaining a type of mucus that is hostile to sperm.

Orgasm Climax of the sexual experience.

Orientation Infant's ability to respond to auditory and visual stimuli in the environment.

Ortolani's maneuver A manual procedure performed to rule out the possibility of congenital hip dysplasia.

Ovarian ligaments Ligaments that anchor the lower pole of the ovary to the cornua of the uterus.

Ovary Female sex gland in which the ova are formed and in which estrogen and progesterone are produced. Normally there are two ovaries, located in the lower abdomen on each side of uterus.

Ovulation Normal process of discharging a mature ovum from an ovary approximately 14 days prior to the onset of menses.

Ovum Female reproductive cell; egg.

Oxygen toxicity Excessive levels of oxygen therapy that result in pathologic changes in tissue.

Oxytocin Hormone normally produced by the posterior pituitary, responsible for stimulation of uterine contractions and the release of milk into the lactiferous ducts.

Oxytocin challenge test (OCT) See *Contraction stress test (CST).*

Papanicolaou (Pap) smear Procedure to detect the presence of cancer of the uterus by microscopic examination of cells gently scraped from the cervix.

Para A woman who has borne offspring who reached the age of viability.

Paracervical block A local anesthetic agent injected transvaginally adjacent to the outer rim of the cervix.

Parametritis Inflammation of the parametrial layer of the uterus.

Parent-newborn attachment Close affectional ties that develop between parent and child. See also *Attachment.*

Passive acquired immunity Transfer of antibodies (IgG) from the mother to the fetus in utero.

Pedigree Graphic representation of a family tree.

Pelvic cavity Bony portion of the birth passages; a curved canal with a longer posterior than anterior wall.

Pelvic cellulitis Infection involving the connective tissue of the broad ligament or, in severe cases, the connective tissue of all the pelvic structures.

Pelvic diaphragm Part of the pelvic floor composed of deep fascia and the levator ani and the coccygeal muscles.

Pelvic floor Muscles and tissue that act as a buttress to the pelvic outlet.

Pelvic inflammatory disease (PID) An infection of the fallopian tubes that may or may not be accompanied by a pelvic abscess; may cause infertility secondary to tubal damage.

Pelvic inlet Upper border of the true pelvis.

Pelvic outlet Lower border of the true pelvis.

Pelvic tilt Also called pelvic rocking; exercise designed to reduce back strain and strengthen abdominal muscle tone.

Penis The male organ of copulation and reproduction.

Percutaneous umbilical blood sampling (PUBS) A technique used to obtain pure fetal blood from the umbilical cord while the fetus is in utero. Also called cordocentesis.

Perimetrium The outermost layer of the corpus of the uterus. Also known as the serosal layer.

Perinatal mortality rate The number of neonatal and fetal deaths per 1000 live births.

Perinatology The medical specialty concerned with the diagnosis and treatment of high-risk conditions of the pregnant woman and her fetus.

Perineal body Wedge-shaped mass of fibromuscular tissue found between the lower part of the vagina and the anal canal.

Perineum The area of tissue between the anus and scrotum in a man or between the anus and vagina in a woman.

Periodic breathing Sporadic episodes of apnea, not associated with cyanosis, that last for about 10 seconds and commonly occur in preterm infants.

Periods of reactivity Predictable patterns of neonate behavior during the first several hours after birth.

Persistant occiput posterior position Malposition of the fetus in which the fetal occiput is posterior in the maternal pelvis.

Persistent pulmonary hypertension of the newborn (PPHN) Respiratory disease resulting from right-to-left shunting of blood away from the lungs and through the ductus arteriosus and patent foramen ovale.

Phenotype The whole physical, biochemical, and physiologic makeup of an individual as determined both genetically and environmentally.

Phenylketonuria A common metabolic disease caused by an inborn error in the metabolism of the amino acid phenylalanine.

Phosphatidylglycerol (PG) A phospholipid present in fetal surfactant after about 35 weeks' gestation.

Phototherapy The treatment of jaundice by exposure to light.

Physiologic anemia of infancy A harmless condition in which the hemoglobin level drops in the first 6 to 12 weeks after birth, then reverts to normal levels.

Physiologic anemia of pregnancy Apparent anemia that results because during pregnancy the plasma volume increases more than the erythrocytes increase.

Physiologic jaundice A harmless condition caused by the normal reduction of red blood cells, occurring 48 or more hours after birth, peaking at the fifth to seventh day, and disappearing between the seventh to tenth day.

Pica The eating of substances not ordinarily considered edible or to have nutritive value.

Placenta Specialized disk-shaped organ that connects the fetus to the uterine wall for gas and nutrient exchange. Also called afterbirth.

Placenta accreta Partial or complete absence of the decidua basalis and abnormal adherence of the placenta to the uterine wall.

Placenta previa Abnormal implantation of the placenta in the lower uterine segment. Classification of type is based on proximity to the cervical os: *total*—completely covers the os; *partial*—covers a portion of the os; *marginal*—is in close proximity to the os.

Platypelloid pelvis An unusually wide pelvis, having a flattened oval transverse shape and a shortened anteroposterior diameter.

Polar body A small cell resulting from the meiotic division of the mature oocyte.

Polycythemia An abnormal increase in the number of total red blood cells in the body's circulation.

Polydactyly A developmental anomaly characterized by more than five digits on the hands or feet.

Positive signs of pregnancy Indications that confirm the presence of pregnancy.

Postconception age periods Period of time in embryonic/fetal development calculated from the time of fertilization of the ovum.

Postmature newborn See *Postterm newborn.*

Postpartal hemorrhage A loss of blood of greater than 500 mL following birth. The hemorrhage is classified as *early* or *immediate* if it occurs within the first 24 hours and *late* or *delayed* after the first 24 hours.

Postpartum After childbirth or delivery.

Postpartum blues A maternal adjustment reaction occurring in the first few postpartal days, characterized by mild depression, tearfulness, anxiety, headache, and irritability.

Postterm newborn Any infant born after 42 weeks' gestation.

Postterm labor Labor that occurs after 42 weeks of gestation.

Postterm pregnancy Pregnancy that lasts beyond 42 weeks' gestation.

Precipitous birth (1) Unduly rapid progression of labor. (2) A birth in which no physician is in attendance.

Precipitous labor Labor lasting less than 3 hours.

Preeclampsia Toxemia of pregnancy, characterized by hypertension, albuminuria, and edema. See also *Eclampsia.*

Pregnancy-induced hypertension (PIH) A hypertensive disorder including preeclampsia and eclampsia as conditions, characterized by the three cardinal signs of hypertension, edema, and proteinuria.

Premature infant See *Preterm infant.*

Premature rupture of the membranes (PROM) See *Rupture of membranes.*

Premenstrual syndrome (PMS) Cluster of symptoms experienced by some women, typically occurring from a few days up to 2 weeks prior to the onset of menses.

Prenatal education Programs offered to expectant families, adolescents, women, or partners to provide education regarding the pregnancy, labor, and birth experience.

Prep Shaving of the pubic area.

Presentation The fetal body part that enters the maternal pelvis first. The three possible presentations are cephalic, shoulder, or breech.

Presenting part The fetal part present in or on the cervical os.

Presumptive signs of pregnancy Symptoms that suggest but do not confirm pregnancy, such as cessation of menses, quickening, Chadwick's sign, and morning sickness.

Preterm infant Any infant born before 38 weeks' gestation.

Preterm labor Labor occurring between 20 and 38 weeks of pregnancy. Also called premature labor.

Primigravida A woman who is pregnant for the first time.

Primipara A woman who has given birth to her first child (past the point of viability), whether or not that child is living or was alive at birth.

Probable signs of pregnancy Manifestations that strongly suggest the likelihood of pregnancy, such as a positive pregnancy test, enlarging abdomen, and positive Goodell's, Hegar's, and Braxton Hicks signs.

Progesterone A hormone produced by the corpus luteum, adrenal cortex, and placenta whose function is to stimulate proliferation of the endometrium to facilitate growth of the embryo.

Progressive relaxation A relaxation technique that involves relaxing first one portion of the body and then another portion, until total body relaxation is achieved; may be used during labor.

Prolactin A hormone secreted by the anterior pituitary that stimulates and sustains lactation in mammals.

Prolapsed cord Umbilical cord that becomes trapped in the vagina before the fetus is born.

Prolonged labor Labor lasting more than 24 hours.

Prostaglandins Complex lipid compounds synthesized by many cells in the body.

Pseudomenstruation Blood-tinged mucus from the vagina in the newborn female infant; caused by withdrawal of maternal hormones that were present during pregnancy.

Psychoprophylaxis (Lamaze) Psychophysical training aimed at preparing the expectant parents to cope with the processes of labor and to avoid concentration on the discomforts associated with childbirth.

Ptyalism Excessive salivation.

Pubic Pertaining to the pubes or pubis.

Pudendal block Injection of an anesthetizing agent at the pudendal nerve to produce numbness of the external genitals and the lower one third of the vagina, to facilitate childbirth and permit episiotomy if necessary.

Puerperal morbidity A maternal temperature of 38C (100.4F) or higher on any 2 of the first 10 postpartal days, excluding the first 24 hours. The temperature is to be taken by mouth at least 4 times per day.

Puerperium The period after completion of the third stage of labor until involution of the uterus is complete, usually 6 weeks.

Quickening The first fetal movements felt by the pregnant woman, usually between 16 to 18 weeks' gestation.

Radiation Heat loss incurred when heat transfers to cooler surfaces and objects not in direct contact with the body.

Rape Sexual activity, often intercourse, against the will of the victim.

Read method Natural childbirth preparation centered on eliminating the fear-tension-pain syndrome.

Reciprocal inhibition The principle that it is impossible to feel relaxed and tense at the same time; the basis for relaxation techniques.

Recommended dietary allowances (RDA) Government-recommended allowances of various vitamins, minerals, and other nutrients.

Regional anesthesia Injection of local anesthetic agents so that they come into direct contact with nervous tissue.

Relaxin A water-soluble protein secreted by the corpus luteum that causes relaxation of the symphysis and cervical dilatation.

Respiratory distress syndrome (RDS) Respiratory disease of the newborn characterized by interference with ventilation at the alveolar level, thought to be caused by the presence of fibrinoid deposits lining the alveolar ducts. Formerly called hyaline membrane disease.

Retinopathy of prematurity Formation of fibrotic tissue behind the lens; associated with retinal detachment and arrested eye growth, seen with hypoxemia in preterm infants.

Rh factor Antigens present on the surface of blood cells that make the blood cell incompatible with blood cells that do not have the antigen.

RhoGAM An anti-Rh (D) gamma-globulin given after delivery to an Rh-negative mother of an Rh-positive fetus or child. Prevents the development of permanent active immunity to the Rh antigen.

Rhythm method The timing of sexual intercourse to avoid the fertile time associated with ovulation.

Risk factors Any findings that suggest the pregnancy may have a negative outcome, either for the woman or her unborn child.

Rooming-in unit A hospital unit where the infant can reside in the same room with the mother after birth and during their postpartal stay.

Rooting reflex An infant's tendency to turn the head and open the lips to suck when one side of the mouth or cheek is touched.

Round ligaments Ligaments that arise from the side of the uterus near the fallopian tube insertion to help the broad ligament keep the uterus in place.

Rugae Transverse ridges of mucous membranes lining the vagina, which allow the vagina to stretch during the descent of the fetal head.

Rupture of membranes (ROM) Rupture may be PROM (premature), SROM (spontaneous), or AROM (artificial). Some clinicians may use the abbreviation RBOW (rupture of bag of waters).

Sacral promontory A projection into the pelvic cavity on the anterior upper portion of the sacrum; serves as an obstetric guide in determining pelvic measurements.

Salpingitis Infection of the fallopian tubes.

Saltatory pattern A fetal heart rate pattern of marked or excessive variability.

Scalp stimulation test (SST) A test used during labor to assess fetal well-being by pressing a fingertip on the fetal scalp. A fetus not under excessive stress will respond to the digital stimulation with heart rate accelerations.

Scarf sign The position of the elbow when the hand of a supine infant is drawn across to the other shoulder until it meets resistance.

Schultze's mechanism Delivery of the placenta with the shiny or fetal surface presenting first.

Self-quieting activity Infant's ability to use personal resources to quiet and console him- or herself.

Semen Thick whitish fluid ejaculated by the male during orgasm and containing the spermatozoa and their nutrients.

Sepsis neonatorum Infections experienced by a neonate during the first month of life.

Sex chromosomes The X and Y chromosomes, which are responsible for sex determination.

Sexually transmitted infection (STI) Refers to infections ordinarily transmitted by direct sexual contact with an infected individual. Also called sexually transmitted disease.

Short-term variability (STV) Refers to the differences between successive heart beats as measured by the R–R wave interval of the QRS cardiac cycle. Measured only by internal electronic fetal monitoring.

Show A pinkish mucous discharge from the vagina that may occur a few hours to a few days prior to the onset of labor.

Simian line A single palmar crease frequently found in children with Down syndrome.

Sinusoidal pattern A wave form of fetal heart rate where long-term variability is present but there is no short-term variability.

Situational contraceptives Contraceptive methods that involve no prior preparation, for instance, abstinence or coitus interruptus.

Skin turgor Elasticity of skin; provides information on hydration status.

Small for gestational age (SGA) Inadequate weight or growth for gestational age; birth weight below the tenth percentile.

Spermatogenesis The process by which mature spermatozoa are formed, during which the number of chromosomes is halved.

Spermatozoa Mature sperm cells of the male animal, produced by the testes.

Spermicides A variety of creams, foams, jellies, and suppositories that, when inserted into the vagina prior to intercourse, destroy sperm or neutralize any vaginal secretions and thereby immobilize sperm.

Spinal block Injection of a local anesthetic agent directly into the spinal fluid in the spinal canal to provide anesthesia for vaginal and cesarean births.

Spinnbarkeit The elasticity of the cervical mucus that is present at ovulation.

Spontaneous abortion Abortion that occurs naturally. Also called miscarriage.

Station Relationship of the presenting fetal part to an imaginary line drawn between the pelvic ischial spines.

Sterility Inability to conceive or to produce offspring.

Stillbirth The delivery of a dead infant.

Striae gravidarum Stretch marks; shiny reddish lines that appear on the abdomen, breasts, thighs, and buttocks of pregnant women as a result of stretching the skin.

Structural-functional framework Defines the family as a social system.

Subconjunctival hemorrhage Hemorrhage on the sclera of a newborn's eye usually caused by changes in vascular tension during birth.

Subdermal implants (Norplant) Silastic capsules containing levonorgestrel; when 6 are implanted in a woman's upper arm, they act as a contraceptive for up to 5 years.

Subinvolution Failure of a part to return to its normal size after functional enlargement, such as failure of the uterus to return to normal size after pregnancy.

Sucking reflex Normal newborn reflex elicited by inserting a finger or nipple in the newborn's mouth, resulting in forceful, rhythmic sucking.

Surfactant A surface-active mixture of lipoproteins secreted in the alveoli and air passages that reduces surface tension of pulmonary fluids and contributes to the elasticity of pulmonary tissue.

Suture Fibrous connection of opposed joint surfaces, as in the skull.

Symphysis pubis Fibrocartilaginous joint between the pelvic bones in the midline.

Syndactyly Malformation of the fingers or toes in which there may be webbing or complete fusion of two or more digits.

Telangiectatic nevi (stork bites) Small clusters of pink-red spots appearing on the nape of the neck and around the eyes of infants; localized areas of capillary dilatation.

Teratogens Nongenetic factors that can produce malformations of the fetus.

Term The normal duration of pregnancy.

Testes The male gonads, in which sperm and testosterone are produced.

Testosterone The male hormone; responsible for the development of secondary male characteristics.

Therapeutic abortion Medically induced termination of pregnancy when a malformed fetus is suspected or when the woman's health is in jeopardy.

Thermal neutral zone (TNZ) An environment that provides for minimal heat loss or expenditure.

Thrombophlebitis Inflammation of a vein wall resulting in thrombus.

Thrush A fungal infection of the oral mucous membranes caused by *Candida albicans*. Most often seen in infants; characterized by white plaques in the mouth.

Tocolysis Use of medications to arrest preterm labor.

Tonic neck reflex Postural reflex seen in the newborn. When the supine infant's head is turned to one side, the arm and leg on that side extend while the extremities on the opposite side flex. Also called the fencing position.

TORCH An acronym used to describe a group of infections that represent potentially severe problems during pregnancy. TO = toxoplasmosis, R = rubella, C = cytomegalovirus, H = herpesvirus.

Total serum bilirubin Sum of conjugated (direct) and unconjugated (indirect) bilirubin.

Touch relaxation A relaxation technique that involves relaxing an area of one's body as another person provides a "touch" cue to that specific area. Touch relaxation is very effective during labor contractions.

Toxic shock syndrome Infection caused by *Staphylococcus aureaus,* found primarily in women of reproductive age.

Transitional milk Breast milk produced from the end of colostrum production until about 2 weeks postpartum.

Transverse diameter The largest diameter of the pelvic inlet; helps determine the shape of the inlet.

Transverse lie A lie in which the fetus is positioned crosswise in the uterus.

Trichomonas vaginalis A parasitic protozoan that may cause inflammation of the vagina, characterized by itching and burning of vulvar tissue and by white, frothy discharge.

Trimester Three months, or one-third of the gestational time for pregnancy.

Trisomy The presence of three homologous chromosomes rather than the normal two.

Trophoblast The outer layer of the blastoderm that will eventually establish the nutrient relationship with the uterine endometrium.

True pelvis The portion that lies below the linea terminalis, made up of the inlet, cavity, and outlet.

Tubal ligation Sterilization of a woman accomplished by transecting or occluding the fallopian tubes.

Turner syndrome A number of anomalies that occur when a woman has only one X chromosome; characteristics include short stature, little sexual differentiation, webbing of the neck with a low posterior hairline, and congenital cardiac anomalies.

Ultrasound High-frequency sound waves that may be directed, through the use of a transducer, into the maternal abdomen. The ultrasonic sound waves reflected by the underlying structures of varying densities allow various maternal and fetal tissues, bones, and fluids to be identified.

Umbilical cord The structure connecting the placenta to the umbilicus of the fetus and through which nutrients from the woman are exchanged for wastes from the fetus.

Uterine atony Relaxation of uterine muscle tone following birth.

Uterine inversion Prolapse of the uterine fundus through the cervix into the vagina; may occur just prior to or during delivery of the placenta; associated with massive hemorrhage requiring emergency treatment.

Uterosacral ligaments Ligaments that provide support for the uterus and cervix at the level of the ischial spines.

Uterus The hollow muscular organ in which the fertilized ovum is implanted and in which the developing fetus is nourished until birth.

Vagina The musculomembranous tube or passageway located between the external genitals and the uterus of a woman.

Vaginal birth after cesarean (VBAC) Practice of permitting a trial of labor and possible vaginal birth for women following a previous cesarean birth for nonrecurring causes such as fetal distress or placenta previa.

Variable deceleration Periodic change in fetal heart rate caused by umbilical cord compression; decelerations vary in onset, occurrence, and waveform.

Vasectomy Surgical removal of a portion of the vas deferens (ductus deferens) to produce infertility.

Vegan A "pure" vegetarian; one who consumes no food from animal sources.

Vena caval syndrome Symptoms of dizziness, pallor, and clamminess that result from lowered blood pressure when a pregnant woman lies supine and the enlarged uterus presses on the vena cava. Also known as supine hypotensive syndrome.

Vernix caseosa A protective cheeselike whitish substance made up of sebum and desquamated epithelial cells that is present on the fetal skin.

Version Turning of the fetus in utero.

Vertex The top or crown of the head.

Vulva The external structure of the female genitals, lying below the mons veneris.

Weaning The process of discontinuing breastfeeding and accustoming an infant to another feeding method.

Wharton's jelly Yellow-white gelatinous material surrounding the vessels of the umbilical cord.

Zona pellucida Transparent inner layer surrounding an ovum.

Zygote A fertilized egg.

Zygote intrafallopian transfer (ZIFT) Retrieval of oocytes under ultrasound guidance followed by in vitro fertilization and laparoscopic replacement of fertilized eggs into fimbriated end of the fallopian tube.

CREDITS

Art Credits

Chapter 2 2–3: Kristin Mount. 2–5: Precision Graphics. 2–8: Kristin Mount. 2–9: Kristin Mount. 2–10: Precision Graphics. 2–11: Kristin Mount. 2–12: Kristin Mount. 2–14: Nea Hanscomb. 2–15: Kristin Mount. 2–17: Kristin Mount.

Chapter 3 3–1: Nea Hanscomb. 3–2: Nea Hanscomb. 3–3*A*: Kristin Mount. 3–4: Precision Graphics. 3–5: Kristin Mount. 3–6: Kristin Mount. 3–7: Kristin Mount. 3–8: Kristin Mount. 3–11: Kristin Mount. 3–12: Kristin Mount. 3–13: Precision Graphics.

Chapter 4 4–1: Nea Hanscomb. 4–2: The Left Coast Group. 4–3*A*: Precision Graphics. 4–4: Nea Hanscomb. 4–13: Precision Graphics. 4–14: Precision Graphics. 4–15: Precision Graphics. 4–16: Kristin Mount. 4–17: Precision Graphics. 4–18: Precision Graphics.

Chapter 5 5–1: Nea Hanscomb. 5–2*B*: Precision Graphics. 5–3*B–D*: Precision Graphics. 5–4: Precision Graphics. 5–6: Nea Hanscomb. 5–8: Precision Graphics. 5–9: Precision Graphics.

Chapter 6 6–1: Nea Hanscomb. 6–2: The Left Coast Group. 6–5: Precision Graphics.

Chapter 7 7–1: Kristin Mount. 7–3: Kristin Mount. 7–4: Kristin Mount. 7–5: Kristin Mount.

Chapter 8 8–1: Nea Hanscomb. 8–3: Kristin Mount. 8–5: Kristin Mount. 8–6: Kristin Mount. 8–7: Kristin Mount.

Chapter 9 9–4: The Left Coast Group. 9–8: Kristin Mount.

Chapter 11 11–1: Robert Voights/Nea Hanscomb. 11–3: The Left Coast Group.

Chapter 13 13–1: Precision Graphics. 13–2: Kristin Mount. 13–5: Kristin Mount.

Chapter 14 14–5: Nea Hanscomb. 14–6: Nea Hanscomb. 14–7: Kristin Mount. 14–8: Nea Hanscomb. 14–9: Kristin Mount.

Chapter 15 15–1: Kristin Mount. 15–2: Kristin Mount. 15–3: Kristin Mount. 15–4: Precision Graphics. 15–5: Precision Graphics. 15–6: Precision Graphics. 15–7: Precision Graphics. 15–8: Precision Graphics. 15–9: Nea Hanscomb. 15–10: Nea Hanscomb. 15–11: Precision Graphics. 15–12: Kristin Mount. 15–13: Kristin Mount. 15–14: Precision Graphics. 15–15: Precision Graphics. 15–16: Precision Graphics.

Chapter 16 16–2: Kristin Mount. 16–3: Kristin Mount. 16–4: Precision Graphics. 16–5: Precision Graphics. 16–6: Precision Graphics. 16–8: Precision Graphics. 16–9: Precision Graphics. 16–10: Nea Hanscomb. 16–11: Nea Hanscomb. 16–12: Nea Hanscomb. 16–13: Nea Hanscomb.

Chapter 17 17–6: Precision Graphics. 17–9: Precision Graphics. 17–11: Precision Graphics.

Chapter 18 18–1: Precision Graphics. 18–2: Kristin Mount. 18–3: Kristin Mount. 18–4: Kristin Mount. 18–5: Kristin Mount. 18–6: Kristin Mount. 18–7: Precision Graphics.

Chapter 19 19–1: The Left Coast Group. 19–2: Precision Graphics. 19–3: Nea Hanscomb. 19–4: Precision Graphics. 19–5: Precision Graphics. 19–6: Precision Graphics. 19–7: Precision Graphics. 19–8: Precision Graphics. 19–9: Precision Graphics. 19–10: Nea Hanscomb. 19–11: Precision Graphics. 19–12: Precision Graphics. 19–14: Nea Hanscomb. 19–15: Precision Graphics. Table 19–1: Nea Hanscomb.

Chapter 20 20–1: Precision Graphics. 20–3: Nea Hanscomb. 20–4: Precision Graphics. 20–5: Precision Graphics. 20–6: Nea Hanscomb.

Chapter 21 21–1: Nea Hanscomb. 21–2: Nea Hanscomb. 21–3: Kristin Mount. 21–4: Nea Hanscomb. 21–5: Precision Graphics. 21–6: Precision Graphics. 21–7: Nea Hanscomb.

Chapter 22 22–1: The Left Coast Group. 22–11: Nea Hanscomb. 22–12: The Left Coast Group. 22–14: Precision Graphics. 22–15: Precision Graphics. 22–24: Kristin Mount. 22–25: Kristin Mount. 22–34: Kristin Mount.

Chapter 23 23–3: Kristin Mount. 23–7: Precision Graphics. 23–8: Precision Graphics. 23–9: Precision Graphics. 23–10: The Left Coast Group. 23–11: Precision Graphics. 23–12: The Left Coast Group.

Chapter 24 24–2: Precision Graphics. 24–4: Precision Graphics. 24–5: Precision Graphics.

Chapter 25 25–1: Nea Hanscomb. 25–7: Precision Graphics. 25–8: Precision Graphics. 25–11: Nea Hanscomb. 25–12: Nea Hanscomb. Table 25–4: Kristin Mount. Table 25–5: Kristin Mount.

Chapter 26 26–2: Precision Graphics. 26–3: Nea Hanscomb. 26–5: Nea Hanscomb. 26–7: Nea Hanscomb. 26–8: Nea Hanscomb. 26–9: Nea Hanscomb.

Chapter 27 27–1: Kristin Mount. 27–5: Precision Graphics. 27–6: Nea Hanscomb.

Chapter 29 29–2: Precision Graphics. 29–5: Precision Graphics.

Chapter 30 30–1: Kristin Mount. 30–2: Kristin Mount.

Photo Credits

Part Openers Part I: Philip Matson/Tony Stone Images/Chicago, Inc. Part II: Laurence Monneret/Tony Stone Images/Chicago, Inc. Part III: Terry Vine/Tony Stone Images/ Chicago, Inc. Part IV: Bruce Ayres/Tony Stone Images/Chicago, Inc. Part V: Tony Fortunato/Tony Stone Images/Chicago, Inc.

Chapter 1 1–1: © Jenny Thomas/ Addison Wesley Longman.

Chapter 3 3–3*B*: © Lennart Nilsson, *A Child is Born*. New York: Dell Publishing, 1990. 3–14: © Petit Format/Nestle/Science Source/Photo Researchers. 3–15: © Petit Format/Nestle/Science Source/Photo Researchers. 3–16: © Lennart Nilsson, *A Child is Born*. New York: Dell Publishing, 1990. 3–17: © Lennart Nilsson, *A Child is Born*. New York: Dell Publishing, 1990. 3–18: © Lennart Nilsson, *A Child is Born*. New York: Dell Publishing, 1990.

Chapter 4 4–3*B*: Courtesy of Lovena Porter. 4–3C: From Speroff, L., et al: *Clinical Gynecological Endocrinology and Infertility,* 5th ed. Baltimore: Williams & Wilkins, 1994. 4–5: Courtesy David Peakman, Reproductive Genetics Center, Denver, CO. 4–6: Courtesy David Peakman, Reproductive Genetics Center, Denver, CO. 4–7: Courtesy Dr. Arthur Robinson, National Jewish Hospital and Research Center, Denver, CO. 4–8: From Jones, K. L.: Smith's *Recognizable Patterns of Human Malformations,* 4th ed. Philadelphia: W. B. Saunders, 1988. 4–9: From Smith, D. W.: Autosomal abnormalities. *Am J Obstet Gynecol* December 1964; 90:1055. 4–10: From Smith, D. W., et al: The D1 trisomy syndrome. *J Pediatr* March 1963; 62:326. 4–11: From Thompson, J. S., Thompson, M. W.: *Genetics in Medicine,* 5th ed. Philadelphia: Saunders, 1991. 4–12: From Thompson, J. S., Thompson, M. W.: *Genetics in Medicine,* 5th ed. Philadelphia: Saunders, 1991.

Chapter 5 5–2*A*: © Kathleen Cameron/ Addison Wesley Longman. 5–3*A*: © Kathleen Cameron/Addison Wesley Longman. 5–5: © Kathleen Cameron/Addison Wesley Longman. 5–7 (top): © Kathleen Cameron/ Addison Wesley Longman. 5–7 (bottom): © Alain McLaughlin/Addison Wesley Longman. 5–10: Courtesy Centers for Disease Control and Prevention. 5–11: Courtesy

Centers for Disease Control and Prevention. 5–12: © D. M. Phillips/Visuals Unlimited. 5–13: © Kenneth Greer/Visuals Unlimited.

Chapter 6 6–3: © Anne Dowie/Addison Wesley Longman. 6–4: © Richard Tauber/Addison Wesley Longman.

Chapter 8 8–2: © Suzanne Arms/Addison Wesley Longman. 8–4: © Richard Tauber/Addison Wesley Longman.

Chapter 9 9–1: © Richard Tauber/Addison Wesley Longman. 9–2: © Richard Tauber/Addison Wesley Longman. 9–3: © Jenny Thomas/Addison Wesley Longman. 9–5 © William Thompson, RN/Addison Wesley Longman. 9–6: © Elena Dorfman/Addison Wesley Longman. 9–7: © Richard Tauber/Addison Wesley Longman.

Chapter 10 10–1: © Amy H. Snyder/Addison Wesley Longman. 10–2: © Jenny Thomas/Addison Wesley Longman. 10–3: © Stella Johnson.

Chapter 11 11–2: Michael Newman/PhotoEdit.

Chapter 12 12–1: © Jenny Thomas/Addison Wesley Longman.

Chapter 13 13–3: © Amy H. Snyder/Addison Wesley Longman. 13–4: © Amy H. Snyder/Addison Wesley Longman.

Chapter 14 14–1: © Richard Tauber/Addison Wesley Longman. 14–2: Courtesy of Diane Roth.14–3: From Cundiff, J. L., Haybrich, K. L., Hinzman, N. G.: "Umbilical Artery Doppler Flow Studies during Pregnancy"; *JOGNN* November/December 1990; 19(6):475, fig 3. 14–4: From Cundiff, J. L., Haybrich, K. L., Hinzman, N. G.: "Umbilical Artery Doppler Flow Studies during Pregnancy"; *JOGNN* November/December 1990; 19(6):475, fig 4.

Chapter 16 16–1: © Stella Johnson. 16–7: © Stella Johnson.

Chapter 17 17–1: © Richard Tauber/Addison Wesley Longman. 17–2: Richard Tauber/Addison Wesley Longman. 17–3: © Stella Johnson. 17–4: © Suzanne Arms/Addison Wesley Longman. 17–5: © Stella Johnson/Addison Wesley Longman. 17–6: © Suzanne Arms/Addison Wesley Longman. 17–8: © Stella Johnson.

Chapter 19 19–13: Courtesy of Dr. Dan Farine, University of Toronto.

Chapter 21 21–9: © Beth Elkin/Addison Wesley Longman. 21–10: © Beth Elkin/Addison Wesley Longman.

Chapter 22 22–2: Reprinted by permission of V. Dubowitz, M. D., Hammersmith Hospital, London, England. 22–3*A*: Courtesy of Barbara Corey, RNC, MSN, MNP. 22–3*B* and *C*: Reprinted by permission of V. Dubowitz, M. D., Hammersmith Hospital, London, England. 22–4*A* and *B*: Reprinted by permission of V. Dubowitz, M. D., Hammersmith Hospital, London, England. 22–4*C*: © Suzanne Arms/Addison Wesley Longman. 22–5*A* and *B*: Reprinted by permission of V. Dubowitz, M. D., Hammersmith Hospital, London, England. 22–5*C*: © Suzanne Arms/Addison Wesley Longman. 22–6*A*: Reprinted by permission of V. Dubowitz, M. D., Hammersmith Hospital, London, England. 22–6*B*: Suzanne Arms/Addison Wesley Longman. 22–6*C*: Reprinted by permission of V. Dubowitz, M. D., Hammersmith Hospital, London, England. 22–7: Reprinted by permission of V. Dubowitz, M. D., Hammersmith Hospital, London, England. 22–8: Reprinted by permission of V. Dubowitz, M. D., Hammersmith Hospital, London, England. 22–9: Reprinted by permission of V. Dubowitz, M. D., Hammersmith Hospital, London, England. 22–10: Reprinted by permission of V. Dubowitz, M. D., Hammersmith Hospital, London, England. 22–13: © Beth Elkin/Addison Wesley Longman. 22–16: © Beth Elkin/Addison Wesley Longman. 22–23: From Korones S. B.: *High Risk Newborn Infants,* 4th ed. St. Louis, C. V. Mosby, 1986. 22–24: Reproduced with permission. From Potter, E. L., Craig, J. M.: *Pathology of the Fetus and Infant,* 3rd ed. © 1975 by Year Book Medical Publishers, Chicago. 22–25: Courtesy of Mead Johnson & Company, Evansville, IN. 22–26: Courtesy of Dr. Ralph Platow. From Potter, E. L., Craig, J. M.: *Pathology of the Fetus and Infant,* 3rd ed. © 1975 by Year Book Medical Publishers, Chicago. 22–27: Courtesy of Mead Johnson & Company, Evansville, IN. 22–28: © Stella Johnson. 22–29: Courtesy of Mead Johnson & Company, Evansville, IN. 22–30: From Korones S. B.: High Risk Newborn Infants 4th ed. St. Louis, C. V. Mosby, 1986. 22–31: © Suzanne Arms/Addison Wesley Longman. 22–32: © Beth Elkin/Addison Wesley Longman. 22–33: Reproduced with permission. From Potter, E. L., Craig, J. M.: *Pathology of the Fetus and Infant, 3rd ed.* © 1975 by Year Book Medical Publishers, Chicago. 22–35*A*: Courtesy of Mead Johnson & Company, Evansville, IN. 22–35*B*: © Stella Johnson. 22–36: © Stella Johnson. 22–37: © Stella Johnson. 22–38: © Stella Johnson. 22–39: © Stella Johnson. 22–40: © Stella Johnson.

Chapter 23 23–1: © Stella Johnson. 23–2: © Beth Elkin/Addison Wesley Longman. 23–4: © Beth Elkin/Addison Wesley Longman. 23–5: © Stella Johnson. 23–6: © Stella Johnson.

Chapter 24 24–1: © Stella Johnson. 24–3: © Stella Johnson. 24–4*B*: © Stella Johnson. 24–6: © Stella Johnson. 24–7: © Elena Dorfman/Addison Wesley Longman. 24–8: © Suzanne Arms Wimberly. From Renfrow, Arms, Fisher: *Breastfeeding: Getting Breastfeeding Right for You,* Celestial Arts, 1990.

Chapter 25 25–4: From Dubowitz, L., Dubowitz, V.: *Gestational Age of the Newborn.* Menlo Park, CA: Addison-Wesley, 1977. Reprinted by permission of V. Dubowitz, MD, Hammersmith Hospital, London, England. 25–5: © Stella Johnson. 25–6: © Stella Johnson. 25–9: Courtesy of Kadlac Medical Center Kangaroo Care Study and Carol Thompson, RN, BSN, NNP. 25–10: Courtesy of Theresa Kledzik, RN, Developmental Nurse, Memorial Hospital. 25–13: © Stella Johnson. Table 25–4: Courtesy of Dr. Paul Winchester.

Chapter 26 26–1: © Stella Johnson. 26–4: © Stella Johnson. 26–6: © Stella Johnson. 26–10: © Beth Elkin/Addison Wesley Longman. 26–11: © Stella Johnson. 26–12: © Stella Johnson.

Chapter 27 27–2: From Bennett, V. R., Brown, L. K.: *Myles Textbook for Midwives,* 11th ed. Edinburgh: Churchill-Livingstone, 1989. p 235 27–04: © Beth Elkin/Addison Wesley Longman. 27–7: © Amy H. Snyder/Addison Wesley Longman.

Chapter 28 28–1: © Anne Dowie/Addison Wesley Longman. 28–2: © Stella Johnson.

Chapter 29 29–1: © Kathy Kieliszewski/Addison Wesley Longman. 29–3: © Stella Johnson. 29–4: © Kathy Kieliszewski/Addison Wesley Longman.

INDEX

NOTE: A *b* following a page number indicates boxed or specially formatted material, a *t* following a page number indicates tabular material; and an *f* following a page number indicates a figure. Drugs are listed under their generic names. When a drug trade name is listed, the reader is referred to the generic name.

Student Tutorial Instructions

This electronic study guide provides you with two study options: Chapter Review and Comprehensive Exam.

Chapter Review Option

The Chapter Review option allows you to practice answering NCLEX style questions. You may continue to try to answer a question until the right answer is selected, and rationales are provided for both correct and incorrect answers. After completing a Chapter Review, you have the option of taking a follow-up test of questions missed.

- To select the Chapter Review option, go to the Main Menu and select File. From the pull-down menu, select New, then Chapter Review. Select a chapter from the table of contents, then click Take.
- Click on your answer choice from the letters (A, B, C, or D) on the bottom of the screen. You will be told if your answer is correct or incorrect and why. Once you have answered a question correctly, click on Next to bring up the next question.
- When you have completed the Chapter Review, click on Done. The performance box monitors your results. To print out these results, go to the Main Menu and select the Test pull-down menu, then select Report Card. Click Print on the Report Card screen.

Comprehensive Exam Option

The Comprehensive Exam option allows you to practice taking a timed exam. You have the option of taking a standard exam or a custom exam. A standard exam consists of 150 randomly generated questions. You select the time allotted for the exam from the column on the right. The custom exam allows you to select the number of questions and the time allotted.

- To select the Comprehensive Exam option, go to the Main Menu and select File. From the pull-down menu, select New, then Comprehensive Exam.
- Select standard or custom exam by clicking on the Standard or Custom box.
- Click on Take at the bottom of the screen when you are ready to take the exam.

Once you have finished answering all the questions, or if the time allotted runs out, a report card will display your exam results. To print out these results, go to the Main Menu and select the Test pull-down menu, then select Results of Exam. Click Print on the Results of Exam screen.

Other Features

Notebook From the Main Menu, go to the Edit pull-down menu, then select Notebook. You can enter any notes you wish by chapter, and you can access these notes during a Chapter Review by clicking on the Notes box.

Preferences This feature allows you to adjust the behavior of the program. From the Main Menu, go to the File pull-down menu, then select Preferences. You may select or unselect any of the preferences listed on the screen.

Help For more information, from the Main Menu go to the Help pull-down menu, then select Instructions, or click the Help box on any screen.